Foundations of Athletic Training

Prevention, Assessment, and Management

Foundations of Athletic Training

Prevention, Assessment, and Management

FOURTH EDITION

Marcia K. Anderson, Ph.D., LATC

Professor

Department of Movement Arts, Health Promotion, and Leisure Studies

Bridgewater State College

Bridgewater, Massachusetts

Gail P. Parr, Ph.D., ATC

Associate Professor

Department of Kinesiology

Towson University

Towson, Maryland

Susan J. Hall, Ph.D.

Professor and Chair

Department of Health and Exercise Sciences

University of Delaware

Newark, Delaware

Wolters Kluwer | Lippincott Williams & Wilkins

Health

Philadelphia · Baltimore · New York · London

Buenos Aires · Hong Kong · Sydney · Tokyo

Acquisitions Editor: Emily J. Lupash
Managing Editor: Jennifer Walsh, Karen Gulliver
Marketing Manager: Christen D. Murphy
Production Editor: Paula C. Williams
Designer: Risa J. Clow

Photographer: Eleanor B. Smith
Medical Illustrator: Tiffany A. Gagnon;
   Imagineering Media Services, Inc.
Compositor: Hearthside and
   Maryland Composition, Inc.

Fourth Edition

Copyright © 2009, 2004, 2000, 1995 Lippincott Williams & Wilkins, a Wolters Kluwer business.

351 West Camden Street
Baltimore, Maryland 21201

530 Walnut Street
Philadelphia, Pennsylvania 19106

Printed in USA

9 8 7 6 5 4 3 2 1

Library of Congress Cataloging-in-Publication Data

Anderson, Marcia K.
  Foundations of athletic training : prevention, assessment, and management / Marcia K. Anderson, Gail P. Parr, Susan J. Hall. -- 4th ed.
      p. cm.
  Includes bibliographical references and index.
  ISBN-13: 978-0-7817-8445-0 (alk. paper)
  ISBN-10: 0-7817-8445-X (alk. paper)
  1. Sports injuries. 2. Sports injuries--Treatment. 3.
Athletes--Health and hygiene. I. Parr, Gail P. II. Hall, Susan J.
(Susan Jean), 1953- III. Title.
  RD97.A53 2009
  617.1'027--dc22

                                                          2007048936

DISCLAIMER

Care has been taken to confirm the accuracy of the information present and to describe generally accepted practices. However, the authors, editors, and publisher are not responsible for errors or omissions or for any consequences from application of the information in this book and make no warranty, expressed or implied, with respect to the currency, completeness, or accuracy of the contents of the publication. Application of this information in a particular situation remains the professional responsibility of the practitioner; the clinical treatments described and recommended may not be considered absolute and universal recommendations.

The authors, editors, and publisher have exerted every effort to ensure that drug selection and dosage set forth in this text are in accordance with the current recommendations and practice at the time of publication. However, in view of ongoing research, changes in government regulations, and the constant flow of information relating to drug therapy and drug reactions, the reader is urged to check the package insert for each drug for any change in indications and dosage and for added warnings and precautions. This is particularly important when the recommended agent is a new or infrequently employed drug.

Some drugs and medical devices presented in this publication have Food and Drug Administration (FDA) clearance for limited use in restricted research settings. It is the responsibility of the health care provider to ascertain the FDA status of each drug or device planned for use in their clinical practice.

To purchase additional copies of this book, call our customer service department at (800) 638-3030 or fax orders to (301) 223-2320. International customers should call (301) 223-2300.

Visit Lippincott Williams & Wilkins on the Internet: http://www.lww.com. Lippincott Williams & Wilkins customer service representatives are available from 8:30 am to 6:00 pm, EST.

Preface

Four major goals were established for the fourth edition of *Foundations of Athletic Training*. The primary goal was to provide the most current and comprehensive content related to the prevention, assessment, and management of injuries and illnesses sustained by physically active individuals. A second goal was to acknowledge the importance and significance of the *Role Delineation Study* (RDS) published by the Board of Certification. The RDS identifies the essential knowledge and skills for the athletic trainer and serves as a blueprint for the development of the certification examination. Acknowledging the importance of the RDS, each chapter begins by identifying the specific RDS competencies covered within that chapter. A third goal was to enhance learning potential through the actual presentation of information. In particular, an extensive color art program is provided. This new format is designed to provide realistic and accurate visualizations of musculoskeletal anatomy, injuries and medical conditions, assessment techniques, and management techniques. The fourth goal also pertained to content presentation. In an effort to continue our tradition of providing special pedagogical features in a visually pleasing format, multicolor borders and formatting have been used to identify critical boxes, field strategies, and tables as a way to highlight key information.

Foundations of Athletic Training has undergone extensive review from leaders in the athletic training field. The review process has been instrumental in enabling us to achieve our goal of developing the most comprehensive text available for athletic training educators and students.

KEY FEATURES IN THIS EDITION

The chapters have been reorganized into seven parts: Foundations of Injury Management, Injury Assessment and Rehabilitation, Axial Region, Upper Extremity, Lower Extremity, Systemic Conditions, and Special Considerations. Many chapters have been expanded to reflect the ever-increasing body of knowledge in the athletic training profession. This expansion is particularly evident in the presentation of information on spinal conditions. Specifically, the chapter "Spinal Conditions" has been divided into two chapters, namely "Cervical and Thoracic Spinal Conditions" and "Lumbar Spinal Conditions."

PEDAGOGICAL FEATURES

Several pedagogical features have been utilized to enhance the text's usefulness as a teaching tool. These in-text features include:

- **Art and Photography Program.** A new color art and photography program supplements the material presented in the text. Using an innovative approach that involves drawings within a human model, the illustration of musculoskeletal anatomy provides a detailed and realistic depiction of structures.

- **BOC Competencies.** As previously noted, the beginning of each chapter includes a list of the BOC competencies addressed in that chapter. This information should be useful to both educators and students.

- **Learning Objectives.** Each chapter opens with a series of learning objectives that identify the key concepts in the chapter.

- **Critical Thinking Scenarios.** Critical thinking scenarios are found at the beginning of most of the major sections in each chapter. These scenarios are intended to encourage the student to critically analyze information and apply decision-making knowledge and skills.

- **Key Terminology.** Important terms are bolded within the text. In addition to the explanation of the term in the chapter, these terms are also defined in the glossary.

- **Critical Information Boxes.** These boxes are interspersed throughout each chapter. They are intended to highlight and summarize important information.

- **Tables.** Several chapters have tables that expand on pertinent information discussed in the text. This format allows a large amount of didactic knowledge to be organized in an easy-to-read summary of information.

- **Field Strategies and Management Algorithms.** In several chapters, field strategies and management algorithms are utilized to present the clinical application of cognitive knowledge.

- **Summary.** Each chapter has a summary of key concepts discussed in the text.

- **References.** Updated references are provided. The majority of the references have been published within the last five years. The exceptions are primarily references to original ground-breaking research.

- **Glossary and Index.** An extensive glossary of terms gathered from the highlighted words in the individual chapters is provided at the end of the book. In addition, a comprehensive index contains cross-references to locate specific information within the text.

ANCILLARY MATERIALS

Online resource centers are available to both athletic training educators and athletic training students on the book's companion website at thePoint.com/Anderson4e.

Instructor's Resource Center

The online resource center is organized by chapters and includes the following:

- **PowerPoint Presentations.** The PowerPoint presentations were developed with an understanding that instructors and students adopt a variety of strategies when using PowerPoint. The slides provide detailed rather than general information, recognizing that it is simpler for an educator to delete rather than add information. In addition, given the tendency of many students to take notes verbatim from a slide, an effort was made to condense the actual wording of statements to streamline the note-taking process. The presentations can be downloaded and customized to meet specific needs.

- **Supporting Lecture Notes.** The lecture notes correspond to the individual slides comprising the PowerPoint presentations. The notes are not intended to serve as an actual lecture. Rather, they are designed to provide the instructor with information that supports the material presented on the slides. As such, the notes include additional explanation and background information, as well as examples of concepts.

- **Teaching Strategies.** The teaching strategies provide additional experiences and instructional methods to complement the learning process. In particular, the teaching strategies provide an active, problem-solving, and critical-thinking approach to learning. For example, Chapters 10–18 contain differential diagnosis problems intended to engage the learner in the analysis of clinical signs and symptoms.

- **Reference Materials.** Each chapter contains a variety of materials intended to supplement the information presented in the text. For example, Chapter 1 provides sample forms pertaining to legal considerations. Chapters 10–18 include handouts that pertain to the injury assessment process (i.e., history, observation/inspection, palpation, and testing). The handouts provide an extensive amount of information in an organized and easy-to-read format.

- **Worksheets.** Utilizing a variety of formats, the exercises in the worksheets require students to demonstrate knowledge and comprehension, as well as apply, analyze, synthesize, and evaluate information. In addition, some exercises incorporate the use of psychomotor skills. Answer sheets are provided for the worksheets.

- **Image Bank.** A bank of the various illustrations contained in the text is provided.

- **Articles and Web Links.** A list of articles and websites that are pertinent to information in various chapters is provided as a supplement for obtaining additional information.

- **Test Bank.** The bank includes more than 1,500 sample test questions composed of multiple choice, matching, true/false, and short answer questions. The program will allow faculty to add/customize their own test questions.

- **WebCT and Blackboard-Ready Cartridges.**

Student Resource Center

The online resource center for students will contain two of the same features available through the instructor's resource center, namely the reference materials and the web links. In addition, the student resource center will include the following:

- **Stedman's Audio Glossary.** The glossary available in the text will also be readily accessible online.

- **Articles and Web Links.** A list of articles and websites that are pertinent to information in various chapters is provided as a supplement for obtaining additional information.

- **Electronic Flash Cards.** Interactive flash cards can be an effective way to study important terms and concepts. Students will have the option to view cards by term/concept or by definition.

- **Reference Materials.** Each chapter contains a variety of materials intended to supplement the information presented in the text. For example, Chapter 1 provides sample forms pertaining to legal considerations. Chapters 9–18 include handouts that pertain to the injury assessment process (i.e., history, observation/inspection, palpation, and testing). The handouts provide an extensive amount of information in an organized and easy-to-read format.

- **Quizzes.** Quizzes will utilize a variety of testing formats, including multiple choice and N-wise multiple choice. These formats are similar to those used on the BOC certification examination.

- **Drag and Drop Figure Labeling.** The images can be labeled by dragging the correct descriptor to the corresponding element of the figure.

In addition, purchasers of the text can access the searchable Full Text On-line by going to the *Foundations of Athletic Training* website at thePoint.com/Anderson4e. See the inside front cover of this text for more details, including the passcode you will need to gain access to the website

Marcia K. Anderson
Bridgewater, Massachusetts

Gail P. Parr
Towson, Maryland

Susan J. Hall
Wilmington, Delaware

Reviewers

Timothy Lee, Diploma SIM, CAT(C)
Certified Athletic Therapist
Ottawa High Performance Centre
Nepean, ON

Stephanie Mazerolle, MS, ATC
Clinical Lab Instructor
University of Connecticut
Storrs, CT

Robin Ploeger, EdD
Athletic Training Curriculum Director
University of Tulsa
Tulsa, OK

Matt Radelet, MS, ATC, CSCS
Associate Athletic Trainer
University of Arizona
Tucson, AZ

Robert Ruhling, PhD
Professor
George Mason University
Manassas, VA

Derek Suranie, MeD, ATC
Assistant Professor/Head Athletic Trainer
North Georgia College and State University
Dahlonega, GA

Lisa Varnum, MA, ATC
Assistant Athletic Trainer/Instructor
University of California, Davis
Davis, CA

Gordon Wilcox, MSc, BEd
Professor
Algonquin College
Ottawa, ON

Acknowledgments

The authors would like to thank the hard-working and talented staff of Lippincott Williams & Wilkins. Emily Lupash and Karen Ruppert provided enthusiastic support, guidance, and innovative ideas for enhancing this edition of the book. Jennifer Walsh was exceptional in overseeing and coordinating the progress of manuscript development and production. A special thank you is extended to both Nancy Peterson and Karen Gulliver for their patience, meticulous attention to detail, and expertise in coordinating the various aspects of this project.

We also want to acknowledge the work of Dr. Kellie Huxel, Assistant Professor at Indiana State University, as a co-author of the online *Instructor's Resource Center* and *Student Resource Center*. Dr. Huxel's experience and insight contributed significantly to the development and enrichment of both resource centers.

PERSONAL ACKNOWLEDGMENT

I would like thank Dr. Victoria Bacon for her continued support and encouragement as we moved through the many stages of the project. I also extend a very special thanks to Tory, my 12-year old faithful companion, continues to wait patiently for her daily walk in the woods as long as she gets an extra treat at the end of the trek. Pets are such devoted friends with unwavering love, as long as their breakfast and supper are on the floor when they are ready to dine. Don't you love them!

MKA

User's Guide

This User's Guide explains all of the key features found in the fourth edition of *Foundations of Athletic Training: Prevention, Assessment, and Management*. Become familiar with them so that you can get the most out of each chapter and then take the information and skills with you into the field as an athletic trainer.

CHAPTER OPENING ELEMENTS

Each chapter begins with the following elements, which will help you get off to the right start.

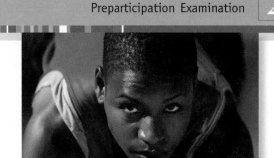

STUDENT OUTCOMES

1. Identify the goals and objectives of a preparticipation examination (PPE).
2. Design a PPE.
3. Identify the specific areas in a PPE that could be examined using a mass station screening process.
4. Identify follow-up questions intended to validate information on a medical history questionnaire.
5. Demonstrate the ability to take vital signs, and identify criteria used to denote abnormal pulse and blood pressure rates.
6. Explain the importance of completing a physical fitness profile as part of the PPE.
7. Demonstrate skinfold measurement at the various sites used to determine body composition.
8. Explain the criteria used to categorize hypermobility and hypomobility.
9. Describe specific methods of measuring strength, power, speed, cardiovascular endurance, agility, balance, and reaction time.
10. Identify specific conditions that could exclude an individual from participating in physical activity or sport.

19

Outcomes

These are the learning objectives that you need to meet after reading the chapter content. (Here's a tip: Read them again after finishing the chapter as a self-test.)

ROLE DELINEATION COMPETENCIES

The following Performance Domains and Tasks defined in the National Athletic Trainers' Association Board of Certification *Role Delineation Study*, 5th Edition are addressed in this chapter:

BOC COMPETENCIES

I. Prevention

F. Maintain clinical and treatment areas by complying with safety and sanitation standards to minimize the risk of injury and illness.

II. Clinical Evaluation and Diagnosis

A. Obtain a history through observation, interview, and/or review of relevant records to assess current or potential injury, illness, or condition.
B. Inspect the involved area(s) visually to assess the injury, illness, or health-related condition.
C. Palpate the involved area(s) using standard techniques to assess the injury, illness, or health-related condition.
D. Perform specific tests in accordance with accepted procedures to assess the injury, illness, or health-related condition.
E. Formulate a clinical impression by interpreting the signs, symptoms, and predisposing factors of the injury, illness, or condition to determine the appropriate course of action.
F. Educate the appropriate individual(s) regarding the assessment by communicating information about the current or potential injury, illness, or health-related condition to encourage compliance with recommended care.
G. Share assessment findings with other health care professionals using effective means of communication to coordinate appropriate care.

III. Immediate Care

A. Employ life-saving techniques through the use of standard emergency procedures in order to reduce morbidity and the incidence of mortality.
B. Prevent exacerbation of non-life threatening condition(s) through the use of standard procedures in order to reduce morbidity.
C. Facilitate the timely transfer of care for conditions beyond the scope of practice of the athletic trainer by implementing appropriate referral strategies to stabilize and/or prevent exacerbation of the condition(s).
D. Direct the appropriate individual(s) in standard immediate care procedures using formal and informal methods to facilitate immediate care.
E. Execute the established emergency action plan using effective communication and administrative practices to facilitate efficient immediate care.

IV. Treatment, Rehabilitation, and Reconditioning

E. Reassess the status of injuries, illnesses, and/or conditions using standard techniques and documentation strategies in order to determine appropriate treatment, rehabilitation, and/or reconditioning and to evaluate readiness to return to a desired level of activity.

V. Organization and Administration

A. Establish action plans for response to injury or illness using available resources to provide the required range of health care services for individuals, athletic activities, and events.
B. Establish policies and procedures for the delivery of health care services following accepted guidelines to promote safe participation, timely care, and legal compliance.
C. Establish policies and procedures for the management of health care facilities and activity areas by referring to accepted guidelines, standards, and regulations to promote safety and legal compliance.
D. Maintain records using an appropriate system to document services rendered, provide for continuity of care, facilitate communication, and meet legal standards.
F. Develop professional relationships with appropriate individuals and entities by applying effective communication techniques to enhance the delivery of health care.

Role Delineation Competencies

Pay close attention to the domains and tasks in this listing. Defined by the *Board of Certification Role Delineation Study, 5th Edition*, these represent the essential knowledge and skills you will need as an athletic trainer—and that you will be expected to master on the certification examination.

SPECIAL FEATURES

The new and unique aspects of this edition are shown and explained here so that you can make the most of them.

Full-Color Design and Artwork

We've completely redesigned this edition —it is now bursting with full color and brand new illustrations and photographs. These will enhance your learning potential by providing accurate and realistic representations of anatomy, common injuries and medical conditions, and assessment and management techniques.

Critical Thinking Questions and Answers

This tried-and-true feature gives you a realistic scenario and then poses a question, which is answered at the end of the section. Use these to practice your critical-thinking, problem-solving, and decision-making skills—they'll serve you well in the future.

---

4   Foundations of Athletic Training

of Certification (BOC) as distinct governing bodies for the profession. In addition, information is presented pertaining to a team approach to the delivery of health care for physically active individuals. Finally, legal liability surrounding injury care is presented relative to reducing the risk of possible litigation.

SPORTS MEDICINE

Should the terms sports medicine and athletic training be used interchangeably?

Sports medicine is a broad and complex branch of health care encompassing several disciplines. Essentially, it is an area of health care and special services that applies medical and scientific knowledge to prevent, recognize, assess, manage, and rehabilitate injuries or illnesses related to sport, exercise, or recreational activity and, in doing so, enhances health fitness and performance of the participant. No single profession can provide the expertise to carry out this enormous responsibility. Rather, professionals from several disciplines play key roles in addressing health care for physically active individuals. These professionals may include certified athletic trainers, team physicians or primary care physicians, orthopaedic physicians, physical therapists, emergency medical technicians, radiologists, nutritionists, exercise physiologists, biomechanists, and sport psychologists.

In many instances, people will refer to "sports medicine" when in fact they should be referring to "athletic training." Athletic trainers are specialists from one of several disciplines within the broader field of Sports Medicine. As such, the terms sports medicine and athletic training should not be used interchangeably.

ATHLETIC TRAINING

Why should individuals involved in pursuing a career as an athletic trainer be familiar with the Role Delineation Study and the Athletic Training Educational Competencies?

As medical experts in the prevention, assessment, treatment, and rehabilitation of injuries resulting from physical activity, certified athletic trainers are uniquely qualified to provide health care services to athletes and physically active individuals. While continuing to have a solid presence in the traditional settings of college/university and secondary school athletic programs, athletic trainers have expanded their medical expertise to include work in clinics (e.g., sports medicine and physical therapy centers), offices (e.g., physicians and hospitals), and industrial/occupational settings. It is estimated that more than 50% of athletic trainers work outside the traditional school athletic setting (1).

National Athletic Trainers' Association

The NATA represents more than 30,000 members in the athletic training profession (1). Since the first meeting in 1950, the NATA has been responsible for the growth and development of the athletic training profession. In establishing standards for professionalism, education, research, and practice settings, the NATA has played a critical role in the evolution of the skills and qualifications of the athletic trainer. The NATA has used a variety of resources, including public relations, scholarship and research grants, governmental affairs, and annual meetings to provide an array of services for

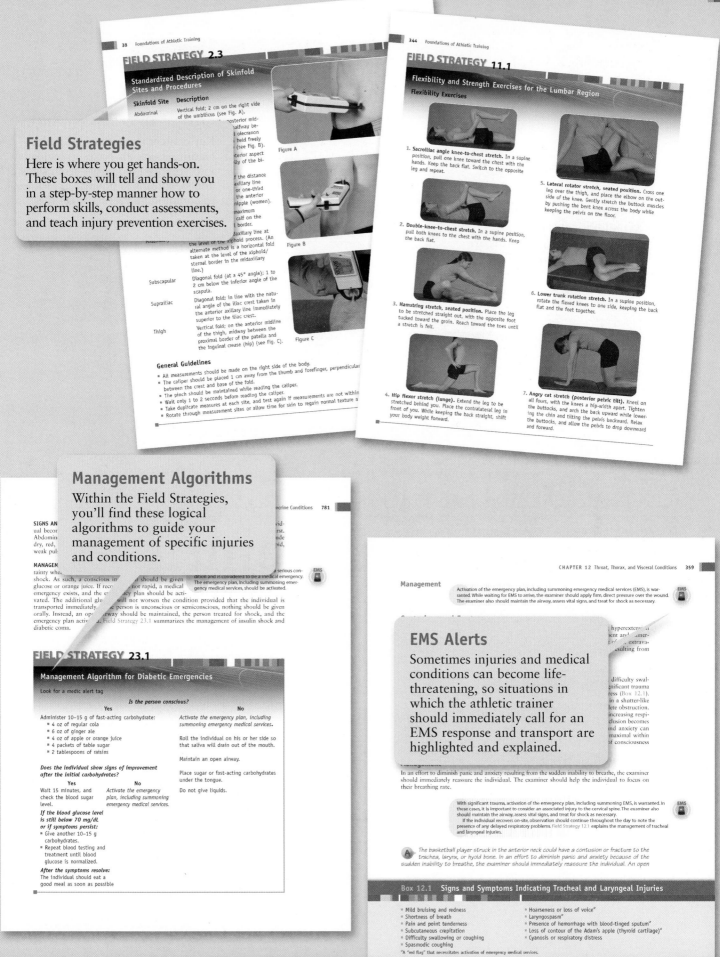

Field Strategies

Here is where you get hands-on. These boxes will tell and show you in a step-by-step manner how to perform skills, conduct assessments, and teach injury prevention exercises.

Management Algorithms

Within the Field Strategies, you'll find these logical algorithms to guide your management of specific injuries and conditions.

EMS Alerts

Sometimes injuries and medical conditions can become life-threatening, so situations in which the athletic trainer should immediately call for an EMS response and transport are highlighted and explained.

Links

The learning doesn't stop with this textbook! Additional tables, boxes, Field Strategies, and sample forms are available to you at the companion website, thePoint. Look for the ☀ so you don't miss these opportunities to expand your knowledge base.

Critical Information Boxes

Key content is summarized in this feature. Look for boxes to highlight info you need to know—from signs and symptoms to practice guidelines to common injuries to safety tips.

ADDITIONAL LEARNING AND TEACHING RESOURCES

This textbook features a power companion website:

http://thepoint.lww.com/anderson4e

thePoint☀

STUDENT RESOURCE CENTER

- Clinically oriented anatomy images
- Drag-and-drop image labeling
- Audio glossary
- Chapter quizzes
- Electronic flashcards
- Web links for supplemental information
- Additional reference material, such as boxes, tables, Field Strategies, and sample forms to support chapters
- **PLUS:** Video clips from Acland's DVD Atlas of Human Anatomy

INSTRUCTOR'S RESOURCE CENTER

- Instructor's Manual with Teaching Strategies, Lecture Notes, Worksheets, Answers, and Handouts
- Test generator
- Image collection
- PowerPoint presentations
- BOC Correlation Chart
- Web links for supplemental information

Contents in Brief

Comprehensive Contents

SECTION IV Upper Extremity 391

SECTION VI   Systemic Conditions 699

Chapter 19   Cardiovascular Disorders 700

Foundations of Sports Injury Care

1

Injury Care and the Athletic Trainer

STUDENT OUTCOMES

1. Describe the mission of the National Athletic Trainers' Association (NATA).

2. Describe the mission of the NATA Board of Certification (BOC).

3. Identify the major performance domains of the entry-level athletic trainer as defined in the *Role Delineation Study* published by the BOC.

4. Identify the requirements for earning the ATC® (certified athletic trainer) credential awarded by the BOC as well as the requirements for maintaining BOC certification.

5. Explain the basic parameters of ethical conduct and standards of professional practice for athletic trainers.

6. Describe potential work settings for individuals holding the ATC credential.

7. Describe a team approach to the delivery of health care to athletes and physically active individuals.

8. Explain standard of care and the factors that must be proved to show legal breach of that duty of care.

9. Describe measures that can reduce the risk of litigation.

ROLE DELINEATION COMPETENCIES

The following Performance Domains and Tasks defined in the National Athletic Trainers' Association Board of Certification *Role Delineation Study*, 5th Edition, are addressed in this chapter:

BOC COMPETENCIES

I. Prevention

A. Educate the appropriate individual(s) about the risks associated with participation and specific activities using effective communication techniques to minimize the risk of injury and illness.

C. Instruct the appropriate individual(s) about standard protective equipment using effective communication techniques to minimize the risk of injury and illness.

F. Maintain clinical and treatment areas by complying with safety and sanitation standards to minimize the risk of injury and illness.

I. Facilitate healthy lifestyle behaviors using effective education, communication, and interventions to reduce the risk of injury and illness and promote wellness.

II. Clinical Evaluation and Diagnosis

D. Direct the appropriate individual(s) in standard immediate care procedures using formal and informal methods to facilitate immediate care.

E. Execute the established emergency action plan using effective communication and administrative practices to facilitate efficient immediate care.

F. Educate the appropriate individual(s) regarding the assessment by communicating information about the current or potential injury, illness, or health-related condition to encourage compliance with recommended care.

G. Share assessment findings with other health care professionals using effective means of communication to coordinate appropriate care.

V. Organization and Administration

A. Establish action plans for response to injury or illness using available resources to provide the required range of health care services for individuals, athletic activities, and events.

B. Establish policies and procedures for the delivery of health care services following accepted guidelines to promote safe participation, timely care, and legal compliance.

C. Establish policies and procedures for the management of health care facilities and activity areas by referring to accepted guidelines, standards, and regulations to promote safety and legal compliance.

E. Maintain records using an appropriate system to document services rendered, provide for continuity of care, facilitate communication, and meet legal standards.

F. Develop professional relationships with appropriate individuals and entities by applying effective communication techniques to enhance the delivery of health care.

VI. Professional Responsibility

A. Demonstrate appropriate professional conduct by complying with applicable standards and maintaining continuing competence to provide quality athletic training services.

B. Adhere to statutory and regulatory provisions and other legal responsibilities relating to the practice of athletic training by maintaining an understanding of these provisions and responsibilities in order to contribute to the safety and welfare of the public.

C. Educate appropriate individuals and entities about the role and standards of practice of the athletic trainer through informal and formal means to improve the ability of those individuals and entities to make informed decisions.

Sport and physical activity, with the inherent risks involved, can lead to injury at one time or another for many participants. Such injuries often are assessed and managed by athletic trainers, who are allied health care professionals involved with the health and safety of sport participants and physically active individuals. This chapter examines the professional practice of athletic trainers, including the function of the National Athletic Trainers' Association (NATA) and the NATA Board of Certification (BOC) as distinct governing bodies for the profession. In addition, information is presented pertaining to a team approach to the delivery of health care for physically active individuals. Finally, legal liability surrounding injury care is presented relative to reducing the risk of possible litigation.

SPORTS MEDICINE

 Should the terms sports medicine and athletic training be used interchangeably?

Sports medicine is a broad and complex branch of health care encompassing several disciplines. Essentially, it is an area of health care and special services that applies medical and scientific knowledge to prevent, recognize, assess, manage, and rehabilitate injuries or illnesses related to sport, exercise, or recreational activity and, in doing so, enhances health fitness and performance of the participant. No single profession can provide the expertise to carry out this enormous responsibility. Rather, professionals from several disciplines play key roles in addressing health care for physically active individuals. These professionals may include certified athletic trainers, team physicians or primary care physicians, orthopaedic physicians, physical therapists, emergency medical technicians, radiologists, nutritionists, exercise physiologists, biomechanists, and sport psychologists.

In many instances, people will refer to "sports medicine" when in fact they should be referring to "athletic training." Athletic trainers are specialists from one of several disciplines within the broader field of Sports Medicine. As such, the terms sports medicine and athletic training should not be used interchangeably.

ATHLETIC TRAINING

Why should individuals involved in pursuing a career as an athletic trainer be familiar with the Role Delineation Study and the Athletic Training Educational Competencies?

As medical experts in the prevention, assessment, treatment, and rehabilitation of injuries resulting from physical activity, certified athletic trainers are uniquely qualified to provide health care services to athletes and physically active individuals. While continuing to have a solid presence in the traditional settings of college/university and secondary school athletic programs, athletic trainers have expanded their medical expertise to include work in clinics (e.g., sports medicine and physical therapy centers), offices (e.g., physicians and hospitals), and industrial/occupational settings. It is estimated that more than 50% of athletic trainers work outside the traditional school athletic setting (1).

National Athletic Trainers' Association

The NATA represents more than 30,000 members in the athletic training profession (1). Since the first meeting in 1950, the NATA has been responsible for the growth and development of the athletic training profession. In establishing standards for professionalism, education, research, and practice settings, the NATA has played a critical role in the evolution of the skills and qualifications of the athletic trainer. The NATA has used a variety of resources, including public relations, scholarship and research grants, governmental affairs, and annual meetings to provide an array of services for its members, health care providers, educational institutions, businesses, and the general public.

A watershed landmark for the NATA came in 1990, when the American Medical Association (AMA) officially recognized athletic trainers as allied health care professionals. Another significant indicator of the progress and trends in the athletic training profession became evident in 1999, when the American Hospital Association assigned uniform billing, or revenue, codes for athletic training. This action was followed in the year 2000 by the AMA's designation of current procedural terminology (CPT) codes for athletic training and reevaluation. In 2005, the creation of the NATA Political Action Committee (NATA-PAC) as an incorporated organization signified another pivotal move in the profession. In promoting its mission to serve as a voice for the athletic training profession among federal legislators, the NATA-PAC aims to heighten awareness of the athletic training profession and, in doing so, to increase opportunities for athletic trainers and the individuals they serve.

Board of Certification

The NATA BOC, a separate governing body from the NATA, is responsible for awarding the ATC® credential. The mission of the BOC includes "identifying for the public, quality health care professionals through a system of certification, adjudication, standards of practice and continuing competency program" (2).

The *Role Delineation Study* (RD) published by the BOC defines the current entry-level knowledge, skills, and abilities required for practice in the profession of athletic training. The RD also serves as a blueprint for the national certification examination. The 5th Edition of the RD defines the major performance domains for the entry-level certified athletic trainer as follows (3):

Prevention

Clinical evaluation and diagnosis

Immediate care

Treatment, rehabilitation, and reconditioning

Organization and administration

Professional responsibility

> A detailed list of athletic training responsibilities within each of these performance domains can be found on the companion website at thePoint.

Prevention

The domain of prevention encompasses a broad spectrum of knowledge and skills that address the risks associated with participation in sport and physical activity. Such risks range in severity from minor to potentially catastrophic injuries or illnesses. In a similar manner, the strategies used to minimize such risks can vary from relatively simple to complex. Examples of injury and illness prevention could involve preparticipation physical examinations; regular safety checks of equipment, facilities, and field areas; designing and implementing year-round conditioning programs to develop and maintain strength, flexibility, agility, and endurance; promoting proper lifting technique and safety in the weight room; following universal safety precautions to prevent the spread of infectious diseases; applying appropriate taping, wrappings, protective devices, or braces; as well as monitoring environmental conditions, such as temperature, humidity, or lightning during thunderstorms, and following guidelines for safe participation in adverse weather.

Clinical Evaluation and Diagnosis

The domain of clinical evaluation and diagnosis addresses the responsibilities of the athletic trainer in using standardized clinical practices to make decisions regarding the nature and severity of an injury or illness. Evaluation, or assessment, can involve several scenarios, including on-field (or on-site) primary assessment (Fig. 1.1), off-field initial assessment, and follow-up assessment. In each situation, the evaluation must follow a systematic format that includes a history of the injury or illness, observation and inspection of the condition, palpation of soft tissues and bony structures, and a variety of tests (e.g., range of motion, muscle strength, sensory and motor neurologic function, ligamentous/capsular integrity, and functional status). This information is essential in making determinations regarding the extent and seriousness of an injury or illness and, ultimately, in deciding the appropriate management of the condition.

Immediate Care

The immediate care domain identifies the role of the athletic trainer subsequent to determining the nature and extent of an injury or illness. Regardless of the setting, the athletic trainer must be prepared to care

■■■■ FIGURE 1.1 **Injury assessment.** Athletic trainers perform assessments in a variety of settings, including on the field.

FIGURE 1.2 Immediate care. Athletic trainers provide immediate care for a variety of conditions, ranging from potentially life-threatening to minor musculoskeletal injuries.

for and prevent further harm in patients with a variety of conditions. As such, immediate care could range from the implementation of standard emergency care for a life-threatening condition (e.g., activating the emergency medical plan) to rendering standard immediate care for a musculoskeletal injury (e.g., immobilizing a possible fracture and applying cold and compression to a sprain or strain) (Fig. 1.2).

Treatment, Rehabilitation, and Reconditioning

The athletic trainer is responsible for the implementation of treatment, rehabilitation, and reconditioning programs appropriate to the diagnosis made during the evaluation and assessment phase (Fig. 1.3). In consultation with a physician, the athletic trainer develops a comprehensive treatment program, including therapeutic goals and objectives, selection of appropriate therapeutic modalities and exercise, use of pharmacologic agents, methods to assess and document progress, and criteria for return to participation. Information gathered and documented during rehabilitation assists the physician in determining when the individual may be cleared for participation.

Organization and Administration

The domain of organization and administration describes the responsibilities of the athletic trainer in developing and executing a series of plans, policies, and procedures to ensure responsive and efficient operation of the athletic training program (3). It is essential that such practices be in keeping with the BOC *Standards of Professional Practice* and the NATA *Code of Ethics*. Some aspects of organization and administration will be similar regardless of the setting, but when developing policies and procedures, consideration must be given to issues specific to the particular environment. General areas that warrant attention in this domain include documentation and maintenance of the health care records, including those pertaining to health services (i.e., preparticipation examinations, injury evaluations, immediate treatment of injuries/illnesses, rehabilitation progress, and medical clearance to participate); other services rendered to an injured party (e.g., counseling, educational programs, and referrals to specialists); confidentiality of medical records; financial, facility, and personnel management; purchase of equipment and supplies; equipment reconditioning records; compliance with defined safety standards; emergency care protocols; public relations; and normal operating procedures.

Professional Responsibility

The domain of professional responsibility focuses on the expectations of the athletic trainer relative to adhering to ethical, legal, and other professional standards (3). The knowledge and skills identified in this area are intended to ensure appropriate care in all aspects of health care delivery (e.g., patient assessment, care, and treatment; knowledge of current best practice; and administrative functions). The BOC addresses professional development primarily in two ways namely, ethical practice and continuing education (3). In both areas, compliance with the BOC *Standards of Professional Practice* is essential to maintaining the ATC® credential.

FIGURE 1.3 Rehabilitation. A major performance domain of the athletic trainer includes the development and implementation of rehabilitation programs.

Box 1.1 Athletic Training Education—Formal Instruction Areas

NATA Professional Course Content Areas
- Risk management and injury/illness prevention
- Pathology of injury/illness
- Assessment of injury/illness
- General medical conditions and disabilities
- Therapeutic exercise; rehabilitative techniques
- Health care administration
- Weight management and body composition
- Psychosocial intervention and referral
- Medical ethics and legal issues
- Pharmacology
- Professional development and responsibilities

Foundational Courses
Human physiology
Human anatomy
Exercise physiology
Kinesiology/biomechanics
Nutrition
Therapeutic modalities
Acute care of injury and illness
Statistics and research design
Strength training and reconditioning

Athletic Training Education

To qualify for certification as an athletic trainer, an individual must earn an undergraduate or graduate degree, having completed an accredited entry-level athletic training education program. Effective July 1, 2006, the recognized accrediting agency is the Commission on Accreditation of Athletic Training Education (CAATE), known formally as the Joint Review Committee on Educational Programs in Athletic Training (JRC-AT) (4). The Education Council of the NATA is responsible for matters pertaining to athletic training education (5).

Using a competency-based approach, athletic training education programs are designed to provide an effective blend of classroom and clinical experience. Education content is based on cognitive (knowledge), psychomotor (skill), affective competencies (professional behaviors), and clinical proficiencies (professional and practice-oriented outcomes) (4). Formal instruction must be provided in designated subject matter areas (Box 1.1)

Completed under the supervision of a clinical instructor, the clinical education experience involves the acquisition and practice of the *Entry-Level Athletic Training Clinical Proficiencies*. The *Proficiencies* define the common set of skills that entry-level athletic trainers should possess (5). As part of the clinical experience, athletic training students complete a field experience designed to provide the opportunity to apply skills in a clinical environment. In addition, the field experience includes opportunities for the athletic training student to implement the policies and procedures of daily health care to participants in sport and physical activity.

The ATC® Credential

To earn the ATC® credential, an individual must complete a CAATE-accredited athletic training education program and pass the national certification examination administered by the BOC. Current and specific information regarding requirements for certification is available on the BOC website (www.bocatc.org).

The ATC® credential holder must demonstrate continuing competence and requalify for certification (2). Specifically, ATC credential holders must complete a predetermined number of continuing education units, including recertification in Emergency Cardiac Care, in a specified 3-year term. Continuing education programs provide an opportunity for athletic trainers to acquire new, innovative skills and techniques and to learn about current research within the profession. Continuing education units may be accumulated in a variety of ways, such as attending workshops, seminars, conferences, and conventions; speaking at a clinical symposium; publishing professional articles; or enrolling in related correspondence or postgraduate education courses. Current standards of continuing education requirements are available on the BOC website (www.bocatc.org).

Standards of Professional Practice

Standards of professional practice are ethical responsibilities that guide one's actions and promote high standards of conduct and integrity to assure high-quality health care (1). A certified athletic trainer should never compromise the health of any individual in his or her care. Decisions made by the athletic trainer in rendering care must be based on sound medical consideration. Individuals should be informed of the risks for injury, protected from injury whenever possible, and if an injury occurs, receive expedient health care and rehabilitation. Participants have a right to confidentiality about their health status. Athletic trainers must be sensitive about dissemination of health information and honor the wishes of an individual not to make the information public.

The NATA has established the Code of Ethics and five basic ethical principles for athletic trainers to follow. These include (1):

1. Members shall respect the rights, welfare, and dignity of all individuals.

2. Members shall comply with the laws and regulations governing the practice of athletic training.

3. Members shall accept responsibility for the exercise of sound judgment.

4. Members shall maintain and promote high standards in the provision of services.

5. Members shall not engage in any form of conduct that constitutes a conflict of interest or reflects adversely on the profession.

A copy of the Code of Ethics is available on the NATA website (www.nata.org).

In addition, the BOC publishes the *Standards of Professional Practice* (2). This document serves as a tool for informing the public, candidates for certification, and ATC credential holders about the standards of professional conduct and disciplinary procedures imposed for the practice of athletic training. A copy of the *Standards* is available on the BOC website (www.bocatc.org).

Registration and Licensure

Athletic trainers, through their state associations, have worked to secure recognition and establish some type of regulation concerning the practice of athletic training within their respective states. States regulate professions to protect the public from harm by unqualified individuals. Without some type of regulation, no legal foundation assures quality of care, because no legal definition exists regarding what an athletic trainer can and cannot do.

Licensure is the strictest form of state regulation and, therefore, is the most effective means of protecting the public. Licensure is necessary to protect the general public, to ensure public safety, to maintain minimum standards in the practice of athletic training, and to promote the highest degree of professional conduct on the part of the athletic trainer (6,7). It is the permission of a governmental body for an individual to practice a profession.

Certification within a state differs from certification as an athletic trainer. Successful completion of the BOC requirements for certification does not automatically qualify an individual for state certification. State certification indicates that a person has the basic knowledge and skills required in the profession and has passed a state certification examination. Many states that offer certification recognize a successful passing score on the BOC examination as a criterion for granting state certification.

Registration, which is used in some states, means that an individual intending to practice athletic training within the state must register with a governmental agency. The state may or may not have educational prerequisites for registration; however, an individual can be removed from the registry for abuse, fraud, or harm to the public or patient. In a few states, athletic trainers are exempt from the licensure requirements of another profession, such as physicians and athletic trainers in Colorado and physical therapists and athletic trainers in Hawaii. A specific scope of practice is defined in the **exemption** statute of the licensing requirement. Athletic trainers do not register with the state but are held to the standards of the scope of practice as defined in the statutes.

A listing of states that regulate athletic trainers can be found on the companion website at thePoint.

To date, 43 states require athletic trainers to meet specific standards of practice within the individual state (1). These laws define the role of the athletic trainer and set the legal parameters under which the athletic trainer can operate within that state. As such, the laws delineate the specific clientele and services that can be provided in various work settings. For information regarding individual state licensure laws or an update on states regulating the practice of athletic training, contact the NATA Government Affairs Committee (www.nata.org).

Although standards vary, in most states, athletic trainers provide services to athletes or physically active individuals under the direct supervision of a physician licensed in that state. Most states accept the successful completion of the BOC examination as a basis for obtaining licensure, although there may or may not be any mechanism for assessing continued competency. Athletic trainers may be restricted in the services they provide in nontraditional settings or in states that do not have licensure laws. Being properly licensed and practicing within the established standards of practice are two of the strongest safeguards against litigation.

Work Settings

Historically, the common work setting for athletic trainers has been organized sports programs (i.e., professional, collegiate, and high school venues). In recent years, as the qualifications of the athletic trainer have evolved, work setting opportunities have expanded outside the athletic arena.

Secondary Schools

The NATA has taken the position that secondary schools should provide a certified athletic trainer to address the health care needs of student athletes (1). Furthermore, it is recommended that the athletic trainer be available both on-site and on a full-time basis. The American Academy of Family Physicians and the AMA support the need to provide appropriate health care to high school student athletes and the role of the athletic trainer as an integral part of a high school athletic program (8,9).

In the secondary school setting, securing the services of an athletic trainer generally occurs in two ways:

1. The athletic trainer is an employee of the school system.

2. The school system develops a contractual agreement with a local hospital or clinic to provide on-campus athletic training services.

In some secondary schools, athletic trainers extend their services to include faculty and students outside the athletic program. In this capacity, the athletic trainer administers care for injuries sustained on school property and provides educational seminars on a variety of health-related topics, such as exercise programs, prevention of injury or illness during physical activity, and proper nutrition.

College/Universities

The responsibilities of the athletic trainer in collegiate settings vary. In some institutions, the athletic trainer functions solely as a member of the athletic health care team. At others, the athletic trainer may be expected to take on additional responsibilities, such as teaching or working in the campus health center.

Professional Sports

Athletic trainers for professional sport teams typically are hired by a single sport team to perform athletic training services throughout the year. During the competitive season, the athletic trainer concentrates on traditional duties. During the off-season, the athletic trainer is involved primarily with developing and supervising rehabilitation and reconditioning programs.

Sports Medicine Clinics

In sports medicine clinics, the athletic trainer is a member of a team comprised of a variety of health care professionals. Under the direction of a physician, the athletic trainer provides services to a diverse patient population. Some clinics specialize in only sport-related injuries, but others deal in cardiac rehabilitation, exercise physiology, biomechanical analysis, or workers' compensation injuries or may serve the general population. In some states, direct billing or licensure standards may restrict the athletic trainer from providing certain services, such as initial patient evaluation or use of electrical modalities.

Industrial/Occupational Settings

In the industrial and occupational setting, athletic trainers provide employees with in-house athletic training services. Working under the direction of a physician, the athletic trainer can perform injury assessment, management, and rehabilitation; develop wellness and fitness programs; and provide education and counseling for employees. This practice has proven to be beneficial for both the company and the employee. Companies that employ an athletic trainer are reporting decreases in the "frequency, severity, and cost of workers' compensation claims for musculoskeletal disorders" (1). In addition, employee productivity has increased subsequent to a decrease in the number of lost or restricted workdays (1).

Physician Practices

In the capacity of physician extender, athletic trainers perform an array of services. In a variety of physician practices (e.g., orthopaedics, osteopathy, family practice, primary care, pediatrics, and occupational medicine), athletic trainers are involved in areas such as triage, patient education, rehabilitation, and exercise prescription. The use of athletic trainers in this capacity can improve the quality of care provided to patients as well as increase physician productivity and efficiency. The patient receives additional personal attention, yet the physician is afforded the opportunity to meet with more patients in relatively the same amount of time. In addition, the potential exists for increased revenue through billing and insurance reimbursement of athletic training services.

A *The Role Delineation Study, published by the BOC, defines the current entry-level knowledge, skills, and abilities of the certified athletic trainer and serves as a blueprint for development of the certification examination. The Athletic Training Educational Competencies, published by the NATA Education Council, defines the educational domains used in preparing entry-level athletic trainers.*

TEAM APPROACH TO DELIVERY OF HEALTH CARE

Q *A member of a high school basketball team was seen by his family physician for an injury sustained during practice. The physician determined that the athlete should not participate in activity for 1 week. After 5 days, the athlete's parents call the school athletic trainer to give approval for their child to play. How should the athletic trainer respond to this situation?*

As members of a health care team, athletic trainers work under the supervision of a licensed physician and with a variety of other professionals. The team approach provides an effective means for ensuring quality health care for physically active individuals.

Team Physician

In organized sport, such as interscholastic, intercollegiate, or professional athletic programs, a team physician may be hired or may volunteer his or her services to direct the primary sports medicine team. This individual supervises the various aspects of health care and is the final authority to determine the mental and physical fitness of athletes in organized programs (10).

The team physician should have an unrestricted medical license and be an MD or DO. The individual should have a fundamental knowledge of emergency care regarding sporting events and a working knowledge of trauma, musculoskeletal injuries, and medical conditions affecting the athlete (10).

In an athletic program, the team physician should administer and review preseason physical examinations; review preseason conditioning programs; assess the quality, effectiveness, and maintenance of protective equipment; diagnose injuries; dispense medications; direct rehabilitation programs; educate the athletic staff regarding emergency policies, procedures, health care insurance coverage, and legal liability; and review all medical forms, policies, and procedures to ensure compliance with school and athletic association guidelines (10). This individual also may serve as a valuable resource in terms of current therapeutic techniques, facilitate referrals to other medical specialists, and provide educational counseling to sport participants, parents, athletic trainers, coaches, and sport supervisors.

A more detailed listing of team physician responsibilities is available at the companion website at thePoint.

In many high school and collegiate settings, financial constraints may prevent hiring a full-time team physician. Instead, several physicians may rotate the responsibility of being present at competitions and are paid a per-game stipend. Primary care physicians, orthopaedists, and other specialists (e.g., osteopaths, internists, general surgeons, and pediatricians) who have a broad and thorough understanding of sports injuries may serve as team physicians. A physician should be present at competitions, particularly those involving high-risk sports, to assess emergency injury and treat any injury or illness.

Primary Care Physician

In some settings, particularly those outside the traditional athletic setting, the primary care or family physician assumes a key role in providing medical care to athletes and physically active individuals of all ages. The services provided by the primary care physician can vary with the background and expertise of the individual. Services performed by a primary care physician can range from completing a preparticipation examination for a young athlete to counseling a middle-aged patient with multiple risk factors for coronary artery disease regarding the parameters for safely beginning an exercise program (10). In some settings, the primary care physician will assume the responsibility for clearing an individual to participate in activity.

The Coach or Sport Supervisor

A coach is responsible for teaching the skills and strategies of a sport. A sport supervisor may not necessarily be a coach but, instead, may be responsible for administering and supervising recreational sport activities or activity areas within health club facilities. Both individuals are responsible for encouraging appropriate behavior and developing an overall awareness of safety and injury prevention. For brevity, coaches and sport supervisors are jointly referred to as coaches.

In the absence of an athletic trainer, the coach must assume a more active role in providing health care to participants. As such, coaches should maintain current certification in emergency cardiac care (i.e., cardiopulmonary resuscitation and automated external defibrillator) and emergency first aid. Coaches should meet with their respective staff to develop an emergency action plan and should periodically practice implementing that plan. In the absence of an athletic trainer, coaches also are expected to evaluate the daily status of participants before any activity, properly fit and use quality safety equipment, teach proper skill development and technique, and constantly reinforce the importance of safety and injury prevention throughout the year (1). In addition, the coach can be responsible for informing the participant of the risk of injury, the strategies for preventing injuries, and the actions to take if an injury is sustained.

Sport/Physical Activity Participant

Individual participants play an essential role in working with the athletic trainer to maximize injury prevention. It is the responsibility of the participant to adhere to prescribed guidelines for the activity. Such responsibilities could include maintaining an appropriate level of fitness, performing within the rules or guidelines of an activity, and maintaining and wearing safety equipment. In the event of an injury, the individual should know where to seek immediate health care and follow medical advice from the physician or athletic trainer. If participants understand and practice safety and preventive measures, the number of injuries or illnesses can be reduced significantly.

Physical Therapist

Physical therapists provide a unique and valuable resource in the overall rehabilitation of an individual. Physical therapists often supervise the rehabilitation of injured participants in a hospital setting, an industrial clinic, or a sports medicine clinic. In some cases, an athletic trainer and physical therapist will combine efforts in designing and implementing rehabilitative care.

Strength and Conditioning Specialist

The use of proper strength and conditioning to improve physical skills, athletic performance, and fitness is the purview of the strength and conditioning specialist. A collaborative effort between the strength and conditioning specialist and an athletic trainer can be advantageous in designing and implementing conditioning programs for injured as well as healthy individuals.

Exercise Physiologist

An exercise physiologist can provide information pertaining to the physiological mechanisms underlying physical activity. As such, the exercise physiologist can offer theoretical and practical suggestions regarding the analysis, improvement, and maintenance of health and fitness as well as the rehabilitation of heart disease and other chronic diseases and/or disabilities (11).

Nutritionist

Nutritionists are concerned primarily with the role of proper dietary care in the prevention and treatment of illnesses but can provide valuable input regarding the specialized needs of athletes and physically active individuals. Examples of particular needs include diets for enhancing performance and preventing injury, effective weight management strategies (e.g., weight gain, loss, or maintenance), physical activity and diabetes, counseling with regard to disordered eating, and nutrient supplementation.

Biomechanist

Applying basic laws of physics in performing mechanical analyses of human movement, a biomechanist can offer practical insight for improving human performance as well as preventing injuries related to sport and physical activity. Information pertaining to kinematics (i.e., the study of spatial and temporal aspects of motion) can provide valuable information pertaining to injury prevention, whereas information regarding kinetics (i.e., the study of forces associated with motion) provides a basis for understanding injury mechanisms.

(A) *The athletic trainer must follow the physician's orders. As such, the athletic trainer should not permit the athlete to return to play and should advise the parent that the family physician is the final authority for determining the athlete's return to play.*

LEGAL CONSIDERATIONS

(Q) *As the athletic trainer at a high school, the athletic director has asked you to speak at the annual preseason meeting attended by the athletes and their parents. What topics should be addressed at this meeting?*

Prevention of injuries and reducing further injury or harm are major responsibilities of athletic trainers. Even with the best possible care, accidents do happen, some of which may result in legal action against several parties, such as athletic trainer, the team physician, or the activity supervisor. Legal action involving the practice of athletic training typically is tried under tort law. A **tort** is a civil wrong done to an individual, whereby the injured party seeks a remedy for damages suffered. Such wrongs may occur from an act of omission, whereby an individual fails to perform a legal duty, or from an act of commission, whereby an individual commits an act that is not their act to perform or an act that is their duty to perform but that is carried out with the wrong procedure, leading to injury or harm. In lawsuits, actions are measured against a standard of care provided by individuals who have a direct duty to provide care.

Standard of Care

Standard of care is measured by what another minimally competent individual educated and practicing in that profession would have done in the same or similar circumstance to protect an individual from harm or further harm. Standard of care is dictated by the profession's duty or **scope of care,** which outlines the role and responsibilities of an individual in that profession and delineates what should be learned in the professional preparation of that individual. In athletic training, the Education Council of the NATA has determined the competencies that define the educational content that students enrolled in a CAATE-accredited athletic training program must master.

By delineating the scope of care for entry-level athletic trainers, the BOC establishes the standard of care that the public can expect to receive from a certified athletic trainer. As such, an individual responsible for providing athletic training services is held to the standard of care expected of an individual holding the ATC credential. Therefore, in states with specific registration, certification, or licensure laws, valid BOC certification and registration or licensure is essential to protect oneself against litigation.

Clearance for Participation

The final authority to clear an individual for activity falls outside the scope of care of a certified athletic trainer. The final authority in measuring an individual's status for participation rests with the physician (e.g., team physician or primary care physician) (10).

Negligence

Athletic trainers are expected to provide a duty of care to participants (12). Failure to provide this care can result in liability, or **negligence.** Negligent torts may occur as a result of **malfeasance, misfeasance, nonfeasance, malpractice,** or **gross negligence** (Box 1.2).

Although participants assume some risk, which is inherent in any physical activity, the individual does not assume the risk that a professional will breach his or her duty of care. To find an individual liable, the injured person must prove that (13):

1. There was a duty of care.

2. There was a breach of that duty.

3. There was harm (e.g., pain and suffering, permanent disability, or loss of wages).

4. The resulting harm was a direct cause from that breach of duty.

For example, if a spectator notices a large hole in the field before a game and a player steps into that hole and fractures an ankle, the spectator is not liable, because that individual has no duty of care for the player. An athletic trainer or coach, however, does have a duty of care to check the field for hazards before competition. As such, the athletic trainer or coach could be held liable for the injury sustained by the participant.

Box 1.2 Definition of Negligent Torts

- **Malfeasance** occurs when an individual commits an act that is not his or her responsibility to perform. For example, if an athletic trainer suspects a neck injury and removes a football helmet, the athletic trainer could be held liable.
- **Misfeasance** occurs when an individual commits an act that is his or her responsibility to perform but either uses the wrong procedure or does the correct procedure in an improper manner. For example, if an athletic trainer suspects a neck injury and improperly secures the head and neck region to the rigid spine board, the athletic trainer could be held liable.
- **Nonfeasance** occurs when an individual fails to perform his or her legal duty of care. For example, if an athletic trainer suspects, or should have suspected, a neck injury and failed to use a rigid back board to stabilize the individual, the athletic trainer could be held liable.
- **Malpractice** occurs when an individual commits a negligent act while providing care.
- **Gross negligence** occurs when an individual has total disregard for the safety of others.

Legal Liabilities

Athletic trainers and coaches can take several precautionary steps to limit the risk of litigation. These may involve:

- Informing the individual about the inherent risks of participation
- Foreseeing the potential for injury. and correcting the situation before harm occurs
- Obtaining informed consent from the individual or their guardian before participation in the sport/activity and before any treatment should an injury occur
- Using quality products and equipment that do not pose a threat to the individual
- Maintaining strict confidentiality of all medical records

Fortunately, the number of lawsuits brought against athletic trainers in the performance of their duties is small (13). Situations that can result in litigation are listed in Box 1.3.

Failure to Warn

Athletic trainers should inform potential participants of the risks for injury during participation. Participants and parents of minor children should understand that risk for injury exists as well as the nature of that risk so that informed judgments can be made about participation. Understanding and comprehending the nature of the risk is determined by the participant's age, experience, and knowledge of pertinent information about the risk. An advanced gymnast, for example, knows and appreciates the risk of injury much more than a novice gymnast. Therefore, it is crucial to warn the novice of any inherent dangers in the activity and continually reinforce that information throughout the entire sport season. Warnings may be communicated at the preseason meeting with parents and participants; during prescreening, when the client is first introduced into the fitness or health facility; and by posting visible warning signs around equipment, requiring protective equipment, and discouraging dangerous techniques. (Other methods that may be used are discussed later in the chapter.)

Foreseeability of Harm

Another duty of care for athletic trainers and coaches is to recognize the potential for injury and then remove that danger before an injury occurs. **Foreseeability of harm** exists when danger is

Box 1.3 Actions That Can Result in Litigation

- Failing to warn an individual about the risks involved in sport participation
- Treating an injured party without his or her consent
- Failing to provide medical information concerning alternative treatments or the risks involved with the needed treatment
- Failing to provide safe facilities, fields, and equipment
- Being aware of a potentially dangerous situation and failing to do anything about it
- Failing to provide an adequate injury prevention program
- Allowing an injured or unfit player to participate, resulting in further injury or harm
- Failing to provide quality training, instruction, and supervision
- Using unsafe equipment
- Negligently moving an injured athlete before properly immobilizing the injured area
- Failing to employ qualified medical personnel
- Failing to have a written emergency action plan
- Failing to properly recognize an injury or illness (both immediate acute care and long-term treatment)
- Failing to immediately refer an injured party to the proper physician
- Failing to keep adequate records
- Treating an injury that did not occur within the school athletic environment

apparent or should have been apparent, resulting in an unreasonably unsafe condition. This potential for injury can be identified during regular inspections of gymnasiums, field areas, swimming pools, safety equipment, and athletic training facilities. For example, unpadded walls under basketball hoops, glass or potholes on playing fields, slippery floors near a whirlpool, exposed wiring, and failure to follow universal safety precautions against the spread of infectious diseases all pose a threat to safety. Unsafe conditions should be identified, reported in writing to appropriate personnel, restricted from use, and repaired or replaced as soon as possible.

Informed Consent

Informed consent implies that an injured party has been reasonably informed of the needed treatment, the possible alternative treatments, and the advantages and disadvantages of each course of action. Valid consent can only be obtained from one who is competent to grant it—that is, an adult who is physically and mentally competent or, in the case of children younger than 18 years, a parent. For minors, exceptions exist in emergency situations when parents are unavailable. Authorization to treat in the absence of the parent, or in the event the individual is physically unable to consent to treatment, should be obtained in writing before the beginning of participation. This consent may be obtained during preparticipation meetings as part of the documentation depicting consent to participate in that activity.

> A sample of an informed consent form is available on the companion website at thePoint.

It is advisable to include an exclusionary clause on the consent form that identifies conditions that will not be treated by the athletic trainer (e.g., injuries not associated with direct participation in a sponsored activity). This can protect the athletic trainer from litigation when refusing to treat a particular injury. For example, suppose an individual is injured in a recreational bicycling accident and fails to seek immediate treatment from an emergency room or physician. Two days later, this individual reports to an athletic trainer with an infected, open wound. In this instance, the athletic trainer should immediately refer this individual to a physician for treatment. In most states, if the athletic trainer attempts to clean the wound and complications arise, the athletic trainer may be held liable for practicing medicine outside the scope of the athletic training profession.

Informed consent must be granted before any treatment. Athletic trainers must be sensitive to cultural and religious beliefs and practices as well—and honor those practices by providing appropriate care consistent with the wishes of the patient. For example, in some cultures, a woman may be taught not to undress or bare skin in the presence of a man other than her husband. Therefore, if a male athletic trainer is assigned to treat a woman with a thoracic injury and she does not feel comfortable, it is better to refer the patient to a female athletic trainer.

Failure to receive informed consent may constitute **battery,** which is any unpermitted or intentional contact with another individual without that individual's consent. Although many courts require that intent to harm be present in an allegation of battery, written documentation of informed consent should be obtained from an individual or parents of minor children before treatment to avoid litigation.

Refusing Help

Although the situation is rare, an injured participant may refuse emergency first aid for a variety of reasons, such as religious beliefs, cultural differences, avoidance of additional pain or discomfort, or the desire to be evaluated and treated by a more medically qualified individual. Regardless of the reason, a conscious and medically competent individual has the right to refuse treatment. An exemption to this standard may occur, however, when failure to move the injured party may result in an increased risk of further injury to the injured party or others in the vicinity of the accident. For example, during an organized bike race, if several bikers collide and fall down onto a busy road, it is appropriate to move any injured individuals off the road so as not to endanger those individuals and any approaching motorists. In this instance, it is best to have another employee summon emergency medical services while the immediate care provider tries to persuade the injured party to accept immediate care until the ambulance arrives. It is helpful to have a witness to the event, because too often, an injured individual may initially refuse consent but later deny having done so.

Product Liability

Individuals often place a high degree of faith in the quality and safety of equipment used in sport and physical activity participation. Manufacturers have a duty of care to design, manufacture, and package safe equipment that will not cause injury to an individual when the equipment is used as intended. This is called an **implied warranty**. An **expressed warranty** is a written guarantee that the product is safe for use. In football, there is an implied warranty that the helmet can protect the head and brain from certain injuries if fitted and used properly. The National Operating Committee on Standards for Athletic Equipment (NOCSAE) has established minimum standards for football helmets to tolerate certain forces when applied to different areas of the helmet. Manufacturers and reconditioners of helmets place a visible expressed warranty on all helmets that meet NOCSAE standards. This statement informs players that the helmet is not intended to be used to butt, ram, or spear an opposing player and that use in this manner could result in serious head, brain, or neck injuries; paralysis; or even death for the player or the opposing player. **Strict liability** makes the manufacturer liable for any and all defective or hazardous equipment that unduly threatens an individual's personal safety.

Any alteration or modification to protective equipment may negate the manufacturer's liability. It is essential that all involved parties understand the potential dangers associated with the use of equipment and that equipment should be used properly and for its intended purpose. For example, the practice of cutting down mouth guards to cover only the front teeth should be strongly prohibited. Furthermore, participants should be continually warned of the inherent dangers if equipment is used in a manner for which it was not intended.

Confidentiality

A major concern of all individuals involved in providing health care is the patient's right to privacy. If the individual is older than 18 years, release of any medical information must be acknowledged in writing by the participant. For individuals younger than 18 years, a parent or legal guardian must provide consent for the dissemination of this information. This permission should identify what, if any, information can be shared with someone other than the individual's physician. In many cases, schools and professional teams have participants give consent that all medical information can be shared between the athletic trainers and supervising physician (12). Information provided to others (e.g., coaches, parents, or supervisors) should be on a need-to-know basis only and given with the full knowledge and consent of the individual, supervising physician, and athletic trainer. Confidentiality extends to all medical records kept within the confines of the athletic training room, including:

- Consent-to-treat form
- Release-of-medical-information form
- Emergency information
- Treatment documentation, including injury report forms, medical referrals, physician evaluations, laboratory reports, surgical reports, and progress notes
- Living will
- Counseling

Legal Defenses

If the threat of litigation exists, many athletic trainers rely on certain conditions to strengthen their case. These include the individual's assumption of risk, Good Samaritan laws, and comparative negligence.

Assumption of Risk

Sport and exercise participants assume some inherent risks in their chosen activity. When individuals agree to participate in competitive activity, they should be informed of the risks of participation, testing, and physical activity and advised that participation is voluntary in nature. Many facilities require that each participant sign an expressed assumption-of-risk form. By signing the form, the individual acknowledges the material risks and that other injuries and even death are a possibility. The form also acknowledges that the individual has had an opportunity to ask questions and have them answered to his

 A sample of an assumption of risk form is available on the companion website at thePoint.

or her complete satisfaction. Finally, the individual affirms a subjective understanding of the risks of their participation in the activity and their voluntary choice to participate, assuming all risks of injury or even death as a result of participation. These forms have successfully aided in the legal defense of individuals involved with providing health care. As stated previously, however, an individual does not assume the risk that a professional will breach the duty of care.

Good Samaritan Laws

Beginning in the early 1960s, several states enacted legislation to protect physicians or other recognized medical personnel from litigation a result of emergency treatment provided to injured individuals at the scene of an accident. These laws, nicknamed "Good Samaritan" laws, were developed to encourage bystanders to assist others in need of emergency care by granting them immunity from potential litigation. Although the laws vary from state to state, immunity generally applies only when the person providing emergency first aid:

1. Acts during an emergency.
2. Acts in good faith to help the victim.
3. Acts without expected compensation.
4. Is not guilty of any malicious misconduct or gross negligence toward the injured party (i.e., does not deviate from acceptable first aid protocol).

Although Good Samaritan laws were intended to protect physicians and medical personnel, several states have expanded the language to include laypersons serving as emergency first aiders. These laws are easy to get around, however, and they should not be relied on by rescuers who erroneously believe the laws will protect them from litigation regardless of their actions. It is essential that sport and fitness coordinators be properly trained in emergency first aid and care of injuries if they are expected to supervise participants and render immediate first aid should a client or athlete sustain an injury during participation.

Comparative Negligence

When an injured person chooses to pursue litigation, several individuals, along with their employers, are named in the suit. These individuals may include the physicians, surgeons, athletic trainers, supervisors, and emergency personnel who provided medical services to the athlete. **Comparative negligence** refers to the relative degree of negligence on the part of the plaintiff and defendant, with damages awarded on a basis proportionate to each person's carelessness. For example, if an individual is found to be 30% at fault for his or her own injury (contributory negligent) and the defendants to be 70% at fault, then on a $100,000 judgment, the defendants are responsible for $70,000 in damages and the individual (i.e., the plaintiff) assumes an equivalent of $30,000 in damages. The courts also weigh the relative degree of negligence on the part of each defendant and awards payment of damages on a basis proportionate to each person's carelessness that leads to the eventual injury.

Preventing Litigation

All members of the sports medicine team should be aware of their duty of care consistent with current state law and should complete that duty of care within established policies and standards of practice. Several steps can reduce the risk of subsequent litigation and include performing regular inspections of athletic fields and facility design, performing safety checks of equipment and facilities, hiring qualified personnel, ensuring proper supervision and instruction, purchasing quality equipment, posting appropriate warning signs, maintaining accurate and complete health care records, and having a well-organized emergency action plan.

> Additional strategies to avoid litigation can be found on the companion website at thePoint.

A *As the athletic trainer at a high school, during a preseason meeting for athletes and their parents, it would be appropriate to attend to the following: explanation of the risks involved in sport participation, completion of an assumption-of-risk form by the athlete and a parent, explanation of procedures for reporting injuries to the athletic trainer, obtaining written informed consent from the parents of minor children before participation, and obtaining emergency contact information.*

SUMMARY

1. Sports medicine is a branch of medicine that applies medical and scientific knowledge to improve sport performance.

2. The NATA establishes standards for professionalism, education, research, and practice settings for athletic trainers. The NATA has played a critical role in the evolution of the skills and qualifications of the athletic trainer to a level that can be used in a variety of fields.

3. The BOC is responsible for awarding the ATC credential. As defined by the BOC, the major performance domains for the entry-level certified athletic trainer are prevention; clinical evaluation and diagnosis; immediate care; treatment, rehabilitation, and reconditioning; organization and administration; and professional responsibility.

4. Work settings for athletic trainers continue to expand as the qualifications of the athletic trainer increase. Work settings include, but are not limited to, secondary school, college/university, or professional athletic programs; sports medicine clinics; industrial/occupational settings; and physician practices.

5. Standards of professional practice are ethical judgments that guide a professional's actions and promote high standards of conduct and integrity.

6. For an athletic trainer, BOC certification and state licensure can help to meet one's duty of care in providing health care.

7. Decisions concerning whether an individual should participate in an activity should be made by the physician based on sound medical consideration and never compromise the health of the individual.

8. To find an individual liable, the injured person must prove duty of care, breach of that duty, harm caused by that breach; and harm as a direct cause of the breach of duty.

9. Steps to reduce the risk of injury and subsequent litigation should include obtaining informed consent; recognizing the potential for injury and correcting it; warning participants of the risk of injury; hiring qualified personnel; providing proper supervision and instruction; purchasing, fitting, and maintaining quality equipment; posting appropriate warning signs; maintaining accurate and complete health care records; protecting confidentiality of medical history; and having a well-organized emergency care system.

REFERENCES

1. National Athletic Trainers' Association. Available at: http://www.nata.org. Accessed 8-24-2007.
2. National Athletic Trainers' Association Board of Certification. Available at: http://www.bocatc.org.
3. National Athletic Trainers' Association Board of Certification, Inc. Role Delineation Study, 5th Ed.. Omaha, NE: National Athletic Trainers' Association Board of Certification, 2004.
4. Joint Review Committee on Educational Programs in Athletic Training. Available at: http://www.jrc-at.org.
5. National Athletic Trainers' Association Education Council. Available at: http://www.nataec.org.
6. Rello MN. The importance of state regulation to the promulgation of the athletic training profession. J Ath Tr 1996;31(2):160–164.
7. Campbell D, Konin J. Regulation of athletic training. In: Konin J. Clinical Athletic Training. Thorofare, NJ: Slack, 1997.
8. American Academy of Family Physicians. Available at: http://www.aafp.org.
9. American Medical Association. Available at: http://www.ama-assn.org.
10. Mellion MB, Walsh WM. The team physician. In: Mellion MB, Walsh WM, Madden C, Putukian M, Shelton GL, eds. The Team Physician's Handbook. Philadelphia: Hanley & Belfus, 2002.
11. American Society of Exercise Physiologists. Available at: http://www.asep.org.
12. Arendt E. What every health care professional should know. NATA News 1996;8(1):20–21.
13. Leverenz LJ, Helms LB. Suing athletic trainers: Part I, a review of the case law involving athletic trainers. Ath Train (JNATA) 1990;25(3):212–216.

Preparticipation Examination

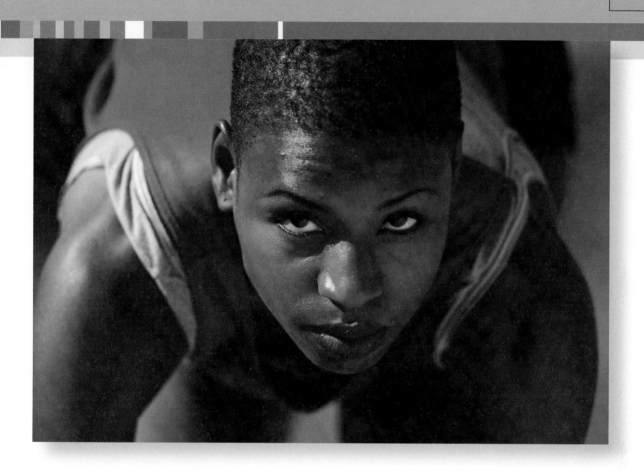

STUDENT OUTCOMES

1. Identify the goals and objectives of a preparticipation examination (PPE).

2. Design a PPE.

3. Identify the specific areas in a PPE that could be examined using a mass station screening process.

4. Identify follow-up questions intended to validate information on a medical history questionnaire.

5. Demonstrate the ability to take vital signs, and identify criteria used to denote abnormal pulse and blood pressure rates.

6. Explain the importance of completing a physical fitness profile as part of the PPE.

7. Demonstrate skinfold measurement at the various sites used to determine body composition.

8. Explain the criteria used to categorize hypermobility and hypomobility.

9. Describe specific methods of measuring strength, power, speed, cardiovascular endurance, agility, balance, and reaction time.

10. Identify specific conditions that could exclude an individual from participating in physical activity or sport.

ROLE DELINEATION COMPETENCIES

The following Performance Domains and Tasks defined in the National Athletic Trainers' Association Board of Certification *Role Delineation Study*, 5th Edition, are addressed in this chapter:

BOC COMPETENCIES

I. Prevention

A. Educate the appropriate individual(s) about risks associated with participation and specific activities using effective communication techniques to minimize the risk of injury and illness.

B. Interpret preparticipation and other relevant screening information in accordance with accepted guidelines to minimize the risk of injury and illness.

VI. Professional Responsibility

B. Adhere to statutory and regulatory provisions and other legal responsibilities relating to the practice of athletic training by maintaining an understanding of these provisions and responsibilities in order to contribute to the safety and welfare of the public.

The preparticipation examination (PPE), often performed annually, helps to ensure an individual's health and safety while participating in physical activity or sport. A PPE can identify preexisting conditions that may place the individual at risk for injury or illness. This chapter examines the PPE process and, following an introduction of the general principles and goals of the PPE, presents information on organizing the PPE using a group format. This includes setting up the examination, gathering a medical history, and conducting the physical examination. Finally, the criteria used to determine if an individual should be allowed to participate, and at what level of intensity, are discussed.

GOALS OF THE PREPARTICIPATION EXAMINATION

Q ▸ *Why is it important to consider the age of the individual when conducting a PPE?*

The basic objective of the PPE is to ensure the health and safety of a physically active individual. This can be accomplished by gathering information regarding the individual's general health, maturity, and fitness level. Those who are at risk for injury or who have conditions that may limit participation can be identified and counseled on health-related issues and steered toward participating in appropriate activities. Many states and sport governing bodies require some type of PPE for competitive athletes; however, states differ greatly regarding specific requirements. Although the frequency and depth of PPEs may vary, most examinations share common goals (Box 2.1).

Because participants range in age from the very young to the very old, the focus of the PPE is dependent on the specific age group. For example, in the prepubescent child (i.e., 6–10 years of age), the focus may be on identifying previously undiagnosed congenital abnormalities. In the pubescent child (i.e., 11–15 years of age), the examination should center on maturation and establishing good health practices for safe participation. In the postpubescent or young adult group (i.e., 16–30 years of age), the history of previous injuries and sport-specific examinations is critical. For individuals with cardiovascular or pulmonary disease, the strenuousness of a sport is an additional consideration.

It is important to acknowledge that limited data exist regarding the relative risks of dynamic and static exercise on various cardiovascular abnormalities (1). For a 16–30 age group, the more strenuous activities and those involving contact or collision sports may require a more extensive examination. Because the adult population (i.e., 30–65 years of age) has a high incidence of overuse injuries, these individuals need an examination based on the nature of the activity in which they intend to engage. The final group, those older than 65 years, often begins or increases activity to prevent a major medical illness. These individuals need an extensive examination based on individual needs,

A table showing classifications of sports based on strenuousness can be found on the companion website at thePoint.

Box 2.1   Goals of the Preparticipation Examination

- Determine general health and current immunization status.
- Detect medical conditions that are not healed or may predispose the individual to injury or illness so that medical treatment can start before sport/activity participation.
- Identify behaviors posing a risk to health that may be corrected through informed counseling.
- Establish baseline parameters for determining when an injured individual may return to activity.
- Assess physical maturity.
- Evaluate level of physical fitness.
- Classify the individual as to readiness for participation.
- Recommend appropriate levels of participation for individuals with medical contraindications to exercise.
- Meet legal and insurance requirements related to participation in physical activity or sport.

taking into consideration not only their physical needs but also any medications being taken and their possible side effects (2).

 Because age can be a factor that influences general health, maturity, and fitness level, it is essential that the focus of the PPE be altered to address issues or concerns specific to the age of the individual.

SETTING UP THE EXAMINATION

 A college soccer athlete has completed the freshman year and is returning to begin the sophomore season. Describe a reevaluation examination for this athlete.

Preparticipation examinations may be set up in a variety of ways. The organizational format depends on factors such as the level of activity (e.g., athlete in an organized competitive sport or individual in an exercise program), the community, the availability of personnel and facilities, the number of individuals being screened, and the personal preference of the evaluator.

Examination Format

The primary care physician (PCP) usually performs PPEs. Typically, the PCP is more knowledgeable about the individual's (and the family's) medical history, congenital or developmental deficiencies, immunization status, and recent injuries or illnesses that could limit participation in physical activity. A PPE administered by the PCP permits a closer examiner/patient relationship, and when the PPE is performed in the physician's office, a more thorough and comprehensive examination can be completed. The office setting provides greater privacy and a more optimal environment for counseling. The expense of the PPE is higher, however, and the time commitment on the part of the physician is more significant.

Because some individuals may have a physician who does not understand the physical demands of a particular sport activity, organized competitive sport programs often use a group or station format to examine a large number of individuals during a limited span of time. A supervising or team physician and several different health care providers perform a series of examinations at different stations. Following the conclusion of the examination, the supervising/team physician determines the individual's readiness for sport participation. This format is more time efficient, reduces costs significantly, and allows athletic trainers and area medical specialists to be involved. This format has several disadvantages, however, including the organizational coordination needed to execute such a comprehensive examination, decreased privacy, brief and often impersonal time spent with each individual, difficulty in following up on any medical concerns that may arise, and inability to have essential communication with parents of those in early and middle adolescence after the examination.

Timing of the Examination

Ideally, a PPE is completed at least 6 weeks before the start of any physical activity. This allows time to evaluate and correct minor problems, such as limited flexibility, muscle weakness, or minor illnesses. It also allows sufficient time for an individual with a potential medical problem to be referred to a specialist (e.g., cardiologist, neurologist, or ophthalmologist). Although many high schools and colleges conduct PPEs during late July or early August for fall sports, PPEs also can be completed during the spring of the year, provided some mechanism exists to report and evaluate any injury or illness that may have occurred during the summer.

Frequency of the Examination

Although an annual complete physical examination is common, it probably is unnecessary unless there is a change in physician or records are not available. A joint publication prepared by the American Academy of Family Physicians, the American Academy of Pediatrics, the American Medical Society of Sports Medicine, and the American Osteopathic Academy of Sports Medicine recommends that an entry-level complete physical examination be performed, followed by a limited annual reevaluation. Many physicians also complete an entry-level examination at each level of participation (e.g., middle school, high school, and college). The entry-level examination is discussed in detail in this chapter. The reevaluation should focus on the medical history and a limited physical examination, including height, weight, blood pressure, pulse, visual acuity, cardiac auscultation, and examination of the skin.

> **A** *A complete PPE is not automatically required on an annual basis. The reevaluation of the soccer athlete should focus on the medical history and a limited physical examination, including height, weight, blood pressure, pulse, visual acuity, cardiac auscultation, and examination of the skin.*

MEDICAL HISTORY

> **Q** *Why should the PPE begin with the medical history?*

A comprehensive medical history can identify a significant percentage of the problems affecting a physically active individual or sport participant. Typically, a written form is completed by the individual, answering in a "yes-no" format. To ensure accuracy, this information should be confirmed in person by the individual or the parents of minor children. A supplemental health history questionnaire can be provided for female athletes to gather information regarding menstrual history, menstrual or vaginal irregularities, urinary tract disorders, and use of birth control pills or hormones.

A sample Medical History Form and Supplemental Health History Questionnaire for Female Participants are available on the companion website at thePoint.

Questions in the medical history might explore current immunization status; past episodes of infectious diseases, loss of consciousness, recurrent headaches, musculoskeletal injuries, heat stroke, chest pains during or after exercise, seizures, breathing difficulties, disordered eating, and chronic medical problems; medication and drug use; allergies; heart murmurs or unusual heart palpitations; use of contact lenses, corrective lenses, dentures, prosthetic devices, or special equipment (e.g., pads, braces, neck rolls, or eye guards); and family history of cardiac problems, vascular problems, sickle cell anemia, diabetes, high blood pressure, sudden death, or neurologic problems. Underweight individuals can be questioned about weight loss, eating patterns, body image, and in the case of females, menses dysfunction.

When using a mass station screening approach, it is advisable to have the medical history station at the start of the examination. This station should have a knowledgeable examiner who can go through each questionnaire and ask detailed follow-up questions. The mass station affords the examiner an opportunity to cross-reference responses on the medical questionnaire. A "red flag" can be noted on specific responses, indicating that the condition warrants further investigation at another station. For example, a history of exercise-induced asthma should be pointed out to the examiner at the pulmonary station. This option allows a more knowledgeable examiner to conduct a thorough examination of the body system most affected by the condition.

A *The medical history establishes a foundation. This information can reveal possible congen-ital, hereditary, or acquired conditions that may put the individual at risk for future prob-lems. By beginning the PPE with the medical history, the information can be validated for accu-racy during the actual examination.*

THE PHYSICAL EXAMINATION

Q *Should a PPE be considered the equivalent of an annual medical examination?*

The PPE is not intended to be all-encompassing. Rather, it is intended to focus on the body systems that are of most concern to the individual depending on the activity or sport of choice. Particular attention should be paid to any areas of concern or red flags identified during the medical history.

Vital Signs

The PPE should establish the individual's baseline physiologic parameters and vital statistics. Height and weight should be taken and compared to standard growth charts. Information such as pulse rate, blood pressure, and body temperature may be recorded at this station by an athletic trainer or other allied health professional (Box 2.2).

Pulse rate usually is taken at the carotid artery by doubling the pulse rate measured during a 30-second period. To further delineate potential cardiovascular problems, the pulse should be taken at the radial and femoral arteries to determine whether the heart rate and rhythm are regu-lar. A weak or nonpalpable pulse at the femoral artery suggests coarctation of the aorta (3). An ir-regular pulse raises suspicion for arrhythmia and requires an electrocardiographic (ECG) evaluation (4).

Following proper guidelines is essential to ensuring accurate readings when measuring blood pressure. It is important that a proper cuff size be used. The bladder should encircle the mid-arm and cover two-thirds of the length of the arm. For an obese arm, a wide cuff (15 cm) should be used. If the arm circumference exceeds 41 cm, a thigh cuff (18 cm wide) should be used. A pediatric cuff may be indicated for a very thin arm. The guidelines for obtaining accurate blood pressure measurements are listed in Field Strategy 2.1.

Individuals with abnormal heart rates or high blood pressure should be rechecked several times at 15- to 20-minute intervals, with the individual lying down between measurements to determine if the high reading is accurate or caused by anxiety (e.g., "white coat syndrome"). If three consec-utive readings are high, the individual should be identified as having hypertension (high blood pressure). Table 2.1 shows hypertension standards by age in children, adolescents, and adults (5).

Individuals with severe degrees of hypertension (i.e., stages 3 and 4) should be further examined by a physician and restricted from high static activities and sports until the condition is controlled

Box 2.2   **Normal Vital Statistics**

- Pulse
Males	60 to 100 bpm
Females	60 to 100 bpm (may increase 10–15 bpm during pregnancy)
Children	120 to 140 bpm
Well-conditioned athletes	Can be as low as 50 bpm

- Blood pressure
Adults	120/80 mg Hg
Children (age, 10 years)	105/70 mm Hg

FIELD STRATEGY 2.1

Measuring Blood Pressure

General Guidelines

- No caffeine should be consumed during the hour before the reading; no smoking should be permitted 30 minutes before the reading.
- Take the measurement in a quiet, warm setting.
- Subject should sit quietly for 5 minutes, with the back supported and the arm supported at the level of the heart, before recording blood pressure.
- The air bladder should encircle and cover two-thirds of the length of the arm. If it does not, the bladder should be placed over the brachial artery (see figure.) If the bladder is too short, misleadingly high readings can result.
- Manometer: Aneroid gauges should be calibrated every 6 months against a mercury manometer.

Technique

- Inflate the bladder quickly to about 200 mm Hg.
- Place the stethoscope over the brachial artery in the cubital fossa.
- Deflate the bladder by 3 mm Hg/second, and listen for the first soft beating sounds (systolic pressure).
- As pressure is reduced, the sound becomes louder and more distinct, then gradually disappears as blood is no longer constricted.
- The pressure at which the sound disappears is the diastolic pressure.
- If the sounds are weak, the patient should be asked to raise the arm and open and close the hand 5 to 10 times. Then, the examiner should reinflate the bladder quickly.
- Record blood pressure, patient position, arm, and cuff size.

Number of Readings and Sites

- Take at least two readings, separated by as much time as is practical. If readings vary by more than 5 mm Hg, take additional readings until two consecutive readings are close.
- If the initial values are elevated, obtain two other sets of readings at least 1 week apart.
- Initially, measure the pressure in both arms; if the pressures differ, use the arm with the higher pressure.
- If arm pressure is elevated, take the pressure in one leg (particularly in patients younger than 30 years).

by lifestyle modification or drug therapy (3). Mild to moderate hypertension in the absence of organ disease or heart disease does not preclude physical activity or sport participation, but this condition should be noted and evaluated on an individual basis. Following the start of an exercise or training program, individuals with hypertension should have their blood pressure checked every 2 to 4 months or more frequently, if indicated, to monitor the impact of exercise.

Body temperature is measured by a thermometer placed under the tongue, in the ear, or under the armpit. Average oral temperature usually is quoted as 37°C (98.6°F), but this can fluctuate considerably. During the early morning hours, temperature may fall as low as 35.8°C (96.4°F), and in the later afternoon or evening, it may rise as high as 37.3°C (99.1°F). Rectal temperatures are higher than oral temperatures by an average of 0.4 to 0.5°C (0.7–0.9°F), although this, too, can be variable. In contrast, axillary temperatures are lower than oral temperatures by approximately 1°F but may take 5 to 10 minutes to register and generally are considered to be less accurate than other measurements (6).

A glass or electronic thermometer may be used for oral temperatures. When using a glass thermometer, the thermometer must initially measure 35°C (96°F) or less. The examiner should insert

TABLE 2.1 Classification of Blood Pressure[a]

AGE AND PHASE	NORMAL (HIGH NORMAL)[B]	PREHYPERTENSIVE	STAGE 1 HYPERTENSION	STAGE 2 HYPERTENSION
6–9 years				
Systolic	111–121	N/A	122–129	:129
Diastolic	70–77		70–85	:85
10–12 years				
Systolic	117–125	N/A	126–133	:133
Diastolic	75–81		82–89	:89
13–15 years				
Systolic	124–135	N/A	136–143	:143
Diastolic	77–85		86–91	:91
16–18 years				
Systolic	127–141	N/A	142–149	:149
Diastolic	80–91		92–97	:97
18 years				
Systolic	<120	120–139	140–159	≥160
Diastolic	<80	80–89	90–99	≥100

[a]Definitions apply to people who are not taking antihypertensive drugs and are not acutely ill. When systolic and diastolic blood pressures fall into different categories, the higher category should be selected to classify blood pressure status. Blood pressure values are based on the average of two or more readings taken at each of two or more visits after the initial screening. For adults age 18 and older, optimal blood pressure is 120/80 mm Hg; prehypertension is blood pressure that is 120–139/80–89 mm Hg. (National Heart, Lung, and Blood Institute. The Seventh Report of the Joint National Committee on Prevention, Detection, Evaluation, and Treatment of High Blood Pressure. Washington DC: U.S. Department of Health and Human Services, 2004.).

[b]Data from Second Task Force on Blood Pressure Control in Children. Bethesda, Maryland: National Heart, Lung, and Blood Institute, 1987.

the thermometer under the individual's tongue, instruct the individual to close the lips, and wait 3 to 5 minutes before removing and reading the temperature (6). If using an electronic thermometer, a disposable cover should be placed carefully over the probe; a digital readout should appear in about 10 seconds. Some electronic thermometers beep when the temperature reaches its maximum.

Infrared tympanic thermometers measure infrared energy emitted by the tympanic membrane and provide a rapid, efficient, and noninvasive method of measuring body temperature. In this method, the external auditory canal must be free of cerumen. The probe is positioned in the canal so that the infrared beam is aimed at the tympanic membrane (if aimed elsewhere, the measurement is invalid). The digital temperature reading should appear in 2 to 3 seconds. This method measures core body temperature, which is higher than the normal oral temperature by approximately 0.8°C (1.4°F) (6).

General Medical Problems

When using the mass station format, general systemic problems should be investigated early in the process to allow follow-up evaluation of any red flags. Information about past surgeries or hospitalizations may lead to facts about a previous injury or an attempt to control a chronic disease. If a previous injury exists, it is necessary to determine if there has been adequate time for optimal healing and if rehabilitation must be completed before clearing the individual for participation.

Recurrent visits to a doctor and/or hospitalization for a chronic disease suggest a poorly controlled chronic condition, such as asthma, diabetes, hypertrophic cardiomyopathy, anemia, or a seizure disorder. General questions regarding these disorders should ascertain the presence, severity, frequency, and control of the condition.

The examiner also should be concerned about problems such as acute infection, malignancy, and progressive diseases (e.g., multiple sclerosis). Acute illnesses (e.g., gastritis, flu, fever, diarrhea, or colds) tend to be self-limiting and usually require only temporary withdrawal from activity.

Inquiries should be made regarding the use of both prescription and over-the-counter medications. In some cases, medications can predispose an individual to certain conditions or illnesses. For example, the use of birth control pills or illicit drugs (e.g., anabolic steroids, amphetamines, or cocaine) may lead to hypertension. In addition, the use of alcohol, tobacco, caffeine, ergogenic aids, or illegal substances should be identified through direct inquiry.

Questions that should be asked regarding general medical conditions include:

1. Are you currently seeing a doctor for a medical problem?

2. Have you ever been diagnosed with a disease or been hospitalized overnight for a disease (e.g., diabetes, epilepsy, anemia, sickle-cell anemia, mononucleosis, or hepatitis)?

3. Have you ever been diagnosed with a progressive disease (e.g., muscular dystrophy, multiple sclerosis, or tuberculosis)?

4. Have you ever been hospitalized for a chronic disease or illness?

5. Have you even been told you have cancer?

6. Are you on any medications or allergic to any medications?

7. Have you ever had surgery?

8. Do you tend to bleed excessively?

9. Are you missing or have function of only one organ (e.g., eye, kidney, lung, or testicle)?

If any of these questions receives a positive response, a plan must be in place to ensure appropriate follow-up assessment.

Cardiovascular Examination

The cardiovascular examination should be completed in a quiet area so that outside noise does not interfere with auscultation of heart sounds. The physician should check for cardiac abnormalities to identify those individuals at risk for sudden death. More than 90% of sudden deaths in exercise and sports involve the cardiovascular system in participants younger than 30 years.

Questions evaluating the cardiovascular system should focus on a history of loss of consciousness, syncope or near-syncope, dizziness, shortness of breath, heart palpitations, and chest pain during or after exercise as well as sudden death occurring in a family member under 50 years of age, which may indicate a predisposition to cardiac anomalies, such as a **prolonged QT syndrome, Marfan's syndrome,** or **mitral valve prolapse** (4,7). Marfan's syndrome should be suspected in an individual who is tall and has an arm span greater than height, long fingers and toes, pectus excavatum chest-wall deformity, and a high arched palate (8).

Questions that should be asked of participants include:

1. Have you ever experienced pain or discomfort in the chest, neck, jaw, or arms during or after being physically active?

2. Have you ever experienced dizziness or passed out during or after physical activity?

3. Have you ever experienced shortness of breath at rest or with mild exercise?

4. When engaged in physical activity, do you tire more quickly than those around you?

5. Have you ever had rheumatic fever, had high or low blood pressure, or been told you have diabetes?

6. Have you ever noticed rapid heart palpitations or felt like your heart "raced"?

Box 2.3   Cardiovascular Red Flags Requiring Further Examination

- Chest pain during exertion
- Unusual fatigue or shortness of breath at rest or with mild exertion
- Dizziness or syncope with activity
- Breathing difficulty while lying down
- Ankle edema
- Heart palpitations or tachycardia
- Known heart murmur
- Abnormal heart rate or arrhythmia
- Uncontrolled hypertension

- Hypertrophic cardiomyopathy
- Congenital coronary artery anomalies
- Marfan's syndrome or aortic coarctation
- Mitral valve prolapse
- Conduction abnormalities
- Arteriosclerotic coronary artery disease
- Anemia
- Enlarged spleen
- Dextrocardia (i.e., heart located on right side of chest)
- Family history of heart problems or sudden death

7. Have you ever been told you have a heart murmur, an irregular heart beat, or any heart disease?

8. Do you have persistent ankle swelling?

9. Has anyone in your family had any heart problems, had a heart attack, or died suddenly before the age of 50?

10. Have any of your relatives had any of the following conditions: hypertrophic cardiomyopathy, dilated cardiomyopathy, Marfan's syndrome, long QT syndrome, or significant heart arrhythmia?

If any of these questions receives a positive response, the individual should be fully evaluated by a cardiologist to determine the presence of conditions such as **hypertrophic cardiomyopathy**, conduction abnormalities, dysrhythmias, valvular problems, and coronary artery defects (Box 2.3). Assessment by a cardiologist will include a variety of techniques. For example, precordial **auscultation** in a supine and standing position can identify heart murmurs consistent with dynamic left ventricular outflow obstruction. Provocative maneuvers help to differentiate functional murmurs from pathologic murmurs. A decrease in venous return can be initiated by having an individual move from a squatting to a standing position while performing a **Valsalva maneuver**; venous return can be increased by having the individual take several deep inspirations, moving from a standing to a squatting position, or performing an isometric hand grip (4). General recommendations for murmurs requiring further evaluation before an individual can participate include:

- Any systolic murmur grade 3 through 6 in severity

- Any diastolic murmur

- Any murmur that gets louder with a Valsalva maneuver

Hypertrophic cardiomyopathy is the most common cause of sudden death in young athletes, followed by congenital coronary artery anomalies, aortic rupture associated with Marfan's syndrome, mitral valve prolapse, and cardiac conduction disorders. In the older physically active individual, arteriosclerosis is almost always the cause of sudden death. If any of these conditions are present, strenuous activity is precluded until an ECG or stress ECG is completed.

Pulmonary Examination

The pulmonary examination may be done in conjunction with the cardiovascular examination. The physician auscultates for clear breath sounds and watches for symmetric movement of the diaphragm. A history of coughing spells or difficulty breathing may indicate exercise-induced bronchospasm. Although easily treated, this condition often goes undetected. In addition, up to 40% of athletes with environmental allergies or seasonal rhinitis experience exercise-induced bronchospasm,

Box 2.4 Pulmonary Red Flags Requiring Further Examination

- Abnormal coughing
- Abnormal shortness of breath at rest or with minimal exertion
- Abnormal breath sounds (e.g., wheezing, rhonchi, rubs, or rales)
- Abnormal or prolonged expiratory phase
- Asthma (uncontrolled or exertional)

- Exercise-induced bronchospasm
- Pulmonary insufficiency
- Pneumothorax
- Severe allergies

and up to 80% of asthmatics are similarly affected. Prolonged symptoms also may indicate possible congenital heart defects, cardiomyopathy, or valvular dysfunction.

The ears, nose, and mouth may be checked at this examination station as well. If any hearing problems are suspected, the individual should be referred to a specialist.

Questions that should be asked include:

1. Have you ever experienced excessive coughing during or after being physically active?

2. Have you ever experienced breathing difficulties or been told you have asthma, bronchitis, or allergies?

3. Have you ever had shortness of breath or heard unusual breath sounds during or after being physically active?

4. Have you ever had a collapsed lung?

If any abnormalities are found (e.g., wheezing, crackles, rhonchi, rubs, rales, or abnormal inspiratory to expiratory ratio), appropriate lung function tests should be ordered. Concerns such as tuberculosis, uncontrolled asthma, exertional asthma, exercise-induced bronchospasm, pulmonary insufficiency resulting from a collapsed lung, or chronic bronchial asthma should be assessed by the physician and discussed with the individual (Box 2.4) (9).

Musculoskeletal Examination

The musculoskeletal examination is critical to the physically active individual and the sport participant. A history of previous fractures, strains, tendinitis, sprains, and dislocations may suggest a predisposition to injury recurrences or potential arthritis. Questions should focus on the nature of any injury sustained, when it occurred, who evaluated it, the duration of the treatment and rehabilitation, and if surgical intervention was necessary. Questions pertaining to the wearing of special protective equipment also may identify injuries or conditions that might otherwise have gone undetected. For example, the use of an ankle brace may indicate a chronic lateral ankle sprain, and the use of a neck roll may indicate previous neurologic impairment of the cervical region.

Questions that might be asked include:

1. Have you ever sprained or dislocated a joint?

2. Have you had repeated backaches?

3. Have you ever strained (pulled) a muscle?

4. Have you ever fractured any bone?

5. Do you experience any persistent swelling of a joint or body region?

6. Have you ever experienced pain in any muscle or joint when you first wake up in the morning?

7. Have you ever been awakened at night because of pain in any joint or muscle?

8. Do you ever have pain during or after activity?

9. What special protective equipment do you use regularly?

FIELD STRATEGY 2.2

Musculoskeletal Examination

Observe:

- Postural symmetry: Note unusual swelling or asymmetry of body segments, including scapular asymmetry, pelvic tilting, and hamstring and calf atrophy.
- Back and spine: Place the individual in a forward flexed/knee extended position to detect scoliosis and to assess hamstring flexibility.
- Lower extremities: Note quadriceps symmetry during contraction and relaxation, genu valgus or varus, pes cavus or pes planus, and excessively pronated or supinated feet.
- Heel standing and toe standing: Assess strength and range of motion in dorsiflexion and plantar flexion, respectively.

Assess Resisted:

- Cervical flexion, extension, lateral flexion, and rotation.
- Shoulder abduction (shrug) to determine trapezius strength.
- Shoulder abduction in the neutral position and in 30° of forward flexion (plane of scapula) with medial (internal) rotation to determine deltoid and supraspinatus strength, respectively.
- Glenohumeral medial and lateral rotation.
- Elbow flexion and extension.
- Wrist flexion, extension, pronation, and supination.
- Finger flexion, extension, abduction, and adduction.
- Hip flexion, extension, abduction, adduction, and internal and external rotation.
- Knee flexion and extension.
- Ankle dorsiflexion, plantar flexion, inversion, and eversion.

The physical examination involves a basic musculoskeletal examination (Field Strategy 2.2). If red flags are noted, a more comprehensive examination of the specific body part should be completed (Box 2.5). It also is recommended that the following tests be performed: apprehension test for possible glenohumeral anterior instability, the patellar grind test to assess patellofemoral function, the Lachman test for anterior cruciate ligament integrity, and the anterior drawer and talar tilt tests for ankle stability (9).

When determining whether an individual should be limited in his or her activity, consideration must be given to the demands of the activity and to the needs of the individual. For example, limited range of motion or instability in the cervical or lumbar region may preclude the individual from participating in a collision or contact sport.

Box 2.5   Musculoskeletal Red Flags Requiring Further Examination

- Chronic joint or spinal instability
- Unhealed fracture, ligament, or muscular injury
- Muscle weakness
- Inflammation or infection of a joint
- Unusual hypomobility or hypermobility

- Growth or maturation disorders
- Symptomatic spondylolysis or spondylolisthesis
- Spear tackler's spine
- Herniated disk with spinal cord compression
- Repetitive stress disorders

TABLE 2.2 Cranial Nerve Assessment

NERVE	NAME	ASSESSMENT
I	Olfactory	Identify familiar odors (e.g., chocolate or coffee)
II	Optic	Test acuity—Snellen chart (blurring or double vision)
III	Oculomotor	Test papillary reaction to light Perform up- and downward gaze
IV	Trochlear	Perform downward and lateral gaze
V	Trigeminal	Touch face to note difference in sensation Clench teeth; push down on chin to separate jaws
VI	Abducens	Perform lateral and medial gaze
VII	Facial	Close eyes tight Smile and show the teeth
VIII	Vestibulocochlear (acoustic nerve)	Identify the sound of fingers snapping near the ear Balance and coordination (stand on one foot)
IX	Glossopharyngeal	Gag reflex; ability to swallow
X	Vagus	Gag reflex; ask the individual to swallow or say "Ahhh"
XI	Accessory	Resisted shoulder shrug
XII	Hypoglossal	Stick out the tongue

Neurologic Examination

The neurologic examination need not be overly complicated. The assessment component of this examination should include pupillary examination and reaction to light (PEARL), cranial nerve assessment (Table 2.2), a brief sensorimotor examination of the upper and lower extremities (see Field Strategy 2.2), and testing of the deep tendon reflexes (Table 2.3).

In the area of history, appropriately designed questions will give a clear indication if the individual is at risk for serious head or nerve injuries. The neurologic history should include questions

TABLE 2.3 Deep Tendon Reflex Testing

REFLEX	SITE OF STIMULATION	NORMAL RESPONSE	NERVE SEGMENT
Jaw	Mandible	Mouth closure	Cranial nerve V
Biceps	Biceps tendon	Biceps contraction	C5-C6
Brachioradialis	Brachioradialis tendon	Elbow flexion and/or pronation	C5-C6
Triceps	Triceps tendon	Elbow extension	C7-C8
Patellar	Quadriceps tendon	Knee extension	L3-L4
Medial hamstrings	Semimembranosus tendon	Knee flexion	L5-S1
Lateral hamstrings	Biceps femoris tendon	Knee flexion	S1-S2
Tibialis posterior	Tibialis posterior tendon behind medial malleolus	Plant flexion with inversion	L4-L5
Achilles	Achilles tendon	Plantar flexion	S1-S2

Box 2.6 Neurologic Red Flags Requiring Further Examination

- More than one concussion
- Cervical spine instability
- Functional cervical spine stenosis
- History of frequent or repeated headaches
- History of seizures

- History of amnesia or tinnitus
- History of head injuries
- History of burners, stingers, or neurapraxia
- History of spinal cord shock or transient quadriplegia
- History of nerve palsy

regarding past head injuries, loss of consciousness, amnesia, or seizures. A history of seizures requires detailed information concerning frequency, treatment, and whether adequate control has been achieved with prescribed medication. Any episodes of brachial plexus injuries (e.g., burners or stingers) or pinched nerves should be documented. A history of transient paresthesia, loss of sensation, or loss of motor function in any region of the body also should be noted. In addition, if an individual has a preexisting narrow cervical spinal canal, a straightened or reversed cervical lordotic curve, and a history of using a spear-tackling technique (**spear tackler's spine**), the individual should be fully evaluated by a neurosurgeon. A detailed examination of the neurologic system, including cervical radiographs, may be warranted before considering participation.

Questions during this phase of the examination may include:

1. Have you ever had a head or neck injury?

2. Have you ever been knocked out or been unconscious?

3. Do you have frequent or repeated headaches?

4. Have you ever had a seizure or been told you have epilepsy?

5. Have you ever had a burner, stinger, or one of your limbs feel numb or fall "asleep" during activity?

6. Have you ever experienced unexplained muscle weakness?

If problems such as recurrent concussions, headaches, or nerve palsies are identified, the individual should be seen by a specialist before being cleared for participation (Box 2.6). If seizure disorders are reported, the examiner should document the initial onset, frequency, and duration of the episodes; the use of medications to control the disorder; and whether the individual is informed of the condition and its side effects and predisposing factors (9). Individuals with epilepsy should be discouraged from activities that may involve recurrent head trauma or the risk of falling, such as rock climbing, football, skiing, scuba diving, or parachuting.

Eye Examination

Visual acuity is best tested using the Snellen or common eye chart (Fig. 2.1). The chart tests the individual's ability to clearly see letters based on a normalized scale. **Emmetropia**, or 20/20 vision, indicates that an individual can read the letters on the 20-foot line of the eye chart when standing 20 feet from the chart, indicating that the light rays are focused precisely on the retina. **Myopia**, or nearsightedness, occurs when the light rays are focused in front of the retina, making only those objects close to the eyes distinguishable. **Hypermetropia**, or farsightedness, occurs when the light rays are focused at a point behind the retina, making only those objects far from the eyes distinguishable. Vision should be assessed monocularly (one eye) and binocularly (both eyes). Individuals who wear corrective glasses or contact lenses should wear them at the time of the vision assessment.

FIGURE 2.1 Snellen eye chart. Visual acuity is measured by the Snellen or common eye chart.

In addition to assessing visual acuity, it may be appropriate to assess other aspects of vision. The presence of involuntary cyclical movement of the eyes (**nystagmus**) is noteworthy. Although it may be normal for an individual, the presence of nystagmus should be documented in the individual's medical file, because it can provide valuable information in the event of head trauma. It also is important to note pupil size. Normally, the pupils are equal in size and shape; however, some individuals may have a congenital difference in pupil size (**anisocoria**). Again, this should be documented in case the individual sustains a head injury. In addition, in some situations, it is beneficial to have information regarding peripheral vision and depth perception.

Questions related to the eye examination might include:

1. Have you ever had problems with blurring or double vision?

2. Have you ever injured your eyes or the area around your eyes?

3. Do you wear glasses, contact lenses, or protective eye wear on a regular basis? What type?

4. Is your vision totally or partially impaired in either eye?

5. Are you color blind?

6. Do you have good peripheral vision?

If any of these questions receives a positive response, corrected vision is poorer than 20/50 (i.e., the individual can read at 20 feet what the average person can read at 50 feet), or one eye is absent, the individual requires further evaluation by an ophthalmologist (Box 2.7). Individuals with sight in only one eye or with limited sight in both eyes may continue to participate in physical activities only if they are informed of the risks involved and understand the dangers associated with loss of depth perception and the potential for injury to the remaining good eye. These individuals should not participate in activities in which the eyes cannot be protected (e.g., boxing, wrestling, and martial arts). An additional consent form specific to eye injuries that outlines the risks involved and the acceptance of those risks should be obtained from the individual (9).

If glasses are worn, the lenses should be made of plastic, polycarbonate, or heat-treated (safety) glass to prevent them from shattering during activity. When possible, contact lenses should be of the soft type; the hard types often become dislodged, are associated more frequently with irritation from foreign bodies, and may shatter.

Myopia should be noted, because such individuals tend to have retinal degeneration, which increases the possibility of retinal detachment. Individuals with retinal detachment may be excluded from contact sports. Those with a healed retinal tear may be allowed to participate in strenuous activity only after being examined and cleared by an ophthalmologist.

Dental Examination

A dental examination usually is performed by a dentist. It is important to determine the number of teeth and the time of the last dental examination. This is critical because of potential liability if teeth are avulsed (knocked out) during participation.

Questions that can be asked include:

1. When did you last see a dentist?

2. Have you ever had any problems with your teeth or gums?

Box 2.7 Ocular Red Flags Requiring Further Examination

- Corrected vision greater than 20/50
- Vision in one eye only
- Severely limited peripheral vision
- Severe myopia (i.e., nearsightedness)
- Retinal detachment or tear

Box 2.8   Dental Red Flags Requiring Further Examination

- Bleeding gums
- Lesions in the mouth
- Loose or displaced teeth
- Loose caps or crowns
- Dental appliances in poor condition

3. Have you ever experienced bleeding gums after brushing or flossing your teeth?

4. Have you ever had any teeth knocked out, damaged, or extracted?

5. Do you wear dentures, crowns, or caps or have a partial plate?

6. Do you wear a mouth guard?

7. Do you smoke cigarettes or chew tobacco?

8. Have you ever had an injury to the jaw or face?

During an examination, the dentist can assess gum condition and the presence of cavities. Dental appliance work should be checked to ensure it is in good condition. The importance of using properly fitted mouth guards as well as the safety and legal issues stemming from cutting down a mouth guard can be stressed. Dental red flags requiring further examination are listed in Box 2.8.

Gastrointestinal Examination

This examination involves evaluating the digestive system, eating habits, and nutrition. During the physical examination, the individual should be supine, with the lower ribs exposed to the antero-superior iliac spines. The examiner palpates for tenderness, masses, or organomegaly (i.e., enlarged organs) to ensure there is no inflammation of the liver (e.g., hepatitis or enlarged liver) or the spleen, especially for individuals involved in contact sports.

General questions about the gastrointestinal system may center on bouts of heartburn, indigestion, diarrhea, or constipation. Any positive responses to the questions should be further investigated (Box 2.9). Questions that may be asked include:

1. Do you eat regularly and have a balanced diet?

2. Do you skip meals?

3. Are there any food groups that you predominantly eat?

4. Do you view yourself as too thin, too fat, or just right?

5. Have you ever tried to control your weight? If so, how was this done?

6. Have you ever had excessive heartburn or indigestion?

7. Have you ever had an ulcer or vomited blood?

Box 2.9   Gastrointestinal Red Flags Requiring Further Examination

- Organomegaly (e.g., enlarged liver or spleen)
- History of hepatitis or infectious mononucleosis
- History of repeated episodes of diarrhea or constipation
- History of gastritis or burning sensation in the stomach (ulcers)
- Extreme tenderness over appendix, liver, or spleen
- Suspicion of anorexia or bulimia

8. Have you ever been constipated or had diarrhea?

9. Have you ever had mononucleosis or hepatitis?

10. Do you have any food allergies or sensitivities?

For activities in which weight control is particularly important (e.g., gymnastics, ballet, crew, boxing, and wrestling), it is advisable to investigate the individual's nutritional status to determine a tendency toward anorexia, bulimia, or disordered eating. This can be accomplished by having the individual record his or her food intake for at least 3 days and then having the record analyzed by a nutritionist.

Genitourinary Examination

Information gained at this station varies depending on the sex of the individual. For females, a complete menstrual history should be gathered. Any responses related to **oligomenorrhea** and **amenorrhea** necessitate further assessment and counseling about the increased risk of bone demineralization (osteopenia), stress fractures, and potential osteoporosis. Gynecologic symptoms that may need further evaluation include **dysmenorrhea**, lower abdominal pain, unusual vaginal discharge, pain during urination, and use of birth control medication. Oral contraceptives may alter the pH of the vagina and increase the risk of pelvic inflammatory disease and hypertension. Discussion surrounding the use of birth control also may promote discussion of safe sexual practices, sexually transmitted diseases (STDs), and pregnancy.

Common questions that may be asked include:

1. Have you ever had problems with your kidneys or genitourinary organs?

2. Have you ever had a kidney or bladder infection?

3. Does it hurt to urinate?

4. Have you ever had an STD? If so, when? What medication was prescribed?

5. Have you noticed any skin lesions on the genitalia or any vaginal or penile discharge?

6. Have you ever been diagnosed as having sugar, albumin, or blood in the urine?

7. *Females:* Have you ever been or are you now pregnant? At what age did menarche occur? How many periods have you had during the last 6 months? When was your last menstrual period? What is the usual length of time between periods? Are the cycles fairly constant or irregular? Do you have a history of abnormal heavy bleeding (menorrhagia), scant bleeding, or intermittent bleeding?

8. *Males:* Are you missing a testicle, or do you have an undescended testicle? Have you ever had a history of testicular pain or a testicular abnormality, such as a hydrocele or varicocele?

As part of the physical examination, the kidney should be assessed by determining the presence of tenderness at the costovertebral angle. Generally, an individual with one kidney should be warned of the risks involved with participating in contact activities, especially if the remaining kidney is abnormally positioned or is diseased. Although not necessarily required in the PPE, a urinalysis should be performed if diabetes or kidney disease is suspected. Conditions such as albuminuria, hematuria, and hemoglobinuria can indicate problems with the urogenital system. These conditions do not preclude activity, but they should be evaluated. The individual should be informed of the potential dangers caused by these conditions. See Box 2.10 for genitourinary red flags requiring further examination.

Dermatologic Examination

Examination of the skin can identify contagious lesions, such as herpes simplex (cold sores), molluscum contagiosum, tinea capitis or corporis, furuncles, impetigo, scabies, and secondary syphilis, which can preclude participation in sports. Skin infections that may be contagious to other participants should be identified and treated. In contrast, lesions such as warts, fungal infections, contact

Box 2.10 Genitourinary Red Flags Requiring Further Examination

- One kidney or diseased kidney
- Absent or undescended testicle
- Hernia (femoral or inguinal)
- Pain with urination
- Possible exercise amenorrhea or pregnancy
- Endometriosis and pelvic inflammatory disease

- Possible sexually transmitted disease
- Hematuria
- Albuminuria
- Hemoglobinuria
- Nephroptosis

dermatitis, psoriasis, seborrhea, and nevi (birthmarks) require further evaluation but do not necessarily mean exclusion from participation. Early treatment typically is effective in managing these conditions.

Questions in this area might include:

1. Have you ever had problems with acne?

2. Have you ever had any skin rashes, itching, or scaling in areas covered by clothing, equipment, or footwear?

3. Do you have any unusual blemishes (e.g., warts or moles) that have changed in size or color over the year?

Any skin lesion associated with a contagious disease or STD warrants immediate referral to a physician for treatment and appropriate counseling. Dermatologic red flags that require further examination are identified in Box 2.11. Chapter 28 provides more detail and photographs of dermatologic conditions.

Examination for Heat Disorders

In activities that take place under conditions of high temperature, high humidity, or a combination of the two, a history should include questions about cramping, syncope, exhaustion, and heat stroke. Questions concerning use of medications also are important, because certain medications can impair the body's ability to release heat (e.g., antihistamines) and place an individual at risk for heat illness (see Chapter 24). It also is advantageous to question the individual regarding regular caffeine consumption, because excessive caffeine can increase the risk for heat disorders.

Specific questions related to heat disorders might include:

1. Have you ever suffered from heat illness or heat cramps?

2. Have you ever participated in an activity in a high-temperature, high-humidity environment?

Box 2.11 Dermatologic Red Flags Requiring Further Examination

- Herpes (e.g., simplex or gladiatorum)
- Impetigo
- Molluscum contagiosum
- Tinea capitis or corporis
- Furuncles
- Secondary syphilis

- Severe acne
- Dermatitis (e.g., contact or clothes)
- Warts
- Fungal infections
- Psoriasis

Box 2.12   Heat-Related Red Flags Requiring Further Examination

- Cardiac disease
- Uncontrolled diabetes
- Hypertension
- Drug use (e.g., amphetamines, cocaine, hallucinogens, laxatives, or narcotics)

- Medication use (e.g., anticholinergics, diuretics, antihistamines, or β-blockers)
- Excessive muscle cramps during participation in heat
- Heat exhaustion
- Heat stroke

3. Have you ever passed out or become dizzy in the heat?

4. Do you have a heart problem, uncontrolled diabetes, hypertension, or poor eating habits?

5. Are you on any medications, such as diuretics, antihistamines, or β-blockers?

6. Do you drink more than two alcoholic or caffeinated beverages (e.g., cola, coffee, or tea) per day?

Individuals at a heightened risk of heat-related disorders include poorly acclimated or poorly conditioned individuals, children, overweight or large individuals, and those with excessive muscle mass. If an individual has a history of heat-related disorders or chronic illnesses, the condition should be investigated thoroughly (Box 2.12).

Laboratory Tests

The use of laboratory testing often is dictated by the focus of the PPE. Laboratory tests are not recommended by the American Academy of Pediatrics as part of a routine PPE, but decisions concerning the use of laboratory testing are at the discretion of the supervising physician and must be consistent with state law (if PPE regulation exists).

When used, the most frequently employed screening test has been the urine dipstick analysis for protein, glucose, and blood. Urine testing has not proven to be effective, however, in detecting renal disease among children. The costs involved, coupled with the low incidence of true renal pathology, do not bear out its use in the PPE.

Similarly, no evidence supports the routine use of blood work, such as **hemoglobin** and **hematocrit**, complete blood count, and blood chemistries. A few states, however, do require particular laboratory tests as a component of the PPE. If certain problems are suspected, information obtained from specific laboratory tests could be advantageous and, as such, should be ordered. For example, if concerns exist relative to the heart, an ECG or stress ECG may be necessary, but these tests should be reserved only for individuals with suggestive positive historical or clinical findings. In addition, drug screening must be performed in some institutions and at certain levels of competition.

A PPE focuses on general systemic conditions as well as on the cardiovascular, pulmonary, musculoskeletal, neurologic, gastrointestinal, genitourinary, and dermatologic systems, but it is not intended to be all-encompassing. It is designed to determine an individual's readiness to participate in a specific sport or physical activity. As such, it should not be considered the equivalent of an annual medical examination.

PHYSICAL FITNESS PROFILE

Following completion of the physical examination, what advantages can be realized from assessing an individual's physical fitness level?

It is critical to assess the physical fitness status of an individual before the start of physical activity to determine whether the individual possesses the attributes, skills, and abilities necessary to meet the demands of the activity. Data from the examination can identify weaknesses that may hinder performance or predispose an individual to injury, and it establishes a baseline of data in the event that an injury is sustained.

A physical fitness profile can assess body composition; maturation and growth; flexibility, strength, power, and speed; agility, balance, and reaction time; and cardiovascular endurance. To be effective, the parameters of the test must be relevant and specific to the participant's selected activity. The test must be easy to perform, measure, and reproduce, and it must be inexpensive. The test should be standardized, controlled, and repeated during the program or season to assess improvement. Results should be explained to participants in a meaningful way so that the significance of those results can be understood.

Anthropometry and Body Composition

Anthropometry is used to determine an individuals' body type (i.e., **mesomorphic**, **endomorphic**, and **ectomorphic**) and suitability for a desired activity, sport, or position played in that sport. Body composition provides detailed information regarding an individual's muscle, fat, and bone mass. The portion of total body weight that is composed of fat tissue is referred to as the percentage of body fat. The total body weight composed of nonfat or lean tissue, which includes muscles, tendons, bones, and connective tissue, is referred to as the lean body weight. Measurements of body composition can provide a reliable means of determining the amount of weight that an individual may safely gain or lose.

Hydrostatic weighing and skinfold measurements often are used to determine body fat measurements. Hydrostatic weighing is more accurate, but skinfold measurement is easier, faster, and nearly as reliable.

In performing skinfold measurements, seven to nine skinfold sites typically are used (Field Strategy 2.3), although many professionals believe that measurement at three sites is adequate (but a different three for males and females) (7). Most male and female athletes should fall between 12 to 17% body fat, although these percentages are only guidelines. Some male athletes may compete at 3 to 5%, whereas other male and female athletes perform very well at higher percentages. Generally, if the percentage of body fat is greater than the upper normal limit of 14% for males and 17% for females, the individual should be put on a weight-loss program or a weight training program to increase lean body mass, but this decision depends on the activity in which the individual wishes to participate. Additional methods of body composition measurement include girth measurements, bone diameter measurements, ultrasound measurement, arm radiograph measurement, and computed tomographic assessment of fat.

Maturation and Growth

Physical maturation refers to the developmental stage of an individual. In adolescents, growth spurts can affect participation in physical activity and may play a role in certain injuries. The growth spurt in girls usually occurs at about age 12; in boys, it occurs around age 14. For example, a growth spurt in a gymnast may adversely affect balance and flexibility, and a growth spurt in the bones of the foot may predispose a young individual to toe deformities if shoes are not repeatedly fitted to the growing foot. Pubertal growth accounts for 20 to 25% of final adult height, and pubertal weight gain accounts for 50% of ideal adult weight.

A common method of measuring maturation in males and females is the Tanner scale (1,10). The five stages of this scale are based on pictorial standards of breast development and pubic hair for females and of genitalia and pubic hair for males. This assessment typically is conducted by a PCP in the privacy of his or her office and in the presence of a parent.

Flexibility

Flexibility is the total range of motion at a joint that occurs pain-free in each of the planes of motion. In most cases, less flexibility is better than too much; however, in certain activities (e.g., gymnastics or wrestling), excessive flexibility is a necessity. Several factors can limit flexibility and range of motion, such as:

- Bony block
- Joint adhesions

FIELD STRATEGY 2.3

Standardized Description of Skinfold Sites and Procedures

Skinfold Site	Description
Abdominal	Vertical fold; 2 cm on the right side of the umbilicus (see Fig. A).
Triceps	Vertical fold; on the posterior midline of the upper arm, halfway between the acromion and olecranon processes, with the arm held freely to the side of the body (see Fig. B).
Biceps	Vertical fold; on the anterior aspect of the arm over the belly of the biceps muscle, 1 cm.
Chest/pectoral	Diagonal fold; one-half the distance between the anterior axillary line and the nipple (men) or one-third the distance between the anterior axillary line and the nipple (women).
Medial calf	Vertical fold; at the maximum circumference of the calf on the midline of its medial border.
Midaxillary	Vertical fold; on midaxillary line at the level of the xiphoid process. (An alternate method is a horizontal fold taken at the level of the xiphoid/ sternal border in the midaxillary line.)
Subscapular	Diagonal fold (at a 45° angle); 1 to 2 cm below the inferior angle of the scapula.
Suprailiac	Diagonal fold; in line with the natural angle of the iliac crest taken in the anterior axillary line immediately superior to the iliac crest.
Thigh	Vertical fold; on the anterior midline of the thigh, midway between the proximal border of the patella and the inguinal crease (hip) (see Fig. C).

Figure A

Figure B

Figure C

General Guidelines

- All measurements should be made on the right side of the body.
- The caliper should be placed 1 cm away from the thumb and forefinger, perpendicular to the skinfold, and halfway between the crest and base of the fold.
- The pinch should be maintained while reading the caliper.
- Wait only 1 to 2 seconds before reading the caliper.
- Take duplicate measures at each site, and test again if measurements are not within 1 to 2 mm.
- Rotate through measurement sites or allow time for skin to regain normal texture and thickness before retesting.

- Muscle tightness

- Tight skin or an inelastic, dense scar tissue

- Muscle bulk

- Swelling

- Pain

- Presence of fat or other soft tissues that block normal motion

- Gender (females tend to be more flexible than males)

- Dominant limb tends to be less mobile than the nondominant limb

- Age (flexibility decreases with age)

- Race (Native Americans are more mobile than blacks, who are more mobile than whites)

- Genetic makeup

■■■ ■ FIGURE 2.2 **Use of a goniometer.** The athletic trainer is using a goniometer to assess range of knee flexion.

Flexibility can be measured with a goniometer, flexometer, or tape measure. Figure 2.2 provides an example of a goniometric measurement of knee flexion. Measurements should be taken to assess flexibility of the hamstrings, quadriceps, gastrocnemius, shoulder, and low back. Hypermobility should be noted and recorded. Hypermobile traits include:

- Passive opposition of the thumb that can reach the flexor aspect of the forearm

- Passive hyperextension of the fingers so that they lie parallel with the extensor aspect of the forearm

- Ability to hyperextend the elbow at least 10°

- Ability to hyperextend the knee at least 10°

- Excessive passive dorsiflexion of the ankle and eversion of the foot

Laxity in one joint does not necessarily mean hypermobility in all joints or in all directions, nor does it identify a pathologic state. Total range of motion can be related to genetic makeup or to the stresses placed on individual joints. Loose-jointed individuals tend to do poorly in strength events and are more susceptible to ligament sprains, dislocations, chronic back pain, disk prolapse, spondylolisthesis, pes planus, joint effusion, and tendinitis (9). If strength and endurance are not at the appropriate level in hypermobile individuals, the joints cannot be supported and may become unstable and subject to injury. These individuals should avoid further stretching exercises and support the joint through proper positioning, balance, and strengthening programs.

In contrast, tight-jointed or hypomobile individuals tend to be more susceptible to muscle strains, nerve pinch syndromes, and overstress tendinitis. If a person is hypomobile, mobilization or manipulation of the affected joint in the direction of tightness may be helpful. Tight supporting structures should be stretched and active exercises used to maintain the restored range of motion. It is important that these individuals retrain their kinesthetic sense so that the acquired range of motion can be maintained or improved.

Strength, Power, and Speed

Strength is the ability of a muscle or group of muscles to produce force in one maximal resistance (1 RM) effort, either statically or dynamically. The demands of a particular sport or activity dictate the level of strength that is needed to perform necessary skills. Strength measures can involve isometric, isotonic, or isokinetic testing through manual muscle testing, grip strength, sit-ups, push-ups, and pull-ups.

Power is the ability of a muscle to produce force in a given time (e.g., to move the body over a distance). Power activities can be measured by throwing a medicine ball, vertical jump and reach, single- or two-legged hop for distance, and stair climbing. As with strength, power measurement should be related to the activity in which the individual will be participating.

Speed is the ability to move body mass over time. It can be assessed by timed sprints (e.g., a 40-, 100-, or 400-meter run).

Agility, Balance, and Reaction Time

Agility is the ability to change directions rapidly when moving at a high rate of speed. Balance is the body's coordinated neuromuscular response to maintain a defined position of equilibrium in response to changing visual, tactile, or kinesthetic stimuli. Agility and balance tests often are measured by time or accuracy (e.g., two correct out of three) and should be developed to be sport/activity specific. Reaction time is measured by the ability to respond to a stimulus. Examples of agility, balance, and reaction tests include run-and-cut drills, carioca steps, shuttle runs, pivoting drills, front-to-back and side-to-side hops, figure-eight running drills, kicking a stationary or moving target, and beam-walking tests.

Cardiovascular Endurance

Cardiovascular endurance, commonly called aerobic capacity, is the body's ability to sustain sub-maximal exercise over an extended period, and it depends on the efficiency of the pulmonary and cardiovascular systems. Several tests may be used to assess cardiovascular endurance. The actual selection of tests should be dependent on the specific demands of the sport/activity. The Harvard step test is commonly used in a physical fitness profile. In this test, the individual is instructed to step up onto an 18-inch platform using a four-step cadence "up-up-down-down" at a rate of about 30 times per minute (a metronome is used for cadence). Following 3.5 minutes at a pace of 2 seconds per step, the individual moves as fast as possible for 30 seconds (total time, 4 minutes). The individual then immediately sits down in a chair and relaxes for 3 minutes while the pulse is determined. The pulse is taken at 30, 60, 120, and 180 seconds after the exercise. The index formula for the pulse is (7):

$$\text{Index} = \frac{[\text{duration of exercise (seconds)} \times 100]}{[2 \times \text{sum of any three pulse counts}]}$$

The higher the index, the better the person's aerobic fitness. If the index is less than 65, the individual is not ready for strenuous activity. Other examples of common endurance tests include the 12-minute walk-run, 1.5-mile run, submaximal ergometer test, and a treadmill test. Although anaerobic fitness is not directly related to the cardiovascular system, if the proposed activity is primarily anaerobic, this measurement involves the ability to move large muscle groups for at least 1 minute but not more than 2 minutes.

Testing the physical fitness of individuals before the start of participation in a program of physical activity or a sport can identify poorly conditioned individuals who may be at risk for certain injuries. By identifying deficits (i.e., excessive body fat percentage, hypermobile joints, or lack of flexibility, strength, power, agility, or endurance), individuals can be started on a corrective program to reduce the risk of injury during the program or season.

CLEARANCE FOR PARTICIPATION

 Can a physician totally exclude an individual from participation in a sport or physical activity?

Subsequent to the conclusion of the PPE, the physician must determine the level of participation based on conditions identified during the examination and knowledge regarding the physical demands of the physical activity. The physician must ask:

1. Will the condition increase the risk of injury to the individual or other participants?

2. Can participation be allowed if medication, rehabilitation, or protective bracing or padding is used? If so, can limited participation be allowed in the interim?

3. If clearance is denied for a particular activity, are there other activities in which the individual can participate safely?

Recent interpretations of the federal Rehabilitation Act and Americans with Disabilities Act have stated that individuals have the legal right to participate in any competitive sport regardless of a preexisting medical condition. For this reason, physicians cannot totally exclude an individual from participation but, rather, can only recommend that the individual not participate because of a medical condition that increases the risk of further injury and/or death as a result of participation (1,11). In these situations, an exculpatory waiver may be used. An exculpatory waiver is based on the individual's assumption of risk and is a release signed by the individual or by the parent of an individual under the age of 18 that releases the physician from liability of negligence.

Most physicians base their recommendations on the American Academy of Pediatrics Committee on Sports Medicine guidelines. Under these guidelines, disqualifying conditions include atlantoaxial instability, severe hypertension, aortic disorders, tuberculosis, severe pulmonary insufficiency, uncontrolled diabetes or convulsive disorders, serious bleeding tendencies, acute infections, enlarged liver or spleen, hernias, symptomatic abnormalities or inflammations, functional instability, previous serious head trauma or surgery, renal disease, or absence of one kidney (11). In general, any individual with only a solitary paired organ (e.g., an eye, a kidney, or a testicle) should be recommended to refrain from participation in contact sports, especially if the remaining organ is abnormal.

> A complete listing of disqualifying conditions for sport participation is available on the companion website at thePoint.

 Subsequent to interpretations of the Rehabilitation Act and Americans with Disabilities Act, a physician cannot totally exclude an individual from participation. The physician can only recommend that the individual not participate because of a medical condition that increases the risk of further injury and/or death as a result of participation.

SUMMARY

1. The basic objective of the PPE is to determine the general health and fitness level of a physically active individual to ensure safe participation in a particular sport/activity.

2. A medical history questionnaire should be completed before the PPE and validated for accuracy during the actual examination.

3. The physical examination involves assessing the vital signs; general medical conditions; and cardiovascular, pulmonary, musculoskeletal, neurologic, gastrointestinal, genitourinary, and dermatologic systems. In addition, the eyes and teeth should be evaluated, and individuals at risk for heat-related illness should be identified.

4. The physical fitness of the individual should be assessed by measuring body composition, maturation, flexibility, strength, power, speed, agility, balance, reaction time, and cardiovascular endurance.

5. At the conclusion of the examination, the physician must ask:

   ▪ Will the abnormality increase the risk of injury to the individual or other participants?

   ▪ Can participation be allowed if medication, rehabilitation, or protective bracing or padding is used? If so, can limited participation be allowed in the interim?

   ▪ If clearance is denied for a particular activity, are there other activities in which the individual can safely participate?

REFERENCES

1. American College of Sports Medicine, American College of Cardiology 26th Bethesda Conference. Mitchell JG, Maron BJ, Raven PB, eds. Recommendations for determining eligibility for competition in athletes with cardiovascular abnormalities. Med Sci Sports Exerc 1994;26(10): S223–S283.

2. Kligman EW, Jewitt MJ, Crowell DL. Recommending exercise to healthy older adults: The preparticipation evaluation and exercise prescription. Phys Sportsmed 1999;27(11):42–62.

3. Seto CK. Preparticipation cardiovascular screening. Clin Sports Med 2003;22(1):22–35.

4. Madden CC, Putukian M. The preparticipation physical evaluation. In: Mellion MB, Walsh M, Madden C, Putukian M, Shelton GL, eds. The Team Physician's Handbook. Philadelphia: Hanley & Belfus, 2002.

5. National Heart, Lung, and Blood Institute. The Seventh Report of the Joint National Committee on Prevention, Detection, Evaluation, and Treatment of High Blood Pressure. Washington DC: U.S. Department of Health and Human Services, 2004.

6. Bickley LS, Szilagyi PG. Bates' Guide to Physical Examination and History Taking. Baltimore: Lippincott Williams & Wilkins, 2003.

7. American College of Sports Medicine. ACSM's Guidelines for Exercise Testing and Prescription, 7th Ed. Baltimore: Williams & Wilkins, 2005.

8. Rockwell PG, Alvarez DJ. Adolescent sports injuries and the preparticipation physical evaluation. Clin Fam Pract 2000;2(4):837–862.

9. Magee DJ. Orthopedic Physical Assessment. Philadelphia: WB Saunders, 2006.

10. Tanner JM. Growth of Adolescence. Oxford, England: Blackwell Scientific, 1962.

11. American Academy of Pediatrics Committee on Sports Medicine and Fitness. Medical conditions affecting sports participation. Pediatrics 2001;107(5):1205–1209.

Protective Equipment

STUDENT OUTCOMES

1. Describe the forces that produce focal and diffuse injuries.

2. State the principles used to design protective equipment.

3. Identify the different types of soft and hard materials used to make protective pads.

4. Explain the athletic trainer's legal duty of care in selecting and fitting protective equipment.

5. List the agencies responsible for establishing material standards for protective devices.

6. Identify the information that should be documented to support an organization's legal duty to provide safe equipment.

7. Demonstrate proper selection and fitting of selected equipment (e.g., football helmets, mouth guards, and shoulder pads).

8. Identify and describe common protective equipment for the head and face, the torso, and the upper and lower body.

ROLE DELINEATION COMPETENCIES

The following Performance Domains and Tasks defined in the National Athletic Trainers' Association Board of Certification *Role Delineation Study*, 5th Edition are addressed in this chapter:

BOC COMPETENCIES

I. Prevention

    C. Instruct the appropriate individual(s) about standard protective equipment using effective communication techniques to minimize the risk of injury and illness.

    D. Apply appropriate prophylactic/protective measures using commercial products or custom-made devices to minimize the risk of injury and illness.

III. Immediate Care

    B. Prevent exacerbation of non–life threatening condition(s) through the use of standard procedures in order to reduce morbidity.

    C. Facilitate the timely transfer of care for conditions beyond the scope of practice of the athletic trainer by implementing appropriate referral strategies to stabilize and/or prevent exacerbation of the condition(s).

    D. Direct the appropriate individual(s) in standard immediate care procedures using formal and informal methods to facilitate immediate care.

IV. Treatment, Rehabilitation, and Reconditioning

    C. Apply braces, splints, or assistive devices in accordance with appropriate standards and practices in order to facilitate recovery, function, and/or performance.

Specialized equipment, when properly used, can protect a participant from accidental or routine injuries associated with a particular sport or physical activity, but limitations exist regarding the effectiveness of protective equipment. A natural outcome of wearing protective equipment is to feel more secure. Unfortunately, this often leads to more aggressive play, which can result in injury to the participant or an opponent. In many cases, it is the shared or sole responsibility of the certified athletic trainer to ensure that protective equipment meets minimum standards of protection, is in good condition, is clean and properly fitted, is used routinely, and is used as intended.

In this chapter, principles of protective equipment and materials used in the development of padding are discussed. This is followed by a review of protective equipment for the head and face and then of equipment commonly used to protect the upper and lower body. When appropriate, guidelines for fitting specific equipment are listed in field strategies. Although several commercial braces and support devices are illustrated, these are intended only to demonstrate the variety of products available to protect a body region.

PRINCIPLES OF PROTECTIVE EQUIPMENT

Q ▸ *What are the advantages of using high-density material in the protection of injuries?*

In events involving impact and collisions, the participant must be protected from high-velocity, low-mass forces and from low-velocity, high-mass forces. High-velocity, low-mass forces occur, for example, when an individual is struck by a ball, puck, bat, or hockey stick. The low mass and high speed of such an impact leads to forces being concentrated in a smaller area, causing **focal injuries** (i.e., injuries concentrated in a small area, such as a contusion). An example of low-velocity, high-mass forces is an individual falling on the ground or ice, or being checked into the sideboards of an ice hockey rink, thereby absorbing the forces over a larger area and leading to **diffuse injuries** (i.e., injuries spread over a larger area, such as a concussion).

Box 3.1 Equipment Design Factors That Can Reduce Potential Injury

- Increase the impact area
- Transfer or disperse the impact area to another body part
- Limit the relative motion of a body part
- Add mass to the body part to limit deformation and displacement
- Reduce friction between contacting surfaces
- Absorb energy
- Resist the absorption of bacteria, fungus, and viruses

Sport-related and physical activity injuries can result from a variety of factors, including:

- Illegal play

- Poor technique

- Inadequate conditioning

- Poorly matched player levels

- A previously injured area that is vulnerable to reinjury

- Low tolerance of an individual to injury

- Inability to adequately protect an area without restricting motion

- Poor quality, maintenance, or cleanliness of protective equipment

Potential means by which equipment can protect an area from accidental or routine injuries associated with a particular activity are listed in Box 3.1. Equipment design extends beyond the physical protective properties to include size, comfort, style, tradition, and both initial and long-term maintenance costs. Individuals responsible for the selection and purchase of equipment should be less concerned about appearance, style, and cost, however, and be most concerned about the ability of the equipment to prevent injury.

Materials Used

The design and selection of protective equipment are based on the optimal level of impact intensity afforded by the given thickness, density, and temperature of the energy-absorbing material. Soft, **low-density material** is light and comfortable to wear, but such material is only effective at low levels of impact intensity. Examples of low-density material include gauze padding, foam, neoprene, Sorbothane™, felt, and moleskin. In contrast, firmer, **high-density material** of the same thickness tends to be less comfortable, offers less cushioning of low-level impact, but can absorb more energy by deformation; as such, it transfers less stress to an area at higher levels of impact intensity. Examples of high-density material include thermomoldable plastics, such as orthoplast and thermoplast, and casting materials, such as fiberglass or plaster.

Another factor to consider in energy-absorbing material is **resilience** to impact forces. Highly resilient materials regain their shape after impact and commonly are used over areas that are subject to repeated impacts. Nonresilient (or slow-recovery resilient) material offers the best protection and is used over areas that are subject to one-time or occasional impacts. It is important to select equipment that will absorb an impact and disperse it before injury occurs to the underlying body part.

Soft Materials

Soft materials are light because of the incorporation of air into the material. Examples include gauze padding, neoprene, Sorbothane, felt, moleskin, and foam. Gauze padding comes in a variety of widths and thicknesses and is used as an absorbent or protective pad. Neoprene sleeves provide uniform compression, therapeutic warmth, and support for a chronic injury, such as a recurrent quadriceps or hamstring strain. The nylon-coated rubber material is comfortable and allows full mobility, better absorption of sweat, less skin breakdown; it also provides the individual with proprioceptive feedback in the affected area. Sorbothane often is used for shoe insoles to absorb and dissipate impact forces during walking and running. Felt is made from matted wool fibers and is pressed into several thicknesses, ranging from ? to 1 inch. Felt can absorb perspiration but, in doing so, has less of a tendency to move under stress. Typically, it is necessary to replace felt daily. Moleskin is a thin felt product with an adhesive bonding on one side that prevents any movement once applied to the skin. This product is used over friction spots to reduce skin irritation or blisters.

Foam, like felt, comes in a variety of thicknesses, ranging from ⅛ to 1 inch, and ranges in density from a very soft, open-cell foam to a denser, closed-cell foam. **Open-cell foam** has cells that are connected to allow the passage of air from cell to cell. Similar to a sponge, this material can absorb fluids and commonly is used to pad bony prominences or to protect the skin under hard edges of protective equipment or custom-fabricated pads. Open-cell foams deform quickly under stress; therefore, they do not have good shock-absorbing qualities. **Closed-cell foam** is used primarily for protection, because air cannot pass from one cell to another. The material rebounds and returns to its original shape quickly, but it offers less cushioning at low levels of impact and is not as comfortable next to the skin.

To use the differing properties of foam effectively, many equipment designers layer materials of varying density. Air management pads combine open- and closed-cell foams encased in polyurethane or nylon to provide maximal shock absorption. Soft, lower-density material is placed next to the skin and is covered by increasingly denser, closed-cell material away from the skin to absorb and disperse higher-intensity blows. The pad is airtight, which prevents quick deformation of the foam so that the energy can be dissipated over the entire surface of the pad. Air management pads often are used in football shoulder pads, but they are more expensive and require extensive maintenance if the nylon covering is torn. If the covering tears, air can pass into the pads, reducing their effectiveness. The liners must then be patched or replaced. Nylon prevents the absorption of perspiration or water, which can help to avoid additional weight, and is easily cleaned with a weak bleach solution.

Some dense foams are thermomoldable; that is, when heated, they can be molded and shaped to fit any body part. When cooled, they retain their shape. These pads can be used repeatedly to immobilize a body structure, deflect an impact, and absorb shock. The pad is secured to the body part with elastic or nonelastic tape.

Hard Materials

Hard materials include thermomoldable plastics, such as orthoplast and thermoplast, and casting materials, such as fiberglass or plaster, which can be used to splint or protect an area. Thermoplastics are divided into two categories: plastic, and rubber. The plastic group uses a polycaprolactone base with varying amounts of inorganic filler, resins, and elastomers to effect the memory, stiffness, and durability of the material. The plastic category tends to conform better than the rubber category and is more appropriate for small splints, such as on the hand. Plastics include materials such as Aquaplast Bluestripe™ (WFR/Aquaplast), Multiform I and II™ (Alimed), Orfit™ (North Coast Medical), and Orthoplast II™ (Johnson & Johnson). Rubber-like materials use a polyisoprene base and include Aquaplast Greenstrip™ (WFR/Aquaplast), Orthoplast™ (Johnson & Johnson), Synergy™ (Roylan), and Ultraform Traditions™ (Sammons).

Most of these materials are heated while lying flat for about 1 minute at temperatures between 150 to 180°F. The material is then shaped for 3 to 4 minutes before returning to a hardened form. Minor changes can be made with a heat gun, but changes should never be performed while the splint is on the patient.

Casting materials, such as fiberglass or plaster, are used to splint a body part, but conditions such as macerations, ulcerations, infections, burns, blisters, rashes, and allergic contact dermatitis can result from extended use. Individuals often report that such casts itch, smell, and are difficult to keep dry. Fiberglass casts with a stockinette or cast padding can limit moisture, but they must be dried (usually with a hair dryer) to prevent maceration, odor, and itching. A new Gore-Tex™ liner developed for use under fiberglass repels water, permits evaporation, and allows bathing, swimming, sweating, and hydrotherapy without any special drying of the cast or skin. The liner comes in 2-, 3-, and 4-inch widths and is applied directly to the skin. Fiberglass casting material is then applied over the liner. Although slightly more expensive than traditional casts, those incorporating this type of liner do not have to be changed as often, because they stay more comfortable throughout the immobilization period.

Construction of Custom Pads and Protective Devices

In some settings, the athletic trainer has access to the soft and hard materials mentioned earlier in this chapter. These materials can be used in constructing a variety of custom pads or protective devices. Custom pads can be advantageous for several reasons, such as cost, design, and availability. In addition, custom pads can be designed to meet the needs of the individual. The athletic trainer should use caution, however, to ensure that custom-made devices are constructed and fit properly. The athletic trainer assumes legal responsibility for use of any custom-made devices.

Rules Regarding Protective Pads

The National Federation of State High School Associations (NFSHSA) and the National Collegiate Athletic Association (NCAA) have specific rules regarding the use of soft and hard materials to protect a body area. The on-site referee must determine that specific fabricated pads are made of soft materials or meet the standards for hard materials established by the NFSHSA or NCAA. Hard, abrasive, or unyielding substances may be used on the hand, wrist, forearm, or elbow if the substance is covered on all exterior surfaces with no less than a ½-inch thick, high-density, closed-cell polyurethane or a material of the same minimum thickness and similar physical properties. In addition, a written authorization form must be signed by a licensed medical physician that indicates the cast or splint is necessary to protect the body part. This form must be available to the referee before the start of competition. The referee must verify that the hard material is properly padded according to the guidelines and has the right to eject the player for using the cast or splint as a weapon.

 High-density materials, such as thermomoldable plastics and casting materials, can absorb more energy by deformation and, in doing so, transfer less stress to an injured area.

LIABILITY AND EQUIPMENT STANDARDS

During football practice, an athletic trainer notices that the quarterback is wearing a helmet with a two-point chin strap. What action or actions should be taken by the athletic trainer, and why?

Legal issues concerning protective equipment are a major concern for every athletic trainer and organized sport program. An organization's duty to ensure the proper use of protective equipment usually is a shared responsibility among the members of the athletic staff. For example, the head coach may be responsible for recommending specific equipment for his or her sport. The athletic director may be responsible for purchasing this recommended equipment. The equipment manager or athletic trainer may then be responsible for properly fitting the equipment based on the manufacturer's guidelines, instructing and warning the individual about proper use of the equipment, regularly inspecting the protective equipment, and keeping accurate records of any repair or reconditioning of the equipment.

Negligence and standard of care for the athletic trainer are discussed in broad terms in Chapter 1. When focusing on protective equipment, the athletic trainer has a duty to:

- Select the most appropriate equipment.

- Properly fit the equipment to the individual.

- Instruct the individual in proper care of the equipment.

- Warn the individual of any danger in using the equipment inappropriately.

- Supervise and monitor the proper use of all protective equipment.

It is the duty of the manufacturer to design, manufacture, and package safe equipment that will not cause injury to an individual when the equipment is used as it was intended. To protect the sport participant from ineffective and poorly constructed athletic equipment, several agencies have developed standards of quality to ensure that equipment does not fail under normal athletic circumstances or contribute to injury. The National Operating Committee on Standards for Athletic Equipment (NOCSAE) sets the standards for football helmets to tolerate certain forces when applied to different areas of the helmet. Currently, baseball, softball, and lacrosse helmets and face masks also must be NOCSAE certified. Other testing agencies for protective equipment include the American Society for Testing and Materials (ASTM) and the Hockey Equipment Certification Council (HECC) of the Canadian Standards Association (CSA). These agencies have established material standards for equipment such as protective eye wear, ice hockey helmets, and face masks.

In addition to agencies that establish standards for the manufacture of equipment, athletic governing bodies establish rules for the mandatory use of specific protective equipment as well as rules governing special protective equipment. These governing bodies include the NFSHSA, the National Association of Intercollegiate Athletics, the NCAA, and the U.S. Olympic Committee. For example, the NCAA requires football players to use a face mask and helmet with a secured, four-point chin strap. In addition, all players must wear helmets that carry a warning label regarding the risk of injury and a manufacturer's or reconditioner's certification indicating that the equipment meets the NOCSAE test standards (1).

After equipment has been purchased, the manufacturer's informational materials, such as brochures and warranties used in the selection process, should be cataloged for reference in the event an injury occurs. This information can document the selection process and particular attributes of the chosen equipment. When an individual provides his or her own protective equipment, the responsibilities of the athletic trainer do not change. The athletic trainer must ensure that the equipment meets safety standards and is fitted correctly, properly maintained and cleaned, and used appropriately. Athletic trainers and coaches should know the dangers involved in using sport equipment and have a duty to properly supervise its fitting and intended use. Athletes should not be allowed to wear or alter any equipment that may endanger the individual or other team members.

> **A** *The athletic trainer should remove from practice any athlete whose helmet does not have a four-point chin strap. Interscholastic and collegiate athletic governing bodies require helmets be secured with a four-point chin strap. As such, the two-point strap does not meet minimum protection standards and should not be allowed on the helmet. If the individual were to sustain an injury while wearing an improper helmet, the athletic trainer could be considered negligent.*

PROTECTIVE EQUIPMENT FOR THE HEAD AND FACE

> **Q** *A high school athletic trainer is concerned about a variety of oral injuries that have occurred on the school's basketball teams. What rationale can be used to convince the administration to purchase mouth guards for the teams?*

Many head and facial injuries can be prevented with regular use of properly fitted helmets and facial protective devices, such as face guards, eye wear, ear wear, mouth guards, and throat protectors. Helmets in particular are required in football, ice hockey, men's lacrosse, baseball, softball, whitewater sports (kayaking), amateur boxing, and bicycling and must be fitted properly to disperse impact forces.

Football Helmets

Football helmet designs typically use a single or double air bladder, closed-cell padding, or a combination of the two. A new helmet designed by Riddell, called the Revolution®, is based on a True-Curve shell shape and is computer-designed around the head's center of gravity. It features increased side and facial protection to lessen the impact in these areas, and it has been found to reduce the incidence of cerebral concussions in high school football players (2).

Air bladders are excellent at absorbing shock, but they must be inspected daily by the players to ensure that adequate inflation is maintained for a proper fit. Helmet shells can be constructed of plastic or a polycarbonate alloy. Polycarbonate is a plastic used in making jet canopies and police riot gear; it is lightweight and both scratch- and impact-resistant. Helmets vary in life expectancy. Typically, the polycarbonate alloy shell has a 5-year warranty; the ABS [**AU: Can ABS be spelled out/defined?**] plastic shell has a 2-year warranty. Manufacturer's guidelines should be followed with regard to the appropriate time for retiring a helmet.

Heat, as an environmental factor, can alter the effectiveness of shock absorption in the liner and some shell materials. As a result, materials compress more easily and absorb less shock at higher compared with lower temperatures. As part of the testing process, the NOCSAE drops the helmet twice within 1 minute from a height of 152 cm (60 inches) on the right frontal boss in ambient temperature. The process is repeated after soaking the helmet for 4 hours at 49°C (120°F). The helmet must meet the same criterion at both temperatures (3). The NOCSAE mark on a helmet indicates that it meets the minimum impact standards and can tolerate forces applied to several different areas. In addition, the NOCSAE includes a warning label regarding the risk of injury on each helmet that states:

> **Warning:** Do not strike an opponent with any part of this helmet or face mask. This is a violation of football rules and may cause you to suffer severe brain or neck injury, including paralysis or death. Severe brain or neck injury may also occur accidentally while playing football. NO HELMET CAN PREVENT ALL SUCH INJURIES. USE THIS HELMET AT YOUR OWN RISK.

This warning label must be clearly visible on the exterior shell of all new and reconditioned helmets. In addition, the athletic trainer should continually warn athletes of the risks involved in football and ensure that the helmet is properly used within the guidelines and rules of the game.

Manufacturer's guidelines should always be followed when fitting a football helmet. Before fitting, the individual should have a haircut in the style that will be worn during the athletic season and wet the head to simulate game conditions.

Once fitted, the helmet should be checked daily for proper fit, which can be altered by hair length, deterioration of internal padding, loss of air from cells, and spread of the face mask. This check is performed by inserting a tongue depressor between the pads and the face. When moved back and forth, a firm resistance should be felt. A snug-fitting helmet should not move in one direction when the head moves in another. In addition, the helmet should be checked weekly by the athletic trainer to ensure proper fit and compliance with safety standards.

Each helmet should have the purchase date and tracking number engraved on the inside. Detailed records should be kept that identify the purchase date, use, reconditioning history, and certification seals. Each individual also should be instructed regarding the proper use, fit, and care of the helmet. In addition, each individual should sign a statement that confirms having read the NOCSAE seal and been informed of the risks of injury through improper use of the helmet or face mask when striking an opponent. This statement should be signed, dated, and kept as part of the individual's medical files.

Field Strategy 3.1: Proper Fitting of a Football Helmet can be found on the companion website at thePoint.

A Weekly Helmet Inspection Checklist is provided on the companion website at thePoint.

Ice Hockey Helmets

Ice hockey helmets must absorb and disperse high-velocity, low-mass forces (e.g., being struck by a stick or puck) and low-velocity, high-mass forces (e.g., being checked into the sideboard or falling on the ice) (Fig. 3.1). As with football helmets, ice hockey helmets reduce head injuries; however, they do not prevent neck injuries caused by axial loading. The use of head protection with a face mask seems to have given many players a sense of invulnerability to injury. Studies have shown that the risk of spinal cord injury and, in particular, quadriplegia may be threefold greater in hockey than in American

███ █ FIGURE 3.1 Ice hockey helmet. Helmets used in ice hockey must absorb and disperse high-velocity, low-mass forces (e.g., being hit by a high stick or a puck) and low-velocity, high-mass forces (e.g., being checked into the boards). Full face guards may be clear or wire mesh.

football (4). The major mechanism for this injury is head-first contact with the boards secondary to a push or a check from behind.

Ice hockey helmet standards are monitored by the ASTM and the HECC, and ice hockey helmets are required to carry the stamp of approval from the CSA. When properly fitted, the helmet should sit level on the head one to two finger widths above the eyebrows. There should be maximum of two finger widths between the neck and chin strap. The face mask should fit properly in the J-clips, and the chin should rest in the chin cup (5). Proper fit is achieved when a snug-fitting helmet does not move, slide, or rotate when the head is turned.

Batting Helmets

Batting helmets are now compulsory in baseball and softball and require the NOCSAE mark (1). Most batting helmets are open-faced with a double ear-flap design and can protect the majority of the superolateral cranium but not the jaw or facial area. Although some studies claim that batting helmets fitted with face shields may prevent or reduce the severity of facial injuries to children, no rigorous data currently support such a claim (6).

It is best to have a thick layer of foam between the primary energy absorber and the head to allow the shell to move slightly and deform. This maximizes its ability to absorb missile kinetic energy from a ball or a bat and prevents excessive pressure on the cranium. The helmet should be snug enough that it does not move or fall off during batting and running bases.

Other Helmets

Lacrosse helmets are mandatory in the men's game and optional in the women's game. These helmets also are worn by field hockey goalies. The helmet is made of a highly resistant plastic or fiberglass shell and must meet NOCSAE standards. The helmet, wire face guard, and chin pad are secured with a four-point chin strap (Fig. 3.2). The helmet should not move in one direction when the head moves in another.

An effective bicycle helmet has a plastic or fiberglass, rigid shell with a chin strap and an energy-absorbing foam liner. Regardless of the type, the helmet can provide substantial protection against injuries to the head and the upper and midface region. A stiffer shell results in better diffusion and resilience to impact. A firmer, dense foam liner is more effective at higher velocities, whereas less stiff foam provides more protection at lower velocities. Increasing the thickness of the liner may lead to a more effective level of protection, but the increased mass and weight of the helmet may make it more uncomfortable. Improved designs have produced helmets that are lightweight and aerodynamic, with an increase in the number of ventilation ports. Wearing a cycling helmet does not increase thermal discomfort to the head or body and has no additional impact on core temperature, head skin temperature, thermal sensation, heart rate, sweat rate, and overall perceived exertion (7).

Although the rate of bicycle helmet usage has increased in the United States, at least one study has found that the overwhelming majority of children, adolescents, and their parents cannot properly fit a bicycle helmet. This increases the potential for exposure of the head's frontal region, which is the most common site of impact in bicycle head injuries (8). Common fitting errors include having the helmet rest too high on the forehead, improper strap position (failure of strap to make a "V" around the ear), and excessive front-to-back movement of the helmet (8,9).

Bicycle helmet fitting should first begin with a properly conditioned helmet (i.e., certified by the Consumer Product Safety Commission, ASTM, American National Standards Institute, or CSA). The helmet should be less than 10 years old, and the plastic cover should be intact, with no visible cracks. When resting on the head, the following guidelines should be used to properly fit the helmet (8):

■■■ FIGURE 3.2 **Lacrosse helmet.** Lacrosse helmets provide full face and neck protection.

■ There should be space of less than two finger breadths in front of, and in the side of, the helmet.

- The helmet should rest two finger breadths above the eyebrows.

- The chin strap should form a "V" around the ear and clip below the ear.

- The helmet front should pull down over the forehead when the mouth is opened.

- Side-to-side, front-to-front, and rotational movement should be 1 inch or less.

Face Guards

Face guards, which vary in size and style, protect and shield the facial region from flying projectiles. The NOCSAE has set standards for strength and deflection for football face guards worn at the high school and college levels. Football face guards are made of heavy-gauge, plastic-coated steel rod designed to withstand impacts from blunt surfaces, such as the turf or another player's knee or elbow. The effectiveness of a football face guard depends on the strength of the guard itself, the helmet attachments, and the four-point chin strap on the helmet. When properly fitted, the face mask should extend two finger widths away from the forehead and allow complete field of vision. No face protection should be less than two bars. If needed, eye shields made of Plexiglas® or polycarbonate can be attached to the face mask.

Ice hockey face guards are made of clear plastic (polycarbonate), steel wire, or a combination of the two and must meet HECC and ASTM standards (see Fig. 3.1). Hockey face guards primarily prevent penetration of the hockey stick, but they also are effective against flying pucks and collisions with helmets, elbows, side boards, and the ice. The use of full-coverage face masks in amateur ice hockey has greatly reduced facial trauma. The use of a single chin strap, however, still allows the helmet to ride back on the head when a force is directed to the frontal region, thus exposing the chin to lacerations. The guard stands away from the nose approximately 1 to 1½ inches. If a wire mesh is used, the holes should be small enough to prevent penetration by a hockey stick.

Lacrosse face guards must meet NOCSAE standards. The wire mesh guard stands away from the face, but the four-point chin strap has a padded chin region in case the guard is driven back during a collision with another player (see Fig. 3.2). Face masks used by catchers and the home-plate umpire in baseball and softball should fit snugly to the cheeks and forehead but should not impair vision. These devices can be used by players in the field and must meet ASTM standards. Men's and women's fencing masks have an adjustable spring to prevent the mask from moving during competition.

Eye Wear

Eye injuries are relatively common and almost always preventable if proper protective wear is used. There are three types of protective eye wear: goggles, face shields, and spectacles.

Goggles have several designs. One is the eyecup design seen in swimming, whereby the eye socket is completely covered. Goggles are made of hard, impact-resistant plastic that is water tight. Because of the streamlined shape and design, contact lenses may be worn during competition when wearing these goggles. Vision may be slightly distorted; however, enhanced vision with the goggles could be a great advantage during flip-turns. Another style of goggles can be worn over spectacles, such as ski goggles. These usually are well ventilated to allow air currents to minimize fogging. A third style of goggles is a sport goggle with a mask design. This type of goggle is relatively lightweight, may or may not include a shield, and is designed to withstand the forces generated by a ball traveling at significant speeds. This type of goggle has become very popular with the U.S. Women's Lacrosse Association, when in 2005, participants were mandated to wear protective eyewear. Goggles worn for women's lacrosse must be ASTM approved (1).

Face shields are secondary protective devices that can be attached to specific helmets. Individuals who wear contact lenses often prefer the shield, because there is less chance that a finger or hand can hit the eye. The shield can be tinted to reduce glare from the sun; however, the plastic can become scratched and may fog up in cold weather.

Spectacles (eyeglasses) contain the lenses, frame, and side shields commonly seen in industrial eye protective wear. The lenses should be 3 mm thick and be made from CR 39 plastic or polycarbonate, both of which can be incorporated with prescription lenses. CR 39 plastic lenses are less expensive, but they scratch more easily, often are thicker and heavier than polycarbonate, and are not impact resistant. In contrast, polycarbonate is lightweight, is scratch-resistant, and can have an anti-fog and ultraviolet inhibitor incorporated into the lens. Of the clear materials developed for protective equipment, polycarbonate has the greatest impact resistance. A disadvantage of the polycarbonate is that static charges cause dust to cling to the lenses more readily than to glass lenses.

The frame should be constructed of a resilient plastic, with reinforced temples, hinges, and nosepiece. Adequate cushioning should protect the eyebrow and nasal bridge from sharp edges. Only polycarbonate eye protectors and eye frames that meet ASTM and parallel CSA standards offer enough protection for a sport participant. Approved eye guards protect the eye when impacted with a racquet ball traveling at 90 mph (40 meters per second) or a racquet going 50 mph (22.2 meters per second). Written acknowledgement that an eye guard meets standards can be found on the product package.

Regardless of the type of protection used, the lenses should be cleaned with warm, soapy water and rinsed with clean water, or a commercially available eyeglass cleaner should be used. A soft cloth should be used to blot dry the lenses. A dry lens should never be wiped or rubbed because of the possibility of scratching the lens by moving foreign particles across the surface. The frames and elastic straps also may be cleaned with soap and water and air-dried. Lenses should be replaced when scratches affect vision or cracks appear at the edges. Protective eye wear always should be stored in a hard case to protect the polycarbonate lenses from being scratched.

Any individual with monocular vision should consult an ophthalmologist before participation in any sport or physical activity because of the resultant reduction of visual fields and depth perception. If a decision is made to participate, the individual should wear maximum eye protection during all practices and competitions. A sweatband should be worn to keep sweat out of the eye guard.

Although participants in physical activity often wear contact lenses because they improve peripheral vision and astigmatism and do not normally cloud during temperature changes, contact lenses do not protect against eye injury. Contact lenses come in two types: a hard or corneal type, which covers only the iris of the eye; and a soft or scleral type, which covers the entire front of the eye. Hard contact lenses often become dislodged and are more frequently associated with irritation from foreign bodies (e.g., corneal abrasions). Dust and other foreign matter may get underneath the lens and damage the cornea, or the cornea may be scratched while inserting or removing the lens.

Soft contact lenses can protect the eye from irritation by chlorine in pools. Although research has shown that pool water causes soft lenses to adhere to the cornea, reducing the risk of loss, wearing soft lenses while swimming is not recommended. Microorganisms found in pool water, especially *Acanthamoeba* sp., are responsible for a rare but serious corneal infection, acanthamoeba keratitis. It is recommended that with or without contact lenses, goggles should always be worn in water to protect against foreign organisms and irritation from chlorine. Swimmers should wait 20 to 30 minutes after leaving the water before removing contact lenses or use saline drops if the lenses must be removed earlier. This allows time for the lenses to stop sticking to the cornea. Lenses should then be immediately disinfected. Removing the lenses too soon may cause corneal abrasions, leaving the cornea susceptible to infection.

Ear Wear

With the exception of boxing, wrestling, and water polo, few sports have specialized ear protection. Repeated friction and trauma to the ear can lead to a permanent deformity, called **hematoma auris** or cauliflower ear (see Chapter 9). For this reason, ear protection should be worn regularly in these sports. Proper fit is achieved when the chin strap is snug and the head gear does not move during contact with another player (Fig. 3.3). The protective ear cup should be deep enough so as not to compress the external ear.

Mouth Guards

An intraoral, readily visible mouth guard is required in all interscholastic and intercollegiate football, ice hockey, field hockey, and

■■■ ■ FIGURE 3.3 **Ear protectors.** Protective ear wear can prevent friction and trauma to the ear that may lead to permanent deformity.

men's and women's lacrosse. The American Dental Association has recommended requiring a mouth guard in acrobatics, basketball, bicycling, boxing, equestrian events, extreme sports, field events, field hockey, football, gymnastics, handball, ice hockey, in-line skating, lacrosse, martial arts, racquetball, rugby, shot putting, skateboarding, skiing, skydiving, soccer, softball, squash, surfing, volleyball, water polo, weight lifting, and wrestling (10).

Properly fitted across the upper teeth, a mouth guard can absorb energy, disperse impact, cushion contact between the upper and lower teeth, and keep the upper lip away from the incisal edges of the teeth. This action significantly reduces dental and oral soft-tissue injuries and, to a lesser extent, jaw fractures, cerebral concussions, and temporomandibular joint injuries. The practice of cutting down mouth guards to cover only the front four teeth invalidates the manufacturer's warranty, cannot prevent many dental injuries, and can lead to airway obstruction should the mouth guard become dislodged. Although some individuals may complain that use of a mouth guard adversely effects speech and breathing, a properly fitted mouth guard should not interfere with either function. The benefits of preventing oral injuries through the use of mouth guards far outweigh any disadvantages.

Three types of mouth guards are commonly available. The most frequently used is the thermally set, mouth-formed mouth guard, which consists of a firm outer shell fitted with a softer inner material. Often referred to as the "boil-n-bite" style, the softer material is thermally or chemically set after being molded to the player's teeth (11). When properly fitted, the mouth-formed guard can virtually match the efficacy and comfort of the custom-made guard. This type of guard is readily available, is inexpensive, and has a loop strap for attachment to a face mask. The loop strap has two advantages: It prevents individuals from choking on the mouth guard, and it prevents the individual from losing the mouth guard when it is ejected from the mouth. These mouth guards often lack full extension into the labial and buccal vestibules. Therefore, they do not provide adequate protection against oral soft-tissue injuries. Furthermore, the thermoplastic inner material loses its elasticity at mouth temperature and may cause the protector to loosen.

Field Strategy 3.2: Fitting Mouth-Formed Mouth Guards is available on the companion website at thePoint.

The most effective type of mouth protector is the custom-fabricated protective mouth guard, which may be a pressure-formed, laminated type or a vacuum-formed type. This protector is expensive and requires special training to obtain the best results. Individuals using this style of protection report that they are more comfortable, do not interfere with breathing or speaking, permit more complete jaw closure, do not cause soft-tissue irritation, and cause less excess salivation (12). Cost of the basic materials is higher than the thermally set mouth guards. The laminated mouth guard uses high heat and pressure to form the material, leading to less deformation of the material when worn for a long period of time. In addition, the mouth guard can be thickened in selected areas as needed and may have inserts added for additional wearer protection. Vacuum-formed mouth guards, on the other hand, are less expensive and easier to design. A triple-layered, ethyl vinyl acetate material (thickness, 5 mm) makes for a sturdier and more protective mouth guard (12). Their fit of vacuum-formed mouth guards, however, can be compromised by an elastic memory because of the low heat used in their construction. After a few minutes of wearing the mouth guard, the warmth from the mouth can trigger the elastic memory, leading to adaptations in the design that make speaking and unrestricted breathing more difficult.

The recommended care of mouth guards is to thoroughly rinse the guard with water after each use and place it in a plastic mouth guard retainer box to air-dry. Periodically, the mouth guard should be soaked over night in a weak bleach solution (i.e., 1 quart of water to 1 tablespoon of bleach).

Throat and Neck Protectors

Blows to the anterior throat can cause serious airway compromise as a result of a crushed larynx and/or upper trachea, edema of the glottic structures, vocal cord disarticulation, hemorrhage, or laryngospasm. The NCAA requires that catchers in baseball and softball wear a built-in or attachable throat guard on their mask (1). Fencing masks and helmets used in field hockey, lacrosse, and ice hockey also provide anterior neck protectors to guard this vulnerable area.

Cervical neck rolls and collars are designed to limit excessive motion of the cervical spine and can be effective in protecting players with a history of repetitive burners or stingers. Properly fitted shoulder pads, however, are perhaps the most critical factor in preventing brachial plexus injuries.

Several commercial collars can be added to the shoulder pads, including the Cowboy collar™ (McDavid), Long Horn neck roll™, LaPorta collar™, and numerous others of similar design.

The Cowboy collar is closed-cell, polyethylene foam that fits underneath the shoulder pads. This collar can be further reinforced by adding a plastic back plate along the posterior aspect of the support. The Long Horn neck roll is larger in diameter than conventional foam collars and can further restrict motion by attaching auxiliary pads over the collar at specific sites. The LaPorta collar is a more rigid, plastic shell secured directly to the shoulder-pad arch. The helmet wedges into the collar, further restricting cervical motion. Cervical collars do not, however, decrease axial loading on the cervical spine when the neck is flexed during a tackle.

 A properly fitted mouth guard will absorb energy, disperse impact, cushion the contact between the upper and lower teeth, and keep the upper lip away from the incisal edges of teeth. As such, a mouth guard will significantly reduce dental and oral soft-tissue injuries and, to a lesser extent, jaw fractures, cerebral concussion, and temporomandibular joint injuries.

PROTECTIVE EQUIPMENT FOR THE UPPER BODY

How does use of a cantilevered system provide protection in football shoulder pads? Is this superior to flat shoulder pads?

In the upper body, special pads and braces often are used to protect the shoulder region, ribs, thorax, breasts, arms, elbows, wrists, and hands. Depending on the activity, special design modifications are needed to allow maximum protection while providing maximal performance.

Shoulder Protection

Shoulder pads should protect the soft- and bony-tissue structures in the shoulder, upper back, and chest. The external shell generally is made of a lightweight yet hard plastic. The inner lining may be composed of closed- or open-cell padding to absorb and disperse the shock; however, use of open-cell padding reduces peak impact forces compared with use of closed-cell pads.

Football shoulder pads are available in two general types: cantilevered, and flat. A channel system, incorporated into both types, uses a series of long, thinner pads attached by Velcro® in the shoulder pads. The pads can be individually fitted so that an air space exists at the acromioclavicular (AC) joint. The impact forces are placed entirely on the anterior and posterior aspect of the shoulder.

Cantilever pads have a hard plastic bridge over the superior aspect of the shoulder to protect the AC joint. These bridges are lightweight, allow maximal range of motion at the shoulder, and can distribute the impact forces throughout the entire shoulder girdle. The cantilevers come in three types: inside, outside, and double. The inside cantilever fits under the arch of the pads and rests against the shoulder. It is more commonly used, because it is less bulky than the outside cantilever, which sits on top of the pad outside of the arch. The outside cantilever is preferred by linemen, because it provides a larger blocking surface and more protection to the shoulder region. The double cantilever is a combination of the inside and outside cantilevers. It provides the greatest amount of protection but is not feasible for all players because of its bulk.

Flat shoulder pads are lightweight, provide less protection to the shoulder region, but allow more glenohumeral joint motion. These pads often are used by quarterbacks or receivers, who must raise their arms above the head to throw or catch a pass. The flat pads often use a belt-buckle strapping to prevent pad displacement, because the elastic webbing straps typically seen in most shoulder pads are inadequate to maintain proper positioning of the flat pads.

In addition to cantilevers, football shoulder pads consist of an arch, two sets of epaulets (shoulder flaps), shoulder cups, and anterior and posterior pads. The arch is shaped to fit the contour of the upper body. The epaulets extend from the edge of the arch and cover the shoulder cups to protect the top of the entire shoulder region. The shoulder cups attach to the arch, run under the epaulets, and should cover the entire deltoid. The anterior pads cover the pectoral muscles and protect the sternum and clavicles. The posterior pads cover the trapezius and protect the scapula and spine.

Football shoulder pads should be selected based on the player's position, body type, and medical history. Linemen need more protection against constant contact and require larger cantilevers. Quarterbacks, offensive backs, and receivers require smaller shoulder cups and flaps to allow greater range of motion in passing and catching.

> *Field Strategy 3.3: Fitting Football Shoulder Pads* can be found on the companion website at thePoint.

Elbow, Forearm, Wrist, and Hand Protection

The entire arm is subjected to compressive and shearing forces in a variety of sports, such as when blocking and tackling an opponent, deflecting projectiles, pushing opponents away to prevent collisions, or breaking a fall. Goalies and field players in many sports are required to have arm, elbow, wrist, and hand protection. In high school and collegiate play, however, no rigid material can be worn at the elbow or below unless covered on all sides by closed-cell foam padding (1).

The use of a counterforce forearm brace may provide some relief for individuals with lateral and medial epicondylitis. These braces are designed to reduce tensile forces in the wrist flexors and extensors, particularly the extensor carpi radialis brevis. Although these braces may relieve pain on return to activity, debate continues about the effectiveness of counterforce forearm braces. These braces should not be used for other causes of elbow pain, such as growth plate problems in children and adolescents or medial elbow instability in adults.

The forearm, wrist, and hand are especially vulnerable to external forces and often are neglected when considering protective equipment. In collision and contact sports, this area should be protected with specialized gloves and pads.

Thorax, Rib, and Abdominal Protection

Many collision and contact sports require special protection of the thorax, rib, and abdominal areas. Catchers in baseball and softball wear full thoracic and abdominal protectors to prevent high-speed blows from a bat or a ball. Individuals in fencing, and goalies in many sports, also wear full thoracic protectors (Fig. 3.4A). Quarterbacks and wide receivers in football often wear rib protectors composed of air-inflated, interconnected cylinders to absorb impact forces caused during tackling (Fig. 3.4B). These protectors should be fitted according to the manufacturer's instructions.

■■■■ FIGURE 3.4 **Chest and rib protection. A,** Several sports require extensive chest protection (e.g., ice hockey). **B,** Rib protectors absorb impact forces caused during tackling.

Sport Bras

Sport bras provide added support to prevent excessive vertical and horizontal breast motion during exercise. Although sport bras are designed to limit motion, few of those currently on the market actually do so, and as a result, many women continue to experience sore or tender breasts after exercise. Sport bras fall into two categories:

1. Bras made from nonelastic material with wide shoulder straps and wide bands under the breasts to provide upward support. Waist-length designs can prevent cutting in below the breasts.

2. Compressive bras that bind the breasts to the chest wall. Women with medium-sized breasts typically prefer this type.

Girls and women with small breasts may not need a special bra. Women with a size C cup or larger need a firm, supportive bra. The bra should have nonslip straps and no irritating seams or fasteners next to the skin, and it should be firm and durable. Choice of fabric depends on the intensity of activity, support needs, sensitivity to fiber, and climatic and seasonal conditions. A cotton/polyester/Lycra® fabric is a popular blend seen in sport bras. In hot weather, an additional outer layer of textured nylon mesh can promote natural cooling of the skin. In sports requiring significant overhead motion, bra straps should stretch to prevent the bra from riding up over the breasts. When overhead motion is not a significant part of the activity, nonstretch straps connected directly to a nonelastic cup are preferable.

Lumbar/Sacral Protection

Lumbar/sacral protection includes weight-training belts used during heavy weight lifting, abdominal binders, and other similar supportive devices (Fig. 3.5). Each should support the abdominal contents, stabilize the trunk, and prevent spinal deformity or injury during heavy lifting. Use of belts or binders can significantly increase proprioception and intra-abdominal pressure to reduce compressive forces in the vertebral bodies and, in doing so, potentially lessen the risk of low back trauma. The use of back belts to prevent occupational low back pain or to reduce lost work time because of occupational low back pain is not supported by the Canadian Centre for Occupational Health and Safety (13) or by the U.S. National Institute for Occupational Safety and Health (14). In contrast, the U.S. Occupational Safety and Health Administration's recent ergonomics regulation classified lumbar supports as personal protective equipment and suggested that they may prevent back injuries in certain industrial settings (14).

A ▶ Cantilever pads have a hard plastic bridge over the superior aspect of the shoulder to protect the AC joint. These lightweight bridges allow maximal range of motion at the shoulder and can distribute the impact forces throughout the entire shoulder girdle. As such, they provide the greatest amount of protection to the shoulder region but are not feasible for all players because of their bulk.

PROTECTIVE EQUIPMENT FOR THE LOWER BODY

Q ▶ A pitcher sustains a thigh contusion after being struck by a hard-driven baseball. What type of padding should be used to protect the thigh from another significant blow?

█ ▌▐ FIGURE 3.5 Lumbar/sacral protection. Abdominal binders support the abdominal contents, stabilize the trunk, and prevent spinal deformity or injury.

In the lower body, commercial braces commonly are used to protect the knee and ankle. In addition, special pads are used to protect bony and soft-tissue structures in the hip and thigh region. Depending on the sport/activity, special design modifications are needed to allow maximum protection while providing maximal performance.

Hip and Buttock Protection

In collision and contact sports, the hip and buttock region require special pads, typically composed of hard polyethylene covered with layers of Ensolite™ to protect the iliac crest, sacrum, coccyx, and genital region. A girdle with special pockets can effectively hold the pads in place (Fig. 3.6). The male genital region is best protected by a protective cup placed in an athletic supporter.

Thigh Protection

Thigh and upper leg pads, such as those illustrated in Figure 3.6, slip into ready-made pockets in the girdle to prevent injury to the quadriceps area. Thigh pads should be placed over the quadriceps muscle group, approximately 6 to 7 inches proximal to the patella. When using asymmetrical thigh pads, the larger flare should be placed on the lateral aspect of the thigh to avoid injury to the genitalia. In addition to thigh pads, neoprene sleeves can provide uniform compression, therapeutic warmth, and support for a quadriceps or hamstring strain.

Knee and Patella Protection

The knee is second only to the ankle and foot in incidence of injury. Knee pads can protect the area from impact during a collision or fall and, in wrestling, can protect the prepatellar and infrapatellar bursa from friction injuries. In football, knee pads reduce contusion and abrasions when falling on artificial turf.

Knee braces fall into three broad functional categories: prophylactic, functional, and rehabilitative. Prophylactic knee braces (PKBs) are designed to protect the medial collateral ligament by redirecting a lateral valgus force away from the joint itself to points more distal on the tibia and femur. Functional knee braces are widely used to provide proprioceptive feedback and to protect unstable anterior cruciate ligament (ACL) injuries or in postsurgical ACL ligament repair or reconstruction (Fig. 3.7A). Rehabilitative braces provide immobilization at a selected angle after injury or surgery, permit controlled range of motion through predetermined arcs, and prevent accidental loading in non–weight bearing patients (Fig. 3.7B).

Decisions to use any of the three major categories of knee braces should rest with the supervising physician or surgeon. Selection should be based on the projected objectives, needs of the participant relative to activity demands, cost-effectiveness, durability, fit, and comfort.

FIGURE 3.6 Hip protection. Girdle pads protect the gluteal and sacral area from high-velocity forces. Thigh pads also can be inserted to protect the quadriceps area.

Prophylactic Knee Braces

Two general types of PKBs are the lateral and bilateral bar designs. The lateral bar PKBs are constructed with single, dual, or polycentric hinge designs. Each model has a knee hyperextension stop and is applied using a combination of neoprene wraps, Velcro straps, and/or adhesive tape. The bilateral bar PKB has a medial and lateral upright bar with biaxial hinges.

After a comprehensive review of the available research, the American Academy of Orthopedic Surgeons concluded that the routine use of available PKBs has not been proven to be effective in reducing either the number or the severity of knee injuries and that, in some instances, it may have been a contributing factor to the injury. As future innovations and design modifications are made in PKBs, benefits in injury prevention may become more cost-effective. Until then, clinicians should base decisions regarding PKB use on the individual needs of the athlete.

Functional Knee Braces

Functional knee braces, commonly called derotation or ACL braces, are designed to control tibial translation and rotational stress relative to the femur with a rigid, snug fit and extension limitations. There are two basic styles of ACL braces: hinge-post-strap, and hinge-post-shell. Performance of

■■■■■ FIGURE 3.7 **Knee braces. A,** Functional knee braces control tibial translation and rotational stress relative to the femur and can provide extension limitations to protect the anterior cruciate ligament. **B,** Rehabilitative braces provide absolute or relative immobilization following surgery.

either brace depends on the magnitude of anterior shear load and the internal torque applied across the tibiofemoral joint, and it may be affected by several factors, including:

- Technique of attachment

- Design of the brace, including hinge design; materials of fabrication; geometry of attachment interface; and mechanism of attachment

- Variables in attachment interface, including how the interface molds around the soft-tissue contours of the limb and how much displacement occurs between the rigid brace and the compliant soft tissues surrounding the distal femur and proximal tibia while loads are applied across the knee.

Derotation braces may be prescribed by a physician for individuals with a mild to moderate degree of instability who participate in activities with low or moderate load potential. Functional knee braces do not guarantee increased stability in those sports requiring cutting, pivoting, or other quick changes in direction. The braces also are used after surgical ACL reconstruction. No consensus exists in the literature relative to whether functional braces have any beneficial muscle activation or proprioceptive effects on the ACL-deficient or -reconstructed limb. It is suggested that patient satisfaction (e.g., symptom reduction or subjective improvement in function) may be positively related to proper fit and hinge alignment along with the maintenance of optimal muscle tone (15,16).

Rehabilitative Braces

Rehabilitative braces come in two distinct designs: a straight immobilizer made of foam with two metal rods running down the side that is secured with Velcro to prevent all motion, and a hinged brace that allows range of motion to be set by tightening a screw control. Early motion prevents joint adhesions from forming, enhances proprioception, and increases synovial nutrient flow to promote healing of cartilage and collagen tissue. The braces are lighter in weight, adjustable for optimal fit, and can be easily removed and reapplied for wound inspection and rehabilitation. As the individual progresses through the rehabilitation program, the allowable range of motion can be adjusted periodically by the clinician. Rehabilitative braces are more effective in protecting against excessive flexion/extension than against anterior/posterior displacement (16).

Patellofemoral Protection

Patella braces are designed to dissipate force, maintain patellar alignment, and improve patellar tracking. A horseshoe-type silicone or felt pad is sewn into an elastic or neoprene sleeve to relieve tension in recurring patellofemoral subluxation or dislocations. These braces relieve anterior knee pain syndrome (17). An alternative brace for treating patellar pain is a strap worn over the infrapatellar tendon (Fig. 3.8).

Lower Leg Protection

Pads for the anterior tibial area should consist of a hard, deflective outer layer and an inner layer of thin foam. Velcro straps and stirrups help to stabilize the pad inside the sock. Many styles also incorporate padding or plastic shells over the ankle malleoli, which often are subject to repeated contusions. Several commercial designs are available.

Ankle and Foot Protection

Commercial ankle braces can be used to prevent or support a postinjury ankle sprain and come in three categories: lace-up brace, semirigid orthosis, or air-bladder brace (Fig. 3.9). A lace-up brace can limit all ankle motions, whereas a semirigid orthosis and air-bladder brace limit only inversion and eversion. Ankle braces have been compared with ankle taping. It is fairly well accepted that maximal loss in taping restriction for both inversion

■■■■ FIGURE 3.8 **Patellofemoral brace.** A strap worn over the infrapatellar ligament may relieve patellar pain.

■■■■ FIGURE 3.9 **Ankle protectors.** Commercial designs include the lace-up brace **(A)**, semirigid orthosis **(B)**, and air-bladder brace **(C)**.

and eversion occurs after 20 minutes or more of exercise. Ankle braces are more effective in reducing ankle injuries, are easier for the wearer to apply independently, do not produce some of the skin irritation associated with adhesive tape, provide better comfort and fit, are more cost-effective, and are comfortable to wear (18–20).

Field Strategy 3.4: Factors in the Selection and Fit of Athletic shoes can be found on the companion website at thePoint.

Selection and fit of shoes also may affect injuries to the lower extremity. Shoes should adequately cushion impact forces and support and guide the foot during the stance and final push-off phase of running. In activities requiring repeated heel impact, additional heel cushioning should be present. Length should be sufficient to allow all toes to be fully extended. Individuals with toe abnormalities or bunions also may require a wider toe box.

In field sports, shoes may have a flat-sole, long-cleat, short-cleat, or a multicleated design. The cleats should be properly positioned under the major weight-bearing joints of the foot and should not be felt through the sole of the shoe. Shoes with the longer, irregular cleats placed at the peripheral margin of the sole, with a number of smaller pointed cleats positioned in the middle of the sole, produce significantly higher torsional resistance and are associated with a significantly higher rate of ACL injury compared with shoes having flat cleats, screw-in cleats, or pivot disks (21). When increased temperature is a factor, such as when playing on turf, only the flat-soled, basketball-style turf shoes are reported to have low-release coefficients at varying elevated temperatures (22). This may lead to a lesser incidence of lower leg injuries. In individuals with arch problems, the shoe should include adequate forefoot, arch, and heel support. In all cases, individuals should select shoes based on the demands of the activity.

Specific foot conditions, such as fallen arches, pronated feet, or medial tibial stress syndrome, can be padded and supported with inner soles, semirigid orthotics, and rigid orthotics. Research has found that a 6.5-mm thick polymeric foam rubber material is more effective in absorbing heel-strike impact than a viscoelastic polymeric shoe insert (23). Antishock heel lifts use a dense silicone mixture to cushion heel impact to relieve strain on the Achilles tendon, and heel cups reduce tissue shearing and shock in the calcaneal region. Other commercially available pads may be used to protect the forefoot region, bunions, and toes, or adhesive felt (moleskin), felt, and foam can be cut to construct similar pads.

Foot Orthotics

Orthotics are devices used in the treatment and prevention of foot and gait abnormalities and related conditions, such as plantar fasciitis, heel pain, shin splints, patellofemoral pain, and low back pain. By changing the angle at which the foot strikes the surface, orthotics can make standing, walking, and running more comfortable and efficient. Orthotics are available in several forms and are constructed of a variety of materials. Foot orthotics fall into three broad categories: orthotics to change foot function, protective orthotics, and those that combine functional control and protection.

Foot orthotics can be rigid, soft, or semirigid. Rigid orthotics are designed to control motion. These orthotics are made from a firm material, such as plastic or carbon fiber, to increase their longevity and decrease the likelihood for changes in their shape. Most often, rigid orthotics are worn in dress or walking shoes. Soft orthotics assist in absorbing shock, improving balance, and relieving painful pressure sites. The use of soft, compressible materials in the construction of soft orthotics readily enables adjustment to changing weight-bearing forces. Eventually, however, the material breaks down; therefore, soft orthotics must be replaced regularly. Semirigid orthotics are used to provide for dynamic balance of the foot while walking or participating in sport and physical activity. This type of orthotic is constructed of layers of soft material that are reinforced with hard, rigid materials.

In addition to the proper selection of the appropriate type of orthotic, accurate fit is an essential component in the use of orthotics. As such, orthotics should be measured and fitted by a qualified medical professional.

The pitcher's thigh should be protected with nonresilient padding made of high-density material, such as orthoplast or thermoplast. The padding should be layered with a soft material that has shock-absorbing qualities, such as closed-cell foam.

SUMMARY

1. Protective equipment is only effective when it is properly fitted and maintained, periodically cleaned and disinfected, and used as intended.

2. The sport participant must be protected from high-velocity, low-mass forces to prevent focal injuries and from low-velocity, high-mass forces to prevent diffuse injuries.

3. Design and selection of protective equipment is based on the following energy-absorbing material factors: thickness, density, resilience, and temperature.

4. The NOCSAE establishes standards for football, baseball, softball, and lacrosse helmets and face masks.

5. The HECC of the CSA establishes standards for ice hockey helmets and face masks.

6. The ASTM establishes standards for protective eyewear, ice hockey helmets and face masks, and other protective equipment.

7. The athletic trainer is ultimately responsible for knowing the rules and standards governing the selection and fitting of protective equipment for each sport.

REFERENCES

1. 2005–06 NCAA Sports Medicine Handbook. Overland Park, KS: The National Collegiate Athletic Association, 2005.
2. Collins M, Lovell MR, Iverson GL, Ide T, Maroon J. Examining concussion rates and return to play in high school football players wearing newer helmet technology: a three-year prospective cohort study. Neurosurgery 2006;58(2):275–286.
3. Hodgson VR. Impact standards for protective equipment. In: Torg JS, ed. Athletic Injuries to the Head, Neck, and Face. St. Louis: Mosby–Year Book, 1991.
4. Reynan PD, Clancy WG Jr. Cervical spine injury, hockey helmets, and face masks. Am J Sports Med 1994;22(2):167–170.
5. Valovich McLeod TC. Proper fit and maintenance of ice-hockey helmets. Ath Ther Today 2005;10(6):54–57.
6. Nicholls RL, Elliott BC, Miller K. Impact injuries in baseball: prevalence, aetiology, and the role of equipment performance. Sports Med 2004;34(1):17–25.
7. Sheffield-Moore M, et al. Thermoregulatory responses to cycling with and without a helmet. Med Sci Sports Exerc 1997;29(6):755–761.
8. Parkinson GW, Hike KE. Bicycle helmet assessment during well visits reveals severe shortcomings in condition and fit. Pediatrics 2003;112(2):320–323.
9. Wellbery C. Proper bicycle helmet fit reduces head injuries. Am Fam Phys 2004;69(5):1271.
10. American Dental Association Division of Communications. The importance of using mouth guards: tips for keeping you smile safe. J Am Dental Ass 2004;135(7):1061.
11. Nathe C. Athletic mouth guards. Access 2005;19(4):22–24.
12. Croll TP, Castaldi CR. Custom sports mouth guard modified for orthodontic patients and children in the transitional dentition. Pediatr Dentistry 2004;26(5):417–420.
13. Canadian Task Force on Preventive Health Care. Use of back belts to prevent occupational low back pain. Can Med Assoc J 2003;169(3):213–214.
14. Occupational Safety and Health Administration. Ergonomic program: final rule. Fed Register 2000;65(220):68261–68870.
15. Vanderuin JF. Grant JA. The role of functional knee braces in managing ACL injuries. Ath Ther Today 2004;9(2):58–62.
16. Mallory N, Kelsbery G, Ketchell D. Does a knee brace decrease recurrent ACL injuries? J Fam Phys 2003;52(10):803–804.
17. BenGal S, et al. The role of the knee brace in the prevention of anterior knee pain syndrome. Am J Sports Med 1997;25(1):118–122.
18. Osborne MD. Rizzo TD Jr. Prevention and treatment of ankle sprain in athletes. Sports Med 2003;33(15):1145–1150.
19. Hume PA, Gerrad DF. Effectiveness of external ankle support: bracing and taping in rugby union. Sports Med 1998;25(5):285–312.
20. Thacker SB, Stroup DF, Brance CM, et al. The prevention of ankle sprains in sports: a systematic review of the literature. Am J Sport Med 1999;27(6):753–760.
21. Lambson RB, Barnhill BS, Higgins RW. Football cleat design and its effect on anterior cruciate ligament injuries: a three-year prospective study. Am J Sports Med 1996;24(2):155–159.
22. Torg JS, Stilwell G, Rogers K. The effect of ambient temperature on the shoe–surface interface release coefficient. Am J Sports Med 1996;24(1):79–82.
23. Shiba N, et al. Shock-absorbing effect of shoe insert materials commonly used in management of lower extremity disorders. Clin Orthop 1995;310(1):130–136.

CHAPTER

4

Protective Taping and Wrapping

STUDENT OUTCOMES

1. Identify uses of prophylactic tape and wraps in the management of musculoskeletal injuries.
2. Explain common principles used in the application of tape and wraps.
3. Describe common taping and wrapping techniques used to prevent or reduce the risk of reinjury.
4. Describe the general principles in applying soft playing casts and hard immobilizing splints or casts.

ROLE DELINEATION COMPETENCIES

The following Performance Domains and Tasks defined in the National Athletic Trainers' Association Board of Certification *Role Delineation Study*, 5th Edition are addressed in this chapter:

BOC COMPETENCIES

I.   Prevention

> D. Apply appropriate prophylactic/protective measures using commercial products or custom-made devices to minimize the risk of injury and illness.

V.   Organization and Administration

> B. Establish policies and procedures for the delivery of health care services following accepted guidelines to promote safe participation, timely care, and legal compliance.

Taping or wrapping a body part can provide support and protection while allowing functional movement. Although these techniques may be used as a prophylactic, or preventative, measure, taping and wrapping are used extensively during rehabilitation to reduce the risk of reinjury. Providing support to an injured body part may allow early return to activity while controlling undesirable movement that may impede the healing process.

   In this chapter, the principles of taping and wrapping as well as the types of tape and wraps that are available, their various uses, and the common techniques of application are addressed. Although many specific skills are illustrated, these are presented as a guide and should not be viewed as the only methods of application. Each technique must be customized for the particular patient and condition.

PRINCIPLES OF TAPING AND WRAPPING

Q   As a prophylactic measure, a basketball player is taped for an inversion ankle sprain. What is the procedure for removing the tape?

Tape and wraps are devices used to:

1. Provide immediate first aid.

2. Limit excessive joint movement.

3. Support an injured body part.

4. Provide compression.

5. Provide proprioceptive feedback.

6. Secure protective pads and dressings.

7. Allow early resumption of activity.

8. Reduce the chance of reinjury.

9. Prevent injury.

An injury must be fully evaluated to determine the pathology and severity of injury before any application of tape or a wrap. Injured anatomic structures must be identified, and an appropriate therapeutic rehabilitation program should be developed to ensure safe return to activity. Too often, premature return to activity can lead to reinjury or a chronic injury. Although tape and wraps may allow the individual to resume early activity, their use should never take the place of a comprehensive rehabilitation program. Only those individuals who are participating in a supervised therapeutic exercise program should be taped or wrapped.

A rehabilitation program, as discussed in Chapter 8, should focus on regaining full range of motion, **proprioception**, strength, endurance, and power in the injured body part while maintaining cardiovascular fitness. The individual should be able to complete, pain-free, all functional tests before being cleared for participation. In each phase of activity, the correct taping or wrapping technique should be selected and properly applied. It also is important to note that when improperly or poorly applied, a taping or wrapping technique can cause damage, including blisters or skin irritation, abnormal stress on body parts, and increased risk of injury to the region.

Types of Tape and Wraps

Many companies manufacture a variety of tapes for the management of musculoskeletal injuries. In general, tape can be made of an elastic or a nonelastic material. Elastic tape can be used to hold protective pads and dressings in place, provide compression, give proprioceptive feedback, and provide support. One advantage of elastic tape is that it allows muscles to contract without impeding circulation or neurologic function. The level of elasticity in tape varies from brand to brand—the more elastic the tape, the easier the application. Elastic tape should be stretched to between one-third and one-half of its elastic capability before application. If it is applied too tightly, the tape can restrict circulation and function of the body part, leading to increased pain or discomfort. Products come in a variety of widths and tensile strengths. A product must be selected according to the pathology of the injury and the desired effect.

Nonelastic tape provides support to joints by restricting excessive motions. The tape may be porous or nonporous. Porous tape allows heat and sweat to pass through minute openings in the tape, which allows the skin to remain cool. Nonporous tape makes the application more occlusive, thus increasing the potential for damage to the underlying skin from friction and retained heat. Like elastic tape, nonelastic tape comes in a variety of widths, primarily ranging from $\frac{1}{2}$ to 3 inches. Nonelastic tape may be bleached or unbleached. Bleached tape tends to be more aesthetically pleasing, but it is more expensive and does not offer better support compared with unbleached tape. Nonelastic tape is more difficult to apply than elastic tape. The body's natural contours increase the potential for wrinkles and excessive pressure from friction on underlying tissues, which can lead to blisters or cuts under the tape if it is applied incorrectly. An effective, wrinkle-free, nonelastic taping technique requires extensive practice and patience.

Wraps come in two major types, elastic and nonelastic. Both types are made of cloth; however, the elastic wrap contains fibers that allow it to be stretched. Elastic wraps can be used to secure pads and dressings, to provide compression and support, and to give proprioceptive feedback. Nonelastic wraps typically are used only to limit joint motion and to provide support. Nonelastic wraps sometimes are used in place of tape for cost-saving reasons; however, they are not as effective. Nonelastic wraps may be used in combination with nonelastic tape for additional support. For example, cloth wraps sometimes are used at the ankle. They do not contour well to the sharp angles in the region, however, nor do they "give" with muscle contractions.

Application of Tape

The body part should be clean, dry, and free of hair before application. Hair should be removed with an electric shaver or disposable razor. Any minor open wounds, such as blisters or cuts, should be cleaned with normal saline and covered with a sterile dressing. Areas sensitive to friction, such as the Achilles tendon or dorsum of the foot, should be protected with a pad and lubricant. Petroleum jelly or a commercial skin lubricant may be applied to a gauze or foam pad.

Occasionally, the patient is required to stand on a table with the hip and knee placed in slight flexion. This can be accomplished by placing the patient's heel on a 1½- to 2-inch heel lift. Old tape cores wound with tape or a commercial taping block may be used. Tape rolls, even those of the appropriate height, compress and become unusable.

When the skin has been prepared appropriately, a light layer of tape adherent is sprayed onto the skin surface and allowed to dry. This provides a sticky surface, permitting the tape to adhere better to the skin and providing a layer of protection for the skin. For individuals who are sensitive to tape, are taped on a daily basis, or are allergic to tape, a single layer of foam underwrap may be applied over the skin before tape application. It is critical that only one layer of underwrap be applied, because several layers may increase sweating under the tape and, in doing so, compromise the effectiveness of the taping technique.

Proper positioning of the athletic trainer is as important as proper positioning of the patient. To avoid unnecessary low back stress, a table of an appropriate height should be used to prevent excessive bending at the waist. If it is necessary to reach above shoulder level, the athletic trainer should stand on a bench or have the patient seated. When several dozen patients must be taped in a short amount of time, proper positioning is critical to prevent overtiring of the athletic trainer.

■ ■ ■ FIGURE 4.1 **Tearing tape.** Hold the tape roll in the dominant hand. Pinch the tear site with the index finger and thumb of both hands. Hold the nondominant hand still as the dominant hand pushes the roll quickly away from the body.

The patient should be placed in a position of function to ensure the desired result. To avoid wrinkles in the tape, only a few inches of tape should be unrolled at one time. As the tape is guided around the contours of the body part, slight tension should be applied. In tearing the tape, the roll should be held in one hand, pinched between the thumb and index finger of each hand (Fig. 4.1). A quick push of the roll away from the body while holding one hand still results in the tape ends being evenly torn.

In most taping techniques, each subsequent strip of tape should overlap the previous strip by one-half to one-third the width of the tape. The tape should be applied snugly but without impairing circulation. Circulation can be assessed by taking a pulse distal to the tape application, feeling for skin temperature, or blanching the nails to check capillary refill. Skin color and temperature should be the same bilaterally above and below the taping. Following application of the tape, the patient should check the body part for support and function.

Removal of Tape

Tape should be removed immediately after activity, because prolonged contact with the skin may cause tissue breakdown and bacteria formation. The tip of the tape cutters or scissors can be dipped in a skin lubricant to facilitate removing the tape from the skin. The scissors or tape cutter should lift the tape up and away from the skin, then advance along the body's natural contours (Fig. 4.2). For example, with an injury to the lateral aspect of the ankle, the initial position of the tape cutter is the posteromedial aspect of the tape application. Next, the cutter is moved distally around the posteromedial malleolus, extending through the arch toward the toes. In this manner, the tape cutter or scissors does not place any undue pressure on sensitive, injured structures. In removing the tape, the skin must be stabilized while the tape is pulled in the direction of the natural hair growth. Tearing tape rapidly off the skin can lead to damaged skin, open wounds, and pain.

■ ■ ■ FIGURE 4.2 **Removing tape.** Lift the tape away from the skin and advance the scissors or tape cutters along the body's natural contours, avoiding sensitive tissues.

Field Strategy 4.1: Application Techniques for Taping a Body Part can be found on the companion website at thePoint.

Following removal of the tape, the skin should be cleansed with a de-adhesive, then washed with soap and water and dried thoroughly. In addition, a skin moisturizer should be applied to prevent skin dryness and breakdown.

The skin should be inspected regularly for signs of irritation, blisters, or infection, including areas that are red, dry, hot, and tender. These signs indicate a possible allergic reaction to the tape or tape adherent. If the skin cannot be protected from irritation, it may be necessary to fit the patient with an appropriate commercial brace rather than risk continued irritation.

Application of Wraps

Field Strategy 4.2: Application Techniques for Wrapping a Body Part is available on the companion website at thePoint.

Application of elastic wraps should begin with the body part in a position of maximum muscle contraction. This ensures that movement and circulation are not impaired during activity. A wrap should be started distal to the injury site and continue to the area proximal to the injury. This prevents any edema formation from settling in the distal digits and provides support against gravitational forces. The wrap should be stretched from one-half to one-third of its total elastic capability before application. Excessive stretching may constrict circulation, compress superficial nerves, and impair function. Each turn of the wrap should overlap at least one-half of the previous, underlying strip. The end of the wrap may be secured with elastic tape for added support.

(A) *Using a tape cutter dipped in a skin lubricant, the tape should be removed immediately after practice. The cutter should follow a path along the body's natural contours; because the injury is an inversion sprain, the cut should take place on the medial side of the ankle. During cutting, the tape should be lifted up and away from the skin. Removing the tape involves slowly pulling it in the direction of the natural hair growth. Following removal, the skin should be cleansed and a skin moisturizer applied.*

COMMON TAPING AND WRAPPING TECHNIQUES

(Q) *An individual has sustained a mild thigh contusion. Immediate management of the injury includes maintaining compression on the injury throughout the remainder of the day. How should the compression be applied, and why?*

The following taping and wrapping techniques are provided as a guide to application. When taping or wrapping a body part, it is appropriate to adapt the technique to the individual's needs.

Taping and Wrapping Techniques for the Lower Extremity

Great Toe Taping

This taping technique is used to limit motion at the first metatarsal-phalangeal joint. Preparation for this taping includes placing an adhesive dressing (e.g., Band-Aid®) over the nail of the great toe for protective purposes. This technique begins with the placement of anchor strips on the great toe and at the midfoot (Fig. 4.3A). If prevention of hyperextension of the toe is desired, a strip of tape is applied from the distal anchor to the proximal anchor on the plantar surface of the foot (Fig. 4.3B). Additional supportive strips are applied until the base of the first metatarsal is covered (Fig. 4.3C). This procedure is completed by reanchoring the strips at the great toe and midfoot (Fig. 4.3D). If the injury involves hyperflexion, the supportive tape strips run on the dorsum of the toe and foot. Occasionally, the patient may have both a hyperextension and a hyperflexion injury; in this case, the two tapings may be combined to limit motion in both directions.

Arch Support

Arch support may be necessary in individuals with plantar fasciitis, high arches, fallen arches, or arch sprains and strains or in those who run or jump excessively. Several techniques can be used to

FIGURE 4.3 Great toe taping. A, Apply anchors. **B,** Apply strip to plantar surface. **C,** Apply additional support strips. **D,** Apply anchors to close.

support the arches of the foot. In taping the arches, the patient's foot should be in a position of slight plantar flexion.

ARCH SUPPORT: TECHNIQUE 1. A simple arch support uses three to four circular strips of tape applied around the midfoot region. The first strip is anchored on the dorsum of the foot and encircles the lateral border of the foot. As the strip moves across the plantar aspect, the strip is secured under the fifth metatarsal with one hand while the other hand applies slight tension in an upward direction through the medial longitudinal arch (Fig. 4.4A). In this manner, tension is applied only through the arch area and does not constrict the blood vessels on the lateral aspect of the foot. Each subsequent strip overlaps the previous, underlying strip by one-half, until the entire arch is covered.

FIGURE 4.4 Arch support: Technique 1. A, Apply tape across the plantar aspect, secure under the 5th metatarsal, apply slight tension in an upward direction through the MLA. **B,** Apply overlapping strips until arch is covered. **C,** A pad can be applied under circular straps for additional support.

FIGURE 4.5 Arch support: Technique 2. X-pattern arch taping. A, Following placement of anchor, apply tape moving from the great toe, along the medial foot, around the heel, and angled back to starting point. **B,** The next strip begins at the 5th metatarsal, moves along the lateral foot, around the heel, and angled back to starting point. **C,** Finish using a simple arch taping.

In addition, by applying the strips from the distal to the proximal aspect of the foot, the exposed edges of the tape do not roll when socks are placed on the foot. An arch pad may be added to this technique for additional support (Fig. 4.4B and C).

ARCH SUPPORT: TECHNIQUE 2. If additional support is required, an alternative "X-arch" technique may be applied. This technique can be particularly useful in providing support for the plantar fascia. An anchor strip is placed at the level of the distal metatarsal heads. Beginning at the base of the great toe, the tape is pulled along the medial aspect of the foot, around the heel, and angled across the arch to end at the starting point (Fig. 4.5A). The second strip begins at the base of the fifth metatarsal, then moves along the lateral aspect of the foot, around the heel, and angled across the arch, back to its point of origin (Fig. 4.5B). Alternating subsequent strips of tape, the same pattern is followed until the entire arch is covered. The technique is closed using the simple arch taping technique (Fig. 4.5C). An alternative closing technique is to use elastic tape.

FIGURE 4.6 Arch support: Technique 3. Alternate arch support taping. A, Following placement of anchor, apply tape moving from the great toe, along the medial foot, around the heel, and angled back to starting point. **B,** Follow same pattern, but angle toward the MLA proximal to previous strip. **C,** Finish using a simple arch taping.

ARCH SUPPORT: TECHNIQUE 3. This technique provides additional support to the medial longitudinal arch. This technique differs from the previous taping in the direction of pull of the support strips. Following the application of the distal anchor, the tape is pulled from the base of the great toe along the medial aspect of the foot, around the heel, and angled across the arch to end at the starting point (Fig. 4.6A). The next strip of tape initially follows the same pattern, but from underneath the foot, the tape is angled toward the medial longitudinal arch proximal to the previous strip (Fig. 4.6B). The process is repeated until the arch is covered. The technique is closed by applying a simple arch taping.

Metatarsal Arch Taping

This technique can be advantageous in the management of metatarsalgia and Morton's neuroma (see Chapter 18). It is designed to provide support for the metatarsal arch. A teardrop-shaped felt pad is placed slightly proximal to the heads of the second through fourth metatarsals (Fig. 4.7A). The pad is held in place by anchoring it with elastic tape (Fig. 4.7B). Caution must be taken to avoid applying the tape too tightly, resulting in restriction of normal foot movement.

Heel Contusion Taping

This taping helps to reinforce the calcaneus fat pad. The patient's ankle should be placed in a neutral position. Anchor strips are applied behind and below the heel (Fig. 4.8A). Using a basket weave technique, strips of tape are applied until the heel is covered (Fig. 4.8B). Anchors are reapplied to close the taping (Fig. 4.8C).

FIGURE 4.7 Metatarsal arch taping for metatarsalgia and Morton's neuroma. A, Apply tear drop pad slightly proximal to the 2nd–4th metatarsal heads. **B,** Anchor using elastic tape.

Open Basket Weave Ankle Taping

The open basket weave is used to control swelling and limit motion associated with an acute inversion, eversion, or syndesmotic ankle sprain. The patient should sit on the table with the ankle flexed at 90°. Using nonelastic tape, one anchor is applied 4 to 6 inches proximal to the ankle joint, and another anchor is applied at the level of the metatarsal heads (Fig. 4.9A). These anchors help to secure the remaining strips of tape to the skin. It is important to apply the anchors without constricting circulation.

FIGURE 4.8 Heel contusion taping. A, Apply anchors behind and below heel. **B,** Using a basket weave technique, apply strips until heel is covered **C,** Reapply anchors to finish.

FIGURE 4.9 Open basket weave ankle taping. A, Apply proximal and distal anchors. **B,** Apply a stirrup strip. **C,** Apply a horseshoe strip. **D,** Continue to alternate stirrups and horseshoes, leaving an opening on anterior aspect and close plantar foot with strips of tape.

The next step is the application of a "stirrup" strip. The tape is placed on the medial aspect of the proximal anchor; extends behind the medial malleolus, under the heel, and behind the lateral malleolus; and is secured back to the proximal anchor (Fig. 4.9B). Next, a "horseshoe" strip of tape is applied. Beginning on the medial aspect of the distal anchor, the horseshoe strip follows the base of the first metatarsal, travels behind the calcaneus, continues to the base of the fifth metatarsal, and ends on the distal anchor (Fig. 4.9C).

This process of alternating stirrups and horseshoes is continued, leaving approximately a ½-inch opening on the anterior aspect of the lower leg and foot. This opening allows some swelling to occur, but it limits gross edema. The plantar aspect is then closed with semicircular strips of tape, and the tape edges are then reanchored (Fig. 4.9D). Two or three horizontal pieces of tape then may be applied to secure the anchors. If further stability is needed, heel locks can be applied (see *Closed Basket Weave Ankle Taping*).

An elastic wrap may be applied over the tape for additional compression; however, it should be removed at night to avoid circulatory compromise. Ideally, the tape should be replaced daily when the individual is performing rehabilitative exercises, but it may be left on for up to 2 days, as long as the skin under the tape is intact and circulation is normal. Application of cold directly over the tape is permissible, but measures should be taken to avoid getting the tape wet. Typically, this can be accomplished by placing the leg in a plastic bag during the cold treatment. Tape that becomes wet from perspiration, ice treatments, or bathing should be removed to avoid skin **maceration**. Any sign of skin maceration or breakdown warrants immediate removal of the tape for further evaluation and treatment.

Closed Basket Weave Ankle Taping

The closed basket weave technique is used to provide external support to ankle ligaments and joint proprioception during activity. Because most ankle sprains are caused by excessive inversion, this explanation focuses on providing support to the lateral ligaments. Adaptations can be made for eversion ankle sprains by neutralizing the pull of the stirrups for support.

The lower leg and foot should be clean, dry, and free of hair. A gauze or foam pad with a lubricant should be applied to the dorsum of the ankle and Achilles tendon area. The patient is placed in a subtalar neutral position with the foot held at 90° of flexion. A proximal anchor should be placed approximately 4 to 6 inches above the ankle joint, distal to the belly of the gastrocnemius. The distal anchor is positioned so that it bisects the styloid process of the fifth metatarsal. Beginning on the medial aspect of the superior anchor, a stirrup strip is applied so that it runs down behind the medial malleolus, under the heel, and behind the lateral malleolus, then pulls up on the lateral aspect and ends on the superior anchor (Fig. 4.10A).

Next, beginning on the medial aspect of the distal anchor, a horseshoe strip of tape is placed along the base of the first metatarsal and behind the heel, following the base of the fifth metatarsal, and ends on the lateral aspect of the distal anchor (Fig. 4.10B). The next stirrup overlaps the first by one-half to two-thirds of the previous, underlying stirrup. A second horseshoe is applied, working again from medial to lateral, overlapping one-half to two-thirds of the previous, underlying strip. This alternation continues until at least three stirrups and three horseshoes are in place (Fig. 4.10C).

The design of this technique gives the tape an appearance of a woven basket and increases the overall strength on the taping. A figure-eight and heel locks are then applied (Fig. 4.10D). The figure-eight starts on the lateral malleolus, crosses over the dorsum of the foot to the medial arch, follows under the foot and up on the lateral aspect of the foot, crosses over the top of the foot to the medial malleolus, and then continues behind the lateral malleolus and back to the starting point. The technique continues by initiating the application of the heel locks (Fig. 4.10E). The tape is directed over the dorsum of the foot and down the medial arch, angled back toward the heel as it crosses the bottom of the foot, and pulled up on the lateral aspect of the heel so that it runs behind the lateral malleolus and around the heel to the medial malleolus. From the medial malleolus, the tape is directed over the dorsum of the foot and down the lateral side, angled back toward the heel as it crosses the bottom of the foot, and pulled up on the medial aspect of the heel so that it moves behind the medial malleolus and around the heel to the lateral malleolus. Finally, the taping technique is closed from

■■ ■■ FIGURE 4.10 **Closed basket weave ankle taping. A,** Apply proximal and distal anchors; apply a stirrup strip. **B,** Apply a horseshoe strip. **C,** Continue to alternate stirrups and horseshoes. **D,** Apply figure of eight. **E,** Apply heel locks. **F,** Close with horizontal anchor strips.

distal to proximal using horizontal anchor strips, which overlap one-half to two-thirds of the previous, underlying strip (Fig. 4.10F). For additional support, a second figure-eight and additional heel locks may be applied.

The most common problem with applying tape is that it can be applied too tightly, resulting in constriction of circulation and discomfort. This is especially true with the distal anchor but can be avoided by placing the distal anchor on the foot without applying tension.

Modified Ankle Taping

This technique is fast and easy to apply, but it provides only a moderate amount of support to the ankle. It commonly is used as both a preventive and a postinjury taping for an individual who has completed the rehabilitation program. Patients who require a more substantial amount of support can combine this taping with a brace or use the closed basket weave technique.

The skin is prepared in the same manner as in closed basket weave taping. The patient is placed in a subtalar neutral position with the foot held at 90° of flexion. Anchors are applied to the foot, bisecting the styloid process of the fifth metatarsal. The second anchor is applied 4 to 6 inches above the ankle joint, slightly distal to the belly of the gastrocnemius. Next, beginning on the medial aspect of the superior anchor, three stirrups are applied (Fig. 4.11A). These strips run posterior to anterior, each overlapping one-half to two-thirds of the previous, underlying stirrup, so that the malleoli are completely covered. The technique continues by applying a figure-eight with heel locks in a continuous fashion (Fig. 4.11B). Caution should be used when crossing behind the Achilles tendon, because tight tape may cause skin irritation and blisters. A second figure-eight is then applied (Fig. 4.11C). Finally, the taping is closed using successive circular strips around the foot, continuing proximal to distal (Fig. 4.11D).

■■■■ FIGURE 4.11 **Modified ankle taping. A,** Apply proximal and distal anchors. **B,** apply 3 stirrup strips.**C,** apply figure-eight with heel locks.**D,** close using successive circular strips around foot, continuing proximal to distal strips.

Achilles Tendon Taping

Taping of the Achilles tendon limits excessive dorsiflexion and, in doing so, reduces the tension placed on the tendon. The patient lies in a prone position on the taping table with the lower leg extended over the table. The foot is passively dorsiflexed to determine the spot of discomfort. This indicates the point to which motion is to be allowed while restricting any further, painful motion. The patient holds the foot in slight plantar flexion, and using nonelastic tape, anchors are applied at the base of the metatarsals and 4 to 6 inches above the ankle joint, slightly distal to the belly of the gastrocnemius (Fig. 4.12A). A heel pad with lubricant is placed over the Achilles tendon. Using 2-inch elastic tape, three to five strips are applied in an X pattern from the distal to proximal anchor, forming a checkrein (Fig. 4.12B and C). The X is reanchored distally and proximally with nonelastic tape (Fig. 4.12D). The patient then moves to a seated position, and using elastic tape, a figure-eight and heel locks are applied (Fig. 4.12E and F). Caution should be taken to avoid applying added pressure over the irritated Achilles tendon area. In addition, a heel lift also may be placed in the shoe to limit dorsiflexion; however, lifts should be placed in both shoes to prevent any undue stress on other body parts.

FIGURE 4.12 Achilles tendon taping. A, Apply anchors. **B,** Apply 3 – 5 strips in an X pattern from distal to proximal anchor. **C,** Form a check rein. **D,** Reanchor the "X" distally and proximally. **E & F,** Apply a figure-eight and heel locks.

Shin Splints Taping

Shin splints is a generic term that refers to pain found on the anterior shin. Often, anterior shin pain is directly related to stress on the medial longitudinal arch; therefore, arch taping may help to alleviate symptoms. If the condition is related to tendinitis of the tibialis posterior muscle, taping the ankle to limit eversion may provide some relief. Stress fractures and compartment syndromes do not benefit from taping—and actually may be aggravated by compression from the tape. This technique should not be applied until the true source of pain has been identified by an experienced health care provider.

The patient stands on a table facing the athletic trainer. A heel lift is placed under the heel of the leg being taped to relax the muscles. Anchors are placed distally above the malleoli and proximally at the tibial tuberosity(Fig. 4.13A). Medial and lateral anchor strips are placed from distal to proximal, lifting up against gravity (Fig. 4.13B). These should follow the line of the malleoli. Tape is applied in an alternating oblique direction, forming an X over the anterior shin, and working distal to proximal until the entire anterior shin is covered (Fig. 4.13C). Next, medial and lateral anchors are applied, followed by the placement of distal and proximal anchors (Fig. 4.13D).

Collateral Ligament Support for the Knee

This taping is designed to provide support and stability to the collateral ligaments of the knee. The patient should be standing on a table with the affected limb resting on a 1½- to 2-inch heel lift. Elastic tape commonly is used because of the dense musculature involved. A distal anchor is applied 2 to 3 inches below the level of the tibial tuberosity; a proximal anchor is placed at the midpoint of the quadriceps muscle group. Lateral and medial supportive strips are applied in an X fashion that outlines the medial and lateral collateral ligaments but keeps the patella exposed (Fig. 4.14A). Successive interlocking X patterns give additional support to the collateral ligaments (Fig. 4.14B). The collateral taping may be further reinforced with nonelastic tape (Fig. 4.14C). Finally, the tape is closed off with successive circular strips, moving from the distal anchor to proximal anchor (Fig. 4.14D).

Rotary Knee Instability Taping

The purpose of this taping is to provide support and stability to the anterior cruciate ligament. The patient stands on the table with the heel elevated. Using elastic tape, anchors are placed 2 to 3 inches

■■■■■ FIGURE 4.13 **Taping for anterior shin pain.** A, Apply anchor distally above malleoli and proximally at tibial tuberosity. **B,** Apply medial and lateral anchor strips distal to proximal. **C,** Apply strips in an alternating oblique direction, forming an X over anterior shin. **D,** Apply medial and lateral anchors; apply distal and proximal anchors.

FIGURE 4.14 Knee collateral ligament support. A, Using elastic tape, apply distal anchor 2 – 3 in. below tibial tuberosity; apply proximal anchor at midpoint of quadriceps. **B,** Apply lateral and medial strips in an X fashion. **C,** Reinforce with nonelastic tape. **D,** Close with strips moving from distal to proximal.

below the tibial tuberosity and at the midquadriceps. A pad with lubricant is placed in the popliteal space. Next, a piece of elastic tape is cut in the middle at both ends and torn to form an X, and the divided ends are placed around the patella and interlocked (Fig. 4.15A). Beginning at the superior anchor, a piece of elastic tape is angled down behind the knee and through the popliteal space, ending on the inferior anchor (Fig. 4.15B). In an opposite direction, a second piece of tape spirals down behind the knee and through the popliteal space, ending on the inferior anchor (Fig. 4.15C). Three to four spirals in each direction provide the necessary support. Once in place, the taping is

FIGURE 4.15 Rotary knee instability strapping. A, Apply distal and proximal anchors; split elastic tape to form an X and interlock the divided ends around the patella. **B,** from superior anchor, apply tape down behind the knee, through the popliteal space, ending on the inferior anchor. **C,** Apply next strip from opposite direction. **D,** Apply 3–4 spirals in each direction and reinforce with nonelastic tape.

closed with strips of tape applied in a circular fashion. Additional support may be provided by using nonelastic tape to reinforce the spiral pattern (Fig. 4.15D). If the collateral ligaments also need support, the collateral taping technique may be applied under the rotary instability technique.

Knee Hyperextension

This taping limits hyperextension of the knee and may be applied with elastic or nonelastic tape. With the patient standing on a table with the heel elevated, a superior anchor is placed at midthigh, encircling the entire thigh, and then an inferior anchor is applied 2 to 3 inches below the tibial tuberosity (Fig. 4.16A). A gauze pad with lubricant is placed in the popliteal space, reducing the friction of the nerves and circulatory supply to the knee. From the inferior anchor, apply tape strips in an X pattern over the gauze in the popliteal space. The X pattern should begin wide and then narrow as the popliteal space is covered. The last strip runs perpendicular to the anchors (Fig. 4.16B). The technique is completed by applying two to three anchors on the lower leg and four to five anchors on the thigh, each overlapping one-half to two-thirds of the previous, underlying strip (Fig. 4.16C). When completed, the taping should allow knee flexion and extension but limit hyperextension.

Patellofemoral Taping: McConnell Technique

This technique is designed to treat patellofemoral pain by correcting patella alignment. The purpose of this taping is to provide a sustained stretch of tight lateral structures and to improve lower limb mechanics. An essential component of this taping is an evaluation of the patella orientation, including the components of gliding, tilt, rotation, and anteroposterior orientation (1).

The area should be shaved and clean, and tape adherent should be applied. The patient should be positioned with the knee in full extension. The two tapes used for this technique are specialty tapes, Fixomull and Leuko Sportape (Biresdorf Australia, Ltd.). The initial step is the application of base strips (Fixomull tape) covering the patellar. This is performed by placing strips on the lateral condyle and extending them across the anterior aspect of the knee to the medial femoral condyle of the knee. For the remainder of the technique, the Leuko Sportape is used.

In correcting a lateral glide, the tape begins on the lateral border of the patella and is pulled medially (Fig. 4.17A). The soft tissue should be lifted over the medial femoral condyle toward the patella to provide more secure fixation. A lateral tilt correction is performed by placing the tape on the middle of the patella. The next step is to pull the tape medially to lift the lateral border (Fig. 4.17B). The soft tissue over the medial femoral condyle should be lifted toward the patella for more

■■■■ FIGURE 4.16 **Knee hyperextension strapping. A,** Apply distal and proximal anchors. **B,** From inferior anchor, apply tape strips in an X pattern; pattern should begin wide and become narrow; the last strip should be perpendicular to the anchors **C,** Apply 2–3 anchors on lower leg and 4 – 5 anchors on thigh.

FIGURE 4.17 Patellofemoral taping using the McConnell technique. A, Lateral glide correction. **B,** Lateral tilt correction. **C,** External rotation correction. **D,** Anterior-posterior correction.

secure fixation. Correction of external rotation is completed by applying the tape to the middle of the inferior border of the patella. Rotating the inferior pole internally and the superior pole externally, the tape is pulled upward and medially (Fig. 4.17C). In correcting an anteroposterior condition, the middle of tape is placed on the superior half of the patella. The tape is attached equally on both sides, lifting the inferior pole (Fig. 4.17D).

The tape is worn by the patient throughout the day. Because the tape is likely to loosen, the patient should be instructed to tighten the strips as necessary.

Quadriceps and Hamstrings Wrap

A thigh strain may involve either the quadriceps or hamstrings muscle group. This technique can be used to provide compression and/or support for either group.

If the quadriceps muscles are involved, the heel of the injured leg should be elevated 2 to 3 inches on a taping block. With the thigh in a neutral position, an elastic wrap is placed on the anterior aspect of the midthigh distal to the painful site (Fig. 4.18A). The wrap is applied in an upward and lateral direction, encircling the thigh (Fig. 4.18B). Elastic tape is then applied over the wrap to provide additional support.

Two techniques may be used if the injury is a hamstring strain. The first technique is appropriate when the

FIGURE 4.18 Quadriceps wrap. A, Place elastic wrap on anterior midthigh distal to painful site. **B,** Apply wrap in an upward and lateral direction, encircling the thigh.

FIGURE 4.19 Hamstrings wrap. A, Encircle thigh several times, pulling from a medial to lateral direction.
B, Pull wrap up across greater trochanter, around lower abdomen to opposite iliac crest, over waist and gluteals,
cross greater trochanter, and end on anterior thigh. **C,** Repeat the pattern and reinforce with nonelastic tape.

strain is to the distal portion of the muscle group. The wrap is applied in a manner similar to the quadriceps wrap. It is directed in an upward and lateral manner, encircling the thigh, and elastic tape is then applied over the wrap to provide additional support. The second technique may be used when the injury occurs in the proximal portion of the muscle group. The wrap is placed on the posteromedial aspect of the thigh, and it encircles the thigh several times, pulling from a medial to lateral direction (Fig. 4.19A). The wrap is then pulled up across the greater trochanter, continues around the lower abdomen, is brought around the opposite iliac crest over the waist and gluteals, and then crosses the greater trochanter, ending back on the anterior thigh (Fig. 4.19B). The thigh is encircled again, moving in a medial to lateral direction. Repeating the same pattern, the wrap is then reinforced with elastic tape (Fig. 4.19C).

Quadriceps Contusion Wrap

This technique can be used to provide compression or protection for a quadriceps contusion. In the management of a contusion if compression is desired, a felt pad of ½-inch thickness should be placed over the injured site. The pad is secured by an elastic wrap (Fig. 4.20A). Beginning at a point distal to the injury, the wrap is applied in an upward and lateral direction, encircling the thigh (Fig. 4.20B). If the desired outcome is to protect the area during activity, a foam pad should be placed over the involved area. Following application of the elastic wrap, the wrap should be covered with elastic tape to provide additional support to the area.

FIGURE 4.20 Quadriceps contusion wrap.
A, Place pad over injured site. **B,** Distal to injury, apply elastic wrap in an upward and lateral direction encircling the thigh.

Groin Wrap

Although groin strains may refer to damage to the hip flexors, hip adductors, or hip abductors, this explanation focuses on preventing stress to the hip adductors. When supporting the adductor muscles, the heel is elevated on a taping block, with the hip internally rotated. The wrap is then placed on the lateral aspect of the thigh and encircles the thigh in a medial direction to draw the thigh further into internal rotation (Fig. 4.21A). The wrap continues around the thigh, crossing over the greater trochanter and continuing across the lower abdomen, covering the iliac crest and around the waist and gluteals, then crossing the greater trochanter and ending

FIGURE 4.21 Groin wrap. A, Place wrap on lateral thigh and encircle thigh in medial direction. **B,** Continue wrap around thigh, over greater trochanter, across lower abdomen, cover iliac crest, around the waist and gluteals, cross greater trochanter, end on thigh. **C,** Reinforce with elastic tape.

back on the thigh (Fig. 4.21B). Following the same pattern, the wrap is then reinforced with elastic tape (Fig. 4.21C).

Hip Contusion Wrap

This technique is designed to provide protection and support to a contused iliac crest. A protective pad should be placed over the iliac crest. The pad is secured by applying an elastic wrap in a spica pattern. The wrap starts at the distal aspect of the anterior thigh and moves over the top of the pad, around the waist, diagonally down toward the lateral thigh, and behind the thigh to the starting point (Fig. 4.22A). This pattern is repeated for the length of the wrap (Fig. 4.22B and C). Application of elastic tape over the wrap provides additional support.

FIGURE 4.22 Hip contusion wrap. A, Place protective pad over iliac crest; apply elastic wrap in spica pattern. **B,** Repeat pattern. **C,** Reinforce with elastic tape.

Taping and Wrapping Techniques for the Upper Extremity

Acromioclavicular Taping

The purpose of this taping is to provide support to the acromioclavicular joint. The patient is positioned with the arm placed in a relaxed position and supported at the elbow. The nipple should be protected with a gauze pad and lubricant to prevent chaffing. Using elastic tape, an anchor is placed at the midbiceps region. A second anchor is placed just below the spine of the scapula, extends over the shoulder through the midclavicular line, and ends just under the nipple. A third anchor is placed just under the nipple and runs horizontally around the trunk, connecting the two ends of the second anchor (Fig. 4.23A). Beginning on the biceps anchor, a strip of tape is pulled from the anchor up and over the acromion process, ending on the midclavicular anchor. A second strip, also originating on the biceps anchor, is pulled up and over the acromion process to anchor on the posterior back. These two strips form an X pattern over the acromion process (Fig. 4.23B). A midclavicular strip is then applied, followed by another horizontal anchor. Each of the anchors should overlap one-half to two-thirds of the previous, underlying piece of tape. The pattern is then repeated, first crossing over the acromion process with the X patterns, then the midclavicular anchor, and finally, the horizontal anchor, until the acromion process is covered (Fig. 4.23C). The horizontal anchors should stop just below the axilla and should not impede arm motion. This taping may be reinforced by covering it with an elastic bandage wrapped as a shoulder spica (Fig. 4.23D).

Shoulder Spica Wrap

This technique can be used to provide support and stabilization for the glenohumeral joint. The patient should hold the injured arm in internal rotation. The technique begins by encircling the arm in a posterior to anterior direction at the midbiceps. Next, the anterior chest is crossed in

■■■■ FIGURE 4.23 **Acromioclavicular taping. A,** Place first anchor at midbiceps; place second anchor below spine of the scapula over shoulder through the midclavicular line; place third anchor under the nipple horizontally around the trunk, connecting the two ends of the second anchor. **B,** Place tape strips in an X pattern moving from biceps anchor up and over acromion process. **C,** Repeat pattern until the acromion process is covered. **D,** Reinforce with elastic bandage wrapped as a shoulder spica.

FIGURE 4.24 Shoulder spica. A, Encircle arm in a posterior to anterior direction at the midbiceps. **B,** Cross anterior chest and bring the wrap under the opposite axilla, across the back, over the acromion process. **C,** Continue wrap through the axilla, around the arm, and again across the anterior chest. **D,** Reinforce with nonelastic tape.

the region of the pectoralis major (Fig. 4.24A). Wrapping in this direction maintains internal rotation of the glenohumeral joint and limits external rotation. The limitation of motion is determined by the amount of internal rotation in which the arm placed initially. The wrap is brought under the opposite axilla, across the back, and over the acromion process in an anterior direction (Fig. 4.24B). The wrap is then continued through the axilla, around the arm, and again, across the anterior chest (Fig. 4.24C). Finally, the wrap is secured with nonelastic tape (Fig. 4.24D).

Elbow Hyperextension

This technique is designed to restrict painful motion while permitting functional movement. The patient should be instructed to clench the fist and hold the elbow in slight flexion with the palm facing up. To determine the degree of flexion, the elbow should be extended to the point of discomfort and then slightly flexed from that point. Using either nonelastic or elastic tape, anchors are applied to the midregion of the forearm and upper arm (Fig. 4.25A). After approximating the distance

FIGURE 4.25 Elbow hyperextension. A, Apply anchors to midregion of forearm and upper arm. **B,** Construct a check rein in an X fan shape. **C,** Attach check rein by applying 3 – 4 additional anchors.

FIGURE 4.26 Elbow sprain taping. A, Apply anchors to midregion of forearm and upper arm. **B,** Place 3–4 strips on nonelastic tape over the ligament in an X pattern. **C,** Secure above and below the joint with elastic tape.

between the two anchors, two strips of tape (the same length as the distance between the anchors) are torn from the roll. A checkrein is constructed by placing these two pieces of tape back to back, then adding five or six additional pieces of tape over the template in an X fan shape (Fig. 4.25B). The checkrein is then attached to the anchors by applying three or four additional anchors. The anchors should overlap each other by one-half to two-thirds. Using an elastic, a figure-eight then may be applied to further secure the taping and prevent slipping during activity (Fig. 4.25C). The radial pulse should be checked and monitored to determine if the tape is too tight.

Elbow Sprain Taping

The purpose of this taping is to provide support for the collateral ligaments of the elbow. The patient's arm is placed in a position of slight flexion. Anchors are applied to the midregion of the forearm and upper arm. If the injury is to the medial collateral ligament, three or four strips of nonelastic tape are placed over the ligament in an X pattern (Fig. 4.26A). The strips are then secured above and below the joint with elastic tape (Fig. 4.26B and C). The cubital fossa should remain open. The same technique can be modified for injury to the lateral collateral ligaments by changing the location of the strips.

Wrist Taping

Hyperextension or hyperflexion of the wrist may damage the ligaments of the wrist. Taping can provide support and stability for the wrist.

FIGURE 4.27 Wrist taping: Technique 1. Apply 3–4 circular strips of tape to the wrist.

WRIST TAPING: TECHNIQUE 1. For a mild sprain, three or four circular strips of tape may be applied to the wrist. The strips should be positioned from distal to proximal and overlap the previous, underlying strip by one-half to two-thirds the width of the tape (Fig. 4.27).

WRIST TAPING: TECHNIQUE 2. This technique can help to limit painful wrist motion. The patient should be instructed to spread his or her fingers. The wrist is positioned in slight flexion or extension, depending on the injury. Anchor strips are placed around the wrist and at the heads of the metacarpals (Fig. 4.28A). If the intent is to limit hyperextension, three or four strips of tape are placed in an X pattern over the palmar aspect of the hand; if the intent is to limit hyperflexion, the X pattern is positioned over the dorsum of the hand (Fig. 4.28B). Next, using either elastic or nonelastic tape, a figure-eight is applied around the wrist and hand (Fig. 4.28C–E). The figure-eight should begin on the radial aspect of the proximal anchor, travel across the dorsum of the hand around the metacarpal heads and across the palm of the hand, and end on the ulnar side

■■■ **FIGURE 4.28 Wrist taping: Technique 2. A,** Place anchor strips around wrist and metacarpal heads. **B,** Place 3–4 tape strips in an X pattern over palmar aspect or dorsum of hand. **C–E,** Apply a figure of eight beginning on the radial aspect of the proximal anchor.

of the proximal anchor (Fig. 4.28F). As the tape is brought through the web space of the thumb and index finger, the tape should be crimped to prevent irritation of the skin.

Thumb Taping

Most thumb injuries occur when the thumb is hyperextended. Thumb taping is designed to provide support and limit extension of the first metacarpophalangeal joint. The thumb is placed in a position of slight flexion and adduction, and an anchor is placed on the wrist. Next, a strip of tape is applied, beginning on the ulnar aspect of the proximal anchor and continuing upward over the palmar aspect of the thenar eminence on the thumb, crossing over the metacarpophalangeal joint, and encircling the thumb (Fig. 4.29A). The strip is then reanchored on the dorsal aspect of the anchor.

■■■ **FIGURE 4.29 Thumb spica. A,** Apply anchor on wrist; apply tape on ulnar aspect of proximal anchor and continue upward over palmar aspect of thenar eminence, cross over MP joint, and encircle thumb; this line of pull makes an X pattern. **B,** Apply 3 – 4 Xs; apply anchor at wrist to finish.

FIGURE 4.30 Buddy taping for the fingers. Apply narrow tape strips around proximal and distal phalanx of two fingers.

This line of pull makes an X pattern. Three or four X patterns should be applied before finishing the taping with additional anchors (Fig. 4.29B).

Finger Taping Technique

Sprains of the interphalangeal joints occur frequently. Taping can assist in providing support for an unstable interphalangeal joint. "Buddy" taping for the fingers involves using an adjacent finger for support. Strips of narrow tape are applied around the proximal phalanx and distal phalanx of the two fingers, leaving the joints uncovered to permit limited flexion and extension of the fingers (Fig. 4.30).

If additional support for the medial and lateral collateral ligaments is needed, anchors can be placed just proximal and distal to the injured joint. Working from distal to proximal, two narrow strips of tape are applied in an X pattern over the collateral ligaments, followed by a longitudinal strip to connect the two anchors (Fig. 4.31A and B). A figure-eight may be applied, using care not to impinge on the circulation. Because the blood supply is very superficial and easily compressed, capillary refill should be checked after taping.

> **A** A felt pad of ½-inch thickness should be placed over the injured site. The wrap should begin distal to the injury site and be applied in an upward and lateral direction, encircling the thigh. This prevents any edema formation from settling in the distal digits and provides support against gravitational forces. The wrap should be stretched from one-half to one-third of its total elastic capability. Excessive stretching may constrict circulation, compress superficial nerves, and impair function. Each turn of the wrap should be overlapped by at least one-half of the previous, underlying strip.

FIGURE 4.31 Collateral ligament taping. A, Apply anchors proximal and distal to injured joint; working from distal to proximal, apply two narrow tape strips in an X pattern over collateral ligaments. **B,** Apply a longitudinal strip to connect the two anchors.

SUMMARY

1. Taping and wrapping a body part provides support and protection while allowing functional movement. Tape and wraps may be used to provide immediate first aid, support an injured body part, or provide pain-free functional movement.

2. Used in conjunction with a comprehensive rehabilitation program, tape or wraps can allow early resumption of activity without the threat of reinjury.

3. When using tape, the skin should be inspected regularly for signs of irritation, blisters, or infection. In particular, skin that is red, dry, hot, and tender suggests an allergic reaction to the tape or tape adherent.

4. If the skin cannot be protected from irritation, it may be necessary to fit the patient with an appropriate brace rather than allow continued irritation.

REFERENCES

1. McConnell J. The management of chondromalacia patella: a long-term solution. Aust J Physiother 1986;32:215.

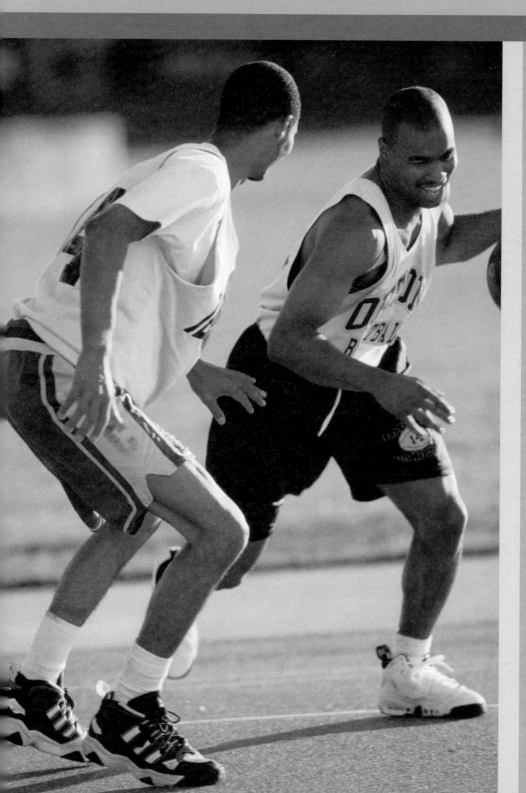

Injury Assessment and Rehabilitation

2

5 Injury Assessment

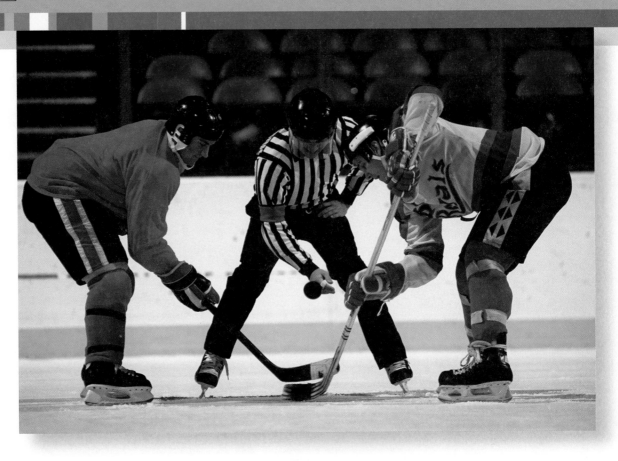

STUDENT OUTCOMES

1. Differentiate between the history of the injury, observation and inspection, palpation, and special tests (HOPS) injury assessment format and the subjective evaluation, objective evaluation, assessment, and plan (SOAP) note format used to assess and manage musculoskeletal injuries.

2. Explain the general components of the history portion of an injury assessment.

3. Describe the processes involved in the visual observation and inspection of an injury.

4. Describe the basic principles that direct the palpation component of an injury assessment.

5. Identify the various types of tests included in the physical examination of an injury.

6. Develop an emergency medical services plan for an athletic training facility.

7. Identify the responsibilities of an emergency response team.

8. List supplies and equipment that should be on-site in case of a medical emergency.

9. Explain the procedures used during an on-site injury assessment.

10. Identify emergency conditions that warrant immediate activation of the emergency medical services system.

11. Demonstrate proper procedures for transporting an injured individual.

12. Describe testing techniques used by medical specialists in diagnosing an injury.

ROLE DELINEATION COMPETENCIES

The following Performance Domains and Tasks defined in the National Athletic Trainers' Association Board of Certification *Role Delineation Study*, 5th Edition are addressed in this chapter:

BOC COMPETENCIES

I. Prevention

F. Maintain clinical and treatment areas by complying with safety and sanitation standards to minimize the risk of injury and illness.

II. Clinical Evaluation and Diagnosis

A. Obtain a history through observation, interview, and/or review of relevant records to assess current or potential injury, illness, or condition.
B. Inspect the involved area(s) visually to assess the injury, illness, or health-related condition.
C. Palpate the involved area(s) using standard techniques to assess the injury, illness, or health-related condition.
D. Perform specific tests in accordance with accepted procedures to assess the injury, illness, or health-related condition.
E. Formulate a clinical impression by interpreting the signs, symptoms, and predisposing factors of the injury, illness, or condition to determine the appropriate course of action.
F. Educate the appropriate individual(s) regarding the assessment by communicating information about the current or potential injury, illness, or health-related condition to encourage compliance with recommended care.
G. Share assessment findings with other health care professionals using effective means of communication to coordinate appropriate care.

III. Immediate Care

A. Employ life-saving techniques through the use of standard emergency procedures in order to reduce morbidity and the incidence of mortality.
B. Prevent exacerbation of non–life threatening condition(s) through the use of standard procedures in order to reduce morbidity.
C. Facilitate the timely transfer of care for conditions beyond the scope of practice of the athletic trainer by implementing appropriate referral strategies to stabilize and/or prevent exacerbation of the condition(s).
D. Direct the appropriate individual(s) in standard immediate care procedures using formal and informal methods to facilitate immediate care.
E. Execute the established emergency action plan using effective communication and administrative practices to facilitate efficient immediate care.

IV. Treatment, Rehabilitation, and Reconditioning

E. Reassess the status of injuries, illnesses, and/or conditions using standard techniques and documentation strategies in order to determine appropriate treatment, rehabilitation, and/or reconditioning and to evaluate readiness to return to a desired level of activity.

V. Organization and Administration

A. Establish action plans for response to injury or illness using available resources to provide the required range of health care services for individuals, athletic activities, and events.
B. Establish policies and procedures for the delivery of health care services following accepted guidelines to promote safe participation, timely care, and legal compliance.
C. Establish policies and procedures for the management of health care facilities and activity areas by referring to accepted guidelines, standards, and regulations to promote safety and legal compliance.
E. Maintain records using an appropriate system to document services rendered, provide for continuity of care, facilitate communication, and meet legal standards.
F. Develop professional relationships with appropriate individuals and entities by applying effective communication techniques to enhance the delivery of health care.

One of the major performance domains for the athletic trainer is clinical assessment and diagnosis. Using standardized clinical practices, the athletic trainer makes decisions relative to the nature and severity of an injury or illness. Because the injury assessment process involves searching for atypical or dysfunctional anatomy, physiology, or biomechanics, a strong understanding of both these areas and the appropriate execution of evaluation techniques is essential to accurate injury assessment. Poor assessment can have a devastating effect on proper treatment and development of appropriate rehabilitation protocols.

This chapter begins with a description of two popular methods of injury assessment—namely, the history of the injury, observation and inspection, palpation, and special tests (HOPS) injury assessment format and the subjective evaluation, objective evaluation, assessment, and plan (SOAP) note format. Information is then presented regarding the various components of the injury assessment process. Next, the principles for developing and implementing an emergency medical plan are discussed, and the components of an "on-site" emergency assessment are presented, with a list of conditions that warrant activation of the emergency medical plan. Details of transporting an injured person from the scene are followed by information concerning several tests and procedures used by medical specialists to diagnose an injury.

Basic first-aid techniques are not included in this book. Rather, the authors assume that students have already completed a basic athletic training or first-aid course and hold current certification in advanced first aid and emergency cardiac care.

THE INJURY EVALUATION PROCESS

Regardless of the type of injury assessment selected by a health care provider, documentation of information on a medical report must be consistent with accepted standards. Abbreviations often are used in writing medical reports. As such, an athletic trainer must have the ability to both write and interpret abbreviations for common medical terms. Apply your knowledge of medical terminology by interpreting the following physician note: Athlete complained of mod knee pain, H/O patella tendonitis, Px revealed, B swelling B AROM painful, Dx B patella tendonitis. NSAID and cryotherapy AOAP.

When evaluating any injury or condition, diagnostic signs and symptoms are obtained and interpreted to determine the type and extent of injury. A diagnostic **sign** is an objective, measurable, physical finding regarding an individual's condition. A sign is what the evaluator hears, feels, sees, or smells when assessing the patient. A **symptom** is information provided by the injured individual regarding his or her perception of the problem. Examples of these subjective feelings include blurred vision, ringing in the ears, fatigue, dizziness, nausea, headache, pain, weakness, and inability to move a body part. Obtaining information about symptoms can determine if the individual has an **acute injury,** resulting from a specific event (**macrotrauma**) leading to a sudden onset of symptoms, or a **chronic injury,** characterized by a slow, insidious onset of symptoms (**microtrauma**) that culminates in a painful inflammatory condition.

Before assessing any injury, the opposite, or noninjured, body part should be assessed. This preliminary step in the injury evaluation process helps to determine the relative dysfunction of the injured body part. If an injury occurs to one of the extremities, the results of individual tests performed on the noninjured body part can be compared with those for the injured body part. Differences can indicate the level and severity of injury. The baseline of information gathered on the noninjured body part also can be used as a reference point to determine when the injured body part has been rehabilitated and, as such, when to allow return to full participation in an activity. Under most circumstances, assessment of the noninjured body part should precede assessment of the injured body part. In some acute injuries, such as fractures or dislocations, assessment of the noninjured body part is not necessary.

The injury evaluation process must include several key components—namely, taking a history of the current condition, visually inspecting the area for noticeable abnormalities, physically palpating the region for abnormalities, and completing functional and stress tests. Although several evaluation models may be used, each follows a consistent, sequential order to ensure that an essential component is not omitted without sufficient reason to do so. Two popular evaluation methods are the HOPS format and the SOAP note format. Each has its advantages, but the SOAP note format is much more inclusive of the entire injury management process.

The HOPS Format

The HOPS format uses both subjective information (i.e., history of the injury) and objective information (i.e., observation and inspection, palpation, and special testing) to recognize and identify problems contributing to the condition. This format is easy to use and follows a basic, consistent format. The HOPS format focuses on the evaluation component of injury management and excludes the rehabilitation process.

The subjective evaluation (i.e., history of the injury) includes the primary complaint, mechanism of injury, characteristics of the symptoms, and related medical history. This information comes from the individual and reflects his or her attitude, mental condition, and perceived physical state.

The objective evaluation (i.e., observation and inspection, palpation, and special tests) provides appropriate, measurable documentation relative to the individual's condition. Measurable factors may include edema, ecchymosis, atrophy, range of motion (ROM), strength, joint instability, functional disability, motor and sensory function, and cardiovascular endurance. This information can be measured repeatedly to track progress from the initial evaluation through final clearance for discharge and return to participation in a sport or other physical activity. A detailed postural assessment and gait analysis also may be documented during the objective evaluation.

The SOAP Note Format

The SOAP note format provides a more detailed and advanced structure for decision making and problem solving in injury management. Used in many physical therapy clinics, sports medicine clinics, and athletic training facilities, these notes document patient care and serve as a vehicle of communication between the on-site clinicians and other health care professionals. These notes are intended to provide information concerning the ongoing status and tolerance of a patient and, in doing so, to avoid duplication of services by health care providers.

The subjective and objective evaluations are identical to those used in the HOPS format; however, two additional components are added to the documentation: assessment, and planning. It is common practice to use abbreviations throughout the notes.

> A listing of commonly used abbreviations is available on the companion website at thePoint.

Assessment

Following the objective evaluation, the examiner analyzes and assesses the individual's status and prognosis. Although a definitive diagnosis may not be known, the suspected site of injury, involved structures, and severity of injury are documented. Subsequently, both long-term and short-term goals are established. Long-term goals should reflect the anticipated status of the individual after a period of rehabilitation and might include pain-free ROM; bilateral strength, power, and muscular endurance; cardiovascular endurance; and return to full functional status. Short-term goals are developed to outline the expected progress within days of the initial injury and might include immediate protection of the injured area and control of inflammation, hemorrhage, muscle spasm, or pain. Short-term goals are updated with each progress note. Progress notes may be written daily, weekly, or biweekly to document progress.

> A sample progress report format is available on the companion website at thePoint.

Plan

The final section of the note lists the therapeutic modalities and exercises, educational consultations, and functional activities used to achieve the documented goals. The action plan should include the following information:

- The immediate treatment given to the injured individual

- The frequency and duration of treatments, therapeutic modalities, and exercises

- Evaluation standards to determine progress toward the goals

- Ongoing patient education

- Criteria for discharge

As the short-term goals are achieved and updated, periodic "in-house review" of the individual's records permits health care providers to evaluate joint ROM; flexibility; muscular strength, power, and endurance; balance or proprioception; and functional status. In addition, these reviews allow health care providers to discuss the continuity of documentation, efficacy of treatment, average time to discharge, and other parameters that may reflect quality of care. When it is determined that the individual can be discharged and cleared for participation, a discharge note should be written to close the file. All information included within the file is confidential and cannot be released to anyone without written approval from the patient.

In a clinical setting, SOAP notes are the sole means of documenting the services provided to the patient. All clinicians have an ethical responsibility to keep accurate and factual records. This information verifies specific services rendered and evaluates the progress of the patient as well as the efficacy of the treatment plan. Insurance companies use this information to determine if services are being appropriately rendered and qualify for reimbursement. More important, this comprehensive record-keeping system can minimize the ever-present threat of malpractice and litigation. In general, the primary error in writing SOAP notes is the error of omission, whereby clinicians fail to adequately document the nature and extent of care provided to the patient. Formal documentation and regular review of records can reduce this threat and minimize the likelihood that inappropriate or inadequate care is being rendered to a patient.

Each component of the subjective and objective assessments are described in detail in the following sections and are repeated throughout each chapter on the various body regions. A brief outline of the steps can be seen in Field Strategy 5.1.

(A) *The physician note states the following: The athlete complains of moderate knee pain and has a history of patella tendonitis. Physical examination reveals bilateral swelling and bilateral painful active range of motion. Diagnosis is bilateral patella tendonitis. Begin non-steroidal anti-inflammatory therapy, and apply cryotherapy as often as possible.*

HISTORY OF THE INJURY

(Q) *A female high school long jumper sustains an ankle injury during practice and immediately reports to the athletic training room. What questions should be asked to identify the cause and extent of this injury?*

Identifying the history of the injury can be the most important step of injury assessment. A complete history includes information regarding the primary complaint, cause or mechanism of the injury, characteristics of the symptoms, and any related medical history that may have a bearing on the specific condition. This information can provide potential reasons for the symptoms and identify injured structures before initiating the physical examination. An individual's medical history file can be an excellent resource for identifying past injuries, subsequent rehabilitation programs, and any factors that may predispose the individual to further injury. Specific to collegiate athletes, the National Collegiate Athletic Association (NCAA) has identified primary components that should be in an intercollegiate athlete's medical record and readily accessible to the athletic trainer (Box 5.1) (1).

History taking involves asking appropriate questions, but it also requires establishing a professional and comfortable atmosphere. When taking a history, the athletic trainer should present a competent manner, listen attentively, and maintain eye contact in an effort to establish rapport with the injured individual. Ideally, this encourages the individual to respond more accurately to questions and instructions.

Often, an unacknowledged obstacle to the evaluation process is the sociocultural dynamics that may exist between the patient and clinician that can hinder communication. It is important for all clinicians to understand and respect each cultural group's attitudes, beliefs, and values as related to health and illness. If English is a second language to the patient, it may be necessary to locate an interpreter. If an interpreter is used, it is important to speak to the client, not to the interpreter. It also may be necessary to speak slower, not louder, and to refrain from using slang terms or jargon. To ensure understanding, the patient should be asked to repeat the instructions.

FIELD STRATEGY 5.1

Injury Assessment Protocol

History of the Injury

1. Primary complaint
   - Current nature, location, and onset of the condition
2. Mechanism of injury
   - Cause of stress, position of limb, and direction of force
   - Changes in running surface, shoes, equipment, techniques, or conditioning modes
3. Characteristics of the symptoms
   - Presence of unusual sensation (i.e., pain, sounds, and feelings)
   - Evolution of the onset, nature, location, severity, and duration of symptoms
4. Disability resulting from the injury
   - Immediate limitations
   - Limitations in occupation and activities of daily living
5. Related medical history
   - Past musculoskeletal injuries, congenital abnormalities, family history, childhood diseases, allergies, or cardiac, respiratory, vascular, or neurologic problems

Observation and Inspection

1. Observation involves analysis of:
   - Overall appearance
   - Body symmetry
   - General motor function
   - Posture and gait
2. Inspection involves observing the injury site for:
   - Deformity, swelling, discoloration, scars, and general skin condition

Palpation

1. Bony structures
   - Determine a possible fracture first
2. Soft-tissue structures:
   - Skin temperature, swelling, point tenderness, crepitus, deformity, muscle spasm, cutaneous sensation, and pulse

Functional Tests

1. Active movement   2. Passive movement and end feel   3. Resisted manual muscle testing

Stress Tests

1. Ligamentous instability tests

Special Tests

Neurologic Tests

1. Dermatomes   2. Myotomes   3. Reflexes   4. Peripheral nerve testing

Activity/Sport-Specific Functional Testing

1. Proprioception and motor coordination

Activity/Sport-Specific Skill Performance

Box 5.1 National Collegiate Athletic Association (NCAA) Guideline 1b: Medical Evaluations, Immunizations, and Records

The following primary components should be included in the athlete's medical record:

1. History of injuries, illnesses, new medications or allergies, pregnancies, and operations, whether sustained during the competitive season or off-season

2. Referrals for and feedback from consultation, treatment, or rehabilitation with subsequent care and clearances

3. Comprehensive entry-year health-status questionnaires and an updated health-status questionnaire each year thereafter, including information on:
   - Illnesses suffered (acute and chronic); athletic and nonathletic hospitalization
   - Surgery
   - Allergies, including hypersensitivity to drugs, foods, and insect bites/stings
   - Medications taken on a regular basis
   - Conditioning status
   - Musculoskeletal injuries (previous and current)
   - Cerebral concussions or episodes involving loss of consciousness
   - Syncope or near-syncope with exercise
   - Exercise-induced asthma or bronchospasm
   - Loss of paired organs
   - Heat-related illness
   - Cardiac conditions and family history of cardiac disease, including sudden death in a family member younger than 50 years and Marfan's syndrome
   - Menstrual history
   - Exposure to tuberculosis

4. Immunization records, including:
   - Measles, mumps, rubella (MMR)
   - Hepatitis B
   - Diphtheria, tetanus, and boosters when appropriate
   - Meningitis

5. Written permission signed by the student-athlete, or by the parent if the athlete is younger than 18 years, that authorizes the release of medical information to others, specifically what information may be released and to whom.

Adapted from Klossner D, ed. NCAA Sports Medicine Handbook: 2005–06. Indianapolis: National Collegiate Athletic Association, 2005; with permission.

When communicating with older clients, a skilled interviewer must consider other issues that may impact the effectiveness of history taking. The client's education and socioeconomic status may affect his or her vocabulary, self-expression, ability to comprehend, and ability to conceptualize questions asked by the interviewer (2). Elderly individuals tend to view the world concretely, think in absolute terms, and may be confused by complicated questions. These individuals also may present with some anxiety if they perceive that the examiner is dismissing the magnitude of their complaints or becoming impatient with the length of time that patients take to answer a question. In addition, patients who may have a hearing loss might feel uncomfortable asking the interviewer to repeat information (2). A skilled examiner takes note of the patient's comfort level by recognizing not only verbal expression but also any emotion behind the expression, such as hidden fears, beliefs, or expectations. Patience, respect, rapport, structure, and reflecting on important information are all useful in conducting a comprehensive medical history.

The history begins by gathering general information, such as the individual's name, sex, age, date of birth, occupation, and activity in which the individual was participating when the injury occurred. Notes regarding body size, body type, and general physical condition also are appropriate.

Although information provided by the individual is subjective, it should still be gathered and recorded as quantitatively as possible. This can be accomplished by recording a number correlating with the described symptoms. For example, the individual can rate the severity of pain using a scale from 1 to 10. The patient also can be asked to quantify the length of time the pain lasts. In using such measures, the progress of the injury can be determined. If the individual reports that pain begins immediately after activity and lasts for 3 or 4 hours, a baseline of information has been established. As the individual undergoes treatment and rehabilitation for the injury, a comparison with the baseline information can determine if the condition is getting better, worse, or remains the same.

Although the intent of taking a history is to narrow the possibilities of conditions causing the injury, the history should always be taken with an open mind. If too few factors are considered, the athletic trainer may reach premature conclusions and fail to adequately address the severity of the injury. It is essential to document in writing the information obtained during the history.

Primary Complaint

The primary complaint focuses on the injured individual's perception of the current injury. Questions should be phrased to allow the individual to describe the current nature, location, and onset of the condition. The following questions could be asked:

- What is the problem?

- What hurts?

- When did the injury occur?

- What activities or motions are weak or painful?

It is important to realize that the individual may not wish to carry on a lengthy discussion about the injury or may trivialize the extent of pain or disability. The examiner must be patient and keep the questions simple and open-ended. It is advantageous to pay close attention to words and gestures used by the patient to describe the condition, because these may provide clues to the quality and intensity of the symptoms.

Mechanism of Injury

After identifying the primary complaint, the next step is to determine the mechanism of injury. This is probably the most important information gained in the history. For an acute injury, questions that might be asked include:

- How did the injury occur? What did you do? How did you do it?

- Did you fall? If so, how did you land?

- Were you struck by an object or another individual? If so, in what position was the involved body part, and in what direction was the force?

For a chronic nature, potential questions include:

- How long has the injury been a problem?

- Do you remember a specific incident that initiated or provoked the current problem?

- Have there been recent changes in running surface, shoes, equipment, techniques, or conditioning modes?

- What activities make the condition feel better? What activities make the condition feel worse?

It is important to visualize the manner in which the injury occurred as a way to identify possible injured structures. The information obtained pertaining to the mechanism of injury directs the objective evaluation.

Characteristics of the Symptoms

The primary complaint must be explored in detail to discover the evolution of symptoms, including the location, onset, severity, frequency, duration, and limitations caused by the pain or disability. The individual's pain perception can indicate which structures may be injured. There are two categories of pain: somatic, and visceral.

Somatic pain arises from the skin, ligaments, muscles, bones, and joints and is the most common type of pain encountered in musculoskeletal injuries. It is classified into two major types: deep, and superficial. Deep somatic pain is described as diffuse or nagging, as if intense pressure is being exerted on the structures, and may be complicated by stabbing pain. Deep somatic pain is longer lasting and usually indicates significant tissue damage to bone, internal joint structures, or muscles. Superficial somatic pain results from injury to the epidermis or dermis and usually is a sharp, prickly type of pain that tends to be brief.

Visceral pain results from disease or injury to an organ in the thoracic or abdominal cavity, such as compression, tension, or distention of the viscera. Similar to deep somatic pain, it is perceived as deeply located, nagging, and pressing, and it often is accompanied by nausea and vomiting. **Referred pain** is a type of visceral pain that travels along the same nerve pathways as somatic pain. It is perceived by the brain as being somatic in origin. In other words, the injury is in one region, but the brain considers it in another. For example, referred pain occurs when an individual has a heart attack and feels pain in the chest, left arm, and sometimes, the neck. Figure 5.1 illustrates cutaneous areas where pain from visceral organs can be referred.

Pain can travel up or down the length of any nerve and be referred to another region. An individual with a low back problem may feel the pain down the gluteal region and into the back of the leg. If a nerve is injured, pain or a change in sensation, such as a numbing or burning sensation, can be felt along the length of the nerve.

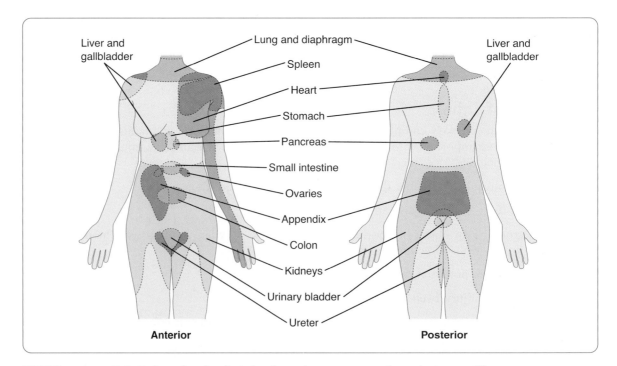

FIGURE 5.1 Referred pain. Certain visceral organs can refer pain to specific cutaneous areas. If all special tests are negative yet the individual continues to feel pain at a specific site, it may be referred pain.

In assessing the injury, the examiner should ask detailed questions about the location, onset, nature, severity, frequency, and duration of the pain. For example, the following questions should be asked:

- Where is the pain?

- Can you point to a specific painful spot?

- Is the pain limited to that area, or does it radiate into other parts of the leg or foot?

- How bad is the pain on a scale from 1 to 10, with 10 being most severe?

- Can you describe the pain (e.g., dull, sharp, or aching)?

In chronic conditions, the following questions should be asked:

- When does the pain begin (e.g., when you get out of bed, while sitting, while walking, during exercise, or at night)?

- How long does the pain last?

- Is the pain worse before, during, or after activity?

- What activities aggravate or alleviate the symptoms?

- Does the pain wake you up at night?

- How long has the condition been present?

- Has the pain changed or stayed the same?

- In the past, what medications, treatments, or exercise programs have improved the situation?

If pain is localized, it suggests that limited bony or soft-tissue structures may be involved. Diffuse pain around the entire joint may indicate inflammation of the joint capsule or injury to several structures. If pain radiates into other areas of the limb or body, it may be traveling up or down the length of a nerve. These responses also can determine if the condition is disabling enough to require referral to a physician. Table 5.1 provides more detailed information regarding pain characteristics and probable causes.

TABLE 5.1 Pain Characteristics and Possible Causes

CHARACTERISTICS	POSSIBLE CAUSES
Morning pain with stiffness that improves with activity	Chronic inflammation with edema, or arthritis
Pain increasing as the day progresses	Increased congestion in a joint
Sharp, stabbing pain during activity	Acute injury, such as ligament sprain or muscular strain
Dull, aching pain aggravated by muscle contraction	Chronic muscular strain
Pain that subsides during activity	Chronic condition or inflammation
Pain on activity relieved by rest	Soft-tissue damage
Pain not affected by rest or activity	Injury to bone
Night pain	Compression of a nerve or bursa
Dull, aching, and hard to localize; aggravated by passive stretching of the muscle and resisted muscle contractions	Muscular pain
Deeply located, nagging, and very localized	Bone pain
Sharp, burning, or numbing sensation that may run the length of the nerve	Nerve pain
Aching over a large area that may be referred to another area of the body	Vascular pain

In assessing the primary complaint of an acute injury, it also is important to determine if the individual experienced other unusual sensations at the time of injury. Specifically, the following questions should be asked:

- Did you hear anything?
- Did you feel anything?

The report of particular sounds and feelings at the time of injury can provide valuable input regarding the type of injury and the structures involved. Hearing a "pop" is characteristic of a rupture to a ligament or tendon, and hearing a snapping or cracking sound may suggest a fracture. Unusual feelings can be presented in a variety of ways. For example, having sustained a tear to the anterior cruciate ligament, an individual may report a feeling of the knee giving way. Following a rupture of the Achilles tendon, an individual may report a feeling of being shot or kicked in the lower leg.

Disability Resulting from the Injury

The examiner should attempt to determine the limitations experienced by the individual because of pain, weakness, or disability from the injury. Questions should not be limited to sport and physical activity but, rather, should determine if the injury has affected the individual's job, school, or daily activities. **Activities of daily living** are actions that most people perform without thinking, such as combing hair, brushing teeth, and walking up or down stairs.

Related Medical History

Information should be obtained regarding other problems or conditions that might have affected the current injury. If a preparticipation examination was conducted, it can be used to verify past childhood diseases; allergies; cardiac, respiratory, vascular, musculoskeletal, or neurologic problems; use of contact lenses, dentures, or prosthetic devices; and past episodes of infectious diseases, loss of consciousness, recurrent headaches, heat stroke, seizures, eating disorders, or chronic medical problems. Previous musculoskeletal injuries or congenital abnormalities may place additional stress on joints and predispose the individual to certain injuries. In some situations, it may be appropriate to ask if the individual is taking any medication. The type, frequency, dosage, and effect of a medication may mask some injury symptoms.

A *In attempting to determine the cause and extent of injury, the female long jumper should be asked questions pertaining to the following: primary complaint (i.e., what, when, and how questions), mechanism of injury (i.e., position of the ankle at the time of injury and the direction of force), characteristics of symptoms (i.e., nature, location, severity, and disability), unusual sensation (i.e., sounds and feelings), related medical history, and past injuries/treatment.*

OBSERVATION AND INSPECTION

Q *A detailed history of the injury has been gathered from the long jumper. The information suggests an inversion sprain of her right ankle. In the continued assessment of this individual, observation and inspection should be performed. What observable factors might indicate the seriousness of injury?*

The objective evaluation during an injury assessment begins with observation and inspection. Although explained as a separate step, observation begins the moment the injured person is seen, and it continues throughout the assessment. **Observation** refers to the visual analysis of overall appearance, symmetry, general motor function, posture, and gait. **Inspection** refers to factors seen at the actual injury site, such as swelling, redness, ecchymosis, cuts, or scars.

Observation

Occasionally, the athletic trainer observes an individual sustain an injury. In many instances, however, the individual comes to the sideline, office, athletic training room, or clinic complaining of pain or discomfort. The athletic trainer should immediately assess the individual's state of consciousness and body language, which may indicate pain, disability, fracture, dislocation, or other conditions. It also is important to note the individual's general posture, willingness and ability to move, ease of motion, and overall attitude.

General observations may focus on the patient's estimated age, physical condition, and personal hygiene. Potential questions to address in the observation include:

- Does the individual appear to be healthy?

- Is the individual's weight appropriate for height, or is the individual underweight or overweight? Is the individual's weight appropriate for the type and level of sport/physical activity participation? Could this be a contributing factor in their injury?

- Is the individual's speech slurred, hoarse, loud, soft, incoherent, slow, fast, or hesitant?

- Is the individual hearing impaired? Is the individual's hearing better through one ear?

- Is the individual oriented to the surroundings or disoriented and unaware of time or place?

- Does the individual seem to be hesitant or avoid eye contact?

By observing these factors, the skilled clinician can more accurately document the patient's characteristics both quickly and accurately (3).

Symmetry and Appearance

The body should be scanned visually to detect **congenital** (i.e., existing at birth) or functional problems that may be a contributing factor. This includes observing any abnormalities in the spinal curves, general symmetry of the various body parts, and general posture of the body from anterior, lateral, and posterior views.

If it is not **contraindicated**, the examiner should observe the normal swing of the individual's arms and legs during walking. By standing behind, in front, and to the side of the individual, observation from all angles is permitted. A shoulder injury may be evident in a limited arm swing or by holding the arm close to the body in a splinted position. A lower extremity injury may produce a noticeable limp, or **antalgic gait**. Running on a treadmill can show functional problems that may have contributed to a lower extremity injury.

> *Field Strategy: Postural Assessment,* a detailed outline of what to look for during this assessment, is available on the companion website at thePoint.

Motor Function

Many clinicians begin observation using a scan examination to assess general motor function. This examination rules out injury at other joints that may be overlooked because of intense pain or discomfort at the primary site of injury. In addition, pain in one area can be referred from another area. Observe the injured person performing gross motor movements of the neck, trunk, and extremities by asking the individual to:

- Extend, flex, laterally flex, and rotate the neck

- Bend forward to touch the toes

- Stand and rotate the trunk to the right and left

- Bring the palms together above the head and then behind the back

- Perform straight leg raises in hip flexion, extension, and abduction

- Flex the knees

- Walk on the heels and toes

Any hesitation by the patient to move a body part or favoring one side over the other should be noted.

Inspection of the Injury Site

Using discretion in safeguarding the person's privacy, the injured area should be fully exposed. This may require the removal of protective equipment and clothing.

The localized injury site should be inspected for any deformity, swelling (i.e., edema or joint effusion), discoloration (e.g., redness, pallor, or ecchymosis), signs of infection (i.e., redness, swelling, pus, red streaks, or swollen **lymph nodes**), scars that might indicate previous surgery, and general skin condition (e.g., oily, dry, blotchy with red spots, sores, or hives). Swelling inside the joint is called localized intra-articular swelling, or joint **effusion**, and this swelling makes the joint appear enlarged, red, and puffy. The amount of swelling should be measured in a quantifiable manner using girth measurements (Field Strategy 5.2). **Ecchymosis** is superficial discoloration of tissue indicative of injury. **Keloids**, which are scars that form at a wound but grow beyond its boundaries, may indicate previous injury. This condition is more common in individuals with dark skin, and it is particularly important to note if surgery may be indicated.

The injured area should be compared to the opposite side if possible. This bilateral comparison helps to establish normal parameters for the individual.

  Observable factors relative to the injured sight that might indicate the seriousness of the injury sustained by the female long jumper include deformity, swelling, discoloration, and signs of previous injury. It is important to perform a bilateral inspection of the injury site as well

FIELD STRATEGY 5.2

Taking Girth Measurements

1. Identify the joint line using prominent bony landmarks. The individual should be non–weight bearing.
2. Using a marked tongue depressor or tape measure, make incremental marks (e.g., 2, 4, and 6 inches) from the joint line. (Do not use a cloth tape measure, because they tend to stretch.)
3. Encircle the body part with the measuring tape, making sure not to fold or twist the tape (Fig. A). If measuring ankle girth, use a figure eight tech-

nique by positioning the tape across the malleoli proximally and around the navicular and base of the fifth metatarsal distally (Fig. B).
4. Take three measurements, and record the average.
5. Repeat these steps for the noninjured body part, and record all findings.
6. Increased girth at the joint line indicates joint swelling. Increased girth over a muscle mass indicates hypertrophy; decreased girth indicates atrophy.

Figure A

Figure B

as of the surrounding area. In addition, observation of general presentation, including the presence of guarding or antalgic gait, will provide important information concerning the nature of the injury.

PALPATION

Q *Inspection of the long jumper's injury revealed mild swelling on the anterolateral aspect of the ankle. Otherwise, no abnormal findings were evident. Observation of the athlete, however, suggests guarding and hesitation to walk. Based on the information provided concerning the long jumper's condition, explain palpation to determine the extent and severity of the injury.*

Informed consent must be granted before making physical contact with a patient. If the patient is younger than 18 years, permission must be granted by the parent or guardian. In some cultures and religions, the act of physically touching an exposed body part may present certain moral and ethical issues. Likewise, some patients may feel uncomfortable being touched by a health care provider of the opposite gender. If a same-gender clinician is not available, the evaluation should be observed by a third party (e.g., another clinician, parent, or guardian).

Bilateral palpation of paired anatomic structures can detect eight physical findings:

1. Temperature
2. Swelling
3. Point tenderness
4. Crepitus
5. Deformity
6. Muscle spasm
7. Cutaneous sensation
8. Pulse

The examiner should have clean, warm hands. Latex examination gloves should be worn as a precaution against disease and infection. Palpation should begin with gentle, circular pressure, followed by gradual, deeper pressure, and it should be initiated on structures away from the site of injury and progress toward the injured area. Palpating the most painful area last avoids any carryover of pain into noninjured areas.

Skin temperature should be noted when the fingers first touch the skin. Increased temperature at the injury site could indicate inflammation or infection, whereas decreased temperature could indicate a reduction in circulation.

The presence of localized or diffuse swelling can be determined through palpation of the injured area. In addition, palpation should assess differences in the density or "feel" of soft tissues that may indicate muscle spasm, hemorrhage, scarring, myositis ossificans, or other conditions.

Point tenderness and crepitus may indicate inflammation when felt over a tendon, bursa, or joint capsule. It is important to note any trigger points that may be found in muscle and, when palpated, refer pain to another site.

Palpation of the bones and bony landmarks can determine the possibility of fractures, crepitus, or loose bony or cartilaginous fragments. Possible fractures can be assessed with percussion, vibrations through use of a tuning fork, compression, and distraction (Fig. 5.2). The region should be immobilized if test results indicate a possible fracture.

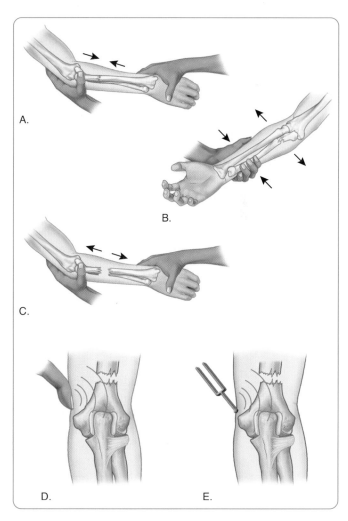

■■■ ■ FIGURE 5.2 **Determining a possible fracture.**
A, Compression (axial and circular). **B,** Distraction.
C, Percussion. **D** and **E,** Vibration.

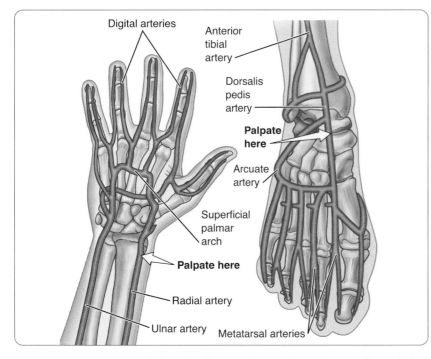

Digital arteries

Anterior tibial artery

Dorsalis pedis artery

Palpate here

Arcuate artery

Superficial palmar arch

Palpate here

Radial artery

Ulnar artery   Metatarsal arteries

■■ ■■ FIGURE 5.3 **Peripheral pulses.** Pulse can be taken at the radial pulse in the wrist (**A**) or the dorsalis pedis on the dorsum of the foot (**B**).

Cutaneous sensation can be tested by running the fingers along both sides of the body part and asking the patient if it feels the same on both sides. This technique can determine possible nerve involvement, particularly if the individual has numbness or tingling in the limb.

Peripheral pulses should be taken distal to an injury to rule out damage to a major artery. Common sites are the radial pulse at the wrist and the dorsalis pedis pulse on the dorsum of the foot (Fig. 5.3).

Palpation of bony and soft-tissue structures will provide information pertaining to several physical findings, including temperature, swelling, point tenderness, crepitus, deformity, muscle spasm, cutaneous sensation, and pulse. In the case of the long jumper, it is important to perform a bilateral palpation of key anatomic structures of the foot, ankle, and lower leg.

PHYSICAL EXAMINATION TESTS

The palpation component of the assessment of the long jumper confirms the presence of swelling over the anterolateral aspect of the ankle. It also reveals point tenderness in the area of the anterior talofibular ligament. Otherwise, no abnormal findings were present. How should testing proceed to determine the integrity of the soft-tissue structures and the extent and severity of injury?

Once fractures and/or dislocations have been ruled out, soft-tissue structures, such as muscles, ligaments, the joint capsule, and bursae, are assessed using a variety of tests. This examination includes functional tests (i.e., active, passive, and resisted ROM), stress tests, special tests, neurologic testing, and sport- or activity-specific functional testing. General principles regarding physical examination are discussed in this chapter; more extensive explanations are provided in the individual joint chapters.

Functional Tests

Functional tests identify the patient's ability to move a body part through the ROM actively, passively, and against resistance. As with all tests, the noninjured side should be evaluated first to establish **normative data**. All motions common to each joint should be tested. Occasionally, it also may be necessary to test the joints proximal and distal to the injury to rule out any referred pain. The available active and passive ROM can be measured objectively using a **goniometer** (Fig. 5.4). The goniometer is a protractor with two rigid arms that intersect at a hinge joint. It is used to measure both joint position and available joint motion, and it can determine when the individual has regained normal motion at a joint.

The arms of the goniometer measure 0° to 180° of motion, or 0° to 360° of motion. Measurements are obtained by placing the goniometer's stationary arm parallel to the proximal bone. The axis of the goniometer should coincide with the joint axis of motion. The goniometer's moving arm is then placed parallel to the distal bone using specific anatomic landmarks as points of reference.

The normal ROM for selected joints is listed in Table 5.2 and in the individual joint chapters. Age and gender may influence ROM. Women in their teens and early twenties tend to have a greater ROM in all planes compared with men. Range of motion decreases after 20 years in both genders, with the decrease occurring to a greater extent in women.

Active Range of Motion

Active range of motion (AROM) is joint motion performed voluntarily by the individual through muscular contraction. Unless contraindicated, AROM should always be performed before **passive range of motion (PROM)**. The AROM indicates the individual's willingness and ability to move the injured body part. Active movement determines possible damage to contractile tissue (i.e., muscle, muscle–tendon junction, tendon, and tendon–periosteal union) and measures muscle strength and movement coordination.

Measurement of all motions, except rotation, starts with the body in anatomic position. For rotation, the starting body position is midway between internal (medial) and external (lateral) rotation. The starting position is measured as 0°. The maximal movement away from the 0° point is the total available ROM. For example, subjective measurement of plantar flexion against gravity involves placing the individual prone on a table with the knees flexed. Next, both thighs are stabilized against the table, and the individual is instructed to plantar flex both ankles. Comparison of movement in both legs indicates if plantar flexion is equal bilaterally.

FIGURE 5.4 Goniometry measurement at the elbow. In anatomic position, the elbow is flexed. The goniometer axis is placed over the lateral epicondyle of the humerus. To accommodate using a goniometer that ranges from 0° to 180°, the stationary arm is held parallel to the longitudinal axis of the radius, pointing toward the styloid process of the radius. The moving arm is held parallel to the longitudinal axis of the humerus, pointing toward the tip of the acromion process. Range of motion is measured at the site where the pointer intersects the scale.

It is important to assess the individual's willingness to perform a movement, the fluidity of movement, and the extent of movement (joint ROM). If symptoms are present, their location in the arc of movement should be noted. Any increase in intensity or quality of symptoms also should be noted. Limitation in motion may result from pain, swelling, muscle spasm, muscle tightness, joint contractures, nerve damage, or mechanical blocks, such as a loose body. If the individual has pain or other symptoms with movement, it can be difficult to determine if the joint, muscle, or both are injured. It is important to assess the following:

- The point during the motion at which pain begins
- The presence of pain in a limited ROM (i.e., painful arc)
- The type of pain and if it is associated with the primary complaint

Anticipated painful movements should be performed last to avoid any carryover of pain from testing one motion to the next.

Passive Range of Motion

If the individual is unable to perform active movements at the injured joint because of pain or spasm, passive movement can be performed. In **passive movement**, the injured limb or body part is moved through the ROM with no assistance from the injured individual (Fig. 5.5). As PROM is performed, the individual should be positioned to allow the muscles to be in a relaxed state. The PROM distinguishes injury to contractile tissues from injury to noncontractile or inert tissues (i.e., bone, ligament, bursae, joint capsule, fascia, dura mater, and nerve roots). If no pain is present during passive motion but is present during active motion, injury to contractile tissue is involved. If noncontractile tissue is injured, passive movement is painful and limitation of movement may be

TABLE 5.2 Normal Ranges of Motion at Selected Joints (No Changes)

JOINT	MOTION	RANGE OF MOTION	JOINT	MOTION	RANGE OF MOTION
Cervical	Flexion	0–80°	Digits 2–5		
	Extension	0–70°	MCP	Flexion	0–90°
	Lateral flexion	0–45°		Extension	0–45°
	Rotation	0–80°		Abduction	0–20°
Lumbar	Forward flexion	0–60°	PIP	Flexion	0–100°
	Extension	0–35°	DIP	Flexion	0–90°
	Lateral flexion	0–20°	Hip	Flexion	0–120
	Rotation	0–50°		Extension	0–30°
Shoulder	Flexion	0–180°		Abduction	0–40°
	Extension	0–60°		Adduction	0–30°
	Abduction	0–180°		Internal rotation	0–40°
	Internal rotation	0–70°		External rotation	0–50°
	External rotation	0–90°	Knee	Flexion	0–135°
	Horizontal abduction/ adduction	0–130°		Extension	0–15°
Elbow	Flexion	0–150°		Medial rotation with knee flexed	0–25°
	Extension	0–10°		Lateral rotation with knee flexed	0–35°
Forearm	Pronation	0–80°	Ankle	Dorsiflexion	0–20°
	Supination	0–80°		Plantar flexion	0–50°
Wrist	Flexion	0–80°		Pronation	0–30°
	Extension	0–70°		Supination	0–50°
	Ulnar deviation	0–30°	Subtalar	Inversion	0–5°
	Radial deviation	0–20°		Eversion	0–5°
Thumb			Toes		
CMC	Abduction	0–70°	1st MTP	Flexion	0–45°
	Flexion	0–15°		Extension	0–75°
	Extension	0–20°	1st IP	Flexion	0–90°
	Opposition	Tip of thumb to tip of 5th finger	2nd to 5th MTP	Flexion	0–40°
MCP	Flexion	0–50°		Extension	0–40°
IP	Flexion	0–80°	PIP	Flexion	0–35°
			DIP	Flexion	0–30°
				Extension	0–60°

CMC, carpometacarpal; DIP, distal interphalangeal; IP, interphalangeal; MCP, metacarpophalangeal; MTP, metatarsophalangeal; PIP, posterior interphalangeal.

■■■■ FIGURE 5.5 **Passive movement.** The body part is moved through the range of motion with no assistance from the injured individual. Any limitation of movement or presence of pain is documented. **A,** Starting position. **B,** End position.

present. Again, any potentially painful motions should be performed last to avoid any carryover of pain from one motion to the next.

A gentle overpressure should be applied at the end of the ROM to determine **end feel.** Overpressure is repeated several times to determine whether an increase in pain occurs, which could signify damage to noncontractile joint structures. The end feel can determine the type of disorder. Three normal end feel sensations (i.e., soft, firm, and hard) and four abnormal end feel sensations (i.e., soft, firm, hard, and empty) exist (Table 5.3).

Differences in ROM between active and passive movements can result from muscle spasm, muscle deficiency, neurologic deficit, contractures, or pain. If pain occurs before the end of the available ROM, it may indicate an acute injury. Stretching and manipulation of the joint are contraindicated. If pain occurs simultaneously at the end of the ROM, a subacute injury may be present, and a mild stretching program may be started cautiously. If no pain is felt as the available ROM is stretched, a chronic injury is present. An appropriate treatment and rehabilitation program should be initiated immediately.

Accessory movements are movements within the joint that accompany traditional active and PROM but cannot be performed voluntarily by the individual. Joint play motions occur within the joint, but only as a response to an outside force and not as a result of any voluntary movement. Joint play motions allow the joint capsule to "give" so that bones can move to absorb an external force. These movements include distraction, sliding, compression, rolling, and spinning of joint surfaces. Joint play movements aid the healing process, relieve pain, reduce disability, and restore full normal ROM. If joint play movement is absent or decreased, this movement must be restored before functional voluntary movement can be accomplished fully (5).

The presence of accessory movement can be determined by manipulating the joint in a position of least strain, called the **loose packed** or **resting position.** The resting position is the position in the ROM in which the joint is under the least amount of stress. It also is the position in which the joint capsule has its greatest capacity. The advantage of testing accessory movements in the loose packed position is that the joint surface contact areas are reduced, proper joint lubrication is enhanced, and friction and erosion in the joints are decreased.

See *Loose Packed Positions of Selected Joints* on the companion website at thePoint.

In contrast, a **close packed position** is the position in which two joint surfaces fit precisely together. In this position, the ligaments and joint capsule are maximally taut. The joint surfaces are maximally compressed and cannot be separated by distractive forces, nor can accessory movements occur. Therefore, if a bone or ligament is injured, pain increases as the joint moves into the close packed position. If swelling is present within the joint, the close packed position cannot be achieved.

See *Closed Packed Positions of Selected Joints* on the companion website at thePoint.

TABLE 5.3 Normal and Abnormal Joint End Feels

END FEEL	STRUCTURE	EXAMPLE
Normal End Feel Sensations		
Soft	Soft-tissue approximation	Elbow flexion (contact between soft tissue of the forearm and anterior arm)
Firm	Muscular stretch	Hip extension (passive stretch of iliopsoas muscle)
	Capsular stretch	External rotation at the shoulder (passive stretch of anterior glenohumeral joint capsule)
	Ligamentous stretch	Forearm supination (tension in the palmar radioulnar ligament of the inferior radioulnar joint, interosseous membrane, oblique cord)
Hard	Bone to bone	Elbow extension (contact between olecranon process and olecranon fossa)
Abnormal End Feel Sensations		
Soft	Occurs sooner or later in the ROM than is usual or in a joint that normally has a firm or hard end feel; feels boggy	Soft-tissue edema Synovitis Ligamentous stretch or tear
Firm	Occurs sooner or later in the ROM than is usual, or in a joint that normally has a soft or hard end feel	Increased muscular tonus Capsular, muscular, ligamentous shortening
Hard	Occurs sooner or later in the ROM than is usual, or in a joint that normally has a soft or firm end feel; a bony grating or bony block is felt	Chondromalacia Osteoarthritis Loose bodies in joint Myositis ossificans Fracture
Empty	No end feel, because the end of the ROM is never reached because of pain; no resistance is felt except for the patient's protective muscle splinting or muscle spasm	Acute joint inflammation Bursitis Fracture Psychogenic in origin

ROM, range of motion.

Resisted Manual Muscle Testing

Resisted manual muscle testing can assess muscle strength and detect injury to the nervous system. Resistance testing is performed by applying an overload pressure in a stationary or static position (sometimes referred to as a **break test**) or throughout the full ROM. Muscle weakness and pain indicate a muscle strain. Muscle weakness in the absence of pain may indicate nerve damage.

In performing a break test, overload pressure is applied with the joint in a neutral position to relax joint structures and reduce joint stress. The muscles are more effectively stressed in this position. When performing a break test, the limb is stabilized proximal to the joint to prevent other motions from compensating for weakness in the involved muscle. Resistance is provided distally on the bone to which the muscle or muscle group attaches; resistance should not be distal to a second joint. In a fixed position, the individual is asked to elicit a maximal contraction while the body part is stabilized to prevent little or no joint movement. For example, when testing the strength of the elbow flexors, the patient's elbow should be positioned at 90°, with the upper arm stabilized against

TABLE 5.4 Grading System for Manual Muscle Testing

NUMERIC	VERBAL	CLINICAL FINDINGS
5	Normal	Complete ROM against gravity with maximal overload
4	Good	Complete ROM against gravity with moderate overload
3+	Fair +	Complete ROM against gravity with minimal overload
3	Fair	Complete ROM against gravity with no overload
3−	Fair −	Some, but not complete, ROM against gravity
2+	Poor +	Initiates motion against gravity
2	Poor	Complete ROM with some assistance and gravity eliminated
2−	Poor −	Initiates motion if gravity is eliminated
1	Trace	Evidence of slight muscular contraction; no joint motion
0	Zero	No muscle contraction palpated

ROM, range of motion.

the body. While the patient maintains the arm in that position, the examiner applies downward overpressure on the distal forearm (Fig. 5.6). Pressure should be held for at least 5 seconds and be repeated five or six times to indicate muscle weakening and the presence or absence of pain. A standardized grading system can be used to measure muscle contraction, but the results are negated if the contraction causes pain (Table 5.4).

Testing resistance throughout the full ROM offers two advantages: First, a better overall assessment of weakness can be determined, and second, a **painful arc** of motion can be located which might otherwise go undetected if the test is only performed in the midrange. When performing resisted testing, the body segment is placed in a specific position to isolate the muscle or muscle group. The muscle or muscle group to be tested is placed in a stretched or elongated position. This position prevents other muscles in the area from performing the movement. Manual pressure is exerted throughout the full ROM and is repeated several times to reveal weakness or pain. The presence of pain during motion should be noted. In this manner, both subjective information (i.e., what the individual feels) and objective information (i.e., weakness) are gathered.

Stress Tests

Each body segment has a series of tests to assess joint function and integrity of joint structures. These tests assess the integrity of noncontractile tissues (e.g., ligaments, intra-articular structures, and joint capsule). Stress tests occur in a single plane and are graded according to severity. Specifically, sprains of ligamentous tissue generally are graded on a three-degree scale after a specific stress is applied to a ligament to test its laxity (Table 5.5). **Laxity** describes the amount of "give" within a joint's supportive tissue. **Instability** refers to a joint's inability to function under the stresses encountered during functional activities.

Ligamentous testing should be done bilaterally and compared with baseline measures. It is essential to perform a test at the proper angle, because a seemingly minor change in the joint angle can significantly alter the laxity of the tissue being stressed. In some instances, it may be appropriate to perform ligamentous stress testing before any other testing. During a stress test, it is important that the patient be able to relax the involved area, because muscle guarding could interfere with the

■■■ ■ FIGURE 5.6 **Resisted manual muscle testing in a static position.** The arm is stabilized against the body. The individual is asked to prevent any movement while downward pressure is applied on the distal forearm.

TABLE 5.5 Grading System for Ligamentous Laxity

GRADE	LIGAMENTOUS END FEEL	DAMAGE
I	Firm (normal)	Slight stretching of the ligament with little or no tearing of the fibers. Pain is present, but the degree of stability roughly compares with that of the opposite extremity.
II	Soft	Partial tearing of the fibers. The joint line "opens up" significantly when compared with the opposite side.
III	Empty	Complete tearing of the ligament. The motion is restricted by other joint structures, such as tendons.

effectiveness of testing. If functional testing causes pain, the patient may find it more difficult to maintain a relaxed position. As such, if a ligamentous injury is suspected, initiating testing with stress tests may be advantageous.

Figure 5.7 demonstrates a **valgus** stress test on the elbow joint to assess the integrity of the joint medial collateral ligaments. During an on-site assessment, tests to determine a possible fracture and major ligament damage at a joint should always be performed before moving an individual who is injured. Only the specific tests deemed to be necessary for the specific injury should be used. Because of the wide variety of stress tests, each is discussed within subsequent chapters.

Special Tests

Special tests have been developed for specific body parts or areas as a means of detecting injury or related pathology. In general, special tests occur across planes and are not graded. For example, Speed's test is used as a technique for assessing pathology related to bicipital tendonitis, and Thompson's test is used to assess potential rupture of the Achilles tendon.

Neurologic Testing

A segmental nerve is the portion of a nerve that originates in the spinal cord and is referred to as a nerve root. Most nerve roots share two components:

1. A somatic portion, which innervates a series of skeletal muscles and provides sensory input from the skin, fascia, muscles, and joints.

2. A visceral component, which is part of the autonomic nervous system.

The autonomic system supplies the blood vessels, dura mater, periosteum, ligaments, and intervertebral disks, among many other structures.

Nerves commonly are injured by tensile or compressive forces, and these injuries are reflected in both motor and sensory deficits. The motor component of a segmental nerve is tested using a **myotome**, a group of muscles primarily innervated by a single nerve root. The sensory component is tested using a **dermatome**, an area of skin supplied by a single nerve root. An injury to a segmental nerve root often affects more than one peripheral nerve and does not demonstrate the same motor loss or sensory deficit as an injury to a single peripheral nerve. Dermatomes, myotomes, and reflexes are used to assess the integrity of the central nervous system (CNS). Peripheral nerves are assessed using manual muscle testing and noting cutaneous sensory changes in peripheral nerve patterns. Neurologic testing is only necessary in orthopaedic injuries when an individual complains of numbness, tingling, or a burning sensation or suffers from unexplained muscular weakness.

■■■ FIGURE 5.7 **Stress tests.** The application of a valgus stress on the elbow joint can assess the integrity of the joint medial collateral ligaments.

Dermatomes

The sensitivity of a dermatome can be assessed by touching a patient with a cotton ball, paper clip, pads of the fingers, or fingernails. In doing so, the examiner should ask the individual about the sensations being experienced. It is important to determine the nature of the sensation (e.g., a sharp or dull sensation) and to assess whether the same sensation was experienced in testing the uninjured body segment. Abnormal responses may be decreased tactile sensation (**hypoesthesia**), excessive tactile sensation (**hyperesthesia**), or loss of sensation (**anesthesia**). **Paresthesia** is another abnormal sensation characterized by a numb, tingling, or burning sensation. Figure 5.8 illustrates dermatome patterns for the segmental nerves.

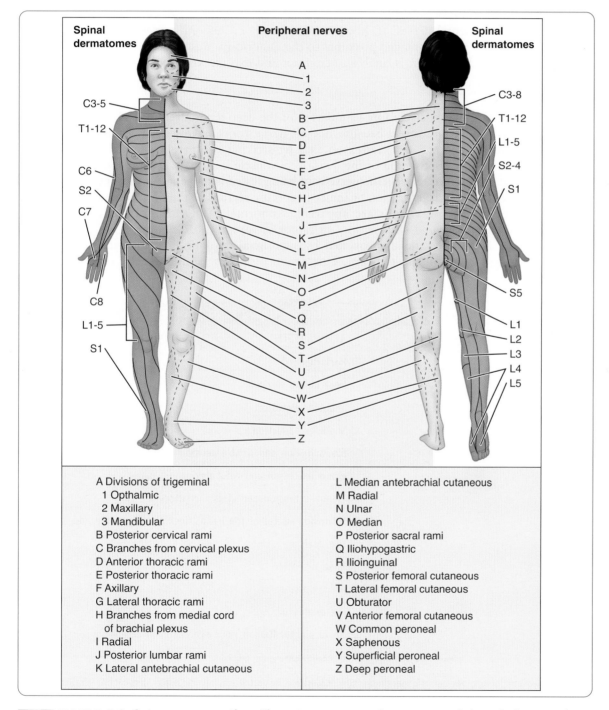

A Divisions of trigeminal
 1 Opthalmic
 2 Maxillary
 3 Mandibular
B Posterior cervical rami
C Branches from cervical plexus
D Anterior thoracic rami
E Posterior thoracic rami
F Axillary
G Lateral thoracic rami
H Branches from medial cord
  of brachial plexus
I Radial
J Posterior lumbar rami
K Lateral antebrachial cutaneous

L Median antebrachial cutaneous
M Radial
N Ulnar
O Median
P Posterior sacral rami
Q Iliohypogastric
R Ilioinguinal
S Posterior femoral cutaneous
T Lateral femoral cutaneous
U Obturator
V Anterior femoral cutaneous
W Common peroneal
X Saphenous
Y Superficial peroneal
Z Deep peroneal

▪▪ ▪▪ FIGURE 5.8 Cutaneous sensation. The cutaneous sensation patterns of the spinal nerves dermatomes differ from the patterns innervated by the peripheral nerves.

Myotomes

The majority of muscles receive segmental innervation from two or more nerve roots. Selected motions, however, may be innervated predominantly by a single nerve root (myotome). Resisted muscle testing of a selected motion can determine the status of the nerve root that supplies that myotome (Table 5.6). In assessing nerve integrity, muscle contractions must be held for at least 5 seconds. A normal response is a strong muscle contraction. Weakness in the myotome indicates a possible injury to the spinal cord nerve root. A weakened muscle contraction may indicate partial paralysis (**paresis**) of the muscles innervated by the nerve root being tested. In a peripheral nerve injury, complete paralysis of the muscles supplied by that nerve occurs. For example, the L3 myotome is tested with knee extension. If the L3 nerve root is damaged at its origin in the spine, a weak muscle contraction occurs. This weakness results because the quadriceps receive innervation from L2 and L4 segmental nerves. If, however, the peripheral femoral nerve, which contains segments of L2, L3, and L4, is damaged proximal to the quadriceps muscle, the muscle cannot receive any nerve impulses; therefore, it is unable to contract and execute knee extension.

Reflexes

Damage to the CNS can be detected by stimulation of the deep tendon reflexes (DTRs) (Table 5.7). Reflex testing is limited, however, because not all nerve roots have a DTR. The most familiar DTR is the patellar, or knee-jerk, reflex elicited by striking the patellar tendon with a reflex hammer, causing a rapid contraction of the quadriceps muscle (Fig. 5.9). Deep tendon reflexes tend to be diminished or absent if the specific nerve root being tested is damaged. Exaggerated, distorted, or absent reflexes indicate degeneration or injury in specific regions of the nervous system. This may be demonstrated before other signs are apparent. Abnormal DTRs are not clinically relevant, however, unless they are found with sensory or motor abnormalities.

Superficial reflexes are reflexes provoked by superficial stroking, usually with a moderately sharp object that does not break the skin. This action produces a reflex muscle contraction. For

TABLE 5.6 Myotomes Used to Test Selected Nerve Root Segments

NERVE ROOT SEGMENT	ACTION TESTED
C1–C2	Neck flexion[a]
C3	Neck lateral flexion[a]
C4	Shoulder elevation
C5	Shoulder abduction
C6	Elbow flexion and wrist extension
C7	Elbow extension and wrist flexion
C8	Thumb extension and ulnar deviation
T1	Intrinsic muscles of the hand (finer abduction and adduction)
L1–L2	Hip flexion
L3	Knee extension
L4	Ankle dorsiflexion
L5	Toe extension
S1	Ankle plantar flexion, foot eversion, hip extension
S2	Knee flexion

[a]These myotomes should not be performed in an individual with a suspected cervical fracture or dislocation, because they may cause serious damage or possibly death.

TABLE 5.7 Deep Tendon Reflexes

REFLEX	STIMULATION SITE	NORMAL RESPONSE	SEGMENTAL LEVEL
Jaw	Mandible	Mouth closes	Cranial nerve V
Biceps	Biceps tendon	Biceps contraction	C5–C6
Brachioradialis	Brachioradialis tendon or just distal to the musculotendinous junction	Flexion of elbow and/or pronation of forearm	C5–C6
Triceps	Distal triceps tendon just superior to olecranon process	Elbow extension/muscle contraction	C7–C8
Patella	Patellar tendon	Leg extension	L3–L4
Medial hamstrings	Semimembranosus tendon	Knee flexion/muscle contraction	L5, S1
Lateral hamstrings	Biceps femoris tendon	Knee flexion/muscle contraction	S1–S2
Tibialis posterior	Tibialis posterior tendon behind medial malleolus	Plantar flexion of foot with inversion	L4–L5
Achilles	Achilles tendon	Plantar flexion of foot	S1–S2

example, the normal response when testing the upper abdominal reflex is for the umbilicus to move up and toward the areas being stroked; this reflex represents segmental level T7–T9. An absence of a superficial reflex indicates a lesion in the cerebral cortex of the brain (upper motor neuron lesion).

> Additional examples of superficial reflexes can be found on the companion website at thePoint.

Pathologic reflexes (Table 5.8) can indicate upper motor neuron lesions if bilateral or lower motor neuron lesions if unilateral. The presence of the reflex often serves as a sign of some pathologic condition.

TABLE 5.8 Pathologic Reflexes[a]

REFLEX	ELICITATION	POSITIVE RESPONSE	PATHOLOGY
Babinski's[b]	Stroke lateral aspect of sole of foot	Extension of big toe; fanning of four small toes	Pyramidal tract lesion
		Test is normal in newborns	Organic hemiplegia
Chaddock's	Stroke lateral side of foot beneath lateral malleolus	Same response as above	Pyramidal tract lesion
Oppenheim's	Stroke anteromedial tibial surface	Same response as above	Pyramidal tract lesion
Gordon's	Squeeze calf muscle firmly	Same response as above	Pyramidal tract lesion
Brudzinski's	Passive flexion of one lower limb	Similar movement occurs in opposite limb	Meningitis
Hoffman's (digital)[c]	"Flicking" of terminal phalanx of index, middle, or ring finger	Reflex flexion of distal phalanx of thumb and of distal phalanx of index or middle finger (whichever one was not "flicked")	Increased irritability of sensory nerve in tetany Pyramidal tract lesion

[a]Bilateral positive response indicates an upper motor neuron lesion. Unilateral positive response may indicate a lower motor neuron lesion.

[b]Test is most commonly performed in the lower limb.

[c]Test is most commonly performed in the upper limb.

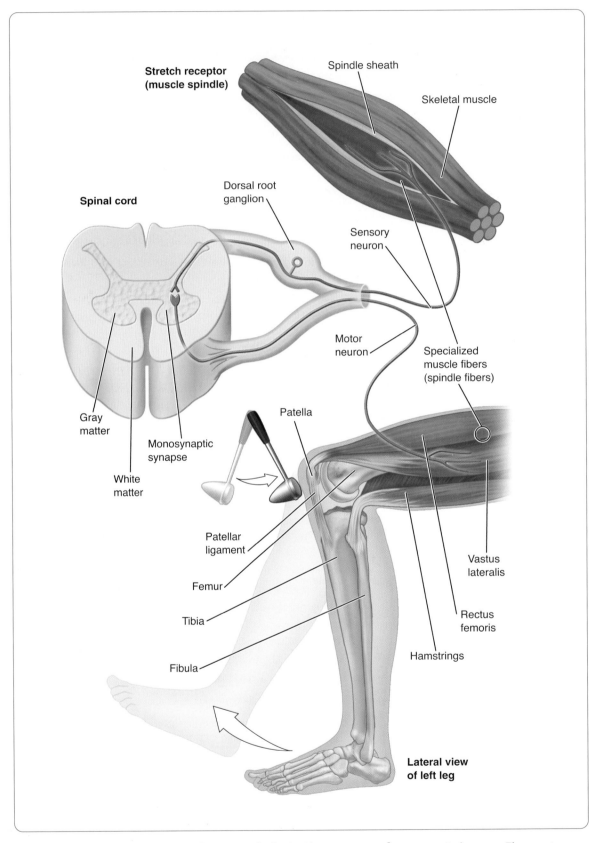

FIGURE 5.9 Reflexes. Reflexes can indicate the presence of nerve root damage. The most familiar stretch reflex is the knee jerk, or patellar reflex, performed by tapping the patellar tendon with a reflex hammer, causing involuntary knee extension.

Peripheral Nerve Testing

Motor function in peripheral nerves is assessed by resisted manual muscle testing throughout the full ROM. Sensory deficits are assessed in a manner identical to that of dermatome testing, except the cutaneous patterns differ (Fig. 5.8). Special compression tests also may be used on nerves close to the skin surface, such as the ulnar and median nerves. For example, the "Tinel sign" test is performed by tapping the skin directly over a superficial nerve (see Fig. 14.16). A positive sign, indicating irritation or compression of the nerve, results in a tingling sensation traveling into the muscles and skin supplied by the nerve.

Activity-Specific Functional Testing

Before permitting an individual to return to sport and physical activity after an injury, the individual's condition must be fully evaluated so that the risk of reinjury is minimal. Activity-specific tests involve the performance of active movements typical of those executed by the individual during sport or activity participation. These movements should assess strength, agility, flexibility, joint stability, endurance, coordination, balance, and activity-specific skill performance. In the rehabilitation process, the individual initially performs these skills at low intensity, then gradually increases the intensity as his or her condition improves. For example, in a lower leg injury, testing should begin by assessing walking, jogging, and then running forward and backward. If these skills are performed pain-free and without a limp, the individual might then be asked to run in a figure-eight or zigzag pattern. Again, each test must be performed pain-free and without a limp. An individual's balance can be tested by performing tasks with the eyes closed (e.g., walking a straight line on the toes and heels, balancing on a wobble board, or walking sideways on the hands while in a push-up position). Any individual who has been discharged from rehabilitation also should be cleared by a physician for participation.

The testing component of an assessment should include functional testing, stress testing, special tests, neurologic testing, and activity-specific functional testing. Given the findings (i.e., history, observation, inspection, and palpation) pertaining to the long jumper, a ligamentous injury should be suspected. As such, it would be appropriate to begin testing by stress testing the ligaments of the ankle. This should be followed by functional testing and neurologic testing. Based on those findings, activity-specific functional testing may or may not be appropriate.

THE EMERGENCY MEDICAL SERVICES SYSTEM

A gymnast slipped off the springboard on an approach to a vault and collided full force into the horse. As the on-site athletic trainer, you observe the gymnast lying motionless on the floor. Based on this information, is it appropriate to activate the institution's emergency medical plan?

Serious injuries can be frightening, particularly if breathing or circulation is impaired. As the first responder on the scene, the athletic trainer is expected to evaluate the situation, assess the severity of injury, recognize life-threatening conditions, provide immediate emergency care, and initiate any emergency procedures to ensure the individual is transported to the nearest medical facility without delay. An **emergency medical services (EMS)** system is a well-developed process that activates the emergency health care services of the athletic training facility and community to provide immediate care to an injured individual. Every athletic training facility should develop a plan that details the activation of their EMS system. The emergency medical plan should be a written document that is comprehensive yet flexible enough to adapt to any emergency situation at any activity venue. The plan should identify the following general principles (6):

- The personnel, with their qualifications, needed to perform responsibilities in executing the plan.

- Equipment needed to carry out the tasks required in the event of an emergency.

- Mechanism of communication to the emergency care providers, and the mode of transportation for the patient.

- The facilities to which the patient will be taken, including how and when those facilities will be notified in advance of the scheduled event or contest.

- Documentation verifying the implementation and evaluation of the emergency plan, actions taken during the emergency, evaluation of the emergency response, and institutional personnel training.

- Documentation of an annual review and rehearsal of the emergency plan, and notations indicating whether the emergency plan was modified and, if so, how the plan was changed.

Every institution/facility should have an emergency response team. The designated emergency response team should meet with representatives from local EMS agencies to discuss, develop, and evaluate the facility's emergency plan. As part of this process, individual responsibilities and protocols for an emergency situation should be determined. In developing the emergency medical plan, it is important to recognize that in any given situation, the members of the emergency response team can vary. For example, a physician may or may not be on-site, the athletic trainer may be working alone or part of an on-site staff, and emergency medical technicians may be present at an event or available only if summoned. The following questions should be addressed relative to each event:

- What emergency equipment must be available?

- What equipment will be provided by the local EMS agency (e.g., spine board and splints) if in attendance at an event?

- Who will be responsible for ensuring that the emergency equipment is operational?

- What type of communication will be used to contact emergency personnel? Who will activate the facility's emergency medical plan?

- Who will assess the injured individual on-site, and under what circumstances will a local EMS agency be called to the site?

- If a physician is present, what are the responsibilities of other medical personnel (e.g., athletic trainer and emergency medical technician)?

- If a physician is not present and the athletic trainer is evaluating the situation, what are the responsibilities of emergency medical technicians responding to the situation?

- If it becomes necessary to stabilize and transport an individual to a medical facility, who will direct the stabilization, and what protocol will be followed for the removal of protective equipment?

- Who will supervise other participants if the athletic trainer is assessing and providing care to an injured individual?

- Who will be responsible for the proper disposal of items and equipment exposed to blood or other bodily fluids?

 Field Strategy: Developing an Emergency Care Plan, available on the companion website at thePoint, summarizes several important issues in developing an emergency medical plan. You also will find a checklist for materials and supplies that should be included in an athletic training medical kit and in the emergency crash kit.

A written emergency plan should be developed for each activity site to address these questions.

The emergency response team should practice the emergency plan through regular educational workshops and training exercises. The use of interactive or simulation practice exercises can better prepare individuals to assume their roles in rendering emergency care.

While the condition of the gymnast may eventually warrant activation of the institution's emergency medical plan, there is not sufficient information at this point to activate the plan. It is important that the athletic trainer assess the athlete's condition to determine whether activation of the emergency medical plan is necessary.

EMERGENCY INJURY ASSESSMENT

Q *In assessing the condition of the injured gymnast, what sequential process can be used to determine if the CNS and/or cardiorespiratory systems are critically injured? What conditions warrant activation of the emergency medical plan, including summoning the local EMS agency?*

Injuries or conditions that impair—or that have the potential to impair—vital function of the CNS and cardiorespiratory system are considered to be emergency situations. In responding to an on-field or on-site injury, the initial assessment performed by the athletic trainer is intended to rule out any life-threatening conditions. The **primary survey** determines level of responsiveness and assesses airway, breathing, and circulation. If at any time during the assessment conditions exist that are an immediate threat to life, or if "red flags" are noted (Box 5.2), the assessment process should be terminated and the emergency medical plan activated.

Occasionally, situations can occur in which more than one individual is injured. **Triage** refers to the rapid assessment of all injured individuals followed by return to the most seriously injured to provide immediate treatment.

Once it has determined that a life-threatening condition does not exist, a secondary survey is performed to identify the type and extent of any injury and the immediate **disposition** of the condition. Decisions must be made regarding the on-field management of the injury (e.g., controlling bleeding or immobilizing a possible fracture or dislocation), the safest method of transportation from the field (e.g., manual conveyance, stretcher, or spine board), and the need for rapid referral of the individual for further medical care.

On-Site History

Regardless of the setting (e.g., on-site or athletic training room), assessment protocols should contain the same basic components. During an on-field (on-site) assessment, the athletic trainer should assume a position close to the injured individual. One hand should be placed on the forehead of the injured individual to stabilize the head and neck and prevent any unnecessary movement. The history of the injury can be obtained from the individual or, if the individual is unconscious, from bystanders who may have witnessed the injury. Questions should be open-ended to allow the person to provide as much information as possible about the injury. The athletic trainer should listen attentively for clues that may indicate the nature of the injury. On-site history taking should be relatively brief as compared to a more comprehensive clinical evaluation. Critical areas of information include:

- **Location of pain.** The site of the injury should be identified; it is important to be aware that several areas may be injured.

- **Presence of abnormal neurologic signs.** The presence of any tingling, numbness, or loss of sensation should be noted.

- **Mechanism of injury.** The position of the injured body part at the point of impact and the direction of force should be identified.

Box 5.2 "Red Flags" Indicating a Serious Emergency and Activation of the Emergency Medical Plan

- Airway obstruction
- Respiratory failure
- Severe shock
- Severe chest or abdominal pains
- Excessive bleeding
- Suspected spinal injury
- Head injury with loss of consciousness
- Severe heat illness
- Fractures involving several ribs, the femur, or pelvis

FIELD STRATEGY 5.3

Determining the History of Injury and Level of Responsiveness

Stabilize the head and neck. Do not move the individual unnecessarily until a spinal injury is ruled out. If nonresponsive:

1. Call the person's name loudly, and gently tap the sternum or touch the arm. If no response, rap the sternum more forcibly with a knuckle, or pinch the soft tissue in the armpit (axillary fold). Note if withdrawal from the painful stimulus occurs. If no response, immediately initiate the primary survey.
2. If airway, breathing, and circulation (ABCs) are adequate, gather a history of the injury. If you did not see what happened, question other players, supervisors, officials, and bystanders. Ask:

   - What happened?
   - Did you see the individual get hit, or did the individual just collapse?
   - How long has the individual been unresponsive?
   - Did the individual become unresponsive suddenly or deteriorate gradually?
   - If it was gradual, did anyone talk to the individual before you arrived?
   - What did the person say? Was it coherent? Did the person moan, groan, or mumble?
   - Has this ever happened before to this individual?

   If conscious, ask:

   1. What happened? Note if the individual is alert and aware of his or her surroundings or has any short- or long-term memory loss. If the individual is lying down, determine if the person was knocked down, fell, or rolled voluntarily into that position.
   2. Are you in pain? Where is the pain? Is it localized, or does it radiate into other areas?
   3. Did you hear any sounds or any unusual sensations when the injury occurred?
   4. Have you ever injured this body part before or experienced a similar injury?
   5. Do you have a headache? Are you experiencing any nausea? Are you dizzy? Can you see clearly?
   6. Are you taking any medication (e.g., prescription, over-the-counter, or vitamins)?

   It is important to avoid leading the individual. Instead, the individual should be encouraged to describe what happened, and the examiner should listen attentively for clues to the nature of the injury.

- **Associated sounds.** A report of hearing a "snap" or a "pop" may indicate a fracture or rupture of a ligament or tendon.

- **History of the injury.** Any preexisting condition or injury may have exacerbated the current injury or may complicate the injury assessment.

The history of the evaluation will enable the athletic trainer to determine the possibility of an associated head or spinal injury, to rule out injury to other body areas, and if necessary, to calm the individual. If the individual cannot open the eyes on verbal command or does not demonstrate withdrawal from painful stimulus, a serious "red flag" injury exists. Field Strategy 5.3 lists several questions to determine a history of the injury and assess the level of responsiveness.

On-Site Observation and Inspection

In an on-site evaluation, the initial observation is completed en route to the injured individual and, therefore, occurs prior to the history taking. Critical areas to observe include:

- **The surrounding environment.** Any equipment or apparatus that may have contributed to the injury should be noted.

- **Body position.** The position of the individual (e.g., prone, supine, or side-lying) should be observed. The appearance of a gross deformity in one of the limbs should be noted. In severe brain injuries, a neurologic sign called "posturing" of the extremities can occur (Fig. 5.10). **Decerebrate rigidity** is characterized by extension of all four extremities. **Decorticate rigidity** is characterized by extension of the legs and marked flexion in the elbows, wrists, and fingers.

- **Movement of the individual.** An individual holding an injured body part and expressing pain indicates consciousness as well as an intact CNS and cardiovascular system. If the individual is not moving or is having a seizure, possible systemic, psychological, or neurologic dysfunction should be suspected.

- **Level of responsiveness.** Sometimes referred to the "shake and shout" stage, the examiner tries to arouse the unconscious individual by gently shaking (without moving the head or neck) and by shouting into each ear. This action will determine whether the person is alert, restless, lethargic, or nonresponsive.

- **Primary survey.** The "ABC technique" should be employed to ensure an open Airway, adequate Breathing, and Circulation.

- **Inspection for head trauma.** The pupils of the eyes should be observed, noting a normal appearance, dilation, or constriction. The facial area and the area behind the ears should be inspected for any redness or ecchymosis. The presence of any clear fluid or bloody discharge from the

A. Decerebrate   B. Decorticate

FIGURE 5.10 Body posturing. A, Decerebrate rigidity is characterized by extension in all four extremities. **B,** Decorticate rigidity is characterized by extension of the legs and flexion of the elbows, wrist, and fingers. Both conditions indicate a severe brain injury.

ears or nose should be noted; this fluid could be cerebrospinal fluid leaking from the cranial area as a result of a skull fracture.

- **Inspection of the injured body part.** The injured area should be checked for joint alignment, redness, ecchymosis, swelling, or cuts. These observations should always be compared to the uninjured body part.

On-Site Palpation

The palpation should include a general head-to-toe assessment. This is done using a gentle, squeezing motion to palpate methodically down the trunk of the body to the fingers and toes. Palpation includes:

- **Bony palpation.**
  - **Possible fractures.** Detected with palpation, percussion, vibration, compression, and distraction (Fig. 5.2).
  - **Crepitus.** Associated with fracture, swelling, or inflammation.
- **Soft-tissue palpation.**
  - **Swelling.** May indicate diffuse hemorrhage or inflammation in a muscle, ligament, bursa, or joint capsule.
  - **Deformity.** An indentation may indicate a rupture in a musculotendinous unit; a protruding, firm bulge may indicate a joint dislocation, ruptured bursa, muscle spasm, or hematoma.
- **Skin temperature.**
  - Normally, the skin is dry, but certain conditions, such as cold, shock, or fever can alter surface blood vessels.
  - Skin temperature is assessed by placing the back of the hand against the individual's forehead or by palpating appendages bilaterally.

On-Site Functional Testing

When not contraindicated, the athletic trainer should identify the individual's willingness to move the injured body part. For a lower extremity injury, this should be expanded to include the willingness to bear weight. Movement is contraindicated, however, in the presence of a possible head or spinal injury, fracture, dislocation, or muscle/tendon rupture. Functional testing includes:

- **Active range of motion.** The individual is asked to move the injured body part through the available ROM. The quantity and quality of movement in the absence of pain should be noted.
- **Passive range of motion.** The examiner moves the injured extremity through the available pain-free ROM, noting any painful arc of motion.
- **Resisted range of motion.** An overpressure (break pressure) should be applied to the involved muscle or muscle group to determine the ability to sustain a forceful contraction.
- **Weight bearing.** If the individual successfully completes active, passive, and resisted motion, walking may be permitted. If the individual is unable to perform these tests, however, or if critical signs and symptoms are apparent, removal from the area should be performed in a non–weight bearing manner.

On-Site Stress Testing

Testing for ligamentous integrity is performed before any muscle guarding or swelling occurs to prevent the extent of injury from being obscured. Typically, only single-plane tests are performed, the results of which are then compared with the noninjured limb.

On-Site Neurologic Testing

Neurologic testing is critical to prevent a catastrophic injury. Although listed as a separate testing phase, neurologic testing, if warranted, may be performed earlier in the evaluation. Critical areas to include are:

- **Cutaneous sensation.** This can be done by running the fingernails along both sides of the injured individual's arms and legs to determine if the same feeling is experienced on both sides of the body part. Pain perception also can be tested by applying a sharp and a dull point to the skin; the ability of the individual to distinguish the difference should be noted.

- **Motor function.** A cranial nerve assessment (see Chapter 9) should be completed. In addition, the ability of the individual to wiggle the fingers and toes on both hands and feet should be assessed, and a bilateral comparison of grip strength should be performed.

Vital Signs

When warranted, the vital signs should be assessed to establish a baseline of information. Vital signs indicate the status of the cardiovascular system and the CNS and include pulse, respiratory rate and quality, blood pressure, and temperature. Although not specifically cited as vital signs, skin color, pupillary response to light, and eye movement also may be assessed to determine neurologic function. Abnormal vital signs indicate a serious injury or illness (Table 5.9).

Pulse

Factors such as age, gender, aerobic physical condition, degree of physical exertion, medications or chemical substances being taken, blood loss, and stress can influence pulse rate and volume. Pulse usually is taken at the carotid artery, because a pulse at that site is not normally obstructed by clothing, equipment, or strappings. Normal adult resting rates range from 60 to 100 beats a minute; for children, the normal resting range is from 120 to 140 beats per minute. Aerobically conditioned athletes may have a pulse rate as low as 40 beats per minute. Pulse rate is assessed by counting the carotid pulse rate for a 30-second period and then doubling it. An assessment of pulse volume, which reflects the sensation of the contraction (e.g., strong/weak), also is important.

Respiration

Breathing rate also varies with gender and age. It averages from 10 to 25 breaths per minute in an adult and from 20 to 25 breaths per minute in a child. Breathing rate is assessed by counting the number of respirations in a 30-second period and then doubling it. The character of the respiration (e.g., rapid, shallow, deep, gasping, or labored) should be noted as well.

Blood Pressure

Blood pressure is the pressure or tension of the blood within the systemic arteries, generally considered to be the aorta. As one of the most important vital signs, blood pressure reflects the effectiveness of the circulatory system. Changes in blood pressure are very significant. **Systolic blood pressure** is measured when the left ventricle contracts and expels blood into the aorta. It is approximately 120 mm Hg for a healthy adult and 125 to 140 mm Hg for healthy children aged 10 to 18 years. **Diastolic blood pressure** is the residual pressure in the aorta between heartbeats and averages 70 to 80 mm Hg in healthy adults and 80 to 90 mm Hg in healthy children aged 10 to 18 years. Blood pressure may be affected by gender, weight, race, lifestyle, and diet. Blood pressure is measured in the brachial artery with a sphygmomanometer and stethoscope (see Field Strategy 2.1).

Temperature

Core temperature can be measured by a thermometer placed under the tongue, in the ear or armpit, or in case of unconsciousness, in the rectum. Average oral temperature usually is quoted at 37°C (98.6°F), but this can fluctuate considerably. During the early morning hours, it may fall as low as

TABLE 5.9 Abnormal Vital Signs and Possible Causes

PULSE

Rapid, weak	Shock, internal hemorrhage, hypoglycemia, heat exhaustion, or hyperventilation
Rapid, bounding	Heat stroke, fright, fever, hypertension, apprehension, hyperglycemia, or normal exertion
Slow, bounding	Skull fracture, stroke, drug use (barbiturates and narcotics), certain cardiac problems, or some poisons
No pulse	Blocked artery, low blood pressure, or cardiac arrest

RESPIRATORY RATE AND QUALITY

Shallow breathing	Shock, heat exhaustion, insulin shock, chest injury, or cardiac problems
Irregular breathing	Airway obstruction, chest injury, diabetic coma, asthma, or cardiac problems
Rapid, deep	Diabetic coma, hyperventilation, or some lung diseases
Frothy blood	Lung damage, such as a puncture wound to the lung from a fractured rib or other penetrating object
Slowed breathing	Stroke, head injury, chest injury, or use of certain drugs
Wheezing	Asthma
Crowing	Spasms of the larynx
Apnea	Hypoxia (lack of oxygen), congestive heart failure, or head injuries
No breathing	Cardiac arrest, poisoning, drug abuse, drowning, head injury, or intrathoracic injuries, with death imminent if action is not taken to correct condition

BLOOD PRESSURE

Systolic < 100 mm Hg	Hypotension caused by shock, hemorrhage, heart attack, internal injury, or poor nutrition
Systolic > 140 mm Hg	Hypertension caused by certain medications, oral contraceptives, anabolic steroids, amphetamines, chronic alcohol use, and obesity

SKIN TEMPERATURE

Dry, cool	Exposure to cold or cervical, thoracic, or lumbar spine injuries
Cool, clammy	Shock, internal hemorrhage, trauma, anxiety, or heat exhaustion
Hot, dry	Disease, infection, high fever, heat stroke, or overexposure to environmental heat
Hot, moist	High fever
Isolated hot spot	Localized infection
Cold appendage	Circulatory problem
"Goose pimples"	Chills, communicable disease, exposure to cold, pain, or fear

SKIN COLOR

Red	Embarrassment, fever, hypertension, heat stroke, carbon monoxide poisoning, diabetic coma, alcohol abuse, infectious disease, inflammation, or allergy
White or ashen	Emotional stress (e.g., fright or anger), anemia, shock, heart attack, hypotension, heat exhaustion, insulin shock, or insufficient circulation
Blue or cyanotic	Heart failure, some severe respiratory disorders, and some poisoning; in dark-skinned individuals, a bluish cast can be seen in the mucous membranes (mouth, tongue, and inner eyelids), lips, and nail beds
Yellow	Liver disease or jaundice

PUPILS

Constricted	Individual is using an opiate-based drug or has ingested a poison
Unequal	Head injury or stroke
Dilated	Shock, hemorrhage, heat stroke, use of a stimulant drug, coma, cardiac arrest, or death

35.8°C (96.4°F), and during the later afternoon or evening hours, it may rise as high as 37.3°C (99.1°F). Rectal temperatures are higher than oral temperatures by an average of 0.4 to 0.5°C (0.7–0.9°F). Although this too can be quite variable, it is considered to be a more accurate measurement of core temperature. In contrast, axillary temperatures are lower than oral temperatures by approximately 1°F. In addition, axillary temperature may take 5 to 10 minutes to register and generally is considered to be less accurate than other measurements (7). Infrared tympanic thermometers measure infrared energy emitted by the tympanic membrane and provide a rapid, efficient, and noninvasive method of measuring body temperature. Infrared tympanic thermometers, however, have failed to detect fever in some patients with AIDS and in neonates, infants, and children, and they are not useful in hypothermic or significantly hyperthermic individuals (8).

Skin Color

Skin color can indicate abnormal blood flow and low blood oxygen concentration in a particular body part or area. Three colors commonly are used to describe light-skinned individuals: red, white or ashen, and blue. The colors and their potential indications also can be seen in Table 5.9. In dark-skinned individuals, skin pigments mask cyanosis; however, a bluish cast can be seen in mucous membranes (e.g., mouth, tongue, and inner eyelids), the lips, and nail beds. Fever in these individuals can be seen by a red flush at the tips of the ears.

Pupils

The pupils are extremely responsive to situations affecting the CNS. Rapid constriction of pupils when the eyes are exposed to intense light is called the **pupillary light reflex**. The pupillary response to light can be assessed by holding a hand over one eye and then moving the hand away quickly, or by shining the light from a penlight into one eye and then observing the pupil's reaction. A normal response would be constriction with the light shining in the eye and dilation as the light is removed. The pupillary reaction is classified as brisk (normal), sluggish, nonreactive, or fixed. The eyes may appear normal, constricted, unequal, or dilated.

Eye movement is tested by asking the individual to focus on a single object. An individual experiencing **diplopia** sees two images instead of one. This condition is attributed to failure of the external eye muscles to work in a coordinated manner. The tracking ability of the eyes can be assessed by asking the individual to follow the examiner's fingers as they move through the six cardinal fields of vision. The individual's depth perception can be assessed by placing a finger several inches in front of the individual and then asking the person to reach out and touch the finger. This assessment should be repeated several times, with the examiner's finger in several different locations.

Disposition

Information gathered during the assessment must be analyzed and decisions made based on the best interests of the injured individual. It is especially important to determine whether the situation can be handled on-site or whether referral to a physician is warranted. As a general rule, the individual should always be referred to the nearest trauma center or emergency clinic if any life-threatening situation is present, if the injury results in loss of normal function, or if no improvement is seen in injury status after a reasonable amount of time. Examples of these injuries are provided in Box 5.2. Other conditions that are not necessarily life-threatening but are serious enough to warrant referral to a physician for immediate care include:

- Eye injuries
- Dental injuries in which a tooth has been knocked loose or knocked out
- Minor or simple fractures
- Lacerations that might require suturing
- Injuries in which a functional deficit is noticeable
- Loss of normal sensation or diminished or absent reflexes
- Noticeable muscular weakness in the extremities
- Any injury if you are uncertain about its severity or nature

Equipment Considerations

One of the primary concerns during an on-site assessment of an injured individual is that of equipment, particularly with regard to removal of an athletic helmet. For an individual with a potential cervical spine injury, removal of a helmet may worsen the condition or lead to additional injury.

Therefore, removal of any helmet should be avoided unless individual circumstances dictate otherwise, especially when the following are considered (1,8):

- Removal of the face mask allows full airway access. The face mask should be removed immediately when the decision is made to transport the injured individual, regardless of his or her current respiratory status.

- Most injuries can be visualized with the helmet in place.

- Neurologic tests can be performed with the helmet in place. The eyes may be examined, the nose and ears checked for fluid or blood, and the level of consciousness determined.

- The individual can be immobilized on a spine board with the helmet in place.

- When both a helmet and shoulder pads are worn, removing the helmet without removing the shoulder pads results in cervical hyperextension.

- Many helmets are radiographically translucent. Therefore, a definitive diagnosis can be made before removal.

Guidelines for removal of any piece of protective equipment should be defined within the emergency medical plan. Situations in which helmets may need to be removed include (1):

- When the helmet and chin strap do not hold the head securely so that immobilization of the helmet does not necessarily immobilize the head.

- When the design of the helmet and chin strap is such that even after removal of the face mask, the airway cannot be controlled.

- When the face mask cannot be removed after a reasonable amount of time.

- When the helmet prevents immobilization for transportation in an appropriate position.

- When extraordinary cases, such as when an automated external defibrillator (AED) is needed, occur.

Use of a defibrillator requires that the individual's chest be fully exposed and dry. Contact points for the defibrillator pads must be placed over the apex of the heart and inferior to the right clavicle. If the defibrillator pads touch wet shoulder pads, the defibrillator's current could arc, leading to decreased effectiveness of the defibrillator; more important, the current could defibrillate the operator. As the use of AEDs becomes more common, standardized protocols for their use must be documented and regularly practiced before their actual use during an emergency situation.

Field Strategy: Removal of Protective Equipment, located on the companion website at thePoint, summarizes the basic steps in removing a face mask, helmet, and shoulder pads.

Regardless of the injured individual's condition, the helmet or shoulder pads must be removed at some point, whether at the site or in the hospital. Because of their familiarity with the equipment, athletic trainers often are asked to assist medical personnel with this procedure.

Face Mask Removal

The face mask should be removed before transportation, regardless of the current respiratory status. Face masks typically are attached to the helmet with four plastic clips. It is recommended that all four clips be cut so that the facemask can be completely removed (9). Several commercial products (e.g., anvil pruner, FM Extractor, Trainer's Angel, PVC pipe cutter, X-Acto knife, and electric screwdriver) can be used to cut the clips or to unscrew the bolts holding the clips. It is important to recognize that older clips harden with age, making them harder to cut, and that screws may become rusted or stripped. Regardless of the manner in which the face mask is removed, it is essential that that in-line stabilization of the head and neck be maintained during the entire procedure.

Helmet Removal

If possible, the helmet should be removed in a controlled environment after radiographs have been obtained—and even then only by qualified medical personnel with training in equipment removal

(9). Two trained individuals are needed to carry out the task. One individual maintains in-line stabilization of the head, neck, and helmet while another person cuts the chin strap. Next, while one assistant continues to maintain stabilization of the chin and back of the neck, the other individual removes any accessible internal helmet padding, such as cheek pads. In removing the pads, a flat object, such as a tongue depressor or the flat edge of tape scissors, can be slid between the helmet and the pad. A slight turn of the inserted object causes the pad to unsnap from the helmet. If an air cell–padding system is present, the system should be deflated by releasing the air at the external port with an inflation needle or large-gauge hypodermic needle. The helmet should then be slid off the occiput with slight forward rotation of the helmet. If the helmet does not move with this action, slight traction can be applied to the helmet as it is carefully rocked anteriorly and posteriorly, with great care being taken not to move the head and neck unit. The helmet should not be spread apart by the ear holes, because this only serves to tighten the helmet on the forehead and occiput region (9).

Shoulder Pad Removal

Shoulder pads should not be removed unless the athlete's life is in danger and this threat outweighs the risk of a possible spinal cord injury that may result from moving the individual. The chest can be exposed without removing the pads to allow the athletic trainer access for evaluation, auscultation of breath and cardiac sounds, chest compression during CPR, and placement of AED pads. The chest is exposed by cutting the shirt from neck to waist and from the midline to the end of each arm sleeve. Next, the rib straps on the sternal portion of the pads should be unfastened or cut. Finally, the halves of the shoulder pads are spread to expose the sternum.

The Inter-Association Task Force recommends that neither the football helmet nor the shoulder pads be removed before transportation (9). Such removal is best done in a controlled environment, such as the emergency room, where several highly trained individuals can assist in simultaneously removing the helmet and shoulder pads. If the pads must be removed, the jersey is first removed using the process described above. Next, all straps securing the shoulder pads to the arms are cut, the laces or straps over the sternum are cut, and the two halves of the shoulder pads are spread apart. All accessories, such as neck rolls or collars, are then cut and/or removed. One individual maintains cervical stabilization in a cephalad direction by placing his or her forearms on the athlete's chest while manually stabilizing the chin and occiput. Assistants should be positioned on each side of the athlete with their hands placed directly against the skin in the thoracic region of the back. Additional support should be provided at other strategic locations down the body as deemed appropriate for the size of the patient. While the patient is lifted, the individual in charge of the head/shoulder stabilization should remove the helmet and then immediately remove the shoulder pads by spreading apart the front panels and pulling them around the head. Next, the remaining jersey and any other accessories are removed, and the patient is lowered, with appropriate immobilization being continued (9).

A *When evaluating the gymnast, a primary survey should be conducted to assess the level of responsiveness, airway, breathing, and circulation. Measurement of vital signs and evaluation of the signs and symptoms gathered during the on-site assessment will determine if the emergency plan should be activated and EMS summoned.*

MOVING THE INJURED PARTICIPANT

Q *What criteria should be used to determine whether an injured individual should be allowed to walk off the field or site of the injury? What is the safest method for transporting an individual with a lower extremity injury?*

Once the extent and severity of the injury have been determined, a decision must be made regarding how to safely remove the individual from the area. Possible methods include ambulatory assistance, manual conveyance, and transport by a stretcher or spine board.

Ambulatory Assistance

Ambulatory assistance is used to aid an injured individual who is able to walk. This implies that the injury is minor and no further harm will occur if the individual is ambulatory. In performing this technique, two individuals of equal or near-equal height should support both sides of the individual. The injured individual drapes his or her arms across the shoulders of the assistants while the arms of the assistants encircle the injured person's back. This position enables the assistants to escort the individual to an appropriate area for further evaluation and treatment.

Manual Conveyance

If the individual is unable to walk or the distance is too great to walk, manual conveyance should be used. The individual continues to drape his or her arms across the assistants' shoulders while one arm of each assistant is placed behind the individual's back and the other arm is placed under the individual's thigh. Both assistants lift the legs up, placing the individual in a seated position. The individual is then carried to an appropriate area. Again, it is essential that the injury be fully evaluated before moving the individual in this manner.

Transport by Spine Board

In the absence of a suspected spinal injury, the safest method to move an individual is with a spine board or stretcher. Ideally, five or six individuals should roll, lift, and carry an injured person. The captain (i.e., the individual with medical seniority) stabilizes the head and gives commands for each person to slowly lift and place the injured individual onto the stretcher. The individual is then secured onto the stretcher. On command, the stretcher is raised to waist level. The individual should be carried feet first so that the captain can constantly monitor the individual's condition. Field Strategy 5.4 describes the process of securing and moving an individual on a spine board.

Pool Extrication

Serious injuries also can occur in a swimming pool environment. If a head or neck injury is suspected, the individual must be placed on a spine board before being removed from the water. Although the principles are the same, carrying out the tasks in water requires practice. Field Strategy 5.5 describes the process of securing and moving an individual in water onto a spine board.

FIELD STRATEGY 5.4

Transporting an Injured Individual on a Spine Board

1. ***Unless ruled out, assume the presence of a spinal injury.*** The captain of the team stabilizes the head and neck in the exact position in which they were found, regardless of the angle. The arms should be placed next to the body, and the legs should be straight. If the individual is lying face down, the individual should be rolled supine. Four or five people are required to "log roll" the individual. The captain should position the arms in the cross-arm technique so that during the log roll, the arms will end in the proper position.
2. The spine board should be placed as close as possible beside the individual. Each person is responsible for one body segment: one at the shoulder, one at the hip, one at the knees, and if needed, one at the feet. On command, the individual should be rolled onto the board in a single motion.
3. Once the injured individual is on the spine board, the captain continues to stabilize the head and neck while another person applies support around the cervical region. The chest is secured to the board first, and then the feet are secured. A helmet should not be removed unless individual circumstances dictate otherwise.
4. When the injured individual is secured, four people lift the stretcher while the captain continues to monitor the individual's condition. The individual should be transported feet first.

FIELD STRATEGY 5.5

Pool Extrication

1. Ease yourself into the water near the individual to avoid any additional wave movement.
2. Face the individual's side, and place one forearm along the length of the individual's sternum. Support the chin by placing the thumb on one side of the individual's chin and the fingers on the other.
3. Place the other forearm along the length of the individual's back, and cradle the head near the base of the skull. Lock both wrists. Press the forearms inward and upward to provide mild traction and stabilization of the neck.
4. Turn the individual supine by slowly rotating the person toward you as you submerge and go under the individual. Avoid any unnecessary movement of the individual's trunk or legs. Slowly tow the individual to the shallow end of the pool. [**Note:** In diving pools without a shallow end, move the individual to the side of the tank. The "captain" lies prone on the deck with arms in the water and takes over the in-line stabilization of the neck.]

5. With the backboard, approach the individual from the side. Glide the foot of the board diagonally under the individual, making sure the board extends beyond the head. Allow the board to rise under the individual.
6. Maintain in-line stabilization while a rigid cervical collar is applied. Secure the individual to the backboard, beginning at the chest and then moving to the hips, thighs, and shins.
7. Before securing the head, it may be necessary to place padding under the head to fill the space between the board and head to maintain stabilization. Place a towel or blanket roll in a horseshoe configuration around the head and neck, and secure to the board.
8. Place the board perpendicular to the pool, and maintain the board in a horizontal position. Remove the board, head first. Tip the board at the head to break the initial suction holding it in the water. Two people should be on the deck to lift and slide the board onto the pool deck. Once on the deck, check vital signs, and assess the individual's condition. Treat for shock, and transport.

A.

B.

C.

D.

E.

F.

G.

H.

An injured individual may walk off the field or site of injury if it is determined that the injury is minor and no further harm will occur if the individual is ambulatory. If the injury is more serious, however, the individual should be non–weight bearing. Manual conveyance or removal by a spine board, stretcher, or chair may be necessary to avoid any additional pain or injury to the individual.

DIAGNOSTIC TESTING

In assessing an injury, what special imaging techniques can be used by the athletic trainer to reach an accurate diagnosis?

Injury recognition is the final step in assessment. A **diagnosis** is the definitive determination of the nature of the injury or illness. Various forms of laboratory tests and imaging techniques may be necessary in establishing a diagnosis. In the majority of cases, these tests can only be ordered by a physician or appropriately licensed medical specialist.

Laboratory Tests

 Additional information about laboratory tests, including synovial fluid classifications, normal ranges for selected blood variables in adults, and normal urine values, is available on the companion website at thePoint.

A variety of laboratory tests can be used in the assessment of an injury and illness (Box 5.3). For example, if an individual has a grossly swollen knee, the physician may draw fluid out of the joint with a hypodermic needle for examination. If the individual reports a sore throat, lethargy, and fever, a throat culture and blood test may be ordered. A complete blood count (CBC) can address several factors; however, other common factors that are tested include hemoglobin, hematocrit, and iron levels. An individual who has blood in the urine likewise requires a urinalysis. Common factors assessed in this laboratory test include pH, glucose, and bacteria.

Radiography

The most common imaging technique is radiography, or the x-ray (Fig. 5.11). A radiograph provides an image of certain body structures and can rule out fractures, infections, and **neoplasms**. The image is formed when a minute amount of radiation passes through the body to expose sensitive film placed on the other side. The ability to penetrate tissues depends on the tissue composition and mass. For example, bones (calcium) restrict rays from passing through; therefore, these images appear white on the film. Lungs or other air-filled structures, however, allow most x-rays to pass through, resulting in the images appearing black. Soft tissues (e.g., heart, kidneys, or liver), allow

Box 5.3 Laboratory Blood Testing

- Red-blood-cell count determines the approximate number of circulating red blood cells (erythrocytes). A decreased count indicates possible anemia, chronic infection, internal hemorrhage, certain types of cancers, or deficiencies in iron, vitamin B_{12}, or folic acid.
- White-blood-cell count determines the approximate number of circulating white blood cells (leukocytes). A decreased count indicates an inability to fight infections.
- Hemoglobin gives the red color to erythrocytes. It transports oxygen to the tissues and carries away the carbon dioxide. A decreased count indicates possible anemia or carbon monoxide poisoning.
- Hematocrit measures the volume of erythrocytes packed by centrifugation in a given volume of blood and is expressed as a percentage. A decreased value indicates anemia.
- Platelets aid in blood clotting. A decreased value indicates decreased clotting ability, internal bleeding, or possible bleeding disorder.

varying degrees of penetration and are difficult to identify on the radiograph. Images are preserved on sheets of film. As film quality and electronic technology have advanced, better imaging has been achieved, and the dose of radiation to the patient has been decreased. The use of radiographs is contraindicated over the thyroid gland, pregnant abdomen, and reproductive organs. If the information gained outweighs the risk, however, these areas can be shielded with a lead drape.

FIGURE 5.11 Radiography. Bone absorbs the x-rays and, therefore, appears white on the radiograph. This radiograph demonstrates a dorsal dislocation of the posterior interphalangeal joint.

Some forms of radiographs use radio-opaque dyes that are absorbed by the tissues, allowing them to be visualized by radiographic examination. A **myelogram** uses an opaque dye that is introduced into the spinal canal through a lumbar puncture. The patient is placed in a tilted position, allowing the dye to flow to different levels of the spinal cord. In viewing the contrasts, physicians can identify pathologies of the spinal canal (e.g., tumors, nerve root compression, and disk disease). Another form of radiographic testing is the **arthrogram**. Again, an opaque dye, air, or a combination of the two is injected into a joint space. The visual study of the joint can detect capsular tissue tears and articular cartilage lesions.

Computed Tomography

Computed tomography (CT) scan is a form of radiography that produces a three-dimensional, cross-sectional picture of a body part (Fig. 5.12). This test is used to reveal abnormalities in bone, fat, and soft tissue and is excellent at detecting tendinous and ligamentous injuries in varying joint positions. Scanners use a beam of light across a "slice" or layer of the body. A special receptor located opposite the beam detects the number of rays passing through the body. The tube emitting the beams of light rotates around the body, and thousands of readings are taken by the receptors. The computer determines the density of the underlying tissues based on the absorption of x-rays by the body, allowing more precision in viewing soft tissues. The computer records the data, analyzes the receptor readings, and calculates the absorption of the light beams at thousands of different points. This information is then converted into a two-dimensional image, or slice, of the body and is displayed on a video screen and/or radiographic film. These slices can be obtained at varying positions and thicknesses, allowing the radiologist or physician to study the area and its surroundings. A CT scan is relatively safe, because the patient is exposed to little radiation during the procedure. A CT scan also yields highly detailed results.

Magnetic Resonance Imaging

Magnetic resonance imaging (MRI) is an excellent tool for visualizing the CNS, spine, and musculoskeletal and cardiovascular systems (Fig. 5.13). One of its assets is the ability to provide soft-tissue differentiation (e.g., ligamentous disruption, such as an anterior cruciate ligament tear). It also is used to demonstrate space-occupying lesions in the brain (e.g., tumor or hematoma) and joint damage (e.g., meniscal tears or osteochondral fractures) as well as to view blood vessels and blood flow without the use of a contrast medium (e.g., cardiac function). In many cases, the MRI has replaced myelography and arthrography.

Images are obtained by placing the patient in an MRI tube that produces the magnetic field. This causes the body's hydrogen

FIGURE 5.12 Computed tomography. A male patient reported increased sleepiness and a change in personality 3 weeks after falling and striking his head. The cranial computed tomographic scan demonstrates a chronic subdural hematoma.

FIGURE 5.13 Magnetic resonance imaging. This magnetic resonance image depicts a large L4–L5 disk herniation.

FIGURE 5.14 Radionuclide scintigraphy. Bone scans can detect stress fractures long before the fracture becomes visible on traditional radiographs. This individual had increased his daily run from 5 to 8 miles per day and included hill climbing over the past few months. He reported increasing pain in his thigh. The bone scan showed increased density in a transverse line, indicating medial periosteal reaction.

nuclei to align with the magnetic axis. The tissues are then bombarded by radio waves, which causes the nuclei to resonate as they absorb the energy. When the energy from the radio waves ceases, the nuclei return to their state of equilibrium by releasing energy, which is then detected by the MRI unit and transformed by a computer into visible images.

Radionuclide Scintigraphy (Bone Scan)

A bone scan is used to detect stress fractures of the long bones and vertebrae, degenerative diseases, infections, or tumors of the bone. A **radionucleotide** material, technetium 99m, is injected into a vein and is slowly absorbed by areas of bone undergoing remodeling. Several hours after the injection, the patient is placed under a recording device that scans radioactive signals and records the images on film. In some scans, active images are recorded on videotape. A total body scan or even a localized scan can take close to an hour. Any areas subject to stress (e.g., fractures or increases of metabolic activity, such as bone marrow centers or tumors) show as areas of greatest uptake and appear darker on the film (Fig. 5.14). Bone scans may be clinically correlated to plain-film radiographs or other diagnostic tests. No special preparation is needed before the bone scan, and the risk to the patient is minimal. The body excretes the radioactive material over a 24-hour period.

Ultrasonic Imaging

Sonography, as it sometimes is called, uses sound waves to view the various internal organs and certain soft-tissue structures, such as tendons. The energy produced is similar to that used during therapeutic ultrasound treatments but has a frequency of less than 0.8 MHz. Although it commonly is used to monitor development of the fetus during pregnancy, it also is used to view tendons and for other soft-tissue imaging. Similar to a sonar device on a submarine, a piezoelectric crystal is used to convert electrical pulses into vibrations that penetrate the body structures. The sound waves are reflected away from the tissues and create a two-dimensional image of the subcutaneous structures.

Electromyography

Certain muscular conditions can be detected using electromyography. This diagnostic tool consists of a thin electrode needle that is inserted into the muscle to determine the level of muscular contraction following an electrical stimulation. Motor unit potentials can be observed on an oscilloscope screen or recorded on an electromyogram. Electromyography is used to detect denervated muscles, nerve root compression injuries, and other muscle diseases.

In some cases, a definitive diagnosis requires laboratory tests or imaging techniques. In the majority of cases, these tests can only be ordered by a physician or appropriately licensed medical specialist. It is essential that athletic trainers be aware of their duty of care consistent with current state law.

SUMMARY

1. In an injury assessment, a problem-solving process incorporates subjective and objective information that is reliable, accurate, and measurable.

2. The HOPS format includes history, observation and inspection, palpation, and special tests.

3. A more popular method of injury management is the SOAP note format, which assesses the individual's status and prognosis and establishes short- and long-term goals for recovery. The format outlines the treatment plan, such as the frequency and duration of treatments, rehabilitation exercises, ongoing patient education, evaluation standards to determine progress, and criteria for discharge.

4. The subjective information gathered during the history taking should include the primary complaint, mechanism of injury, characteristics of the symptoms, disabilities resulting from the injury, and related medical history.

5. The objective assessment should include observation and inspection, bony and soft-tissue palpation, functional tests, stress tests for specific joints or structures, neurologic testing, and activity-specific functional tests.

6. In consultation with the supervising physician and local EMS agencies, the athletic trainer should coordinate the development of an emergency plan. The purpose of this plan is to ensure rapid and complete emergency care to an injured individual. The plan should be evaluated annually and practiced by all parties on a regular basis.

7. In an emergency injury assessment, the presence of a head or spinal cord injury should be assumed. As such, the head and neck should be stabilized before proceeding. Assessment of all injuries, no matter how minor, should include a primary injury assessment to determine level of responsiveness and to assess the ABCs. A secondary assessment determines the presence of moderate to severe injuries.

8. As a general rule, an individual should always be referred to the nearest trauma center or emergency clinic if any life-threatening situation is present or if the injury results in loss of normal function.

9. The use of a variety of laboratory tests and imaging techniques can be instrumental in establishing an accurate diagnosis of an injury or illness. In the majority of cases, these tests can only be ordered by a physician or appropriately licensed medical specialist.

REFERENCES

1. Klossner D, ed. NCAA Sports Medicine Handbook: 2005–06. Indianapolis: National Collegiate Athletic Association, 2005.
2. Lesser JM, Hughes SV, Jemelka JR, Kumar S. Compiling a complete medical history: challenges and strategies for taking a comprehensive history in the elderly. Geriatrics 2005;60(11):22–25.
3. Documenting general observations. Nursing 2006; 36(2):25.
4. Norkin CC, White DJ. Measurement of Joint Motion: A Guide to Goniometry. Philadelphia: FA Davis, 2003.
5. Magee, DJ. Orthopedic Physical Assessment. Philadelphia: WB Saunders, Elsevier Science, 2002.
6. Anderson JC, Courson RW, Kleinert DM, McLoda TA. National Athletic Trainers' Association Position Statement: emergency planning in athletics. J Ath Tr 2002;37(1):99–104.
7. Bickley LS, Szilagyi PG. Bates' Guide to Physical Examination and History Taking. Baltimore: Lippincott Williams & Wilkins, 2003.
8. Guertler AT. The clinical practice of emergency medicine. Emerg Med Clin North Am 1997;15(2):303–313.
9. Kleiner DM, Almquist JL, Bailes J, et al. Prehospital Care of the Spine-Injured Athlete: A Document from the Inter-Association Task Force for Appropriate Care of the Spine-Injured Athlete. Dallas, TX: Inter-Association Task Force for Appropriate Care of the Spine-Inured Athlete; 2001.

Tissue Healing and Wound Care

STUDENT OUTCOMES

1. Describe the major mechanical forces that produce injury to biologic tissues—namely, compression, tension, shear, stress, strain, bending, and torsion.

2. Explain the effect of the material constituents and structural organization of skin, tendon, ligament, muscle, and bone on their ability to withstand the mechanical loads to which each is subjected.

3. List common injuries of skin, muscles and tendons, joints, and bone.

4. Describe the processes by which tissue healing occurs in skin, tendons, muscles, ligaments, and bone.

5. Explain wound care for both superficial and deep soft-tissue injuries.

6. Describe the appropriate immediate management of bone injuries.

7. Explain the mechanisms by which nerves are injured and the processes by which nerves can heal.

8. Describe the types of altered sensation that can result from a nerve injury.

9. Describe the appropriate immediate management of nerve injuries.

10. Explain the neurologic basis of pain, including factors that mediate pain.

ROLE DELINEATION COMPETENCIES

The following Performance Domains and Tasks defined in the National Athletic Trainers' Association Board of Certification *Role Delineation Study*, 5th Edition are addressed in this chapter:

BOC COMPETENCIES

I.   Prevention

    C. Instruct the appropriate individual(s) about standard protective equipment using effective communication techniques to minimize the risk of injury and illness.

    D. Apply appropriate prophylactic/protective measures using commercial products or custom-made devices to minimize the risk of injury and illness.

II.   Clinical Evaluation and Diagnosis

    E. Formulate a clinical impression by interpreting the signs, symptoms, and predisposing factors of the injury, illness, or condition to determine the appropriate course of action.

    F. Educate the appropriate individual(s) regarding the assessment by communicating information about the current or potential injury, illness, or health-related condition to encourage compliance with recommended care.

III.   Immediate Care

    B. Prevent exacerbation of non–life threatening condition(s) through the use of standard procedures to reduce morbidity.

IV.   Treatment, Rehabilitation, and Reconditioning

    B. Administer therapeutic modalities using standard techniques and procedures to facilitate recovery, function, and/or performance.

    C. Apply braces, splints, or assistive devices in accordance with appropriate standards and practices to facilitate recovery, function, and/or performance.

Human movement during sport and exercise typically is faster and produces greater force than activities of daily living. As a result, the potential for injury also is heightened. Understanding the different ways in which forces act on the body is necessary in comprehending techniques to prevent injuries. Likewise, knowing the material and structural properties of skin, tendon, muscle, ligament, bone, and nerve can lay a foundation for understanding the response of these tissues to applied forces and can facilitate an individual's safe return to sport participation.

This chapter begins with a general discussion of injury mechanisms, including descriptions of force and torque as well as their effects. This is followed by sections on soft tissues, bone, and nerve addressing the mechanical characteristics of these tissues, classification of injuries, processes by which the specific tissues heal, and general wound care for these injuries. A more detailed explanation of wound care for specific injuries is discussed in individual chapters.

INJURY MECHANISMS

Q *When the human body sustains force, the potential exists to strengthen body tissues or to injure them. A previously sedentary, middle-aged adult wants to initiate a running program as a way to improve his cardiovascular fitness. What advice should be provided to this individual for reducing the risk of sustaining a mechanical stress–related injury? Why?*

Analyzing the mechanics of injuries to the human body is complicated by several factors. First, potentially injurious forces applied to the body act at different angles, over different surface areas, and over different periods of time. Second, the human body is composed of many different types of tissue, which respond differently to applied forces. Finally, injury to the human body is not an all-or-nothing phenomenon—that is, injuries range in severity. This section introduces the types of mechanical loading that can cause injury and describes the basic mechanical responses of biologic tissues to these forms of loading.

Force and Its Effects

Force may be thought of as a push or a pull acting on a body. A multitude of forces act on our bodies routinely during the day. The forces of gravity and friction enable us to move about in predictable ways when muscles produce internal forces. During participation in sport and physical activity, force is applied to balls, bats, racquets, clubs, and other objects, and force is absorbed from impact with the ground or floor, the object used, and in contact sports, even other participants.

When a force acts, two potential effects on the target object exist. The first is acceleration, or change in velocity, and the second is deformation, or change in shape. For example, when a racquetball is struck with a racquet, the ball is both accelerated (i.e., put in motion in the direction of the racquet swing) and deformed (i.e., flattened on the side that is struck). The greater the stiffness of the material to which a force is applied, the greater the likelihood that the deformation will be too small to be easily seen. The more elastic the material to which a force is applied, the greater the likelihood that the deformation will be temporary, with the material springing back to regain its original shape.

When tissues sustain a force, two primary factors dictate whether injury occurs—namely, the size, or magnitude, of the force, and the material properties of the involved tissues (Box 6.1). A load-deformation curve demonstrates the deformation of a structure in response to progressive loading, or force application. If a load is relatively small, the response of the structure is elastic. As such, when the load is removed, the material will return to its original size and shape. Within the elastic region of the load-deformation curve, the greater the stiffness of the material, the steeper the slope of the line becomes. Therefore, greater stiffness translates to less deformation in response to a given load. If a load exceeds the material's **yield point**, or **elastic limit**, however, the response of the structure is plastic. In this situation, when the load is removed, some amount of deformation will remain. Loads exceeding the ultimate failure point on the load-deformation curve result in mechanical **failure** of the structure, which translates to fracturing of bone or rupturing of soft tissues.

The direction of an applied force also has important implications for injury potential. Many tissues are **anisotropic**, meaning that the structure is stronger in resisting force from certain directions compared with others. The anatomic makeup of many of the joints of the human body also means they are more susceptible to injury from a given direction. For example, lateral ankle sprains are much more common than medial ankle sprains because ligamentous support of the ankle is much stronger on the medial side. Consequently, when discussing injury mechanisms, force commonly is categorized according to the direction from which the force acts on the affected structure.

Force acting along the long axis of a structure is termed **axial force**. When the opponent in fencing is touched with the foil, the foil is loaded axially. When the human body is in an upright standing position, body weight creates axial loads on the femur and tibia.

Axial loading that produces a squeezing or crushing effect is termed **compressive force**, or compression (Fig. 6.1A). The weight of the human body constantly produces compression on the

Box 6.1   Factors Affecting the Likelihood of Injury

- Size or magnitude of the force
- Direction in which the force is applied (i.e., axial compression, tensile, or shear force)
- Area over which the force is applied
- Magnitude of stress produced by the force

- The force's moment arm, which determines the amount of torque generated
- Material properties of the tissues affected and their ability to sustain strain

A. Compression   B. Tension   C. Shear

■■■■ FIGURE 6.1 **Mechanisms of injury.** Compression **(A)** and tension **(B)** are directed along the longitudinal axis of a structure, whereas shear **(C)** acts parallel to a surface.

bones that support it. The fifth lumbar vertebra must support the weight of the head, trunk, and arms when the body is erect, producing compression on the intervertebral disk below it. When a football player is sandwiched between two opposing players, the force acting on that player is compressive. In the absence of sufficient padding, compressive forces often result in bruises or contusions.

Axial loading in the direction opposite that of compression is called **tensile force**, or tension (Fig. 6.1B). Tension is a pulling force that tends to stretch the object to which it is applied. Muscle contraction produces tensile force on the attached bone, enabling movement of that bone. When the foot and ankle are inverted, the tensile forces applied to the lateral ligaments may result in an ankle sprain.

Whereas compressive and tensile forces are directed, respectively, toward and away from an object, a third category of force, termed **shear force**, acts parallel or tangent to a plane passing through the object (Fig. 6.1C). Shear force tends to cause one part of the object to slide or displace with respect to another part of the object. For example, shear forces acting on the spine can cause spondylolisthesis, a condition involving anterior slippage of a vertebra with respect to the vertebra below it.

When the human body sustains force, another important factor related to the likelihood of injury is the magnitude of the **stress** produced by that force. Mechanical stress is defined as force divided by the surface area over which the force is applied (Fig. 6.2). When a given

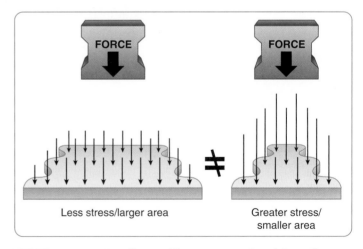

■■■■ FIGURE 6.2 **Stress.** The stress produced by a force depends on the area over which the force is spread. For example, the stress sustained by the superficial tissues of the arm would be lower than that with the force distributed directly over a small, bony landmark. The risk of injury increases when force is sustained over smaller areas.

force is distributed over a large area, the resulting stress is less than if the force were distributed over a smaller area. Alternatively, if a force is concentrated over a small area, the mechanical stress is relatively high. A high magnitude of stress, rather than a high magnitude of force, is what tends to result in injury to biologic tissues. One of the reasons that participants in contact sports wear pads is because a pad dissipates force across its entire area, thereby reducing the stress acting on the player.

Strain may be thought of as the amount of deformation an object undergoes in response to an applied force. Application of compressive force to an object produces shortening and widening of the structure, whereas tensile force produces lengthening and narrowing of the structure. Shear results in internal changes in the structure on which the force is acting. The ultimate strength of biologic tissues determines the amount of strain that a structure can withstand without fracturing or rupturing.

Injury to biologic tissues can result from a single traumatic force of relatively large magnitude or from repeated forces of relatively smaller magnitude. When a single force produces an injury, the injury is called an **acute injury,** and the causative force is termed **macrotrauma.** An acute injury, such as a ruptured anterior cruciate ligament or a fractured humerus, is characterized by a definitive moment of onset followed by a relatively predictable process of healing. When repeated or chronic loading over a period of time produces an injury, that injury is called a **chronic injury** or **stress injury,** and the causative mechanism is termed **microtrauma.** A chronic injury, such as glenohumeral bursitis or a metatarsal stress fracture, develops and worsens gradually over time, typically culminating in a threshold episode in which pain and inflammation become evident. Chronic injuries may persist for months or years.

Many tissues, including tendon, ligament, muscle, and bone, tend to respond to gradually increased mechanical stress by becoming larger and stronger. According to the basic principle of overload, the tissues of the body when stressed at tolerable limits will adapt and improve their function. Accordingly, in designing an exercise program, it is important to ensure a gradual increase in the intensity and duration of activities. For example, when a runner's training protocol incorporates progressively increasing mileage, it is important that this occur in a deliberate and carefully planned manner so that the body can adapt to the increased mechanical stress and, thereby, prevent a potential injury. Overuse syndromes and stress fractures result from the body's inability to adapt to an increased training regimen.

Torque and Its Effects

When a swinging door is opened, a hand applies force to the door, causing it to rotate about its hinges. Two factors influence whether the door will swing in response to the force. One factor is the force's **magnitude.** Equally important, however, is the force's **moment arm,** which is the perpendicular distance from the force's line of action to the axis of rotation. The product of a force and its moment arm is called **torque,** or moment. Torque may be thought of as a rotary force. It is the amount of torque acting on an object that determines whether a rotating body, such as a door, will move.

In the human body, torque produces rotation of a body segment about a joint. When a muscle develops tension, it produces torque at the joint that it crosses. The amount of torque produced is the product of muscle force and the muscle's moment arm with respect to the joint center (Fig. 6.3). For example, the torque produced by the biceps brachii is the product of the tension developed by the muscle and the distance between its attachment on the radius and the center of rotation at the elbow.

Excessive torque can produce injury. Such torque usually is generated by forces external to the body rather than by the muscles. The simultaneous application of

FIGURE 6.3 Movement and torque. Torque is the product of the magnitude of muscle force and the muscle's moment arm (perpendicular distance of the muscle's line of action to the axis of rotation at the joint center).

forces from opposite directions at different points along a structure, such as a long bone, generates a torque known as a bending moment, which can cause **bending** and, ultimately, fracture of the bone. For example, if a football player's leg is anchored to the ground and the player is tackled on that leg from the front while being pushed into the tackle from behind, a bending moment is created on the leg. When bending is present, the structure is loaded in tension on one side and in compression on the opposite side (Fig. 6.4A). Because bone is stronger in resisting compression compared with tension, the side of the bone loaded in tension will fracture if the bending moment is sufficiently large.

The application of torque about the long axis of a structure such as a long bone can cause **torsion**, or twisting of the structure (Fig. 6.4B). Torsion results in the creation of shear stress throughout the structure. This often is seen in skiing accidents in which one boot and ski are firmly planted as the skier rotates during a fall. The result is a torsion load that can cause a spiral fracture of the tibia.

According to the overload principle, the body, when stressed at tolerable limits, will adapt and improve its function. As such, the runner should be advised to incorporate gradual and progressive increases in mileage and time so that the body can adapt to the new training and, thereby, reduce the likelihood of injury.

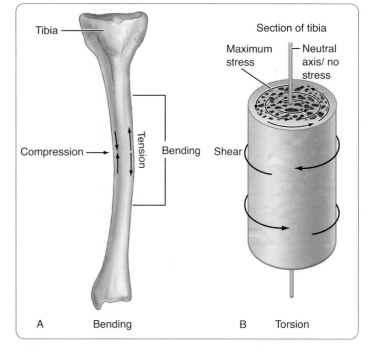

FIGURE 6.4 Bone injury mechanisms. A, Bones loaded in bending are subject to compression on one side and tension on the other. **B,** Bones loaded in torsion develop internal shear stress, with maximal stress at the periphery.

SOFT-TISSUE INJURIES

Two weeks into a new running program, a previously sedentary, middle-aged man reports pain along the distal third of the posteromedial border of the tibia of his lower left leg. He indicates that 5 days ago, he began experiencing pain while running, but it did not restrict his performance. He reports that for the past 2 days, however, the pain has restricted his performance. Based on this information, what actions, if any, should be taken with regard to this individual? Why?

Skin, tendon, muscle, and ligament are soft (nonbony) tissues that behave in characteristic ways when subjected to different forms of loading. Anatomic structure and material composition influence the mechanical behavior of each tissue.

Anatomic Properties of Soft Tissue

The major building block of skin, tendons, and ligaments is collagen, a protein that is strong in resisting tension. Collagen fibers have a wavy configuration in a tissue that is not under tension (Fig. 6.5). This enables collagenous tissues, which are inelastic, to stretch slightly under tensile loading as these fibers straighten. As such, collagen fibers provide strength and flexibility to tissues, but they are relatively inelastic. Elastin, another protein substance, provides added elasticity to some connective tissue structures.

Skin

The integumentary system comprises the skin, hair, nails, and glands of the skin and is the largest organ in the body. It provides protection and sensation, regulates fluid balance and temperature,

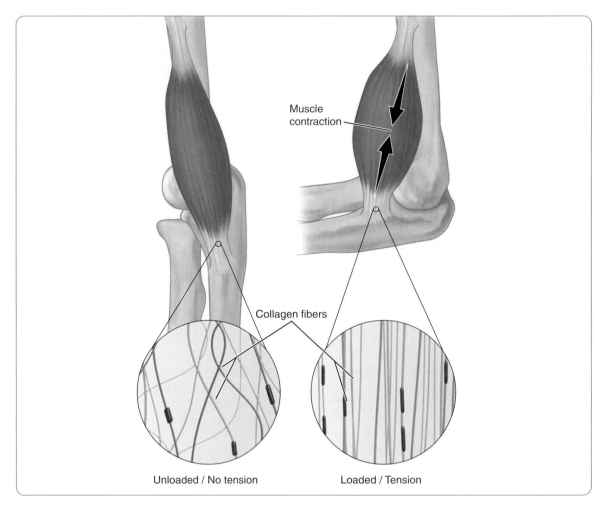

Muscle contraction

Collagen fibers

Unloaded / No tension

Loaded / Tension

▮▮▮ ▮ **FIGURE 6.5 Collagen fibers.** Collagen fibers have a wavy configuration when unloaded and a straightened configuration when loaded in tension.

and produces vitamins (vitamin D) and immune system components. The skin is composed of three regions. The outer region, known as the epidermis, has multiple layers containing the pigment melanin, along with the hair, nails, sebaceous glands, and sweat glands (Fig. 6.6). The outer surface, made up of dead epithelial cells, is replaced every 3 to 4 weeks by new cells pushed up from the dermis. The dermis is the largest portion of the skin and provides both strength and structure. It contains blood vessels, nerve endings, hair follicles, sebaceous glands, and sweat glands and is beneath the epidermis. The dermis is composed of dense, irregular connective tissue, which is characterized by a loose, multidirectional arrangement of collagen fibers. This fiber arrangement enables resistance to multidirectional loads, including compression, tension, and shear. This type of tissue also forms fascia, which are fibrous sheets of connective tissue that surround muscles. Dense, irregular connective tissue also covers internal structures, such as the liver, lymph nodes, and testes, as well as bone, cartilage, and nerves. The innermost layer of skin is the subcutaneous or hypodermal layer. The primary tissue is adipose, which provides cushioning between the skin layers, muscle, and bone and is instrumental in regulating body temperature because of its insulating properties.

Elastic fibers and reticular fibers are other components of the skin. Elastic fibers provide the skin with some elasticity. Reticular fibers are composed of a type of collagen known as reticulin. These fibers function like collagen fibers but are much thinner, and they provide support for internal structures, such as the lymph nodes, spleen, bone marrow, and liver.

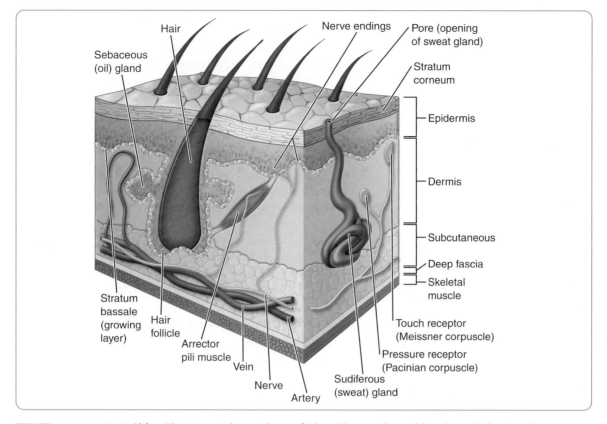

Hair
Nerve endings
Pore (opening of sweat gland)
Sebaceous (oil) gland
Stratum corneum
Epidermis
Dermis
Subcutaneous
Deep fascia
Skeletal muscle
Stratum bassale (growing layer)
Hair follicle
Arrector pili muscle
Vein
Nerve
Artery
Sudiferous (sweat) gland
Pressure receptor (Pacinian corpuscle)
Touch receptor (Meissner corpuscle)

FIGURE 6.6 Skin. The two major regions of the skin are the epidermis and the dermis.

Tendons, Aponeuroses, and Muscles

Tendons connect muscle to bone. They are composed of dense, regular connective tissue that consists of tightly packed bundles of unidirectional collagen fibers (Fig. 6.7). The collagen fibers are arranged in a parallel pattern, enabling resistance to high, unidirectional tensile loads when the attached muscle contracts. By virtue of their collagenous composition, tendons are about twice as strong as the muscles to which they attach.

The aponeuroses are another set of structures formed by dense, regular connective tissue. These are strong, flat, sheet-like tissues that attach muscles to other muscles or bones.

Muscle is a highly organized structure. A sheath known as the endomysium surrounds each muscle cell, or fiber. Small numbers of fibers are bound up into fascicles by a dense connective tissue sheath called the perimysium. A muscle is composed of several fascicles surrounded by the epimysium (Fig. 6.8).

The structure and composition of muscle enable it to function in a **viscoelastic** fashion—that is, with both elasticity and time-dependent extensibility. **Extensibility** is the ability to be stretched or increase in length, whereas **elasticity** is the ability to return to normal length after either lengthening or shortening has taken place. The viscoelastic aspect of muscle extensibility enables muscle to stretch to greater lengths over time in response to a sustained tensile force. This means that a static stretch maintained for 30 seconds is more effective than a series of short, ballistic stretches for increasing muscle length.

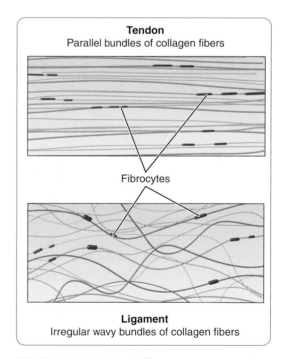

Tendon
Parallel bundles of collagen fibers

Fibrocytes

Ligament
Irregular wavy bundles of collagen fibers

FIGURE 6.7 Collagen arrangements in tendon and ligament tissue. The arrangement of collagen in tendons and ligaments differs, producing differences in their ability to resist tensile loads.

FIGURE 6.8 **Muscle tissue.** Skeletal muscle is composed of muscle cells, connective tissue, blood vessels, and nerves.

Another of muscle's characteristic properties, **irritability**, is the ability to respond to a stimulus. Stimuli affecting muscles can be either electrochemical, such as an action potential from the attaching nerve, or mechanical, such as an external blow to the muscle. If the stimulus is of sufficient magnitude, muscle responds by developing tension. The ability to develop **tension** is a property unique to muscle. Although some sources refer to this ability as contractility, a muscle may or may not shorten when tension is developed. For example, isometric "contraction" involves no joint movement and no change in muscle length, and eccentric "contraction" actually involves lengthening of the muscle developing tension. Only when a muscle develops tension concentrically does it also shorten. When a stimulated muscle develops tension, the amount of tension present is the same throughout the muscle and tendon and at the site of the tendon attachment to bone.

Joint Capsule and Ligaments

A joint capsule is a membrane that encloses a joint. It functions to hold the bones firmly in place. The outer portion of the capsule is fibrous and composed primarily of collagen. The inner lining of the capsule consists of a synovial membrane, which secretes a clear, slightly yellow liquid, called synovial fluid, that provides lubrication inside the articular capsule at synovial joints. (Joints are explained in more detail later in this chapter.)

Ligaments connect bone to bone. Similar to tendons, they are composed of dense, regular connective tissue that consists of tightly packed bundles of unidirectional collagen fibers. In ligaments, however, the parallel collagen fibers also are interwoven. This arrangement is well suited to ligament function, providing resistance to large tensile loads along the long axis of the ligament but also providing resistance to smaller tensile loads from other directions.

Ligaments contain more elastin than tendons and, as such, are somewhat more elastic. This is critical from a functional standpoint, because ligaments are connected at both ends to bones whereas tendons attach on one end to muscle, a tissue with some elasticity.

Bursa

Bursa are membranous sacs that contain small amounts of synovial fluid and serve to reduce friction. Common sites for bursa are in the tissues where friction develops, including the area between tendons and bone, tendons and skin, and ligaments and bone.

Anatomic Properties of Joints

A joint is the site at which two bones connect. The study of joints is call **arthrology**. Joints can be classified by structure, function, or number of axes present that permit motion.

Classification of Joints

The structural classification of joints focuses on the material binding the bones together. In this case, joints are classified as fibrous, cartilaginous, or synovial. Functionally, joints are classified as synarthrodial (i.e., immovable joints), amphiarthrodial (i.e., slightly moveable joints), or diarthrodial (i.e., freely movable joints). Human movement often is described in three dimensions based on a system of planes and axes. Based on movement potential, joints are classified as nonaxial (i.e., slipping movements only, because the joint has no axis around which movement can occur), uniaxial (i.e., movement in one plane), biaxial (i.e., movement in two planes), or multiaxial (i.e., movement in or around three planes).

FIBROUS JOINTS. The fibrous joints of the bones are held together by fibrous tissue. The amount of movement at a fibrous joint (**synarthrosis**) depends on the length of the fibers uniting the bones. A fibrous joint can absorb shock, but it permits little or no movement of the articulating bones. **Sutures,** which are seen only in the skull, involve irregularly grooved, articulating bone sheets tightly bound by fibers that are continuous with the periosteum. **Syndesmoses** are joints that are joined by dense fibrous tissue that permit extremely limited motion. The tissue may be a ligament or a fibrous membrane (e.g., the inferior tibiofibular joint or the interosseous membrane between the interosseous borders of the radius and ulna). A unique joint, a **gomphosis** joint, is found between a tooth and the bone in its alveolus (socket) where the fibrous tissue of the periodontal ligament firmly anchors the tooth.

CARTILAGINOUS JOINTS. The cartilaginous joints (amphiarthroses) unite bones by either hyaline cartilage or fibrocartilage. The sternocostal joints and the epiphyseal plates before ossification are examples of a primary cartilaginous joint, or a **synchondrosis**, whereby the articulating bones are held together by a thin layer of hyaline cartilage. In a secondary cartilaginous joint, the articular surfaces of the bones are covered with hyaline cartilage, which in turn is fused to an intervening pad, or plate, of fibrous tissue or fibrocartilage. These are strong, slightly movable joints designed for strength and shock absorption. Examples of secondary cartilaginous joints are the pubic symphysis (**symphyses**), intervertebral joints, and manubriosternal joint (between the manubrium and the body of the sternum).

SYNOVIAL JOINTS. From a functional perspective, synovial joints (**diarthroses**) are the most common and most important type of joint. They normally provide free movement between the articulating bone surfaces. Freely movable joints predominantly are seen in the limbs, whereas immovable and slightly movable joints largely are restricted to the axial skeleton. Diarthrodial joints are classified according to their shape, which dictates the type and range of motion permitted. The classifications are as follows:

- **Plane.** The articulating surfaces are nearly flat, and the only movement permitted is nonaxial gliding or short slipping movement. Examples include the intermetatarsal, intercarpal, and facet joints of the vertebrae.

- **Hinge.** One articulating bone surface is concave, and the other is convex. Strong collateral ligaments restrict motion to a single plane (uniaxial). Hinge joints permit flexion and extension only and can be seen at the elbow and interphalangeal joints.

- **Pivot.** A rounded or conical end of one bone rotates within a sleeve or ring composed of bone (and, possibly, ligaments), allowing uniaxial rotation of one bone around its own long axis or against another. The atlantoaxial joint and both the proximal and distal radioulnar joints are examples of this type of joint.

- **Condyloid.** The oval (ellipsoidal) articular surface of one bone fits into a reciprocal concavity of another. These biaxial joints permit all angular motions—namely, flexion, extension, abduction, adduction, and circumduction. The key characteristic of these joints is that both articulating surfaces are oval. The radiocarpal (wrist) joint and the metacarpophalangeal (knuckle) joints are typical condyloid joints.

- **Saddle.** These biaxial joints resemble a condyloid joint; however, saddle joints allow greater freedom of movement. Each articular surface has both concave and convex areas; that is, it is shaped like a saddle. The carpometacarpal joint of the thumb is an example of this type of joint.

- **Ball-and-socket.** The spherical or hemispherical head of one bone articulates with the cup-like socket of another. These joints are multiaxial and the most freely moving synovial joints in that

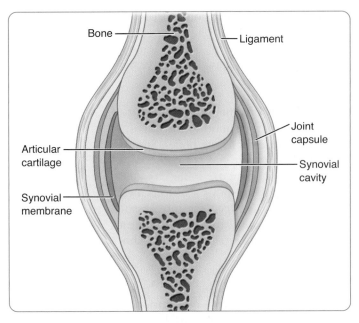

FIGURE 6.9 Joint capsule. Synovial joints have articular cartilage, a joint (synovial) cavity, an articular capsule, synovial membrane, synovial fluid, and reinforcing ligaments.

they permit universal movement in all axes and planes, including rotation. Examples include the shoulder and hip joints.

General Structure of Synovial Joints

Diarthrodial joints are distinguished by five features (Fig. 6.9):

1. **Articular cartilage.** Glassy-smooth hyaline cartilage covers the ends of the bony surfaces. These cushions absorb compression placed on the joint and, thereby, protect the bone ends from being crushed. The cartilage has no nerves or blood vessels; it is nourished by the synovial fluid covering its free surface. The nutrients in the synovial fluid come from the capillaries in the synovial membrane.

2. **Joint (synovial) cavity.** Unique to synovial joints, the joint cavity is filled with synovial fluid.

3. **Articular capsule.** The joint cavity is enclosed by a double-layered capsule. The external layer is a tough, flexible, fibrous capsule that is continuous with the periosteum of the articulating bones. The capsule functions to help hold the bones of the joint in place. The inner layer is a synovial membrane composed of loose connective tissue, which covers all internal joint surfaces that are not hyaline cartilage. The synovial membrane produces synovial fluid that lubricates the joint.

4. **Synovial fluid.** A small amount of synovial fluid occupies all free spaces within the joint capsule. This fluid is derived largely by filtration from blood flowing through the capillaries in the synovial membrane. Synovial fluid has a viscous, egg-white consistency because of its content of hyaluronic acid secreted by cells in the synovial membrane, but it thins and becomes less viscous as it warms during joint activity. Synovial fluid also is found within the articular cartilages, providing a slippery, weight-bearing film that reduces friction between the cartilages. In a weeping action, the fluid is forced from the cartilages when a joint is compressed. As pressure on the joint is relieved, the synovial fluid seeps back into the articular cartilages like water into a sponge. Synovial fluid also contains phagocytic cells that clear the joint cavity of microbes or cellular debris.

5. **Reinforcing ligaments.** Synovial joints are reinforced by a number of ligaments. More commonly, the ligaments are intrinsic, or capsular; that is, they are thickened parts of the fibrous capsule. In some cases, ligaments may remain distinct and are found outside the capsule (extracapsular) or deep to it (intracapsular). Because intracapsular ligaments are covered with synovial membrane, they do not actually lie within the joint cavity (extrasynovial).

Some synovial joints have other distinguishing features besides those listed above. **Articular disks** are present in some synovial joints where the articulating surfaces are incongruous (e.g., the articular disk of the wrist joint). These fibrocartilaginous pads help to protect and hold the bones together. In some joints, they are attached to only one of the bones (e.g., the menisci in the knee). Articular disks have no nerves except at the attached margins. Some synovial joints have a fibrocartilaginous ring, called a **labrum,** which deepens the articular surface of one of the bones (e.g., the acetabular labrum in the hip joint). In other synovial joints, a tendon passes within the capsule of the joint (e.g., the long head of the biceps brachii muscle runs within the shoulder joint capsule).

Classification of Skin Injuries

Forces applied to the body in different ways and from different directions result in different types of injury. Because the skin is the body's first layer of defense against injury, it is the most frequently injured body tissue.

Box 6.2 Signs and Symptoms of Contusions

- History of acute onset is present.
- Mechanism is usually a compressive force.
- Pain is localized over the injury site.
- Ecchymosis may be present if hemorrhage is superficial.
- Range of motion may be limited because of swelling and hemorrhage.
- Swelling may compress nerves, leading to pain and temporary paralysis.
- If the compressive force is great enough, injury also may occur in muscle tissue (strain).

Abrasions are common, minor skin injuries caused by shear when the skin is scraped with sufficient force, usually in one direction, against a rough surface. The greater the applied force, the more layers of skin are scraped away.

Blisters are minor skin injuries caused by repeated application of shear in one or more directions, as happens when a shoe rubs back and forth against the foot. The result is the formation of a pocket of fluid between the epidermis and dermis as fluid migrates to the site of injury.

Skin bruises are injuries resulting from compression sustained during a blow. Damage to the underlying capillaries causes the accumulation of blood within the skin.

Incisions, lacerations, avulsions, and punctures are breaks in the skin resulting from injury. An incision is a clean cut produced by the application of a tensile force to the skin as it is stretched along a sharp edge. A laceration is an irregular tear in the skin that typically results from a combination of tension and shear. An avulsion is a severe laceration that results in complete separation of the skin from the underlying tissues. A puncture wound results when a sharp, cylindrical object penetrates the skin and underlying tissues with tensile loading.

Classification of Muscle/Tendon Injuries

Injuries to the soft tissues below the skin also are dependent on the nature of the causative force, the location of the force, and the material properties of the involved tissues. Muscle **contusions,** or bruises, result from a direct compressive force sustained from a heavy blow. Such injuries vary in severity in accordance with the area and depth over which blood vessels are ruptured (Box 6.2). **Ecchymosis,** or tissue discoloration, may be present if the hemorrhage is superficial. As blood and lymph flow into the damaged area, swelling occurs, often resulting in the formation of a hard mass composed of blood and dead tissue called a **hematoma.** This mass may restrict joint motion. Nerve compression usually accompanies such injuries, leading to pain and, sometimes, temporary paralysis.

Muscle contusions are rated in accordance with the extent to which associated joint range of motion is impaired (Table 6.1). A first-degree contusion causes little or no restriction in range of

TABLE 6.1 Classifications of Contusions

	FIRST DEGREE	SECOND DEGREE	THIRD DEGREE
Damage to tissue	Superficial tissues are crushed	Superficial and some deep tissues are crushed	Deeper tissues are crushed (fascia surrounding muscle may rupture, allowing swollen tissues to protrude)
Weakness	None	Mild to moderate	Moderate to severe
Muscle spasm	None	None	Possible
Loss of function	Mild	Moderate	Severe
Ecchymosis	Mild	Moderate	Severe
Swelling	Mild	Moderate	Severe
Range of motion	No restriction	Decreased	Significantly decreased because of swelling

Box 6.3 Signs and Symptoms of Strains and Sprains

Strains

- History of acute onset is present.
- Mechanism of injury results from overstretch or overload.
- Pain is localized over the injury site, which tends to be at or near a musculotendinous junction.
- Discoloration, in severe cases, is caused by blood pooling distal to the site of trauma.
- If moderate, muscle weakness is evident.

Sprains

- History of acute onset is present.
- Mechanism of injury may result from overstretch or overload.
- Pain is localized over the injury site.
- Joint instability is detectable, if assessed before joint effusion.
- If severe, injury may result in subluxation or dislocation of the joint.

movement, a second-degree contusion causes a noticeable reduction in range of motion, and a third-degree contusion causes severe restriction of motion. With a third-degree contusion, the fascia surrounding the muscle may be ruptured, causing swollen muscle tissues to protrude.

Traumatic injury to muscles and tendons, termed **strains**, are caused by indirect forces (i.e., abnormally high tensile forces) that produce rupturing of the tissue and subsequent hemorrhage and swelling (Box 6.3). The likelihood of strains depends on the magnitude of the force and the structure's cross-sectional area. The greater the cross-sectional area of a muscle, the greater its strength, meaning it can produce more force and translate that force to the attached tendon. In a similar manner, the larger the cross-sectional area of the tendon, the greater the force it can withstand. The increased cross-sectional area translates to reduced stress. Because tendons are stronger than their attached muscle, the muscle portion of the musculotendinous unit almost always ruptures first. Muscle strains tend to be located near the musculotendinous junction, where muscle cross-sectional area is smallest. A tendon begins to develop tears when it is stretched approximately 5 to 8% beyond its normal length (1).

Strains are categorized as first, second, and third degree (Table 6.2). First-degree strains involve only microtearing of the collagen fibers. They are characterized by mild pain and local tenderness, but they may present with no readily observable symptoms. In a first-degree strain, no loss of function in activities of daily living occurs. Second-degree injuries involve an extensive rupturing of the tissue and are characterized by moderate pain, muscle weakness, and loss of function. Third-degree injuries produce a major loss of tissue continuity that results in a significant loss of function or movement. Severe pain followed by decreased pain attributed to nerve separation is typical in a third-degree strain. The tearing of muscle tissue can damage small blood vessels, which results in bleeding that may present as swelling and ecchymosis, particularly if the damage is superficial rather than deep.

Although typically not associated with injury, muscle **cramps** and **spasms** are painful, involuntary muscle contractions common to participation in sport and physical activity. A cramp is a painful, involuntary contraction that may be **clonic**, with alternating contraction and relaxation, or **tonic**, with continued contraction over a period of time. Cramps appear to be brought on by a biochemical imbalance, sometimes associated with muscle fatigue. A muscle spasm is an involuntary contraction of short duration caused by reflex action that can be biochemically derived or initiated by a mechanical blow to a nerve or muscle.

Myositis and **fasciitis** refer, respectively, to inflammation of a muscle's connective tissues and inflammation of the sheaths of fascia surrounding portions of muscle. These are chronic conditions that develop over time as the result of repeated body movements that irritate these tissues.

TABLE 6.2 Classifications of Strains

	FIRST DEGREE	SECOND DEGREE	THIRD DEGREE
Damage to muscle	Few fibers of muscle are torn	Nearly half of muscle fibers are torn	All muscle fibers are torn (rupture)
Weakness	Mild	Moderate to severe (reflex inhibition)	Moderate to severe
Muscle spasm	Mild	Moderate to severe	Moderate to severe
Loss of function	Mild	Moderate to severe	Severe (reflex inhibition)
Swelling	Mild	Moderate to severe	Moderate to severe
Palpable defect	No	No	Yes (if early)
Pain on contraction	Mild	Moderate to severe	None to mild
Pain with stretching	Yes	Yes	No
Range of motion	Decreased	Decreased	May increase or decrease depending on swelling

Tendinitis and **tenosynovitis** involve, respectively, inflammation within the tendon itself or of the tendon sheath. Tendinitis is closely related to the process of normal aging and degenerative changes within tendons (tendinosis), and it is characterized by pain and swelling with tendon movement (Box 6.4). Tenosynovitis may be acute or chronic. Acute tenosynovitis is characterized by a grating sound (crepitus) with movement, inflammation, and local swelling. Chronic tenosynovitis has the additional symptom of nodule formation in the tendon sheath.

Prolonged chronic inflammation of a muscle or tendon can result in the accumulation of mineral deposits resembling bone in the affected tissues, a process known as **ectopic calcification**. Accumulation of mineral deposits in muscle is known as **myositis ossificans**. A common site for this condition is the quadriceps region. The muscle typically is very tender, and as the ossificans develops, a hardened mass can be palpated within the muscle mass. In tendons, the condition is called **calcific tendinitis**.

Overuse injuries may result from intrinsic factors (e.g., malalignment of limbs, muscular imbalances, and other anatomic factors) or extrinsic factors (e.g., training errors, faulty technique, incorrect surfaces and equipment, and poor environmental conditions). Typically, overuse injuries are classified in four stages based on pain and dysfunction:

Stage 1: Pain after activity only.

Stage 2: Pain during activity, does not restrict performance.

Stage 3: Pain during activity, restricts performance.

Stage 4: Chronic, unremitting pain, even at rest.

Box 6.4   Signs and Symptoms of Tendinitis

- History of chronic onset is present.
- Mechanism of injury is caused by overuse or by repetitive overstretch or overload.
- Pain exists throughout the length of the tendon and increases during palpation.
- Swelling may be minor to major, and thickening of the tendon may be present.
- Crepitus may be present.
- Pain occurs at the extremes of motion during passive range of motion and active range of motion.
- Pain increases during stretching and resisted range of motion; strength decreases with pain.

Joint Injury Classifications

Sprains are traumatic injury to ligaments. Abnormally high tensile forces produce a stretching or tearing of tissues that compromises the ability of the ligament to stabilize the joint (Box 6.3). The tissue tearing also results in the flow of blood and lymph into the damaged area, producing swelling and restricting the range of motion.

Sprains are categorized as first, second, and third degree (Table 6.3). First-degree sprains involve only microtearing of the collagen fibers. Signs and symptoms include mild discomfort, mild point tenderness, minimal or no swelling, but minimal or no loss of function. Second-degree injuries involve tearing of nearly half the ligament fibers that result in a moderate loss of function and detectable joint instability. They are characterized by moderate pain, moderate swelling, and ecchymosis. Third-degree sprains produce a major loss of tissue continuity that results in a significant loss of function, severe instability, and severe pain.

A dislocation is a traumatic injury that occurs when the bones that comprise a joint are forced beyond their normal position, resulting in the displacement of one joint surface on another. A partial or incomplete dislocation is called a **subluxation**. The resultant damage includes rupturing of the joint capsule and ligaments as well as potential tearing of surrounding muscle–tendon units. In addition, many acute dislocations have an associated fracture or nerve injury. Signs and symptoms associated with a dislocation include pain, swelling, point tenderness, deformity, and loss of limb function.

Because of extensive stretching of the connective tissues surrounding a joint associated with a traumatic dislocation, susceptibility to chronic or recurrent dislocations is increased. Less force is required to sustain a recurrent dislocation. Whereas recurrent dislocations may be less painful, the subsequent damage to joint structures can be extensive and lead to chronic joint problems. The most common sites for dislocations are the fingers and the glenohumeral joint of the shoulder.

Osteoarthritis is a type of arthritis attributed to degeneration of the articular cartilage in a joint. Individuals with osteoarthritis experience pain and limited movement at the involved joint. Osteoarthritis has no definitive cause; rather, it is attributed to a combination of factors, including stresses sustained during certain types of physical activity, joint trauma, and the aging process. It is one of the leading causes of disability among American adults. It should be noted, however, that physical activity is being promoted as a potential strategy for managing arthritis (2).

Bursitis involves irritation of one or more bursae. It may be acute or chronic, depending on whether it is brought on by a single traumatic compression or by repeated compressions associated with overuse of the joint. Local swelling of a bursa can be very pronounced, particularly at the

TABLE 6.3 Classifications of Sprains

	FIRST DEGREE	SECOND DEGREE	THIRD DEGREE
Damage to ligament	Few fibers of ligament are torn	Nearly half of fibers are torn	All ligament fibers are torn (rupture)
Distraction with stress tests	<5 mm distraction	5-10 mm distraction	>10 mm distraction
Weakness	Mild	Mild to moderate	Mild to moderate
Muscle spasm	None	None to minor	None to minor
Loss of function	Mild	Moderate to severe	Severe (instability)
Swelling	Mild	Moderate	Moderate to severe
Pain on contraction	None	None	None
Pain with stretching	Yes	Yes	No
Range of motion	Decreased	Decreased	May increase or decrease depending on swelling; dislocation or subluxation possible

olecranon bursa of the elbow and the prepatellar bursa of the knee. An inflamed bursa is point tender and can be warm to the touch.

A *The runner's symptoms suggest a stage 3 overuse injury. He should be advised to stop running until a complete assessment can be performed. Because the pain is only present on the left leg, the assessment should include attention to both intrinsic and extrinsic factors that could contribute to injury.*

SOFT-TISSUE HEALING

Q *An assessment of the middle aged male runner suggests a possible lower leg strain. Clearly, identification of the type of injury is advantageous in making decisions concerning management, but such identification is only part of the process. Why is an understanding of the healing of soft tissue essential in determining the management of injury?*

The reparative process for injured soft tissues involves a complex series of interrelated physical and chemical activities. Because the normal healing process takes place in a regular and predictable fashion, knowledge of the various signs and symptoms exhibited at the injury site is essential for monitoring the progress of healing. Ultimately, this information is critical to decisions regarding appropriate rehabilitation and return to participation.

Healing of soft tissues is a three-phase process involving inflammation, proliferation, and maturation. Although it is useful to discuss the healing phenomenon in terms of these different stages, it should be recognized that these processes usually overlap, both spatially and temporally, within injured tissues.

Inflammatory Phase (Days 0–6)

The familiar symptoms of inflammation have long been recognized and, in fact, were documented by early Greek and Roman physicians as rubor (redness), calor (local heat), tumor (swelling), dolor (pain), and in severe cases, functio laesa (loss of function). Although inflammation can be produced by an adverse response to chemical, thermal, and infectious agents, the focus of this explanation is the characteristic course of the inflammatory response following injury.

Depending on the nature of the causative forces, inflammation can be acute or chronic. Acute inflammatory response is of relatively brief duration and involves a characteristic hemodynamic activity that generates **exudate**, a plasma-like fluid that exudes out of tissue or its capillaries and is composed of protein and granular leukocytes (white blood cells). Alternatively, chronic inflammatory response is of prolonged duration and is characterized by the presence of nongranular leukocytes and the production of scar tissue.

The beginning of the acute inflammatory phase involves the activation of three mechanisms that act to stop blood loss from the wound. The first mechanism involves local vasoconstriction that lasts from a few seconds to as long as 10 minutes. Larger blood vessels constrict in response to signals from neurotransmitters, and the capillaries and smaller arterioles and venules constrict because of the influence of serotonin and catecholamines released from the platelets and serum during injury. The resulting reduction in the volume of blood flow in the region promotes increased blood viscosity or resistance to the flow, which further reduces blood loss at the injury site.

A second response to the loss of blood is the platelet reaction. The platelet reaction provokes clotting as individual cells irreversibly combine with each other and with fibrin to form a mechanical plug that occludes the end of a ruptured blood vessel. As the fibrin forms the blood clot or scab, this covering mechanism on the skin surface protects the underlying tissues from harmful bacterial invasion. The platelets also produce an array of chemical mediators that play significant roles in the inflammatory and proliferation phases of healing. These mediators include serotonin, adrenaline, noradrenaline, and histamine, all of which are primary agents in the inflammatory response. The enzyme adenosine triphosphatase, which is central in supplying the energy needed for healing, also is found in platelets.

The third response is the activation of the coagulation cascade. A cascade is a heightened physiologic response consisting of several different, interrelated processes. Fibrinogen molecules are converted into fibrin for clot formation through two different pathways. The extrinsic pathway is activated by thromboplastin, which is released from damaged tissue. The intrinsic pathway, inside the blood vessels, is enabled by the interaction between platelets and the Hageman factor. Both paths result in the formation of prothrombin activator that converts prothrombin into thrombin.

Following vasoconstriction, vasodilation is brought on by a local axon reflex and the complement and kinin cascades. In the complement cascade, approximately 20 proteins that normally circulate in the blood in inactive form become active to promote a variety of activities essential for healing. One process activated is the attraction of neutrophils and macrophages to rid the injury site of debris and infectious agents through **phagocytosis**. As the flow of blood to the injured area slows, these cells are redistributed to the periphery, where they begin to adhere to the endothelial lining. Mast cells and basophils also are stimulated to release histamine, further promoting vasodilation. The kinin cascade provokes the conversion of the inactive enzyme kallikrein to the activated bradykinin in both blood and tissue. Bradykinin promotes vasodilation and increases permeability of the blood vessel wall, contributing to the formation of tissue exudate.

In addition, increased blood flow to the region causes swelling. Blood from the broken vessels and damaged tissues forms a hematoma, which in combination with necrotic tissue forms the **zone of primary injury**.

Approximately 1 hour postinjury, swelling, or **edema**, occurs as the vascular walls become more permeable, and increased pressure within the vessels forces a plasma exudate out into the interstitial tissues (Fig. 6.10). This increased permeability or porosity of the blood vessel walls typically exists for only a few minutes in cases of mild trauma, with a return to normal permeability in 20 to 30 minutes. More severe trauma can result in a prolonged state of increased permeability and, sometimes, in delayed onset of increased permeability, with swelling not becoming apparent until some time after the original injury. The tissue exudate provides a critically important part of the body's defense, both by diluting toxins present in the wound and by enabling delivery of the cells that remove damaged tissue and enable reconstruction.

The complement and kinin cascades act to speed the arrival of reparative cells in the exudate. **Mast cells** are connective tissue cells that carry heparin, which prolongs clotting, and histamine. Platelets and basophil leukocytes also transport histamine, which serves as a vasodilator and increases blood vessel permeability. The leukocytes release enzymes that interact with phospholipids in the

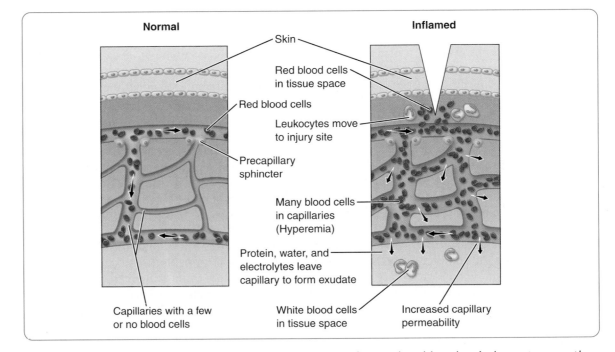

FIGURE 6.10 Acute inflammatory process. Edema forms when histochemical agents open the pores in the vascular walls, allowing plasma to migrate into the interstitial space.

cell membranes to produce arachidonic acid. Arachidonic acid activates further inflammation of the affected cells through production of chemical mediators, including prostaglandins and leukotrienes. Bradykinin, a major plasma protease present during inflammation, increases vessel permeability and stimulates nerve endings to cause pain. This chain of chemical activity produces the **zone of secondary injury**, which includes all the tissues affected by inflammation, edema, and hypoxia. After the debris and waste products from the damaged tissues are ingested through phagocytosis, the leukocytes re-enter the bloodstream, and the acute inflammatory reaction subsides.

The Proliferative Phase (Days 3–21)

The proliferative phase involves repair and regeneration of the injured tissue and takes place from approximately 3 days following the injury through the next 3 to 6 weeks, overlapping the later part of the inflammatory phase. The proliferative processes include the development of new blood vessels (angiogenesis), fibrous tissue formation (fibroplasia), generation of new epithelial tissue (re-epithelialization), and wound contraction.

This stage begins when the size of the hematoma is sufficiently diminished to allow room for the growth of new tissue. Although the skin has the ability to regenerate new skin tissue, the other soft tissues replace damaged cells with scar tissue.

Healing through scar formation begins with the accumulation of exuded fluid containing a large concentration of protein and damaged cellular tissues. This accumulation forms the foundation for a highly vascularized mass of immature connective tissues that include fibroblasts, which are capable of generating collagen. The fibroblasts begin to produce immature collagen through the process known as fibroplasia.

Fibroplasia and angiogenesis are interdependent processes, with the deposition of the new connective tissue matrix fueled by nutrients from the blood supply and the newly forming blood vessels reliant on mechanical support and protection from the matrix. The developing connective tissue at the wound site is primarily type I and III collagen, cells, blood vessels, and a matrix containing glycoproteins and proteoglycans. Type III collagen is particularly useful at this stage because of its ability to rapidly form cross-links that contribute to stabilization at the wound site. It is fibroblasts that have been chemically drawn to the region that secrete the collagen. The enzymatic reactions involved in collagen production are dependent on specific concentrations of oxygen, ascorbate, ferrous ions, and lactate within the microenvironment of the wound.

Fibroblasts also produce attachment factors that promote angiogenesis by helping the growing vessels attach to basement membrane collagen. The primary driving force for angiogenesis, however, comes from the platelet response and the hypoxic wound environment. New vessel formation begins with activation of enzymes by a potent growth factor, which acts on the existing vessels to dissolve their basement membranes and liberate endothelial cells. These cells are then chemically drawn to hypoxic sites within a wound, where they fuse and form new vessels.

Other characteristics of the proliferation stage include an increase in the number of blood vessels present, increased water content in the injury zone, and re-epithelialization at the surface caused by epithelial cells migrating from the periphery and toward the center of the wound.

Maturation Phase (Up to 1+ Year)

The final phase of soft-tissue wound repair is known as the maturation, or remodeling, phase. This period involves maturation of the newly formed tissue into scar tissue. The associated processes include decreased fibroblast activity, increased organization of the extracellular matrix, decreased tissue water content, reduced vascularity, and a return to normal histochemical activity. In soft tissue, these processes begin approximately 3 weeks postinjury, overlapping the proliferative phase. Type I and III collagen continue to increase, replacing immature collagen and resulting in contraction of the wound.

Although the epithelium typically has regenerated completely by 3 to 4 weeks postinjury, the tensile strength of the wound at this time is only approximately 25% of normal (3). After several more months, strength may still be as much as 30% below the preinjury level (4). This is partly because of the orientation of the collagen fibers, which tends to be more vertical during this period of time than in normal tissue, where their orientation usually is horizontal. The collagen turnover rate in a newly healed scar also is very high, so failure to provide appropriate support for the wound site can result in a larger scar. Excessive scar tissue is called keloid tissue.

Because scar tissue is fibrous, inelastic, and nonvascular, it is less strong and less functional than the original tissues. In addition, the development of the scar typically causes the wound to shrink, resulting in decreased flexibility of the affected tissues following the injury. This explains why someone, such as a person with paraplegia who has a healed pressure sore from a wheelchair seat in poor condition, can easily redevelop breakdown in the same area if the pressure stresses reoccur in that same area (5).

See *Phases of Soft-Tissue Wound Healing* on the companion website at thePoint for a summary of the three stages of the healing process.

Remodeling continues for a year or more as collagen fibers become oriented along the lines of mechanical stress to which the tissue usually is subjected. The tensile strength of scar tissue may continue to increase for as long as 2 years postinjury.

Muscle fibers are permanent cells that do not reproduce or proliferate in response to either injury or training. Reserve cells in the basement membrane of each muscle fiber, however, are able to regenerate muscle fiber following injury. Severe muscle injury can result in scarring or the formation of **adhesions** within the muscle, which inhibits the potential for fiber regeneration from the reserve cells. Consequently, following severe injury, muscle may regain only approximately 50% of its preinjury strength (1).

Because tendons and ligaments have few reparative cells, healing of these structures is a slow process that can take more than a year. Regeneration is enhanced by proximity to other soft tissues that can assist with supplying the chemical mediators and building blocks required. For this reason, isolated ligaments, such as the anterior cruciate, have poor chances for healing (6). If tendons and ligaments undergo abnormally high tensile stress before scar formation is complete, the newly forming tissues can be elongated. If this occurs in ligaments, joint instability may result.

Because tendons, ligaments, and muscles **hypertrophy** and **atrophy** in response to levels of mechanical stress, complete immobilization of the injury leads to atrophy, loss of strength, and decreased rate of healing in these tissues. The amount of atrophy generally is proportional to the time of immobilization. As such, although immobilization may be necessary to protect the injured tissues during the early stages of recovery, strengthening exercises should be implemented as soon as appropriate during rehabilitation of the injury. Increased risk for reinjury exists as long as the strength of affected tissues is less than the preinjury level.

The Role of Growth Factors

Growth factors are proteins that play crucial roles during all three phases of the healing process. Their functions include attracting cells to the wound, stimulating their proliferation, and directing the deposition of the extracellular matrix.

First discovered in the granules of platelets, platelet-derived growth factor (PDGF) also is released from macrophages, endothelial cells, vascular smooth cells, and fibroblasts. The presence of PDGF is one of the most important factors in the success of the first two stages of healing. Platelet-derived growth factor acts as a chemical attractant for fibroblasts, neutrophils, and macrophages and also promotes the replication of fibroblasts and vascular smooth muscle cells. It also activates macrophages and stimulates fibroblasts to secrete types I and III collagen.

Another important growth factor, transforming growth factor–β, is actually a group of several different proteins with similar structural and chemical properties. Transforming growth factor–β is produced by platelets, macrophages, bone cells, monocytes, and lymphocytes and is capable of both stimulating and inhibiting fibroblasts. Transforming growth factor–β also stimulates angiogenesis and accelerates collagen deposition.

Another group of proteins with a common high affinity for heparin is called basic fibroblast growth factor. The platelet-derived enzyme heparitinase chemically separates this factor from heparin. Basic fibroblast growth factor stimulates proliferation of endothelial cells and is distributed in endothelial cells, macrophages, and fibroblasts. It is critically important in angiogenesis, releasing the basement membrane–degrading enzymes that separate endothelial cells before new vessel formation.

Two closely related growth factors are epidermal growth factor and transforming growth factor–α. Both originate from transmembrane proteins, and both act on the epidermal growth factor receptor. Whereas both of these growth factors facilitate the development of granulation tissue, transforming growth factor–α also regulates angiogenesis and promotes epidermal regrowth (7).

 Fortunately, the normal healing process takes place in a regular and predictable fashion. Knowledge of the various signs and symptoms exhibited at the injury site from the time of injury and its subsequent progression is essential for monitoring the progress of healing and for making appropriate decisions regarding management of the injury. If the runner's condition is not managed properly, it could result in both delayed and less-than-optimal healing, exacerbation of the condition, and development of additional injuries.

SOFT-TISSUE WOUND CARE MANAGEMENT

Initial management of the runner's condition involves reducing pain and inflammation. Describe a strategy for accomplishing this goal.

As discussed, soft-tissue injuries may involve open wounds (e.g., abrasions, blisters, lacerations, and puncture wounds) or closed wounds (e.g., contusion, strains, sprains, and bursitis). This section explains the immediate care of both broad categories of soft-tissue injuries.

Care of Open Soft-Tissue Injuries

In providing wound care for open soft-tissue injuries, it is critical to follow universal precautions and infection control standards. In addition to using safety equipment, disinfecting equipment and materials used during wound care, and properly discarding contaminated materials, several steps in general wound care should be followed:

- If possible, wash hands before beginning treatment.

- Apply gloves.

- Apply direct pressure to the wound with sterile gauze or a nonstick material.

- Cleanse the wound and the area around the wound (at least twice the size of the wound) with saline water or a similar antiseptic agent, such as povidone-iodine (Betadine).

- Dress and bandage the wound site securely for continued activity.

- Creams or ointments may or may not be used with occlusive dressings. If used, dressings should be covered beyond their borders with underwrap and elastic adhesive tape where possible.

> See *Field Strategy: General Guidelines for Preventing Spread of Bloodborne Pathogens,* on the companion website at thePoint.

- Change dressings as necessary, and look for signs of infection (i.e., local heat, swelling, redness, pain, pus, and elevated body temperature).

Wounds must be covered with an appropriate dressing. The decision about what type of dressing to use depends on the location, size, type/depth of wound, amount of drainage/exudate expected, presence of infection, need for debridement, and expected frequency and difficulty in dressing change, costs, and patient comfort (5). Common gauze dressings are relatively inexpensive, but they must be changed frequently, which increases its cost factor. Dry gauze prevents contamination, but it can lock in exudate and does not keep the wound moist. Wet gauze strips are used to pack wounds with tunnels or fistulas to aid in drainage. Nonadherent gauze, such as Telfa™, Xeroform™, or Vaseline Gauze™, absorbs some drainage or allows drainage through it but prevents any outer gauze dressing from adhering to the wound or sutures/staples and, thereby, prevents further injury when the dressing is removed (5).

Several choices exist beyond the traditional gauze dressing, including hydrocolloids, hydrogels, transparent films, collagen, alginates, foams, and antimicrobials. Hydrocolloids are indicated for use on partial- and full-thickness wounds with or without necrotic tissue and are useful on areas that require contouring, such as the heels or ears. Hydrogel dressings may be used on wounds with necrotic tissue, such as minor burns or tissue damaged by radiation. Transparent films are used on partial-thickness wounds with little or no exudate, on wounds with necrosis, or as a primary or secondary dressing over lacerations, abrasions, and second-degree burns. Collagen dressings typically are indicated for pressure ulcers, venous ulcers, surgical wounds, diabetic ulcers, abrasions, second-degree burns, and traumatic wounds, but they usually require a secondary dressing. Alginates are indicated for wounds with moderate to heavy exudate, such as over infected wounds, diabetic ulcers, and pressure ulcers, and also require a secondary dressing. Foam dressings have small, open cells capable of holding fluids. The area of the dressing directly over the wound is nonadherent (for easy removal) and is available with an adhesive border that can act as a bacterial barrier. Antimicrobial dressings are indicated for wounds that would benefit from topical antimicrobial agents. These dressings reduce the risk of infection in wounds, sites with percutaneous lines, and surgical incisions (8). In all cases, regardless of the dressing selected, a moist—not wet—environment is best to ensure adequate healing (9).

Field Strategy 6.1 explains the basic care for common skin injuries. It is assumed that the examiner is already gloved. These techniques can be adapted for use with other open wounds as well.

FIELD STRATEGY 6.1

Care of Open Wounds

Abrasions

1. Clean and remove visible contaminants with a fluid flush using water and sweeps of gauze.
2. Clean the wound site and area around the wound with antiseptic solution.
3. Dress and bandage the wound securely for continued play.
4. For dirty abrasions, or when it has been at least 5 years since a tetanus booster, refer for medical care.

Blisters

1. Clean both the wound site and the area around the wound with antiseptic solution.
2. Leave the roof of the blister intact for at least 24 hours, and cover the area with a topical antibiotic and a dry, sterile dressing. Do *not* aspirate a blood-filled blister.
3. If the blister is large and subject to continued compression, use a small, sterile needle to aspirate the clear fluid, or incise the skin of clear blisters according to physician protocol.
4. Once the fluid is removed, cleanse the area again with an antiseptic solution.
5. Pad the nontender skin around the blister with an adhesive, soft-foam material (donut pad), New Skin®, or 2nd Skin®.
6. Dress and bandage the wound site securely for continued play.

Incisions and Lacerations

1. Clean both the wound site and the area around the wound with antiseptic solution.

2. Spray tape adherent on a cotton-tipped applicator, and apply above and below the wound.
3. Beginning in the middle of the wound, bring the edges together, and secure the Steri-Strips® below the wound. Lift up and secure above the wound. Make sure the edges of the wound are approximated.
4. Apply a second Steri-Strips® in a similar manner immediately adjacent to one side of the original strip. Apply a third strip on the other side. Alternate sides until the entire wound is covered.
5. Dress the wound with an adhesive tincture base covered with an occlusive or nonstick, sterile dressing.
6. Sutures may be desirable for any depth of laceration, especially around the face. Any wound open to the full-thickness of the dermis, however, should be sutured within 10 hours of the injury.
7. Refer for medical care if it has been more than 5 years since a tetanus booster or if signs of infection appear.

Care of Closed Soft-Tissue Injuries

Closed wound care focuses on immediately reducing inflammation, pain, and secondary hypoxia. Several initial steps should be followed in providing general acute care:

- Apply crushed-ice packs for 30 minutes directly to the skin as quickly as possible following the injury (40 minutes for a large muscle mass, such as the quadriceps). Do not place a towel or elastic wrap (dry or wet) between the crushed-ice pack and skin, because this will reduce the effectiveness of the treatment.

- Apply the crushed-ice cold pack for 30 minutes. Elevate the body part at least 6 to 10 inches above the level of the heart.

- Following the initial ice treatment, remove the ice pack, apply a compression wrap, and continue elevation.

- Reapply the crushed-ice pack every 2 hours (every hour if the individual is active between applications, such as walking on crutches or showering) until bedtime.

- Instruct the individual to wear the compression wrap throughout the night.

> See *Field Strategy: Care of Closed Wounds* on the companion website at thePoint for information regarding the basic care of closed soft-tissue injuries after the acute protocol has been followed. Because the severity of injuries can range from mild to severe, these guidelines are provided as a general guide. Each injury must be assessed and treated on an individual basis.

A *An accepted strategy for managing the runner's pain and inflammation is the application of cold to the area. Cold, ideally in the form of a crushed-ice pack, should be applied directly to the site and surrounding area for 30 minutes and then reapplied every 2 hours throughout the day.*

BONE INJURIES

Q *Following a period of rehabilitation, including abstaining from running for a period 3 weeks, the runner is symptom free. He is given clearance from his physician to resume his running program with some modifications (i.e., a more gradual increase in time and intensity of running sessions). Within 4 weeks, however, he returns complaining of localized pain in the same area (i.e., posteromedial tibia approximately 3 inches proximal to the ankle joint). The pain has been present for 1 week and is particularly noticeable during weight-bearing activities. What injury should be suspected? What are the implications for the individual's continued training?*

In keeping with its material constituents and structural organization, bone behaves predictably in response to stress. The composition and structure of bone make it strong for its relatively light weight.

Anatomic Properties of Bone

The primary constituents of bone are calcium carbonate, calcium phosphate, collagen, and water. The minerals, making up 60 to 70% of bone weight, provide stiffness and strength in resisting compression. Collagen provides bone with some degree of flexibility and strength in resisting tension. Aging causes a progressive loss of collagen and increase in bone brittleness. As such, the bones of children are more pliable than those of adults.

Longitudinal bone growth continues only as long as the bone's epiphyseal plates, or growth plates, continue to exist (Fig. 6.11). Epiphyseal plates are cartilaginous disks near the ends of the long bones. Longitudinal bone growth takes place on the diaphysis (central) side of the plates. During or shortly after adolescence, the plate disappears, and the bone fuses, terminating longitudinal growth. Most

■■ ■■ FIGURE 6.11 Epiphyseal growth plate. The epiphyseal plates of the femur and tibia are visible in this radiograph. Note that the individual has a mild irregularity of the tibial tubercle characteristic of Osgood-Schlatter disease.

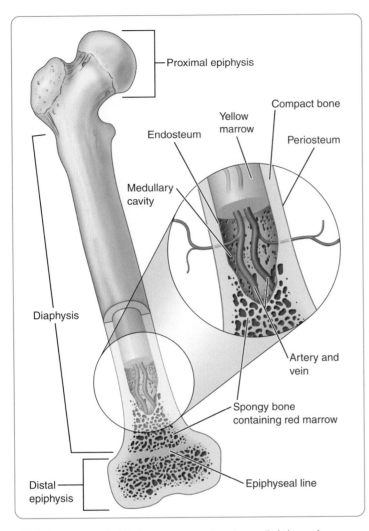

Proximal epiphysis

Compact bone

Yellow marrow

Endosteum

Periosteum

Medullary cavity

Diaphysis

Artery and vein

Spongy bone containing red marrow

Distal epiphysis

Epiphyseal line

FIGURE 6.12 Bone macrostructure. Epiphyseal growth lines are found at both ends of the bone. Cortical bone surrounds the cancellous bone and the medullary cavity. Cancellous bone is more porous than cortical bone.

epiphyses close by age 18, but some may be present until approximately age 25.

Although the most rapid bone growth occurs before adulthood, bones continue to grow in diameter throughout most of a person's life span. The internal layer of the periosteum builds new, concentric layers of bone tissue on top of the existing ones. At the same time, bone is resorbed or eliminated around the sides of the medullary cavity so that the diameter of the cavity is continually enlarged. The bone cells that form new bone tissue are called **osteoblasts**, and those that resorb bone are known as **osteoclasts**. In healthy adult bone, the activity of osteoblasts and osteoclasts, referred to as bone turnover, is largely balanced. The total amount of bone remains approximately constant until women reach 40 years of age and men reach 60 years, when a gradual decline in bone mass begins. As such, physically active individuals past these ages may be at increased risk for bone fractures; however, regular participation in weight-bearing exercise has been shown to be effective in reducing age-related bone loss.

Regardless of age, some bones are more susceptible to fracture as a result of their internal composition. Bone tissue is categorized as either **cortical**, if the porosity is low (with 5–30% nonmineralized tissue), or **cancellous**, if the porosity is high (with 30 to >90% of nonmineralized tissue) (Fig. 6.12). Most human bones have outer shells of cortical bone, with cancellous bone underneath. Cortical bone is stiffer, which means that it can withstand greater stress but less strain than cancellous bone; however, cancellous bone has the advantage of being spongier than cortical bone, which means that it can undergo more strain before fracturing. The mineralization of cancellous bone varies with the individual's age and with the location of the bone in the body. Both cortical and cancellous bone is anisotropic. As such, they exhibit different strengths and stiffnesses in response to forces applied from different directions. Bone is strongest in resisting compressive stress and weakest in resisting shear stress.

Bone size and shape also influence the likelihood of fracture. The direction and magnitude of the forces to which they are habitually subjected largely determine the shape and size of the bone. The direction in which new bone tissue forms is in response to the adaptation required in resisting encountered loads, particularly in regions of high stress, such as the femoral neck. The mineralization and girth of bone increases in response to increased levels of stress. For example, the bones of the dominant arm of professional tennis players and professional baseball players have been found to be larger and stronger than the bones of their nondominant arms (10,11).

Classification of Bone Injuries

A **fracture** is a disruption in the continuity of a bone (Fig. 6.13). Signs of fracture include swelling and bruising (discoloration), deformity or shortening of the limb, point tenderness, grating or crepitus, guarding or disability, and exposed bone ends.

The type of fracture that is sustained depends on the type of mechanical loading that caused it as well as on the health and maturity of the bone at the time of injury. Fractures are considered to

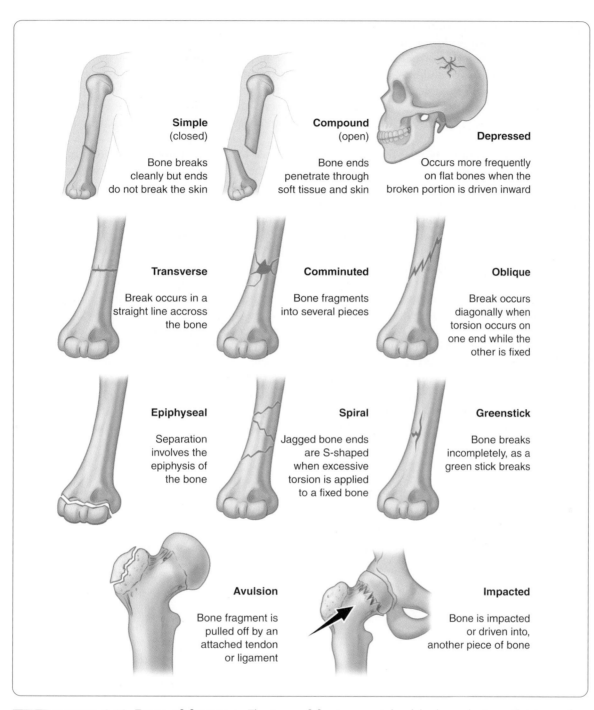

Simple
(closed)

Bone breaks
cleanly but ends
do not break the skin

Compound
(open)

Bone ends
penetrate through
soft tissue and skin

Depressed

Occurs more frequently
on flat bones when the
broken portion is driven inward

Transverse

Break occurs in a
straight line accross
the bone

Comminuted

Bone fragments
into several pieces

Oblique

Break occurs
diagonally when
torsion occurs on
one end while the
other is fixed

Epiphyseal

Separation
involves the
epiphysis of
the bone

Spiral

Jagged bone ends
are S-shaped
when excessive
torsion is applied
to a fixed bone

Greenstick

Bone breaks
incompletely, as a
green stick breaks

Avulsion

Bone fragment is
pulled off by an
attached tendon
or ligament

Impacted

Bone is impacted
or driven into,
another piece of bone

◼◼◼◼ FIGURE 6.13 **Types of fractures.** The type of fracture sustained is dependent on the type of mechanical load that causes the injury.

be closed when the bone ends remain intact within the surrounding soft tissues and to be open, or compound, when one or both bone ends protrude from the skin.

Excessive torsional and bending loads, as exemplified by tibial fractures resulting from skiing accidents, often produce spiral fractures of the long bones. Such fractures are the result of a combined loading pattern of shear and tension, producing failure at an oblique angle to the long axis of the bone.

Because bone is stronger in resisting compression than in resisting tension and shear, acute compression fractures of bone are rare. Under combined loading, however, a fracture resulting from a torsional load may be affected by the presence of a compressive load. An **impacted** fracture is one in which the opposite sides of the fracture are compressed together. Fractures that result in depression of bone fragments into the underlying tissues are termed **depressed**.

Because the bones of children contain relatively larger amounts of collagen compared with adult bones, they are more flexible and more resistant to fracture under day-to-day loading than adult bones are. Consequently, **greenstick** fractures, or incomplete fractures, are more common in children than in adults. A greenstick fracture is an incomplete fracture typically caused by bending or torsional loads.

Avulsions are another type of fracture caused by tensile loading that involve a tendon or ligament pulling a small chip of bone away from the rest of the bone. Explosive throwing and jumping movements may result in avulsion fractures. When loading is very rapid, a fracture is more likely to be **comminuted**, meaning that it contains multiple fragments.

Stress fractures, also known as fatigue fractures, result from repeated, low-magnitude forces. Stress fractures differ from acute fractures in that they can worsen over time, beginning as a small disruption in the continuity of the outer layers of cortical bone and ending as a complete cortical fracture, with possible displacement of the bone ends. Stress fractures of the metatarsals, femoral neck, and pubis have been reported among runners who have apparently overtrained. Stress fractures of the pars interarticularis region of the lumbar vertebrae occur with higher-than-normal frequencies among football linemen and female gymnasts.

Osteopenia, a condition of reduced bone mineral density, predisposes an individual to all types of fractures but particularly to stress fractures. The condition is found primarily among adolescent female athletes, especially distance runners, who are amenorrheic. Although **amenorrhea** among this group is not well understood, it appears to be related to a low percentage of body fat and/or high training mileage. The link between cessation of menses and osteopenia also is not well understood. Possible contributing factors include hyperactivity of osteoclasts, hypoactivity of osteoblasts, hormonal factors, and insufficiencies of dietary calcium or other minerals or nutrients.

Classification of Epiphyseal Injuries

The bones of children and adolescents are vulnerable to epiphyseal injuries, including injuries to the cartilaginous epiphyseal plate, articular cartilage, and apophysis. The apophyses are sites of tendon attachments to bone, where bone shape is influenced by the tensile loads to which these sites are subjected. Both acute and repetitive loading can injure the growth plate, potentially resulting in premature closure of the epiphyseal junction and termination of bone growth. "Little League elbow," for example, is a stress injury to the medial epicondylar epiphysis of the humerus. Salter (12) has categorized acute epiphyseal injuries into five distinct types (Fig. 6.14):

Type I: Complete separation of the epiphysis from the metaphysis with no fracture to the bone.

Type II: Separation of the epiphysis and a small portion of the metaphysis.

Type III: Fracture of the epiphysis.

Type IV: Fracture of a part of the epiphysis and metaphysis.

Type V: Compression of the epiphysis without fracture, resulting in compromised epiphyseal function.

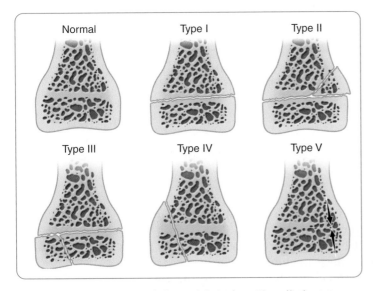

FIGURE 6.14 Epiphyseal injuries. Five distinct types of injuries involve the epiphysis.

Another category of epiphyseal injuries is referred to collectively as **osteochondrosis.** Osteochondrosis results from disruption of blood supply to an epiphysis, with associated tissue necrosis and potential deformation of the epiphysis. Because the cause of the condition is poorly understood, it typically is termed idiopathic osteochondrosis. Osteochondroses most commonly occur between the ages of 3 and 10 and are more prevalent among boys than girls (12). Specific disease names have been given to sites where osteochondrosis is common, such as Legg-Calvé-Perthes disease, which is osteochondrosis of the femoral head.

The apophyses also are subject to osteochondrosis, particularly among children and adolescents. These conditions, referred to as **apophysitis,** may be idiopathic; however, they can be associated with traumatic avulsion-type fractures. Common sites for apophysitis are the calcaneus (i.e., Sever disease) and the tibial tubercle at the site of the patellar tendon attachment (i.e., Osgood-Schlatter disease).

Bony Tissue Healing

Healing of acute bone fractures is a three-phase process, as is soft-tissue healing. The acute inflammatory phase lasts approximately 4 days. The formation of a hematoma in the medullary canal and surrounding tissues causes damage to the periosteum and surrounding soft tissues. The ensuing inflammatory response involves vasodilation, edema formation, and histochemical changes associated with soft-tissue inflammation.

During repair and regeneration, osteoclasts resorb damaged bone tissues, whereas osteoblasts build new bone. Between the fractured bone ends, a fibrous, vascularized tissue, known as a **callus,** is formed (Fig. 6.15). The callus contains weak, immature bone tissue that strengthens with time through bone remodeling. The process of callus formation is known as enchondral bone healing. An alternative process, known as direct bone healing, can occur when the fractured bone ends are immobilized in direct contact with one another. This enables new, interwoven bone tissue to be deposited without the formation of a callus. Unless a fracture is fixed by metal plates, screens, or rods, healing normally takes place through the enchondral process. Because noninvasive treatment generally is preferred, a fixation device is only implanted when it appears unlikely that the fracture will heal acceptably without one.

Maturation and remodeling of bone tissue involves osteoblast activity on the concave side of the fracture, which is loaded in compression, and osteoclast activity on the convex side of the fracture, which is loaded in tension. The process continues until normal shape is restored and bone strength is commensurate with the loads to which the bone is routinely subjected.

Because stress fractures continue to worsen as long as the site is overloaded, it is important to recognize these injuries as early as possible. Elimination or reduction of the repetitive mechanical stress causing the fracture is the primary factor necessary for healing. This allows a gradual restoration of the proper balance of osteoblast and osteoclast activity in the bone.

Management of Bone Injuries

Possible fractures can be detected with palpation, percussion, use of a tuning fork (vibrations), compression, and distraction (see Fig. 5.2). Palpation can detect deformity, crepitus, swelling, or increased pain at the fracture site. Percussion uses a tapping motion of the finger over a bony structure. A tuning fork works in the same manner; vibrations travel through the bone and cause increased pain at a fracture site. Compression is performed by gently compressing the distal end of the bone toward the proximal end or by encircling the body part (e.g., a foot or a hand) and gently squeezing, thereby compressing the heads of the bones together. Again, if a fracture is present, pain increases at the fracture site. Distraction employs a tensile force, whereby the application of traction to both ends of the fractured bone helps to relieve pain.

A suspected fracture should be splinted before the individual is moved to avoid damage to surrounding ligaments, tendons, blood vessels, and nerves. Field Strategy 6.2 explains the immediate management of fractures.

FIGURE 6.15 **Bone healing.** The process of endochondral bone healing involves callus formation.

Pain localized over a bone that is particularly painful during weight-bearing activities is a classic symptom of a stress injury. The runner should be referred to a physician for further evaluation. In addition, he should be advised to stop running and to reduce weight-bearing activities as much as possible.

FIELD STRATEGY 6.2

Management Algorithm for Bone Injuries

1. Remove clothing and jewelry from around the injury site. (Cut clothing away with scissors to avoid moving the injured area.)
2. Check distal pulse and sensation. If either is abnormal, activate **EMS**.
3. Cover all wounds, including open fractures, with sterile dressings, and secure them.
4. Do not attempt to push bone ends back underneath the skin.
5. Pad the splint to prevent local pressure.
6. Apply minimal in-line traction, and maintain it until the splint is in place and secured.
7. Immobilize the joints above and below the fracture site.
8. Splint in the position found if:
   - Pain increases with gentle traction or the limb resists positioning.
   - The fracture is severely angulated.
9. Do not straighten unless it is absolutely necessary to incorporate the limb into the splint; move as little as possible.
10. Splint firmly, but do not impair circulation.
11. Recheck distal pulse and sensation after applying splint.
12. Check vital signs, treat for shock, and transport to medical facility.

NERVE INJURIES

Q *The runner is diagnosed with a tibial stress fracture. If the runner had continued his running program rather than seeking medical attention, would he have been susceptible to a nerve injury?*

The nervous system is divided into the central nervous system, consisting of the brain and spinal cord, and the peripheral nervous system, which includes 12 pairs of cranial nerves and 31 pairs of spinal nerves, along with their branches (Fig. 6.16). The human body has eight pairs of cervical spinal nerves (C1–C8), 12 pairs of thoracic nerves (T1–T12), five pairs of lumbar nerves (L1–L5), five pairs of sacral nerves (S1–S5), and one pair of tiny coccygeal nerves (designated C0). Injuries to any of these nerves can be devastating to the individual, potentially resulting in temporary or even permanent disability.

Anatomic Properties of Nerves

Each spinal nerve is formed from anterior and posterior roots on the spinal cord that unite at the intervertebral foramen. The posterior branches are the **afferent** (sensory) **nerves** that transmit information from sensory receptors in the skin, tendons, ligaments, and muscles to the central nervous system. The anterior branches are the **efferent** (motor) **nerves** that transmit control signals to the muscles. The nerve fibers are heavily vascularized and are encased

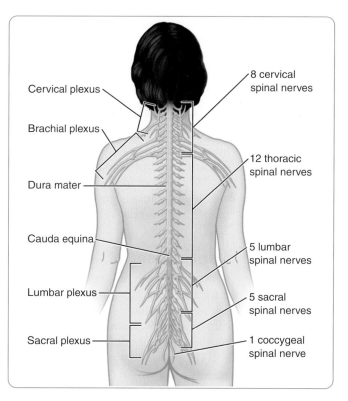

■■■■ FIGURE 6.16 **Spinal nerves.** Each spinal nerve is formed from anterior and posterior roots on the spinal cord. The posterior branches are afferent nerves; the anterior branches are efferent nerves.

in a multilayered, segmental protective sheath called the myelin sheath. Myelin protects and electrically insulates fibers from one another, and it increases the speed of transmission of nerve impulses. Myelinated fibers (axons bearing a myelin sheath) conduct nerve impulses rapidly, whereas unmyelinated fibers tend to conduct impulses quite slowly.

Classification of Nerve Injuries

Tensile or compressive forces most commonly injure nerves. Tensile injuries are more likely to occur during severe, high-speed accidents, such as automobile accidents or impact collisions in contact sports. When a nerve is loaded in tension, the nerve fibers tend to rupture before the surrounding connective tissue sheath. Because the nerve roots on the spinal cord are not protected by connective tissue, they are particularly susceptible to tensile injury, especially in response to stretching of the brachial plexus or cervical nerve roots.

Nerve injuries caused by tensile forces typically are graded in three levels. Grade I injuries represent **neurapraxia,** the mildest lesion. A neurapraxia is a localized conduction block that causes temporary loss of sensation and/or motor function from selective demyelination of the axon sheath without true axonal disruption. Recovery usually occurs within days to a few weeks. Grade II injuries are called **axonotmesis injuries,** which produce significant motor and mild sensory deficits that last at least 2 weeks. Axonotmesis disrupts the axon and myelin sheath but leaves the epineurium intact. The epineurium is the connective tissue that encapsulates the nerve trunk and binds the fascicles together. Axonal regrowth occurs at a rate of 1 to 2 mm/day; full or normal function usually is restored. Grade III injuries represent **neurotmesis injuries,** which disrupt the endoneurium. These severe injuries have a poor prognosis, with motor and sensory deficit persisting for up to 1 year. Surgical intervention often is necessary to avoid poor or imperfect regeneration.

Compressive injuries of nerves are more complex, because their severity depends on the magnitude and duration of loading and on whether the applied pressure is direct or indirect. Because nerve function is highly dependent on oxygen provided by the associated blood vessels, damage to the blood supply caused by a compressive injury results in damage to the nerve.

Nerve injuries can result in a range of afferent symptoms, from severe pain to complete loss of sensation. Terms used to describe altered sensation include **hypoesthesia** (a reduction in sensation), **hyperesthesia** (heightened sensation), and **paresthesia** (a sense of numbness, prickling, or tingling). Pinching of a nerve can result in a sharp wave of pain that is transmitted through a body segment. Irritation or inflammation of a nerve can result in chronic pain along the nerve's course, known as **neuralgia.**

Nerve Healing

When a nerve is completely severed, healing does not occur, and loss of function typically is permanent. Unless such injuries are repaired surgically, random regrowth of the nerve occurs, resulting in the formation of a **neuroma,** or nerve tumor.

When nerve fibers are ruptured in a tensile injury but the surrounding myelin sheath remains intact, it sometimes is possible for a nerve to regenerate along the pathway provided by the sheath. Such regeneration is relatively slow, however, proceeding at a rate of less than 1 mm/day, or approximately 2.5 cm/month (1).

Management of Nerve Injuries

If nerves are injured, cutaneous sensation or muscle movement may become impaired. Neurologic testing is explained and demonstrated in Chapter 5. Sensation is assessed by touching the person with a cotton ball, paper clip, pads of the fingers, and fingernails to determine if the individual can differentiate between sharp and dull. It also is important to determine if the sensation feels the same on the injured body segment as it does on the uninjured body segment.

The motor component can be tested with manual muscle testing. In testing a myotome, a normal response is a strong muscle contraction. A weakened muscle contraction may indicate partial paralysis of the muscles innervated by the nerve root being tested. A peripheral nerve injury results in complete paralysis of the muscles supplied by that nerve. If a muscle strain is present, a weakened muscle contraction is accompanied by pain.

It is critical that a possible nerve injury be identified and the individual referred immediately to a physician for advanced evaluation and care.

See *Field Strategy: Management of Nerve Injuries* on the companion website at thePoint for basic principles used in the management of nerve injuries.

> Nerve injuries typically are the result of tension or compression forces. As such, the runner was not likely to sustain a nerve injury. If left untreated, however, a stress fracture can become an acute fracture. The fractured ends of the bones and the swelling associated with an acute fracture pose a possible danger to nerves in the involved area.

PAIN

> Observation of two individuals involved in rehabilitation programs for similar lower leg injuries reveals different patient responses. One patient avoids exercises because of excessive pain; the other patient performs workouts without complaint. What variables may explain the different responses?

Pain is a negative sensory and emotional experience associated with actual or potential tissue damage. It also is a universal symptom common to most injuries. An individual's perception of pain is influenced by various physical, chemical, social, and psychological factors.

The Neurologic Basis of Pain

Pain can originate from somatic, visceral, and psychogenic sources. Somatic pain originates in the skin as well as internal structures of the musculoskeletal system. Visceral pain, which often is diffuse or referred rather than localized to the problem site, originates from the internal organs. Psychogenic pain involves no apparent physical cause of the pain, although the sensation of pain is felt.

Stimulation of specialized afferent nerve endings, called **nociceptors**, produces the pain sensation. The name *nociceptor* is derived from the word *noxious*, meaning physically harmful or destructive. Nociceptors are prevalent in the skin, meninges, periosteum, teeth, and some internal organs.

In most acute injuries, pain is initiated by **mechanosensitive** nociceptors responding to the traumatic force that caused the injury. In chronic injuries and during the early stages of healing of acute injuries, pain persists because of the activation of **chemosensitive** nociceptors. Bradykinin, serotonin, histamines, and prostaglandins are all chemicals transported to the injury site during inflammation that activate the chemosensitive nociceptors. Thermal extremes also can stimulate other specialized nociceptors to produce pain.

Two types of afferent nerves transmit the sensation of pain to the spinal cord. Small-diameter, slow-transmission, unmyelinated C fibers transmit low-level pain that might be described as dull or aching. Sharp, piercing types of pain are transmitted by larger, faster, thinly myelinated A fibers. Pain can be transmitted along both types of afferent nerves from somatic and visceral sources. Activity involving A and C fibers from the visceral organs also can provoke autonomic responses, such as changes in blood pressure, heart rate, and respiration.

Afferent nerves carrying pain impulses, along with those transporting sensations such as touch, temperature, and proprioception, articulate with the spinal cord through the substantia gelatinosa of the cord's dorsal horn. Specialized T cells then transmit impulses from all the afferent fibers up the spinal cord to the brain, with each T cell carrying a single impulse. Within the brain, the pain impulses are transmitted to the thalamus (primarily to its ventral posterior lateral nucleus) as well as to the somatosensory cortex, where pain is perceived.

According to the gate control theory of pain proposed by Melzack and Wall (13), the substantia gelatinosa acts as a gatekeeper by allowing either a pain response or one of the other afferent sensations to be transported by each T cell. This theory is substantiated by the observation that increased sensory input can reduce the sensation of pain. For example, extreme cold often can numb pain. Because hundreds or thousands of "gates" are in operation, however, added sensory input more commonly reduces rather than eliminates the feeling of pain, because pain impulses get through to some of the T cells.

Factors That Mediate Pain

Some brain cells have the ability to produce narcotic-like, pain-killing compounds known as opioid peptides, including β-endorphin and methionine enkephalin. Both compounds work by blocking neural receptor sites that transmit pain. Several different sites in the brain produce endorphins. Stressors, such as physical exercise, mental stress, and electrical stimulation, provoke the release of endorphins into the cerebrospinal fluid. A phenomenon called "runner's high," which is a feeling of euphoria that occurs among long-distance runners, has been attributed to endorphin release. The brainstem and pituitary gland produce enkephalins. Enkephalins block pain neurotransmitters in the dorsal horn of the spinal cord.

The central nervous system also imposes a set of **cognitive** (i.e., quality of knowing or perceiving) and **affective** (i.e., pertaining to feelings or a mental state) filters on both the perception of pain and the subsequent expression of perceived pain. Social and cultural factors can powerfully influence the level of pain tolerance. For example, in American society, it is much more acceptable for females than males to express feelings of pain. Individual personality and a state of mental preoccupation also can be significant modifiers of pain.

Referred and Radiating Pain

Referred pain is perceived at a location remote from the site of the tissues actually causing the pain. A proposed explanation for referred pain begins with the fact that neurons carrying pain impulses split into several branches within the spinal cord. Although some of these branches connect with other pain-transmitting fibers, some also connect with afferent nerve pathways from the skin. This cross-branching can cause the brain to misinterpret the true location of the pain. In some instances, referred pain behaves in a logical and predictable fashion. Pain from internal organs typically is projected outward to corresponding **dermatomes** of the skin. For example, heart attacks can produce a sensation of pain in the superior thoracic wall and medial aspect of the left arm. In most cases, the affected internal organ and corresponding dermatome receive innervation from the same spinal nerve roots.

Referred pain should not be confused with radiating pain, which is pain that is felt both at its source and along a nerve. Pinching of the sciatic nerve at its root may cause pain that radiates along the nerve's course down the posterior aspect of the leg.

Differences in pain perception and tolerance can be caused by differences in chemical, social, and psychological influences as well as by differences in the severity of the original injury and the progression of the healing process.

SUMMARY

1. When a force acts, two effects occur on the target tissue: acceleration, or change in velocity, and deformation, or change in shape.

2. Two factors determine if injury occurs to a tissue: the magnitude of the force, and the material properties of the tissues involved.

3. Biologic tissues are strongest in resisting the form of loading to which they most commonly are subjected.

4. Force exceeding a structure's yield point causes rupture or fracture.

5. Most common mechanisms of injury include compressive force from axial loading, which compresses or crushes an object; tensile force from tension or traction on an object; and shearing force, which acts parallel or tangent to a plane passing through the object.

6. In tendons, the collagen fibers are arranged in a parallel pattern, enabling resistance to high, unidirectional tensile loads when the attached muscle contracts.

7. In ligaments, the collagen fibers are largely parallel but also interwoven, providing resistance to large tensile loads along the long axis of the ligament and to smaller tensile loads from other directions.

8. The viscoelastic aspect of muscle extensibility enables muscles to stretch to greater lengths over time in response to a sustained tensile force.

9. Injury to soft tissue and joints can be acute or chronic. Strains and sprains are common acute injuries associated with participation in sport and physical activity. Tendinitis and osteoarthritis are common chronic or overuse injuries.

10. Wound healing entails three overlapping phases: inflammation, proliferation, and maturation (remodeling). During the inflammatory phase, blood loss is curtailed, clotting takes place, and histochemical cascades promote coagulation, vasodilation, and attraction of specialized cells to rid the wound site of foreign or infectious agents. The proliferative phase includes angiogenesis, bioplasia, re-epithelialization, and wound contraction. The maturation phase involves remodeling of the newly formed tissue.

11. Growth factors are proteins that attract cells to the wound, stimulate their proliferation, and direct the deposition of the extracellular matrix.

12. The mineralization and girth of bone increases in response to increased levels of stress.

13. Because bone is stronger in resisting compressive forces than in resisting both tension and shear forces, acute compression fractures are rare. Most fractures occur on the side of the bone placed in tension.

14. Maturation of bone tissue involves osteoblast activity on the concave side of the fracture, which is loaded in compression, and osteoclast activity on the convex side of the fracture, which is loaded in tension.

15. Nerve injuries caused by tensile forces are graded in three levels: neurapraxia injury, with temporary loss of sensation or motor function; axonotmesis injury, with significant motor and sensory deficits that last at least 2 weeks; and neurotmesis injury, with significant motor and sensory deficits persisting for up to 1 year.

16. Pain associated with injury is transmitted by specialized afferent nerve endings called nociceptors. Mechanosensitive nociceptors respond to traumatic forces that cause the injury. Chemosensitive nociceptors respond to chronic injuries and are activated during the early states of healing in acute injuries.

17. Pain is transmitted along two types of afferent nerves: small-diameter, slow-transmission, unmyelinated C fibers, which transmit low-level pain, and larger, faster, finely myelinated A fibers, which transmit sharp, piercing types of pain.

18. Afferent nerves carry nerve impulses to the spinal cord through the substantia gelatinosa of the cord's dorsal horn up to the thalamus as well as to the somatosensory cortex, where pain is perceived.

19. Stressors, such as physical exercise, mental stress, and electrical stimulation, provoke the release of endorphins into the cerebrospinal fluid and can mediate the perception of pain.

REFERENCES

1. Schenck RC ed. Athletic Training and Sports Medicine, 3rd Ed. Park Ridge, IL: American Academy of Orthopaedic Surgeons, 2000.
2. National Center for Chronic Disease Prevention and Health Promotion. Physical activity: the arthritis pain reliever. Available at: http://www.cdc.gov/arthritis/campaigns/physical_activity/download_general.htm. Accessed July 18, 2005.
3. Wong ME, Hollinger JO, Pinero GJ. Integrated processes responsible for soft-tissue healing. Oral Surg Oral Med Oral Pathol 1996;82(5):475–492.
4. Orgill D, Demling RH. Current concepts and approaches to wound healing. Crit Care Med 1988;16:899.
5. Harvey C. Wound healing. Ortho Nurs 2005;24(2):143–159.
6. Hefti F, Stoll TM. Healing of ligaments and tendons. Orthopedics 1995;24(3):237–245.
7. Rappolee DA, Mark D, Banda MJ, et al. Wound macrophages express TGF-α and other growth factors in vivo: analysis by mRNA phenotyping. Science 1988;241:708.
8. Mendez-Eastman S. Wound dressing categories. Plastic Surg Nurs 2005;25(2):95–99.
9. Reiman P. Wound care management update. Dermatology 2005;26(9):34.
10. Jones HH, Priest JD, Hayes WC, et al. Humeral hypertrophy in response to exercise. J Bone Joint Surg Am 1977;59:204–208.
11. Watson RC. Bone growth and physical activity. In: Mazess RB, ed. International Conference on Bone Measurements. DHEW Pub No. NIH 75-683. Washington, DC: Department of Health, Education, & Welfare, 1973.
12. Salter RB. Textbook of Disorders and Injuries of the Musculoskeletal System. Baltimore: Lippincott Williams & Wilkins, 1999.
13. Melzack R, Wall PD. Pain mechanisms: a new theory. Science 1965;150(699):971–979.

7 Therapeutic Modalities

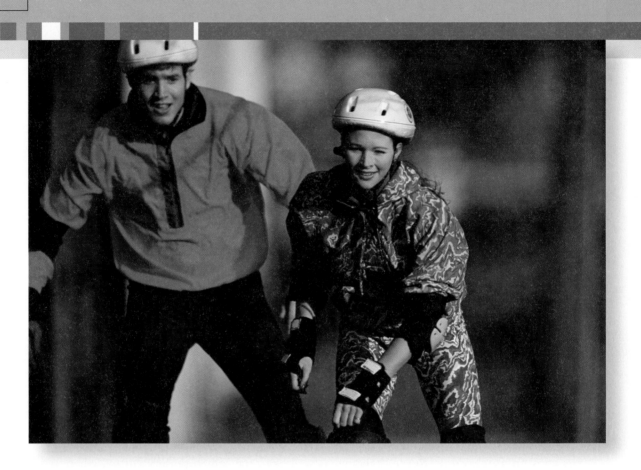

STUDENT OUTCOMES

1. Explain the principles associated with the electromagnetic spectrum, and identify the types of energy found in the non-ionizing range of the spectrum.

2. Explain the transfer of energy from one object to another, and identify the factors that can affect this transfer.

3. Describe the physiologic effects of cryotherapy and thermotherapy.

4. List the indications and contraindications for the various methods of cold and heat treatments, including ultrasound and diathermy.

5. Explain the principles that govern ultrasound, including the physiologic effects and modes of application.

6. Explain the principles of electricity, and describe the different types of current.

7. Describe the various parameters that can be manipulated in electrotherapy to produce the desired effects.

8. Explain the various types of electrical stimulating units and the use of each.

9. Describe the benefits attained in each of the five basic massage strokes, and explain their application.

10. Explain the principles that govern traction and continuous passive motion.

11. Identify and describe the various categories of therapeutic medications used to promote healing, and give examples of common drugs in each category.

ROLE DELINEATION COMPETENCIES

The following Performance Domains and Tasks defined in the National Athletic Trainers' Association Board of Certification *Role Delineation Study*, 5th Edition are addressed in this chapter:

BOC COMPETENCIES

IV.   Treatment, Rehabilitation, and Reconditioning

B. Administer therapeutic modalities using standard techniques and procedures in order to facilitate recovery, function, and/or performance.

F. Educate the appropriate individual(s) in the treatment, rehabilitation, and reconditioning of injuries, illnesses, and/or conditions using applicable methods and materials to facilitate recovery, function, and/or performance.

The ultimate goal of rehabilitation is to return the injured participant to activity in a pain-free and fully functional condition. The rehabilitation process must focus on controlling pain and inflammation and on regaining normal joint range of motion (ROM), flexibility, muscular strength, muscular endurance, coordination, and power. Therapeutic modalities and medications are used to create an optimal environment for injury repair by limiting the inflammatory process and breaking the pain-spasm cycle. Use of any modality depends on the supervising physician's exercise prescription as well as on the injury site and the type and severity of injury. An **indication** is a condition that could benefit from a specific modality, whereas a **contraindication** is a condition that could be adversely affected by a particular modality. In some cases, a modality may be indicated and contraindicated for the same condition. For example, thermotherapy may be contraindicated for tendinitis during the initial phase of the exercise program; however, once acute inflammation is controlled, heat therapy may be indicated. Frequent evaluation of the individual's progress is necessary to ensure that the appropriate modality is being used.

This chapter initially addresses the basic principles associated with the electromagnetic spectrum and the factors affecting the transfer of energy. Then, the more common therapeutic modalities used in injury management are discussed. The material presented is a general overview of the various modalities. Because of the extensive information and clinical skills that are needed to adequately comprehend and apply therapeutic modalities in a clinical setting, this chapter should not be used in lieu of a specialized course on therapeutic techniques. It is essential that such a course be a part of the professional preparation of an athletic trainer.

ELECTROMAGNETIC SPECTRUM

> **Q▶** *During practice, a lacrosse player sustains a contusion to the posterior aspect of the upper arm. A bag of crushed ice is applied to the injured area using a compression wrap. Should the ice bag be applied directly to the skin or over a layer of towel covering the skin? Explain the process of energy transmission between the ice bag and the underlying soft tissues.*

On a daily basis, the environment is impacted by a variety of energy forms. Each form of energy falls under the category of **electromagnetic radiation** and can be located on an **electromagnetic spectrum** based on its wavelength or frequency (Fig. 7.1). Electrical therapeutic modalities are part of the electromagnetic spectrum, which is divided into two major zones: the ionizing range, and the nonionizing range. Regardless of the range, electromagnetic energy has several common characteristics:

- Electromagnetic energy is composed of pure energy and does not have a mass.
- Energy travels at the speed of light (300 million meters per second).
- Energy waveforms travel in a straight line and can travel in a vacuum.
- Energy requires no transmission medium.

FIGURE 7.1 Electromagnetic spectrum. The electromagnetic spectrum covers a wide range of wavelengths and frequencies.

Ionizing Range

Energy in the ionizing range can readily alter the components of atoms (i.e., electrons, protons, and neutrons). This radiation can easily penetrate tissue to deposit energy within the cells. If the energy level is high enough, the cell loses its ability to regenerate, leading to cell death. Used diagnostically in radiography (i.e., in x-ray dosages below that required for cell death) and therapeutically to treat certain cancers (i.e., above the threshold), the level is strictly controlled and monitored to prevent injury to the patient. It is not used by athletic trainers or physical therapists.

Non-Ionizing Range

Energy in the non-ionizing range commonly is used in the management of musculoskeletal injuries. This portion of the spectrum incorporates ultraviolet, visible, and infrared light. Electromagnetic waves are produced when the temperature rises and the electron activity increases. Ultraviolet light has a shorter wavelength than visible light; therefore, it is undetectable by the human eye. This energy source causes superficial chemical changes in the skin and is used to treat certain skin conditions; sunburns are an example of excessive exposure to ultraviolet rays. Wavelengths greater than visible light are called infrared light, or intrared energy. The infrared wavelengths closest to visible light are called near-infrared energy and can produce thermal effects 5 to 10 mm deep in tissue. The infrared wavelengths farthest from the visible are called far-infrared energy and result in more superficial heating of the skin (<2 mm deep). Energy forms with much longer wavelengths are collectively known as diathermy and can increase tissue temperature through a process called conversion. Microwave and shortwave diathermy are examples of this energy source.

Transfer of Energy

Electromagnetic energy can travel through a vacuum with no transfer medium. Energy moves from an area of high concentration to an area of lower concentration by energy carriers, such as mechanical waves, electrons, photons, and molecules. This energy flow in the form of heat involves the exchange of kinetic energy, or energy possessed by an object by virtue of its motion, and is transferred via radiation, conduction, convection, conversion, or evaporation.

Radiation

Radiation is the transfer of energy in the form of infrared waves (radiant energy) without physical contact. All matter radiates energy in the form of heat. Usually, body heat is warmer than the environment, and radiant heat energy is dissipated through the air to surrounding solid, cooler objects. When the temperature of surrounding objects in the environment exceeds skin temperature, radiant heat is absorbed. Shortwave and microwave diathermy are examples of both radiant energy transfer, but they can also heat by conversion.

Conduction

Conduction is the direct transfer of energy between two objects in physical contact with each other. A difference in temperature is necessary to initiate the movement of kinetic energy from one molecule to another, and the energy moves from an area of high temperature to an area of lower temperature. Examples of conductive thermal agents are ice bags, ice packs, moist hot packs, and paraffin.

Convection

Convection, a more rapid process than conduction, occurs when a medium such as air or water moves across the body, creating temperature variations. The effectiveness of heat loss or heat gain by conduction depends on the speed at which the air or water next to the body is moved away once it becomes warmed. For example, if air movement is slow, the air molecules next to the skin are warmed and act as insulation. In contrast, if warmer air molecules are continually replaced by cooler molecules (e.g., on a breezy day or in a room with a fan), heat loss increases as the air currents carry heat away. Fluidotherapy and whirlpools are examples of therapeutic modalities that exchange energy by convection.

Conversion

Conversion involves the changing of another energy form (e.g., sound, electricity, or a chemical agent) into heat. In ultrasound therapy, mechanical energy produced by high-frequency sound waves is converted to heat energy at tissue interfaces. In microwave diathermy, high electromagnetic energy is converted into heat, which can heat deep tissues. Chemical agents, such as liniments or balms, create heat by acting as counterirritants to superficial sensory nerve endings, thus reducing the transmission of pain from underlying nerves.

Evaporation

Heat loss can occur during evaporation as well. Vapo-coolant sprays, for example, spread a liquid over the skin surface. The heat absorbed by the liquid cools the skin surface as the liquid changes into a gaseous state. Evaporation also is the means by which the body cools itself on a hot day through the evaporation of sweat.

Factors Affecting Energy Transfer

When electromagnetic energy is transmitted in a vacuum, it travels in a straight line. When traveling through a physical medium, however, the path is influenced by the density of the medium, and the energy may be reflected, refracted, or absorbed by the material or may continue to pass through

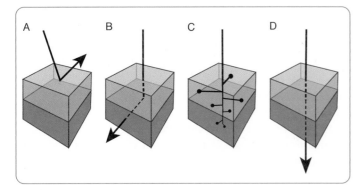

FIGURE 7.2 Factors affecting the transmission of energy. A, Reflection. The energy wave may be partially or fully reflected by the tissue layer. **B,** Refraction. The energy wave is bent as it strikes an interface between two different tissue layer densities. **C,** Absorption. Energy can be absorbed by one layer reducing the energy available to deeper tissues. **D,** Transmission. Any energy that is not reflected or absorbed by a tissue layer will continue to pass through the medium to the next layer, where it can again be reflected, refracted, absorbed, or transmitted through the tissue.

the material, unaffected by its density (Fig. 7.2). **Reflection** occurs when the wave strikes an object and is bent back away from the material. An echo is an example of a reflected sound. The reflection itself may be complete or partial. **Refraction** is the deflection of waves because of a change in the speed of absorption as the wave passes between media of different densities. If energy passes through a high-density layer and enters a low-density layer, its speed increases. In contrast, if energy passes through a low-density layer and enters a high-density layer, its speed decreases. **Absorption** occurs when the wave passes through a medium and its kinetic energy is either partially or totally assimilated by the tissue. Any energy that is not reflected or absorbed by a tissue layer passes through the layer until it strikes another layer with a different density, where it may again be reflected, refracted, absorbed, or transmitted through the medium. Each time the wave is partially reflected, refracted, or absorbed, the remaining energy available to the deeper tissues is reduced. This inverse relationship is called the **law of Grotthus-Draper:** The more energy the superficial tissues absorb, the less energy is available to be transmitted to the underlying tissues.

Effect of Energy on Tissue

To be effective, therapeutic modalities must be capable of producing the desired effects at the intended tissue depth. When energy is applied to the body, the maximal effect occurs when energy rays strike the body at a right angle (90°). As the angle deviates from 90°, some of the energy is reflected away from the target site, thereby reducing the level of absorption. The **cosine law** (Fig. 7.3) states that as the angle deviates from 90°, the energy varies with the cosine of the angle:

$$\text{Effective energy} = \text{Energy} \times \text{Cosine of the angle of incidence}$$

With radiant energy, a difference of ±10° from the right angle is considered to be within acceptable limits (1). Another law that affects energy absorption is the **inverse square law** (Fig. 7.4), which states that the intensity of radiant energy striking the tissues is directly proportional to the square

FIGURE 7.3 The cosine law. When energy is applied to a body part, the maximal effect occurs when energy rays strike the body at a right angle (90°). As the angle deviates from 90°, some of the energy is reflected away from the targeted site, thereby reducing the level of absorption. This concept is critical in the application of ultrasound.

of the distance between the source of the energy and the tissues:

$$E = \frac{E_S}{D^2}$$

where

ES = amount of energy produced by the source

D^2 = square of the distance between the target and the source

E = resulting energy absorbed by the tissue

This means that each time the distance between the energy and the tissue is doubled, the intensity of the energy received by the tissue is reduced by a factor of four.

 The bag of crushed ice should be applied directly to the skin of the lacrosse player. Because the thermal energy is being transferred via conduction, application directly to the skin promotes a more efficient and effective transfer of cold to the injured area.

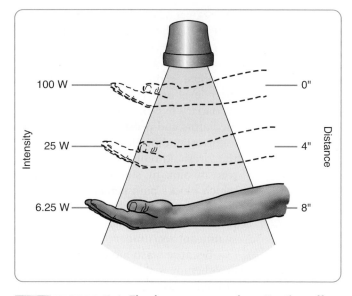

■■ ■■ FIGURE 7.4 The inverse square law. Heating effect equals x(a). When the distance between the energy source and the skin is reduced by half, the heating effect is increased by fourfold (inverse of ½ = equals 2, and 2^2 = 4).

CRYOTHERAPY

In treating the lacrosse player's contusion, for how long a period of time should the ice bag be applied? What contraindications may prohibit the use of cold in this case?

Cryotherapy describes multiple types of cold application that use the kind of electromagnetic energy classified as infrared radiation. When cold is applied to skin, which is a warmer object, heat is removed or lost; this is referred to as heat abstraction, or cooling. The most common modes of heat transfer with cold application are conduction and evaporation. Cold application for less than 15 minutes causes immediate skin cooling, cooling of subcutaneous tissue after a slight delay, and cooling in muscle tissue after a longer delay. This leads to decreased cell metabolism, inflammation, circulation, pain perception, muscle spasm, muscle force production, and increased tissue stiffness (2). Depth of cold penetration can reach 4 to 5 cm and is dependent on the duration of treatment: The longer the treatment, the greater the depth of cooling, and the greater the decrease in temperature. The magnitude of temperature change depends on:

- Type of cooling modality (e.g., ice massage versus ice slush, where treatment temperature differs)
- Temperature difference between the cold object and soft tissue
- Use of a compression wrap to secure the cold agent
- Insulating medium between the skin and cold agent
- Amount of subcutaneous insulation (adipose tissue/fat)
- Depth of the target tissue
- Vascularity and thermal conductivity of the area being cooled
- Limb circumference
- Sympathetic nervous system
- Duration of the application

The greater the temperature gradient between the skin and cooling source, the greater the resulting temperature change in the tissue. Likewise, the deeper the tissue, the more time is required to lower the temperature. Adipose tissue acts as an insulator and resists heat transfer, both heat gain and heat loss. The amount of adipose tissue influences the degree and rate at which muscle is cooled and, conversely, the return to its precooled temperature.

Cold therapy is used to lower the temperature in soft tissues (e.g., subcutaneous tissue, muscle, or joints), reduce pain, and control edema. Cold application leads to vasoconstriction at the cellular level and decreases tissue metabolism (i.e., decreases the need for oxygen), which reduces secondary hypoxia. Capillary permeability and pain are decreased, and the release of inflammatory mediators and prostaglandin synthesis is inhibited. As the temperature of peripheral nerves decreases, a corresponding decrease occurs in nerve conduction velocity across the nerve synapse, increasing the threshold required for nerves to fire. The gate theory of pain hypothesizes that cold inhibits pain transmission by stimulating large-diameter neurons in the spinal cord, acting as a counterirritant, which blocks pain perception. Because of the inhibition of nerves and muscle spindle activity, muscles in spasm are relaxed, breaking the pain-spasm cycle and leading to an **analgesic**, or pain-free, effect. During ice application, a decline in fast-twitch muscle fiber tension occurs, resulting in a more significant recruitment of slow-twitch muscle fibers, thereby increasing muscle endurance (3).

Because vasoconstriction leads to a decrease in metabolic rate, inflammation, and pain, cryotherapy is the modality of choice during the acute phase of an injury. The therapeutic application of cold cools the surface skin temperature between 1° to 10°C (33–50°F) (4); however, researchers have identified that maximal decreases in localized blood flow can occur at temperatures ranging from 12.83° to 15°C (55–59°F) (5,6). The desired therapeutic range of cooling can be obtained through the use of ice bags (e.g., crushed or cubed), commercial ice packs, ice cups (e.g., ice massage), cold water baths (e.g., immersion or whirlpool), and vapo-coolant sprays. Recent technology also has provided new forms of cold application, such as the Cryocuff or controlled cold therapy (CCT) units.

Cryotherapy is usually applied for 20 to 30 minutes several times a day for maximum cooling of both superficial and deep tissues. Treatment times may vary depending on the thickness of the adipose layer. When using ice packs, it was found that the time required to lower deep tissue temperature for selected skinfold thicknesses of 0 to 10, 11 to 20, 21 to 30, and 31 to 40 mm were 12, 30, 40, and 60 minutes, respectively (7). Barriers used between the ice application and skin also can affect heat abstraction. Research has shown that a dry towel or dry elastic wrap should not be used in treatment times of 30 minutes or less; rather, the cold agent should be applied directly to the skin for optimal therapeutic effects (4,8). Using an elastic wrap to secure the cold agent (e.g., ice pack) to the body part, however, produces a significant reduction in subcutaneous tissue temperatures as compared with simply placing the cold agent on the skin (9). Ice application is continued during the first 24 to 72 hours after injury or until acute bleeding and capillary leakage have stopped, whichever is longer.

Another consideration is the length of time required to rewarm the injured area. Knight (4) has shown that except for the fingers, the rewarming time to approach normal body temperature is at least 90 minutes. This results in a treatment protocol of applying an ice pack for 20 to 30 minutes, followed by 90 minutes of rewarming. Fingers can rewarm more quickly, even following a 20- to 30-minute ice treatment, presumably because of their increased circulation. Fingers need only 20 to 30 minutes to rewarm.

Certain methods of cryotherapy also may be used before ROM exercises and at the conclusion of an exercise bout (Box 7.1). Use of cold treatments before exercise is called **cryokinetics**. Cryokinetics alternates several bouts of cold using ice massage, ice packs, ice immersion, or iced towels with active exercise. The injured body part is numbed by applying cold for 10 to 20 minutes, and the individual is instructed to perform various progressive exercises. These exercises may begin with simple, non–weight bearing ROM activities and progress to more complex, weight-bearing activities. All exercise bouts must be pain-free. As the mild anesthesia from the cold wears off, the body part is renumbed with a 3- to 5-minute cold treatment. The exercise bout is repeated three to four times each session. The session ends with exercise if the individual is able to participate in activity or with cold if the individual is not able to participate in activity.

Methods of cryotherapy include cold packs, ice massage, ice immersion, and vapo-coolant sprays. Regardless of the methods of application, the individual feels four progressive sensations: cold, burning, aching, and **analgesia**.

Box 7.1   Cryotherapy Application

Indications

Acute or chronic pain
Acute or chronic muscle spasm/guarding
Acute inflammation or injury
Postsurgical pain and edema
Neuralgia
Superficial first-degree burns
Used with exercises to:
  ▪ Facilitate mobilization
  ▪ Relieve pain
  ▪ Decrease muscle spasticity

Contraindications

Decreased cold sensitivity and/or hypersensitivity
Cold allergy/cold-induced urticaria
Circulatory or sensory impairment
Raynaud's phenomenon
Advanced diabetes
Hypertension
Uncovered open wounds
Cardiac or respiratory disorders
Nerve palsy
Arthritis
Lupus

Cold Packs

Cold packs are administered in four common methods: plastic bags filled with crushed, flaked, or cubed ice; reusable cold gel packs; CCT units; and instant (chemical) cold packs. Most methods are inexpensive and maintain a constant temperature, making them very effective in cooling tissue.

Ice Bags

When filled with flaked ice or small cubes, ice bags can be safely applied to the skin for 30 to 40 minutes without danger of frostbite. Furthermore, ice packs can be molded to the body's contours, held in place by a cold compression wrap, and elevated above the heart to minimize swelling and pooling of fluids in the interstitial tissue spaces (Fig. 7.5A). During the initial treatments, the skin should be checked frequently for wheal or blister formation (Fig. 7.5B). A disadvantage of this application method is the cost of the ice machine, which can be expensive.

Reusable Cold Packs

Reusable commercial gel packs contain silica gel enclosed in a strong vinyl or plastic case, and they come in a variety of sizes to conform to the body's natural contours (Fig. 7.6). Used with compression

■■■■ FIGURE 7.5 **Ice treatments. A,** Ice, compression, and elevation can reduce acute inflammation. **B,** A slightly raised wheal formation may appear shortly after cold application in individuals who are sensitive to cold or have cold allergies.

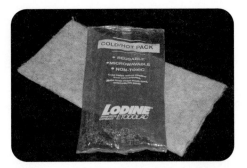

FIGURE 7.6 Commercial gel packs. Commercial gel packs come in a variety of sizes to conform to the body's natural contours.

and elevation, they are an effective method of cold application. The packs should be stored at a temperature of approximately −5°C (−23°F) for at least 2 hours before application (2). Because the packs are stored at sub-zero temperatures, they may cause frostbite if used improperly. A wet towel or cloth should be placed between the pack and skin to prevent frostbite and to maintain a hygienic surface for the reusable packs. Treatment time ranges from 15 to 20 minutes.

Controlled Compression Therapy (CCT) Units

Controlled compression therapy units use static, external compression and cold application to decrease blood flow to an extremity and assist venous return, decrease edema, and increase the effective depth of cold penetration. In doing so, both pain and recovery time are decreased. Commercial circulating-cold-water wraps, such as Cryo/Cuff (Aircast, Inc., Summit, NJ) and Polar Care (Breg, Inc., Vista, CA) use ice water placed in an insulated thermos. When the thermos is raised above the body part, water flows into the pad wrapped around the injured extremity, maintaining cold compression for 5 to 7 hours (Fig. 7.7A). These often are applied after surgery over dressings and casts. Some CCT units provide a motorized, intermittent compression treatment when cooled water is circulated through a boot or sleeve around the injured body part and the sleeve is inflated intermittently. This is done for 20 to 30 minutes, several times a day, to pump edematous fluid from the extremity (Fig. 7.7B). During deflation, the patient can perform active ROM exercises to enhance blood flow to the injured area. The unit can be used several times a day, but never with a suspected compartment syndrome or fracture or in an individual with a peripheral vascular disease or impaired circulation.

Instant Cold Packs

Instant (chemical) cold packs are convenient to carry in an athletic training kit, can be disposed of after a single use, and can conform to a body part. Each bag contains two chemicals separated by a plastic barrier. When the barrier is ruptured, the chemicals mix, producing cold. Disadvantages of this type of application are the short duration of the cold application, the expense in using the pack only once, and the potential of the pack to tear or leak. The chemical substance that produces the cold has an alkaline pH, which can cause burns if the liquid substance comes in contact with the skin. As such, the packs should never be squeezed or used in front of the face and, if possible, should be placed inside another plastic bag. Treatment ranges from 15 to 20 minutes. In longer treatments, the pack warms and becomes ineffective. Some commercial packs can be refrozen and reused.

FIGURE 7.7 Cold compression therapy units. A, These devices provide circumferential cold compression around a specific body part. When the thermos is raised above the body part, water flows throughout the unit, maintaining cold compression for 5 to 7 hours. **B,** Some units have a motorized unit that can provide pressure or intermittent compression to an injured area to decrease edema.

Ice Massage

Ice massage is an inexpensive and effective method of cold application. Performed over a relatively small area, such as a muscle belly, tendon, bursa, or trigger point, it produces significant cooling of the skin and a large, reactive **hyperemia**, or increase of blood flow into the region, once the treatment has ended. As such, it is not the treatment of choice in cases of acute injury. Ice massage is particularly useful for its analgesic effect in relieving pain that may inhibit stretching of a muscle, and it has been shown to decrease muscle soreness when combined with stretching (2). It commonly is used before ROM exercises and deep friction massage when treating chronic tendinitis and muscle strains.

◼◼◼◼ FIGURE 7.8 **Ice immersion.** This technique quickly reduces temperature over the entire surface area of a distal extremity. Toe caps may be used to prevent frostbite of the toes during the treatment.

Treatment consists of water frozen in a cup, which is rubbed over an area 10 × 15 cm using small, overlapping, circular motions for 5 to 10 minutes. A continuous motion is used to prevent tissue damage. If this treatment is applied properly, skin temperature usually will not drop below 15°C (59°F); therefore, the risk of damaging tissue and producing frostbite is minimal (2). A wooden tongue depressor frozen in the cup can provide a handle for easy application. During ice massage, the stages of cold, burning, and aching pass rapidly, within approximately 1 to 2 minutes. A prolonged aching or burning sensation may result if the area covered is too large or if a hypersensitive response occurs.

Ice Immersion

Ice immersion (ice slush bath) is used to reduce temperature quickly over the entire surface of a distal extremity (e.g., forearm, hand, ankle, or foot). A variety of containers or basins may be used. Because of the analgesic effect and the buoyancy of water, ice immersion and cold whirlpools often are used during the inflammatory phase to reduce edema formation after blunt injury. If the goal is to reduce edema, placing the body part in a stationary position below the level of the heart keeps fluid in the body segment and is contraindicated. This can be avoided by placing a compression wrap over the body part before submersion and performing active muscle contractions. Neoprene toe caps may be used to reduce discomfort on the toes.

A bucket or cold whirlpool is filled with water and ice (Fig. 7.8). Bucket immersion in 40° to 50°F (4–10°C) water or a 50° to 60°F (10–15.6°C) whirlpool cools tissues as effectively as an ice pack. The lower the temperature, the shorter the duration of immersion. Treatment lasts from 10 to 15 minutes. When pain is relieved, the part is removed from the water, and functional movement patterns are performed. As pain returns, the area is reimmersed. The cycle continues three or four times.

Cold whirlpool baths also provide a hydromassaging effect. The intensity of the effect is controlled by the amount of air that is emitted through the electrical turbine. The turbine can be moved up and down or directed at a specific angle and locked in place. The whirlpool turbine should not be operated unless water totally covers the impeller. In addition to controlling acute inflammation, cold whirlpools can be used to decrease soft-tissue trauma and increase active ROM after prolonged immobilization.

Vapo-Coolant Sprays

Fluoromethane is a nonflammable, nontoxic spray that uses rapid evaporation of chemicals on the skin to cool the area before treatment of trigger points (Fig. 7.9). The effects are temporary and superficial. When using a vapo-coolant spray to increase ROM in an area where no trigger point is present, the patient should be comfortably positioned with the muscle maintained on passive stretch. The bottle of vapo-coolant spray is then inverted, held at a 30° to 45° angle, and sprayed approximately 12 inches

◼◼◼◼ FIGURE 7.9 **Vapo-coolant sprays.** These sprays temporarily freeze superficial tissues and can reduce the pain-spasm cycle before stretching exercises.

away from the skin. The entire length of the muscle is sprayed two or three times in a unidirectional, parallel sweeping pattern as a gradual stretch is applied by the clinician up to, but not exceeding, the point of pain. Allow the tissue to rewarm. Repeat the process with two or three more sweeps, with increasing stretch placed on the muscle. The treatment may be followed by a moist heat treatment or massage.

(A) *The ice bag should be applied to the lacrosse player's injured upper arm for a period of 20 to 30 minutes. After a maximum of 90 minutes, intended to allow rewarming of the area, another cold treatment should be initiated. This process should be followed throughout the remainder of the day. If the individual experiences any skin blanching, numbness, burning, or tingling sensations, the cold treatment should be stopped.*

THERMOTHERAPY

(Q) *Following 5 days using cold treatments for the upper arm contusion, the lacrosse player shows significant improvement. The only significant finding is a slight decrease in strength as compared bilaterally with the uninvolved arm. Can the application of heat be advantageous during this stage in the healing process? What criteria would indicate that it is safe to use a heat modality at this time?*

Thermotherapy, or heat application, typically is used during the second phase of rehabilitation to increase blood flow and promote healing in the injured area (Box 7.2). If used during the acute inflammatory stage, heat application may overwhelm the injured blood and lymphatic vessels, leading to increased hemorrhage and edema. When applied at the appropriate time, however, heat can increase circulation and cellular metabolism; produce an analgesic, or sedative, effect; and assist in the resolution of pain and muscle-guarding spasms. Vasodilation and increased circulation result in an influx of oxygen and nutrients into the area to promote healing of damaged tissues. Debris and waste products are removed from the injury site. Used before stretching exercises, joint mobilization, or active exercise, thermotherapy can increase the extensibility of connective tissue, leading to increased ROM. In the same manner as cold application, heat flow through tissue also varies with the type of tissue and is called thermal conductivity.

Superficial heating agents involve the transfer of heat through conduction, convection, and radiation. Common examples of superficial thermotherapy are warm whirlpools or immersion, moist heat packs, paraffin baths, fluidotherapy, and infrared lamps. Penetrating thermotherapy, including ultrasound, phonophoresis, and diathermy, are discussed in more detail later in the chapter.

To attain therapeutic effects from vigorous heating, tissue temperature must be elevated to between 40° and 45° C (104–113°F). Within these temperatures, hyperemia, which indicates increased blood flow, occurs. Potential tissue damage can occur with temperatures above this range; temperatures

Box 7.2 Thermotherapy Application

Indications

Subacute or chronic injuries, to:
- Reduce swelling, edema and ecchymosis
- Reduce muscle spasm/guarding

Subacute or chronic muscle spasm

Increase blood flow to:
- Increase range of motion prior to activity
- Resolve hematoma
- Facilitate tissue healing
- Relieve joint contractures
- Fight infection

Contraindications

Acute inflammation or injuries
Impaired or poor circulation
Subacute or chronic pain
Advanced arthritis
Impaired or poor sensation
Impaired thermal regulation
Malignancy/neoplasms
Thrombophlebitis

below this range are considered to be only mild heating and insufficient to stimulate cellular metabolism enough to cause therapeutic effects (10,11). Changes in surface tissue temperature caused by superficial heating agents depend on the intensity of heat applied, time of heat exposure, volume of tissue exposed, and thermal medium for surface heat.

The greatest degree of elevated temperature occurs in the skin and subcutaneous tissues within 0.5 cm of the skin surface. In areas with adequate circulation, temperature increases to its maximum within 6 to 8 minutes of exposure. Muscle temperature at depths of 1 to 2 cm increase to a lesser degree and require a longer duration of exposure (i.e., 15–30 minutes) to reach peak values (11). After peak temperatures are reached (i.e., approximately 7–9 minutes), a plateau effect or slight decrease in skin temperature is seen over the rest of the heat application. As mentioned, fat is an insulator and has a low thermal conductivity value. Therefore, tissues under a large amount of fat are minimally affected by superficial heating agents. To elevate deep tissues to the desired thermal levels without burning the skin and subcutaneous tissue, a deep-heating agent, such as continuous ultrasound or shortwave diathermy, should be selected.

Whirlpool Tanks

Whirlpool and immersion tanks combine warm or hot water with a hydromassaging effect to increase superficial skin temperature (Fig. 7.10). Tanks may be portable or fixed and include the more common extremity tanks and full-body therapeutic tubs, such as the Hubbard tank or walk tank.

Whirlpools are analgesic agents that relax muscle spasms, relieve joint pain and stiffness, provide mechanical debridement, and facilitate ROM exercises after prolonged immobilization. As with cold whirlpools and immersion baths, buoyancy facilitates increased ROM, and the hydromassaging effect is controlled by the amount of air that is emitted through the electrical turbine. The more agitation, the greater the water movement. The turbine can be moved up and down or directed at a specific angle and locked in place. Treatment time ranges from 20 to 30 minutes. Total body immersion exceeding 20 to 30 minutes can dehydrate the individual, leading to dizziness and a high body core temperature. Only the body parts being treated should be immersed.

> See *Field Strategy: Techniques for Using a Whirlpool Bath* on the companion website at thePoint for an explanation of the use of this modality.

For safety reasons, ground-fault circuit interrupters (GFCIs) should be installed in all receptacles or in the circuit breaker box in the hydrotherapy area. They should be no more than 1.5 meters away from the tanks. A sensor located within the GFCI monitors current in the hot and neutral lines that feed the receptacle. Because the maximum safe transthoracic current (through intact skin) is deemed to be 5 mA, the GFCI activates at this level and immediately trips the circuit to disconnect all current to the receptacle. These receptacles should be inspected annually to ensure proper operation.

Contrast Baths

A contrast bath alternates cold and hot tubs or whirlpools. This elicits a local vasoconstriction–vasodilation fluctuation to reduce edema and restore ROM in subacute or chronic injuries. Two whirlpools or containers are placed next to each other. One is filled with cold water and ice at 10° to 18°C (50–65°F), and the other is filled with hot water at 38° to 44°C (100–111°F) (12). The injured extremity is alternated between the two tubs. One treatment method involves a hot water to cold water ratio of 3:1 or 4:1 for approximately 20 minutes. In subacute conditions, the treatment begins and ends in cold water before starting therapeutic exercise. In chronic conditions, the treatment more often is concluded in warm immersion. A second method is to base treatment on a variable time frame. During the first cycle, 75% of the time is in cold water and 25% in hot water. The second cycle moves to 50% in cold water and 50% in hot water, with the third cycle moving to 25% in cold water and 75% in hot water. Research, however, has failed to demonstrate any significant physiologic effect on intramuscular

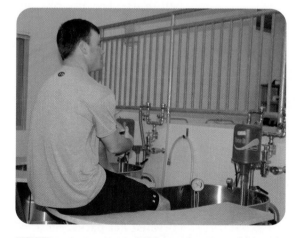

FIGURE 7.10 Whirlpools. Hot whirlpools increase superficial skin temperatures, leading to an analgesic effect that can reduce muscle spasm and pain, facilitate range of motion exercises, and promote healing.

tissue temperature 1 cm below the skin and subcutaneous fat (13,14). Therefore, contrast therapy may need to be reconsidered as a viable therapeutic modality.

Hot Tub and Jacuzzis

Although not a common modality in the athletic training room, many individuals have access to a hot tub or jacuzzi. Because organic contaminants, high water temperature, and turbulence reduce the effectiveness of chlorine as a bacterial agent, infection with *Pseudomonas aeruginosa* causing folliculitis is an alarming and increasing problem associated with use of hot tubs and jacuzzis. If infection is to be prevented, these tubs must have an effective filtration and chlorination system. Chlorine and pH levels should be monitored hourly during periods of heavy use, and calcium hardness should be evaluated weekly (12). The water should be drained, superchlorinated, and refilled once every 3 months. The water temperature should not exceed 38.9°C (102°F).

Moist Heat Packs

Heat packs provide superficial heat, transferring energy to the individual's skin by way of conduction. Each subsequent underlying tissue layer is heated through conduction from the overlying tissue, reaching a slightly deeper tissue level than occurs with a whirlpool. Like other forms of superficial heating, deeper tissues, including the musculature, are not significantly heated. The heat transfer is inhibited by subcutaneous fat, which acts as a thermal insulator, and by the increased blood flow through the area, which carries away externally applied heat. Hot packs most often are used to promote soft-tissue healing, reduce pain and superficial muscle spasm while promoting general relaxation, and improve tissue extensibility.

The pack consists of a canvas or nylon case filled with a hydrophilic silicate (or other hydrophilic substance) or with sand. The packs are stored in a hot water unit at a temperature ranging from 70° to 75°C (158–170°F) (Fig. 7.11). When removed from the water, a pack should be wrapped in a commercial padded cover or in six to eight layers of toweling and then placed directly over the injury site for 20 to 30 minutes. Commercial hot pack covers may need additional layers of toweling to ensure adequate insulation for the hot pack.

The pack should be secured and completely cover the area being treated. As with other forms of heat application, the patient should only feel a mild to moderate sensation of heat. The patient should never lie on top of the pack, because this may accelerate the rate of heat transfer, leading to burns on sensitive skin. Following 5 minutes of treatment, the area should be checked for any redness or signs of burning. At the conclusion of the treatment, the hot pack should be replaced in the heating unit for rewarming. It is strongly recommended that hot pack temperature be measured before use, because rewarming varies depending on the temperature of the hot pack before its return to the heating unit, on size of the heating unit, and on the number of used packs simultaneously returned for reheating (15).

The hot packs should be checked regularly for leaks, and a hot pack should be discarded if any leaking occurs. This may become evident when cleaning the unit on a monthly basis. Hydrophilic silicate may accumulate on the bottom of the unit and should be removed so as not to interfere with the heating element.

FIGURE 7.11 Moist hot packs. Moist heat treatments can burn sensitive skin. As such, the pack should be placed in a commercial padded towel or in six to eight layers of toweling, and the skin surface should be checked periodically for redness or signs of burning.

Paraffin Bath

Paraffin baths provide heat to contoured bony areas of the body (e.g., feet, hands, or wrists). They are used to treat subacute or chronic rheumatoid arthritis associated with joint stiffness and decreased ROM as well as other common chronic injuries and diseases, such as systemic sclerosis (16). A paraffin and mineral oil mixture (6:1 or 7:1 ratio) is heated in a unit at 45° to 54°C (113–129°F). The purpose of adding mineral oil is to lower the melting temperature of paraffin from 54°C (129°F) to between 45° and 50°C (113–122°F), making the mixture more comfortable for patients during the treatment.

Several methods of paraffin application may be employed; however, two principal methods of application are used: dip and wrap, and dip and reimmerse. For both methods, the body part should be thoroughly cleansed and dried, and all jewelry should be removed. The body part should be placed in a relaxed position and then dipped into the bath several times, each time allowing the previous coat to dry (Fig. 7.12). The patient should not move the fingers or toes so as not to break the seal of the glove being formed. In addition, outer layers of paraffin should not extend over new skin, because burning may occur. When completed, the body part should be wrapped in a plastic bag and towel to maintain heat and then elevated for 15 to 20 minutes (or until heat is no longer generated).

When using the dip and reimmerse method, after the formation of a wax glove, the body part covered by the glove is put back into the wax container for 10 to 20 minutes without moving it. This method results in a more vigorous response relative to temperature elevation and changes in blood flow. This technique should not be used in individuals predisposed to edema, however, or in those who cannot sit in the position required for treatment.

When the treatment is completed, the wax should be peeled off and returned to the bath, where it can be reused. The mineral oil in the wax helps to keep the skin soft and pliable during massage when treating a variety of hand and foot conditions. In comparison with other heat modalities, paraffin wax is not significantly better at decreasing pain or increasing joint ROM. It should not be used in patients with decreased sensation, open wounds, thin scars, skin rashes, or peripheral vascular disease.

FIGURE 7.12 Paraffin bath. A thoroughly cleansed limb is dipped several times into the paraffin solution. The body part is then wrapped in plastic and a towel to maintain heat, or it can be reimmersed into the solution and held motionless for the duration of the treatment.

Fluidotherapy

Fluidotherapy is a dry thermal modality that transfers its energy (i.e., heat) to soft tissues by forced convection. Heat is transferred through the forced movements, or agitation (blower action), in the unit chamber of heated air and Cellex particles, which are then circulated around the treated body part, making the fluidized bed behave with properties similar to those of liquids. Used to treat acute injuries and wounds, decrease pain and swelling, and increase ROM and inadequate blood flow, this modality is more effective than paraffin wax baths and warm whirlpool tubs at inducing absolute temperature increases in peripheral joint capsules and muscles (17). Both temperature and the amount of particle agitation can be varied. Treatment temperature ranges from 46° to 51°C (115°–124°F) (10).

For optimal heating, the patient should remove all jewelry and wash the treated body parts before positioning the body area in the fluidotherapy chamber. A skin sensory heat discrimination test of the patient is mandatory before considering application of this modality. This test consists of setting the amount of heat needed, the speed of particle agitation required, and the total treatment session duration.

Advantages of this superficial heating modality include that exercise can be performed during the treatment, higher treatment temperatures can be tolerated, and heat is distributed over the entire limb surface area with minimal to no pressure applied to the treated site. If a body part has an open wound, a plastic barrier or bag can be placed over the wound to prevent any fine cellulose particles from becoming embedded in the wound and to minimize the risk of cross-contamination. Treatment duration ranges from 15 to 20 minutes.

A. *The lacrosse player's upper arm contusion showed significant improvement after 5 days of ice treatments. As long as the individual does not report point tenderness at the involved area, it probably is safe to move to a heat treatment. Heat can increase the local circulation and, in doing so, promote healing. It also can be used in conjunction with stretching and mild exercise to strengthen the injured muscle.*

ULTRASOUND

Two weeks after injury, the lacrosse player is pain-free. There is a small, palpable, swollen area in the triceps at the spot where the force was sustained. What type of heat treatment would be most effective at this point in the healing process?

Superficial heating agents were discussed in the previous section. These agents produce temperature elevations in skin and underlying subcutaneous tissues to a depth of 1 to 2 cm. Ultrasound uses high-frequency acoustic (sound) waves rather than electromagnetic energy to elicit thermal and non-thermal effects in deep tissue to depths of 3 cm or more. This transfer of energy takes place in the deep structures without causing excessive heating of the overlying superficial structures. The actual mechanism of ultrasound, produced via the **reverse piezoelectric effect**, converts electrical current to mechanical energy as it passes through a piezoelectric crystal (e.g., quartz, barium titanate or lead zirconate titanate) housed in the transducer head. The vibration of the crystal results in organic molecules moving in longitudinal waves that move the energy into the deep tissues to produce temperature increases (i.e., thermal effects) as well as mechanical and chemical alterations (i.e., non-thermal effects). Thermal effects increase collagen tissue extensibility, blood flow, sensory and motor neuron velocity, and enzymatic activity and decrease muscle spasm, joint stiffness, inflammation, and pain. Nonthermal effects (i.e., mechanical effect) increase skin permeability, thus decreasing the inflammatory response, reducing pain, and facilitating the soft-tissue healing process. Both pulsed and continuous ultrasound reduces nerve conduction velocity of pain nerve fibers.

The Ultrasound Wave

Unlike electromagnetic energy, sound cannot travel in a vacuum. Sound waves, such as those produced by a human voice, diverge in all directions. This principle allows people to hear others talking while standing or positioned behind them. As the frequency increases, the level of divergence decreases. Like sound waves, the frequencies used in therapeutic ultrasound produce collimated cylindrical beams, similar to a light beam leaving a flashlight, that have a width slightly smaller than the diameter of the transducer head. The **effective radiating area** is the portion of the transducer's surface area that actually produces the ultrasound wave.

Frequency and Attenuation

The frequency of ultrasound is measured in megahertz (MHz) and represents the number of waves (in millions) that occur in 1 second. Frequencies range between 0.75 and 3.3 MHz. For any given source of sound, the higher the frequency, the less the emerging sound beam diverges. For example, low-frequency ultrasound produces a more widely diverging beam compared with high-frequency ultrasound, which produces a collimated beam. The more commonly used 1.0-MHz ultrasound heats tissue from 3 to 5 cm deep, whereas 3-MHz ultrasound heats tissue less than 2 cm deep but may have an affect on tissues 2.5 to 3.0 cm deep (18,19).

Energy contained within a sound beam decreases as it travels through tissue. The level of absorption depends on the type of tissues to which it is applied. Tissues with high protein content (e.g., nerve and muscle tissue) absorb ultrasound readily. Deflection (i.e., reflection or refraction) is greater at heterogeneous (different or unrelated) tissue interfaces, especially at the bone–muscle interface. This deflection creates standing waves that increase heat. Ultrasound that is not absorbed or deflected is transmitted through the tissue.

Absorption of sound (and, therefore, attenuation) increases as the frequency increases. The higher the frequency, the more rapidly the molecules are forced to move against this friction. As the absorption increases, less sound energy is available to move through the tissue. The 1-MHz machine most often is used on individuals with a high percentage of subcutaneous body fat and whenever the desired effects are in the deeper structures. This ultrasound unit also has been used to stimulate collagen synthesis in tendon fibroblasts after an injury as well as cell division during periods of rapid cell proliferation (20). In addition, it has been used on tendons on the second and fourth days after surgery to increase tensile strength. After the fifth day, however, application decreases tensile strength (21).

The high-frequency, 3-MHz machine provides treatment to superficial tissues and tendons, with a depth of penetration between 1 and 2 cm (⅓ to ¼ inch). The low penetration depth is associated with limited transmission of energy, rapid absorption of energy, and higher heating rate in a relatively limited tissue depth.

Types of Waves

Sound waves can be produced as a continuous or pulsed wave. A continuous wave is one in which the sound intensity remains constant, whereas a pulsed wave is intermittently interrupted. Pulsed waves are further delineated by the fraction of time the sound is present over one pulse period, or duty cycle. This is calculated with the following equation:

$$\text{Duty cycle} = \frac{\text{Duration of pulse (time on)} \times 100}{\text{Pulse period (time on + time off)}}$$

Typical duty cycles in the pulse mode range from 0.05 (5%) to 0.5 (50%), with the most commonly used duty cycle being 0.02 (20%) (22). Continuous ultrasound waves provide both thermal and nonthermal effects and are used when a deep, elevated tissue temperature is advisable. Pulsed ultrasound and low-intensity, continuous ultrasound produce primarily nonthermal effects and are used to facilitate repair and soft-tissue healing when a high increase in tissue temperature is not desired.

Intensity

Therapeutic intensities are expressed in Watts per square centimeter (W/cm^2) and range from 0.25 to 2.0 W/cm^2. The greater the intensity, the greater the resulting temperature elevation. Thermal temperature can increase 7° to 8°F up to 2.5 cm deep in the muscle after the application of ultrasound at 1.5W/cm^2 for 10 minutes (23). As mentioned, ultrasound waves are absorbed in those tissues that are highest in collagen content, and they are reflected at tissue interfaces, particularly between bone and muscle.

Clinical Uses

Ultrasound is used to manage several soft-tissue conditions, such as tendinitis, bursitis, and muscle spasm; to reabsorb calcium deposits in soft tissue; and to reduce joint contractures, pain, and scar tissue (Box 7.3). In other areas, musculoskeletal ultrasound frequently is used to determine the presence or absence of tendon tears or the extent of dermal injuries (24,25). Wound healing is enhanced

Box 7.3 Ultrasound Application

Indications
Deep tissue heating
Acute inflammatory conditions (pulsed)
Chronic inflammatory conditions (pulsed or continuous)
Spasticity/muscle spasm
Trigger areas
Increase extensibility of collagen tissue
Joint adhesions/contractures
Neuroma
Postacute myositis ossificans

Contraindications
Acute and postacute hemorrhage (continuous)
Infection
Thrombophlebitis
Areas of impaired circulation/sensation
Over stress fracture sites or osteoporosis
Over suspected malignancy/cancer
Over the pelvic or lumbar areas during menstruation or pregnancy
Over epiphyseal growth plates
Over the eyes, heart, skull, spine, or genitals
Over active sites of infection or sepsis
Over an implanted pacemaker
Over exposed metal that penetrates the skin

with low-intensity, pulsed ultrasound. It is recommended that ultrasound treatment begin 2 weeks after injury, during the proliferative phase of healing. Earlier treatment may increase inflammation and delay healing time. Tissue healing is thought to occur predominantly through nonthermal effects. An intensity of 0.5 to 1.0 W/cm^2 pulsed at 20% is recommended for superficial wounds. For skin lesions and ulcers, a frequency of 3 MHz or higher is recommended (22).

Ultrasound often is used with other modalities. When used in conjunction with hot packs, muscle spasm and muscle guarding may be reduced. The hot pack produces superficial heating, and the ultrasound, using a 1-MHz ultrasound frequency, produces heating in the deeper tissues. Because ultrasound can increase the blood flow to deep tissues, this modality often is used with electrical stimulation units. The electrical current produces a muscle contraction or modulates pain; the ultrasound increases circulation and provides deep heating. This combination of treatment protocols can be effective in treating both trigger and acupuncture points.

Application

Because ultrasound waves cannot travel through air, a coupling agent is used between the transducer head and skin to facilitate passage of the waves. Coupling gels are applied liberally over the area to be treated. The transducer head is then stroked slowly over the area (Fig. 7.13). Strokes are applied in small, continuous circles or longitudinal patterns to distribute the energy as evenly as possible at a rate of 4 cm/s to prevent **cavitation** (gas bubble formation) in deep tissues (26). The total area covered usually is two- to threefold the size of the transducer head for every 5 minutes of exposure. If a larger area is covered, the effective dosage and elevated temperature changes that are delivered to any one region decrease. A firm, uniform amount of pressure exerted on the transducer head maximizes the transmission of acoustic energy between the sound head and tissue interface.

A common alternate method for irregularly shaped areas (e.g., wrist, hand, ankle, or foot) is application under water. A rubber-type basin should be used for these treatments. For several reasons, metal containers and whirlpools should not be used for underwater treatments. If the treatment is given in a metal basin or whirlpool, some of the ultrasound energy is reflected off the metal, thus increasing the intensity in certain areas near the metal. In addition, water in a whirlpool often has a large number of air bubbles, which tend to reduce the transmission of ultrasound. This problem is even more pronounced if the turbine was used before the ultrasound treatment. Water treatments are indirect and generally have a 0.5- to 3-cm space between the patient and the sound head. Intensity is increased by 0.5 W/cm^2 to compensate for air and minerals in the water. Small air bubbles tend to accumulate on the face of the transducer head and the skin surface when this method is used. The clinician should quickly wipe off the accumulated bubbles during the treatment. No jewelry should be worn under the water surface. In addition, the clinician should hold the transducer head so that his or her hand is out of the water.

If for some reason the injured area cannot be immersed in water, a bladder technique may be used. A small balloon is filled with water or aqueous gel. To prevent blockage of the ultrasound energy, all air pockets must be eliminated. The ultrasound energy is transmitted from the transducer to the injured site through this bladder. Both sides of the balloon should be coated with gel to ensure good contact.

Research has shown that ultrasound treatments using gel in direct contact with the patient produce more heat than ultrasound administered indirectly underwater produces (27–31). A reusable gel pad is another method of application over bony protuberances or irregular surfaces. These pads, when used with ultrasound gel, have been found to be more effective than using the traditional water bath immersion method (31). Intensity for both gel and underwater treatment is determined by the stage of injury, mode used (i.e., pulsed or continuous), desired depth of penetration, and patient tolerance. The patient may feel a mild, warm sensation.

FIGURE 7.13 Ultrasound. A coupling agent is used between the transducer head and area being treated. The head is then moved in small circles or longitudinal strokes to distribute the energy as evenly as possible to prevent damage to the underlying tissues.

When the goal of treatment is to elevate tissue temperature over a large quantity of soft tissue (e.g., hip or back), a continuous-wave mode with intensities as high as 1.5 to 2.0 W/cm^2 typically is used. A lower intensity (0.5–1.0 W/cm^2) and a higher frequency are used over areas with less soft-tissue coverage and where bone is closer to the skin surface. At tissue–bone interfaces, approximately 35% of the ultrasound beam is reflected, resulting in an increased intensity in the soft tissue overlying the bone, particularly the periosteum (27). Elevated temperatures should be maintained at least 5 minutes after the patient reports the sensation of gentle heat to allow an increase in extensibility. If heat production in tissues greater than 3 cm deep is the desired effect, 10 minutes of treatment after the patient reports the sensation of heat is the minimum (30).

Phonophoresis

Phonophoresis is a technique in which the mechanical effects of ultrasound are used to enhance percutaneous absorption of anti-inflammatory drugs (e.g., cortisol, dexamethasone, and **salicylates**) and local analgesics (e.g., lidocaine) through the skin to the underlying tissues. One advantage of this modality is that the drug is delivered directly to the site where the effect is sought. Phonophoresis is believed to accelerate functional recovery by decreasing pain and promoting healing. High ultrasound intensities have been used to deliver these medications to depths of 5 to 6 cm subcutaneously, into skeletal muscle and peripheral nerves (32). Pulsed-waved ultrasound appears to be more effective than continuous-wave ultrasound (33).

This technique is used during the postacute stage in conditions to treat painful trigger points, bursitis, contusions, or other chronic soft-tissue conditions, such as epicondylitis (22,34). Phonophoresis also may be helpful in treating neuropathic pain, including phantom pain and central pain (35). The standard coupling gel is replaced by a gel or cream containing the medication. Commercial chem-pads impregnated with the medication also are readily available and may be used in lieu of the traditional medicated ointment applicators. Continuous ultrasound is used, because tissue permeability is increased by the thermal effects and, therefore, the medication is more easily absorbed. Treatment occurs at a lower intensity (i.e., 1.0–1.5 W/cm^2) for 5 to 15 minutes.

A *Ultrasound would be an accepted treatment for the small, palpable, swollen area in the triceps. Ultrasound can provide both thermal and nonthermal effects to increase circulation, blood flow, and tissue extensibility and to reduce hematoma formation and optimize the healing process.*

SHORTWAVE DIATHERMY

Q *In treating the lacrosse player's triceps contusion, would diathermy be an accepted treatment?*

Diathermy, which literally means "to heat through," uses electromagnetic energy from the nonionizing radio frequency part of the spectrum. Because the duration of the impulses is so short, no ion movement occurs. The result is no stimulation of motor or sensory nerves.

Two types of generators are used for heating. One places two condenser plates (capacitive or condenser field) on either side of the injured area, thus placing the patient in the electrical circuit. The other method uses an induction coil (induction field) wrapped around the body part that places the patient in an electromagnetic field. Heating is uneven, because different tissues resist energy at different levels, an application of **Joule's law**, which states that the greater the resistance or impedance, the more heat is developed. Tissues with a high fluid content, such as skeletal muscle and areas surrounding joints, absorb more of the energy and are heated to a greater extent, whereas fat is not heated as much. Because the applicators are not in contact with the skin, this method can be used for heating skeletal muscle when the skin is abraded so long as edema is not present.

Shortwave diathermy can be delivered as either a continuous or a pulsed form. Rapid vibration of the continuous shortwave diathermy (CSWD) waves is absorbed by the body and converted into heat by the resisting tissues. This elicits deep, penetrating thermal effects and is used primarily in chronic conditions. When these waves are interrupted at regular intervals, pulsed (or bursts of) radio frequency energy are delivered to the tissues and are referred to as pulsed radio frequency radiation (PRFR). Pulsed radio frequency radiation may produce either thermal or nonthermal effects on tissues. Low power produces nonthermal effects, and high power produces thermal effects. Pulsed shortwave diathermy may be used in acute and subacute conditions, preventing tissue temperatures from rising too fast or too high.

Therapeutic devices that deliver CSWD and PRFR use high-frequency alternating currents to oscillate at specified radio frequencies between 10 and 50 MHz. The most commonly used radio frequency is 27.12 MHz. Microwave diathermy, another form of electromagnetic radiation, can be directed toward the body and reflected from the skin; it uses ultrahigh frequencies (UHF) at 2,450 MHz. Microwave diathermy is seldom used today, however, and is not discussed in this section.

Continuous Shortwave Diathermy

The goal of CSWD is to raise tissue temperature to within the physiologically effective range of 37.5° to 44°C (99.5–111.2°F) in deeper tissues (2.5–5.0 cm). This is done by introducing a high-frequency electrical current with a power output of 80 to 120 W. The depth of penetration and extent of heat production depends on wave frequency, the electrical properties of the tissues receiving the electromagnetic energy, and the type of applicator used.

The physiologic effects known to occur with other therapeutic heat treatments also are produced with CSWD. Mild heating usually is desired in acute musculoskeletal conditions, whereas vigorous heating may be needed in chronic conditions. Because the effects occur in deeper tissue, CSWD is used to increase extensibility of deep collagen tissue, decrease joint stiffness, relieve deep pain and muscle spasm, increase blood flow, assist in the resolution of inflammation, and facilitate healing of soft-tissue injuries in the postacute stage (Box 7.4).

Pulsed Shortwave Diathermy

Pulsed shortwave diathermy (PSWD) is known by several names, including pulsed electromagnetic fields, pulsed electromagnetic energy, and PRFR. A relatively new type of diathermy, it uses a timing circuit to electrically interrupt the 27.12-MHz waves and produce bursts, or pulse trains, containing a series of high-frequency, sine wave oscillations. Each pulse train has a preset "time on" and is separated from successive pulse trains by a "time off" determined by the pulse repetition rate, or frequency. The pulse frequency can be varied from 1 to 700 pulses per second by turning the pulse-frequency control on the equipment operation panel.

Box 7.4   Diathermy Applications

Indications
Chronic inflammation (bursitis, tendinitis, myositis, osteoarthritis, etc.)
Joint capsule contractures
Degenerative joint disease
Sacroiliac strains
Acute or chronic pain
Subacute inflammation
Deep muscles spasms
Ankylosing spondylitis
Osteoarthritis
Chronic pelvic inflammatory disease
Epicondylitis

Contraindications
Over internally and externally worn metal objects
Over metal surgical implants
Metal objects within immediate area
Unshielded cardiac pacemaker
Peripheral vascular disease
Patients with hemophilia
Sensitive areas, including over:
- Lumbar, pelvic, or abdominal areas in women with metallic intrauterine devices
- Ischemic, hemorrhagic, malignant, and acutely inflamed tissues
- Eyes, face, skull, genitals, and swollen joints
- Moist wound dressings, clothing, or perspiration
- Pregnant abdomen
- Epiphyseal plates in children

The production of heat in tissues depends on the manipulation of peak pulse power, pulse frequency, and pulse duration. The measure of heat production is the mean power, which is lower than the power that is delivered (80–120 W) during most CSWD treatments. Nonthermal effects may be produced at mean power levels below 38 W; thermal effects are produced when mean power levels exceed 38 W. Mean power levels between 38 and 80 W are appropriate for treatment of acute and subacute inflammatory conditions and have been shown to assist in the absorption of hematomas, reduce ankle swelling, and stimulate collagen formation. Pulsed shortwave diathermy is applied to the patient in the same manner as CSWD. Most PSWD devices have the drum type of inductive applicator. Therefore, one could expect less heating of superficial fat and more heating of tissues such as superficial muscle, which has a high electrolyte level. Indications and contradictions are the same for PSWD as for CSWD.

A *Shortwave diathermy can provide deep heating to tissues with a higher water content, such as muscle. It is important to recognize, however, that the extent of muscle heating can be inhibited by the thickness of the subcutaneous fat layer. As such, other modalities may be more effective in providing a deep heat treatment.*

ELECTROTHERAPY

Q *In conjunction with a heat treatment for the lacrosse player's upper arm contusion, what type of electrotherapy could be used to elicit a muscle contraction and, in doing so, decrease muscle guarding and atrophy?*

Electrical therapy is a popular therapeutic modality that can be applied to injured or immobilized muscles during the early stages of a therapeutic exercise program, when the muscle is at its weakest. The various forms of electrotherapy are used to decrease pain; increase blood flow, ROM, and muscle strength; re-educate muscle; facilitate absorption of anti-inflammatory, analgesic, or anesthetic drugs to the injured area; and promote wound healing. An understanding of the clinical use of electrical stimulation requires an understanding of the basic principles of electricity.

Principles of Electricity

Electrical energy flows between two points. In an atom, protons are positively charged, electrons are negatively charged, and neutrons have no charge. Equal numbers of protons and electrons produce balanced neutrality in the atom. Transfer of energy from one atom to the next involves the movement of electrons only from the nucleus, thereby creating an electrical imbalance. This subtraction and addition of electrons causes atoms to become electrically charged, and such atoms are then called ions. An ion that has more electrons is said to be negatively charged; an ion that has more protons is said to be positively charged. Ions of similar charge repel each another, whereas ions of dissimilar charge attract one another. The strength of the force and the distance between ions determine how quickly the transfer of energy occurs.

Types of Currents

Four types of electrical current can be applied to tissues (Fig. 7.14). Two types fall under the category of continuous current: direct, and alternating. Direct current (DC) is a continuous, one-directional flow of ions and is used to

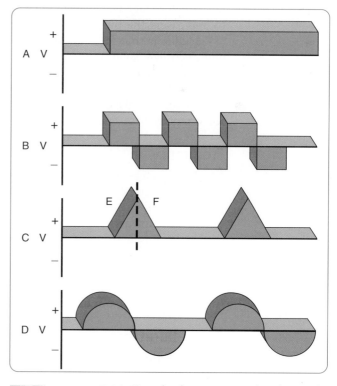

FIGURE 7.14 Four basic currents. The shape of the waveforms can be altered by changing the rate of rise and the rate of decay. **A,** Direct current (DC) with square wave. **B,** Alternating current (AC) with square wave. **C,** Monophasic with triangular wave. e = rate of rise; f = rate of decay. **D,** Biphasic with sine wave.

modulate pain, elicit a muscle contraction, or produce ion movement. Alternating current (AC) is a continuous, two-directional flow of ions used to modulate pain or elicit a muscle contraction. A third classification, pulsed current, represents a type of current that has been modulated to produce specific biophysical effects. With this type of current, a flow of ions in DC or AC is briefly interrupted. The current may be one-directional (monophasic), two-directional (biphasic), or polyphasic (pertains to pulsed currents that usually contain three or more pulses grouped together). These groups of pulses are interrupted for short periods of time and repeat themselves at regular intervals. Pulsed currents are used in interferential and so-called Russian currents. In therapeutic use, each current can be manipulated by altering the frequency, intensity, and duration of the wave or pulse.

Current Modifications

See *Parameter Modification for Neuromuscular Electrical Stimulation (NMES)* on the companion website at thePoint for guidelines to achieving therapeutic effect with this technology.

Once the basic current type is known, several parameters can be manipulated for the desired effects. The more common parameters include the amplitude, frequency, pulse duration, pulse charge, electrode setup, polarity, mode, duty cycle, and duration of treatment (36). An electrical unit with the prescribed current type should be selected, and then the modifications indicated for the desired effect should be applied.

Amplitude

Amplitude is a measure of the force, or intensity, that drives the current. The maximum amplitude is the top, or highest, point of each phase. The term is synonymous with **voltage** and is measured in millivolts (mV), although some units use milliamperage (mA) as a measure of amplitude. Voltage causes the ions to move, but the actual movement is called **current**. If the current is presented graphically, the voltage is represented by the magnitude of the wave. If resistance remains the same, an increase in voltage will increase the amperage (i.e., rate of current flow). Average current can be increased by increasing the pulse duration, increasing the pulse frequency, or some combination of the two.

Mediums that facilitate movement of the ions are called **conductors** and include water, blood, and electrolyte solutions (e.g., sweat). Mediums that inhibit movement of the ions are called **resistors** and include skin, fat, and lotion. The combination of voltage, current, and resistance is measured in ohms (Ω). **Ohm's law** ($I = V/R$) states that current (I) in a conductor increases as the driving force (V) becomes larger or as resistance (R) is decreased. For example, 1 volt is the amount of electrical force required to send a current of 1 amp through a resistance of 1 ohm.

Frequency

Frequency refers to the number of waveform cycles per second (cps) or hertz (Hz) with AC, the number of pulses per second (pps) with monophasic or biphasic current, or the number of bursts per second (bps) with Russian stimulation. One purpose in altering frequency is to control the force of muscle contractions during neuromuscular stimulation. Low-frequency stimulation (<15 pps) causes the muscle to twitch with each pulse, cycle, or burst. As the frequency increases (15–40 pps), stimulation minimizes the relaxation phase of the muscle contraction. At higher frequencies (>40 pps), the stimulation is so fast that no relaxation occurs and a sustained, maximal contraction (tetany) is generated. Therefore, if the intent is to fatigue a muscle, the clinician can choose the appropriate frequency to bring about this effect.

Pulse Duration

Phase duration, or current duration as it is sometimes called, refers to the length of time that current is flowing. Pulse duration is the length of a single pulse of monophasic or biphasic current. In biphasic current, the sum of the two phases represents the pulse duration, whereas in monophasic current, the phase and pulse duration are synonymous. The time between each subsequent pulse is called the interpulse interval. The combined time of the pulse duration and interpulse interval is referred to as the pulse period. More powerful muscle contractions are generated with a pulse duration of 300 to 500 microseconds (µs). Duration of less than 1 millisecond will not stimulate denervated muscle, regardless of the current's amplitude.

Pulse Charge

In a single phase, the pulse charge, or the quantity of an electrical current, is the product of the phase duration and amplitude and represents the total amount of electricity being delivered to the individual during each pulse. Amplitude, pulse duration, interpulse interval, phase duration, and phase charge are illustrated in Fig. 7.15.

Electrode Setup

Electrical currents are introduced into the body through electrodes and a conducting medium. The smaller active pad has the greatest current density and brings the current into the body. The active electrode ranges from a very small pad to one that is 4 inches square. Water or an electrolyte gel is used to obtain high conductivity. The arrangement of the pads depends on the polarity of the active pad, not on the number or size. If only one active electrode is used, or if the active electrodes are of the same charge, the arrangement is monopolar. This pattern requires the use of a large dispersal pad to take on the charge opposite that of the active pad and, in doing so, complete the circuit. The dispersal pad, from which the electrons leave the body, should be as large as possible to reduce current density. With the low current density, no sensation should be felt beneath the dispersal pad. When the active pads are of opposite charges, the arrangement is bipolar. Because this arrangement provides a complete circuit, no dispersal pad is necessary. Interferential stimulation requires a quadripolar electrode arrangement; this is nothing more than a bipolar arrangement from two channels where the currents cross at the treatment site. This electrode arrangement can be seen in Fig. 7.16.

The pads should be placed at least one pad width apart. The closer the pads are, the shallower and more isolated the contraction; the farther apart the pads are, the deeper and more generalized the contraction. The physiologic effects can occur anywhere between the pads but usually occur at the active electrode, because current density is greatest at this point.

Polarity

Polarity refers to the direction of current flow and can be toward either a positive or a negative pole. During DC and monophasic stimulation, the active electrode(s) can be either positive or negative, and current will flow in a predetermined direction (away from the negative electrode). During AC or biphasic stimulation, the polarity of the active pads alternates between positive and negative with each phase of the current.

Mode

In a monopolar arrangement, the term mode refers to the alternating (reciprocating) or continuous flow of current through the active electrodes. The term alternating means that the active electrodes receive current on an alternating basis, whereas with continuous flow, each electrode receives current throughout the treatment period. In neuromuscular stimulation, another popular mode is ramped, or surge, amplitude. The amplitude builds gradually to the desired level, which improves patient comfort and safety by preventing sudden, powerful muscle contractions.

Duty Cycle

Duty cycle refers to the ratio of the amount of time that current is flowing (i.e., on time) to the amount of time it is not flowing (i.e., off time). Used in neuromuscular stimulation, the duty cycle

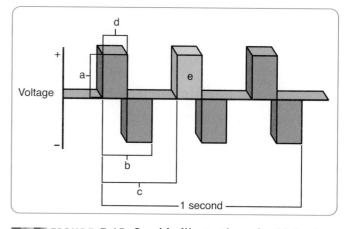

FIGURE 7.15 Graphic illustration of a biphasic current. a, amplitude (intensity); b, pulse duration; c, interpulse interval; d, phase duration; e, phase charge. Frequency= 3 pulses per second.

FIGURE 7.16 Transcutaneous electrical nerve stimulation. A transcutaneous electrical nerve stimulation unit is used to decrease acute and chronic pain to an injured area.

simulates repetitions and rest so as to delay the onset of fatigue. In edema formation, it creates a muscle pump. With neuromuscular stimulation, the recommended duty cycle should be 1:4, or 20%, initially (i.e., 10 seconds on and 40 seconds off) and should gradually increase as fatigability decreases. Manual control of the duty cycle is necessary to prevent discomfort for the patient.

Duration of Treatment

Duration of treatment is the total time during which the patient is subjected to electrical stimulation. Many units have internal timers. Treatment duration typically is 15 to 30 minutes.

Electrical Stimulating Units

Several different types of electrical stimulating units are available (Box 7.5). Although it would be much easier to name the units based on the types of current that characterize the stimulation devices, this is not the case. Names often are used to show distinction between the characteristics, indications, and parameters of the various units. Unfortunately, many units could fall under the same general title. To complicate matters further, many common names, such as Galvanic, Faradic, and Russian stimulation, are still used.

Transcutaneous Electrical Nerve Stimulation

By varying the selection and setting of pulse duration, pulse/burst frequency, and current amplitude, clinicians can program transcutaneous electrical nerve stimulation (TENS) units to deliver one of the five basic therapeutic modes (10):

1. Conventional TENS units typically are portable, biphasic generators with parameters that allow pain control via electrical pulses having short duration, high frequency, and low to comfortable current amplitude.

2. Acupuncture-like TENS has electrical pulses of long duration, low frequency, and comfortable to tolerable current amplitude. It is called acupuncture-like, because the pulse frequency is low, resembling that used in acupuncture therapy.

3. Brief-intense TENS has electrical pulses of long duration, high frequency, and comfortable to tolerable current amplitude. It gets its name because the duration of application is briefer and the current amplitude higher than in the other modes, triggering a somewhat brief yet intense stimulation during treatment.

4. Burst TENS delivers bursts of pulses, not individual pulses, of low frequency at comfortable current amplitude.

5. Modulation TENS delivers random electronic modulation of pulse duration, pulse frequency, and current amplitude.

See *The Five Classic Modes of TENS Therapy and Their Respective Biophysical and Physiological Characteristics* on the companion website at thePoint.

The units can produce analgesia and decrease acute and chronic pain as well as pain associated with delayed-onset muscle soreness, although the duration of analgesia is unpredictable. Often, TENS is used continuously after surgery in a 30- to 60-minute session, several times a day. It is thought that TENS works to override the body's internal signals of pain (gate theory of pain) or to stimulate the release of endorphins, a strong, opiate-like substance produced by the body. The unit uses small, carbonized silicone electrodes to transmit electrical pulses through the skin (Fig. 7.16). Most units are small enough to be worn on a belt and are battery powered. The electrodes are taped on the skin over or around the painful site, but they also may be secured along the peripheral or spinal nerve pathways. For individuals who have allergic reactions to the tape adhesive or who develop skin abrasions from repeated applications, electrodes with a self-adhering adhesive are available.

High-Voltage Pulsed Stimulation

High-voltage pulsed stimulation uses a monophasic current with a twin-peak waveform, a relatively short pulse duration and long interpulse interval, and an amplitude range above 150 mV. The short

Box 7.5   Application of Neuromuscular Electrical Stimulation

TENS	Indications	Contraindications
	↓ Posttraumatic pain, acute and chronic	Patients with pacemakers
	↓ Postsurgical pain	Pregnancy (abdominal and/or pelvic area)
	↑ Analgesia	Pain of unknown origin

High-voltage pulsed	Indications	Contraindications
	↑ Circulation and joint mobility	Pacemakers
	↑ Muscle re-education and strength	Pain of unknown origin
	↑ Wound and fracture healing	Pregnancy (abdominal and/or pelvic area)
	↑ Nonunion fracture healing	Thrombophlebitis
	↓ Muscle spasm/spasticity	Superficial skin lesions or infections
	↓ Pain and edema	Cancerous lesions over suspected fracture sites
	↓ Disuse atrophy	
	Denervation of peripheral nerve injuries	

Interferential	Indications	Contraindications
	↑ Circulation and wound healing	Pacemakers
	↓ Pain, acute and chronic	Pregnancy (abdominal and/or pelvic area)
	↓ Reduction of muscle spasm/guarding	Thrombophlebitis
	↓ Posttraumatic and chronic edema	Pain of unknown origin
	↓ Abdominal organ dysfunction	Prolonged use (may increase muscle soreness)

Low-intensity stimulation	Indications	Contraindications
	↑ Nonunion wound healing	Malignancy
	↑ Fracture healing	Hypersensitive skin
	Iontophoresis	Allergies to certain drugs

TENS, transcutaneous electrical nerve stimulation.

phase duration activates sensory and type II motor nerves without stimulating pain fibers. High-voltage pulsed stimulation often is used to re-educate muscle, increase joint mobility, promote dermal wound healing, and decrease pain, edema, muscle spasm, and muscle atrophy, but it is ineffective in reducing the soreness, loss of ROM, and loss of strength associated with delayed-onset muscle soreness (37).

Neuromuscular Electrical Stimulation

Neuromuscular electrical stimulation (NMES) units are designed to elicit a muscle contraction of moderately high intensity with relatively little patient discomfort, and they typically involve biphasic currents with a duty cycle. High-voltage electrical stimulation uses an output of 100 to 500 volts to reduce edema, pain, and muscle spasm during the acute phase. It also is used to exercise muscle and delay atrophy, maintain muscle size and strength during periods of immobilization, re-educate muscles, and increase blood flow to tissues (Fig. 7.17). Direct current is used primarily to stimulate denervated muscle and enhance wound healing as well as during iontophoresis.

FIGURE 7.17 Electrical muscle stimulation. These units are used to stimulate muscle to maintain muscle size and strength during immobilization, re-educate muscles, prevent muscle atrophy, and increase blood flow to tissues and, thereby, decrease pain and spasm.

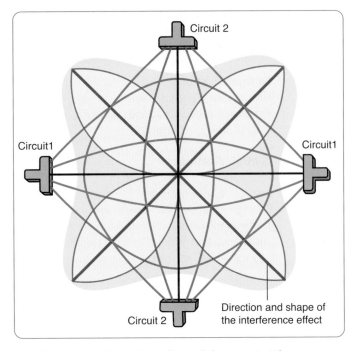

Circuit 2

Circuit1

Circuit1

Circuit 2

Direction and shape of the interference effect

FIGURE 7.18 Interferential current. When arranged in a square alignment, the quadripolar electrode setup actually is a bipolar arrangement from two channels. An electric field is created where the currents cross between the lines of electrical current flow. The maximum interference effect takes place near the center over the treatment site.

Interferential Stimulation

Interferential current uses two separate generators and a quadripolar electrode arrangement to produce two simultaneous AC electrical currents acting on the tissues. The two paired pads are placed perpendicular to each other, and the current crosses at the midpoint (Fig. 7.18). A predictable pattern of interference occurs as the interference effects branch off at 45 angles from the center of the treatment in the shape of a four-leaf clover. Tissues within this area receive the maximal treatment effect. When the electrodes are placed properly, the stimulation should be felt only between the electrodes, not under the electrodes. Most medium-frequency, sinusoidal currents used to generate interferential current have a medium-frequency range of 3,000 to 5,000 Hz and are programmable to deliver beats (or envelopes) of interferential current at a low-frequency range of approximately 1 to 200 beats per second (bps) (10). The higher frequencies lower skin resistance, thus eliciting a stronger response with less current intensity. Furthermore, sensory perception is decreased between the pads, allowing the use of a higher current, which increases stimulation. The amplitude and/or beat frequency can be modulated throughout the treatment by selecting the scan or sweep mode, respectively. Interferential stimulation is used to decrease pain, acute and chronic edema, and muscle spasm; strengthen weakened muscles; improve blood flow to an area; heal chronic wounds; and relieve abdominal organ dysfunction.

Low-Intensity Stimulation

Low-intensity stimulation (LIS) is the current term to replace the units originally called microcurrent electrical nerve stimulators (MENS) units. Low-intensity stimulation units are available in a variety of waveforms, from modified monophasic to biphasic square waves. The units tend to be applied at a subsensory or very low sensory level. with a current operating at less than 1,000 μA. The devices deliver an electrical current to the body with approximately 1/1,000 the amperage of TENS but with a pulse duration that may be up to 2,500-fold longer. The stimulation pathway is not designed to stimulate peripheral nerves to elicit a muscle contraction but, rather, is used to reduce acute and chronic pain and inflammation, reduce edema, and facilitate healing in superficial wounds, sprains, strains, fractures, and neuropathies. The efficacy of microcurrent therapy and, subsequently, of LIS units is based primarily on anecdotal evidence rather than on valid research. It is posited that the current mimics the normal electrical current within the body, which is disrupted with injury, and, in doing so, reduces pain and spasm and improves healing (38). Several studies have shown that microcurrent is ineffective in reducing pain and increasing muscle function associated with delayed-onset muscle soreness (39,40).

Galvanic Stimulation

Galvanic stimulation is the common name for any stimulator using DC.

Russian Current

Russian current is a type of neuromuscular stimulation that uses AC, with frequencies ranging from 2,000 to 10,000 Hz. The current is generated in bursts, with interburst intervals. The number of bps can be manipulated within the therapeutic range. For example, a high-frequency AC current easily penetrates the skin and provides a high-amplitude, low-frequency (bps) current to the muscle.

Russian electrical stimulation is designed to produce an isometric contraction and is useful in muscle re-education. Because it induces an isometric rather than an isotonic contraction, strength gains do not transfer across the entire joint but, instead, are restricted to a narrow arc on either side of the joint angle at which the muscle is stimulated. Russian current, however, does permit the individual to contract actively along with the stimulation, provides an adequate work-to-rest interval, and usually is comfortable for the individual.

Faradic Current

Faradic current is a specialized, asymmetrical biphasic wave. Although popular in the past, it now is thought to have little benefit over symmetrical waves (38).

Iontophoresis

Iontophoresis uses a DC monophasic waveform with a peak current amplitude of up to 5 mA. The current drives charged molecules from certain medications, such as anti-inflammatories (dexamethasone), anesthetics (lidocaine), or analgesics (aspirin or acetaminophen), into damaged tissue. It is used as a local anesthetic to treat inflammatory conditions, such as arthritis, myositis ossificans, plantar fasciitis; myofascial pain syndrome; and skin conditions by reducing edema. It also is used for the management of hyperhidrosis, Peyronie's disease, and temporomandibular disorders (10). Contraindications include allergy to the ion being used, decreased sensation, and placement of electrodes directly over unhealed or partially healed skin wounds or new scar tissue. No contact should exist between metal or carbon–rubber electrode components and the skin, and electrodes should never be removed or rearranged until the unit has been turned off.

Iontophoresis is noninvasive and painless, uses a sterile application, and is excellent for those patients who fear injections. It yields tissue concentrations that are lower than those achieved with injections but greater than those with oral administration, because it avoids enzymatic breakdown in the gastrointestinal tract. A major disadvantage of this treatment is the electrolysis of NaCl in the body by DC. Electrolysis produces an increased pH (acidic) condition at the cathode (positive electrode) and a decreased pH (alkaline) condition at the anode (negative electrode). These pH changes can lead to tissue burns, especially with high intensities or prolonged application. Therefore, the negative electrode should be large, perhaps twice the size of the positive electrode, to reduce current density. With the newer controlled generators and buffered electrodes, clinicians can selectively decrease the current density under the anode to decrease the incidence of burns.

Before treatment, the skin must be thoroughly cleansed. Next, well-saturated electrodes are applied over the most focal point of tissue inflammation or pain unless skin irritation is visible. The polarity of the medication determines which electrode is used to drive the molecules into the skin. The medication is placed under the active (delivery) electrode with the same polarity. The return electrode is placed 4 to 6 inches away. When the current is applied, the molecules are pushed away from the active electrode and into the skin toward the injured site. The medication can penetrate 6 to 20 mm below the skin surfaces and, in many instances, can reach the depth of tendinous structures, although the dose of the medication reaching this depth is not universally accepted. This localized treatment often is preferred over more disruptive systemic treatments.

A *The use of ultrasound and a high-voltage pulsed stimulator or interferential stimulation will increase blood flow to the involved muscle. The electrical current can stimulate a muscle contraction to produce muscle pumping, retard atrophy, and strengthen the muscle.*

OTHER TREATMENT MODALITIES

Q *Electrical modalities are not always available for use by athletic trainers. What other treatment modalities might be used to promote healing of the lacrosse player's upper arm contusion?*

Many of the electrotherapeutic modalities are costly and may not be readily available in all clinical settings. In addition, state licensure laws may prohibit an athletic trainer from using certain modalities in some settings. As such, it becomes necessary to use other treatment modalities to achieve the same results.

Massage

Massage involves manipulation of the soft tissues to increase cutaneous circulation, cell metabolism, and venous and lymphatic flow to assist in the removal of edema; stretch superficial scar tissue; alleviate soft-tissue adhesions; and decrease neuromuscular excitability (Box 7.6). As a result, relaxation, pain relief, edema reduction, and increased ROM can be achieved. To reduce friction between the patient's skin and hand, particularly over hairy areas, lubricants (i.e., massage lotion, peanut oil, coconut oil, or powder) often are used. These lubricants should have a lanolin base or be alcohol free. Massage involves five basic strokes:

1. Effleurage (stroking)

2. Pétrissage (kneading)

3. Tapotement (percussion)

4. Vibration

5. Friction.

> The various techniques used in therapeutic massage, including their uses and methods of application, are outlined in *Techniques of Massage* on the companion website at thePoint.

Effleurage is a superficial, longitudinal stroke to relax the patient. When applied toward the heart, it reduces swelling and aids in venous return. It is the most commonly used stroke, and it begins and ends each massage. Effleurage permits the clinician to evaluate the condition, distribute the lubricant, warm the skin and superficial tissue, and promote relaxation.

Pétrissage consists of pressing and rolling the muscles under the fingers and hands. This "milking" action over deep tissues and muscle increases venous and lymphatic return and removes metabolic waste products from the injured area. Furthermore, it breaks up adhesions within the underlying tissues, loosens fibrous tissue, and increases elasticity of the skin.

Tapotement uses sharp, alternating, brisk hand movements, such as hacking, slapping, beating, cupping, and clapping, to increase blood flow and stimulate peripheral nerve endings. Because this technique is used for stimulation and not for relaxation, it is not used in most massage treatments.

Vibration consists of finite, gentle, and rhythmic movement of the fingers to vibrate the underlying tissues. It is used for relaxation or stimulation.

Friction is the deepest form of massage and consists of deep, circular motions performed by the thumb, knuckles, or ends of the fingers at right angles to the involved tissue. These deep circular movements can loosen adherent fibrous tissue (scar), aid in the absorption of edema, and reduce localized muscular spasm. Transverse friction massage is a deep friction massage that is performed across the grain of the muscle, tendon sheath, or ligament. Cross-friction massage is the most

Box 7.6   Application of Therapeutic Massage

Indications
Increase local circulation
Increase venous and lymphatic flow
Reduce pain (analgesia)
Reduce muscle spasm
Stretch superficial scar tissue
Improve systemic relaxation
Chronic myositis, bursitis, tendinitis, tenosynovitis, fibrositis

Contraindications
Acute contusions, sprains, and strains
Over fracture sites
Over open lesions or skin conditions
Conditions such as acute phlebitis, thrombosis, severe varicose veins, cellulites, synovitis, arteriosclesis, and cancerous regions

Box 7.7 Application of Traction

Indications
Herniated disk protrusions
Spinal nerve impingement
Spinal nerve inflammation
Joint hypomobility
Narrowing of intervertebral foramen
Degenerative joint disease
Spondylolisthesis
Muscle spasm and guarding
Joint pain

Contraindications
Unstable vertebrae
Acute lumbago
Gross emphysema
S4 nerve root signs
Temporomandibular dysfunction
Patient discomfort

effective technique and is used to break up adhesions and promote healing of muscle and ligament tears.

One recent study found that blood flow did not significantly increase with effleurage, pétrissage, and tapotement on either a small or large muscle mass (41). Another study found that manual massage did not have a significant impact on the recovery of muscle function following exercise or on any of the physiologic factors associated with the recovery process (42). In both studies, the researchers concluded that light exercise of the affected muscles probably is more effective than massage in improving muscle blood flow (thereby enhancing healing) and temporarily reducing muscle soreness. Because the types and duration of massage typically are based on the preference of the individual and clinician, its use in athletic settings for these purposes should be questioned.

Traction

Traction is the process of drawing or pulling tension on a body segment. The most common forms involve lumbar and cervical traction. Spinal traction more commonly is used to treat small, herniated disk protrusions that may result in spinal nerve impingement, although it also may be used to treat a variety of other conditions (Box 7.7). The effects of spinal traction include distraction of the vertebral bodies, widening of the vertebral foramen, a combination of distraction and gliding of vertebral facets, and stretching and relaxation of the paraspinal muscles and ligamentous structures of the spinal segment.

A distractive force commonly is applied using a mechanical device or manually by a clinician. Traction may be applied continuously, through a low, distracting force for up to several hours; statically, with a sustained distracting force applied for the entire treatment time, usually 30 minutes; or intermittently, with a distracting force applied and released for several seconds repeatedly over the course of the treatment time. For example, in lumbar traction, a split table is used to eliminate friction. A special nonslip harness lined with vinyl is used to transfer the distractive force comfortably to the patient and stabilize the trunk and thoracic area while the lumbar spine is placed under traction. A distractive force, usually up to half the patient's body weight, is applied for 30 minutes daily for 2 to 4 weeks. Although intermittent traction tends to be more comfortable for the patient, sustained traction is more effective in treating lumbar disk problems. In cervical traction, the patient may be either supine or seated. Again, a nonslip cervical harness is secured under the chin and back of the head to transfer the distractive force comfortably to the patient. Recommended force ranges from 10 to 30 pounds.

With manual traction, the clinician applies the distractive force for a few seconds or, sometimes, with a quick, sudden thrust. This method has been effective in reducing joint pain when the traction is applied within the normal range of joint movement. Because the clinician can feel the relaxation or resistance, it is possible to instantaneously change the patient's position, direction of the force,

Box 7.8 Application of Continuous Passive Motion

Indications
Postoperative rehabilitation to:
- Reduce pain
- Improve general circulation
- Enhance joint nutrition
- Prevent joint contractures
- Benefit collagen re-modeling

Following knee manipulation
Following joint debridement
Following meniscal or osteochondral repair
Tendon lacerations

Contraindications
Noncompliant patient
If use would disrupt surgical repair, fracture fixation, or lead to hemorrhage in postoperative period
Malfunction of device

magnitude of the force, or duration of the treatment, making manual traction more flexible and adaptable than mechanical traction.

Continuous Passive Motion

Continuous passive motion is a modality that applies an external force to move the joint through a preset arc of motion. It primarily is used postsurgically at the knee, after knee manipulation, or after stable fixation of intra-articular and extra-articular fractures of most joints, such as the hand, wrist, hip, shoulder, elbow, and ankle. It also may be used to improve wound healing, accelerate clearance of a **hemarthrosis**, and prevent cartilage degeneration in septic arthritis (Box 7.8). The application is relatively pain-free and has been shown to stimulate the intrinsic healing process, maintain articular cartilage nutrition, reduce disuse effects, retard joint stiffness and the pain-spasm cycle, and benefit collagen remodeling, joint dynamics, and pain reduction (1,43).

 Massage may be used after the acute phase has ended. Stroking and kneading toward the heart may provide some beneficial effects; however, mild exercise may be just as beneficial.

MEDICATIONS

In managing the lacrosse player's injury, can the athletic trainer recommend and dispense medications?

Therapeutic drugs are either prescription or over-the-counter medications used to treat an injury or illness. Common drugs used to control pain, inflammation, and muscle spasm include anesthetics, analgesics, nonsteroidal anti-inflammatory drugs (NSAIDs), adrenocorticosteroids, and muscle relaxants. A more detailed presentation of therapeutic drugs can be found in Chapter 27.

Local anesthetics eliminate short-term pain sensation in a specific body part or region by blocking afferent neural transmissions along peripheral nerves. Many of these drugs can be identified by their "-caine" suffixes (e.g., lidocaine, procaine, and benzocaine). The drugs may be applied topically to skin for minor irritations (e.g., burns, abrasions, or mild inflammation), introduced into subcutaneous tissues (e.g., bursitis, tendinitis, or contusions) via phonophoresis or iontophoresis, injected by a physician into soft tissue around a laceration for surgical repair (i.e., suturing), or injected by a physician near a peripheral nerve to interrupt nerve transmission (i.e., nerve block).

Aspirin is the most commonly used drug to relieve pain and inflammation. Because of its anti-clotting properties, it is not used during the acute phase of healing. Aspirin is associated with a number of adverse side effects, including gastrointestinal irritation. Stomach distress can be limited by using coated aspirin to delay release of the drug until it reaches the small intestine or by taking a buffered aspirin to blunt the acidic effects of aspirin in the stomach. Chronic use or high doses (i.e., 10–30 g) can lead to renal problems, liver toxicity, congestive heart failure, hypertension, aspirin intoxication, or poisoning may occur. Normal dosage is 325 to 650 mg every 4 hours.

Acetaminophen (e.g., Tylenol) is an analgesic and an **antipyretic**, but it does not have any appreciable anti-inflammatory or anticlotting effects. Unlike aspirin, acetaminophen is not associated with gastrointestinal irritation; however, high doses can be toxic to the liver and even may be fatal.

Nonsteroidal anti-inflammatory drugs commonly are used to dilate blood vessels and inhibit production of prostaglandins. Certain prostaglandins increase local blood flow, capillary permeability, erythema, and edema associated with inflammation and are believed to decrease the sensitivity of pain receptors to the effects of other pain-producing substances, such as bradykinin (1,21). Therefore, these drugs decrease inflammation, relieve mild to moderate pain, decrease body temperature associated with fever, increase collagen strength, and inhibit coagulation and blood clotting. The most important time to administer NSAIDs is during the early stages of healing, when prostaglandins produce the most detrimental effects of pain and edema. Prolonged use (i.e., ≥2 weeks) actually may retard the healing process. Examples of NSAIDs include ibuprofen (e.g., Advil, Nuprin, Motrin, and Rufen), naproxen sodium (e.g., Aleve), indomethacin (e.g., Indocin), and piroxicam (e.g., Feldene).

> See *Nonsteroidal Anti-Inflammatory Drugs (NSAIDs)* on the companion website at thePoint for a listing of common NSAIDs and suggested dosages.

Ibuprofen and the other NSAIDs are administered primarily for pain relief and anti-inflammatory effects; however, they are more expensive than aspirin. Although many are still associated with some stomach discomfort, they provide better effects in many patients. Taking the medication after a meal or with a glass of milk or water greatly reduces stomach discomfort.

Adrenocorticosteroids are steroid hormones produced by the adrenal cortex. Higher doses, referred to as a pharmacologic dose, typically are used to treat endocrine disorders but also can be used to decrease edema, inflammation, **erythema**, and tenderness in a region. These drugs may be applied topically, given orally, or injected by a physician into a specific area, such as a tendon or a joint. Examples of these drugs include cortisone, prednisone, and hydrocortisone. Because many of these drugs can lead to breakdown and rupture of structures, long-term use can depress the adrenal glands and increase the risk of osteoporosis.

Skeletal muscle relaxants are used to relieve muscle spasms, which can result from certain musculoskeletal injuries or inflammation. When involuntary tension in the muscle cannot be relaxed, it leads to intense pain and a buildup of pain-mediating metabolites (e.g., lactate). A vicious cycle is created, with the increased pain leading to more spasm, leading to more pain, leading to still more spasm. Skeletal muscle relaxants break the pain-spasm cycle by depressing the neural activity causing the continuous muscle contractions, thus reducing muscle excitability. Muscle relaxants do not prevent muscle contraction but, rather, attempt to normalize muscle excitability to decrease pain and improve motor function. Examples of muscle relaxants include Flexeril, Soma, and Dantrium.

Because of legal liability, athletic trainers cannot recommend, prescribe, or dispense medications. The individual can be seen by the team physician, who may prescribe certain NSAIDs to promote healing, or the individual may voluntarily take over-the-counter medications as needed. The athletic trainer should monitor the individual, however, to ensure his or her compliance with manufacturer's suggested guidelines.

SUMMARY

1. Rehabilitation begins immediately after injury assessment with the use of therapeutic modalities to limit pain, inflammation, and loss of ROM.

2. Therapeutic modalities, with the exception of ultrasound, fall within the electromagnetic spectrum based on their wavelength or frequency. All electromagnetic energy is pure energy that travels in a straight line at the speed of light (300 million meters per second) in a vacuum.

3. Depending on the medium, energy can be reflected, refracted, absorbed, or transmitted.

4. Common therapeutic modalities include cryotherapy, thermotherapy, ultrasound, diathermy, electrical stimulation, massage, traction, continuous passive motion, and medications to promote healing. Although many are used every day in treating musculoskeletal injuries, many others must be used under the direction of a physician or a licensed health care provider. Being a technician and merely applying a modality is not an acceptable athletic training practice.

5. Cryotherapy is used to decrease pain, inflammation, and muscle guarding and spasm as well as to facilitate mobilization.

6. Thermotherapy is used to treat subacute or chronic injuries to reduce swelling, edema, ecchymosis, and muscle spasm; increase blood flow and ROM; facilitate tissue healing; relieve joint contractures; and fight infection.

7. Ultrasound produces both thermal and nonthermal effects. Thermal effects include increased blood flow, extensibility of collagen tissue, sensory and motor nerve conduction velocity, and enzymatic activity as well as decreased muscle spasm, joint stiffness, inflammation, and pain. Nonthermal effects include decreased edema; increased blood flow, cell membrane and vascular wall permeability, protein synthesis, and tissue regeneration; and promotion of healing.

8. Diathermy is used to treat joint inflammation (e.g., bursitis, tendinitis, and synovitis), joint capsule contractures, subacute and chronic inflammatory conditions in deep-tissue layers, osteoarthritis, ankylosing spondylitis, and chronic pelvic inflammatory disease.

9. Electrotherapy is used to decrease pain, re-educate peripheral nerves, delay denervation and disuse atrophy by stimulating muscle contractions, reduce posttraumatic edema, and maintain ROM by reducing muscle spasm, inhibiting spasticity, re-educating partially denervated muscle, and facilitating voluntary motor function.

10. Iontophoresis is used to introduce ions into the body tissues by means of a direct electrical current. This treatment is beneficial in reducing inflammation, muscle spasm, ischemia, and edema.

11. Massage involves manipulation of the soft tissues to increase cutaneous circulation, cell metabolism, and venous and lymphatic flow to assist in the removal of edema; stretch superficial scar tissue; alleviate soft-tissue adhesions; and decrease neuromuscular excitability. Strokes include effleurage, pétrissage, tapotement, vibration, and friction massage.

12. Traction is the process of drawing or pulling tension on a body segment and commonly is used on the spine to treat herniated disk protrusion, spinal nerve inflammation or impingement, narrowing of intervertebral foramen, and muscle spasm and pain.

13. Continuous passive motion applies an external force to move the joint through a preset arc of motion and primarily is used postsurgically at the knee, after knee manipulation, or after stable fixation of intra-articular and extra-articular fractures of most joints.

14. Nonsteroidal anti-inflammatory drugs commonly are used to dilate blood vessels and inhibit production of prostaglandins to decrease inflammation, relieve mild-to-moderate pain, decrease body temperature associated with fever, increase collagen strength, and inhibit coagulation and blood clotting.

15. Because of the complexity of each of the therapeutic modalities, students should enroll in a separate therapeutic modalities class, permitting practice and demonstration of proper clinical skills associated with the application of therapeutic modalities.

16. While using any modality, if the individual begins to show signs of pain, swelling, discomfort, tingling, or loss of sensation, the treatment should be stopped and the individual re-evaluated to determine if the selected modality is appropriate for the current phase of healing.

REFERENCES

1. Starkey C. Therapeutic Modalities for Athletic Trainers. 3rd Ed. Philadelphia: FA Davis, 2004.
2. Nolan TP Jr. Technical aspects of therapeutic modalities. In: Michlovitz SL, Nolan TP Jr, eds. Modalities for Therapeutic Intervention. Philadelphia: FA Davis, 2005.
3. Kimura IF, Gulick DT, Thompson GT. The effect of cryotherapy on eccentric plantar flexion peak torque and endurance. J Ath Train 1997;32(2):124–126.
4. Knight KL. Cryotherapy in Sport Injury Management. Champaign, IL: Human Kinetics, 1995.

5. Knight KL, Bryan KS, Halvorsen JM. Circulatory changes in the forearm in 1, 5, 10, and 15°C water. Int J Sports Med 1981;4:281.

6. Ho SS, Illgen RL, Meyer RW, et al. Comparison of various icing times in decreasing bone metabolism and blood flow in the knee. Am J Sports Med 1995;23(1):74–76.

7. Otte, JW, Merrick MA, Ingersoll CD, Cordova ML. Subcutaneous adipose tissue thickness alters cooling time during cryotherapy. Arch Phys Med Rehabil 2002; 83(11): 1501–1505.

8. Tsang KK, Buxton BP, Guion WK, et al. The effects of cryotherapy applied through various barriers. J Sport Rehab 1997;(4):343–354.

9. Danielson R, Jaeger J, Rippetoe J, et al. Differences in skin surface temperature and pressure during the application of various cold and compression devices. J Ath Train 1997; 32(2):S34.

10. Bélanger AY. Thermotherapy. In: Evidence-Based Guide to Therapeutic Physical Agents. Philadelphia: Lippincott Williams & Wilkins, 2003.

11. Michlovitz SL, Rennie S. Heat therapy modalities: beyond fake and bake. In: Michlovitz SL, Nolan TP Jr, eds. Modalities for Therapeutic Intervention. Philadelphia: FA Davis, 2005.

12. Walsh MT. Hydrotherapy: the use of water as a therapeutic agent. In: Michlovitz SL, ed. Thermal Agents in Rehabilitation. Philadelphia: FA Davis, 1996.

13. Myrer JW, Draper DO, Durrant E. Contrast therapy and intramuscular temperature in the human leg. J Ath Train 1994;29(4):318–322.

14. Myrer JW, Measom M, Durrant E, et al. Cold- and hot-pack contrast therapy: subcutaneous and intramuscular temperature change. J Ath Train 1997;32(3):238–241.

15. Kaiser DA, Knight KL, Huff JM, Jutte LS, Carlson P. Hot-pack warming in 4- and 8-pack Hydrocollator® units. J Sport Rehabil, 2004;13(s):103–113.

16. Sandqvist G, Åkesson A, Eklund M. Evaluation of paraffin bath treatment in patients with systemic sclerosis. Disabil Rehabil 2004;26(16):981–987.

17. Borrel RM, Parker R, Henley EJ, Masley D, Repinecz M. Comparison of in vivo temperatures produced by hydrotherapy, paraffin wax treatment, and fluidotherapy. Phys Ther 1980;60(10):1273–1276.

18. Hayes BT, Sandrey MA, Merrick MA, Cordova ML. The differences between 1-MHz and 3-MHz ultrasound in the heating of subcutaneous tissues. J Ath Train 2001;36(2):S-92.

19. Schneider NC, Walsh CT, Lemley SF, et al. 3 MHz continuous ultrasound can elevate tissue temperature at 3-cm depth. Phys Ther 2001;81:A8.

20. Ramirez A, Schwane JA, McFarland C, et al. The effect of ultrasound on collagen synthesis and fibroblast proliferation in vitro. Med Sci Sports Exerc 1997;29(3):326–332.

21. Houglum PA. Soft tissue healing and its impact on rehabilitation. J Sport Rehab 1992;1(1):19–39.

22. Sparrow KJ. Therapeutic ultrasound. In: Michlovitz SL, Nolan TP Jr, eds. Modalities for Therapeutic Intervention. Philadelphia: FA Davis, 2005.

23. Draper, DO, Sunderland S. Examination of the law of Grotthus-Draper: does ultrasound penetrate subcutaneous fat in humans. J Ath Train 1993;28(3):246–250.

24. Grant TH, Kelikian AS, Jereb SE, McCarthy RJ. Ultra-sound diagnosis of peroneal tendon tears. J Bone Joint Surg Am 2005;87(8):1788–1794.

25. Loudon JK, Cagle PE, Dyson M. High-frequency ultrasound: an overview of potential uses in physical therapy. Phys Ther Rev 2005;10(4):209–215.

26. Klucinec B. Effectiveness of the Aquaflex gel pad in transmission of acoustic energy. J Ath Train 1996;31(4):313–317.

27. Draper DO, Castel JC, Castel D. Rate of temperature increase in human muscle during 1-MHZ and 3-MHZ continuous ultrasound. J Orthop Sports Phys Ther 1995; 22(4):142–149.

28. Forest G, Rosen K. Ultrasound treatments in degassed water. J Sport Rehab 1992;1(4):284–289.

29. Merrick MA, Mihalyov MR, Roethemeier JL, Cordova ML, Ingersoll CD. A comparison of intramuscular temperature during ultrasound treatments with coupling gel or gel pads. J Orthop Sports Phys Ther 2002;32(5):216–220.

30. Draper DO. Ten mistakes commonly made with ultrasound use: current research sheds light on myths. Athletic Training: Sports Health Care Perspective 1996;2:95.

31. Klucinec B, Scheidler M, Denegar C, Domholdt, Burgess S. Transmissivity of coupling agents used to deliver ultrasound through indirect methods. J Orthop Sports Phys Ther 2000;30(5):263–269.

32. Ciccone CD, Leggin BG, Callamoro JJ. Effects of ultrasound and trolamine salicylate phonophoresis on delayed-onset muscle soreness. Phys Ther 1991;71(9):666–675.

33. Gagnie G, Vinck E, Rimbaut S, Vanderstraeten G. Phonophoresis versus topical application of ketoprofen: comparison between tissue and plasma levels. Phys Ther 2003;83(8):707–712.

34. Baskurt F, Özcan A, Algun C. Comparison of effects of phonophoresis and iontophoresis of naproxen in the treatment of lateral epicondylitis. Clin Rehabil 2003;17(1):l96–100.

35. Hsieh YL. Effects of ultrasound and diclofenac phonophoresis on inflammatory pain relief: suppression of inducible nitric oxide synthase in arthritis rats 2006;86(1):39–49.

36. Johnston TE. Muscle weakness and loss of motor performance. In: Michlovitz SL, Nolan TP Jr, eds. Modalities for Therapeutic Intervention. Philadelphia: FA Davis, 2005.

37. Butterfield DL, Draper DO, Ricard MD, et al. The effects of high-volt pulsed current electrical stimulation on delayed-onset muscle soreness. J Ath Train1997;32(1):15–20.

38. Holcomb WR. A practical guide to electrical therapy. J Sport Rehab 1997;6(3):272–282.

39. Bonacci JA, Higbie EJ. Effects of microcurrent treatment on perceived pain and muscle strength following eccentric exercise. J Ath Train 1997;32(2):119–123.

40. Denegar CR, Yoho AP, Borowicz AJ, et al. The effects of low-volt, microamperage stimulation on delayed onset muscle soreness. J Sport Rehab 1992;1(2):95-102.

41. Shoemaker JK, Tiidus PM, Mader R. Failure of manual massage to alter limb blood flow: measures by Doppler ultrasound. Med Sci Sports Exerc 1997;29(5):610–614.

42. Tiidus PM. Manual massage and recovery of muscle function following exercise: a literature review. J Orthop Sports Phys Ther 1997;25(2):107–112.

43. Chiarello CM, Gundersen L, O'Halloran R. The effect of continuous passive motion duration and increment on ROM in total knee arthroplasty patients. J Orthop Sports Phys Ther 1997;25(2):119–127.

8 Therapeutic Exercise Program

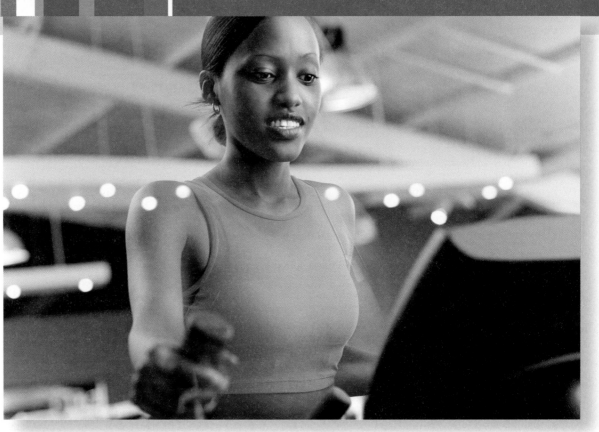

STUDENT OUTCOMES

1. Explain the principles of the cognitive model used to describe an individual's adjustment to injury.

2. Identify various psychological influences that can affect an injured individual, and describe strategies or intervention techniques used to overcome these influences.

3. Explain the importance of dealing with the psychological concerns that an individual may develop during a therapeutic exercise program.

4. Identify key factors in the development of a therapeutic exercise program.

5. Describe the four phases of a therapeutic exercise program, including the goals of these phases and the methodology of implementation.

6. List the criteria used to clear an individual to return to full participation in sport and physical activity.

ROLE DELINEATION COMPETENCIES

The following Performance Domains and Tasks defined in the National Athletic Trainers' Association Board of Certification *Role Delineation Study*, 5th Edition are addressed in this chapter:

BOC COMPETENCIES

I. Prevention

H. Facilitate physical conditioning by designing and implementing appropriate programs to minimize the risk of injury and illness.

IV. Treatment, Rehabilitation, and Reconditioning

A. Administer therapeutic and conditioning exercise(s) using standard techniques and procedures in order to facilitate recovery, function, and/or performance.
C. Apply braces, splints, or assistive devices in accordance with appropriate standards and practices in order to facilitate recovery, function, and/or performance.
F. Educate the appropriate individual(s) in the treatment, rehabilitation, and reconditioning of injuries, illnesses, and/or conditions using applicable methods and materials to facilitate recovery, function, and/or performance.
G. Provide guidance and/or counseling for the appropriate individual(s) in the treatment, rehabilitation, and reconditioning of injuries, illnesses, and/or conditions through communication to facilitate recovery, function, and/or performance.

V. Organization and Administration

A. Establish action plans for response to injury or illness using available resources to provide the required range of health care services for individuals, athletic activities, and events.
B. Establish policies and procedures for the delivery of health care services following accepted guidelines to promote safe participation, timely care, and legal compliance.
F. Develop professional relationships with appropriate individuals and entities by applying effective communication techniques to enhance the delivery of health care.

The ultimate goal of therapeutic exercise is to return the injured participant to pain-free and fully functional activity. To accomplish this, attention must focus on modulating pain and restoring normal joint range of motion (ROM), kinematics, flexibility, muscular strength, endurance, coordination, and power. Furthermore, cardiovascular endurance and strength in the unaffected limb must be maintained.

Psychological influences can inhibit or enhance an individual's progress during a therapeutic exercise program. As such, an awareness of the physical, psychological, emotional, social, and performance factors that may affect the individual during rehabilitation is essential. An understanding of each component is necessary within a well-organized, individualized therapeutic exercise program.

In this chapter, emotional and psychological factors that may affect injured individuals and their progress through the rehabilitation program are presented. Next, a therapeutic exercise program following the SOAP (Subjective evaluation, Objective evaluation, Assessment, and Plan) note format is explained. Phases of a therapeutic exercise program are presented, including criteria used to determine when an individual is ready to progress in the program and, ultimately, to participate in sport or physical activity. Practical application of the material for the various body segments is included in Chapters 10 through 17.

PSYCHOLOGICAL ASPECTS OF THE INJURED PARTICIPANT

> *A female distance runner is diagnosed with plantar fasciitis a week before an Olympic qualifying race. She has been training for this race and a potential spot on the Olympic team for the past 3 years. The injury will prevent her from competing at her desired level for approximately 1 month, eliminating any chance of a position on the Olympic team. How might this athlete react to the inability to race competitively? What impact will this reaction have on her motivation to improve? How can the athletic trainer help this person cope with the physical, psychological, and emotional effects that may hinder progress in the therapeutic exercise program?*

For many individuals, the development and maintenance of a physically fit body provides a focal point for social and economic success that is important for self-esteem. When participation in a sport or physical activity is integral to one's lifestyle, sustaining an injury can be a devastating experience. Therefore, a therapeutic exercise program must address not only the physical needs but also the emotional and psychological needs of the individual.

In general, two models categorize an individual's adjustment to injury—namely, stage and cognitive models. The stage perspective often is linked to the Kubler-Ross stages of grieving through which an individual progresses when confronted with loss. These stages include denial and isolation, anger, bargaining, depression, and acceptance. Although this model has some intuitive appeal, the stereotypic linear pattern of distinct emotional responses has not stood up to empirical scrutiny (1). Furthermore, if an individual reacts to injury in a linear manner, then clinicians should be able to predict a patient's progress during rehabilitation; however, this rarely is the case.

More recently, cognitive models have been used to explain the psychological aspects of injury and the athlete's perception of injuries. This perspective suggests that each person reacts differently to an injury, depending on his or her personality traits, coping mechanisms, and both personal and situational factors. Personal factors include performance anxiety, self-esteem/motivation, extroversion/introversion, psychological investment in the sport or physical activity, coping resources, history of past stressors (e.g., previous injuries, academics, and family life events), previous intervention strategies, and social support. In comparison, situational factors may involve the type of sport or physical activity, relationship with the coach/supervisor, characteristics of the injury (e.g., severity, history, and type), timing of the injury (e.g., preseason, in-season, or playoffs), level and intensity of the injury, period in the individual's career, and the individual's role on a team. Each of these factors interacts with the cognitive, emotional, psychological, and behavioral responses of the individual to influence the success or failure of a therapeutic exercise program.

Strategies to Assist Athletes and Physically Active Individuals Cope with Injury

A number of strategies can be employed to assist athletes and physically active individuals cope effectively with injury.

Education

It is imperative that the clinician inform the individual about the injury and recovery process. The use of a specific treatment, the intended goal, and any side effects or sensations that may be experienced should be explained. This helps the individual understand the management and rehabilitation process, avoids any surprises, and hopefully, reduces any anxiety being experienced (2).

Goal Setting

Goal setting is an effective technique used to provide guidance and increase motivation during a recovery program. This practice helps to guide the individual's effort; provides a sense of control that may enhance motivation, persistence, and commitment; and facilitates the incorporation of new strategies to improve performance. Individuals who set specific personal goals in each rehabilitation session exhibit an increase in self efficacy, or the sense of having the power to produce intended outcomes, and experience greater satisfaction with their performance (3–6).

The process begins by establishing a strong and supportive rapport between the clinician and the patient as they work in partnership to return the patient to preinjury status. To achieve success, the

Box 8.1   Guide to Goal Setting for Therapeutic Exercise

Goals should be:

- **Specific and Measurable.** The patient must know exactly what to do and be able to determine if gains are made.
- **Stated in Positive versus Negative Language.** Knowing what to do guides behavior, whereas knowing what to avoid creates a focus on errors without providing a constructive alternative.
- **Challenging but Realistic.** Overly difficult goals set up the individual for failure and pose a threat to the individual. The lower the individual's self-confidence, the more important success becomes, and the greater the importance of setting attainable goals.
- **Established on a Timetable for Completion.** This allows a check on progress and evaluation of whether realistic goals have been set.
- **Integrated as Short-, Intermediate-, and Long-Term Goals.** A comprehensive program links daily activities with expectations for specific competitions as well as for season and career goals.
- **Personalized and Internalized.** The patient must embrace goals as their own, not as something from the outside.
- **Monitored and Evaluated.** Feedback must be provided to assess goals, and the goals should be modified based on progress.
- **Linked to Life Goals.** This identifies sport and rehabilitation as learning experiences in life, and it helps the individual put sport/physical activity in a broader perspective. This is especially important for individuals whose return to sport/activity is doubtful.

clinician must form a genuine relationship with the patient and listen intently for clues that indicate what the individual is or is not feeling. Goals should be realistic, objective, measurable, and attainable.

Long-term goals can reduce the individual's fears of the unknown but do little to motivate the individual on a day-to-day basis. Therefore, short-term goals should be established to serve as daily motivators. Goals should be personalized, challenging, yet realistic. A timetable for completion should be established and measured to monitor progress. Box 8.1 shows guidelines for goal setting during therapeutic exercise.

Plateaus and setbacks usually occur because something is blocking the individual's progress. These barriers fall under four general categories: lack of knowledge, lack of skill, lack of risk-taking ability, and lack of social support.

Fear of Risk-Taking

Most individuals experience some level of fear and anxiety of the unknown. In a therapeutic exercise program, such emotions can block the individual's ability to work hard at meeting the challenges of the exercise program. For example, fear of increased pain, discomfort, or reinjury during an exercise may limit the individual's motivation to exert full effort. Constant positive feedback from the clinician can help to overcome many of these obstacles.

Social Support

The injured patient needs to feel as important as noninjured individuals and not feel alone or isolated. Friends, colleagues, coaches/supervisors, and the athletic trainer can provide emotional, challenging material, and informational support to help the individual recognize their progress and value to others. It is important to stress the individual's value as a person and maintain his or her connections to friends, family, a team, and any other supportive entities.

Psychological Influences

Five major factors can significantly influence the rehabilitation process: confidence, motivation, anxiety, focus, and management of pain.

Confidence

Confidence is perhaps the most critical factor to a complete and timely recovery. Low confidence can lead to a host of negative thinking and talk, which in turn can lead to increasing anxiety, negative emotions (e.g., bitterness, confusion, anger, or guilt), and low motivation, which can interfere with the individual's focus. Four main types of confidence can affect recovery: program, adherence, physical, and return to sport. **Program confidence** refers to the strength of the individual's belief that the rehabilitation program will enable recovery and is significantly influenced by the clinician's confidence in the effectiveness of the program. **Adherence confidence** refers to the individual's belief that the prescribed exercise program can be completed. This factor can be enhanced by informing the individual that application of skills learned in other areas, such as goal setting, can heighten success in the rehabilitation program. **Physical confidence** is knowing that one's body is capable of handling the demands placed on it during rehabilitation and subsequent competition. Responding well to the rigors of the exercise program, maintaining a positive attitude about the ups and downs of rehabilitation, and using imagery can enhance this factor. **Return-to-activity confidence** relates to the individual's belief that his or her return to competition is at a level equal to or better than the preinjury status (7).

Motivation

Motivation has the greatest influence on adherence in rehabilitation. Low motivation can result in poor attendance, incomplete exercises, low effort and intensity, lack of attentiveness to instructions, undefined goals, using unspecified pain to avoid exercise, and insupportable excuses. Motivation can be enhanced through goal setting by reminding the individual that rehabilitation is a type of physical performance, improving commitment, providing clear direction and the means to achieve full recovery, and offering deliberate steps to recovery. High motivation builds confidence, reduces anxiety and the perception of pain, and refocuses the individual's attention on the positive rather than the negative aspects of rehabilitation (4,6).

Anxiety

Anxiety is the negative and threatening psychological and physical reaction to the injury. It produces a wide range of physical, cognitive, emotional, social, and performance problems. Table 8.1 lists many of these signs and symptoms.

Anxiety can be caused by a number of factors, such as pain, slow healing, low confidence, pressure from others, and lack of familiarity, predictability, and control. Anxiety can restrict oxygen intake and blood flow, increase muscle tension and pain, reduce confidence and motivation, and lead the individual to focus on the negative rather than the positive aspects of rehabilitation. Physically active individuals can control anxiety by using deep breathing, passive and active relaxation, soothing music, smiling, and therapeutic massage. A rehabilitation routine can benefit recovery by encompassing all the activities necessary for total preparation, including a review of the goals for that day; mental preparation to ensure prime confidence, motivation, intensity, and focus; and physical preparation, such as stretching and warm-up (7).

TABLE 8.1 Signs and Symptoms of Anxiety in Rehabilitation

CATEGORY	SIGNS AND SYMPTOMS
Physical	Muscle tension and bracing; short, choppy breathing; decreased coordination; fatigue; rushed speech; minor secondary injuries or nagging illness with recurrent physical complaints; and sleeping problems
Cognitive	Excessive negativity and overly self-critical statements of low confidence in rehabilitation, extreme thinking and unrealistic expectations, and very narrow focus
Emotional	Anger, depression, irritability, moodiness, and impatience
Social	Decreased communication, social withdrawal, intolerance, and abruptness with others
Performance	Overall decline in motivation and enjoyment in rehabilitation, loss of interest in sports and other activities, nervousness and physical tension during therapy, trying too hard in therapy or "giving up" in response to obstacles and setbacks, and decrease in school or work performance

Focus

Often misunderstood and ignored, focus is critical to the rehabilitation process. In essence, **focus** is the ability to perceive and address various internal cues (e.g., thoughts, emotions, and physical responses) and external cues (e.g., sights and sounds) and, when needed, to shift focus to other cues in a natural, effortless manner. Focus differs from concentration in that concentration usually is linked to the ability to attend to one thing for a long period of time. In contrast, focus is the ability to attend to various cues occurring simultaneously and to shift focus when the need arises. For example, an individual may be executing an exercise and have to shift focus externally to listen to the instructions for an exercise. The individual then needs to focus internally to consciously monitor the intensity of any pain being experienced. The ability to focus often is compared with the beam of a Mag-Lite flashlight in that the beam can be adjusted to illuminate a wide area or focused to brighten a narrow area (7).

Cues that interfere with rehabilitation include negative thoughts, anxiety, pain (as an inhibitor), preoccupation with the injury after returning to participation in sport or physical activity, peer pressure to recover quickly, any distraction during physical therapy, and comparisons to others on return to activity. Facilitating cues may include pain (as information), proprioceptive responses, physical dimensions such as ROM and strength, information that the clinician provides, support from others, and feedback from the therapeutic exercise equipment. To maintain one's prime focus, the patient must balance his or her focus on short- and long-term goals and pay attention to the four principles of focus. In general, the individual should be encouraged to focus on:

Positive rather than negative attributes of the rehabilitation

Present time rather than the past

Process and what needs to be done on a day-to-day basis to enhance recovery

Progress while moving through the rehabilitation program

It is important that the individual avoid being distracted during the exercise session. Too often, distractions in the room (e.g., noise, talking, or music) can result in individuals redirecting their eyes and attention toward something else rather than focusing internally on the exercise. It is important to learn to control the eyes and process only beneficial information, such as instructions on proper execution of an exercise. The use of keywords and rehabilitation imagery also may be helpful. For example, if muscle tension is present, a keyword might be *relax,* or the individual could imagine the muscle relaxing and elongating. These cues can help an individual focus on the task at hand.

Pain Management

Pain is the most debilitating obstacle to overcome during rehabilitation. It can have significant physical, psychological, and emotional consequences. Physically active individuals must be able to differentiate between benign and harmful pain. **Benign pain** usually is characterized as dull, generalized, not long-lasting after exertion, and not associated with swelling, localized tenderness, or long-term soreness. In contrast, **harmful pain** is characterized as sharp, localized to the injury site, experienced during and persisting after exertion, and usually associated with swelling, localized tenderness, and prolonged soreness.

Although pain can be controlled with medication, nonpharmacologic methods, such as pain reduction and pain focusing, can be used to control pain (Table 8.2). Pain reduction techniques (e.g., muscle relaxation training, deep breathing, meditation, and therapeutic massage) directly affect the physiologic aspects of pain by decreasing the actual amount of pain that is present. Pain focusing directs attention onto (association) or away from (dissociation) the pain by reducing or altering the perception of pain. Strategies for focusing pain include external focus, such as emotionally powerful or intellectually absorbing activities, pleasant or neutral imaging, rhythmic cognitive activity, dramatic coping, and situational assessment (7).

Mental Skills Training

Knowing that an individual may be very concerned about the physical, psychological, social, and performance ramifications of an injury, the clinician can help the individual confront and overcome

TABLE 8.2 Pain Management Techniques	
TECHNIQUE	**EXAMPLES**
Pain Reduction	
Deep breathing	Emphasize slow, deep, rhythmic breathing
Muscle relaxation	Passive or progressive relaxation
Meditation	Repetitive focusing on mantra or breathing
Therapeutic massage	Manual manipulation of muscles, tendons, and ligaments
Pain Focusing	
External focus	Listening to relaxing or inspiring music, watching a movie, or playing chess
Soothing imagery	Generating calming images (e.g., lying on a beach or floating in space)
Neutral imaginings	Imagining playing chess or building a model airplane
Rhythmic cognitive activity	Saying the alphabet backward or meditation
Pain acknowledgment	Giving pain a "hot" color, such as red, and then changing it to a less painful, "cool" color, such as blue
Dramatic coping	Seeing pain as being part of an epic challenge to overcome insurmountable odds
Situational assessment	Evaluating the causes of pain to take steps to reduce it

these concerns by using mental skills training. Mental skills training has been successful for enhancing performance as well as facilitating recovery from injury. Specifically, the use of relaxation, positive self-talk, and imagery are useful during rehabilitation.

Relaxation

An individual's reaction to injury often evokes fear and anxiety along with physical pain. Relaxation is an effective technique to help reduce pain and the effects of anxiety. Relaxation training can help injured persons learn to reduce tension, slow their breathing, and lower their heart rate. Two general methods of relaxation training exist—namely, mind to muscle and muscle to mind. Mind to muscle often is accomplished with the aid of meditation; muscle to mind involves the active contraction of various muscles to achieve relaxation (e.g., Jacobsonian method).

Imagery

Imagery has long been used in the training process as a way to enhance performance. It involves the mental execution of a skill before the actual performance of the skill. In the rehabilitation process, imagery can be used to mentally practice the skills or processes that will expedite and promote a safe return to activity, such as envisioning healing, soothing (i.e., pain management), or performance (i.e., proper technique of an exercise). Imagery also can be enhanced by preceding it with relaxation exercises, such as passive or progressive relaxation. Relaxation can reduce anxiety and the physical manifestations of pain and increase the vividness and control in imagery. Mental imagery can serve to motivate the individual to realize that this technique can facilitate their performance on return to activity.

Positive Self-Talk

Injured individuals often express negative feelings about the injury, themselves, and occasionally, their coaches or supervisors. These negative feelings inhibit the individual and produce a self-defeating attitude. These thoughts and feelings can be redirected into positive, task-oriented thoughts, however, that direct and motivate the individual to succeed in the rehabilitation process.

Role of the Athletic Trainer

A team approach to injury rehabilitation is key to achieving success. It is essential that the athletic trainer involve the patient in all phases of treatment as well as provide education about the many challenges the individual will face during the rehabilitation process. Seriously injured individuals may experience a variety of fears, social isolation, and loss of income or potential scholarships. This fear of the unknown may lead to increased tension, anger, and depression during the exercise period. If the individual does not perceive a gradual rate of recovery, the resulting frustration and boredom may deter a successful outcome. The athletic trainer should encourage the injured individual to develop a positive attitude by using social support networks and psychological skills to manage pain and, in doing so, direct the individual's energies into compliance with the treatment protocols. Positive encouragement may allow the individual to feel better about working at a higher intensity despite discomfort, fatigue, or pain.

Including the individual as an integral part of the rehabilitation process is especially important when goals are established that direct the exercise program. The goals must be realistic and provide some means to measure progress so that the individual can perceive a gradual rate of recovery. Whenever possible, the rehabilitation program should mirror the individual's regular training program, including the level of intensity, frequency, and duration. In some cases, activity modification and creativity may enable the physically active individual to do limited exercise or activity with others (e.g., practice with a team). For an athlete, this may reduce the feelings of isolation and loss of daily interaction with the coach and other players. Using graphs or charts to document progress also can help the individual see improvement. The athletic trainer must develop a positive professional relationship with the patient to assist the individual in recovering physically and psychologically from the injury.

Referral for Psychological Problems

Athletic trainers seldom have the necessary professional training required for the assessment and treatment of mental health issues. In a recent survey of athletic trainers, 90% indicated that addressing the psychological aspects of an injury is important. Fewer than 25% had ever referred an individual for counseling because of an injury, however, and only 8% had a standard procedure for referral (8). A clearly defined and well-organized procedural plan should be developed to guide the athletic trainer's actions and to ensure confidentiality. Initially, criteria should be developed that establish when psychological distress or clinical issues are evident. During rehabilitation, several psychological factors can arise, including anxiety, depression, anger, pain, and treatment noncompliance. Box 8.2 lists common signs and symptoms associated with psychological distress.

As a general rule, an individual with any psychological difficulty that persists for more than a few days and interferes with the progress of rehabilitation should be referred to a licensed mental health professional (e.g., psychologist, psychiatrist, or counselor). Failure to address these issues can lead to an escalation in the distress and frustration of the patient. When a concern arises, the athletic trainer should consult with a mental health professional to discuss patient symptoms and determine the need or benefits of engaging in professional counseling. If the athletic trainer and licensed mental health professional determine that a referral is necessary, the athletic trainer should meet with the patient to share these concerns and educate the individual concerning the benefits of counseling. The athletic trainer should point out that the referral is a positive step in helping the individual to recover and return to sport and participation in physical activity. If possible, it may be advantageous to mention the previous use of a psychologist having helped other individuals recover. In this manner, the patient is likely to view the referral as a normal and positive aspect of the rehabilitation process (8,9).

Once a referral has been made, it is important for the athletic trainer to follow up with the mental health professional and continue to provide support for the patient. It is important to remember that ethical considerations prohibit mental health professionals from discussing cases with third parties unless the patient gives explicit written permission. In cases involving athletes, it is beneficial to get this permission in advance, allowing the mental health professional and athletic trainer to discuss the individual's condition and develop strategies to facilitate the rehabilitation process.

In locating a licensed mental health professional with the qualifications and clinical experience to work with physically active individuals, it may be helpful to investigate the availability of

Box 8.2 Common Signs and Symptoms Associated with Psychological Distress

Any sudden change in behavior or the continued presence of signs and symptoms of psychological distress may warrant a referral to a licensed mental health professional. The more of the following signs and symptoms that an individual demonstrates, the greater the need for a referral:

- Denying the seriousness or extent of injury
- Displaying signs of depression
- Displaying angry outbursts
- Displaying signs and symptoms of anxiety
- Lack of commitment to one's own rehabilitation
- Not adhering to the rehabilitation program
- Exercising beyond the recommended plan
- Not cooperating with the rehabilitation professional
- Bargaining with the rehabilitation professional over treatment or time out of competition
- Poor focus and/or inconsistent effort or intensity during the rehabilitation program
- Unconfirmed reports of pain
- Change in mood or inappropriate affect

personnel in college and university settings. Area hospitals also may be a resource, because many have a department of psychiatry or psychology, with a clinical psychologist specializing in various rehabilitation issues.

A *The distance runner will not be able to try out for a position on the next Olympic team. Clearly, her emotional and psychological state will have a direct impact on the success or failure of the therapeutic exercise program. Goal setting and mental skills training can be beneficial in addressing psychological influences that may inhibit the program. If progress is inhibited for several days because of suspected psychological issues, the athletic trainer should consult with a licensed mental health professional.*

DEVELOPING A THERAPEUTIC EXERCISE PROGRAM

Q *The female distance runner diagnosed with plantar fasciitis complains of pain with weight bearing that radiates up the medial side of the heel as well as across the lateral side of the foot. In addition, passive extension of the great toe and dorsiflexion of the ankle increase pain and discomfort. What short- and long-term goals could the athletic trainer and the athlete establish for the therapeutic exercise program? How should progress be measured?*

In designing an individualized therapeutic exercise program, several sequential steps help to identify the needs of the patient:

1. Assess the present level of function and dysfunction from girth measurements, goniometric assessment, strength tests, neurologic assessment, stress tests, and functional activities.

2. Organize and interpret the assessment to identify primary and secondary structural or functional deficits.

3. Establish short- and long-term goals to return the individual safely to participation.

4. Develop and supervise the treatment plan, incorporating therapeutic exercise, therapeutic modalities, and medication.

5. Reassess the progress of the plan, and adjust as needed.

The process is dependent on the patient's progress and adaptation to the therapeutic exercise program.

Assess the Patient

The subjective evaluation (i.e., history of the injury) is recorded in the **Subjective**, or S, portion of the SOAP note. This information should include the primary complaint, mechanism of injury, characteristics of the symptoms, functional impairments, previous injuries to the area, and family history. The objective evaluation (i.e., observation and inspection, palpation, and physical examination tests) establishes a baseline of measurable information and is recorded in the **Objective**, or O, portion of the SOAP note. This information documents the visual analysis of the injury site, symmetry, and appearance; determines the presence of a possible fracture; identifies abnormal clinical findings in the bony and soft-tissue structures; and measures functional testing (i.e., active, passive, and resisted ROM), ligamentous and capsular integrity, neurologic testing, and sport-specific functional testing. In paired body segments, the dysfunction of the injured body part is always compared with the noninjured body part to establish standards for bilateral functional status.

Interpret the Assessment

When an assessment is completed, the data must be interpreted to identify factors outside the normal limits for an individual of the same age and fitness level. Specifically, primary deficits or weaknesses must be defined. These deficits, along with secondary problems resulting from prolonged immobilization, extended inactivity, or lack of intervention, are organized into a priority list of concerns. Examples of major concerns may include decreased ROM, muscle weakness or stiffness, joint contractures, sensory changes, inability to walk without a limp, or increased pain with activity. Physical assets are then identified to determine the individual's present functional status. For example, normal gait and bilateral equal ROM should be documented. Specific problems are then recorded in a section called the problem list, which is a part of the **Assessment**, or A, portion of the SOAP note.

Establish Goals

Next, long-term goals are established for the individual's expected level of performance at the conclusion of the exercise program. These goals typically focus on functional deficits in performing activities of daily living and might include bilateral equal ROM, flexibility, muscular strength, endurance, and power; relaxation training; and restoration of coordination and cardiovascular endurance. Then, short-term goals are developed to address the specific component skills needed to reach the long-term goals. The athletic trainer and patient should discuss and develop the goals. The individual must feel a part of the process, because this may educate and motivate the individual to work harder to attain the stated goals. Many sport-specific factors, such as the demands of the sport; position played; time remaining in the season; regular-season versus post-season or tournament play; game rules and regulations regarding prosthetic braces or safety equipment; location, nature, and severity of injury; the mental state of the individual, may affect goal development.

The short-term goals are developed in a graduated sequence to address the list of problems identified during the assessment. For example, a high-priority short-term goal is the control of pain, inflammation, and spasm. Each short-term goal should be moderately difficult yet realistic. Specific subgoals should include an estimated timetable for attaining each one. These subgoals are time-dependent but not fixed, because it is important to consider individual differences in preinjury fitness and functional status, severity of injury, motivation to complete the goals, and subsequent improvement. Constant reinforcement from the athletic trainer to achieve the subgoals can be an incentive to continually progress toward the long-term goals. Long- and short-term goals may be recorded in the **Assessment**, or A, portion of the SOAP note; however, many athletic trainers choose to begin the **Treatment Plan**, or P, portion of the SOAP note with the objectives.

An example of short-term goals can be seen on the companion website at thePoint.

Develop and Supervise the Treatment Plan

Any therapeutic exercise and modality used to achieve the goals is recorded in the **Plan**, or P, section of the SOAP note along with any medications prescribed by the physician. To return the individual safely to participation, the therapeutic exercise program is divided into four phases. The termination of one phase and initiation of the next may overlap; however, each phase has a specific role.

Box 8.3 Phases of the Therapeutic Exercise Program

Phase 1: Control Inflammation
- Control the inflammatory stage, and minimize scar tissue with cryotherapy using **PRICE** principles (**P**rotect, **R**estrict activity, **I**ce, **C**ompression, and **E**levation).
- Instruct the patient on relaxation and coping techniques.
- Maintain range of motion (ROM), joint flexibility, strength, endurance, and power in the unaffected body parts.
- Maintain cardiovascular endurance.

Phase 2: Restore Motion
- Restore ROM to within 80% of normal in the unaffected limb.
- Restore joint flexibility to that observed in the unaffected limb.
- Begin proprioceptive stimulation through closed isotonic chain exercises.
- Begin pain-free, isometric strengthening exercises on the affected limb.
- Begin unresisted, pain-free functional patterns of sport/activity-specific motion.
- Maintain muscular strength, endurance, and power in unaffected muscles.
- Maintain cardiovascular endurance.

Phase 3: Develop Muscular Strength, Power, and Endurance
- Restore full ROM and proprioception in the affected limb.
- Restore muscular strength, endurance, and power using progressive resisted exercise.
- Maintain cardiovascular endurance.
- Initiate minimal to moderate resistance in sport/activity-specific functional patterns.

Phase 4: Return to Sport/Physical Activity
- Analyze skill performance, and correct biomechanical inefficiencies in motion.
- Improve muscular strength, endurance, and power.
- Restore coordination and balance.
- Improve cardiovascular endurance.
- Increase sport/activity-specific functional patterns, and return to protected activity as tolerated.

In phase 1, the inflammatory response, pain, swelling, and ecchymosis are controlled. Phase 2 focuses on regaining any deficits in ROM at the affected joint and restoring proprioception. Phase 3 involves restoring muscle strength, endurance, and power in the affected limb. Phase 4 prepares the individual to return to activity and includes sport-specific skill training, regaining coordination, and improving cardiovascular conditioning. These phases and their expected outcomes are discussed in more detail later in the chapter, and Box 8.3 lists the various phases of a therapeutic exercise program.

Each phase of the exercise program must be supervised and documented. In addition, progress notes should be completed on a weekly or biweekly basis. In many health care settings, these records also are used for third-party reimbursement of services rendered and, should litigation occur, provide documentation of services rendered.

Reassess the Progress of the Program

Short-term goals should be flexible enough to accommodate the progress of the individual. For example, if therapeutic modalities or medications are used and the individual attains a short-term goal sooner than expected, a new short-term goal should be written. Some conditions, however, such as edema, hemorrhage, muscle spasm, atrophy, or infection, may impede the healing process and delay attainment of a short-term goal. Periodic measurement of girth, ROM, muscle strength, endurance, power, and cardiovascular fitness determine whether progress occurs. If progress is not seen, the individual should be re-evaluated. The athletic trainer must determine if the delay is caused by physical problems, noncompliance, or psychological influences, necessitating referral to the appropriate specialist (e.g., physician or clinical psychologist). The individual should continue to progress through the short-term goals until the long-term goals are attained and the individual is cleared for full activity.

A *Long-term goals for the distance runner might include pain-free ROM, flexibility, muscle strength, endurance, and power; maintenance of cardiovascular endurance; restoration of normal joint biomechanics; increased proprioception and coordination; restoration of bilateral function of activities of daily living; and pain-free, unlimited motion in sport-specific skills.*

PHASE 1: CONTROLLING INFLAMMATION

Q *Given the acute nature of the distance runner's plantar fasciitis, the acute care protocol was followed, including submersion of the foot in an ice bath. Would it be appropriate to begin any rehabilitation exercises during this initial phase of injury management?*

Phase 1 of the exercise program begins immediately after injury assessment. The primary goal is to control inflammation by limiting hemorrhage, edema, effusion, muscle spasm, and pain. The individual can move into phase 2 when the following criteria have been attained:

- Control of inflammation with minimal edema, swelling, muscle spasm, and pain

- Range of motion, joint flexibility, muscular strength, endurance, and power are maintained in the non-injured areas of the body

- Cardiovascular fitness is maintained at the preinjury level

Collagenous scar formation, a natural component of the repair and regeneration of injured soft tissue, is less efficient and tolerant of tensile forces compared with the original mature tissue. The length of the inflammatory response is a key factor influencing the ultimate stability and function of scar tissue: The longer the inflammatory process progresses, the more likely the resulting scar tissue will be less dense and weaker in yielding to applied stress. Furthermore, immobilization for more than 2 or 3 weeks may lead to joint adhesions that inhibit the regeneration of muscle fiber. Therefore, all inflammatory symptoms need to be controlled as soon as possible. **PRICE**, a well-known acronym for **P**rotect, **R**estrict activity, **I**ce, **C**ompression, and **E**levation, is used to reduce acute symptoms at an injury site.

Control of Inflammation

Following trauma, hemorrhage and edema at the site of injury lead to a pooling of tissue fluids and blood products that increases pain and muscle spasm. The increased pressure decreases the flow of blood to the injury site, leading to hypoxia (i.e., deficiency of oxygen). As pain continues, the threshold for pain is lowered. These events lead to the cyclical pattern of pain-spasm-hypoxia-pain. For this reason, cryotherapy (i.e., ice, compression, and elevation) is preferred during the acute inflammation stage to decrease circulation, cellular metabolism, need for oxygen, and conduction velocity of nerve impulses to break the pain-spasm cycle. An elastic compression wrap can decrease hemorrhage and hematoma formation yet still expand in cases of extreme swelling. Elevation uses gravity to reduce the pooling of fluids and pressure inside the venous and lymphatic vessels and, thereby, prevent fluid from filtering into the surrounding tissue spaces. The result is less tissue necrosis and local waste, leading to a shorter inflammatory phase. Field Strategy 8.1 explains acute care of soft-tissue injuries using the PRICE principle.

Cryotherapy, intermittent compression, and electrical muscle stimulation (EMS) may be used to control hemorrhage and eliminate edema. Electrical therapy also has been shown to decrease pain and muscle spasm, strengthen weakened muscles, improve blood flow to an area, and enhance the healing rate of injured tendons. Transcutaneous electrical nerve stimulation (TENS) also may be used to limit pain (see Chapter 7). The modality of choice is determined by the size and location of the injured area, availability of the modality, and preference of the supervising health care provider.

FIELD STRATEGY 8.1

Acute Care of Soft-Tissue Injuries

Ice Application

- Apply crushed ice for 30 minutes directly to the skin (40 minutes for a large muscle mass, such as the quadriceps).
- Ice applications should be repeated every 2 hours when awake (every hour if the athlete is active) and may extend to more than 72 hours postinjury.
- Skin temperature can indicate when acute swelling has subsided. For example, if the area (compared bilaterally) feels warm to the touch, swelling continues. If in doubt, extend the time of a cold application.

Compression

- On an extremity, apply the wrap in a distal-to-proximal direction to avoid forcing extracellular fluid into the distal digits.
- Take a distal pulse after applying the wrap to ensure that the wrap is not overly tight.
- Felt horseshoe pads placed around the malleolus may be combined with an elastic wrap or tape to limit ankle swelling.
- Maintain compression continuously on the injury for the first 24 hours.

Elevation

- Elevate the body part 6 to 10 inches above the level of the heart.
- While sleeping, place a hard suitcase between the mattress and box spring, or place the extremity on a series of pillows.

Restrict Activity and Protect the Area

- If the individual is unable to walk without a limp, fit the person for crutches, and apply an appropriate protective device to limit unnecessary movement of the injured joint.
- If the individual has an upper extremity injury and is unable to move the limb without pain, fit the person with an appropriate sling or brace.

A decision to discontinue treatment and move to another modality should be based on the cessation of inflammation. Placing the back of the hand over the injured site shows any temperature change as compared with an uninjured area. Increased heat may indicate that inflammation and edema are still present, and a cooler area may indicate diminished circulation in an area.

Effects of Immobilization

The effects of immobilization on the various tissues of the body have been extensively covered in the literature. It is well accepted that muscle tension, muscle and ligament atrophy, decreased circulation, and loss of motion prolong the repair and regeneration of damaged tissues.

Muscle

Immobilization can lead to a loss of muscle strength within 24 hours. This is manifested by decreases in muscle fiber size, total muscle weight, size and number of mitochondria (the energy source of the cell), muscle tension produced, and resting levels of glycogen and adenosine triphosphate, which reduces muscle endurance. Motor nerves become less efficient in recruiting and stimulating muscle fibers. Immobilization also increases muscle fatigability as a result of decreased oxidative capacity. The rate of loss appears to be more rapid during the initial days of immobilization; however, after

5 to 7 days, the loss of muscle mass diminishes (10). Although both slow-twitch (type I) and fast-twitch (type II) muscle fibers atrophy, it generally is accepted that greater degeneration occurs in slow-twitch fibers with immobilization, and that muscles immobilized in a lengthened or neutral position maintain muscle weight and fiber cross-sectional area better than muscles immobilized in a shortened position. When shortened, the length of the fibers decreases, leading to increased connective tissue and reduced muscle extensibility. Muscles immobilized in a shortened position atrophy faster and have a greater loss of contractile function.

Articular Cartilage

The greatest impact of immobilization occurs in the articular cartilage, where adverse changes appear within 1 week of immobilization. The specific effects depend on the length of immobilization, position of the joint, and joint loading. Intermittent loading and unloading of synovial joints is necessary to ensure the proper metabolic exchange necessary for normal function. Constant contact with opposing bone ends can lead to pressure necrosis and cartilage cell (chondrocyte) death. In contrast, noncontact between two surfaces promotes growth of connective tissue into the joint. Diminished weight bearing, as well as loading and unloading, also can increase bone resorption. In general, articular cartilage softens and decreases in thickness. Immobilization for longer than 30 days can lead to progressive osteoarthritis.

Ligaments

Similar to bone, ligaments adapt to normal stress by remodeling in response to the mechanical demands that are placed on them. Stress leads to a stiffer, stronger ligament, whereas immobilization leads to a weaker, more compliant structure. This causes a decrease in the tensile strength, thus reducing the ability of ligaments to provide joint stability.

Bone

Mechanical strain on a bone affects the osteoblastic (bone cell formation) and osteoclastic (bone cell resorption) activity on the bone surface. Accordingly, the effects of immobilization on bone are similar to those on other connective tissues. Limited weight-bearing and muscle activity lead to bone loss, which can be detected as early as 2 weeks after immobilization (10). As immobilization time increases, bone resorption occurs, resulting in the bones becoming more brittle and highly susceptible to fracture. Disuse atrophy appears to increase bone loss at a rate 5- to 20-fold greater than that resulting from metabolic disorders affecting bone (11). Therefore, non–weight bearing immobilization should be limited to as short a time as possible.

Effects of Remobilization

Early controlled mobilization can speed the healing process. Bone and soft tissue respond to the physical demands that are placed on them, causing the formation of collagen to remodel or realign along the lines of stress and, thereby, promoting healthy joint biomechanics (**Wolff's law**). Continuous passive motion can prevent joint adhesions and stiffness and decrease joint hemarthrosis (blood in the joint) and pain. Early motion, as well as loading and unloading of joints, through partial weight-bearing exercise maintain joint lubrication to nourish articular cartilage, menisci, and ligaments. This leads to an optimal environment for proper collagen fibril formation. Tissues recover at different rates with mobilization: Muscle recovers more quickly, and articular cartilage and bone respond least favorably.

Muscle

Muscle regeneration begins within 3 to 5 days after mobilization. Both fast-twitch and slow-twitch muscle fibers can completely recover after 6 weeks. Muscle contractile activity rapidly increases protein synthesis; however, maximal isometric tension may not return to normal until 4 months after mobilized activity. The use of electrotherapy (i.e., EMS) may be helpful in re-educating muscles, limiting pain and spasm, and decreasing effusion through the pumping action of the contracting muscle. Unfortunately, neither EMS nor isometric exercise has been shown to prevent disuse atrophy.

Articular Cartilage

The effects of immobilization, whether with contact or with loss of contact between joint surfaces, can adversely interfere with cartilage nutrition. Articular cartilage generally responds favorably to mechanical stimuli, with structural modifications noted after exercise. Soft-tissue changes are reversible if immobilization does not exceed 30 days; these structural changes may not be reversible if immobilization exceeds 30 days.

Ligaments

The bone–ligament junction recovers more slowly than the mechanical properties in the midportion of the ligament. In addition, other nontraumatized ligaments weaken with disuse. Recovery depends on the duration of immobilization. Studies have shown that following 12 weeks of immobilization, a recovery of 50% of normal strength in a healing ligament is found after 6 months, 80% after 1 year, and 100% after 1 to 3 years, depending on the type of stresses placed on the ligament and on the prevention of repeated injury (12). Although the properties of ligaments return to normal with remobilization, the bone–ligament junction takes longer to return to normal. This factor must be considered when planning a rehabilitation program.

Bone

Although bone lost during immobilization may be regained, the period of recovery can be several-fold greater than the period of immobilization. In disuse osteoporosis, a condition involving reduced quantity of bone tissue, bone loss may not be reversible on remobilization of the limb. Isotonic and isometric exercises during the immobilization period can decrease some bone loss and hasten recovery after returning to a normal loading environment.

Protection After Injury

See *Field Strategy: Fitting and Using Crutches and Canes* on the companion website at thePoint.

The type of protection selected and the length of activity modification depend on the severity of injury, the structures damaged, and the philosophy of the supervising health care provider. Several materials, including elastic wraps, tape, pads, slings, hinged braces, splints, casts, and crutches, can be used to protect the area; many of these items were discussed and illustrated in Chapter 4. If an individual cannot walk without pain or walks with a limp, crutches should be recommended.

Restricted activity does not imply cessation of activity but, rather, means "relative rest"—that is, decreasing activity to a level below that required in sport but tolerated by the recently injured tissue or joint. **Detraining**, or loss of the benefits gained in physical training, can occur after only 1 to 2 weeks of nonactivity, with significant decreases measured in both metabolic and working capacities (13). Strengthening exercises in a weight-lifting program can be alternated with cardiovascular exercises, such as jogging, swimming, or use of a stationary bike or upper body ergometer. These exercises can prevent the individual from experiencing depression as a result of inactivity and can be done simultaneously with phase 1 exercises as long as the injured area is not irritated or inflamed.

In addition to cold treatments for control of inflammation, it would be appropriate to initiate gentle stretching exercises during this phase. The particular areas that should be stretched include the Achilles tendon and the toe flexor tendons. In addition, general body strength and cardiovascular endurance exercise can be performed as long as the injured area is not irritated.

PHASE 2: RESTORATION OF MOTION

The acute inflammatory symptoms associated with the plantar fasciitis have subsided. In the ongoing treatment of the plantar fasciitis, what type of exercises should be encouraged at this point during the rehabilitation process? Are there any modalities that could be used to supplement the exercise program?

Phase 2 begins immediately after the inflammation is controlled. This phase focuses on restoring ROM and flexibility at the injured site as well as on continuing to maintain general body strength and cardiovascular endurance. This phase may begin as early as 4 days after the injury, when swelling has stopped, or may have to wait until several weeks after the injury. The injured site may still be tender to touch, but it is not as painful as in the earlier phase. Also, pain is much less evident on passive and active ROM (AROM). If the patient is in an immobilizer or splint, the splint should be removed for treatment and exercise. The splint then can be replaced to support and protect the injured site. The individual can move into phase 3 when the following criteria have been completed:

- Inflammation and pain are under control.

- Range of motion is within 80% of normal in the unaffected limb.

- Bilateral joint flexibility is restored, and proprioception is regained.

- Cardiovascular endurance and general body strength are maintained at the preinjury level.

Assessment of normal ROM should be done with a goniometer on the paired, uninjured joint (see Chapter 5). Cryotherapy may be used before exercise to decrease perceived pain, or EMS or thermotherapy may be used to warm the tissues and increase circulation to the region. When the tissue is warmed, friction massage or joint mobilization may be helpful to break up scar tissue to regain normal motion.

Progression in this phase begins gradually, with restoration of ROM, proprioception, and total joint flexibility. Factors that limit joint motion include bony block; joint adhesions; muscle tightness; tight skin or inelastic, dense scar tissue; swelling; pain; and fat or other soft tissues that block normal motion. Prolonged immobilization can lead to muscles losing their flexibility and assuming a shortened position, which is referred to as a **contracture**. Connective tissue around joints has no contractile properties; connective tissue is supple and elongates slowly with a sustained stretch. Similar to muscle tissue, however, connective tissue adaptively shortens if immobilized. Connective tissue and muscles may be lengthened through passive and active stretching as well as proprioceptive neuromuscular facilitation exercises.

Passive Range of Motion

Two types of movement must be present for normal motion to occur about a joint. Physiologic motion, measured by a goniometer, occurs in the cardinal movement planes of flexion-extension, abduction-adduction, and rotation. Accessory motion, also referred to as **arthrokinematics**, is involuntary joint motion that occurs simultaneously with physiologic motion, but it cannot be measured precisely. Accessory movements involve the spinning, rolling, or gliding of one articular surface relative to another. Normal accessory movement must be present for full physiologic ROM to occur. If any accessory motion component is limited, normal physiologic motion will not occur.

Limited passive ROM (PROM) is called **hypomobility**. These discrete limitations of motion prevent pain-free return to competition and predispose an individual to microtraumatic injuries that reinflame the original injury. Restoring PROM prevents degenerative joint changes and promotes healing.

Joint Mobilization

Joint mobilization uses various oscillating forces, applied in the open packed position, to "free up" stiff joints. The oscillations produce several key benefits in the healing process:

- Breaking up adhesions, and relieving capsular restrictions

- Distracting impacted tissues

- Increasing lubrication for normal articular cartilage

- Reducing pain and muscle tension

- Restoring full ROM, and facilitating healing

Box 8.4 Contraindications to Joint Mobilization

- Acute inflammation
- Advanced osteoarthritis
- Congenital bone deformities
- Fractures
- Hypermobility
- Infections
- Malignancy
- Neurologic signs
- Osteoporosis
- Premature stressing of surgical structures
- Rheumatoid arthritis
- Vascular disease

Joint mobilization is contraindicated in several instances (Box 8.4). Maitland (14) described five grades of mobilization:

- **Grade I:** A small-amplitude movement at the beginning of the ROM. Used when pain and spasm limit movement early in the ROM.

- **Grade II:** Large-amplitude movement within the mid-ROM. Used when spasm limits movement sooner with a quick oscillation than with a slow one, or when slowly increasing pain restricts movement halfway into the range.

- **Grade III:** A large-amplitude movement up to the pathologic limit in the ROM. Used when pain and resistance from spasm, inert tissue tension, or tissue compression limit movement near the end of the ROM.

- **Grade IV:** A small-amplitude movement at the very end of the ROM. Used when resistance limits movement in the absence of pain and spasm.

- **Grade V:** A small-amplitude, quick thrust delivered at the end of the ROM, usually accompanied by a popping sound called a manipulation. Used when minimal resistance limits the end of the ROM. Manipulation is most effectively accomplished by the velocity rather than the force of the thrust.

In performing joint mobilization, the individual is placed in a comfortable position, with the joint placed in an open packed position. This allows the surrounding tissues to be as lax as possible and the intracapsular space to be at its largest. The direction of force is dependent on the contour of the joint surface of the structure being mobilized. The concave–convex rule states that when the concave surface is stationary and the convex surface is mobilized, a glide of the convex segment should be in the direction opposite to the restriction of joint movement. If the convex articular surface is stationary and the concave surface is mobilized, however, gliding of the concave segment should be in the same direction as the restriction of joint movement (Fig. 8.1). Typical treatment involves a series of three to six mobilizations lasting for up to 30 seconds, with one to three oscillations per second (14). Figure 8.2 demonstrates joint mobilization technique.

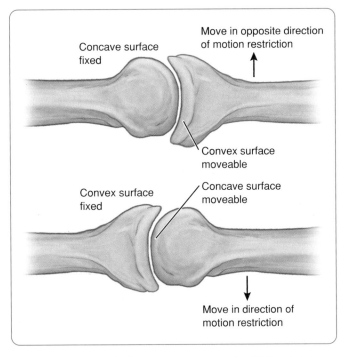

FIGURE 8.1 Concave–convex rule. If the joint surface to be moved is convex, it should be mobilized in the direction opposite that of the motion restriction. If the joint surface of the body segment being moved is concave, it should be moved in the direction of the motion restriction.

Flexibility

Flexibility is the total ROM at a joint that occurs pain-free in each of the planes of motion. Joint flexibility is a combination of normal joint mechanics, mobility of soft tissues, and muscle extensibility. For example, the hip joint may have full PROM, but when doing active hip flexion from a seated position, as in touching one's toes, resistance from tight hamstrings may limit full hip flexion. This type of resistance may be generated from tension in muscle fibers or connective tissue.

Muscles contain two primary proprioceptors that can be stimulated during stretching—namely, the muscle spindles and the Golgi tendon organs. Because muscle spindles lie parallel to muscle fibers, they stretch with the muscle. When stimulated, the spindle sensory fibers discharge and, through reflex action in the spinal cord, initiate impulses to cause the muscle to contract reflexively, thus inhibiting the stretch. Muscles that perform the desired movement are called **agonists**. Unlike muscle spindles, Golgi tendon organs are connected in a series of fibers located in tendons and joint ligaments, and they respond to muscle tension rather than to muscle length. If the stretch continues for an extended time (i.e., longer than 6–8 seconds),

FIGURE 8.2 Joint mobilization technique. Posterior humeral glide uses one hand to stabilize the humerus at the elbow while the other hand glides the humeral head in a posterior direction (arrow) to increase flexion and medial rotation at the joint.

the Golgi tendons are stimulated. This stimulus, unlike the stimulus from muscle spindles, causes a reflex inhibition in the **antagonist** muscles, and this sensory mechanism protects the musculotendinous unit from excessive tensile forces that could damage muscle fibers.

Flexibility can be increased through ballistic or static stretching techniques. **Ballistic stretching** uses repetitive bouncing motions at the end of the available ROM. Muscle spindles are repetitively stretched, but because the bouncing motions are of short duration, the Golgi tendon organs do not fire. As such, the muscles resist relaxation. Because generated momentum may carry the body part beyond the normal ROM, the muscles being stretched often remain contracted to prevent overstretching, leading to microscopic tears in the musculotendinous unit. In a **static stretch**, movement is slow and deliberate; Box 8.5 outlines guidelines for static stretching to improve flexibility. Golgi

Box 8.5   Guidelines for Static Stretching to Improve Flexibility

1. Stretching is facilitated by warm body tissues; therefore, a brief warm-up period is recommended. If it is not possible to jog lightly, stretching could be performed after a superficial heat treatment.
2. In the designated stretch position, the individual should move to a position in which a sensation of tension is felt.
3. No bouncing should be associated with the stretch. The stretch position should be held for 10 to 30 seconds, until a sense of relaxation occurs. The individual should be aware of the feeling of relaxation or "letting go." A stretch should be repeated six to eight times.
4. Breathing should be performed rhythmically and slowly. The individual should exhale during the actual stretch.
5. It is important to avoid being overly aggressive in stretching. Increased flexibility may not be noticed for 4 to 6 weeks.
6. If an area is particularly resistant to stretching, then partner stretching or proprioceptive neuromuscular facilitation may be used.
7. Vigorous stretching of tissues should be avoided in the following conditions:
    - After a recent fracture
    - After prolonged immobilization
    - With acute inflammation or infection in or around the joint
    - With a bony block that limits motion
    - With muscle contractures or when joint adhesions limit motion
    - With acute pain during stretching

FIGURE 8.3 Proprioceptive neuromuscular facilitation. In performing proprioceptive neuromuscular facilitation stretching techniques, the athletic trainer passively stretches a muscle group. In this picture, the hip flexors are being stretched. When slight tension is felt, the individual isometrically contracts the muscle group against resistance for 3, 6, or 10 seconds. The muscle is then passively stretched. This process is repeated four or five times.

tendon organs are able to override impulses from the muscle spindles, leading to a safer, more effective muscle stretch. When the muscle is stretched to the point at which a mild burn is felt, the joint position is maintained statically for approximately 15 seconds and then is repeated several times.

Proprioceptive neuromuscular facilitation promotes and hastens the response of the neuromuscular system through stimulation of the proprioceptors (Fig. 8.3). The patient should be taught how to perform the exercise through cutaneous and auditory input. Often, the individual looks at the moving limb while the examiner moves the limb from the starting to terminal position. Verbal cues are used to coordinate voluntary effort with reflex responses. Words such as "push" or "pull" commonly are used to ask for an isotonic contraction. "Hold" may be used for an isometric or stabilizing contraction, followed by "relax." Manual (cutaneous contact) helps to influence the direction of motion and to facilitate a maximal response, because reflex responses are greatly affected by pressure receptors.

These exercises increase flexibility in one muscle group (i.e., agonist) and simultaneously improve strength in another muscle group (i.e., antagonist). Furthermore, if instituted early in the exercise program, proprioceptive neuromuscular facilitation stretches can aid in elongating scar tissue. As scar tissue matures and increases in density, it becomes less receptive to short-term stretches and may require prolonged stretching to achieve deformational changes in the tissue.

The proprioceptive neuromuscular facilitation techniques recruit muscle contractions in a coordinated pattern as agonists and antagonists move through a ROM. One technique uses **active inhibition,** whereby the muscle group reflexively relaxes before the stretching maneuver. Common methods include contract-relax, hold-relax, and slow reversal-hold-relax (Box 8.6). The examiner stabilizes the limb to be exercised. Alternating contractions and passive stretching of a group of muscles are then performed. Contractions may be held for 3, 6, or 10 seconds, with similar results obtained (15).

A second technique, known as **reciprocal inhibition,** uses active agonist contractions to relax a tight antagonist muscle. In this technique, the individual contracts, against resistance, the muscle opposite the tight muscle. This causes a reciprocal inhibition of the tight muscle, leading to muscle lengthening. An advantage to proprioceptive neuromuscular facilitation exercise is the ability to stretch a tight muscle that may be painful or in the early stages of healing. In addition, movement can occur in a single plane or in a diagonal pattern that mimics actual skill performance.

Active Assisted Range of Motion

Frequently, PROM at the injured joint may be greater than active motion, perhaps because of muscle weakness. A person may be able to sit on top of a table and slide the leg across the tabletop away from the body to fully extend the knee. If, however, the individual sits at the edge of the table with the legs hanging over the edge and then attempts to straighten the knee, the individual may be unable to move the limb voluntarily into full extension. In this situation, normal joint mechanics exist, and full PROM is present. To attain full AROM, however, the individual may require some assistance from an athletic trainer, a mechanical device, or the opposite limb (active assisted ROM). Working the limb through available pain-free motion with assistance restores normal AROM more quickly than working the limb within limited voluntary motion.

Box 8.6 Active Inhibition Techniques

To stretch the hamstring group on a single leg using the three separate proprioceptive neuromuscular facilitation techniques, the following guidelines should be followed:

Contract-Relax
1. The thigh is stabilized and the hip passively flexed into the agonist pattern until limitation is felt in the hamstrings.
2. The individual performs an isotonic contraction with the hamstrings through the antagonist pattern.
3. A passive stretch is applied into the agonist pattern until limitation is felt, and the sequence is repeated.

Hold-Relax
1. The leg is passively moved into the agonist pattern until resistance is felt in the hamstrings.
2. The individual performs an isometric contraction to "hold" the position for approximately 10 seconds.
3. The individual should relax for approximately 5 seconds.
4. A passive stretch is applied into the agonist pattern until limitation is felt, and the sequence is repeated.

Slow Reversal-Hold-Relax
1. The individual consciously relaxes the hamstring muscles while doing a concentric contraction of the quadriceps muscles into the agonist pattern.
2. The individual performs an isometric contraction, against resistance, into the antagonist pattern for 10 seconds.
3. The individual should relax for approximately 10 seconds..
4. The individual actively moves the body part further into the agonist pattern, and the sequence is repeated.

Active Range of Motion

Active ROM exercises performed by the individual enhance circulation through a pumping action during muscular contraction and relaxation. Full, pain-free AROM need not be achieved before strength exercises are initiated; however, performance of skills and drills, such as throwing or full squats, requiring full functional motion or certain agility drills must be delayed until proper joint mechanics are restored. Active ROM exercises should be relatively painless and may be facilitated during certain stages of the program by completing the exercises in a whirlpool to provide an analgesic effect and relieve the stress of gravity on sensitive structures. Examples of AROM exercises include spelling out the letters of the alphabet with the ankle and using a wand or cane with the upper extremity to improve joint mobility.

See *Field Strategy: Range of Motion Exercises for the Lower and Upper Extremities* on the companion website at thePoint.

Resisted Range of Motion

Resisted ROM may be either static or dynamic. Static movement is measured with an isometric muscle contraction and can be used during phases 1 and 2 of the exercise program in a pain-free arc of motion. Dynamic resisted motion (dynamic strengthening) is discussed in the next section.

Isometric training measures a muscle's maximum potential to produce static force. The muscle is at a constant tension, whereas muscle length and joint angle remain the same. For example, standing in a doorway and pushing outward against the door frame produces a maximal muscle contraction, but joints of the upper extremity do not appear to move. In performing an isometric contraction, a maximal force is generated against an object, such as the examiner's hand, for approximately 10 seconds and is repeated 10 times per set. Contractions, performed every 20° throughout the available ROM, are called multiangle isometric exercises.

Isometric exercise is useful when motion:

1. Is contraindicated by pathology or bracing.

2. Is limited because of muscle weakness at a particular angle, called a **sticking point**.

3. When a painful arc is present.

Isometric strength exercises are the least effective training method, because although circumference and strength increase, strength gains are limited to a range of 10° on either side of the joint angle. In addition, during isometric exercise, an adverse, rapid increase in blood pressure can occur when the breath is held against a closed glottis. This occurrence, referred to as the **Valsalva effect**, can be avoided with proper breathing.

Proprioception

Proprioception is a specialized variation of the sensory modality of touch that encompasses the sensation of joint movement (**kinesthesia**) and joint position. Sensory receptors located in the skin, muscles, tendons, ligaments, and joints provide input into the central nervous system relative to tissue deformation. Visual and vestibular centers also contribute afferent information to the central nervous system regarding body position and balance. The ability to sense body position is mediated by cutaneous, muscle, and joint mechanoreceptors.

Joint Mechanoreceptors

Joint mechanoreceptors are found in the joint capsule, ligaments, menisci, labra, and fat pads, and they include four types of nerve endings: Ruffini's corpuscles, Golgi receptors, pacinian corpuscles, and free nerve endings. Ruffini's corpuscles are sensitive to intra-articular pressure and stretching of the joint capsule. Golgi receptors are intraligamentous and become active when the ligaments are stressed at the end ranges of joint movement. Pacinian corpuscles are sensitive to high-frequency vibration and pressure. Free nerve endings are sensitive to mechanical stress and the deformation and loading of soft tissues that comprise the joint.

Muscle Mechanoreceptors

As mentioned, the receptors found in muscle and tendons are the muscle spindles and Golgi tendon organs. Muscle spindles are innervated by both afferent and efferent fibers and can detect not only muscle length but also, and more importary, the rate of change in muscle length. Golgi tendon organs respond to both contraction and stretch of the musculotendinous junction. If the stretch continues for an extended time (i.e., longer than 6–8 seconds), the Golgi tendons are stimulated, causing a reflex inhibition in the antagonist muscles. This sensory mechanism protects the musculotendinous unit from excessive tensile forces that could damage muscle fibers.

Regaining Proprioception

Balance involves positioning the body's center of gravity over a base of support through the integration of information received from the various proprioceptors within the body. Even when the body appears motionless, a constant postural sway is caused by a series of muscle contractions that correct and maintain dynamic equilibrium in an upright position. When balance is disrupted, as in falling forward or stumbling, the response is primarily automatic and reflexive. An injury or illness can interrupt the neuromuscular feedback mechanisms. Restoration of the proprioceptive feedback is necessary for promoting dynamic joint and functional stability to prevent reinjury.

Proprioceptive exercises must be specific to the type of activity that the individual will encounter during participation in a sport and physical activity. In general, the progression of activities to develop dynamic, reactive neuromuscular control is achieved through a progression that moves from slow speed to high speed, low force to high force, and controlled to uncontrolled activities. A patient might begin with Romberg's test, which requires the individual to stand with the feet together, arms at the sides, and eyes closed. The examiner looks for any tendency to sway or fall to one side. A single-leg stance test (e.g., stork stand) requires the individual to maintain balance while standing on one leg for a specified time with the eyes closed. In the next stage, with the eyes open, the patient can progress to playing catch with a ball. This exercise can be made more difficult by having the patient balance on a trampoline while playing catch with a ball. Use of a biomechanical ankle platform system (BAPS) board might begin with bilateral balancing and progress to one-legged balancing, dribbling a basketball, or playing catch with a ball. Many of these exercises can be adapted to the upper extremity. An individual can begin in a push-up position and shift his or her weight from one hand to another or perform isometric or isotonic press-ups, balance on one hand, balance on a BAPS board or ball, or walk on the hands over material of different densities or heights.

Open Versus Closed Kinetic Chain Exercises

A common error in developing an exercise program is failure to assess the proximal and distal segments of the entire extremity, or kinetic chain. A **kinematic chain** is a series of interrelated joints that constitute a complex motor unit, constructed so that motion at one joint will produce motion at the other joints in a predictable manner. Whereas kinematics describes the appearance of motion, **kinetics** involves the forces, whether internal (e.g., muscle contractions or connective tissue restraints) or external (e.g., gravity, inertia, or segmental masses) that affect motion. Initially, a closed kinetic chain (CKC) was characterized as the distal segment of the extremity in an erect, weight-bearing position, such as the lower extremity when a person is weight bearing. Subsequently, when the distal segment of the extremity is free to move without causing motion at another joint, such as when non–weight bearing, the system was referred to as an open kinetic chain (OKC). When force is applied, the distal segment may function independently or in unison with the other joints. Movements of the more proximal joints are affected by OKC and CKC positions. For example, the rotational components of the ankle, knee, and hip reverse direction when moving from an OKC to CKC position.

Because of incongruities between the lower and upper extremity, particularly in the shoulder region, several authors have challenged the traditional definition of OKC and CKC positions (16–18). Stabilizing muscles in the scapulothoracic region produces a joint compression force that stabilizes the glenohumeral joint in much the same manner as a CKC in the lower extremity. Although debate continues on defining CKC and OKC relative to the upper extremity, there remains general agreement that both CKC and OKC exercises should be incorporated into an upper and lower extremity rehabilitation program.

Injury and subsequent immobilization can affect the proprioceptors in the skeletal muscles, tendons, and joints. In rehabilitation, it is critical that CKC activities be used to retrain joints and muscle proprioceptors to respond to sensory input. Closed kinetic chain exercises are recommended because they:

- Stimulate and re-educate the proprioceptors.

- Increase joint stability and congruity.

- Provide greater joint compressive forces.

- Exercise multiple joints through weight-bearing and muscular contractions.

- Better control velocity and torque.

- Reduce shear forces.

- Increase muscle coactivation.

- Allow better use of the SAID (Specific Adaptations to Imposed Demands) principle.

- Permit more functional patterns of movement (including spiral and diagonal) and greater specificity for athletic activities.

- Facilitate postural and dynamic stabilization mechanics.

In contrast, OKC exercises can isolate a specific muscle group for intense strength and endurance exercises. In addition, they can develop strength in very weak muscles that may not function properly in a CKC system because of muscle substitution. Although OKC exercises may produce great gains in peak force production, these exercises usually are limited to one joint in a single plane (uniplanar) and have greater potential for joint shear, limited functional application, and limited eccentric and proprioceptive retraining. Open kinetic chain exercises, however, can assist in developing a patient–athletic trainer rapport through uniplanar and multiplanar manual therapeutic techniques. Figure 8.4 illustrates OKC and CKC chain exercises for the lower extremity.

FIGURE 8.4 Open and closed chain exercises for the lower extremity. A, Open chain exercise for the hamstrings. **B**, Closed chain exercise for the hip and knee extensors.

When ROM has been achieved, repetition of motion through actual skill movements can improve coordination and joint mechanics as the individual progresses into phase 3 of the program. For example, a pitcher may begin throwing without resistance or force application in front of a mirror to visualize the action. This also can motivate the individual to continue to progress in the therapeutic exercise program.

> *During phase 2, passive stretching and AROM exercises should be conducted. In particular, stretching and strengthening of both the intrinsic and extrinsic muscles of the foot and ankle should be major parts of the rehabilitation plan. Cryotherapy, thermotherapy, EMS, or massage can complement the exercise program as needed.*

PHASE 3: DEVELOPING MUSCULAR STRENGTH, ENDURANCE, AND POWER

> *The distance runner has full, pain-free ROM. She wants to resume her running workouts. Is it advisable for her to so at this time? What is the likelihood that reinjury will occur?*

Phase 3 focuses on developing muscular strength, endurance, and power in the injured extremity as compared with the uninjured extremity. The individual can move into phase 4 when the following criteria have been completed:

- Bilateral ROM and joint flexibility are restored.

- Muscular strength, endurance, and power in the affected limb are equal or near equal to those in the unaffected limb.

- Cardiovascular endurance and general body strength are equal to or better than the preinjury levels.

- Sport-specific functional patterns are completed using mild to moderate resistance.

- The individual is psychologically ready to return to protected activity.

Muscular Strength

Strength is the ability of a muscle or a group of muscles to produce force in one maximal effort. Although static strength (isometric strengthening) is used during phases 1 and 2 in a pain-free arc of motion, dynamic strengthening is preferred during phase 3 of the program. Two types of contractions occur in dynamic strength: **concentric**, in which a shortening of muscle fibers decreases the angle of the associated joint, and **eccentric**, in which the muscle resists its own lengthening so that the joint angle increases during the contraction. Concentric and eccentric contractions also may be referred to as positive and negative work, respectively. Concentric contractions work to accelerate a limb; for example, the gluteus maximus and quadriceps muscles concentrically contract to accelerate the body upward from a crouched position. In contrast, eccentric contractions work to decelerate a limb and provide shock absorption, especially during high-velocity dynamic activities. For example, the shoulder external rotators decelerate the shoulder during the follow-through phase of the overhead throw.

Eccentric contractions generate greater force than isometric contractions, and isometric contractions generate greater force than concentric contractions. In addition, less tension is required in an eccentric contraction. One major disadvantage of eccentric training, however, is delayed-onset muscle soreness, which is defined as muscular pain or discomfort 1 to 5 days following unusual muscular exertion. Delayed-onset muscle soreness is associated with joint swelling and weakness, which may last after the cessation of pain. This differs from acute-onset muscle soreness, in which pain during exercise ceases after the exercise bout is completed. To prevent the onset of delayed-onset muscle soreness, eccentric exercises should progress gradually. Dynamic muscle strength is gained through isotonic or isokinetic exercise (Fig. 8.5).

Isotonic Training (Variable Speed/Fixed Resistance)

A more common method of strength training is isotonic exercise or, as it sometimes is called, **progressive resistive exercise**. In this technique, a maximal muscle contraction generates a force to move a constant load throughout the ROM at a variable speed. Both concentric and eccentric

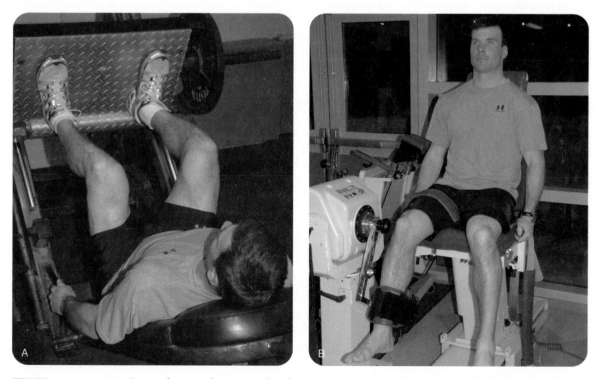

FIGURE 8.5 Dynamic muscle strengthening. Dynamic strength may be gained through (**A**) isotonic exercise or (**B**) isokinetic exercise.

contractions are possible with free weights, elastic or rubber tubing, and weight machines. Free weights are inexpensive and can be used in diagonal patterns for sport or activity-specific skills, but adding or removing weights from the bars can be troublesome. In addition, a spotter may be required for safety purposes to avoid heavy weights being dropped. Thera-Band, or surgical tubing, is inexpensive and easy to set up, can be used in diagonal patterns for sport or activity-specific skills, and can be adjusted to the patient's level of strength using bands of different tension. Weights on commercial machines can be changed quickly and easily. Using several stations of free weights and commercial machines, an individual can perform circuit training to strengthen multiple muscle groups in a single exercise session. Typically, however, the machines are large and expensive, work in only a single plane of motion, and may not match the biomechanical makeup or body size of the individual.

Isotonic training permits exercise of multiple joints simultaneously, both eccentric and concentric contractions, and weight-bearing CKC exercises. A disadvantage is that when a load is applied, the muscle can only move that load through the ROM with as much force as the muscle provides at its weakest point. Nautilus and Eagle equipment are examples of variable resistance machines with an elliptical cam. The cam system provides minimal resistance where the ability to produce force is comparatively lower (i.e., early and late in the ROM) and greatest resistance where the muscle is at its optimal length-tension and mechanical advantage (i.e., usually the midrange). The axis of rotation generates an isokinetic-like effect, but angular velocity cannot be controlled.

Isokinetic Training (Fixed Speed/Variable Resistance)

Isokinetic training, or accommodating resistance, allows an individual to provide muscular overload and angular movement to rotate a lever arm at a controlled velocity or fixed speed. Theoretically, isokinetic training should activate the maximum number of motor units, which consistently overloads muscles and achieves maximum tension-developing or force-output capacity at every point in the ROM, even at the relatively "weaker" joint angles. Cybex, Biodex, and Kin Com are examples of equipment that use this strength training method. Coupled with a computer and appropriate software, torque-motion curves, total work, average power, and measures of torque to body weight can be instantaneously calculated to provide immediate, objective measurement to the individual and examiner.

Two advantages of isokinetic training are that a muscle group can be exercised to its maximum potential throughout the full ROM and that the dynamometer's resistance mechanism essentially disengages if pain is experienced by the patient. As the muscles fatigue, however, isokinetic resistance decreases. In contrast, with an isotonic contraction, because the resistance is constant as the muscle fatigues, the muscle must either recruit additional motor units, thus increasing muscle force, or fail to perform the complete repetition. It is hypothesized that during rehabilitation, isotonic training is more effective than isokinetic training in achieving rapid gains in strength during training using the daily adjusted progressive resistance exercise (DAPRE) technique (19). Two other disadvantages are the cost of the machine, computer, and software package (ranging from $25,000–60,000) and the fact that most available machines permit only OKC exercises. For this reason, isokinetic training should be used in conjunction with other modes of resistance training.

Muscular Endurance

Muscular endurance is the ability of muscle tissue to exert repetitive tension over an extended period of time. The rate of muscle fatigue is related to the endurance level of the muscle (i.e., the more rapidly the muscle fatigues, the lower the muscle endurance). A direct relationship exists between muscle strength and muscle endurance. As muscle endurance is developed, density in the capillary beds increases, providing a greater blood supply and, thus, a greater oxygen supply to the working muscle. Increases in muscle endurance may influence gains in strength; however, development of strength has not been shown to increase muscle endurance. Muscular endurance is gained by lifting low weights at a faster contractile velocity with more repetitions in the exercise session or with the use of stationary bikes or aquatic therapy, Stair Master, Nordic Track, or Slide Board.

Muscular Power

Muscular power is the ability of muscle to produce force in a given time. Power training is started after the injured limb has regained at least 80% of the muscle strength in the unaffected limb.

Regaining power involves weight training at higher contractile velocities or using plyometric exercises.

Plyometric training employs the inherent stretch–recoil characteristics of skeletal muscle through an initial, rapid eccentric (loading) prestretching of a muscle, thereby activating the stretch reflex to produce tension before initiating an explosive concentric contraction of the muscle. This stretch produces a strong stimulus at the level of the spinal cord, which causes an explosive reflex concentric contraction. The greater the stretch from the muscle's resting length immediately before the concentric contraction, the greater the load the muscle can lift or overcome. Injury can result if the individual does not have full ROM, flexibility, and near-normal strength before beginning these exercises. Examples of plyometric exercises include a standing jump, multiple jumps, box jumps or drop jumping from a height, single- or double-leg hops, bounding, leaps, and skips. In the upper extremity, a medicine ball, surgical tubing, plyoback, and boxes can be used. Performing jumping and skipping exercises on grass reduces the impact on the lower extremity during landing. These exercises should be performed every 3 days to allow the muscles to recover from fatigue.

Functional Application of Exercise

Strength, endurance, and power can only be increased by using the **overload principle**, which states that physiologic improvements occur only when an individual physically demands more than normally is required of the muscles. This philosophy is based on the SAID principle, which states that the body responds to a given demand with a specific and predictable adaptation. Overload is achieved by manipulating intensity, duration, frequency, specificity, speed, and progression in the exercise program.

Intensity

Intensity reflects both the caloric cost of the work and the specific energy systems that are activated. Strength gains depend primarily on the intensity of the overload, not on the specific training method used to improve strength. The DAPRE of Knight (20) is an objective method of increasing resistance as the individual's strength increases or decreases. A fixed percentage of the maximum weight for a single repetition is lifted during the first and second sets. Maximum repetitions of the resistance maximum are lifted during the third set. Adaptations to the amount of weight lifted are then increased or decreased accordingly during the fourth set and during the first set of the next session. The DAPRE guidelines are based on the concept that if the working weight is ideal, the individual can perform six repetitions when told to perform as many as possible. If the individual can perform more than six repetitions, the weight is too light. Conversely, if the individual cannot lift six repetitions, the weight is too heavy.

See *Daily Adjusted Progressive Resistance Exercise Program* on the companion website at thePoint.

For individuals with chronic injuries or early postoperative rehabilitation, the DAPRE method may not be appropriate. Instead, a high-repetition, low-weight exercise may be more productive, particularly during the early phases. High weights potentially can cause a breakdown of the supporting soft-tissue structures and exacerbate the condition. Use of smaller weights and submaximal intensities can stimulate blood flow and limit tissue damage. To gain strength and endurance, higher repetitions are required. The individual begins with two or three sets of 10 repetitions, progressing to five sets of 10 repetitions as tolerated. When the individual can perform 50 repetitions, 1 pound may be added and the repetitions reduced to three sets of 10 repetitions. All exercises should be performed slowly, concentrating on proper technique. As strength increases, the DAPRE method or other type of progressive resistance exercise schedule may be used.

Duration

Duration refers to the estimated time that it will take to return the individual to full (100%) activity; more commonly, however, duration refers to the length of a single exercise session. This time can shorten if pain, swelling, or muscle soreness occurs. In general, the individual must participate in at least 20 minutes of continuous activity, with the heart rate elevated to at least 70% of maximal. This is particularly important when increasing cardiovascular endurance, which will be explained later in the chapter.

Frequency

Frequency refers to the number of exercise sessions per day or week. Although exercise performed twice daily yields greater improvement than exercise performed once daily, in most cases the exercise program should be conducted three to four times per week. It is critical not to work the same muscle groups on successive days to allow recovery from fatigue and muscle soreness. If daily bouts are planned, strength and power exercises may be alternated with cardiovascular conditioning, or exercises for the lower extremity may alternate with exercises for the upper extremity.

Specificity

An exercise program must address the specific needs of the patient. For example, exercises that mimic the throwing action will benefit a baseball pitcher but are not applicable to a football lineman. If exercises simulate actual skills used in the individual's sport or activity, the patient is more likely to be motivated and compliant with the exercise program. The type of exercise (e.g., isometric, isotonic, or isokinetic) also is important. Individuals who rely on eccentric loading also must include eccentric training in their rehabilitation program. Rhythm, or velocity, also has been shown to be specific to that required for the sport skill, with the greatest gains in strength consistently occurring at training speeds (21).

Speed

Speed refers to the rate at which the exercise is performed. Initially, exercises should be performed in a slow, deliberate manner, at a rate of approximately 60° per second, with emphasis placed on concentric and eccentric contractions. The individual should exercise throughout the full ROM, pausing at the end of the exercise. Large muscle groups should be exercised first, followed by the smaller groups. In addition, the exercise speed should be varied. As strength, endurance, and power increase, functional movements should increase in speed. Surgical tubing can be used to develop a high-speed regimen to produce concentric and eccentric synergistic patterns, and isokinetic units also may be used at the highest speeds.

Progression

See *Field Strategy: Power and Strength Exercises* on the companion website at thePoint.

In an effort to maintain motivation and compliance, an objective improvement should occur each day, whether this is an increase in repetitions or intensity. Muscular strength is improved with a minimum of 3 days per week of training that includes 12 to 15 repetitions per bout of 8 to 10 exercises for the major muscle groups (13). If the individual complains of pain, swelling, or residual muscle soreness, the program may need to be decreased or varied in intensity. An orderly progression should move from ROM exercises to isometric, isotonic, isokinetic, and functional activities, however, progressing from low to high intensity with ever-increasing demands on the patient as the healing process allows.

A *Before permitting the distance runner to resume running workouts, her muscle strength, endurance, and power in the affected limb, in addition to full and pain-free ROM, must be at or near the levels of the unaffected limb to prevent reinjury.*

PHASE 4: RETURN TO SPORT/PHYSICAL ACTIVITY

Q *The distance runner has full ROM and near-normal strength in the affected limb. She has maintained cardiovascular endurance by swimming and using an upper body ergometer. What additional factors need to be considered to prepare this individual for return to full activity?*

The individual can return to their sport activity as soon as muscle strength, endurance, and power are restored. During phase 4, the individual also should correct any biomechanical inefficiency in motion; restore coordination and muscle strength, endurance, and power in sport-specific skills; and improve cardiovascular endurance. The individual may be returned to activity if the following goals are attained:

- Coordination and balance are normal.

- Sport-specific functional patterns are restored in the injured extremity.

- Muscle strength, endurance, and power in the affected limb are equal to those in the unaffected limb.

- Cardiovascular endurance is equal to or greater than the preinjury level.

- The individual receives clearance to return to participation by the supervising physician.

Coordination

Coordination refers to the body's ability to execute smooth, fluid, accurate, and controlled movements. Simple movement, such as combing hair, involves a complex muscular interaction using the appropriate speed, distance, direction, rhythm, and muscle tension to execute the task. Coordination may be divided into two categories: gross motor movements involving large muscle groups, and fine motor movements using small groups. Gross motor movements involve activities such as standing, walking, skipping, and running. Fine motor movements are seen in precise actions, particularly with the fingers, such as picking up a coin off a table, clutching an opponent's jersey, or picking up a ground ball with a glove. Coordination and proprioception are directly linked. When an injury occurs and the limb is immobilized, sensory input from proprioceptors and motor commands are disrupted, resulting in an alteration of coordination.

Performing CKC activities during phase 2 of the exercise program can help to restore proprioceptive input and improve coordination. Constant repetition of motor activities using sensory cues (i.e., tactile, visual, or proprioceptive) or increasing the speed of the activity over time can continue to develop coordination during phases 3 and 4. A wobble board, teeter board, ProFitter, or BAPS board often is used to improve sensory cues and balance in the lower extremity. Proprioceptive neuromuscular facilitation patterns and the ProFitter also may be used to improve sensory cues in the upper and lower extremities.

See *Field Strategy: Lower Extremity Exercises to Improve Balance and Proprioception* on the companion website at thePoint.

Sport/Activity-Specific Skill Conditioning

Because different sports require different skills, therapeutic exercise should progress to the load and speed that are expected for the individual's sport or physical activity. For example, a baseball player performs skills at different speeds and intensities than a football lineman. Therefore, exercises must be coupled with functional training or with specificity of training related to the physical demands of the sport.

As ROM, muscular strength, and coordination are restored, the individual should work the affected extremity through functional diagonal and sport-specific patterns. For example, during phase 3, a baseball pitcher may have been moving the injured arm through the throwing pattern with mild to moderate resistance. During phase 4, the individual should increase resistance and speed of motion. Working with a ball attached to surgical tubing, the individual can develop a kinesthetic awareness in a functional pattern. When controlled motion is done without pain, actual throwing can begin. Initially, short throws with low intensity can be used, progressing to longer throws with low intensity. As the player feels more comfortable and is pain-free with the action, the number of throws and their intensity are increased. Similar programs can be developed for other sports or physical activities. Other sport/activity-specific skills that can be performed at this level include sprint work, agility runs, figure-eights, side stepping, shuttle runs, and interval training (i.e., alternating periods of intense work and active recovery).

Cardiovascular Endurance

Cardiovascular endurance, commonly called aerobic capacity, is the body's ability to sustain submaximal exercise over an extended period and depends on the efficiency of the pulmonary and cardiovascular systems. When an injured individual is unable to continue or chooses to stop aerobic training, detraining occurs within 1 to 2 weeks (13). If the individual returns to activity without a high cardiovascular endurance level, fatigue sets in quickly, which places the individual at risk for reinjury.

Similar to strength training, maintaining and improving cardiovascular endurance is influenced by an interaction of frequency, duration, and intensity. The American College of Sports Medicine (ACSM) recommends that aerobic training be moderate–intensity aerobic physical activity for a minimum of 30 minutes per exercise session on 5 or more days per week or vigorous–intensity aerobic activity for a minimum of 20 minutes on 3 or more days (13,22). If added consideration is needed to preserve bone health during adulthood, the ACSM recommends 30 to 60 minutes of weight-bearing cardiovascular exercises three to five times per week in addition to resistance exercises two or three times per week (23). Targeted heart rate can be calculated in two manners:

1. An estimated HRmax for both men and women is approximately 220 beats per minute. Heart rate is related to age, with HRmax decreasing as an individual ages. A relatively simple calculation is

$$HRmax = 220 - Age$$

   With a 20-year-old individual working at 80% of maximum, the calculation is $0.8 \times (220 - 20)$, or 160 beats per minute.

2. Another commonly used formula (Karvonen formula) assumes that the targeted range of heart rate is between 60 and 90% of HRmax. This calculation is

$$Target\ HR\ range = [(HRmax - HRrest) \times 0.60\ and\ 0.90] + HRrest$$

   where HRrest is the individual's resting heart rate. If an individual's HRmax is 180 beats per minute and the HRrest is 60 beats per minute, this method yields a target HR range of between 132 and 168 beats per minute.

See *Field Strategy: Cardiovascular Conditioning Exercises* on the companion website at thePoint.

Non–weight bearing exercises, such as swimming, rowing, biking, or use of the upper body ergometer, can be helpful early during the therapeutic program, particularly if the individual has a lower extremity injury. Walking, cross-country skiing, jumping rope, or running can be performed as the condition improves.

A *In preparing the distance runner for return to her sport, modifications in running workouts must be addressed, because it would not be appropriate for the athlete to continue at her previous level of training. Ongoing management of the condition should be addressed as well. In particular, the athlete should be informed about signs and symptoms that would warrant a decrease in activity and a return to more intensive rehabilitation. Finally, the documentation needed to clear the distance runner for return to activity, including a doctor's medical clearance, should be completed. It is important to remember that all written documentation of the exercise program and written medical clearance should be placed in the individual's file and stored in a safe, secure location for a minimum of 3 to 5 years.*

SUMMARY

1. A therapeutic exercise program must address not only the physical needs of the individual but also the emotional and psychological needs.

2. Several factors can affect an individual's reaction to the rehabilitation process, including performance anxiety, self-esteem/motivation, extroversion/introversion, psychological investment in the sport, coping resources, history of past stressors (previous injuries, academic, family, and life events), and previous intervention strategies.

3. Goal setting is a common practice used by athletic trainers to motivate patients in the recovery program.

4. Psychological influences that may affect an individual's success in the rehabilitation process include confidence, motivation, anxiety, focus, and management of pain.

5. As a general rule, any psychological difficulty that persists for more than a few days and interferes with the progress of rehabilitation should be referred to a licensed mental health professional.

6. Rehabilitation begins immediately after injury assessment and includes the following:

   ■ The level of function and dysfunction is assessed.

   ■ Results are organized and interpreted.

   ■ A list of patient problems is formulated.

   ■ Long- and short-term goals are established.

   ■ A treatment plan is developed, including therapeutic exercises, modalities, and medications.

   ■ The program is then supervised and periodically reassessed with appropriate changes made.

7. Phase 1 of the therapeutic exercise program should focus on patient education and control of inflammation, muscle spasm, and pain.

8. Phase 2 should regain any deficits in ROM and proprioception at the affected joint as compared with the unaffected joint.

9. Phase 3 should regain muscular strength, endurance, and power in the affected limb.

10. Phase 4 prepares the individual to return to activity and includes analysis of motion, sport/activity-specific skill training, regaining coordination, and cardiovascular conditioning.

11. At the conclusion of the rehabilitation program, the supervising physician determines if the individual is ready to return to full activity. This decision should be based on a review of the individual's ROM and flexibility; muscular strength, endurance, and power; biomechanical skill; proprioception and coordination; and cardiovascular endurance.

12. If additional protective bracing, padding, or taping is necessary to enable the individual to return safely to activity, this should be documented in the individual's file. In addition, it should be stressed that use of any protective device should not replace a maintenance program of conditioning exercises.

13. The athletic trainer should keep a watchful eye on the individual as he or she returns to activity. If the individual begins to show signs of pain, swelling, or discomfort or if skill performance deteriorates, the individual should be re-evaluated to determine whether activity should continue or the therapeutic exercise program needs to be reinstituted.

REFERENCES

1. Wagman D, Khelifa M. Psychological issues in sport injury rehabilitation: current knowledge and practice. J Ath Train 1996;31(3):257–261.
2. Petitpas AJ. Going for the goal. Ath Ther Today 1997; 2(4):30–31.
3. Scherzer CB, Brewer BW, Cornelius AE, et al. Psychological skills and adherence to rehabilitation after reconstruction of the anterior cruciate ligament. J Sport Rehab 2001;10(3):165–172.
4. Shelley GA, Trowbridge CA, Detling N. Practical counseling skills for athletic therapists. Ath Ther Today 2003; 8(2):57–62.
5. Theodorakis Y, Malliou P, Papaioannou A, et al. The effect of personal goals, self-efficacy, and self-satisfaction on injury rehabilitation. J Sport Rehab 1996;5(3):214–223.
6. Theodorakis Y, Beneka A, Malliou P, et al. Examining psychological factors during injury rehabilitation. J Sports Rehab 1997;6(4):355–363.
7. Taylor J, Taylor S. Psychological Approaches to Sports Injury Rehabilitation. Gaithersburg, MD: Aspen, 1997.
8. Larson GA, Starkey C, Zaichknowsky LD. Psychological aspects of athletic injuries as perceived by athletic trainers. Sport Psychologist 1996;10(1):37–47.
9. Heil J. Psychology of Sport Injury. Champaign, IL: Human Kinetics, 1993.
10. Mangine B, Harrelson GL. Physiologic factors of rehabilitation. In: Andrews JR, Harrelson GL, Wilk KE, eds. Physical Rehabilitation of the Injured Athlete. Philadelphia: WB Saunders, 2004.
11. Mazess RB, Whedon GD. Immobilization and bone. Calcif Tissue Int 1983;35:265–267.
12. Konin JG, Harrelson GL, Leaver-Dunn D. Range of

motion and flexibility. In: Andrews JR, Harrelson GL, Wilk KE, eds. Physical Rehabilitation of the Injured Athlete. Philadelphia: WB Saunders, 2004.

13. McArdle WD, Katch FI, Katch VL. Exercise Physiology: Energy, Nutrition, and Human Performance. Baltimore: Lippincott Williams & Wilkins, 2007.

14. Maitland GD. Extremity Manipulation. London: Butterworth, 1977.

15. Nelson KC, Cornelius WL. The relationship between isometric contraction durations and improvement in shoulder joint ROM. J Sports Med Phys Fit 1991;31(3):385–388.

16. Wilk KE, Arrigo CA, Andrews JR. Closed and open kinetic chain exercise for the upper extremity. J Sports Rehab 1996;5(1):88–102.

17. Lephart SM, Henry TJ. Functional rehabilitation for the upper and lower extremities. Orthop Clin North Am 1995;26(3):579–592.

18. Dillman CH, Murray TA, Hintermeister RA. Biomechanical differences of open and closed chain exercises with

respect to the shoulder. J Sports Rehab 1994;3(3):228–238.

19. Knight KL, Ingersoll CD, Bartholomew J. Isotonic contractions might be more effective than isokinetic contractions in developing muscle strength. J Sports Rehab 2001;10(2)124–131.

20. Knight KL. Rehabilitating chondromalacia patellae. Phys Sportsmed 1979;7(10):147–148.

21. Dale RB, Harrelson GL, Leaver-Dunn D. Principles of rehabilitation. In: Andrews JR, Harrelson GL, Wilk KE, eds. Physical Rehabilitation of the Injured Athlete. Philadelphia: WB Saunders, 2004.

22. Haskell et al. Physical Activity and Public Health: Updated recommendation for adults from the American College of Sports Medicine and the American Heart Association. Circulation 2007; 116.

23. American College of Sports Medicine. Position stand: physical activity and bone health. Med Sci Sports Exerc 2004;36(11):1985–1996.

PART

Conditions to the Axial Region

3

Chapter 9
Head and Facial Conditions

Chapter 10
Cervical and Thoracic
Spinal Conditions

Chapter 11
Lumbar Spinal Conditions

Chapter 12
Throat, Thorax, and
Visceral Conditions

Head and Facial Conditions

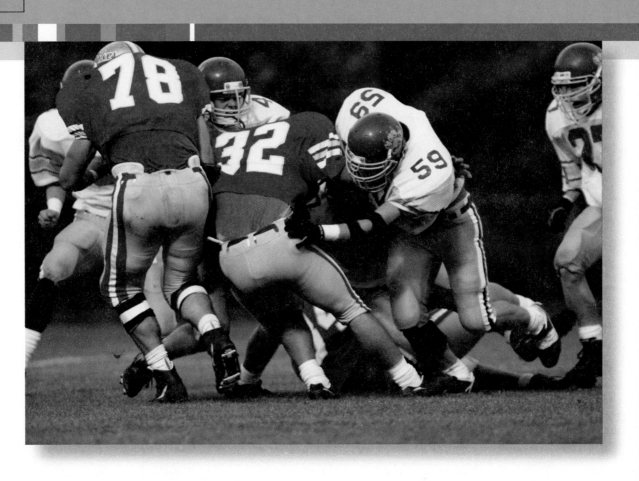

STUDENT OUTCOMES

1. Locate the major bony and soft-tissue structures of the head and facial region.

2. Explain the importance of wearing protective equipment to prevent injury to the head and facial region.

3. Describe the forces responsible for cranial injuries.

4. Identify the signs and symptoms associated with a possible skull fracture.

5. Recognize the critical signs and symptoms that indicate a focal or diffuse cranial injury.

6. Describe the evaluation and management of a cranial injury.

7. Identify the signs and symptoms associated with a possible facial fracture.

8. Describe the signs and symptoms of epistaxis, deviated septum, and fractured nose.

9. Describe the differences in managing a loose versus a fractured or dislocated tooth.

10. Recognize common external and internal ear conditions, and explain their management.

11. Describe the use of an otoscope to assess nose and ear conditions.

12. Identify the signs and symptoms of serious nasal, ear, or eye injuries that warrant immediate referral to a physician.

13. Describe the evaluation of an eye injury and the use of an ophthalmoscope.

ROLE DELINEATION COMPETENCIES

The following Performance Domains and Tasks defined in the National Athletic Trainers' Association Board of Certification *Role Delineation Study*, 5th Edition are addressed in this chapter:

BOC COMPETENCIES

II.   Clinical Evaluation and Diagnosis

A. Obtain a history through observation, interview, and/or review of relevant records to assess current or potential injury, illness, or condition.
B. Inspect the involved area(s) visually to assess the injury, illness, or health-related condition.
C. Palpate the involved area(s) using standard techniques to assess the injury, illness, or health-related condition.
D. Perform specific tests in accordance with accepted procedures to assess the injury, illness, or health-related condition.
E. Formulate a clinical impression by interpreting the signs, symptoms, and predisposing factors of the injury, illness, or condition to determine the appropriate course of action.

III.   Immediate Care

A. Employ life-saving techniques through the use of standard emergency procedures in order to reduce morbidity and the incidence of mortality.
B. Prevent exacerbation of non–life threatening condition(s) through the use of standard procedures in order to reduce morbidity.
C. Facilitate the timely transfer of care for conditions beyond the scope of practice of the athletic trainer by implementing appropriate referral strategies to stabilize and/or prevent exacerbation of the condition(s).

IV.   Treatment, Rehabilitation, and Reconditioning

E. Reassess the status of injuries, illnesses, and/or conditions using standard techniques and documentation strategies in order to determine appropriate treatment, rehabilitation, and/or reconditioning and to evaluate readiness to return to a desired level of activity.
F. Educate the appropriate individual(s) in the treatment, rehabilitation, and reconditioning of injuries, illnesses, and/or conditions using applicable methods and materials to facilitate recovery, function, and/or performance.

The head and facial area are frequent sites for minor injuries, including lacerations, contusions, and mild concussions. Although intracranial injuries have been associated with sport-related fatalities, increased standards for protective equipment, rule changes that prohibit leading with the head for contact, and development and use of the face mask have significantly decreased the incidence of injuries since the mid-1970s. In addition, a significant decrease in eye, ear, and dental injuries has been seen when protective equipment is worn.

This chapter begins with a general anatomical review of the head and facial region. Discussion concerning preventive measures is followed by information regarding the mechanisms of injury most commonly linked to cranial injuries. The signs, symptoms, and management of the more common focal and diffuse cranial injuries are discussed, followed by steps to include in a thorough assessment of a head injury. The final section discusses the more common facial, nasal, ear, and eye injuries and their management.

ANATOMY OF THE HEAD AND FACIAL REGION

Q *While playing racquetball, a 40-year-old man collides with the back wall of the court and hits his head. He sustains a superficial cut to the back of the head that is bleeding profusely. What anatomical structure(s) are likely to have been injured, and is this a potentially serious injury?*

This review of anatomy focuses on the brain and its coverings; the facial area, including the eyes, ears, and nose; and the nerve and blood supply to the region. Although the numerous muscles of the face and jaw enable speaking, chewing, and facial expression, these muscles are not commonly involved in injuries attributed to participation in sport and physical activity and, therefore, are not discussed.

Bones of the Skull

The skull is composed primarily of flat bones that interlock at immovable joints called sutures (Fig. 9.1). The bones that form the portion of the skull referred to as the cranium protect the brain. The thin bones of the cranium include the frontal, occipital, sphenoid, and ethmoid bones as well as two parietal and two temporal bones. The material properties and thickness of the cranial bones vary, with the strongest being the occipital bone and the weakest the temporal bones. The facial bones provide the structure of the face and form the sinuses, orbits of the eyes, nasal cavity, and the mouth; these bones include the paired maxilla, zygomatic, palatine, nasal, lacrimal, vomer, and inferior nasal concha bones, along with the bridge and mandible. The large opening at the base of the skull that sits atop the spinal column is called the foramen magnum.

The Scalp

The scalp is composed of three layers: the skin, the subcutaneous connective tissue, and the pericranium. The protective function of these tissues is enhanced by the hair and by the looseness of the scalp, which enable some dissipation of force when the head sustains a glancing blow. The scalp and face have an extensive blood supply; as a result, superficial lacerations tend to bleed profusely.

The Brain

The four major regions of the brain are the cerebral hemispheres, diencephalon, brainstem, and cerebellum. The entire brain and spinal cord are enclosed in three layers of protective tissue known collectively as the meninges (Fig. 9.2). The outermost membrane is the dura mater, a thick, fibrous tissue containing dural sinuses that act as veins to transport blood from the brain to the jugular veins of the neck. The arachnoid mater is a thin membrane internal to the dura mater; it is separated from the dura mater by the subdural space. Beneath the arachnoid mater is the subarachnoid space, which is filled with cerebrospinal fluid (CSF) and contains the largest of the blood vessels supplying the brain. The arachnoid mater is connected to the inner pia mater by web-like strands of connective tissue. The dura mater and arachnoid mater are rather loose membranes; in comparison, the pia mater is in direct contact with the cerebral cortex and contains numerous small blood vessels.

The Eyes

The eye is a hollow sphere, approximately 2.5 cm (1 inch) in diameter in adults (Fig. 9.3). The anterior eye surface receives protection from the eyelids, eyelashes, and attached conjunctiva. The conjunctiva lines the eyelids and the external surface of the eye and secretes mucus to lubricate the external eye. The lacrimal glands, which are located above the lateral ends of the eyes, continually release tears across the eye surface through several small ducts. The lacrimal ducts, which are located at the medial corners of the eyes, serve as drains for the moisture. These ducts funnel the moisture into the lacrimal sac and, eventually, into the nasal cavity.

The eye is surrounded by three protective tissue layers called tunics. The outer tunic is a thick, white, connective tissue called the sclera and forms the "white of the eye." The cornea, which is found in the central anterior part of the sclera, is clear to permit the passage of light into the eye. The choroid, or the middle covering, is a highly vascularized tissue that usually appears blue or brown on the anterior eye and contains the pupil. The inner protective layer is the retina, which contains light-sensitive photoreceptor cells that stimulate nerve endings to provide sight.

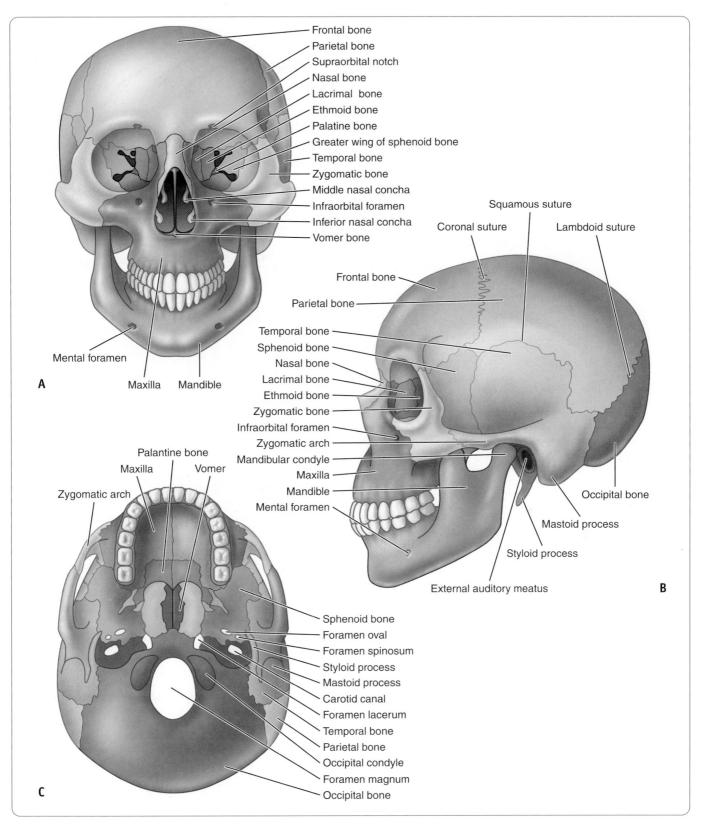

Frontal bone
Parietal bone
Supraorbital notch
Nasal bone
Lacrimal bone
Ethmoid bone
Palatine bone
Greater wing of sphenoid bone
Temporal bone
Zygomatic bone
Middle nasal concha
Infraorbital foramen
Inferior nasal concha
Vomer bone

Mental foramen

A   Maxilla   Mandible

Squamous suture
Coronal suture   Lambdoid suture

Frontal bone
Parietal bone
Temporal bone
Sphenoid bone
Nasal bone
Lacrimal bone
Ethmoid bone
Zygomatic bone
Infraorbital foramen
Zygomatic arch
Mandibular condyle
Maxilla
Mandible
Mental foramen

Occipital bone
Mastoid process
Styloid process
External auditory meatus   **B**

Palantine bone
Maxilla   Vomer
Zygomatic arch

Sphenoid bone
Foramen oval
Foramen spinosum
Styloid process
Mastoid process
Carotid canal
Foramen lacerum
Temporal bone
Parietal bone
Occipital condyle
Foramen magnum
C   Occipital bone

■■■■ FIGURE 9.1 **Bones of the skull. A,** Frontal view. **B,** Lateral view. **C,** Inferior view.

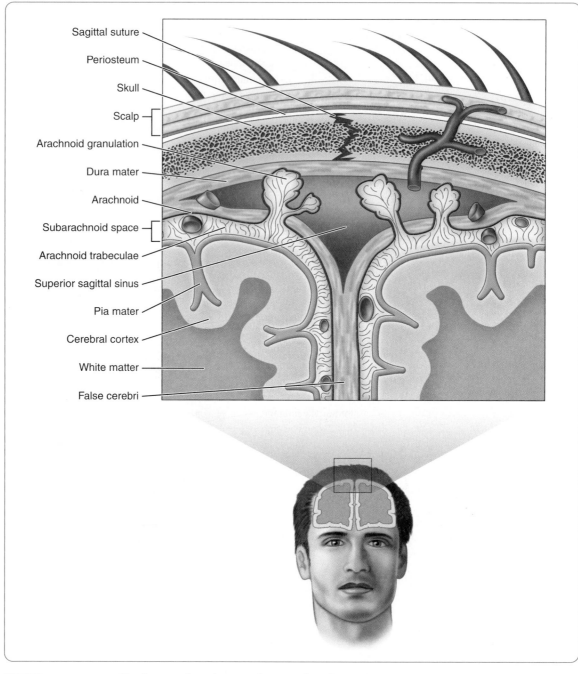

Sagittal suture
Periosteum
Skull
Scalp
Arachnoid granulation
Dura mater
Arachnoid
Subarachnoid space
Arachnoid trabeculae
Superior sagittal sinus
Pia mater
Cerebral cortex
White matter
False cerebri

▣▣▣▣ FIGURE 9.2 **Meninges.** Three layers of protective tissue, known as the meninges, enclose the brain and spinal cord.

The Nose

The nose is composed of bone and hyaline cartilage. The roof is formed by the cribriform plate of the ethmoid bone. The nasal bones form the bridge of the nose. Inferiorly, the lateral walls are shaped by the superior and middle conchae of the ethmoid bone, the vertical plates of the palatine bones, and the inferior nasal conchae (Fig. 9.4). The nasal cavity is separated into right and left halves by the nasal septum, which is made of cartilage and can be deviated or fractured if struck by a blunt object. A deviated septum can complicate the assessment and treatment of soft-tissue injuries.

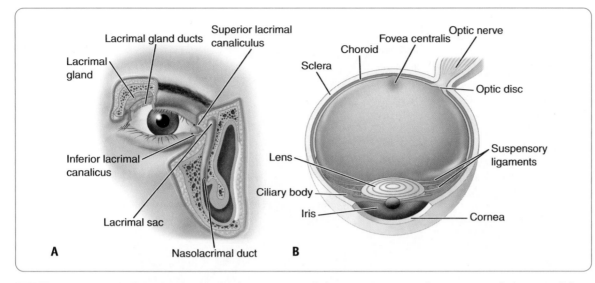

FIGURE 9.3 Eye. A, The lacrimal structures of the eye. **B,** Internal structures of the eye globe.

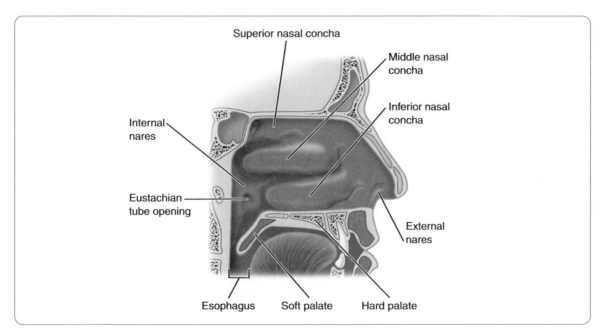

FIGURE 9.4 The nose. The nose is composed of bone and cartilage.

The Ear

The ear is divided into three major areas: the outer ear (auricle and external auditory canal), the middle ear (tympanic membrane), and the inner ear (labyrinth) (Fig. 9.5). Assisting the middle and inner ear in the process of hearing and equalizing pressure between the two areas is the eustachian tube, a canal that links the nose and middle ear.

Nerves of the Head and Face

Twelve pairs of cranial nerves emerge from the brain. These nerves have motor functions, sensory functions, or both. The cranial nerves are numbered and named according to their functions and are listed in Table 9.1.

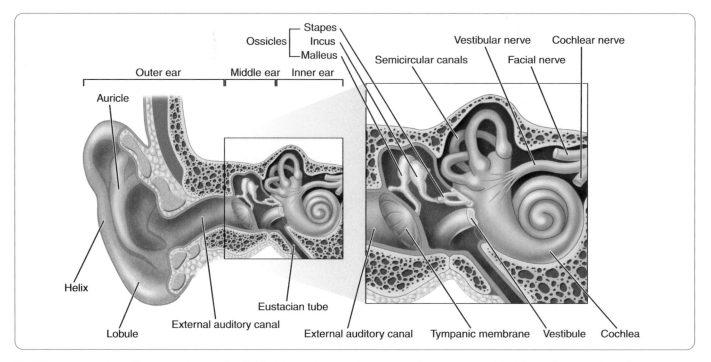

FIGURE 9.5 The ear. The ear is divided into three major areas: the outer ear (auricle and external auditory canal), the middle ear (tympanic membrane), and the inner ear (labyrinth).

TABLE 9.1 The Cranial Nerves

NUMBER	NAME	SENSORY	MOTOR	FUNCTION
I	Olfactory	X (smell)		Sense of smell
II	Optic	X (vision)		Vision
III	Oculomotor		X	Control of some of the extrinsic eye muscles
IV	Trochlear		X	Control of the remaining extrinsic eye muscles
V	Trigeminal	X (general sensation)	X	Sensation of the facial region and movement of the jaw muscles
VI	Abducens		X	Control of lateral eye movement
VII	Facial	X (taste)	X	Control of facial movement, taste, and secretion of tears and saliva
VIII	Vestibulocochlear	X (hearing and balance)		Hearing and equilibrium (acoustic)
IX	Glossopharyngeal	X (taste)	X	Taste, control of the tongue and pharynx, and secretion of saliva
X	Vagus	X (taste)	X	Taste and sensation to the pharynx, larynx, trachea, and bronchioles
XI	Accessory		X	Control of movements of the pharynx, larynx, head, and shoulders
XII	Hypoglossal		X	Control of tongue movements

Blood Vessels of the Head and Face

The major vessels supplying the head and face are the common carotid and vertebral arteries (Fig. 9.6). The common carotid artery ascends through the neck on either side to divide into the external and internal carotid arteries just below the level of the jaw. The external carotid arteries and their branches supply most regions of the head external to the brain. The middle meningeal artery supplies the skull and dura mater; if this artery is damaged, serious epidural bleeding can result. The internal carotid arteries send branches to the eyes and supply portions of the cerebral hemispheres and the parietal and temporal lobes of the cerebrum. The left and right vertebral arteries and their branches supply blood to the posterior region of the brain.

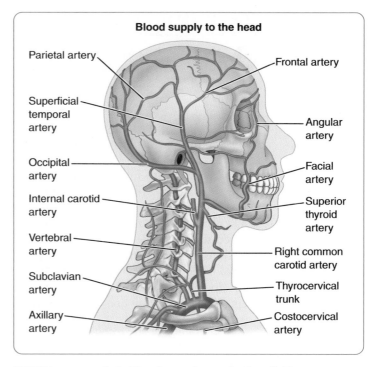

Because the scalp and face have an extensive blood supply, superficial lacerations of the head tend to bleed profusely. Given the mechanism of injury, however, it is important to rule out cerebral trauma. If no signs of a cerebral trauma (discussed later in this chapter) are present, the scalp injury is not serious as long as bleeding is controlled.

 FIGURE 9.6 Blood supply to the head. The common carotid and vertebral arteries are the major vessels supplying blood to the brain.

PREVENTION OF HEAD AND FACIAL INJURIES

A high school athletic director is faced with making budget cuts. He requests justification for purchasing mouth guards for teams other than football (i.e., soccer, basketball, lacrosse, and field hockey). Provide a rationale for ensuring that athletes in any sport involving contact should be provided with mouth guards.

The most important preventive measure for the head and facial area is the use of protective equipment. Many sports, such as baseball/softball, competitive bicycling, fencing, field hockey, football, ice hockey, lacrosse, and wrestling, require some type of head or facial protective equipment for participation. When used properly, protective equipment can protect the head and facial area from accidental or routine injuries. It is important to recognize, however, that protective equipment cannot prevent all injuries. To be effective, equipment must be properly fitted, clean, in good condition, and used in the manner for which it was designed.

Protective equipment may include a helmet, face guard, mouth guard, eyewear, earwear, and throat protector. Helmets protect the cranial portion of the skull by absorbing and dispersing impact forces, thereby reducing cerebral trauma. Face guards protect and shield the facial region. Mouth guards have been shown to reduce dental and oral soft-tissue injuries as well as cerebral concussions, jaw fractures, and temporomandibular joint (TMJ) injuries. Eyewear, earwear, and throat protectors reduce injuries to their respective regions. Chapter 3 provides information regarding protective equipment for the head and face.

 A properly fitted mouth guard can help to prevent dental and oral soft-tissue injuries, but it also can help to reduce the incidence and severity of cerebral concussions, jaw fractures, and TMJ injuries.

SCALP INJURIES

In attempting to keep a ball from going out of bounds, a basketball player collides with the bleachers. As the athletic trainer approaches the player, she notices bleeding from the scalp. Explain the immediate management of this injury.

The scalp is the outermost anatomical structure of the cranium and the first area of contact in head trauma. The scalp is highly vascular and bleeds freely, making it a frequent site for abrasions, lacerations, contusions, or hematomas between the layers of tissue. The primary concerns with any scalp laceration are to control bleeding, prevent contamination, and assess for a possible skull fracture.

In keeping with universal precautions, latex gloves should be worn during the management of any open wound. Mild direct pressure should be applied to the area with sterile gauze until bleeding has stopped. The wound should be inspected for any foreign bodies or signs of a skull fracture. If a skull fracture is ruled out, the wound should be cleansed with surgical soap or saline solution, covered with a sterile dressing, and the individual referred to a physician for possible suturing.

Abrasions and contusions should be treated with gentle cleansing, topical antiseptics, and ice to control hemorrhage. Hematomas, or "goose eggs," involve a collection of blood between the layers of the scalp and the skull. Crushed ice and a pressure bandage should be used to control hemorrhage and edema. If the condition does not improve in 24 hours, the individual should be referred to a physician.

In managing the bleeding scalp, it would be appropriate for the athletic trainer to hand sterile gauze to the athlete and direct the individual to apply gentle pressure to the area while the athletic trainer puts on latex gloves. Once gloved, the athletic trainer should inspect the area and continue to apply pressure until the bleeding has stopped. If a skull fracture is ruled out, the area should be cleansed with surgical soap or saline solution and covered with a sterile dressing. Depending on the nature of the wound, referral to a physician may be required for possible suturing.

CRANIAL INJURY MECHANISMS

Explain the mechanism for a contrecoup cerebral injury.

The occurrence of a skull fracture or intracranial injury is dependent on the material properties of the skull, the thickness of the skull in the specific area, the magnitude and direction of impact, and the size of the impact area. Direct impact causes two phenomena to occur—namely, deformation and acceleration. When a blow impacts the skull, the bone deforms and bends inward, placing the inner border of the skull under tensile strain while the outer border is compressed (Fig. 9.7A). If

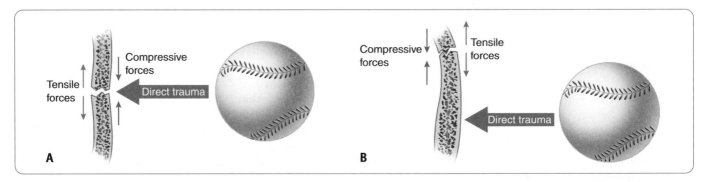

FIGURE 9.7 **Mechanical failure in bone.** When a blow impacts the skull, the bone deforms and bends inward, placing tensile stress on the inner border of the skull. **A,** If an impact is of sufficient magnitude and the skull is thin in the region of the impact, a skull fracture occurs at the impact site. **B,** If the skull is thick and dense enough at the area of impact, it may sustain bending without fracture; however, the fracture may occur some distance from the impact zone, in a region where the skull is thinner.

the impact is of sufficient magnitude and the skull in the region of impact is thin, a skull fracture occurs at the site where tensile loading occurs. In contrast, if the skull is thick and dense enough at the area of impact, it may sustain inward bending without fracture. A fracture then may occur some distance from the impact zone in a region where the skull is thinner (Fig. 9.7B).

On impact, shock waves pass through the skull to the brain, causing it to accelerate. This acceleration can lead to shear, tensile, and compression strains within the brain substance, with shear being the most serious. Axial rotation coupled with acceleration can lead to **contrecoup injuries** (Fig. 9.8), which are injuries located away from the actual impact site.

Cerebral trauma can lead to **focal injuries**, involving only localized damage (i.e., epidural, subdural, or intracerebral hematomas), or **diffuse injuries**, involving widespread disruption and damage to the function and/or structure of the brain. Although diffuse injuries account for only one-quarter of the fatalities caused by head trauma, they tend to be a more prevalent cause of long-term neurologic deficits. If cerebral injuries are recognized and treated immediately, the severity can potentially be limited to the initial structural damage; however, if other factors, such as ischemia, hypoxia, cerebral swelling, and hemorrhaging around the brain occur, additional damage and possible neurologic dysfunction result. Therefore, accurate assessment of head injuries is essential to ensure prompt medical attention to rule out serious underlying problems that may complicate the original injury. A conscious, ambulatory individual should not be considered to have only a minor injury but, rather, should be assessed continually to determine if posttraumatic signs or symptoms indicate a more serious underlying condition.

■■ ■■ FIGURE 9.8 **Contrecoup injury.** Axial rotation coupled with acceleration can result in a contrecoup injury.

 Subsequent to impact to the skull, the brain accelerates. In some case, this acceleration results in injury away from the site of impact (contrecoup). In particular, axial rotation coupled with acceleration can lead to contrecoup injury.

SKULL FRACTURES

While driving toward the basket, a basketball player is undercut. She falls sideways and strikes her head sharply on the floor. The individual complains of an intense headache, disorientation, and blurred vision. Do these signs and symptoms indicate that a skull fracture may be present?

Skull fractures may be linear (i.e., in a line), comminuted (i.e., in multiple pieces), depressed (i.e., fragments driven internally toward the brain), or basilar (i.e., involving the base of the skull) (Fig. 9.9). With a break in the skin adjacent to the fracture site and a tear in the underlying dura mater, an individual has a high risk of bacterial infection into the intracranial cavity, which can result in **septic meningitis**. When a severe blow to the head occurs, a skull fracture should always be suspected. Often, however, it is difficult to detect the presence of a deep scalp hematoma.

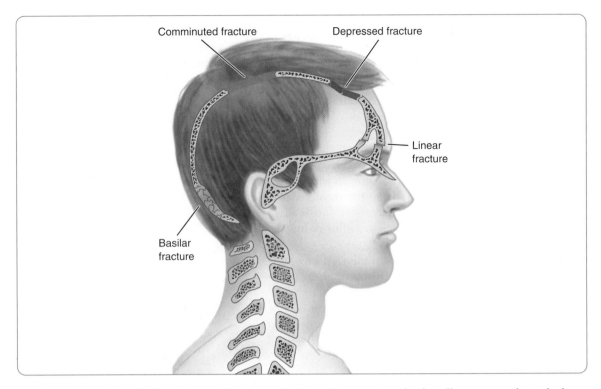

█ █ █ █ FIGURE 9.9 Skull fractures. Fractures of the skull are categorized as linear, comminuted, depressed, or basilar.

Signs and Symptoms

Depending on the fracture site, different signs may appear (Box 9.1). For example, a fracture at the eyebrow level may travel into the anterior cranial fossa and sinuses, leading to discoloration around the eyes (**raccoon eyes**). Bony fragments may damage the optic or olfactory cranial nerves, leading to blindness or loss of smell. A basilar fracture above and behind the ear may lead to **Battle's sign**, which is a discoloration that can appear within minutes behind the ear. In some cases, blood or CSF may leak from the nose or ear canal. Identification of the type of leaking fluid can be assessed by gently absorbing some of it with a gauze pad and then observing the pad for possible separation of clear fluid from blood. This action is called "targeting," or the "halo test," and it is important to note that this test is not always reliable. A hearing loss or facial paralysis also may be present. A fracture to the temple region may damage the meningeal arteries, causing epidural bleeding between

Box 9.1   Possible Signs and Symptoms of a Skull Fracture

- Visible deformity (do not be misled by a "goose egg" [a fracture may be under the site])
- Deep laceration or severe bruise to the scalp
- Palpable depression or crepitus
- Unequal pupils
- Discoloration under both eyes (raccoon eyes) or behind the ear (Battle's sign)

- Bleeding or clear fluid (cerebrospinal fluid) from the nose and/or ear
- Loss of smell
- Loss of sight or major vision disturbances
- Unconsciousness for more than 2 minutes after direct trauma to the head

FIELD STRATEGY 9.1

Evaluation and Management of a Suspected Skull Fracture

Evaluation

1. Stabilize the head and neck.
2. Check the airway, breathing, and circulation.
3. Take vital signs (i.e., pulse, respiration, and blood pressure).
4. Observe for:
   - Swelling or discoloration around the eyes or behind the ears
   - Blood or cerebrospinal fluid leaking from the nose or ears
   - Pupil size, pupillary response to light, and eye movement
5. Palpate for depressions, blood, and crepitus. Palpate cervical vertebrae for associated neck injury.

Management

6. Activate the emergency plan, including summoning emergency medical services.
7. Cover any open wounds with a sterile dressing, but do not apply pressure to the area.
8. Elevate the upper body and head if there is no evidence of shock or of neck or spinal injury. If such evidence is present, keep the individual lying flat.
9. Treat for shock.
10. Recheck vital signs and symptoms every 5 minutes until emergency medical services arrives.

the dura mater and the skull (epidural hematoma). This can be life-threatening and is discussed in more detail in the section on focal cerebral injuries.

Management

A skull fracture can be a life-threatening condition. If any of the signs and symptoms mentioned in Box 9.1 become apparent, activation of the emergency plan, including summoning emergency medical services (EMS), is warranted. Field Strategy 9.1 summarizes management of a suspected skull fracture.

Signs that indicate a possible skull fracture include deformity, unequal pupils, discoloration around both eyes or behind the ears, bleeding or CSF leaking from the nose and/or ear, and any loss of sight or smell. The basketball player did not exhibit any of these "red flags." Even so, the individual should be thoroughly evaluated for head trauma. If any of the signs appear during the assessment, the emergency plan should be activated.

FOCAL CEREBRAL CONDITIONS

After colliding with another player, a lacrosse player is lying down on the field and complaining of a headache and dizziness. Following 15 minutes of ice application to the region, the individual complains of increasing headache, dizziness, and nausea. There also is increased mental confusion. What do these symptoms indicate, and how should this injury be managed?

Focal cerebral injuries usually result in a localized collection of blood or hematoma. The skull has no room for additional accumulation of blood or fluid; as such, any additional foreign matter within the cranial cavity increases pressure on the brain, leading to significant alterations in neurologic function. Depending on the location of the accumulated blood relative to the dura mater, these hematomas are classified as epidural (outside the dura mater) or subdural (deep to the dura mater). A cerebral contusion also is classified as a focal injury; however, no mass-occupying lesion is associated with this condition.

Epidural Hematoma

An epidural hematoma is very rare during participation in sport and physical activity. Typically, the condition is caused by a direct blow to the side of the head and almost always is associated with a skull fracture (Fig. 9.10A). If the middle meningeal artery or its branches are severed, the subsequent arterial bleeding leads to a "high-pressure" epidural hematoma. The middle meningeal vein also may be damaged, leading to a more insidious onset of symptoms.

Signs and Symptoms

The individual may experience an initial loss of consciousness (LOC) at the time of injury, followed by a lucid interval during which the individual feels relatively normal and asymptomatic. Within 10 to 20 minutes, however, a gradual decline in mental status occurs as the hematoma outside the brain reaches a critical size and compresses the underlying brain. Other signs and symptoms may include increased headache, drowsiness, nausea, and vomiting as well as decreased level of consciousness; an ipsilateral dilated pupil on the side of the hematoma; and subsequently, contralateral weakness and decerebrate posturing. This triad of symptoms, however, is only present in one-third of individuals with epidural hematomas (1).

Management

EMS Activation of the emergency plan, including summoning EMS, is warranted. The examiner should continue to maintain the airway, breathing, and circulation (ABCs), assess vital signs, and treat for shock. This condition may require immediate surgery to decompress the hematoma and control arterial bleeding.

Subdural Hematoma

A subdural hematoma is approximately threefold more frequent than an epidural hematoma and is the leading cause of catastrophic death in football players (1). Hemorrhage occurs when the bridging

FIGURE 9.10 Cerebral hematomas. A, This epidural hematoma resulted from a fracture that extended into the orbital roof and sinus area, leading to rapid hemorrhage in the right frontal lobe of the brain. **B,** The subdural hematoma on the right side of the brain is fairly evident. A chronic subdural hematoma can be seen on the left side of the brain.

veins between the brain and the dura mater are torn. It is caused by acceleration forces of the head rather than by the impact of the force. A subdural hematoma may be classified as either acute, which presents 48 to 72 hours after injury, or chronic (Fig. 9.10B), which occurs in a later time frame with more variable clinical manifestations, and either simple or complicated. In a simple subdural hematoma, blood collects in the subdural space, but no underlying cerebral injury occurs. Complex subdural hematomas are characterized by contusions of the brain's surface and associated cerebral swelling that increase intracerebral pressure. The mortality rate for simple subdural hematomas is approximately 20%, whereas complicated subdural hematomas have a mortality rate of 50% (2).

Signs and Symptoms

In a simple subdural hematoma, the individual is less likely to be rendered unconscious. These individuals seldom demonstrate deterioration in level of consciousness, and fewer than 15% have a lucid interval. In a complicated subdural hematoma, the individual typically is knocked out and remains unconscious. Signs and symptoms of increasing intracranial pressure include:

- Pupillary dilation and retinal changes on the affected side
- Irregular eye tracking or eye movement
- Severe headache
- Nausea and/or vomiting
- Confusion and/or drastic changes in emotional control
- Progressive or sudden impairment of consciousness
- Rising blood pressure
- Falling pulse rate
- Irregular respirations
- Increased body temperature

Signs and symptoms may not become apparent for hours, days, or even weeks after injury, subsequent to the clot absorbing fluid and expanding.

Management

Early diagnosis of a subdural hematoma is essential for a successful recovery. Loss of consciousness implies a poor prognosis, with an overall mortality rate of 35 to 50% (3).

> Activation of the emergency plan, including summoning EMS, is warranted. The examiner should continue to maintain the ABCs, assess vital signs, and treat for shock.

EMS

Cerebral Contusion

A cerebral contusion is a focal injury, but a mass-occupying lesion is not present. Instead, microhemorrhage, cerebral infarction, necrosis, and edema of the brain occur. This condition is visible on a computed tomographic (CT) scan as an area of high-density blood interspersed with brain tissue.

Cerebral contusions most often occur as a result of an acceleration–deceleration mechanism from the inward deformation of the skull at the impact site. For example, an acceleration force is generated when another individual or an object (e.g., a ball or hockey puck) hits an individual's head. In this situation, the site of maximal injury usually is at the point of impact (i.e., coup injury). In comparison, deceleration forces are generated when an individual's head strikes the ground, and the subsequent site of maximal injury is opposite the point of impact (i.e., contrecoup injury). Injury results from the brain rebounding against the skull or from vacuum phenomena existing within the parenchyma at that location. The contrecoup lesions lead to hemorrhage in the cerebral tissue directly opposite the impact site, typically at the inferior surfaces of the frontal and temporal lobes. Although the contusion can occur in any portion of the cortex, brainstem, or cerebellum, these lobes, because of the close anatomical relationship between bony ridges and the frontal lobes, are particularly susceptible to this type of injury. The injury may be limited to small, localized areas or involve large, extensive areas.

Signs and Symptoms

Clinical signs and symptoms vary greatly, depending on the location, number, and extent of the hemorrhagic lesions. A cerebral contusion injury may evolve over hours or days after the injury. The individual may present with essentially normal function or may experience any type of neurologic deterioration, including coma. Frequently, behavioral or mental status changes are present because of the involvement of the frontal or temporal lobes (4). A danger flag exists when an individual has a normal neurologic examination but persistent symptoms such as headaches, dizziness, or nausea.

Management

 Activation of the emergency plan, including summoning EMS, is warranted. The examiner should continue to maintain the ABCs, assess vital signs, and treat for shock.

Dizziness, headache, nausea, and increased mental confusion are "red flags" indicating serious intracranial hemorrhage. The management of this condition involves activating the emergency plan (including summoning EMS), monitoring vital signs, and treating for shock.

DIFFUSE CEREBRAL CONDITIONS

After colliding with an opponent, a football player was momentarily stunned, "saw stars," and had blurred vision for approximately 30 seconds. After 3 or 4 minutes, the individual reports feeling much better, except for a slight headache. Can this individual return to activity?

Diffuse cerebral injuries involve trauma to widespread areas of the brain rather than one specific site. The range of these injuries can vary from mild to severe, involving impairment of neural function, structural damage, or both.

Concussions

In November 2001, the First International Symposium on Concussion in Sport was held in Vienna to provide recommendations to improve the safety and health of athletes who suffer concussive injuries. Several issues were discussed, including protective equipment, epidemiology, basic and clinical science, grading systems, cognitive assessment, and management. A second international symposium was held in 2004 in Prague (5). Subsequently, sport-related concussions have been defined as a complex pathophysiological process affecting the brain and induced by traumatic biomechanical forces (6). Common features that incorporate clinical, pathological, and biomechanical injury constructs that may be used to further define the nature of a concussive head injury include:

- Concussions may be caused by a direct blow to the head, face, neck, or elsewhere on the body causing an impulsive force to be transmitted to the head. These injuries typically result in the rapid onset of short-lived impairment of neurologic function that resolves spontaneously.

- Neuropathological changes may occur, but the acute clinical symptoms typically reflect a functional disturbance rather than a structural injury.

- Concussions may or may not involve LOC but, instead, may lead to a gradient of clinical symptoms that are associated with grossly normal structural neuroimaging studies.

- Resolution of the clinical and cognitive symptoms usually follows a sequential course (5,6).

The injury may cause an immediate and transient impairment of neural function, such as alteration of consciousness and disturbance of vision and equilibrium. Under normal conditions, the brain balances a series of electrochemical events in billions of brain cells. When the brain is shaken or jarred, brain function can be disrupted temporarily without causing injury or damage to brain tissue. For example, mild trauma can result in interruption of cerebral function. Signs and symptoms range from mild to moderate and are transient and reversible. This can be attributed to the minimal damage to soft-tissue structures. As the impact magnitude increases with an acceleration injury, both cerebral function and structural damage may occur, resulting in more serious signs and symptoms. These include varying degrees of LOC, headache, confusion, memory loss, nausea, **tinnitus**, pupillary changes, dizziness, and loss of coordination.

Classifications of Concussions

More than 16 different classification schemes attempt to define the various degrees of brain dysfunction in cerebral concussions. None of the scales, however, has been universally accepted and followed, which has led to much confusion over determining the severity of a traumatic brain injury. It is critical to understand that no two concussions will be identical, nor will the signs and symptoms be the same. Each injury will vary depending on the magnitude of force to the head, the level of metabolic dysfunction, the tissue damage and duration of time needed to recover, the number of previous concussions, and the time between injuries.

Currently, three main approaches to grading sports-related concussions are used. One approach is to grade the traumatic brain injury at the time of injury based on the existing signs and symptoms within 15 minutes of injury. The American Academy of Neurology Concussion Grading Scale (Table 9.2) is widely used in this approach (7). Although confusion and amnesia remain the most frequently cited symptoms, not all injuries behave as expected in the initial evaluation, making the decision concerning return to play more challenging.

Another popular approach is the Cantu Evidence-Based Grading Scale, which grades the injury only after all signs and symptoms of concussion have resolved (8). Less emphasis is placed on LOC as a predictor of potential impairment, and additional weight is placed on overall symptom duration.

The third approach in grading a concussion is not to use any grading scale but, rather, attend to the individual's recovery based on their symptoms, neuropsychological tests, and postural-stability tests. This allows the supervising health care provider to determine when the patient is symptomatic or asymptomatic. Once asymptomatic, the individual can begin a progressive regimen of activity that increases in its demands over several days. This progression will differ in individuals who are withheld from activity for only a few days versus individuals who are withheld for several weeks. This multitiered approach was summarized and supported by consensus at the 2001 Vienna Conference on Concussion in Sport and reaffirmed at the 2004 Conference. Their recommendation was to abandon the continued use of grading scales in favor of combined measures of recovery to determine injury severity (and/or prognosis) and, hence, individually guide ROT decisions (5,6).

The usefulness of a clinical examination and a signs and symptom checklist (available at the companion website on thePoint) is well established in athletic training to assess a concussion. These guidelines may be used to define the level of injury and describe the actions that should be taken if such injuries are suspected. Box 9.2 lists several signs and symptoms seen in cases of concussion.

Simple Concussion

SIGNS AND SYMPTOMS. Although a simple concussion is the most common concussion, it is the most difficult to recognize. The individual may simply report "I had my bell rung." Use of this phrase or

TABLE 9.2 Grading Scales for Athletic Head Injury

	GRADE I/MILD	GRADE II/MODERATE	GRADE III/SEVERE
AAN	Transient confusion; no LOC; symptoms and mental status resolve < 15 min	Transient confusion; no LOC; symptoms and mental status resolve > 15 min	Any LOC
Cantu	No LOC; PTA < 30 min; PCSS < 24 h	LOC < 1 min or PTA ≥ 30 min but < 24 h or PCSS ≥ 24 h but < 7 days	LOC ≥ 1 min. or PTA ≥ 24 h or PCSS ≥ 7 days

AAN, American Academy of Neurology; LOC, loss of consciousness; PTA, posttraumatic amnesia (anterograde/retrograde); PCSS, postconcussion signs and symptoms other than amnesia.

Box 9.2 Typical Signs and Symptoms of a Concussion

- Vacant stare (e.g., befuddled facial expression; glassy eyed)
- Visual problems (e.g., seeing stars or flashing lights; double vision)
- Headache or pressure in the head
- Delayed verbal and motor responses (e.g., slow to answer questions or follow instructions)
- Confusion and inability to focus attention (e.g., easily distracted; unable to follow through with normal activities)
- Disorientation (e.g., walking in the wrong direction; unaware of time, date, and place)
- Slurred or incoherent speech (e.g., making disjointed or incomprehensible statements)
- Gross observable incoordination with balance of dizziness (e.g., stumbling; inability to walk tandem/straight line)
- Emotions out of proportion to circumstances (e.g., distraught; crying for no apparent reason; laughing)
- Memory deficits (e.g., exhibited by the individual repeatedly asking the same question that has already been answered; or inability to memorize and recall three of three words or three of three objects in 5 minutes)
- Any period of loss of consciousness (e.g., paralytic coma; unresponsiveness to arousal)

the term "ding" should not be used to determine the severity of injury, as it carries a connotation that may underestimate the severity of injury. The individual is not rendered unconscious, and the only neurologic deficit is a brief period of posttraumatic confusion (e.g., inattentiveness, poor concentration, and an inability to process information or sequence tasks) or posttraumatic amnesia. Usually, the concussion symptoms or mental status abnormalities that are observed on examination resolve within a 30-minute period (8). If significant disorientation, confusion, memory disturbance, dizziness, headache, or other neurologic abnormality persists after 30 minutes of observation, a more serious concussion is present (4). In a simple concussion, the injury progressively resolves, without complications, over 7 to 10 days.

MANAGEMENT. The individual should be removed from competition and examined immediately as well as at 5-minute intervals to detect amnesia or postconcussion symptoms at rest or with exertion (see *Assessment of Cranial Conditions*). If activity provokes early postconcussion symptoms (e.g., **vertigo**, headache, nausea, and **photophobia**), the individual should be disqualified from returning to activity. Individuals who remain free of symptoms for at least 15 minutes may return to activity. A second simple concussion during the same activity, however, eliminates the individual from further activity that day. Return to activity after a concussion follows a sequential process (5):

1. No activity; complete rest. Once asymptomatic, proceed to step 2.
2. Light aerobic exercise, such as walking or stationary cycling; no resistance training.
3. Sport-specific exercise (e.g., skating in hockey and running in soccer); progressive addition of resistance training at steps 3 and 4.
4. Noncontact training drills.
5. Full-contact training after medical clearance.
6. Game play.

The individual may not proceed to the next step until he or she is asymptomatic at the current level. Apart from limiting play or physical training while the individual is symptomatic, no further intervention is required during the period of recovery, and the individual resumes activity without further problems. If any postconcussion symptoms occur, the individual should drop back to the previous asymptomatic level and try to progress again after 24 hours (5,6).

Complex Concussion

SIGNS AND SYMPTOMS. In a complex concussion, the individual suffers persistent symptoms (including persistent symptom recurrence with exertion), specific sequelae (e.g., prolonged LOC [>1 minute]), or prolonged cognitive impairment following the injury. This classification also includes those individuals who suffer multiple concussions over time or repeated concussions with progressively less force of impact (6). Less frequently, no LOC occurs; however, the individual experiences a protracted period of posttraumatic amnesia lasting more than 30 minutes but less than 24 hours. This posttraumatic amnesia may involve loss of memory for events immediately preceding the injury (**retrograde amnesia**) or for events following the injury (**anterograde amnesia**). This memory loss may diminish somewhat, but the individual will always have some degree of permanent (although short) memory loss about the injury. Other signs that may be present include moderate dizziness and unsteady gait, blurred vision, tinnitus, and headache.

MANAGEMENT. An individual with a complex concussion should be removed from activity and should not be allowed to return that day. Frequent on-site examinations should look for signs of evolving intracranial pathology. Formal neuropsychological testing and other assessment tests should be considered with a multidisciplinary approach by physicians or neurologists who have expertise in the management of concussive injuries. Either CT or magnetic resonance imaging is recommended but may contribute little to the evaluation; however, these modalities should be employed whenever suspicion of an intracerebral structural lesion exists. Such instances may include prolonged disturbance of conscious state, focal neurologic deficit, or worsening symptoms (6,9).

Rehabilitation will be more prolonged, and return to activity may be less prescriptive. Complex cases should be managed by a physician with specific expertise in concussive injuries. Additionally, individuals with complex concussions not only should be symptom free but also should not be taking any pharmacological agents or medications that may affect or modify the symptoms of concussion. In professional sports, team physicians are experienced in concussion management and have access to immediate (i.e., sideline) neurocognitive assessment, so return-to-play management often is more rapid in this setting. Even so, full clinical and cognitive recovery must be present before clearance for play is given (5,6).

Posttraumatic Headaches

Posttraumatic vascular headaches can be confused with a simple concussion or postconcussive headache. A vascular headache is a result of vasospasm and does not usually occur with impact but, rather, develops shortly afterward.

Signs and Symptoms

Symptoms, such as a localized area of blindness, may follow the appearance of brilliantly colored, shimmering lights (scintillating scotoma). Posttraumatic migraine headaches, also referred to as footballer's migraine, have been reported in soccer players after repetitive heading of the ball. In addition, migraines are characterized by recurrent attacks of severe headache with sudden onset, with or without visual or gastrointestinal problems.

Management

This individual should be immediately referred to a physician for further evaluation and care.

Postconcussion Syndrome

Postconcussion syndrome may develop after any concussion and tends to occur more frequently in women than in men. A myriad of cognitive impairments may extend from the time of injury to 48 hours after trauma and last for several weeks to months after injury. The extended duration of symptoms is thought to be related to altered neurotransmitter function.

Signs and Symptoms

The syndrome is characterized by decreased attention span, persistent headaches, blurred vision, vertigo, memory loss, irritability, and inability to concentrate on even the simplest task. Exercise may lead to headache, dizziness, and premature fatigue. These symptoms may predispose the individual to second-impact syndrome.

Management

The individual can undergo CT, but the scan generally is normal. No definitive treatment exists other than symptomatic measures to control the headaches. A physician should supervise the level of activity—and prohibit the individual from returning to activity until symptoms resolve both at rest and on exertion.

Second-Impact Syndrome

Second-impact syndrome occurs when an individual who has sustained an initial head injury, usually a concussion, sustains a second head injury before the symptoms associated with the previous one have totally resolved.

Signs and Symptoms

With the initial injury, visual, motor, or sensory changes occur, and the individual may have difficulty with thought and memory. Before these symptoms resolve, which may take days or even weeks, the individual returns to activity and sustains a second head trauma. This second trauma may be relatively minor and does not have to be the result of direct contact. Following the trauma, the individual may appear to be stunned but often completes the current action or play and, in some cases, can walk unassisted. As the vascular engorgement within the cranium increases intracranial pressure, the brainstem becomes compromised. Subsequently, the individual collapses with rapidly dilating pupils, progressing to loss of eye movement, coma, and respiratory failure.

Management

The usual interval from second impact to brainstem failure is short (typically 2–5 minutes). Management involves immediate activation of the emergency care plan, including summoning EMS, and maintenance of basic life support.

During efforts to prevent second–impact syndrome, it is imperative that any individual who complains of a headache, light-headedness, visual disturbances, or other neurologic symptoms not be allowed to participate in any physical activity with the potential for head trauma until he or she is totally asymptomatic.

The individual was momentarily stunned, "saw stars," and had blurred vision. This is not uncommon in a simple concussion. A lingering headache should signal caution, however, and return to activity should not be permitted. This individual should be carefully watched for increased headache intensity, unsteady gait, nausea, photophobia, or mood swings, which dictate immediate evaluation by a physician.

ASSESSMENT OF CRANIAL CONDITIONS

A rugby player comes off the field complaining of what appears to have been a "bell ringer." What questions should be asked as part of the history component during the assessment of this individual?

Any individual who receives a blow, or any significant acceleration–deceleration type of force to the head, should be evaluated thoroughly. This encompasses gathering a history, observing and inspecting the head and facial area for signs of trauma, and assessing mental status, neurologic integrity, and external provocative tests. These components are not separate and distinct but, rather, occur simultaneously. For matters of clarity, these components are presented in separate parts of this section.

Because significant head trauma also may cause neck injury, it should always be assumed that a cervical injury is present. In approaching this individual, the examiner should gather a brief history of the mechanism of injury, duration of unconsciousness, and any other pertinent information from those at the scene. As part of the evaluation process, it is important to establish and maintain an open airway. If the individual is face down, the head and neck should be stabilized and the individual log rolled into a supine position while continuing to stabilize the cervical spine. Any mouth guard, dentures, or partial plates should be removed to prevent occlusion of the airway. Rescue breathing and cardiopulmonary resuscitation should be initiated as needed.

Vital Signs

Vital signs should be taken early in the assessment to establish a baseline of information that can be rechecked periodically to determine if the individual's status is improving or deteriorating. Vital signs include pulse, respiration, blood pressure, and body temperature. With head trauma, however, body temperature is not as critical as the other signs. Any abnormal variations, such as falling pulse rate, rising blood pressure, or irregular breathing, indicate increasing intracranial pressure.

1. **Pulse:**

   - *Small weak pulse*—Pulse pressure is diminished, and the pulse feels weak and small; causes include decreased stroke volume and increase peripheral resistance.

   - *Short, rapid, weak pulse*—Indicates heart failure or shock.

   - *Slow, bounding pulse*—Indicates increasing intracranial pressure.

   - *Accelerated pulse*—A rapid pulse (i.e., :150 beats per minute) may indicate pressure on the base of the brain.

2. **Respiration:**

   - *Slow breathing (bradypnea)*—Breathing at less than 12 breaths per minute indicates increased intracranial pressure.

   - *Cheyne-Stokes breathing*—Periods of deep breathing alternating with periods of apnea (no breathing) indicates brain damage.

   - *Ataxic (Biot's) breathing*—Characterized by unpredictable irregularity; breaths may be shallow or deep and stop for short periods, indicating respiratory depression and brain damage, typically at the medullary level.

   - *Apneustic breathing*—Characterized by prolonged inspirations unrelieved by attempts to exhale, which indicates trauma to the pons.

3. **Blood pressure:** An increase in systolic blood pressure or decrease in diastolic blood pressure indicates rising intracranial pressure. Low blood pressure rarely occurs in a head injury; however, it may indicate a possible cervical injury or serious blood loss from an injury elsewhere in the body.

4. **Pulse pressure:** The normal difference between diastolic and systolic pressure is approximately 40 mm Hg. A pulse pressure of greater than 50 mm Hg indicates increased intracranial bleeding.

History and Mental Status Testing

Amnesia and confusion, including a heightened distractibility, inability to maintain a coherent stream of thought, and inability to carry out a sequence of goal-directed movements, are hallmark signs of a concussion. The confusion and memory dysfunction may be immediate after injury, or it may be a delayed process, taking several minutes to fully evolve. As such, close observation and assessment repeated over a period of time are necessary to determine if the evolving neuropathologic change associated with a concussion leads to physical signs and symptoms or to the development of memory dysfunction. Initially, the examiner should call the person's name and gently tap the individual on the cheek or arm to get a response. Slurred speech, difficulty in constructing sentences, or inability to understand commands must be noted. The examiner should continue to stabilize the head and neck throughout the assessment. The following examples may be used to gather the history of the injury and test the mental status of the injured participant:

1. **Orientation:** Ask the individual about the time, place, person, and situation (e.g., the circumstances surrounding the mechanism of injury).

2. **Concentration:** Recite three digits, and ask the individual to recite them backward. Move to four digits, and then to five digits (e.g., 3-1-7, 4-6-8-2, and 5-3-0-7-4). Ask the individual to list the months of the year in reverse order.

3. **Memory:** Name three words or identify three objects for the individual, and ask the person to recall these words or objects. Every 5 minutes, ask the individual to do so again. Additionally, ask the individual to recall recent newsworthy events or provide details of the current activity (e.g., plays, moves, and strategies).

4. **Behavior:** The individual's behavior, attitude, and demeanor may change after head trauma. This may present as irrational and inappropriate behavior, belligerence, or verbal or physical abuse directed at others.

5. **Symptoms:** Headache is one of the most reported symptoms (86%) with a concussion (10). Progressive headaches indicate increasing intracranial pressure and signal danger. It is important to note if the individual is experiencing nausea, because intracranial pressure can stimulate the reflex onset of nausea and vomiting. If this symptom is present, it indicates a fairly serious intracranial injury. Other common symptoms that may be reported include dizziness, confusion, disorientation, blurred vision amnesia, neck pain, and fatigue (10).

6. **Loss of consciousness:** Less than 8.9% of all concussions involve LOC (10). It is important to determine if the individual is totally unresponsive, confused, or disoriented. If LOC occurred, it is important to note whether it occurred immediately on direct impact or whether the person progressed to unconsciousness. In addition, the length of time of unconsciousness should be recorded. The individual's response to painful stimuli (e.g., squeezing the trapezius, pinching soft tissue between the thumb and index finger in the axilla, knuckle to the sternum, or squeezing the Achilles tendon) should be assessed. The occurrence of a seizure also should be noted.

Observation and Inspection

Observation of facial expression and function should be performed throughout the evaluation (see Table 9.3 *Cranial Nerve Assessment*). The following areas and conditions should be assessed in the observation component of the evaluation:

1. **Leakage of CSF:** Cerebrospinal fluid is a clear, colorless fluid that protects and cushions the brain and spinal cord. A basilar skull fracture may result in blood and CSF leaking from the ear. A fracture to the cribriform plate in the anterior cranial area may result in blood and CSF leaking from the nose.

2. **Signs of trauma:** Discoloration around the eyes (raccoon eyes) and behind the ears (Battle's sign) may indicate a skull fracture. A depression, elevation, or bleeding may indicate a skull fracture, laceration, or hematoma. Snoring, which may result from a fracture to the anterior cranial floor, should be noted.

3. **Skin color:** Skin color and the presence of moisture or sweat should be assessed. If shock is developing, the skin may appear ashen or pale and be moist and cool.

4. **Loss of emotional control:** Irritability, aggressive behavior, or uncontrolled crying for no apparent reason indicates cerebral dysfunction.

5. **Graded symptom checklist:** A standardized graded symptom checklist has been recommended by the National Athletic Trainers' Association for use during the initial evaluation of a head injury and each subsequent follow-up assessment until all signs and symptoms have returned to normal both at rest and during physical exertion. The supervising health care provider can quantify or score the severity of the symptom on a scale of 0 to 6, where 0 = not present, 1 = mild, 3 = moderate, and 6 = more severe (9).

A sample graded symptom checklist can be found on the companion website at thePoint.

Palpation

Palpation can help to determine possible skull or facial fractures. The examiner should palpate for point tenderness, crepitus, depressions, elevations, swelling, blood, or changes in skin temperature. The following sites should be palpated:

1. Scalp and hair

2. Base of the skull (occiput), external ear, and periauricular area

3. TMJ

4. Cervical spinous processes

5. Hyoid bone and cartilages

6. Mandible

7. Maxilla

8. Teeth

9. Zygomatic arch (cheek)

10. Frontal bone and entire eye orbit

11. Nasal bones and nasal cartilage

Neurologic Tests

Tests should be used that assess upper motor neuron function of the brain through coordination, sensation, and agility and should include a combination of cognition, postural stability, and self-reported symptoms. Evaluation of myotomes and dermatomes is not an effective tool in assessing cranial injuries, because they address lower motor neuron function associated with the spinal column and spinal nerves.

1. **Cranial nerve assessment:** Integrity of the cranial nerves can be assessed quickly by sense of smell, vision, eye tracking, smiling, clenching the jaw, hearing, balance, sense of taste, speaking, and strength of shoulder shrugs (Table 9.3).

TABLE 9.3 Cranial Nerve Assessment

NUMBER	NERVE	MOTOR FUNCTION
I	Olfactory	Identify familiar odors (chocolate, coffee)
II	Optic	Test visual fields: Snellen chart (blurring or double vision)
III	Oculomotor	Test pupillary reaction to light
		Perform upward and downward gaze
IV	Trochlear	Perform downward and lateral gaze
V	Trigeminal	Touch face to note difference in sensation
		Clench teeth; push down on chin to separate jaws
VI	Abducens	Perform lateral and medial gaze
VII	Facial	Close eyes tight
		Smile and show the teeth
VIII	Vestibulocochlear (acoustic nerve)	Identify the sound of fingers snapping near the ear
		Balance and coordination (stand on one foot)
IX	Glossopharyngeal	Gag reflex; ask the athlete to swallow
X	Vagus	Gag reflex; ask athlete to swallow or say "Ahhh"
XI	Accessory	Resisted shoulder shrug
XII	Hypoglossal	Stick out the tongue

2. **Pupil abnormalities:** Pupil size and accommodation to light should be equal in both eyes. A dilated pupil on one side may indicate a subdural or epidural hematoma. Dilated pupils on both sides indicate severe cranial injury with death imminent. The examiner should ask the individual to look up, down, and sideways (six cardinal planes of vision). The coordinated and fluid motion of both eyes should be noted. The individual should be asked about blurred or double vision or the presence of "stars" or flashes of light on impact. Blurred or double vision, abnormal oscillating movements of the eye (**nystagmus**), or uncoordinated gross movement through the cardinal planes indicate disturbance of the cranial nerves that innervate the eyes and eye muscles.

3. **Babinski's reflex:** The individual should be lying down with the eyes closed and the leg held in a slightly elevated and flexed position. A pointed object is stroked along the plantar aspect of the foot. A normal sign is for the toes to curl downward in flexion and adduction (Fig. 9.11A). A positive sign suggests an upper motor neuron lesion and is demonstrated by extension of the big toe and abduction (splaying) of the other toes (Fig. 9.11B).

4. **Strength:** A bilateral comparison of grip strength should be performed by having the examiner place his or her hands inside the individual's hands and then asking the individual to squeeze.

5. **Neuropsychological assessments:**

   ■ **Standardized Assessment of Concussion:** Standardized Assessment of Concussion (11–14) is an abbreviated neurocognitive test designed for medical personnel with no previous expertise in psychometric testing. The Standardized Assessment of Concussion requires approximately 5 minutes to administer, and it evaluates four key mental functions (i.e., orientation, immediate memory, concentration, and delayed recall), summing to a total composite score of 30 points. A standard neurologic screening is included to assess deficits in strength, sensation, and coordination that result from head trauma. The form, which is used to record baseline information and subsequent testing, however, has no definitive guidelines or cutoff scores established for interpreting performance on the examination. The critical part of using the instrument is to collect baseline normative data that can be used for comparison purposes in the event of a concussion to determine the severity of injury and follow the individual's recovery.

   ■ **Paper-and-pencil tests:** A number of assessment tools focus on verbal learning, verbal scanning, attention, concentration, short-term memory, visual perception and tracking, and general brain function. These include the Hopkins Verbal Learning Test (John Hopkins University, Baltimore, MD), Trail Making Test A & B (Reitan Neuropsychological Laboratory, Tucson, AZ), Wechsler Digit Span Test (Psychological Corporation, San Antonio, TX), Stroop Color-Word Interference Test (Stoelting Co., Wood Dale, IL), Symbol Digit Modalities Test (Western Psychological Services, Los Angeles, CA), and Controlled Oral Word Association Test (COWAT; Psychological Assessment Resources, Inc. Odessa, FL) (15).

The Standardized Assessment of Concussion is available on the companion website on thePoint.

■ **Computerized neuropsychological tests:** Recently, a number of computerized neuropsychological tests have been developed to test individuals who have sustained a concussion. Advantages in administering these tests is their ease of administration, ability to baseline test a large number of athletes in a short period of time, and multiple forms used with the testing paradigm, which reduces the practice effects (9). Examples of the more common tests include the Automated Neuropsychological Assessment Metrics (National Rehabilitation Hospital Assistive Technology and Neuroscience Center, Washington, DC), CogSport (CogState Ltd., Victoria, Australia), Concussion Resolution Index (HeadMinder, Inc., New York, NY), and the Immediate Postconcussion Assessment and Cognitive Testing (ImPACT; University of Pittsburg Medical Center, Pittsburgh, PA) (9).

■■■■ FIGURE 9.12 **Finger-to-nose test.** The individual should be standing with his or her eyes open and arms out to the side. The examiner instructs the individual to touch his or her index finger to the nose and then alternate with the other hand to the nose. Inability to perform this test indicates physical disorientation and lack of coordination and should preclude reentry to activity.

6. **Coordination and balance:**

■ **Finger-to-nose test:** This test can assess balance, depth perception, and ability to focus on an object. While the individual's eyes are open and his or her arms are out to the side, the examiner should instruct the individual to touch the index finger of one hand to the nose and then alternate with the other hand to the nose. The examiner should observe for any swaying or inability to touch the nose. Then, standing a few feet from the person, the examiner should hold a finger in front of the injured individual. The individual should alternate between the right and left hand to reach out and touch the examiner's finger (Fig. 9.12). The examiner can change the position of the finger after two or three touches. A variation is to have the individual touch his or her nose between each touch of the examiner's finger. The speed of touch between the nose and finger is then progressively increased.

■ **Gait:** Observing the individual walking in a straight line, the examiner should note any swaying or unsteadiness of gait. Heel-to-toe walking (tandem walking) also may be performed.

■ **Romberg test:** The individual is asked to stand with the feet together, arms at the side, and eyes closed while maintaining balance (Fig. 9.13). While standing lateral or posterior to the individual—to support the patient, if needed—the examiner observes for any body

■■■■ FIGURE 9.13 **Romberg test. A,** The individual should be standing with his or her eyes closed and arms at the side. The examiner instructs the individual to maintain a standing position. Any sway indicates lack of balance and sensation and should preclude reentry to activity. **B,** A variation may include having the individual tilt the head backward and lift one foot off the ground while trying to maintain balance.

FIGURE 9.14 One-legged (stork) stand. The examiner instructs the individual to stand and balance on one leg. If this is accomplished, the individual should be instructed to lean backward. Inability to perform this task indicates lack of balance and should preclude reentry to activity.

sway, indicating a positive test. Variations include the individual raising his or her arms to 90°, standing on the toes, touching the nose with the hand while the eyes are closed (finger-to-nose test), standing in a tandem position on a foam surface, and tilting the head backward while lifting one foot off the ground. Recently, the standard Romberg test has been criticized for its lack of sensibility and objectivity, because a considerable amount of stress is required to produce a positive test.

- **One-legged stand (stork stand):** The individual is instructed to stand on one foot and lean backward with the eyes closed. The examiner notes any difficulties in performing the action (Fig. 9.14).

- **Balance Error Scoring System (BESS):** This clinical tool is designed to assess impairment of balance and coordination in the physically active population. The assessment involves three different stances (i.e., double leg, single leg, and tandem leg), with each stance being completed twice, once while standing on a firm surface and again while standing on a foam surface (Fig. 9.15). The battery of tests is performed before the start of participation in an activity or sport (e.g., as part of the preparticipation examination) to establish a baseline of information. Following head injury, the BESS can be administered on-site or in an office/clinic setting to compare the current results with the initial findings.

External Provocative Tests

These tests require the individual to perform exertional activities, such as running or push-ups. Any appearance of associated symptoms (e.g., headaches, dizziness, nausea, unsteadiness, photophobia, blurred or double vision, loss of emotional control, or mental status changes) is abnormal. If the assessment has already determined a possible intracranial injury, the individual should not be subjected to these tests. If, however, a possible intracranial injury has not yet been determined, the following tests can be performed:

- 40-yard sprint
- Five jumping jacks
- Five sit-ups
- Five push-ups
- Five knee bends

Determination of Findings

If the individual is not in a crisis situation, an evaluation of vital signs, mental status, and neurologic tests should be completed every 5 to 7 minutes to determine progress of the condition.

If the individual has been evaluated by a physician on-site and the signs and symptoms linger but appear to be minor, it is essential to ensure ongoing monitoring of the individual. An individual close to the injured party, such as a parent, spouse, or roommate, should be informed of the injury and told to look for problematic signs, including changes in behavior, unsteady gait, slurring of speech, a progressive headache or nausea, restlessness, mental confusion, or drowsiness. These danger signs should be fully explained to the observer and provided on an information sheet.

A sample *Information Sheet on Follow-up Care for a Head Injury* is available on the companion website at thePoint.

Field Strategy 9.2 summarizes an assessment of a cranial injury.

FIGURE 9.15 Balance error scoring system (BESS). This test involves three different stances (double leg, single leg, and tandem leg), each completed twice (once while standing on a firm surface and again while standing on a foam surface).

FIELD STRATEGY 9.2

Cranial Injury Evaluation

1. Stabilize head and neck.
2. Check airway, breathing, and circulation. (If a helmet is worn, remove the face mask, but do not remove the helmet or chin strap.)
3. Determine the initial level of consciousness.
4. Activate the emergency plan, including summoning emergency medical services if necessary.
5. Take vital signs (i.e., pulse, respiration, and blood pressure).
6. History and mental status testing:
   - Orientation (e.g., time, place, person, and situation)
   - Concentration (e.g., count digits backward or recite the months of the year in reverse order)
   - Memory (e.g., names of teams in previous contests, recall of three words and three objects, recent newsworthy events, or details of the contest)
   - Symptoms (e.g., headache, nausea, or tinnitus)
7. Observation and inspection:
   - Leakage of cerebrospinal fluid
   - Signs of trauma (e.g., deformity, body posturing, or discoloration around the eyes and behind the ears)
   - Loss of emotional control (e.g., irritability, aggressiveness, or uncontrolled crying)
8. Palpate bony and soft-tissue structures for point tenderness, crepitus, depressions, elevations, swelling, blood, or changes in skin temperature.
9. Neurologic examination:
   - Cranial nerve assessment
   - Pupil abnormalities (e.g., pupil size, response to light, eye movement, nystagmus, or blurred or double vision)
   - Babinski's reflex
   - Strength
   - Neuropsychological assessments
   - Coordination and balance (e.g., finger-to-nose test, gait, Romberg test, one-legged stork stand, or balance error scoring system)
10. External provocative test:
    - 40-yard sprint
    - Five sit-ups
    - Five push-ups
    - Five knee bends
11. Take vital signs, and recheck every 5 to 7 minutes.

In evaluating the head trauma sustained by the rugby player, a history that includes questions pertaining to LOC, headache, confusion, memory loss, nausea, tinnitus, and loss of coordination should be completed.

FACIAL CONDITIONS

A hockey player was taking a shot on goal when his stick hit the jaw of the player guarding him. That player comes off the ice bleeding from the mouth and unable to close the jaw. He is having difficulty articulating his words. Explain the palpation of this condition. What type of injury should be suspected, and why?

Injuries to the cheek, nose, lips, and jaw are very common in sports that involve moving projectiles (e.g., sticks, balls, bats, or racquets), in contact sports (e.g., football, rugby, or ice hockey), and in sports that involve collisions with objects (e.g., diving, skiing, ice hockey, or swimming). Many of these injuries can be prevented by wearing properly fitted face masks and mouth guards. Because the facial area has a vast arterial system, lacerations bleed freely, and rapid swelling often hides the true extent of injury. Box 9.3 identifies the signs and symptoms of serious facial injuries that warrant further examination by a physician.

Facial Soft-Tissue Conditions

Facial contusions, abrasions, and lacerations are managed in the same manner as those located elsewhere on the body. Contusions, which are the most commonly encountered facial injury, usually result from blunt trauma (16). Ice is applied to control swelling and hemorrhage. If an abrasion or laceration is present, the wound should be cleansed with a saline solution, an antibiotic ointment used, and an occlusive dressing of gauze or tape applied. In minor lacerations (<1 inch long and one-eighth of an inch deep), application of butterfly bandages or Steri-strips can facilitate wound closure. The area requires protection with sterile gauze and tape. The individual can return to participation, but at the conclusion of the event, the individual should see a physician to determine if sutures are needed. Lacerations older than 12 hours should not be sutured but, rather, should be allowed to heal by secondary intention because of the increased risk of wound infection (16). Larger and more complicated injuries, such as those with jagged edges or damage to nerves, veins, or bony structures, should be referred immediately to a physician.

Temporomandibular Joint Conditions

The TMJ is a sliding hinge joint that is stabilized by ligaments and is separated into upper and lower compartments by a fibrocartilage meniscus. Injury occurs when a blow to the mandible transmits the force to the condyles. Injuries may involve intracapsular bleeding (hemarthrosis), inflammation of the capsular ligaments (capsulitis), meniscal displacement, subluxation/dislocation of the condyles, or fracture.

Signs and Symptoms

Common signs and symptoms include an inability to open the mouth (normal opening, 40 mm), deviation of the jaw to the side of the injury on opening, pain on opening and biting, **malocclusion** (change in bite), joint noise (i.e., clicking, popping, or crepitus), or an inability to close the mouth (17).

Box 9.3 Facial "Red Flags" Requiring Further Examination by a Physician

- Obvious deformity or crepitus
- Appearance of a long face
- Increased pain on palpation

- Irregular eye movement or failure to accommodate to light
- Malocclusion of the teeth

Management

A crushed ice pack should be placed over the area to control swelling. The examiner may elect to temporarily immobilize the jaw with an elastic bandage wrapped under the chin and over the top of the head. Subsequent management of TMJ injuries often involves refraining from opening the mouth for 7 to 10 days and eating a soft diet. Anti-inflammatory medication may assist in reducing pain and inflammation. During the acute period, lifting of heavy weights should be restricted.

Facial Fractures

Direct impact can fracture the facial bones, including the mandible (jaw), maxilla (upper jaw), zygomatic bone (cheek), or nasal bones. The most common fractures occur to the nasal bones, followed by the zygomatic bone and the mandible, respectively (18).

Zygomatic Fractures

SIGNS AND SYMPTOMS. Direct impact to the zygomatic bone results in a flat or depressed appearance of the cheek. Swelling and ecchymosis about the eye may occlude vision and hide damage to the orbit. Occasionally, the eye on the side of the fracture may appear to be sunken, or the eye opposite the fracture may appear to be raised. Double vision is common, and paresthesia or anesthesia (numbness) may be present on the affected cheek.

MANAGEMENT. A crushed-ice pack should be placed over the area to control swelling, but it is important to avoid pressure or compression over the fracture site. The individual should be referred immediately to a physician. In most cases, the condition can easily be reduced surgically and may not require internal fixation. An exception occurs when the fracture involves the eye orbit and surgical repair becomes more extensive. Healing usually occurs within 6 to 8 weeks. Special facial protection should be worn for 3 to 4 months. A complication of this condition includes blurred vision over an extended period. As such, individuals in activities requiring eye–hand coordination may not return to their previous level of participation for some time.

Mandibular Fractures

SIGNS AND SYMPTOMS. This injury seldom occurs as an isolated, single fracture; it more often is a double fracture or a fracture-dislocation. The most common fracture sites are the mandibular angle and condyles, both of which lead to malocclusion (Fig. 9.16). Because the articulation of words is impossible, changes in speech are apparent. Oral bleeding may occur even though a mouth guard is properly fitted and worn. Pain, discoloration, swelling, and facial distortion may be present. The individual is unable to maintain a firm bite on a tongue depressor placed in his or her mouth (Fig. 9.17).

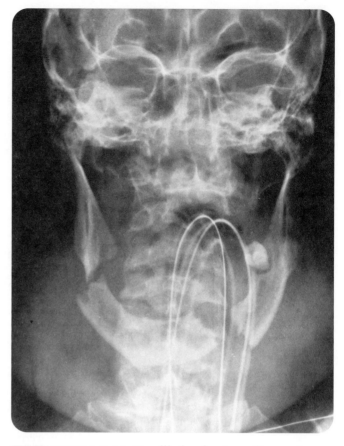

■■ ■ ■ FIGURE 9.16 **Mandibular fracture.** The most common site for a mandibular fracture is near the angle of the jaw, which leads to malocclusion of the teeth.

■■ ■ ■ FIGURE 9.17 **Tongue blade test.** In a suspected mandibular fracture, a tongue blade (tongue depressor) is placed in the individual's mouth. The individual is instructed to hold the blade in place as the examiner rotates or twists the blade. A positive sign is the inability to hold a firm bite on the blade or increased pain on movement of the blade.

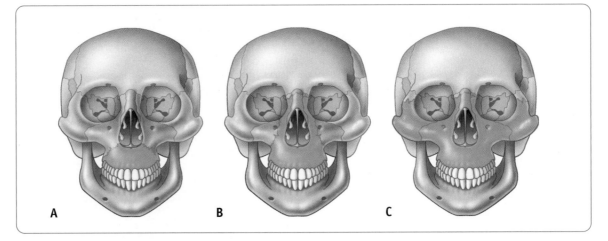

FIGURE 9.18 Maxillary fractures. Fractures to the maxilla may involve separation of the palate **(A)**, may extend into the nasal region **(B)**, or may involve complete craniofacial dissociation **(C)**. These midface fractures are commonly referred to as LeFort fractures.

MANAGEMENT. It is important with this type of fracture for the examiner to maintain an open airway, because the tongue may occlude the airway. Management involves dressing any open wounds and immobilizing the jaw with an elastic bandage wrapped under the chin and over the top of the head. A crushed-ice pack may be placed over the area to control swelling; however, pressure or compression over the fracture site should be avoided. The individual should be referred immediately to a physician. Repair involves internal fixation (i.e., wiring the jaw closed) or using bone plates, which may allow some individuals to return to sport participation. During the healing period, a high-protein, high-carbohydrate, liquid diet is required. A weight loss of 5 to 10% is not uncommon. Mild activities, such as stationary bicycling, swimming, and use of light weights, to maintain muscle tone and conditioning are recommended.

Maxillary Fractures

SIGNS AND SYMPTOMS. If the upper jaw, or midface, is fractured (LeFort fractures), the maxilla may be mobile, giving the appearance of a longer face (Fig. 9.18). Nasal bleeding, ecchymosis in the cheek or buccal region, malocclusion, nasal deformity, or a flattening and splaying of the naso-orbital region may be present.

MANAGEMENT. Treatment involves maintaining the airway. A forward-sitting position allows adequate drainage of saliva and blood. A crushed-ice pack may be placed over the area to control swelling, but it is important to avoid pressure or compression over the fracture site. The individual should be referred immediately to a physician. Although reduction and internal fixation often are used to immobilize the region, extensive surgery and possible secondary reconstruction occasionally are necessary to treat the condition.

A *Because the individual is bleeding, universal precautions should be followed during palpation of the maxilla, mandible, zygomatic bone, nasal bone, and TMJ. As indicated by the apparent malocclusion and inability to close the jaw, the hockey player may have a fractured jaw.*

NASAL CONDITIONS

Q *A basketball player received a lateral blow to the nose from an opposing player's elbow. The nose is bleeding and has a flattened appearance. What signs and symptoms indicate that this individual needs to be referred immediately to a physician?*

Box 9.4   Nasal "Red Flags" Requiring Further Examination by a Physician

- Bleeding or cerebrospinal fluid from the nose
- Loss of smell
- Nasal deformity or fracture
- Nosebleed that does not stop within 5 minutes
- Foreign objects that cannot be removed easily

Nasal injuries are common in sports during which protective face guards are not worn. Epistaxis, deviated septum, and nasal fractures are common injuries to the nasal region. Box 9.4 identifies the signs and symptoms of nasal conditions that warrant further examination by a physician.

Epistaxis

Signs and Symptoms

Epistaxis, or nosebleed, can be either anterior or posterior. Anterior bleeding originates from superficial blood vessels on the anterior septum (Klesselbach's area) and is more common than posterior bleeding from the lateral wall.

Management

Most nosebleeds stop spontaneously after applying mild pressure at the nasal bone for 5 to 10 minutes. In addition, ice could be applied to the back of the neck to assist in producing a reflex vasoconstriction. The head should be tilted slightly forward, reducing the risk of blood traveling down the oropharynx. A nasal plug or pledget may be used but seldom is needed; if used, however, the plug can be coated with topical astringents or soaked with vasoconstrictors, such as tannic acid or a 1% phenylephrine hydrochloride solution (as long as the individual is not allergic to them). The plug should extend externally for at least half an inch. If bleeding continues for more than 5 minutes despite manual pressure and ice, the individual should be referred to a physician.

Individuals should be instructed not to blow their nose following significant bouts of epistaxis. Recurrent bouts may need to be treated with nasal cauterization, chemically with silver nitrate sticks, or with electrocautery under local anesthesia.

Deviated Septum

The nasal septum is the partition between the right and left sides of the nose. A deviated septum may be congenital and asymptomatic; however, nasal trauma, such as a nasal fracture or lateral compression on the nasal region, can displace the septum, leading to difficulty in breathing. Under normal circumstances, when an individual closes one nostril and attempts to breathe through the other, that nostril closes during inhalation, and breathing is unobstructed. Expiration should be easy and smooth.

Signs and Symptoms

The most obvious sign is a consistent difference in airflow between the two sides of the nose when one nostril is blocked. Inspection with an otoscope can confirm the presence of a deviated septum. If trauma was involved in the injury, a septal hematoma may be visible through the otoscope.

See *Field Strategy: Use of an Otoscope to Inspect the Nose and Ear*, available on the companion website at thePoint.

Management

If a deviated septum is suspected, the individual should be referred to a physician for further care. Surgery often is indicated to drain a septal hematoma and repair the deviated septum; this may involve reshaping the nasal cartilage and bone (i.e., septoplasty or submucous resection). Correction of a deviated septum usually does not change the outer appearance of the nose.

Nasal Fractures

Persistent or profuse bleeding may indicate a complex nasal fracture with an injury to the ethmoid artery that requires direct visualization.

Signs and Symptoms

Epistaxis usually is present, and the nose may appear to be flattened and lose its symmetry, particularly with a lateral force. Because of its prominence, the nose is particularly susceptible to lateral displacement (17). Severity can range from a slightly depressed, greenstick fracture (seen in adolescents) to total displacement and/or disruption in the bony and cartilaginous parts of the nose. The nasal airway can be obstructed with bony fragments, or the fracture can extend into the cranial region and cause a loss of CSF. There may be crepitus over the nasal bridge and ecchymosis under the eyes.

Management

If the only injury is to the nose, the individual should be evaluated to ensure that no septal hematoma (i.e., blood from an acute injury that accumulates beneath the septal perichondrium) has formed, which would require immediate referral to a physician for incision and drainage. The nose should then be viewed by standing behind and above the individual while looking down an imaginary line to determine if the nose is centered. Using a small mirror, the injured individual should look at the nose to determine if it appears to be normal. Treatment involves controlling bleeding, applying ice to limit swelling and hemorrhage, and referring the individual to a physician for further examination. A custom acrylic face shield, helmet with face mask, or other protective device should be worn during contact sports for 4 weeks after injury (16). Field Strategy 9.3 provides guidelines for the assessment and care of a nasal injury.

A *Signs and symptoms that indicate a serious nasal injury include excessive bleeding or CSF from the nose, loss of smell, nasal deformity or fracture, or a nosebleed that does not stop within 5 minutes. If present, the individual should be referred immediately to a physician.*

FIELD STRATEGY 9.3

Evaluation and Management of a Nasal Injury

1. Check airway, breathing, and circulation. Bony fragments may occlude the airway.
2. Determine responsiveness.
3. Check for signs of a concussion and/or skull fracture.
4. History:
   - Primary complaint (e.g., pain, dizziness, disorientation, nausea, vision disturbances, or tinnitus)
   - Mechanism of injury
   - Disability from injury (inability to breathe through one side of nose)
5. Observation and inspection:
   - Obvious deformity or abnormal deviation
   - Bleeding and/or cerebrospinal fluid from the nose
   - Check pupil size, pupillary response to light, eye movement, nystagmus, or blurred or double vision, which may indicate an associated cranial injury
   - Abnormal breathing rate and pattern
   - Stand behind the individual and look down an imaginary line to see if the nose is deviated
6. Palpation:
   - Palpate the two nasal bones with the forefinger and thumb (checking for swelling, depressions, crepitus, mobility, etc.)
   - Check the internal structures of the nasal area for any abnormalities
7. After bleeding is controlled, inspect the internal structures for any abnormalities.
8. Apply ice to control hemorrhage, and refer the individual to a physician for further care.

ORAL AND DENTAL CONDITIONS

Following a collision during a high school soccer game, an athlete complains of significant pain after being hit in the mouth. The inside of the upper lip is bleeding, and one tooth is intruded. How should this injury be managed?

The most commonly injured tooth is the maxillary central incisor, which is positioned front and center and receives 80% of all dental trauma (20). During sport and physical activity, nearly all such injuries are preventable through regular use of mouth protectors. Mouth protectors prevent injury to the lips, teeth, cheek, tongue, mandible, neck, TMJ, and brain by absorbing shock, spreading impact, cushioning the contact between the upper and lower jaws, and keeping the upper lip away from the incisal edges of the teeth. Although certain sports (e.g., football, boxing, field hockey, and lacrosse) require mouth guards, few coaches or league officials require these devices in other contact and collision sports. Box 9.5 identifies the signs and symptoms of oral and dental conditions that warrant further examination by a physician.

Periodontal Disease

Periodontal disease (gum disease) ranges from **gingivitis**, or mild inflammation of the gums, to **periodontitis**, or inflammation of the deeper gum tissues that normally hold the teeth in place. Approximately 80% of American adults have some form of gum disease. Gingivitis usually is caused by bacteria that irritate the gums, leading to swelling and bleeding. Bacteria, along with minerals in the saliva, form tartar (calculus), which provides an environment for additional bacteria to accumulate and irritate the gums. If left unchecked, gingivitis can lead to the more serious form of gum disease, periodontitis. This long-term infection eventually can result in loss of the teeth. Thorough daily brushing, regular flossing, and frequent professional cleaning reduce the risk of developing serious gingivitis.

Signs and Symptoms

Initial signs of gingivitis include tender, swollen, or bleeding gums, particularly when the teeth are brushed. There also may be a change in color of the gums from pink to dusky red. Plaque, which is the soft, white form of salivary salts, protein, and bacteria that covers the teeth and leads to gingivitis, is not readily visible. Signs and symptoms of periodontitis may include swollen or recessed gums; an unpleasant taste in the mouth; bad breath; tooth pain, especially when eating hot, cold, or sweet foods; loose teeth; change in the bite; and drainage or pus around one or more teeth.

Management

Gingivitis usually clears after a professional cleaning by a dentist or hygienist, followed by proper daily oral hygiene. The cleaning involves the removal of all tartar and plaque from the teeth. Removing the tartar and plaque eliminates the source of irritation to the gums, allowing the gums to heal. If gingivitis has progressed to periodontitis, more extensive treatment is necessary; the dentist may try to remove the pockets of bacteria between the gums and teeth and may recommend antibiotics. Other nonsurgical treatments may include scaling, sometimes done with an ultrasonic device, to remove tartar and bacteria from the tooth surfaces and beneath the gums. A technique

Box 9.5   Oral and Dental "Red Flags" Requiring Further Examination by a Physician

- Lacerations involving the lip, outer border of the lip, or tongue
- Loose teeth either laterally displaced, intruded, or extruded
- Chipped, cracked, fractured, or dislodged teeth
- Any individual complaining of persistent toothache or sensitivity to heat and cold
- Inability to close the jaw
- Malocclusion of the teeth

known as root planing is used to smooth the root surfaces, discouraging further accumulation of tartar. In advanced stages of periodontitis, surgery may be necessary.

Dental Caries (Tooth Decay)

Dental caries, also known as tooth decay and cavities, are caused primarily by plaque. When plaque collects and hardens, tartar is formed. Bacteria within the plaque contain acids that begin to dissolve the tooth enamel. These problems can cause openings in the tooth enamel, which then allow bacteria to infect the center of the tooth (the pulp). This condition can be accelerated by ingesting acid-rich foods or foods that are high in sugar and starch. Combined with poor oral hygiene, this condition can lead to a painful tooth cavity. If neglected, the infection can spread from the pulp to the root of the tooth and, finally, to the bones supporting the tooth. An **abscessed tooth** is a painful infection at the root of a tooth or between the gum and a tooth. Although primarily caused by severe tooth decay, the condition also can result from gingivitis or trauma to the tooth, such as when a tooth is broken or chipped.

Signs and Symptoms

A tooth with a cavity typically presents with pain during chewing and sensitivity to hot or cold foods and beverages. If a tooth abscess is present, a throbbing pain or a sharp or shooting pain is common. Other symptoms may include fever, bitter taste in the mouth, bad breath, swollen neck glands, general discomfort, uneasiness or ill feeling, redness and swelling of the gums, swollen area of the upper or lower jaw, or an open, draining sore on the side of the gum. If the root of the tooth dies as a result of infection, the toothache may stop. this does not mean the infection has healed, however; the infection remains active and continues to spread and destroy tissue. If any symptoms are present, the individual should be referred immediately to a dentist.

Management

In mild tooth decay, the dentist scrapes the region and applies a filling. If a more serious condition is present, a radiograph may be obtained to assess the presence of a tooth abscess and bone erosion. To eliminate infection, the abscess may need to be drained via a procedure known as a root canal. Root canal surgery also may be recommended to remove any diseased root tissue after the infection has subsided; subsequently, a crown may be placed over the tooth. The tooth also may be extracted, allowing drainage through the socket, and a third way to drain the abscess is by incision into the swollen gum tissue. Antibiotics are prescribed to help fight the infection. Warm saltwater rinses and over-the-counter pain-reducing medication can be used to relieve pain and discomfort associated with an abscessed tooth.

Mouth Lacerations

Management

Treatment of minor lacerations is the same as in cases with other lacerations. This includes applying direct pressure to stop bleeding, cleaning the area with a saline solution, applying Steri-strips if needed, and covering the wound with a dry, sterile dressing. Lacerations that extend completely through the lip or that involve the outer lip or large tongue lacerations require special suturing. A badly scarred tongue can affect taste and interfere with speech patterns. Tongue lacerations require cleansing with water or mouthwash and referral to a physician for possible suturing. The individual should not be permitted to return to participation until the wound is healed. If sutures are applied, protection is continued for at least 7 days.

Loose Teeth

Management

A loosened tooth may be partially displaced, **intruded**, **extruded**, or avulsed (Fig. 9.19). When the tooth has been displaced outwardly or laterally displaced, the examiner should try to place the tooth back into its normal position without forcing it. Teeth that are intruded should be left alone; any

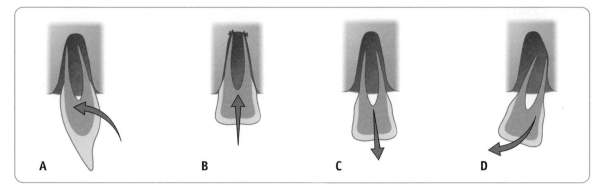

■■ ■ FIGURE 9.19 **Loose teeth.** Loose teeth may involve partial displacement **(A)**, intrusion **(B)**, extrusion **(C)**, or avulsion **(D)**.

attempt to move the tooth may result in permanent loss of the tooth or damage to any underlying permanent teeth. The individual should be referred to a dentist immediately. A dental radiograph can rule out damage under the gum line and ensure the tooth is properly replaced. The damaged tooth is then splinted to the surrounding teeth for 2 to 3 weeks.

Fractured Tooth

Signs and Symptoms

Fractures may occur through the enamel, dentin, pulp, or root of the tooth. Fractures involving the enamel cause no symptoms and can be smoothed by the dentist to prevent further injury to the lips and inner lining of the oral cavity. Fractures extending into the dentin cause pain and increased sensitivity to cold and heat. Fractures exposing the pulp or root of the tooth lead to severe pain and sensitivity.

Management

The individual should be referred to a dentist who will apply a sedative dressing over the exposed area and, later, attach a permanent, composite resin crown. Fractures exposing the pulp involve more extensive dental work. If the pulp exposure is small, a pulp-capping procedure, placing calcium hydroxide on the area, can bridge the exposed area and, if successful, eliminate the need for a root canal. Another treatment involves removing a portion of the pulp in the root canal, leaving the uninjured pulp in the root. This has been successful in younger patients whose roots have not yet fully formed. The final method of treatment is a total root canal.

Dislocated Tooth

Management

Teeth that have been totally avulsed from their sockets often can be located in the individual's mouth or on the ground. These teeth can be saved, but time is of the essence. A dislocated tooth should be held by the crown. It is important not to rub the tooth or remove any dirt. If the tooth is rinsed in milk or saline and replaced intraorally in the tooth socket within 30 minutes, the prognosis for a successful replanting is 90%. It should be noted that tap or drinking water can damage the periodontal ligament cells on the root surface and compromise implantation procedures. Implantation that occurs after 2 hours results in a 95% failure rate (21). Semirigid fixation for 7 to 10 days may be followed by root canal therapy. Contact drills and competition are restricted during this period of time, and an appropriate face or mouth guard should be worn to prevent further injury.

 The examiner should not attempt to move the intruded tooth, because the action could result in permanent loss of the tooth or damage to any underlying permanent teeth. The individual should be referred immediately to a dentist.

EAR CONDITIONS

Q *A wrestler was not wearing protective headgear during practice. He is now complaining about a burning, aching sensation on the outer ear. It appears to be somewhat inflamed and sensitive to touch, but no swelling is apparent. How should this injury be managed, and what signs might indicate a more serious problem?*

Several conditions may affect the ear. Foreign bodies in the ear usually are harmless and easily removed with a speculum. Trauma to the ear can lead to auricular hematoma, and infection to the ear can lead to localized inflammation of the auditory canal (otitis externa), impacted cerumen, swimmer's ear (otitis media), or a tympanic membrane rupture. Box 9.6 identifies the signs and symptoms of ear conditions that warrant further examination by a physician.

External Ear Conditions

Signs and Symptoms

Auricular hematoma, or "cauliflower ear," is a relatively minor injury caused when repeated blunt trauma pulls the cartilage away from the perichondrium. A hematoma forms between the perichondrium and cartilage of the ear and compromises blood supply to the cartilage, leading to a painful and throbbing injury. If left untreated, the hematoma forms a fibrosis in the overlying skin, leading to necrosis of the auricular cartilage that results in the characteristic "cauliflower ear" appearance (Fig. 9.20). This condition, which is common in wrestlers, can be prevented by wearing proper headgear.

Management

Immediate treatment involves icing the region to reduce pain and swelling. An ice pack should be applied for 20 minutes. If the swelling is still present, the hematoma must be aspirated by a physician to avoid pressure and permanent cartilage damage. Once aspirated, a pressure dressing should be applied for 7 to 14 days. The individual should not take aspirin or nonsteroidal anti-inflammatory drugs for several days; however, antibiotics are recommended for 7 to 10 days (16). It is imperative that the individual wear protective headgear to prevent reoccurrence.

Internal Ear Conditions

A blow to the ear, pressure changes (as seen in diving and scuba diving), and infection may injure the external auditory meatus and eardrum. Although typically seen in water sports, damage to the internal ear may occur in any sport, such as in soccer when a player is hit on the ear by a ball. Any individual with intense pain in the ear, a feeling of fullness, nausea, tinnitus, dizziness, or hearing loss should be evaluated immediately by a physician. Most minor ruptures of the eardrum heal spontaneously; larger ruptures may require surgical repair.

FIGURE 9.20 Cauliflower ear deformity. The hematoma results in the skin being pulled away from the ear cartilage.

Box 9.6 Ear "Red Flags" Requiring Further Examination by a Physician

- Bleeding or cerebrospinal fluid from the ear canal
- Bleeding or swelling behind the ear (Battle's sign)
- Hematoma or swelling that removes the creases of the outer ear
- Tinnitus or hearing impairment
- Feeling of fullness in the ear; vertigo
- Foreign body in the ear that cannot be easily removed
- "Popping" or itching in the ear
- Pain when the ear lobe is pulled

Impacted Cerumen

Cerumen, or ear wax, is produced by the ceruminous glands, which are modified apocrine glands in the external auditory canal. Cerumen is a sticky substance thought to trap insects and foreign material in the ear canal. In many individuals, the ear is naturally cleansed as the cerumen dries and then falls out of the external auditory canal. In others, however, cerumen builds up excessively and becomes compacted, a condition that can impair hearing.

SIGNS AND SYMPTOMS. Impacted cerumen causes some degree of hearing loss or muffled hearing. Pain generally is not present, because no infection is present.

MANAGEMENT. Removal of the excess ear wax can be accomplished by irrigating the ear canal with warm water. A cotton tip applicator should not be used, because this may increase the impaction or damage the eardrum. If irrigation is not successful, referral to a physician is necessary to remove the cerumen with a curette.

Otitis Externa

Otitis externa is a bacterial infection that involves the lining of the external auditory canal. Because of its prevalence among individuals who participate in water activities, it is commonly termed "swimmer's ear." Otitis externa frequently occurs in individuals who fail to dry the ear canal after being in water, resulting in a change of the pH of the ear canal's skin.

SIGNS AND SYMPTOMS. In acute conditions, pain is the predominant symptom. In chronic cases, such as those seen with excessive use of cotton swabs, itching is a more common complaint, with discomfort and pain being secondary. There may or may not be a discharge of pus. Gentle pressure around the external auditory opening and pulling on the pinna causes increased pain. If left untreated, the infection can spread to the middle ear, causing balance disturbances or hearing loss. Commercial ear plugs may not be helpful in preventing this condition.

MANAGEMENT. Custom ear plugs from an audiologist or otolaryngologist may be necessary. The condition also can be prevented by using eardrops to dry the canal. The majority of ear drops contain an acidifying agent, either aluminum acetate or vinegar. An effective homemade remedy is equal parts of white vinegar (acetic acid), 70% alcohol, and water. One or two drops after water exposure or showering is the standard recommendation. If no improvement is seen, the individual should be referred to a physician, who may prescribe drops containing broad-spectrum antibiotics.

Otitis Media

Localized infections of the middle ear (**otitis media**) can occur secondary to upper respiratory infections. These infections often are caused by bacteria but also may be caused by viruses. Bacterial and viral infections have the same signs and symptoms.

SIGNS AND SYMPTOMS. When the mastoid area is pressed, the individual will complain of pain and a sense of fullness in the ear. Swelling of the mucous membranes may cause a partial or complete block of the eustachian tube (the connection between the middle ear and pharynx), resulting in inhibition of hearing. The tympanic membrane may appear red and bulging. Serous otitis often is associated with otitis media and upper respiratory infection; an amber-colored or bloody fluid is seen through the eardrum and is associated with complaints of "ears popping."

MANAGEMENT. A physician may prescribe an antibiotic for 10 days if there is an infection, or decongestants may be used to shrink the swollen mucous membranes. If the middle ear of an individual with otitis media is completely filled with fluid, air travel should be discouraged. If the ear is filled with fluid and air and the eustachian tube is not working properly, the air bubbles will expand on ascent and contract on descent. Both ascent and descent cause severe pain and may rupture the eardrum. In addition, rupture of the membranes separating the middle ear from the inner ear could occur—with catastrophic results. Therefore, air travel is not recommended until the middle ear has returned to normal appearance and function.

Tympanic Membrane Rupture

The tympanic membrane vibrates when sound waves strike it, starting the process of converting sound waves into nerve impulses that travel to the brain. Damage to the eardrum interrupts the hearing process and may impair hearing. The eardrum also acts as a barrier to keep outside material, such as bacteria, from entering the middle ear. A rupture (perforated) eardrum is a tear or a hole in the eardrum, which can allow bacteria to more easily reach the middle ear and cause infection. A ruptured eardrum may be caused by an infection (e.g., otitis media); direct trauma (e.g., being slapped or being hit by a ball on the external ear); changes in pressure (e.g., rapid ascent or descent in a plane or underwater); loud, sudden noises (e.g., explosion); or foreign objects in the ear (e.g., cotton swab or bobby pin pushed too far into the ear canal).

SIGNS AND SYMPTOMS. A ruptured eardrum can be very painful initially. Other signs and symptoms include sharp, sudden ear pain or discomfort; tinnitus; clear, pus-filled, or bloody drainage from the ear; sudden decrease in ear pain followed by drainage; and hearing loss. Use of an otoscope may identify the damaged area.

MANAGEMENT. The individual should be referred immediately to a physician for further care. Most small to moderate perforations of the tympanic membrane heal without treatment within a few weeks, although some may take months. If the tear or hole in the eardrum does not heal by itself, treatment may involve an eardrum patch or surgery. Closing the perforation is essential to prevent water from entering the ear while showering, bathing, or swimming, which could cause middle ear infection. Hearing is improved, and any tinnitus is diminished. Repair of the perforation also prevents development of a skin cyst in the middle ear (cholesteatoma), which can cause chronic middle ear infections and damage the ear structure.

 Ice should be placed on the wrestler's ear to control swelling. If any hemorrhage or edema between the perichondrium and cartilage appears to flatten the wrinkles or creases of the ear, the individual should be referred immediately to a physician for follow-up care. Protective earwear should be worn by all wrestlers at every practice and competition.

EYE CONDITIONS

While moving through the circuit training area in an exercise facility, an adult exerciser received a significant blow to the eye from another exerciser's elbow. What signs and symptoms indicate a serious condition?

The eyes are exposed daily to potential trauma and injury, yet many eye injuries could be prevented by wearing protective eyewear. This is especially true in racquetball and squash, in which players are confined to a limited space with swinging racquets and balls traveling at high speeds. Individuals who require corrective lenses should use strong plastic or semirigid rubber frames and impact-resistant lenses. If glasses are not required, the American Academy of Pediatrics and the American Academy of Ophthalmology recommend that protective eyewear and/or face masks should be worn during participation in sports with a high risk of injury (22). Sport participants with only one good eye should consult an ophthalmologist to determine what mandatory protective eyewear should be worn to prevent further injury. Box 9.7 identifies the signs and symptoms of eye conditions that necessitate further examination by a physician.

Periorbital Ecchymosis

Signs and Symptoms

Impact forces can cause significant swelling and hemorrhage into the surrounding eyelids. This discoloration is called **periorbital ecchymosis** or, more commonly, a black eye.

Management

Trauma to the eye requires inspection for obvious abnormalities, palpation of the orbit for a possible orbital fracture, and assessment of pupillary response to light by shining a concentrated light

Box 9.7   Eye "Red Flags" Requiring Further Examination by a Physician

- Visual disturbances or loss of vision
- Unequal pupils or bilateral, dilated pupils
- Irregular eye movement or failure to accommodate to light
- Severe ecchymosis and swelling (raccoon eyes)
- Suspected corneal abrasion or corneal laceration

- Blood in the anterior chamber
- Embedded foreign body
- Individual complaining of floaters, light flashes, or a "curtain falling over the eye"
- Itching, burning, watery eye that appears pink
- Displaced contact lens that cannot be easily removed

beam into the eye and noting the bilateral rate of constriction. The ability of an individual to focus clearly on an object must be assessed. The anterior chamber of the eye should be inspected for any obvious bleeding (see *Hemorrhage into the Anterior Chamber*). Treatment involves controlling the swelling and hemorrhage by using crushed ice or ice water in a latex surgical glove; it is essential that the glove does not have rosin or other powdered substances on it. Because of possible leakage, chemical ice bags should not be used. This condition requires referral to an ophthalmologist for further examination to rule out an underlying fracture or injury to the globe.

Foreign Bodies

Signs and Symptoms

Dust or dirt in the eyes can lead to intense pain and tearing. The individual may resist any attempt to open the eyelids to view the eye.

Management

The foreign body, if not embedded or on the cornea, should be removed and the eye inspected for any scratches, abrasions, or lacerations (Field Strategy 9.4).

A foreign object that is impaled or embedded should not be touched, and removal should not be attempted. Activation of the emergency plan is warranted, including summoning of EMS. Medically trained individuals will stabilize the object and provide rigid protection for the orbit. In the cornea, a fluorescein stain may reveal the object's location, and topical anesthetics may be necessary to facilitate the physician's examination.

Sty

Signs and Symptoms

A sty (hordeolum) is an infection of the sebaceous gland of an eyelash or eyelash follicle. The condition starts as a red nodule that will progress into a painful pustule within a few days.

FIELD STRATEGY 9.4

Removing a Foreign Body from the Eye

1. Examine the lower lid by gently pulling the skin down below the eye. Ask the individual to look up, and inspect the lower portion of the globe and eyelid for any foreign object.
2. Examine the upper lid by asking the individual to look downward.
3. Grasp the eyelashes and pull downward.
4. Place a cotton-tipped applicator on the outside portion of the upper lid.
5. Pull the lid over the applicator, and hold the rolled lid against the upper bony ridge of the orbit.
6. Remove the foreign body with a sterile, moist gauze pad. If you are unable to successfully remove the foreign object, patch both eyes with a sterile, nonpressure, oval gauze pad, and refer the individual to a physician for immediate care.

Management

Treatment involves application of warm, moist compresses. If the pustule does not improve within 2 days, physician referral is required, because a prescription topical ointment may be necessary.

Conjunctivitis (Pinkeye)

Signs and Symptoms

Conjunctivitis is an inflammation, often resulting from chlorine irritation or bacterial infection of the conjunctiva. The condition leads to itching, burning, and watering of the eye, causing the conjunctiva to become inflamed and red and giving a "pink eye" appearance.

Management

This bacterial condition can be highly infectious, so the individual should be referred immediately to a physician for medical treatment.

Corneal Abrasion

Signs and Symptoms

Occasionally, a foreign body scratches the cornea, resulting in a sudden onset of pain, tearing, and photophobia. Blinking and movement of the eye only aggravate the condition. Examination may not reveal a foreign object, but the individual continues to complain that something is in the eye.

Management

Initial management involves covering the eye with a dry, sterile dressing. A corneal abrasion is best seen by using a fluorescein dye strip. Soft contact lenses should be removed before applying the dye, because these lenses absorb the dye and can be ruined. The orange color of the dye is augmented by using a blue light, changing the orange dye to a bright green and illuminating the abrasion. Treatment usually involves a topical ointment, such as 2% homatropine, to reduce pain, relax ciliary muscle spasms, and prevent secondary bacterial infection. It may be advantageous to wear an eye patch for 24 to 48 hours. If used, the patch must be tight enough to ensure that the lids are closed beneath the patch and firm enough to prevent the lids from opening and closing.

Corneal Laceration

Signs and Symptoms

Lacerations to the cornea are caused by sharp objects, such as fingernails, darts, skate blades, or broken glass. Signs and symptoms include severe pain, discomfort, decreased visual acuity, and distortion or displacement of the pupil. The pupil should be inspected for symmetry with the opposite eye. Lacerations of the cornea often incarcerate iris tissue, causing distortion and displacement of the pupil.

Management

If a laceration is suspected, any pressure on the globe should be avoided to prevent extrusion of the intraocular contents. The eye should be covered using a protective shield with the pressure exerted on the bony orbit, not on the soft tissue. This condition warrants immediate referral to a physician. The individual should be moved in either a supine or upright position. (Avoid a prone or head-down position.) As such, it may be necessary to activate the emergency plan, including summoning EMS, for transportation to the nearest medical facility.

Subconjunctival Hemorrhage

Signs and Symptoms

Direct trauma also can lead to **subconjunctival hemorrhage**. Several small capillaries rupture, making the white sclera of the eye appear red, blotchy, and inflamed. This condition is not as serious as it may appear to be.

Management

This relatively harmless condition requires no treatment and resolves spontaneously in 1 to 3 weeks. If blurred vision, pain, limited eye movement, or blood in the anterior chamber is present, however, immediate referral to an ophthalmologist is warranted.

Hemorrhage into the Anterior Chamber

Hemorrhage into the anterior chamber (**hyphema**) usually results from blunt trauma caused by a small ball (e.g., squash or racquetball), hockey puck, stick (e.g., field hockey or ice hockey), or swinging racquet (e.g., squash or racquetball). The small size of the object enables it to fit within the confines of the eye orbit, thereby inflicting direct damage to the eye.

■■■■ FIGURE 9.21 **Hyphema.** Blood in the anterior chamber of the eye signals a serious eye injury.

Signs and Symptoms

Initially, a red tinge in the anterior chamber may be present, but within a few hours, blood begins to settle into the anterior chamber, giving a characteristic meniscus appearance (Fig. 9.21). Frequently, it occurs in microscopic quantities, and visual acuity may not be affected. Such bleeding indicates that an intraocular injury has occurred, however, and the source of the bleeding must be identified to prevent recurrent bleeding, which can lead to both massive and destructive results.

Management

Both eyes should be patched. Because this condition necessitates immediate referral to a physician, it may be necessary to activate the emergency plan, including summoning EMS, so that the individual can be transported in a semireclining or a seated position. The condition requires hospitalization, bed rest, bilateral patching of the eyes, and sedation. The initial hemorrhage usually resolves in a few days, with good prognosis for full recovery.

Detached Retina

Damage to the posterior segment of the eye can occur with or without trauma to the anterior segment. A **detached retina** occurs when fluid seeps into the retinal break and separates the neurosensory retina from the retinal epithelium. This can occur days or even weeks after the initial trauma.

Signs and Symptoms

Detachment almost always begins at the retinal periphery, resulting in a positive scotoma (a blind spot perceived by the patient) at the edge of the visual field. As the detachment progresses and the scotoma enlarges, the individual frequently describes the condition with phrases like "a curtain fell over my eye" or "I keep seeing flashes of lights going on and off." An ophthalmoscope may be used to view the optic disc and retinal vessels.

See *Field Strategy: Using the Ophthalmoscope*, found on the companion website at thePoint.

Management

If a detached retina is suspected, both eyes should be patched. Immediate referral to an ophthalmologist is required, because surgery often is necessary.

Orbital "Blowout" Fracture

A blowout fracture is caused by the impact from a blunt object (one usually larger than the eye orbit). On impact, forces drive the orbital contents posteriorly against the orbital walls. This sudden increase in intraorbital pressure is released in the area of least resistance, typically the orbital floor (roof of maxillary sinus). The result is that the globe descends into the defect in the floor.

FIGURE 9.22 Orbital "blowout" fracture. An orbital fracture can entrap the inferior rectus muscle, leading to an inability to elevate the eye.

Signs and Symptoms

Examination may reveal **diplopia**, absent eye movement, numbness on the side of the fracture below the eye, and a recessed, downward displacement of the globe. The lack of eye movement becomes evident when the individual is asked to look up and only one eye is able to move (Fig. 9.22).

Management

Ice should be applied to the area to limit swelling; however, do not add additional compression or pressure over the suspected fracture site. The individual should be referred immediately to a physician. Tomograms or radiographs are necessary to confirm a fracture, and surgery may be indicated to repair the defect in the orbital floor.

Displaced Contact Lens

Hard contact lenses can slow the progression of **myopia** (nearsightedness). In sports, however, soft contact lenses are preferred, both because eye accommodation and adjustment time are less and because the lenses can be easily replaced and worn for longer periods of time.

Hard contact lenses frequently are involved in corneal abrasions. Foreign objects get underneath the lens and damage the cornea, or the cornea may be injured while putting in or taking out the lens. If irritation is present, the lens should be removed and cleaned. In an eye injury, individuals may be able to remove the lens themselves. Pain or photophobia may preclude them from doing this, however, and it may become necessary to assist them. Field Strategy 9.5 demonstrates a full assessment of an eye injury.

Dilated pupils, any abnormal eye movement, throbbing pain or headache, and vision disturbances such as diplopia, sensitivity to light, and loss of all or part of a field of vision indicate a serious eye injury that warrants immediate referral.

SUMMARY

1. Wearing protective equipment can significantly reduce the incidence and severity of head and facial injuries.

2. Minor injuries, such as nosebleeds, contusions, abrasions, lacerations, and minor concussions, can be handled easily on the field by the examiner. If complications arise or the condition does not improve within a reasonable amount of time, the examiner should immediately consult a physician about the injury.

3. Signs that indicate a possible skull fracture include deformity, unequal pupils, discoloration around both eyes or behind the ears, bleeding or CSF leaking from the nose and/or ear, and any loss of sight or smell.

4. Signs or symptoms of increasing intracranial pressure following head trauma include severe headache, pupil irregularity or irregular eye tracking, confusion or progressive or sudden impairment of consciousness, rising blood pressure and falling pulse rate, and drastic changes in emotional control.

5. Signs and symptoms of a concussion include headache, dizziness or vertigo, lack of awareness of surroundings, nausea and vomiting, deteriorating level of consciousness, disturbance of vigilance with heightened distractibility, inability to maintain coherent thought patterns, and inability to carry out a sequence of goal-directed movements.

6. Injuries that indicate increasing intracranial pressure, memory dysfunction, or gross observable incoordination require immediate referral to a physician.

FIELD STRATEGY 9.5

Eye Evaluation

1. Check airway, breathing, and circulation.
2. Determine responsiveness.
3. History:
   - Determine primary complaint. Ask about the level of pain, discomfort, extent of voluntary eyelid movement, and extent of vision.
   - Determine mechanism of injury. Objects larger than the eye orbit may lead to orbital fracture. Objects smaller than the eye orbit may lead to direct trauma to the eye globe. Did the trauma result from blunt trauma, a sharp object, or a projectile?

4. Observation and inspection:
   - Look for obvious deformity or abnormal deviation in the surrounding eye orbit.
   - Observe ecchymosis and extent of swelling in the eyelids and surrounding tissue. If the eyelid is swollen shut and the individual cannot voluntarily open it, do not force it open, which may cause further damage.
   - Observe any bleeding from deep lacerations of the eyelid.
   - Observe the level of both pupils and the eye globe for anterior or posterior displacement, presence of any corneal lacerations, and bleeding in the anterior chamber.
   - Inspect pupil size, accommodation to light, and sensitivity to light with a penlight.

5. Palpation:
   - Carefully palpate the bony rim of the eye orbit and cheek bone for any swelling, depressions, crepitus, or mobility.
   - Control any bleeding.

6. Special tests:
   - Determine eye vision. Compare the vision of the uninjured eye to the injured eye. Is it blurred or sensitive to light? Does the individual have double vision? Can the individual distinguish how many fingers you are holding up in all four quadrants of vision? Can the individual distinguish objects that are close from objects that are far away?
   - Determine eye movement. Move your finger through the six cardinal planes of vision. Do the eyes move in a coordinated manner? If one eye moves upward and the other remains in a stationary position, the inferior rectus muscle may be entrapped because of an orbital fracture.
   - Vision disturbances, such as persistent blurred vision, diplopia, sensitivity to light, loss of all or part of a field of vision, dilated pupils, any abnormal eye movement, and throbbing pain or headache, indicate a serious eye injury that warrants immediate referral.

7. Fractures to the facial bones often result in malocclusion.

8. The nose is particularly susceptible to lateral displacement from trauma. Simultaneously, the trauma also may lead to a concussion.

9. When a loose tooth has been displaced outwardly or laterally, the examiner should try to place the tooth back into its normal position without forcing it. Teeth that are intruded should be left alone; any attempt to move the tooth may result in permanent loss of the tooth. The individual should be referred to a dentist immediately.

10. A dislocated tooth should be located, rinsed in milk or a saline solution, and replaced intra-orally within the tooth socket. The individual should be seen by a dentist within 30 minutes for replacement of the tooth.

11. Cauliflower ear is common in wrestlers but is completely preventable by wearing proper headgear at all times when on the mat.

12. Otitis externa is a bacterial infection involving the lining of the external auditory meatus, commonly called swimmer's ear. Otitis media is a localized infection of the middle ear.

13. A foreign body in the eye, if not embedded or on the cornea, should be removed and the eye inspected for any scratches, abrasions, or lacerations.

14. Direct trauma to the eye can lead to corneal laceration, rupture of the globe, hemorrhage into the anterior chamber, detached retina, or orbital fracture. Loss of visual acuity, abnormal eye movement, diplopia, numbness below the eye, or a downward displacement of the globe should signal a serious condition. The individual should be referred to an ophthalmologist immediately.

REFERENCES

1. Ghiselli G, Schaadt G, McAllister DR. On-the-field evaluation of an athlete with a head or neck injury. Clin Sports Med 2003;22(3):445–465.

2. Logan SM, Bell GW, Leonard JC. Acute subdural hematoma in a high school football player after two unreported episodes of head trauma: a case report. J Ath Train 2001;36(4):433–436.

3. Putukian M, Madden CC. Head injuries. In: Mellion MB, Walsh WM, Madden C, Putukian M, Shelton GL, eds. The Team Physician's Handbook. Philadelphia: Hanley & Belfus, 2002.

4. Bailes JE, Hudson V. Classification of sport-related head trauma: a spectrum of mild to severe injury. J Ath Train 2001;36(3):236–243.

5. Aubry M, Cantu RC, Dvorak J, et al. Summary and agreement statement of the First International Conference on Concussion in Sport, Vienna, 2001: Recommendations for the improvement of safety and health of athletes who may suffer concussive injuries. Phys Sportsmed 2002;30(2):57–63.

6. McCrory P, Johnston K, Meeuwisse W, et al. Summary and agreement statement of the Second International Conference on Concussion in Sport, Prague, 2004. Phys Sportsmed 2005;33(4):29–44.

7. Quality Standards Subcommittee of the American Academy of Neurology. Practice parameter: the management of concussion in sports. Neurology 1997;48(3):581–585.

8. Cantu RC. Posttraumatic retrograde and anterograde amnesia: pathophysiology and implications in grading and safe return to play. J Ath Train 2001;36(3):244–248.

9. Guskiewicz KM, Bruce SL, Cantu RC, et al. National Athletic Trainers' Association position statement: management of sport-related concussion. J Ath Train 2004;39(3):280–297.

10. Guskiewicz KM, Weaver NL, Padua DA, Garrett WE. Epidemiology of concussion in collegiate and high school football players. Am J Sports Med 2000;28(5):643–650.

11. McCrea M, Kelly JP, Randolph C. Standardized Assessment of Concussion (SAC): Manual for Administration, Scoring, and Interpretation. Waukesha, WI: CHS, 1996.

12. McCrea M, Kelly JP, Kluge J, et al. Standardized assessment of concussion in football players. Neurology 1997;48(3):586–588.

13. McCrea M, Kelly JP, Randolph C. Standardized Assessment of Concussion (SAC): Manual for Administration, Scoring, and Interpretation (2nd ed.). Waukesha, WI: CHS, 2000.

14. McCrea M. Standardized mental status testing on the sideline after sport-related concussion. J Ath Train 2001;36(3):274–279.

15. Guskiewicz KM. Concussion in sport: the grading-system dilemma. Ath Ther Today 2001;6(1):18–27.

16. Romeo SJ, Hawley CJ, Romeo MW, et al. Facial injuries in sports. Phys Sportsmed 2005;33(4):45–53.

17. Tu HK, Davis LF, Nique TA. Maxillofacial injuries. In: Mellion MB, Walsh WM, Madden C, Putukian M, Shelton G, eds. The Team Physician's Handbook. Philadelphia: Hanley & Belfus, 2002.

18. Iida S, Kogo M, Sugiura T, et al. Retrospective analysis of 1,502 patients with facial fractures. Int J Oral Maxillofac Surg 2001;30(4):286–290.

19. Bickley LS, Szilagyi PG. Bates' Guide to Physical Examination and History Taking. Philadelphia: Lippincott Williams & Wilkins, 2003.

20. Woodmansey KF. Athletic mouth guards prevent orofacial injuries. Col Health 1997;45(5):179–182.

21. Kumamoto DP, Jacob M, Nickelsen D. Oral trauma: on-field assessment. Phys Sportsmed 1995;23(5):53–62.

22. American Academy of Pediatrics and American Academy of Ophthalmology. Policy statement: protective eyewear for young athletes. Pediatrics 2004;113(3):619–622.

Cervical and Thoracic Spinal Conditions

STUDENT OUTCOMES

1. Locate and explain the functional significance of the bony and soft-tissue structures of the cervical and thoracic regions of the spine.

2. Describe the motion capabilities in the cervical and thoracic regions of the spine.

3. Identify the factors that contribute to mechanical loading on the cervical and thoracic regions of the spine.

4. Describe specific strategies in activities of daily living to reduce stress in the cervical and thoracic regions.

5. Identify the anatomical variations that can predispose individuals to cervical and thoracic injuries.

6. Explain the measures used to prevent injury to the cervical and thoracic spinal regions.

7. Describe the common injuries and conditions found in the cervical and thoracic regions.

8. Describe a thorough assessment of the cervical and thoracic spinal regions.

9. List the rehabilitative exercises for the cervical and thoracic spinal regions.

ROLE DELINEATION COMPETENCIES

The following Performance Domains and Tasks defined in the National Athletic Trainers' Association Board of Certification *Role Delineation Study*, 5th Edition are addressed in this chapter:

BOC COMPETENCIES

II. Clinical Evaluation and Diagnosis

A. Obtain a history through observation, interview, and/or review of relevant records to assess current or potential injury, illness, or condition.

B. Inspect the involved area(s) visually to assess the injury, illness, or health-related condition.

C. Palpate the involved area(s) using standard techniques to assess the injury, illness, or health-related condition.

D. Perform specific tests in accordance with accepted procedures to assess the injury, illness, or health-related condition.

E. Formulate a clinical impression by interpreting the signs, symptoms, and predisposing factors of the injury, illness, or condition to determine the appropriate course of action.

III. Immediate Care

A. Employ life-saving techniques through the use of standard emergency procedures in order to reduce morbidity and the incidence of mortality.

B. Prevent exacerbation of non–life threatening condition(s) through the use of standard procedures in order to reduce morbidity.

C. Facilitate the timely transfer of care for conditions beyond the scope of practice of the athletic trainer by implementing appropriate referral strategies to stabilize and/or prevent exacerbation of the condition(s).

IV. Treatment, Rehabilitation, and Reconditioning

E. Reassess the status of injuries, illnesses, and/or conditions using standard techniques and documentation strategies in order to determine appropriate treatment, rehabilitation, and/or reconditioning and to evaluate readiness to return to a desired level of activity.

F. Educate the appropriate individual(s) in the treatment, rehabilitation, and reconditioning of injuries, illnesses, and/or conditions using applicable methods and materials to facilitate recovery, function, and/or performance.

The spine is a complex linkage system that transfers loads between the upper and lower extremities, enables motion of the trunk in all three planes, and protects the delicate spinal cord. Most injuries to the neck and upper back are relatively minor, consisting of contusions, muscle strains, and ligament sprains. Acute spinal fractures and dislocations in this region are extremely serious, however, and can lead to paralysis or death. Annually, sports-related cervical injuries account for 27% of all spinal cord injuries occurring in children, with the most common victim being an older adolescent male and the most commonly involved sport being football (1). Prompt and accurate on-site assessment is essential for optimizing the outcomes of these potentially devastating injuries (2).

This chapter begins with a review of the intricate anatomical structures that make up the cervical and thoracic regions of the spine, followed by a discussion of the kinematics and kinetics of these regions. A discussion concerning the identification of anatomical variations that may predispose individuals to cervical and thoracic spinal conditions leads into the strategies used to prevent injury. Information regarding common injuries sustained within these regions of the spinal column during participation in sport and physical activity is followed by a presentation of techniques used in spinal injury assessment. Finally, examples of general rehabilitation exercises for the cervical and thoracic regions are provided.

ANATOMY OF THE CERVICAL AND THORACIC SPINE

The five regions of the spine—namely, the cervical, thoracic, lumbar, sacral, and coccygeal regions—are structurally and functionally distinct. The spine includes four normal curves (Fig. 10.1). As viewed from the side, the thoracic and sacral curves are convex posteriorly, and the lumbar and cervical curves are concave posteriorly. These curves constitute posture and can be modified by a host of factors, including heredity, disease, and forces acting on the spine. Abnormal spinal curves are referred to as curvatures. Exacerbated curvature of the thoracic region is discussed later in this chapter.

Cervical and Thoracic Spinal Column and Vertebrae

The human body has seven cervical vertebrae and 12 thoracic vertebrae (Figs. 10.2 and 10.3). A typical vertebra consists of a body, a hollow ring known as the vertebral arch, and several bony processes (see Fig. 10.3). The superior and inferior articular processes mate with the articular processes of adjacent vertebrae to form the **facet joints**. The right and left pedicles have notches on their superior and inferior borders that provide openings between adjacent pedicles and are called intervertebral foramina. The spinal nerves pass through these foramina. The spinous and transverse processes serve as handles for muscle attachments. Forming a stacked column, the neural arches, posterior sides of the bodies, and intervertebral disks form a protective passageway for the spinal cord and associated blood vessels. The thinnest part of the neural arch is called the **pars interarticularis**. The pars region of the vertebrae is susceptible to stress fractures.

The first cervical vertebra is called the **atlas**, because it bears the weight of the head. Articulating with the occipital condyles, the atlanto-occipital joint permits the nodding of the head (see Fig. 10.2).

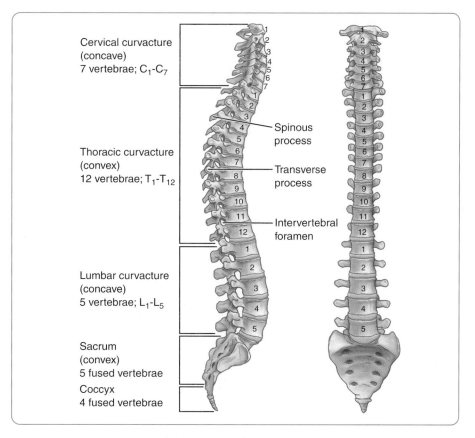

Cervical curvacture
(concave)
7 vertebrae; C_1-C_7

Thoracic curvacture
(convex)
12 vertebrae; T_1-T_{12}

Lumbar curvacture
(concave)
5 vertebrae; L_1-L_5

Sacrum
(convex)
5 fused vertebrae

Coccyx
4 fused vertebrae

Spinous process

Transverse process

Intervertebral foramen

FIGURE 10.1 Vertebral column. Four characteristic curves of the spine can be viewed from the lateral aspect.

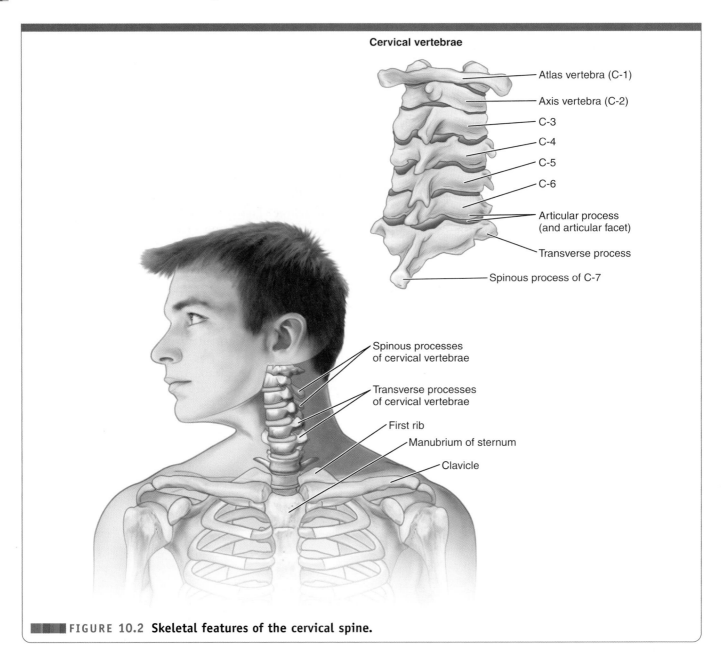

Cervical vertebrae

Atlas vertebra (C-1)

Axis vertebra (C-2)

C-3

C-4

C-5

C-6

Articular process
(and articular facet)

Transverse process

Spinous process of C-7

Spinous processes
of cervical vertebrae

Transverse processes
of cervical vertebrae

First rib

Manubrium of sternum

Clavicle

FIGURE 10.2 Skeletal features of the cervical spine.

The atlas does not have a body or a spinous process. Instead, it has anterior and posterior arches and a thick, lateral mass. The second cervical vertebra, or **axis**, is characterized by a tooth-like process called the dens or odontoid process, which projects upward from its body. This process is held in place against the inner surface of the atlas by the transverse ligament. This joint allows the head to rotate and pivot on the neck. The transverse processes of the cervical vertebrae have a foramen (**transverse foramen**), through which the vertebral artery, vein, and a plexus of sympathetic nerves pass. The spinous processes of the cervical vertebrae C_2–C_6 often are bifid. The seventh cervical vertebra, or vertebra prominens, has a large spinous process with a somewhat bulbous tip.

The thoracic vertebrae have extra facets (costal facets) on the transverse processes and the body for articulation with the ribs (see Fig. 10.3). The spinous processes of the thoracic vertebrae tend to be long and slender, and they direct markedly downward so that they overlap each other. Those of the lower thoracic vertebrae are broader and directed more posteriorly, in this respect being transitional between typical thoracic and typical lumbar vertebrae.

Vertebral size progressively increases from the cervical region down through the lumbar region. This serves a functional purpose, because when the body is in an upright position, each vertebra

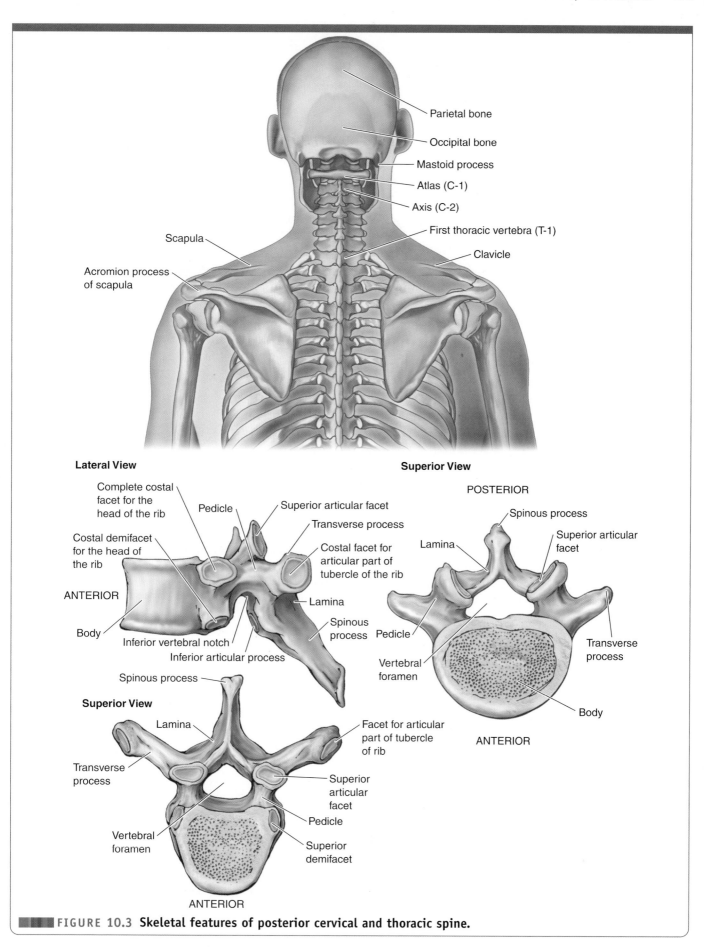

FIGURE 10.3 Skeletal features of posterior cervical and thoracic spine.

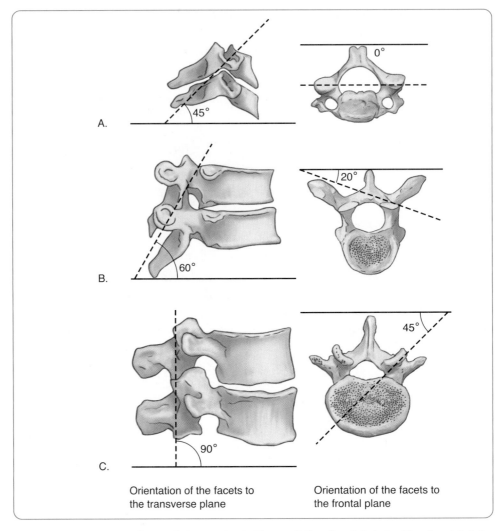

A.

45°

0°

B.

60°

20°

C.

90°

45°

Orientation of the facets to
the transverse plane

Orientation of the facets to
the frontal plane

FIGURE 10.4 Approximate orientations of the facet joints. The facet joint
orientation in both the sagittal plane (lateral view) and transverse plane (superior
view) shifts progressively throughout the length of the spinal column. **A,** Cervical vertebrae (C₃–C₇). **B,** Thoracic vertebrae. **C,** Lumbar vertebrae.

must support the weight of the trunk positioned above it as well as that of the arms and head. The
size and angulation of the vertebral processes also vary throughout the spinal column. This changes
the orientation of the facet joints, which limit range of motion (ROM) in the different spinal
regions (Fig. 10.4).

Within the cervical, thoracic, and lumbar regions, any two adjacent vertebrae and the soft tissues
between them are collectively referred to as a motion segment. The motion segment is referred to
as the functional unit of the spine (Fig. 10.5).

Intervertebral Disks

Fibrocartilaginous disks provide cushioning between the articulating vertebral bodies. In the intervertebral disk consists a thick ring of fibrous cartilage referred to as the **annulus fibrosus,** which
surrounds a gelatinous material known as the **nucleus pulposus.** The disks have a dual function:
They serve as shock absorbers and allow the spine to bend. Because the disks receive no blood
supply, they must rely on changes in posture and body position to produce a pumping action that
brings in nutrients and flushes out metabolic waste products with an influx and outflux of fluid.
Because maintaining a fixed body position curtails this pumping action, sitting in one position for
a long period of time can negatively affect disk health.

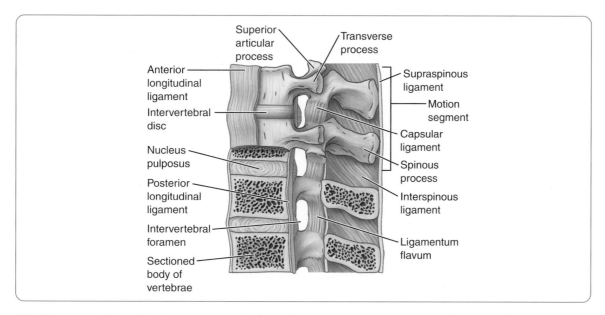

■■■■ FIGURE 10.5 **Motion segment of the spine.** A motion segment includes two adjacent verte-brae and the intervening soft tissues. It is considered to be the functional unit of the spine.

Ligaments of the Spine

A number of ligaments support the spine (Fig. 10.6). Anterior and posterior longitudinal ligaments connect the vertebral bodies of the motion segments. The supraspinous ligament attaches to the spinous processes throughout the length of the spine and is enlarged in the cervical region, where it is known as the ligamentum nuchae (or "ligament of the neck"). Another major ligament, the

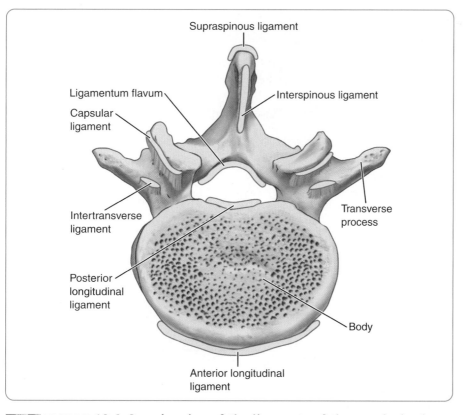

■■■■ FIGURE 10.6 **Superior view of the ligaments of the vertebral column.**

ligamentum flavum, connects the pedicles of adjacent vertebrae. This ligament contains a high proportion of elastic fibers that keep it constantly in tension, contributing to spinal stability. The interspinous ligaments, intertransverse ligaments, and ligamentum flava link the spinous processes, transverse processes, and laminae of adjacent vertebrae, respectively.

See *Muscles of the Spine,* found on the companion website at thePoint, for the attachments, actions, and innervations of the major muscles of the upper trunk.

Muscles of the Cervical and Thoracic Regions of the Spine and Trunk

The muscles of the neck and trunk are paired, with one on the left and one on the right side of the body (Figs. 10.7 and 10.8). These muscles produce lateral flexion and/or rotation of the trunk when they act unilaterally and trunk flexion or extension when they act bilaterally. Collectively, the primary movers for back extension are called the erector spinae muscles.

Spinal Cord and Spinal Nerves

The brain and spinal cord make up the central nervous system. The spinal cord extends from the brainstem to the level of the first or second lumbar vertebrae. Like the brain, the spinal cord is encased in the three meninges. The spinal cord serves as the major neural pathway for conducting sensory impulses to the brain and motor impulses from the brain. It also provides direct connections between sensory and motor nerves inside the cord, enabling reflex activity. Deep tendon reflexes are used consistently during injury assessment to determine possible spinal nerve damage. Exaggerated, distorted, or absent reflexes indicate damage to the nervous system, often before other signs are apparent.

Thirty-one pairs of spinal nerves emanate from the cord, including eight cervical and 12 thoracic. Many of the spinal nerves converge (combine) and diverge (separate) to form a complex network of interjoining nerves, called a nerve plexus.

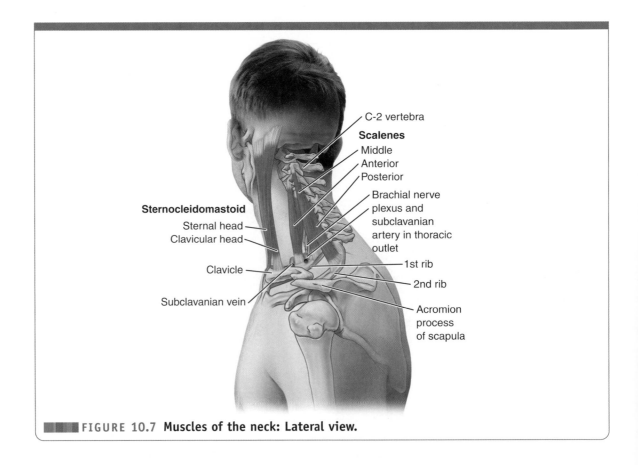

FIGURE 10.7 Muscles of the neck: Lateral view.

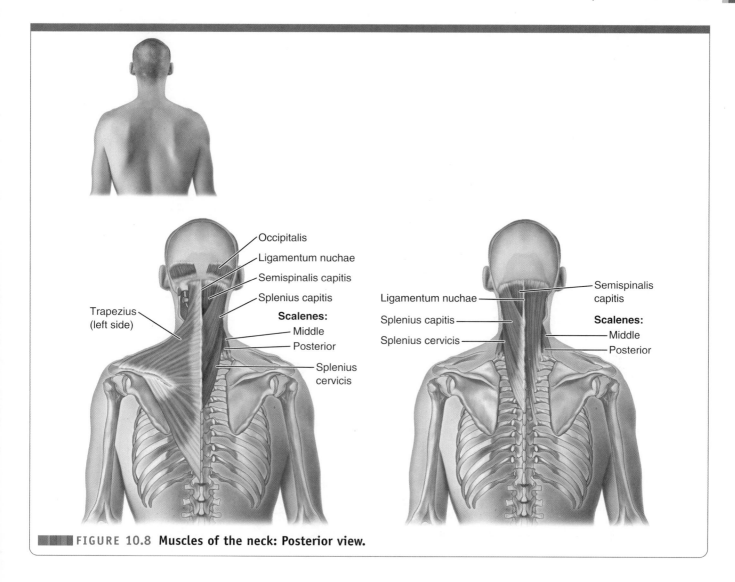

■■■■FIGURE 10.8 **Muscles of the neck: Posterior view.**

The Cervical Plexus

The cervical plexus consists of the ventral rami of spinal nerves C_1–C_4. These nerves innervate muscles of the neck, shoulder, and diaphragm (phrenic nerves, C_3–C_5) and supply sensation for the skin of the ear, neck, and upper chest. The plexus lies lateral in relation to the first three cervical vertebrae, ventrolateral to the levator scapulae and scalenus medius, and deep to the sternocleidomastoid muscle. Impingement of the plexus results in headaches, neck pain, and breathing difficulties and most often results from pressure on the nerves by the suboccipital and sternocleidomastoid muscles.

The Brachial Plexus

The shoulder region and upper extremity receive sensory and motor innervation from the brachial plexus, which originates from the C_5 through T_1 nerve roots. These nerve roots converge and diverge to form three trunks, followed by three divisions and then by three cords. This complex structure terminates in distal branches that form the musculocutaneous, median, ulnar, axillary, and radial nerves, which innervate the arm, forearm, and hand (Fig, 10.9). The C_5 and C_6 nerve roots form the upper trunk, the C_7 forms the middle trunk, and the C_8 and T_1 form the lower trunk. Each trunk then divides into anterior and posterior divisions. The posterior divisions converge to form the posterior cord. The anterior divisions of the upper and middle trunk form the lateral cord, whereas the anterior division of the lower trunk forms the medial cord.

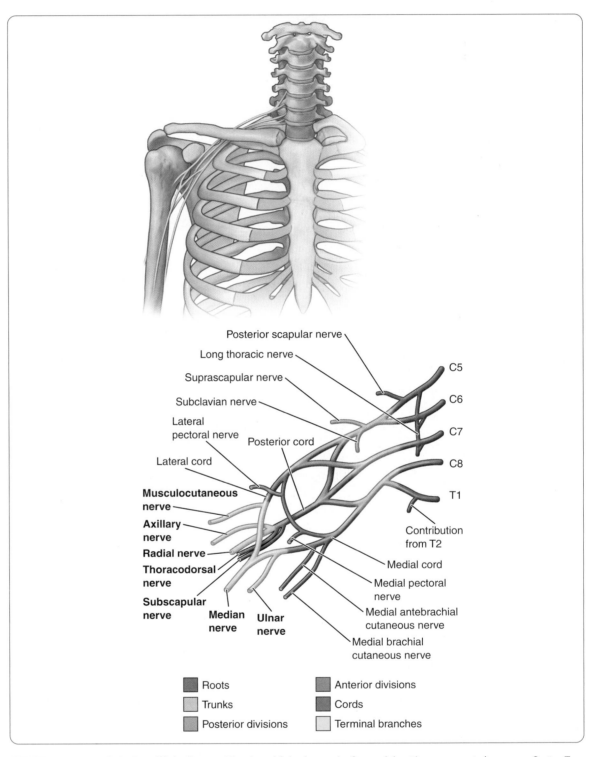

Posterior scapular nerve

Long thoracic nerve

Suprascapular nerve

Subclavian nerve

Lateral pectoral nerve

Posterior cord

Lateral cord

Musculocutaneous nerve

Axillary nerve

Radial nerve

Thoracodorsal nerve

Subscapular nerve

Median nerve

Ulnar nerve

C5

C6

C7

C8

T1

Contribution from T2

Medial cord

Medial pectoral nerve

Medial antebrachial cutaneous nerve

Medial brachial cutaneous nerve

Roots

Trunks

Posterior divisions

Anterior divisions

Cords

Terminal branches

■■■■ FIGURE 10.9 **Brachial plexus.** The brachial plexus is formed by the segmental nerves C_5 to T_1.

The posterior cord branches into the axillary and radial nerves, which innervate the shoulder, elbow, wrist, and finger extensors. Placing the arm in anatomical position, the lateral half of the medial cord joins with the medial half of the lateral cord to form the large median nerve that innervates most of the wrist and finger flexors. The remaining portion of the medial cord terminates as the ulnar nerve, which innervates the flexor carpi ulnaris and the intrinsic muscles of the hand. The remaining portion of the lateral cord terminates as the musculocutaneous nerve, which innervates

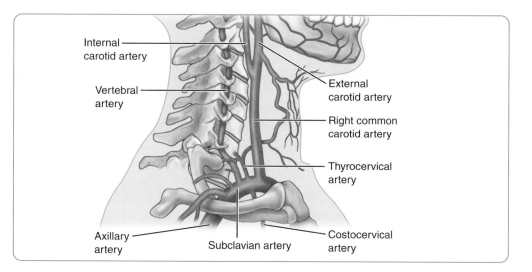

FIGURE 10.10 Blood vessels to the spine. Cervical vertebrae receive a large portion of their blood supply from the vertebral artery, a branch off of the subclavian artery.

the main elbow flexors. Minor branches from the medial and lateral cords innervate the pectoral muscles and cutaneous nerves on the medial arm and forearm. Variations in the length and quality of the components of the brachial plexus often occur, adding to its complexity (3).

Blood Vessels

The largest blood vessels coursing through the neck are the common carotid arteries (Fig. 10.10). The common carotid arteries divide into external and internal carotid arteries, which provide the major blood supply to the brain, head, and face. The vertebral arteries, which are located in the posterior neck, are a source of blood supply for the spinal cord.

KINEMATICS AND MAJOR MUSCLE ACTIONS OF THE CERVICAL AND THORACIC SPINE

Kinematics is the study of the spatial and temporal aspects of motion, which translates to movement, form, or technique. Evaluation of the kinematics of a particular movement can provide information about the timing and sequencing of movement, which can then yield important clues for injury prevention. This section describes the kinematics of the cervical and thoracic spine and identifies the muscles responsible for specific movements.

The vertebral joints enable motion in all planes of movement and permit circumduction. The motion allowed between any two adjacent vertebrae is small, so spinal movements always involve a number of motion segments. The ROM allowed at each motion segment is governed by anatomical constraints, which vary throughout the cervical, thoracic, and lumbar regions of the spine.

Flexion, Extension, and Hyperextension

Spinal flexion is anterior bending of the spine in the sagittal plane, with extension being the return to anatomical position from a position of flexion. The flexion-extension capability of the motion segments at different levels of the spine varies, with approximately 40° cumulatively allowed in the cervical region (4). Flexion-extension in the thoracic region is restricted by the rib cage, with a flexion-extension capability of only approximately 4° in the upper thoracic segments, of approximately 6° in the midthoracic segments, and of up to 12° in the two lower thoracic segments.

When the spine is extended backward past anatomical position in the sagittal plane, the motion is termed **hyperextension**. The ROM for spinal hyperextension is approximately 24° in the cervical region and 22° in the thoracic region (4).

Lateral Flexion and Rotation

Movement of the spine away from anatomical position in a lateral direction in the frontal plane is termed lateral flexion. In the thoracic region, the cumulative ROM for lateral flexion to each side is approximately 31°, with 49° permitted in the cervical region (4). Spinal rotation capability is greatest in the cervical region, with approximately 105° of motion allowed between the base of the skull and C_7 (4). In the thoracic region, approximately 9° of rotation is permitted among the upper six motion segments; however, from T_7–T_8 downward, the ROM in rotation progressively decreases.

KINETICS OF THE SPINE

Kinetics is the study of the forces associated with motion. Because force ultimately is the cause of injury, understanding the kinetics pertaining to the spine is an important foundation for understanding mechanisms of injury.

Forces acting on the spine include body weight, tension in the spinal ligaments and paraspinal muscles, intra-abdominal pressure, and any applied external loads. When the body is in an upright position, the major form of loading on the spine is axial. In this position, body weight, the weight of any load held in the hands, and the tension in the surrounding ligaments and muscles contribute to spinal compression. Although most of the axial compression load on the spine is borne by the vertebral bodies and disks, the facet joints also assist with load bearing. When the cervical spine is in hyperextension, the facet joints may bear up to approximately 30% of the load.

Effect of Loading

The primary axial load on the cervical spine during nonimpact situations is caused by the weight of the head. Holding the head in other than an upright position tends to elevate the tension required of the cervical paraspinal muscles. The compression load on the thoracic spine is affected by the weight of the body positioned above the thoracic spine and by the weight of any load held in the hands. External loads generally create more compression on the thoracic spine than changes in body position (5).

Effect of Impact

For individuals participating in high-speed collision and contact sports, impact forces are an inherent risk in terms of potential spinal injuries. Because the ROM in the cervical spine is greatest in flexion, a head position of extreme flexion generates the largest bending moment. When combined with axial compression loading, this generates the leading mechanism of injury for severe cervical spine injuries. For example, when a football tackle is executed with the head in a flexed position, the cervical spine is aligned in a segmented column and is subjected to both large compressional forces, generated by the cervical muscles, and axial impact forces (Fig. 10.11). Impact causes loading along the longitudinal axis of the cervical vertebrae, leading to compression deformation. The intervertebral disks can absorb some energy initially; however, as continued force is exerted, further deformation and buckling occurs, leading to failure of the intervertebral disks, cervical vertebrae, or both (Fig. 10.12). The potential results include subluxation, disk herniation, facet dislocation, or fracture-dislocation at one or more spinal levels. In soccer, heading the ball does not typically cause traumatic injury, but players may develop degenerative changes to the cervical spine earlier than the normal population because of the repetitive stress (6).

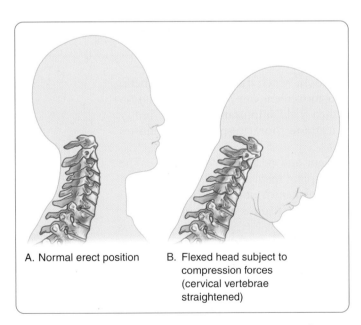

A. Normal erect position

B. Flexed head subject to compression forces (cervical vertebrae straightened)

■■■■■ FIGURE 10.11 **Axial loading. A,** In a normally erect position, the cervical spine is slightly extended. **B,** When a football tackle is executed with the head flexed at about 30°, the cervical vertebrae are aligned in a column and subjected to compression forces, generated by the cervical muscles, and to axial loading.

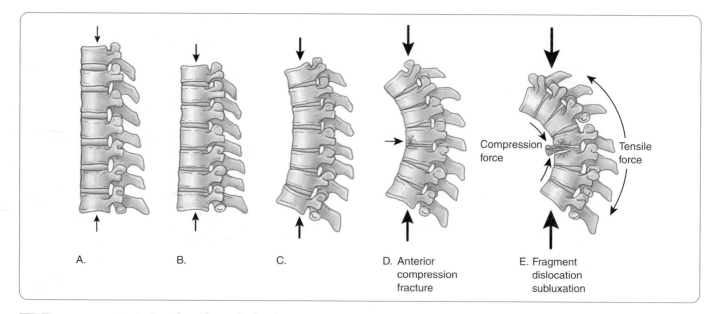

■■■■ FIGURE 10.12 **Results of cervical spine compression deformation. A** and **B,** Axial loading on the vertebral column causes compressive deformation of the intervertebral disks. **C,** Angular deformation and buckling occurs as the load continues and the maximum compression deformation is reached. **D** and **E,** Continued force results in an anterior compression fracture, subluxation, or dislocation.

ANATOMICAL VARIATIONS PREDISPOSING INDIVIDUALS TO SPINAL CONDITIONS

Mechanical stress derived from lateral spinal muscle imbalances or from sustaining repeated impact forces can cause back pain and/or injury. Excessive spinal curvatures can be congenital or acquired through weight training or sport participation.

Kyphosis

Accentuation of the thoracic curve is called **kyphosis** (Fig. 10.13A). The cause of kyphosis can be congenital, idiopathic (unknown), or secondary to osteoporosis. Congenital kyphosis arises from deficits in the formation of either the vertebral bodies or the anterior and posterior vertebral elements. Idiopathic kyphosis, also known as **Scheuermann's disease** or osteochondritis of the spine, is common among adolescents and involves development of one or more wedge-shaped vertebrae in the thoracic or lumbar regions through abnormal behavior of the epiphyseal plate. The individual typically has a round-shouldered appearance, with or without back pain. Weight lifters, gymnasts, and football linemen, who overdevelop the pectoral muscles, also are prone to this condition. In addition, it may be caused by overtraining with the butterfly stroke, hence the nickname "swimmer's back."

Scoliosis

Lateral curvature of the spine is known as **scoliosis** (Fig. 10.13B). The lateral deformity, coupled with rotational deformity of the involved vertebrae, may range from mild to

■■■■ FIGURE 10.13 **Spinal anomalies. A,** Thoracic kyphosis. **B,** Scoliosis.

severe. Scoliosis may appear as either a C- or an S-shaped curve involving the thoracic spine, lumbar spine, or both. Scoliosis can be structural or nonstructural. Structural scoliosis involves an inflexible curvature that persists with lateral bending of the spine. Nonstructural scoliosis curves are flexible and are corrected with lateral bending. Although congenital abnormalities, certain cancers, and leg length discrepancy may lead to scoliosis, approximately 70 to 90% of all cases are idiopathic. Idiopathic scoliosis most commonly is diagnosed between the ages of 10 and 13 years but can be seen at any age and is more common in females.

Symptoms associated with scoliosis vary with the severity of the condition. Mild cases (curvature < 20°) usually are asymptomatic and self-limiting. If scoliosis presents during childhood, reassessment should occur every 3 to 4 months until the adolescent has skeletally matured. Active treatment is not necessary as long as the curve is nonprogressive. If the individual is skeletally immature and the curve is moderate (20–45°) and progressive, bracing is necessary. In many instances, the treatment allows enough time out of the brace for daily participation in sport and physical activity. In general, relatively unrestricted physical activity is recommended for almost all adolescents with scoliosis. Mild to moderate cases can be treated with strength, flexibility, and general fitness activities. Severe scoliosis, which is characterized by extreme lateral deviation and localized rotation of the spine, can be painful and deforming, and it may require surgery (fusion with spinal instrumentation).

PREVENTION OF SPINAL CONDITIONS

Although most of the load on the spine is borne by the vertebral bodies and disks, the facet joints assist with some load bearing. Protective equipment can prevent some injuries to the cervical and thoracic regions; however, physical conditioning plays a more important role in preventing injuries to the overall region.

Protective Equipment

Several pieces of equipment can be used to protect the spine. In the cervical region, a neck roll or posterolateral pad made of a high, thick, and stiff material can be attached to shoulder pads to limit excessive motion of the cervical spine. Such restraints have been shown to reduce the incidence of repetitive burners and stingers; however, they also may increase the risk of cervical spine injuries by limiting the natural flexibility of the neck. In the upper body, shoulder pads extend over and protect the upper thoracic region. Rib protectors composed of air-inflated, interconnected cylinders can protect a limited region of the thoracic spine. Many of these protective devices are discussed and demonstrated in Chapter 3.

Physical Conditioning

Strengthening of the back muscles is imperative to stabilize the spinal column. Strengthening exercises for the cervical region may involve isometric contractions, manual resistance, or weight training with free weights or specialized machines. Exercises should include neck flexion, extension, lateral flexion, and rotation as well as scapular elevation. Stabilization of the cervical spine is particularly important for wrestlers and football lineman, who are consistently subjected to extremes of motion at the neck. Exercises to strengthen the thoracic region should involve back extension, lateral flexion, and rotation; abdominal strengthening; and exercises for the lower trapezius and latissimus dorsi.

Normal ROM is essential in stabilizing the spine and preventing injury. If warranted, stretching exercises should be used to promote and maintain normal ROM in the cervical and thoracic regions.

Proper Skill Technique

Proper skill technique is vital in preventing spinal injuries. Helmets are designed to protect the cranial region from injury but do not prevent axial loading on the cervical spine. It is critical that proper techniques be taught and reinforced in an effort to reduce the potential for injury. Since the 1976 rule change banning spearing in high school football, a large reduction in the incidence of catastrophic spinal injuries has occurred, although the practice of spearing continues (7).

CERVICAL SPINE CONDITIONS

Q *The major concern with cervical injuries is the potential involvement of the spinal cord and nerve roots. What specific signs and symptoms of a cervical injury suggest neural involvement and, as such, a potentially catastrophic injury?*

The relatively small size of the cervical vertebrae, combined with the nearly horizontal orientation of the cervical facet joints, makes the cervical spine the most mobile region of the spinal column. As such, this area is especially vulnerable to injury.

Torticollis

Torticollis, or scoliosis of the cervical spine, is a deformity of the neck in which the head tilts toward one shoulder and, simultaneously, the chin rotates toward the opposite shoulder. It is a symptom as well as a disease, and it has a host of underlying pathologies. Torticollis can be divided into two types, congenital and acquired. Infants who are born with torticollis appear to be healthy at delivery but, within 2 to 8 weeks, develop soft-tissue swelling over an injured sternocleidomastoid. Injury may result from birth trauma or intrauterine malpositioning (breech positioning).

In children, acquired torticollis may result from trauma or be secondary to infection of the throat, pharynx, or cervical adenitis. In adults, the condition may result from a muscular strain, viral infection, psychogenic etiology, vertebral or clavicular fractures, or traumatic unilateral facet subluxation or impingement.

The common "wry neck" as a result of a muscular strain often follows exposure to cold air-currents or, occasionally, sleeping with the neck in an abnormal position, which leads to painful, tender cervical muscles. The individual maintains the head in a position toward the side of the involved muscle to provide for a potential state of relaxation of that muscle. A ligamentous or capsular injury occurs when the neck is completely extended, flexed, or rotated and the individual turns the head abruptly, which exceeds the yield point of the tissues. This results in a rotary subluxation when one or more pairs of facets move beyond their normal ROM. As a result of this excess motion, the articular surfaces lose their physical relationship and are "jammed" together, with resultant separation of the anatomically opposite joints. As a result of capsular tearing and stretching as well as impingement along with traumatic edema of the synovium and capsular tissue, unilateral narrowing of the intervertebral foramen, with resultant pain, occurs.

Signs and Symptoms

The patient presents with the head tilted to one side and the chin pointed toward the opposite shoulder. For example, if the head tilts right and the chin points left, the muscles on the right side are affected. Subsequently, ROM is limited. In addition, a palpable lump or swelling may be found in the involved muscle.

Management

In acquired torticollis, symptoms usually resolve spontaneously within 2 weeks. Treatment is symptomatic and consists of cryotherapy, heat, massage, supportive cervical collar, muscle relaxants, interferential muscle stimulation, and analgesics. Range-of-motion exercises should allow normal motion to be regained relatively quickly. Continued care will enhance the ability of the individual to resume normal activities.

Cervical Sprains

Cervical sprains typically occur at the extremes of motion or in association with a violent muscle contraction or external force. Injury can occur to any of the major ligaments traversing the cervical spine as well as to the capsular ligaments surrounding the facet joints. Minor activity, such as maintaining the head in an uncomfortable posture or sleeping position, also can produce sprains of the neck.

Signs and Symptoms

Symptoms include pain, stiffness, and restricted ROM, but no neurologic or osseous injury exists. Unlike cervical strains, the symptoms of a severe sprain can persist for several days.

Management

Initial treatment includes rest, cryotherapy, prescribed nonsteroidal anti-inflammatory drugs (NSAIDs), and use of a cervical collar for support. Follow-up treatment may involve continued cryotherapy or superficial heat, gentle stretching, and isometric exercises. Return to competition should not occur until the individual is free of neck pain, with and without axial compression, and when ROM and neck strength are normal. This decision should be made collaboratively with the physician.

Cervical Strains

Cervical strains usually involve the sternocleidomastoid or upper trapezius, although the scalenes, levator scapulae, and splenius muscles may be involved as well. The same mechanisms that cause cervical sprains also cause cervical strains, and in many instances, both injuries occur simultaneously.

Signs and Symptoms

Symptoms include pain, stiffness, and restricted ROM. Palpation reveals muscle spasm and increased pain during active contraction or passive stretching of the involved muscle.

Management

Cryotherapy, prescribed NSAIDs, gentle stretching and isometric exercises of the involved muscle, and use of a cervical collar for support facilitate symptoms subsiding within 3 to 7 days. Follow-up treatment may involve continued cryotherapy or superficial heat as well as strengthening the neck muscles through appropriate resistance exercise. Return to competition should not occur until the individual is free of neck pain, with and without axial compression, and when ROM and neck strength are normal. This decision should be made collaboratively with the physician.

Cervical Spinal Stenosis

Structural spinal stenosis is defined as a narrowing of the sagittal diameter of the cervical spinal canal compared to the diameter of the corresponding vertebral body (Torg ratio) (8). Recently, the ratio method has been shown to have low predictive value. Functional spinal stenosis, a more accurate measure of stenosis, is defined as a loss of cerebrospinal fluid (CSF) around the cord or, in more extreme cases, as a deformation of the spinal cord. This is documented by magnetic resonance imaging, contrast-enhanced computed tomographic scans, or myelography. As a result of the reduced CSF, the ability of the spinal cord to decompress itself is limited, potentially leading to more acute and severe symptoms.

Individuals may remain asymptomatic until a direct blow to the forehead (forced hyperextension) or occiput (hyperflexion) produces neurologic signs. Lateral blows causing rapid lateral flexion with or without rotation also can lead to acute symptoms. The most commonly affected cervical segments are C_5 and C_6.

Signs and Symptoms

On impact, the individual may develop immediate quadriplegia with sensory changes or motor deficits in both arms, both legs, or all four extremities. Sensory changes may include burning pain, numbness, tingling, or total loss of sensation. Motor changes may include weakness or complete paralysis, with arm weakness being greater than leg weakness, secondary to contusion (bruising) of the central portion of the spinal cord (central cord syndrome). The changes are always bilateral, differentiating this condition from a nerve root injury, which is always unilateral. The episode may be transient, with full recovery in 10 to 15 minutes, although in some cases, complete recovery does not occur for 36 to 38 hours (9). This condition often is called a **neurapraxia**, because neural changes are only temporary.

Management

Structural spinal stenosis may be discovered during routine radiographs, but a magnetic resonance image often is needed to determine the presence of functional stenosis. An individual who has had an episode of structurally related cervical spinal neurapraxia, with or without transient quadriplegia, is not necessarily predisposed to permanent neurologic injury. Individuals with developing spinal stenosis or spinal stenosis associated with congenital abnormalities have returned safely to partic-

Because of the serious nature of this injury, the emergency plan, including summoning emergency medical services (EMS), should be activated. This individual requires transport on a spine board.

ipation. A growing number of physicians, however, have concluded that individuals who have functional stenosis of the cervical spine with associated cervical spine instability, or acute or chronic intervertebral disk disease, should be advised to discontinue participation in contact sports.

Spear Tackler's Spine

Flexion of the neck, as seen in spear tackling, produces a straightened cervical spine that acts like a segmental column, predisposing the spine to permanent neurologic injury with further axial loading. Spear tackler's spine originally was described in 1993, after a review of data from the National Football Head and Neck Injury Registry (10). The registry reported that four athletes who suffered permanent neurologic injury had the following common characteristics:

- Developmental narrowing of the cervical spinal canal
- Straightening or reversal of the normal cervical lordotic curve
- Preexisting minor posttraumatic radiographic evidence of bony or ligamentous injury
- History of using spear-tackling techniques

Signs and Symptoms

As with any catastrophic neck injury, the individual may develop immediate pain with sensory changes and motor deficits distal to the injury site. Sensory changes may include burning pain, numbness, tingling, or total loss of sensation. Motor changes may include weakness or complete paralysis.

Management

Controversy still exists regarding the criteria for returning an injured individual to participation. Some neurosurgeons believe that if the normal cervical lordosis is restored by treatment and the individual refrains from further spear-tackling techniques, a high degree of risk for reinjury does not exist (11). The majority of neurosurgeons, however, believe that the condition is an absolute contraindication to further participation in contact/collision sports (10,12).

Because of the serious nature of this injury, the emergency plan, including summoning EMS, should be activated. This individual requires transport on a spine board.

Cervical Disk Injuries

Less common than lumbar disk injuries, cervical disk injuries usually affect older, physically active individuals. The primary mechanisms involve sustained, repetitive cervical compression, axial loading, or hyperflexion injuries during contact sports. Disk disease may be classified as either soft- or hard-disk disease. Soft-disk herniation refers to an acute process in which the nucleus pulposus herniates through the posterior annulus, resulting in signs and symptoms of cord or nerve root compression. In sports participation, acute cervical disk herniations are thought to result from uncontrolled lateral bending of the neck (12). In contrast, hard-disk disease refers to a more chronic, degenerative process, with a diminished disk height and the formation of marginal osteophytes. The condition usually begins early in life and proceeds through a series of defined steps preceding most, if not all, symptomatic disk herniations.

Signs and Symptoms

Individuals with degenerative disk disease and acute disk herniations usually present with varying degrees of neck or arm pain that may radiate into the shoulder or arm. Pain often is exacerbated by Valsalva maneuvers (e.g., breath-holding, straining, or coughing) and neck movement. Spurling's maneuver (i.e., turning the head with the neck extended) often reproduces sharp radicular pain

■■■■■ FIGURE 10.14 **Cervical fracture/ dislocation.** The mechanism of axial loading and violent neck flexion can result in a cervical fracture/dislocation.

into the affected extremity in the distribution of the compressed nerve root. If the spinal cord is compressed, a positive Babinski's sign often is present. Severe cases may involve complete loss of motor function below the level of injury, including arm and leg paralysis. Symptoms in the physically active population tend to be more pronounced because of the demands of their sport.

Management

Initial treatment for the majority of all herniated cervical disk injuries is nonoperative. Treatment consists of rest, immobilization in a cervical collar for 1 to 3 days, activity modification, anti-inflammatory medication, cervical traction, and occasionally, therapeutic injections (13). Therapeutic exercise may be instituted as symptoms improve, emphasizing isometric strengthening and cervical ROM, followed by sport/activity-specific exercises and drills. The individual may return to sport/activity participation once he or she is asymptomatic and has regained full strength and mobility.

Cervical Fractures and Dislocations

Unsafe practices, such as diving into shallow water, spearing in football, or landing on the posterior neck during gymnastic or trampoline activities, can lead to cervical fractures and dislocations from the axial loading and violent neck flexion (Fig. 10.14). Some fractures, such as those of the spinous process or unilateral laminar fractures, may require only immobilization in a cervical collar. Others, such as a bilateral pars interarticularis fracture of C_2 ("hangman's fracture"), may require a cervical collar or Halo vest immobilization.

Signs and Symptoms

In sports, serious injuries commonly occur at the fourth, fifth, and sixth cervical vertebrae. Because neural damage can range from none to complete severance of the spinal cord, there is a range of accompanying symptoms (Box 10.1). Painful palpation over the spinous processes, muscle spasm, or palpable defect indicates a possible fracture or dislocation. Radiating pain, numbness, weakness in a myotome, paralysis, and loss of bladder or bowel control are all critical signs of neural damage. If a unilateral cervical dislocation is present, the neck is visibly tilted toward the dislocated side, with muscle tightness resulting from stretch on the convex side and muscle slack on the concave side.

Management

 Because of the serious nature of this injury, the emergency plan, including summoning EMS, should be activated. This individual requires transport on a spine board.

Because spinal cord damage can lead to paralysis or death, a suspected unstable neck injury should be treated as a medical emergency. An unstable neck injury should be suspected in an unconscious individual, an individual who is awake but has numbness and/or paralysis, and in a neurologically

Box 10.1   Red Flags Indicating a Possible Cervical Spine Injury

- Pain over the spinous process, with or without deformity
- Unrelenting neck pain or muscle spasm
- Abnormal sensations in the head, neck, trunk, or extremities
- Muscular weakness in the extremities
- Loss of coordinated movement

- Paralysis or inability to move a body part
- Absent or weak reflexes
- Loss of bladder or bowel control
- Mechanism of injury involving violent axial loading, flexion, or rotation of the neck

intact individual who has neck pain or pain with neck movement. Without moving the head or neck out of alignment, light cervical traction should be applied while the neck is being stabilized, and airway, breathing, and circulation (ABCs) should be assessed for any life-threatening situation.

A *Critical signs of neural damage include sensory changes (i.e., burning pain, numbness, tingling, or total loss of sensation), motor changes (i.e., weakness in a myotome complete paralysis), and loss of bladder or bowel control are critical signs of neural damage.*

BRACHIAL PLEXUS CONDITIONS

Q *While throwing a two-handed overhead pass, a basketball player is hit on the right arm. The arm is forced into excessive external rotation, abduction, and extension. The player experiences an immediate burning pain and a prickly sensation that radiates down the arm and into the hand as well as an inability to raise the arm. What injury should be suspected, and is this a serious injury?*

The brachial plexus is a complex neural structure that innervates the upper extremity and that typically is damaged in two manners (Fig. 10.15). A stretch injury may be caused when a tensile force leads to forceful, downward traction of the clavicle while the head is distracted in the opposite direction, such as when an individual is tackled and subsequently rolls onto the shoulder with the head turned to the opposite side. A stretch injury also may occur when the arm is forced into excessive external rotation, abduction, and extension. The injury usually affects the upper trunk (C_5, C_6) of the brachial plexus, which leads to a sensory loss or paresthesia in the thumb and index finger. A second mechanism of injury involves compression of the fixed plexus between the football shoulder pad and the superior medial scapula, where the brachial plexus is most superficial. This site, called the Erb's point, is located 2 to 3 cm above the clavicle at the level of the transverse process of the C_6 vertebra.

Burners are graded in three levels (Table 10.1). Grade I burners represent neurapraxia, the mildest lesion. A neurapraxia is a localized conduction block that causes temporary loss of sensation and/or loss of motor function from selective demyelination of the axon sheath without true axonal disruption. Recovery usually occurs within days to a few weeks. Grade II burners are axonotmesis injuries that produce significant motor and mild sensory deficits that last for at least 2 weeks. Axonotmesis disrupts the axon and myelin sheath, but it leaves the epineurium intact. Axonal regrowth occurs at a rate of 1 to 2 mm per day; full or normal function usually is restored. Grade III

FIGURE 10.15 Common mechanisms of a brachial plexus stretch. A, A blow to the head causing lateral flexion and shoulder depression may lead to a traction injury to the upper trunk of the brachial plexus. **B,** An injury also can occur when a blow to the supraclavicular region causes lateral flexion with rotation and extension of the cervical spine away from the blow. **C,** Compression over Erb's point, representing the most superficial passage of the brachial plexus, also can lead to pain and paresthesia radiating into the upper extremity.

GRADE	INJURY	SIGNS	PROGNOSIS
TABLE 10.1 Classifications of Burners			
I	Neurapraxia	Temporary loss of sensation and/or loss of motor function	Recovery within a few days to a few weeks
II	Axonotmesis	Significant motor and mild sensory deficits	Deficits last at least 2 weeks Regrowth is slow, but full or normal function usually is restored
III	Neurotmesis	Motor and sensory deficits persist for up to 1 year	Poor prognosis Surgical intervention often is necessary

burners are neurotmesis injuries, which disrupt the endoneurium. These severe injuries have a poor prognosis, with motor and sensory deficit persisting for up to 1 year. Surgical intervention often is necessary to avoid poor or imperfect regeneration.

Acute Burners

Signs and Symptoms

The individual notices an immediate, severe, burning pain and prickly paresthesia that radiates from the supraclavicular area down the arm and into the hand, hence the nickname "burner" or "stinger." Pain usually is transient and subsides in 5 to 10 minutes, but tenderness over the supraclavicular area and shoulder weakness may persist for hours or even days after the injury. Often, the individual tries to shake the arm to "get the feeling back." Muscle weakness is evident in actions involving shoulder abduction and external rotation.

Management

When weakness is present, the individual should be removed from activity. A brief nerve root screening should be performed. The myotomes should be tested bilaterally:

- Shoulder abduction for the C_5 nerve root
- Elbow flexion for C_6
- Elbow extension for C_7
- Thumb extension for C_8
- Finger abduction and adduction for T_1

The brachial plexus traction test also may be performed (see *Assessment of Spinal Conditions*). The test is performed by passively flexing the individual's head to one side while applying a downward pressure on the opposite shoulder. If pain increases or radiates into the upper arm that is being depressed, it indicates stretching of the brachial plexus.

If strength and function return completely within 5 minutes, the individual can return to activity. If any neurologic symptoms persist after this time, however, the individual should not be allowed to return to activity until the following criteria for return to play after a burner have been met:

- No neck pain, arm pain, or dysesthesia (impairment of sensation)
- Full pain-free ROM in the neck and upper extremity
- Normal strength on manual muscle testing as compared to preseason measurements
- Normal deep tendon reflexes
- Negative brachial plexus traction test

It also is imperative to follow the individual closely with a postactivity examination and with successive examinations for several days to detect any recurrence of weakness.

Treatment may involve ice massage to the upper trapezius and shoulder to decrease pain and inflammation of a secondary muscle strain. A sling may be necessary, particularly for individuals with weakness in the rotator cuff muscles.

Following a grade II or III burner, strength training is contraindicated during early rehabilitation, because immature motor end plates may be damaged during resistance training. Range-of-motion exercises for the cervical spine should begin in the supine position and progress to a seated position. Isometric strengthening exercises can progress to diagonal flexion and extension, then to exercises using machines or free weights. When shoulder ROM is near normal in all planes, closed chain strengthening should be initiated, with progression into isotonic and isodynamic exercise. Scapulothoracic motion should be smooth and isolated, avoiding any muscle substitution. Concentric and eccentric strengthening exercises should be conducted in external and internal rotation (45° abduction), adduction, and extension.

Chronic Burners

Signs and Symptoms

In contrast, chronic burners are characterized by more frequent acute episodes that may not produce areas of numbness. Muscle weakness in the shoulder muscles may develop hours or even days after the initial injury and may result in a dropped shoulder or visible atrophy of the shoulder muscles.

Management

These individuals should be examined after activity, during the week, and again the following week, because weakness may not become apparent until days after the initial injury. Initial treatment follows the same parameters of acute burners. In football, the use of lifters, a supplemental pad at the base of the neck, or a modified A-frame shoulder pad supplemented by a cervical collar attached to the posterior aspect of the shoulder pads may limit excessive lateral neck flexion and extension to prevent reoccurrence.

Suprascapular Nerve Injury

The suprascapular nerve also may be damaged with the same mechanisms. This nerve innervates the supraspinatus, infraspinatus, and glenohumeral joint capsule. During motions such as those in pitching, spiking, or overhead serving, extreme velocity and torque forces generated during the cocking, acceleration, and release phases subject this nerve and its adjoining artery to rapid stretching.

Signs and Symptoms

Both the supraspinatus and infraspinatus muscles may appear to be weak and atrophied. Infraspinatus wasting usually is more apparent, however, because it is not hidden under the trapezius muscle. Because the supraspinatus and infraspinatus are not functioning properly, other problems, such as rotator cuff tendinitis, impingement syndrome, bicipital tenosynovitis, or bursitis of the shoulder, may be present and overshadow this condition.

Management

If an individual with chronic shoulder problems does not respond well to standard treatment, the individual should be referred to a physician for further evaluation. Once identified, the condition responds well to a ROM and strengthening program.

The basketball player experienced a brachial plexus stretch injury. The paresthesia (i.e., burning and prickling) and muscle weakness should resolve in a few minutes, at which time the individual can return to activity. If neurologic symptoms persist, the individual should not be allowed to return to activity, and referral to a physician is warranted.

THORACIC SPINE CONDITIONS

> **Q** *A 15-year-old, butterfly-stroke swimmer is complaining of localized pain and tenderness in the midback region over the thoracic spine. The pain came on gradually and only hurts during execution of the stroke. Fracture tests are negative. What other condition(s) might be suspected?*

The protective rib cage limits movement in the thoracic motion segments; however, the thoracolumbar junction is a region of potentially high stress during flexion-extension movements of the trunk. Injuries to this area may include contusions, strains, sprains, fractures, and apophysitis.

Thoracic Contusions, Strains, and Sprains

Direct blows to the back during contact sports frequently yield contusions to the muscles in the thoracic region. Such injuries range in severity but generally are characterized by pain, ecchymosis, spasm, and limited swelling.

Signs and Symptoms

Thoracic sprains and strains result from either overloading or overstretching muscles in the region through violent or sustained muscle contractions. Painful spasms of the back muscles serve as a protective mechanism to immobilize the injured area and may develop as a sympathetic response to sprains. The presence of such spasms, however, makes it difficult to determine whether the injury is actually a sprain or a strain. Dramatic improvement in a thoracic sprain can be seen in 24 to 48 hours. In contrast, severe strains may require 3 to 4 weeks to heal.

Management

Initial treatment consists of cryotherapy, NSAIDs, and activity modification. Follow-up management may include application of superficial heat, ultrasound, massage, and appropriate stretching and resistance exercise as needed to recondition the individual.

Thoracic Spinal Fractures and Apophysitis

The rib cage stabilizes and limits motion in the thoracic spine and, in doing so, lessens the likelihood of injury to this area. Thoracic fractures tend to be concentrated at the lower end of the thoracic spine, in the transitional region between the thoracic and lumbar curvatures.

Large compressive loads, such as those sustained during heavy weight lifting, head-on contact in football or rugby, or landing on the buttock area during a fall, can fracture the vertebral end plates or lead to a **wedge fracture**, which is named after the shape of the deformed vertebral body (Fig. 10.16A). Females with **osteopenia**, a condition of reduced bone mineralization, are particularly susceptible to these fractures. More commonly, compressive stress during small, repetitive loads in an activity such as running leads to a progressive compression fracture of a weakened vertebral body. As with any fracture, pain and muscle guarding are present in the region of the fracture site. Referral to a physician is warranted.

Another leading cause of thoracic fractures among adolescents and young adults is **Scheuermann's disease**. This condition, which appears to be related to mechanical stress, involves degeneration of the epiphyseal end plates of the vertebral bodies and typically includes at least three adjacent motion segments. The vertebral end plates have a wavy appearance, and the intervertebral disk spaces are narrowed. If the end plate is sufficiently compromised, additional compression from axial and flexion overload forces cause prolapse of the intervertebral disk into the vertebral body (Fig. 10.16B). The result is a decrease in spinal height and an accentuation of the thoracic curve, leading to kyphosis. Onset typically occurs in the late juvenile period, from 8 to 12 years of age; more severe fixed deformities are seen in individuals from 12 to 16 years of age. The condition is twice as common in girls as in boys. A high incidence of Scheuermann's disease has been documented among gymnasts, trampolinists, cyclists, wrestlers, and rowers. Following referral to a physician, treatment involves modification of activity in proportion to the pain. Stretching exercises for the shoulder, neck, and

■■■■ FIGURE 10.16 **Thoracic fracture and apophysitis. A,** Radiograph of a compression wedge fracture in the thoracic region as a result of several compressed motion segments. **B,** Scheuermann's disease occurs when end plate changes lead to erosion in the anterior vertebral body, which drives a herniated disk forward into the body. In this radiograph, several end plate changes can be seen leading to erosion of the vertebral bodies.

back muscles should be coupled with strengthening the abdominal and spinal extensor muscles. If the kyphosis continues to progress, bracing may be included with the exercise program.

Repeated flexion-extension of the thoracic spine can cause inflammation of the apophyses, which are the growth centers of the vertebral bodies. Like Scheuermann's disease, apophysitis is a progressive condition that is characterized by local pain and tenderness. After referral to a physician, treatment for apophysitis includes elimination of the flexion-extension stress as well as strengthening abdominal and other trunk muscles.

 The swimmer may have developed apophysitis because of the repeated flexion-extension motions that are executed during the butterfly stroke. This individual should be referred to a physician for follow-up examination.

ASSESSMENT OF SPINAL CONDITIONS

Before the start of an afternoon practice, a college field-hockey player reports to the athletic training room with a "stiff neck." She reports that she did not experience any neck pain or discomfort during or after practice the previous day.

Injury assessment of the spine is complex and cannot be rushed. In a traumatic episode, if a fully conscious person is not experiencing severe pain, spasm, or tenderness, it is rare that the individual has sustained a significant spinal injury. More likely, the individual has experienced a minor injury, such as a muscular strain or sprain. Even so, it is essential that injury assessment be performed in a deliberate manner, taking as much time as necessary.

Box 10.2 Red Flags that Warrant Immobilization and Immediate Referral to a Physician

- Severe pain, point tenderness, or deformity along the vertebral column
- Loss or change in sensation anywhere in the body
- Paralysis or inability to move a body part
- Diminished or absent reflexes
- Muscle weakness in a myotome

- Pain radiating into the extremities
- Trunk or abdominal pain that may be referred from the visceral organs
- Any injury for which you are uncertain about the severity or nature

The severity of pain and the presence or absence of neurologic symptoms, neck spasm, and tenderness can indicate when a backboard and neck stabilization are needed. When in doubt, it should be assumed that a severe spinal injury is present, and the emergency care plan should be activated. The individual's head, neck, or spine should not be moved, and the helmet should not be removed. Once a significant physical finding indicates possible nerve involvement, immobilization and immediate transportation to the nearest medical facility are warranted, regardless of whether a total assessment is completed. Box 10.2 identifies several signs and symptoms that necessitate activating the emergency care plan and, potentially, summoning EMS.

See *Field Strategy: Cervical Spine Injury Evaluation*, available on the companion website at thePoint, for a summary of the assessment procedure.

For cases in which the individual walks into an examination room complaining of neck or upper back pain, it is relatively safe to assume that a serious spinal injury is not present. The assessment that follows focuses on a cervical and thoracic spinal assessment in a conscious individual. Specific information related to an acute injury is included where appropriate.

HISTORY

What basic information needs to be obtained from the field-hockey player as part of the history component of this injury assessment?

A history of the injury should include information regarding the primary complaint, mechanism of injury, characteristics of the symptoms, disability resulting from the injury, previous injuries to the area, and any family history that may have some bearing on this specific condition. In a spinal injury, questions should be asked about the location of pain (i.e., localized or radiating), type of pain (i.e., dull, aching, sharp, or burning), presence of sensory changes (i.e., numbness, tingling, or absence of sensation), and possible muscle weakness or paralysis. If the injury is to the neck, questions should be asked to determine any long- and short-term memory loss, which may indicate an associated concussion or subdural hematoma. It is important to note the length of time it takes the individual to respond to the questions.

See *Field Strategy: Developing a History for a Cervical Spine Injury*, available on the companion website at thePoint, for general questions related to a spinal injury.

In attempting to determine the cause and extent of injury, the field-hockey player should be asked questions pertaining to the primary complaint (i.e., what, when, and how questions), mechanism of injury(e.g., potential mechanism the previous day), characteristics and onset of symptoms (i.e., nature, location, severity, or disability), unusual sensation, related medical history (i.e., past injuries/treatment).

OBSERVATION AND INSPECTION

Q *The field-hockey player cannot recall a specific mechanism of injury but states that she was involved in a collision during practice the previous day. She reports pain and stiffness on the left side of the neck on waking up this morning, which has continued throughout the day. She does not report any previous history of injury to the cervical spine, and no evidence of sensory or motor deficits is found. What specific factors should be observed and inspected in the on-going assessment of the field hockey player, and is it appropriate to perform a scan examination?*

Observation should begin as soon as the examiner sets eyes on the individual. Body language can signal pain, disability, and muscle weakness. It is necessary to note the individual's willingness or ability to move, general posture, ease in motion, and general attitude. Clothing and protective equipment may prevent visual observation of abnormalities in the spinal alignment. As such, the individual should be suitably dressed so that the back is as exposed as possible; for girls and women, a bra, halter top, or swimsuit can be worn. Observation should begin with a postural assessment, progress through a scan examination and gait analysis, and end with an inspection of the injury site.

Posture

Posture assessment can detect congenital or functional problems that may contribute to the injury. The examination should begin by asking the individual to sit down and then stand. The head and neck posture should be observed. It is important to note whether the head is held erect or is carried in a forward position. The presence of any abnormal spinal curvatures should be recorded as well. Normal presentation includes a smooth cervical lordosis with gentle transition into thoracic kyphosis. If a cervical injury is present, the head tends to be tilted and rotated away from the pain, and the head is tilted upward. A "forward" head (i.e., ear forward of the acromion) or accentuated cervicothoracic hump creates a constant flexion moment of the head over the spine. It also is appropriate to determine if the chin is directly in line with the throat. Unilateral spasm of the cervical muscles results in lateral flexion of the head toward the involved side. The chin also may be rotated to the side opposite the tilt, indicating **torticollis** ("wry neck").

The individual should be instructed to lean forward and touch the toes while keeping the knees straight (i.e., Adam's position). The vertebrae and contour of the back should be observed. The presence of a hump or raised scapula on one side (convex side of curve) and a hollow (concave side of curve) on the other indicates scoliosis. The combination of the hump and the hollow is caused by vertebral rotation. If a lateral curve is present while standing but disappears on flexion, a nonstructural scoliosis curve is present. If the condition is structural scoliosis, the curve remains.

Identification of any noticeable asymmetries, including discrepancies in the height of the shoulder or scapula, hip, or patella, should be recorded. A flexed posturing at the hips from tight hip flexors results in a compensatory increase in the lumbar and cervical lordoses. Obesity with rounded shoulders or a hunched posture, as typically occurs in individuals with overdeveloped anterior chest muscles, can predispose to thoracic outlet syndrome or other chronic strain patterns. The bilateral muscle mass, tone, and hypertrophy/atrophy should be observed. Atrophy of the deltoid muscle may indicate axillary nerve palsy. Atrophy of the posterior scapular muscles may result from impingement of a cervical nerve root or a brachial plexus injury.

The presence of any dark areas of skin pigmentation, such as café-au-lait spots, should be noted. This could indicate a possible collagen disease or abnormal growth of neural tissues (neurofibromatosis 1).

See *Field Strategy: Postural Assessment of the Cervical and Upper Thoracic Spine,* available on the companion website at thePoint, for specific postural factors to observe in the head and spinal region.

Scan Examination

Active movement should not be performed when pain is present over the vertebrae or when motor/sensory deficits are present. If that is not the case, a scan examination can be used to assess general motor function (Box 10.3). It can potentially rule out injury at other joints that may be overlooked because of intense pain or discomfort at the primary injury site. Active movement of

Box 10.3   Scan Examination for a Cervical Spine Injury

The athletic trainer should instruct the athlete to perform the skills listed in the following. During these movements, observe for signs of pain, hesitation to move a body part, or abnormal movement. If these signs are present, complete a more thorough evaluation of the affected body part, and if necessary, immobilize the area and refer the athlete to a physician for further care.

- Touch the chin to the chest.
- Look up at the ceiling while keeping the back straight.
- Turn the head sideways in both directions.
- Try to touch each ear to the shoulder.
- Rotate the trunk sideways while keeping the hips stabilized.
- Lean forward, and touch the toes.
- Look up at the ceiling with hyperextension of the trunk.

- Lean sideways, and do lateral flexion of the trunk.
- While placing a hand on a table for support:
  - Do a single straight-leg raise forward, backward, and sideways.
  - Flex the knee.
  - Rise up on the toes.
  - Balance on the heels.

the spine may be included in this step and need not be repeated with functional tests. It is important to note any hesitation in moving a body part or preference for using one side over the other.

Gait Assessment

The individual should be asked to walk several yards while the examiner observes normal body movement. The examiner should stand behind, in front of, and to the side of the individual to observe from all angles. Subtle posture abnormalities, such as kyphosis or scoliosis, should be noted.

Injury Site Inspection

Local inspection of the injury site should include observation for deformity, swelling, discoloration, muscle spasm, atrophy, hypertrophy, scars that might indicate previous surgery, and general skin condition. It is important to note any altered coloration of the skin, ulcers, or vein distention as evidence of upper limb ischemia.

Gross Neuromuscular Assessment

With an acute injury, a posture and scan examination is not possible; however, it is beneficial to perform a neuromuscular assessment before palpation to detect any motor and/or sensory deficits. The individual should not be moved but, rather, asked to perform submaximal, bilateral hand-squeeze, and ankle dorsiflexion. These two actions assess the cervical and lumbar spinal nerves, respectively. Muscle weakness and/or diminished sensation over the hands and feet indicate a serious injury. If any deficits are noted, the emergency plan, including summoning EMS, should be activated. If no deficits are noted, it does not rule out possible neurologic involvement or fracture. Therefore, palpation should be done with the individual maintained in the position in which he or she was found.

(A) *Observation should note the individual's willingness or ability to move, general posture, ease in motion, and general attitude. Observation should begin with a postural assessment, progress through a scan examination and gait analysis, and end with an inspection of the injury site.*

PALPATION

(Q) *A postural examination reveals a slight head tilt to the left side, with the chin pointed toward the opposite shoulder. An inspection of the area reveals no abnormal findings. Because the individual is experiencing pain on the left side and not over the vertebrae, a scan* *examination is performed and reveals limited ROM on the involved side because of pain. Describe the appropriate progression of the palpation component in the assessment of the field-hockey player.*

With injuries that do not involve neural damage, fracture, or dislocation, palpation can proceed in the following manner. Bony and soft-tissue structures are palpated to detect temperature, swelling, point tenderness, trigger points, deformity, crepitus, muscle spasm, and cutaneous sensation. Palpation may be done in a seated, standing, supine, or prone position. To relax the neck and spinal muscles, the individual should lie on a table. When the examiner is palpating posterior neck structures, the individual should be supine. The examiner should reach around the neck with both hands and palpate either side of the spine with the fingertips. Muscle spasms in the erector spinae, sternocleidomastoid muscles, scalene muscles, and/or upper trapezius may indicate dysfunction of the cervical spine. In palpating the thoracic region, the individual should be prone. A pillow or blanket should be placed under the hip region to tilt the pelvis back and relax the lumbar curvature. Muscle spasm in the lower erector spinae, lower trapezius, serratus posterior, quadratus lumborum, latissimus dorsi, or gluteus maximus may indicate dysfunction of the thoracic or lumbar spine. Surface landmarks can facilitate palpation (Table 10.2); the following structures should be palpated:

Anterior Aspect

1. Hyoid bone, thyroid cartilage, first cricoid ring, and trachea.

2. Sternocleidomastoid muscle, manubrium, clavicle, and supraclavicular fossa.

3. Sternum, ribs, and costal cartilage.

4. Abdomen and inguinal area. Note any abnormal tenderness or masses indicating internal pathology that is referring pain to the spinal region.

Posterior Aspect

1. External protuberance of the occiput.

2. Mastoid processes.

3. Spinous processes. The spinous processes of C_2, C_6, and C_7 are the most prominent. Note any tenderness, crepitus, or deviation from the norm. A noticeable discrepancy can indicate a fracture or vertebral subluxation. Pain and tenderness without positive findings on muscle movement may indicate that the problem is not musculoskeletal in origin.

4. Facet joints. The facet articulations are approximately a thumb's breadth (2–3 cm or 0.8–1.2 inches) to either side of the spinous process. Point tenderness, especially with

TABLE 10.2 Surface Landmarks on the Back	
VERTEBRA	**BONY LANDMARK**
C_2	One finger's breadth inferior to the mastoid process
C_6	Posterior to the cricoid cartilage
C_7 and T_1	Prominent spinous processes in neck
T_2	Top of scapula
T_4	Base of spine of scapula
T_7	Inferior angle of scapula
T_{12}	Lowest floating rib
L_4	Top of iliac crest
L_5	Demarcated by bilateral dimples
S_2	Level of posterior superior iliac spines

extension and rotation to the same side, suggests facet joint pain. In the thoracic area, it is difficult to palpate these joints because of the overlying musculature. Muscle spasm and tenderness may indicate pathology in the gallbladder (spasm on the right side around the eighth and ninth costal cartilages, spleen (spasm at the left side at the level of ribs 9–11), and kidneys (posterior spasm at the level of ribs 11–12).

5. Interspinous and supraspinous ligaments, ligamentum flavum, paraspinal muscles, and quadratus lumborum. Trigger points of the paraspinal and shoulder girdle regions refer pain to a more distal area. Tender points that increase with muscular contraction indicate a localized muscle strain. An area that is tender to palpation but not painful during muscle contraction may indicate referred pain from another area.

6. Scapula, trapezius, latissimus dorsi, and paravertebral muscles. Tightness or spasms in the paravertebral muscles increases lordosis in the lumbar spine.

Lateral Aspect

1. Transverse process of cervical vertebrae.

2. Lymph nodes and carotid arteries. The lymph nodes will only be palpable if they are swollen. The nodes are palpated along the line of the sternocleidomastoid muscle, and the carotid pulse may be palpated between the sternocleidomastoid muscle and the trachea.

3. Temporomandibular joints, mandible, and parotid glands. The parotid gland lies over the angle of the mandible. If the gland is swollen, it is palpable as a soft, boggy structure.

A *Both bony and soft-tissue structures should be palpated to determine the presence of swelling, spasm, and crepitus as well as to detect point tenderness, temperature, or trigger points.*

PHYSICAL EXAMINATION TESTS

Q *Palpation of the field-hockey player reveals spasm in the musculature on the involved side. What tests should be performed in the ongoing assessment of the field-hockey player?*

It is imperative to work slowly through the different tests, because injuries to the spinal region can be very complex. If, at any time, movement leads to increased acute pain or to change in sensation or if the individual resists moving the spine, a significant injury should be assumed to exist. As such, the emergency plan should be activated, including summoning EMS.

Functional Tests

Goniometry measurements of the spine are not typically taken because of the difficulty in measuring individual regional motions. Completion of gross movement patterns is adequate to determine normal ROM. Further assessment can be conducted if motion is limited.

Active Movement

If active movement of the spine was conducted during the scan examination, it need not be repeated. The individual's willingness to perform the movement as well as the smoothness and completeness of the movement should be noted. It is important to determine whether pain, spasm, or stiffness block the full ROM. Movements to the left and right should be compared bilaterally, and cervical and thoracic movement should be tested in the standing position. Spinal movements include:

1. Cervical flexion (80–90°)

2. Cervical extension (70°)

3. Lateral cervical flexion (left and right; 20–45°)

4. Cervical rotation (left and right; 70–90°)

5. Forward thoracic trunk flexion (20–45°)

6. Thoracic trunk extension (25–45°)

7. Lateral trunk flexion (left and right; 20–40°)

8. Trunk rotation (35–50°)

Passive Range of Motion

Passive movement should not be performed in an individual with an acute injury when motor and sensory deficits are present. These deficits indicate a spinal injury, and any movement could be catastrophic. In other injuries involving the presence of motor and sensory deficits, passive ROM can be performed if the individual does not have full ROM. In performing passive motion, the individual is placed in a supine position. The cervical region is moved passively through the various movements. The normal end feel for the cervical spine is tissue stretch in all four movements. Thoracic passive movement seldom is performed in a gross fashion. Individual movement may be tested by palpating over and between the spinous processes of the lower cervical and upper thoracic spines as the patient performs the motions. Normal motion between the spinous processes include flexion (move apart), extension (move together), rotation (one side moves forward, and the other moves back), and lateral flexion (one side moves apart, and one side moves together). The normal end feels for thoracic movements also are tissue stretch.

Resisted Muscle Testing

Resisted movement is performed throughout the full ROM in the same movements as active muscle testing. It is important to stabilize the hip and trunk during cervical testing to avoid muscle substitution. This can be accomplished by having the individual in the seated position and the examiner using one hand to stabilize the shoulder or thorax while the other hand applies manual overpressure. When testing the thoracic region, the weight of the trunk stabilizes the hips. The individual should be instructed not to allow the examiner to move the body part that is being tested. Maximal force must be applied when testing the major muscle groups to detect early weakness. By repetitively loading the resisting muscle with rapid, consecutive impulses, more subtle weakness can be detected. The assessed cervical and thoracic movements are demonstrated in Figures 10.17 and 10.18, respectively.

■■■■■■ FIGURE 10.17 **Active movements of the cervical spine. A,** Flexion. **B,** Extension. **C,** Lateral flexion. **D,** Rotation.

▪▪▪▪ FIGURE 10.18 **Active movements of the thoracic region. A,** Flexion. **B,** Extension. **C,** Lateral flexion. **D,** Rotation.

Stress and Functional Tests

Several stress tests can be used in spinal assessment. Only those deemed to be relevant should be performed. If any increased pain or change of sensation occurs, the individual should be immobilized, and the emergency plan should be activated, including summoning EMS.

Cervical Spine Tests

BRACHIAL PLEXUS TRACTION TEST. This test should not be performed until the possibility of bony trauma has been ruled out. While standing behind the patient, the athletic trainer passively flexes the individual's head to one side while applying a downward pressure on the opposite shoulder (Fig. 10.19). If pain increases or radiates into the upper arm that is being depressed, it indicates

■■ ■ FIGURE 10.19 **Brachial plexus traction test.** The examiner applies downward pressure during lateral bending away from the involved shoulder while simultaneously depressing the involved shoulder. Radiating pain or a burning sensation indicates injury to the brachial plexus. If pain increases on the side toward the lateral bending, it indicates irritation or compression of the nerve roots between two vertebrae.

stretching of the brachial plexus. If pain increases on the side toward the lateral bending, it indicates irritation or compression of the nerve roots between two vertebrae.

BRACHIAL PLEXUS TENSION TEST. While seated, the individual is asked to abduct and laterally rotate the arms, with the elbows extended and the forearms pronated, until symptoms appear (Fig. 10.20A). Next, the individual is asked to lower the arms until the symptoms disappear. The examiner then holds this position. Finally, the individual flexes the elbows, interlocking the individual's hands behind the head (Fig. 10.20B). If radicular pain is reproduced with the elbows flexed, this is a positive result for stress on the ulnar nerve and the C_8 and T_1 nerve roots.

■■ ■ FIGURE 10.20 **Brachial plexus tension test. A,** The examiner instructs the patient to pronate the forearm and abduct and then laterally rotate the arm until symptoms are felt. Next, the patient is instructed to lower the arm until the symptoms disappear. **B,** While the examiner holds the arms in this position, the patient flexes the elbows and places his or her hands behind the head. A positive test is indicated by return of symptoms.

■■■■ FIGURE 10.21 **Compression test.** The neck should be in a neutral position. The examiner carefully pushes straight down on the individual's head. Increased pain or altered sensation is a positive sign, indicating pressure on a nerve root. The test also can be performed with the neck slightly flexed to one side.

■■■■ FIGURE 10.22 **Spurling's test.** The individual is instructed to extend, rotate, and laterally bend the neck. Next, the examiner carefully applies downward pressure on the individual's head. Increased pain indicates cervical nerve root involvement.

CERVICAL COMPRESSION TEST. The compression test can detect pressure on a cervical nerve root as a result of degeneration or narrowing of a neural foramen. While the patient is sitting on a stable chair or table, the examiner applies compression straight down on the individual's head (Fig. 10.21). Increased pain or altered sensation is a positive sign, indicating pressure on a nerve root. The distribution of the pain and altered sensation can indicate which nerve root is involved.

SPURLING'S TEST (FORAMINAL COMPRESSION TEST). The Spurling's test is a variation of the cervical compression test. The individual extends the neck, then rotates and laterally bends the head to the same side while the examiner applies downward pressure to the top of the head (Fig. 10.22). If this position, with or without pressure, reproduces radiating pain into the upper limb, a nerve root impingement caused by a narrowing of the neural foramina is suggested. The distribution of the pain and altered sensation can indicate which nerve root is involved.

CERVICAL DISTRACTION TEST. This test is performed by having the examiner place one hand under the individual's chin and the other hand around the occiput, then slowly lifting the head (Fig. 10.23). The test is positive if pain decreases or is relieved as the head is lifted; this indicates that pressure on the nerve root is relieved. Pain that is increased with distraction indicates ligamentous injury.

SHOULDER ABDUCTION TEST. The individual may be seated or standing and is asked to abduct the shoulder, resting the hand on the top of the head (Fig. 10.24). A decrease in symptoms may indicate a nerve root compression, possibly resulting from a herniated disk, epidural vein compression, or nerve root compression, usually in the C_4-C_5 or C_5-C_6 area.

VERTEBRAL ARTERY TEST. The individual should be supine. The examiner is seated at the head of the patient and supports the occiput in both hands. The examiner passively extends and laterally flexes and rotates the cervical spine in the same direction, then holds the position for 30 seconds (Fig. 10.25). If the patient experiences any dizziness, confusion, abnormal movement of the eyes (nystagmus), unilateral pupil changes, or nausea, occlusion of the cervical vertebral artery should be suspected, and the individual should be referred to a physician immediately, without performing additional tests.

■■ ■■ FIGURE 10.23 **Distraction test.** The examiner lifts the head slowly. The test is positive if pain is decreased or relieved as the head is lifted, indicating that pressure on the nerve root is relieved. Pain that increases with distraction indicates ligamentous injury.

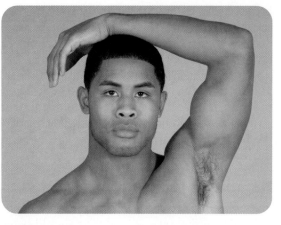

■■ ■■ FIGURE 10.24 **Shoulder abduction test.** The patient actively abducts the arm and places the hand on top of the head. If symptoms are relieved, a nerve root compression or herniated disk may be present.

Spring Test for Facet Joint Mobility

Hypomobility of the vertebrae, especially at the facet joint, may be assessed with the spring test (Fig. 10.26). With the patient prone, the examiner stands over the patient with the thumbs placed over the spinous process to be tested. The examiner carefully pushes the spinous process anteriorly, feeling for a springing of the vertebrae. The test is positive if pain is elicited or if the vertebra does not move ("spring").

Nerve Root Impingement

VALSALVA'S TEST. Valsalva's maneuver is used to determine the presence of space-occupying lesions (e.g., herniated disk, tumor, or osteophytes). While supine, the individual is asked to take a deep

■■ ■■ FIGURE 10.25 **Vertebral artery test.** While supporting the patient's head, the examiner passively extends, laterally flexes, and rotates the head, then holds this position for 30 seconds. If the patient becomes dizzy, confused, or nauseated or has abnormal eye movement, the individual should be referred immediately to a physician to determine if the vertebral artery is occluded.

■■ ■■ FIGURE 10.26 **Facet joint spring test.** While placing the thumbs directly over the spinous process, the examiner carefully pushes the spinous process anteriorly, feeling for the springing of the vertebrae. If pain is elicited or the vertebra is hypomobile, facet joint pathology is present.

breath and then hold it while bearing down, as if moving the bowels. Caution should be used with this test, however, because the maneuver increases intrathecal pressure, which can slow the pulse, decrease venous return, and increase venous pressure, each of which may cause fainting. A positive test is indicated by increased pain.

FIRST THORACIC NERVE ROOT STRETCH. The individual should be positioned with the forearm pronated to 90°. Then, the individual is instructed to abduct the arm to 90° and flex the elbow; no symptoms should be elicited in this position. Next, the individual must place his or her hand behind the head, fully flexing the elbow. This action stretches the ulnar nerve and T_1 nerve root. Pain in the scapular area or arm is indicative of a positive test for T_1 nerve root pathology.

Neurologic Tests

Because trauma to the brain or spinal cord can be reflected in **hyperreflexia**, muscle weakness, loss of sensation, and ataxia, several tests should be performed to assess for upper and lower motor neuron lesions. Upper quarter neurologic screening tests for trauma to the C_5–T_1 nerve roots, whereas lower quarter neurologic screening tests the L_1–S_2 nerve roots. In addition, loss of bowel and bladder control can be a sign of upper motor neuron lesions. Neurologic integrity can be assessed through special tests, myotomes, reflexes, segmental dermatomes, and peripheral nerve cutaneous patterns.

Upper Motor Neuron Tests

OPPENHEIM TEST. The individual should be supine. Using the edge of his or her fingernail, the examiner strokes the crest of the anteromedial tibia (Fig. 10.27). A positive sign is extension of the big toe and abduction (splaying) of the other toes or hypersensitivity to the test and suggests an upper motor neuron lesion.

BABINSKI TEST. The individual should be supine, with the eyes closed and the leg held in a slightly elevated and flexed position. A pointed object is stroked along the plantar aspect of the foot (see Fig. 9.11). A normal sign is for the toes to curl downward in flexion and adduction. A positive sign is extension of the big toe and abduction (splaying) of the other toes, which suggests an upper motor neuron lesion.

HOFFMANN'S SIGN. Hoffman's sign is the upper limb equivalent of the Babinski test. The examiner holds the patient's middle finger and briskly flicks the distal phalanx. A positive sign occurs if the interphalangeal joint of the thumb of the same hand flexes.

■■■ FIGURE 10.27 **Oppenheim test.** The patient is supine. The examiner runs a fingernail along the crest of the antero-medial tibia. A positive test result is seen when the great toe extends and the other toes splay or when the individual reports hypersensitivity to the test.

TABLE 10.3 Myotomes Used to Test Selected Nerve

NERVE ROOT SEGMENT	ACTION TESTED
C_1–C_2	Neck flexion[a]
C_3 and cranial nerve XI	Lateral neck flexion[a]
C_4 and cranial nerve XI	Shoulder elevation
C_5	Shoulder abduction
C_6	Elbow flexion and/or wrist extension
C_7	Elbow extension and/or wrist flexion
C_8	Thumb extension and/or ulnar deviation
T_1	Finger abduction and adduction

[a] These myotomes should not be performed if a cervical fracture or dislocation is suspected, because they may cause serious damage or even death.

Myotomes

Isometric muscle testing is performed in the neck and upper extremities to test specific myotomes (Table 10.3). Myotomes were originally discussed in Chapter 5. Maximal force should be applied when testing the major muscle groups to detect weakness.

Reflexes

Repetitive tapping of the reflexes may show a gradual decline in the reflex response not otherwise noted with a singe tap. Absent or decreased reflexes are not necessarily pathologic, especially in individuals who have well-developed muscles. Upper limb reflexes can be increased by having the individual perform an isometric contraction, such as squeezing the knees together during the test. Reflexes in the upper extremity include the biceps (C_5–C_6), brachioradialis (C_6), and triceps (C_7). Asymmetry between sides should raise suspicion of an abnormality.

Cutaneous Patterns

The wide variation of dermatomal innervation and the subjectivity of the test make it less useful than motor or reflex testing; however, the test is useful to check for a sensory loss in a peripheral nerve distribution if an upper limb peripheral nerve entrapment is suspected. The segmental nerve dermatome patterns and peripheral nerve cutaneous patterns were shown in Figure 5.8. Bilaterally testing for altered sensation with sharp and dull touch is performed by running the open hand and fingernails over the head, neck, back, thorax, abdomen, and upper and lower extremities (front, back, and sides). The patient is asked if the sensation feels the same on one body segment as compared to the other.

Referred Pain

Pain can be referred to the thoracic spine from various abdominal organs. Figure 5.1 shows cutaneous areas of the thorax where pain from visceral organs is referred.

Activity-Specific Functional Testing

Before return to sport/activity, the individual must have a normal neurologic examination with pain-free ROM, normal bilateral muscle strength, cutaneous sensation, and reflexes. Axial head compression can be performed on the sideline as an additional safety check. If pain is present, the individual should not return to sport/activity. The sport/activity-specific functional tests that should be performed include walking, bending, lifting, jogging, running, figure-eight running, karioka running, and sport/activity-specific skills. Tests must be performed pain-free and with unlimited movement.

> **A** The testing component of an assessment should include functional testing, stress testing, special tests, neurologic testing, and activity-specific functional testing. Given the findings (i.e., history, observation, inspection, and palpation) pertaining to the field-hockey player, a "wry" neck (torticollis) should be suspected. Functional testing (i.e., active, passive, and resisted ROM) is warranted.

REHABILITATION

> **Q** The findings from the testing component of the assessment are as follows: active ROM of the cervical spine limited on the involved side because of pain, resisted ROM of the cervical spine, grade IV flexion and extension, left lateral flexion and rotation, and right lateral flexion and rotation that could not be graded because of pain. The assessment of the field-hockey player suggests acute torticollis. Should she be permitted to participate in practice on a limited basis? Explain the management of this condition and the criteria for return to play.

Rehabilitation programs must be developed on an individual basis and address the specific needs of the individual. Exercises to relieve pain related to postural problems may not address pain related to an acute injury; therefore, a variety of exercises are listed in this section to allow selection of those most appropriate for the individual. The program should relieve pain and muscle tension; restore motion and balance; develop strength, endurance, and power; and maintain cardiovascular fitness. Patient education also is critical in teaching the skills and techniques that are needed to prevent recurrence.

Relief of Pain and Muscle Tension

Maintaining a prolonged posture can lead to discomfort. This can be avoided by doing active ROM exercises to relieve stress on supporting structures, promote circulation, and maintain flexibility. For example, exercises, including neck flexion, extension, lateral flexion and rotation, shoulder rolls, and glenohumeral circumduction, can be beneficial for relieving tension in the cervical and upper thoracic region. Conscious relaxation training can relax an individual who generally is tense or release tension in specific muscle groups, such as the upper trapezius. Grade I and II mobilization exercises can be initiated early in the program to relieve pain and stretch tight structures to restore accessory movements to the joints.

Restoration of Motion

Flexibility exercises and mobilization techniques can be used to increase the ROM of specific structures in the cervical and thoracic spine. Flexibility exercises can include passive and active stretching techniques. The intensity and duration of the exercise will vary relative to the site of the inflamed tissue. Examples of ROM exercises for the cervical spine are illustrated in Field Strategy 10.1.

Joint mobilization techniques for the cervical and thoracic spine can be used to restore motion. As a general rule, grade III and IV mobilization exercises can begin as soon as pain and muscle guarding are relieved.

Restoration of Proprioception and Balance

Restoring proprioceptive awareness of balanced posture and positioning is essential for maintaining normal alignment of the spine. Proprioceptive exercises should be initiated at the same time as the strengthening program. Exercises for the cervical and thoracic spines should focus on patient awareness of correct alignment and active control of posture.

Muscular Strength, Endurance, and Power

Isometric contractions to strengthen the neck musculature can progress to manual resistance, self-resistance, and commercial machines as available and tolerated. In addition, functional exercises

FIELD STRATEGY 10.1

Flexibility Exercises for the Cervical Spine

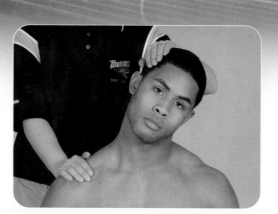

- Flexibility exercises can be performed actively and passively to increase range of motion in the cervical spine. A stretch should be held for approximately 20 seconds and the action repeated four or five times. The patient should feel a slight stretch in the absence of any pain.

- Initially, the exercises should be performed actively. Additional stretching can be provided by having the patient or the clinician use his or her hands to apply light pressure as the motion reaches its end range. Again, it is important that the motion be free of pain.

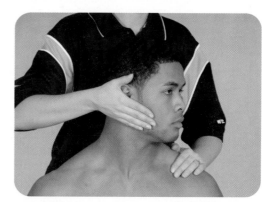

- The motions of cervical flexion, extension, lateral flexion, and rotation should be preformed as necessary. Stretching exercises can be performed in a seated position and should begin with the patient in a position of axial extension (i.e., with the chin tucked and the neck straight).

- Joint mobilization techniques also can be used to improve flexibility; however, specific techniques for the cervical spine are not within the scope of this textbook.

specific to the needs of the individual are advantageous. For example, neck strength is particularly important for wrestlers and football linemen, who need added stability and strength in the cervical region.

Cardiovascular Fitness

In selecting exercises to maintain and improve cardiovascular fitness, one should be aware of the potential problems with specific exercises. For example, aquatic exercises offer a variety of benefits, but a cervical spine injury could be aggravated by performing the freestyle stoke. Specifically, the continuous cervical rotation may have an adverse effect on the cervical spine. In a similar manner, cycling as a means of aerobic training could present problems depending on the type of bike that is used. A bike that enables an upright position typically would be more appropriate, because less stress is transmitted to both the cervical and thoracic spine as compared with other bikes.

The field-hockey player should not be permitted to practice until she has complete ROM and normal strength in all ranges of motion. Treatment is symptomatic and includes cryotherapy or application of heat as well as ROM exercises.

SUMMARY

1. The spine is a linkage system that transfers loads between the upper and lower extremities, enables motion in all three planes, and protects the delicate spinal cord. Although most injuries to the back are relatively minor and can be managed successfully using the PRICE principles (protect, restrict activity, ice, compression, and elevation), spinal fractures and nerve conditions do occur.

2. Two adjacent vertebrae and the soft-tissues between them are collectively referred to as a motion segment. The motion segment is the functional unit of the spine. The intervertebral disk is a fibrocartilaginous disk that provides cushioning between the articulating vertebral bodies.

3. The interspinous ligaments, intertransverse ligaments, and ligamentum flava link the spinous processes, transverse process, and laminae, respectively, of adjacent vertebrae. Collectively, the primary movers for back extension are called the erector spinae muscles.

4. The spinal cord extends from the brainstem to the level of the first or second lumbar vertebrae. Thirty-one pairs of spinal nerves emanate from the cord, with the distal bundle of spinal nerves known as the cauda equina.

5. Anatomical variations in the cervical and thoracic regions that can predispose an individual to spinal injuries include kyphosis and scoliosis.

6. Functional spinal stenosis is defined as a loss of CSF around the cord or, in more extreme cases, as a deformation of the spinal cord. The cervical segments most commonly affected are C_5 and C_6.

7. Signs and symptoms that indicate a serious cervical spine injury include pain over the spinous process, with or without deformity; unrelenting neck pain or muscle spasm; abnormal sensations in the head, neck, trunk, or extremities; muscular weakness in the extremities; paralysis or inability to move a body part; and absence of weak reflexes.

8. Because spinal cord damage can lead to paralysis or death, a suspected unstable neck injury should be treated as a medical emergency. The emergency care plan should be activated, including summoning EMS.

9. Brachial plexus injuries are graded in three levels:
   - *Neurapraxia injuries*—temporary loss of sensation and/or loss of motor function that recovers within 2 weeks
   - *Axonotmesis injuries*—significant motor and mild sensory deficits that last for at least 2 weeks
   - *Neurotmesis injuries*—severe motor and sensory deficits that persist for up to 1 year with poor prognosis

10. Thoracic fractures tend to be concentrated at the lower end of the thoracic spine. Large compressive loads can lead to a wedge fracture, or Scheuermann's disease can lead to degeneration of the epiphyseal end plates of the vertebral bodies, causing the intervertebral disk to prolapse into the vertebral body.

11. Assessment of a spinal injury should begin with a thorough history of the injury and include neurologic tests to determine possible nerve involvement. The severity of pain and the

presence or absence of neurologic symptoms, neck spasm, and tenderness can indicate when backboard and neck stabilization are needed.

12. If, at any time, an individual complains of acute pain in the spine, change in sensation anywhere on the body, or resistance to moving the spine, a significant injury should be assumed and the emergency care plan activated, including summoning EMS.

13. A rehabilitation program should focus on reduction of pain and spasm; restoration of motion and balance; development of strength, endurance, and power; and maintenance of cardiovascular fitness.

REFERENCES

1. Brown RL, Brunn MA, Garcia VF. Cervical spine injuries in children: a review of 103 patients treated consecutively at a level 1 pediatric trauma center. J Pediatr Surg 2001; 36(8):1107–1114.
2. Banerjee R, Palumbo MA, Fadale PD. Catastrophic cervical spine injuries in the collision sport athlete. Part 1: Epidemiology, functional anatomy, and diagnosis. Am J Sports Med 2004;32(4):1077–1087.
3. Leinberry CF, Wehbe MA. Brachial plexus anatomy. Hand Clin 2004;20(1):1–5.
4. Moskovich R. Biomechanics of the cervical spine. In: Nordin M, Frankel VH, eds. Basic Biomechanics of the Musculoskeletal System, 3rd Ed. Philadelphia: Lippincott Williams & Wilkins, 2001.
5. Polga DJ, Beaubien BP, Kallemeier PM, et al. Measurement of in vivo intradiskal pressure in healthy thoracic intervertebral disks. Spine 2004;29(12):1320–1324.
6. Kartal A, Yildiran I, Senkoylu A, Korkusuz F. Soccer causes degenerative changes in the cervical spine. Eur Spine J 2004;13(1):76–82.
7. Heck JF. The incidence of spearing during a high school's 1975 and 1990 football seasons. J Ath Train 1996;31(1): 31–37.
8. Torg JS, Pavlov H, Genuario SE, et al. Neurapraxia of the cervical spinal cord with transient quadriplegia. J Bone Joint Surg Am 1986;68: 1354–1370.
9. Moore J, Rice EL, Moore JM. Neck injuries. In: Mellion MB, Walsh WM, Madden C, Putukian M, Shelton GL, eds. The Team Physician's Handbook, 3rd ed. Philadelphia: Hanley & Belfus, 2005.
10. Torg JS, Sennett B, Pavlov H, et al. Spear tackler's spine: an entity precluding participation in tackle football and collision activities that expose the cervical spine to axial injury inputs. Am J Sports Med 1993;21(5):640–649.
11. Wilberger JE. Athletic spinal cord and spine injuries: guidelines for initial management. Clin Sport Med 1998; 17(1):111–120.
12. Torg JS, Ramsey-Emrheim JA. Cervical spine and brachial plexus injuries: return-to-play recommendation. Phys Sportsmed 1997;25(7):61–88.
13. Zmurko MG, Tannoury TY, Tannoury CA, Anderson DG. Cervical sprains, disk herniations, minor fractures, and other cervical injuries in the athlete. Clin Sports Med 2003;22(3):513–521.

Lumbar Spinal Conditions

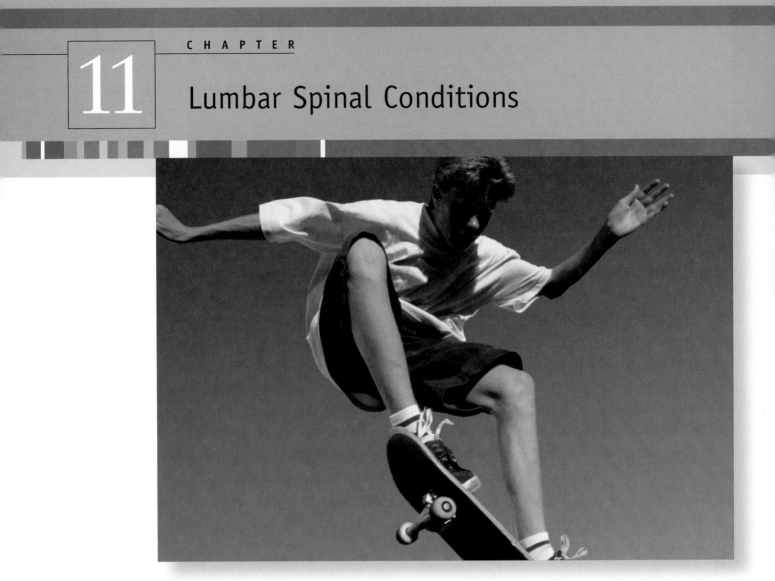

STUDENT OUTCOMES

1. Locate and explain the functional significance of the bony and soft-tissue structures of the lumbar spine.

2. Describe the motion capabilities of the lumbar spine.

3. Identify the factors that contribute to mechanical loading on the spine.

4. Describe specific strategies in activities of daily living to reduce spinal stress in the lumbar region.

5. Identify anatomical variations that can predispose individuals to lumbar spine injuries.

6. Explain the measures used to prevent injury to the lumbar spinal region.

7. Describe the common injuries and conditions of the lumbar spine and low back area in physically active individuals.

8. Describe a thorough assessment of the lumbar spine.

9. Identify rehabilitative exercises for the lumbar region.

ROLE DELINEATION COMPETENCIES

The following Performance Domains and Tasks defined in the National Athletic Trainers' Association Board of Certification *Role Delineation Study*, 5th Edition are addressed in this chapter:

BOC COMPETENCIES

II. Clinical Evaluation and Diagnosis

A. Obtain a history through observation, interview, and/or review of relevant records to assess current or potential injury, illness, or condition.
B. Inspect the involved area(s) visually to assess the injury, illness, or health-related condition.
C. Palpate the involved area(s) using standard techniques to assess the injury, illness, or health-related condition.
D. Perform specific tests in accordance with accepted procedures to assess the injury, illness, or health-related condition.
E. Formulate a clinical impression by interpreting the signs, symptoms, and predisposing factors of the injury, illness, or condition to determine the appropriate course of action.

III. Immediate Care

A. Employ life-saving techniques through the use of standard emergency procedures in order to reduce morbidity and the incidence of mortality.
B. Prevent exacerbation of non–life threatening condition(s) through the use of standard procedures in order to reduce morbidity.
C. Facilitate the timely transfer of care for conditions beyond the scope of practice of the athletic trainer by implementing appropriate referral strategies to stabilize and/or prevent exacerbation of the condition(s).

IV. Treatment, Rehabilitation, and Reconditioning

E. Reassess the status of injuries, illnesses, and/or conditions using standard techniques and documentation strategies in order to determine appropriate treatment, rehabilitation, and/or reconditioning and to evaluate readiness to return to a desired level of activity.
F. Educate the appropriate individual(s) in the treatment, rehabilitation, and reconditioning of injuries, illnesses, and/or conditions using applicable methods and materials to facilitate recovery, function, and/or performance.

Low back pain is a widespread problem that affects both the athletic and nonathletic populations. Nearly 30% of children have experienced low back pain at some time, with the incidence increasing with age until approximately 16 years, when the adult incidence of 75 to 80% is reached (1). Low back pain is more common in boys than in girls, and it is associated with increased physical activity and stronger back flexor muscles (2,3). Although the main causes of low back pain in athletes are musculotendinous strains and ligamentous sprains, chronic or recurring pain often is a symptom of lumbar disk degeneration or stress injuries to the bony articulations of the lumbar spine (4). Pain emanating from the lumbar disks most commonly affects the low back, buttocks, and hips and may result from progressive damage to the annular fibers, particularly the pain fibers that reside in the outer third of the annulus (5). Low back problems are especially common in equestrian sports, weight lifting, ice hockey, gymnastics, diving, football, wrestling, and aerobics.

This chapter begins with a review of the anatomical structures in the lumbar spine, followed by a discussion of the kinematics and kinetics of the region. Identification of anatomical variations that may predispose individuals to lumbar spinal conditions leads into strategies used to prevent injury. Information regarding common injuries sustained within the lumbar spine during participation in sport and physical activity is followed by a presentation of lumbar spinal injury assessment. Finally, examples of general rehabilitation exercises are provided.

ANATOMY OF THE LUMBAR SPINE

As mentioned in Chapter 10,[AU/ED: Please confirm chapter x-ref.] the lumbar and sacral regions of the spine are anatomically and functionally unique. Normal lumbar curvature is concave, and sacral curvature is convex, from the posterior perspective.

Lower Spinal Column

The lower spinal column, which forms a convex curve anteriorly, includes five lumbar, five fused sacral, and four small, fused coccygeal vertebrae (Fig. 11.1). The sacrum articulates with the ilium to form the sacroiliac (SI) joint.

Supporting the weight of the head, trunk, and upper extremities, the lumbar vertebral bodies have larger articulating surface areas and greater depth than those of any other spinal region. In addition, the orientation of the facet joints varies in comparison to the cervical and thoracic spines

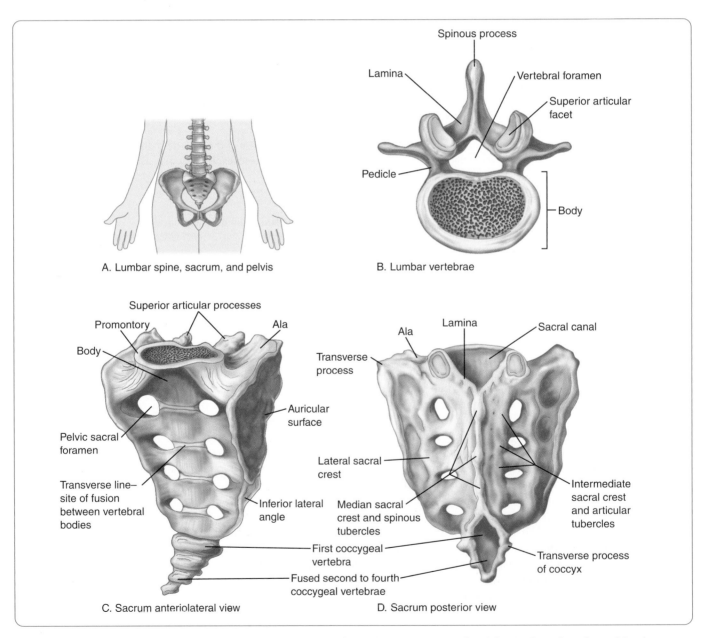

A. Lumbar spine, sacrum, and pelvis

B. Lumbar vertebrae

C. Sacrum anteriolateral view

D. Sacrum posterior view

■■■■ FIGURE 11.1 **Bones of the lumbar region. A**, Lumbar spine, sacrum, and pelvis. **B**, Superior view of lumbar vertebra. **C**, Anterolateral view of sacrum and coccyx. **D**, Posterior view of sacrum and coccyx.

(see Fig. 10.4). Information concerning the general structures of the spinal vertebrae and intervertebral disks is presented in Chapter 10.

Ligaments of the Lumbar Spine and Trunk

General information regarding the spinal ligaments is presented in Chapter 10. Specific to the lumbar spine, several ligaments, including the iliolumbar ligaments, posterior SI ligaments, sacrospinous ligament, and the sacrotuberous ligament, are responsible for maintaining its articulation with the sacrum (Fig. 11.2).

Muscles of the Lumbar Spine and Trunk

The muscles of the trunk are paired, with one on the left side and one on the right side of the body (Fig. 11.3). These muscles produce lateral flexion and/or rotation of the trunk when acting unilaterally and trunk flexion or extension when acting bilaterally. Collectively, the primary movers for back extension are called the erector spinae muscles.

See *Muscles of the Lumbar Spine,* available on the companion web site at thePoint, for the attachments, actions, and innervations of the major muscles of the lumbar region.

Spinal Cord and Spinal Nerves

The lumbar plexus and sacral plexus are prominent in the lower trunk. The distal end of the spinal cord, at approximately L_1–L_2, includes a bundle of spinal nerves that extends downward through the vertebral canal and is known collectively as the cauda equina, after its resemblance to a horse's tail.

The Lumbar Plexus

Supplying the anterior and medial muscles of the thigh region is the lumbar plexus, formed by the T_{12}–L_5 nerve roots (Fig. 11.4). The posterior branches of the L_2–L_4 nerve roots form the femoral

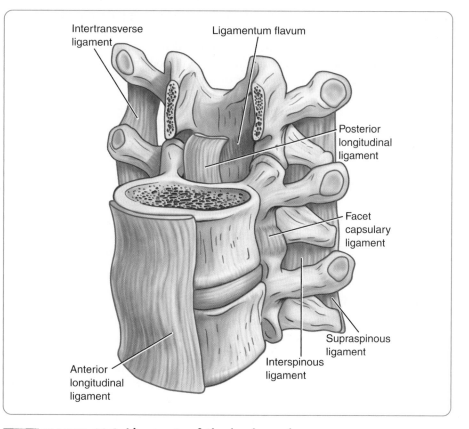

Intertransverse ligament

Ligamentum flavum

Posterior longitudinal ligament

Facet capsulary ligament

Supraspinous ligament

Interspinous ligament

Anterior longitudinal ligament

■■■■ FIGURE 11.2 **Ligaments of the lumbar spine.**

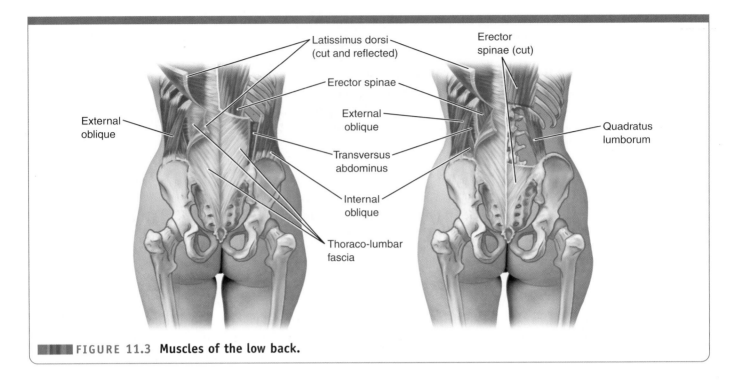

FIGURE 11.3 Muscles of the low back.

nerve, innervating the quadriceps, whereas the anterior branches form the obturator nerve, innervating most of the adductor muscle group.

The Sacral Plexus

A portion of the lumbar plexus (L_4–L_5) forms the lumbosacral trunk and courses downward to form the upper portion of the sacral plexus (Fig. 11.5). This plexus supplies the muscles of the buttock region and, through the sciatic nerve, the muscles of the posterior thigh and entire lower leg. The sciatic nerve is composed of two distinct nerves, the tibial nerve and the common peroneal nerve. The tibial nerve, formed by the anterior branches of the upper five nerve roots, innervates all the muscles on the posterior leg with the exception of the short head of the biceps femoris. The common peroneal nerve, formed by the posterior branches of the upper four nerve roots, innervates the short head of the biceps femoris, then divides in the vicinity of the head of the fibula into the deep peroneal nerve and the superficial peroneal nerve. These nerves innervate the anterior compartment of the lower leg and lateral compartments of the lower leg, respectively.

KINEMATICS AND MAJOR MUSCLE ACTIONS OF THE LUMBAR SPINE

The vertebral joints enable motion in all planes of movement as well as circumduction. Because the motion allowed between any two adjacent vertebrae is small, spinal movements always involve a number of motion segments. The ROM allowed at each motion segment is governed by anatomical constraints that vary through the lumbar region of the spine.

Flexion, Extension, and Hyperextension

The flexion-extension capability of the motion segments ranges from 12 to 20° in the lumbar region (6). It is important to avoid confusing spinal flexion with hip flexion or with forward pelvic tilt, although all three motions occur during an activity such as touching the toes. Hip flexion consists of anteriorly directed, sagittal plane rotation of the femur with respect to the pelvic girdle (or vice versa), and forward pelvic tilt is anteriorly directed movement of the anterior superior iliac spine (ASIS) with respect to the pubic symphysis.

When the spine is extended backward past anatomical position in the sagittal plane, the motion is termed **hyperextension**. The ROM for spinal hyperextension is considerable in the lumbar region,

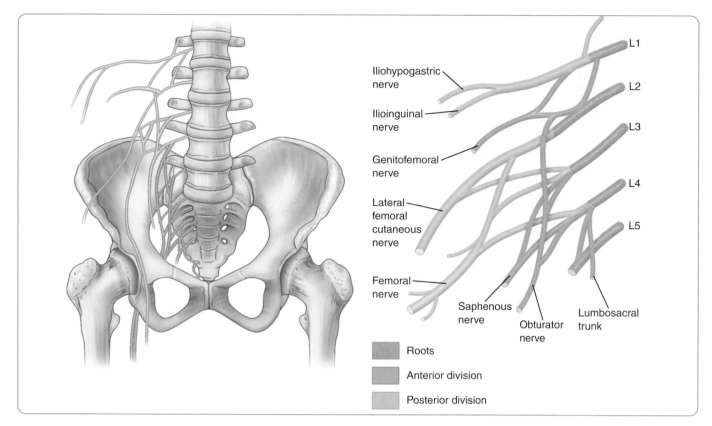

Iliohypogastric
nerve

Ilioinguinal
nerve

Genitofemoral
nerve

Lateral
femoral
cutaneous
nerve

Femoral
nerve

Saphenous
nerve

Obturator
nerve

Lumbosacral
trunk

L1
L2
L3
L4
L5

Roots

Anterior division

Posterior division

FIGURE 11.4 Lumbar plexus. The lumbar plexus is formed by the segmental nerves T_{12}–L_5. The lower portion of

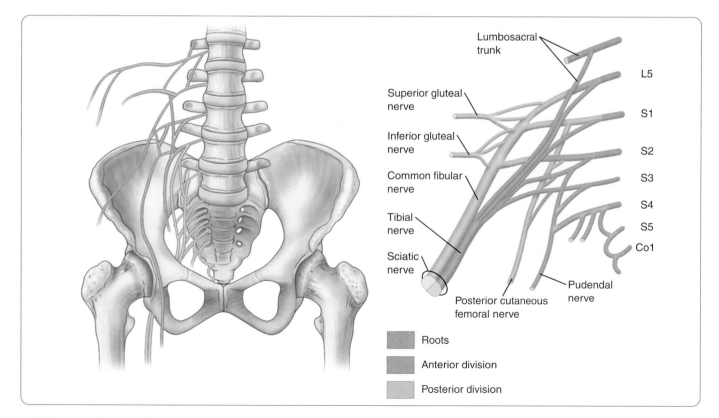

Lumbosacral
trunk

Superior gluteal
nerve

Inferior gluteal
nerve

Common fibular
nerve

Tibial
nerve

Sciatic
nerve

Posterior cutaneous
femoral nerve

Pudendal
nerve

L5
S1
S2
S3
S4
S5
Co1

Roots

Anterior division

Posterior division

FIGURE 11.5 Sacral plexus. The sacral plexus is formed by the segmental nerves L_4–S_5. This plexus innervates the lower leg, ankle, and foot via the tibial and common peroneal nerves.

ranging as high as 21° at L₅–S₁. The cumulative ROM for hyperextension is 54° in the lumbar region. Lumbar hyperextension is required in many sport skills, including several swimming strokes, the high jump and pole vault, wrestling, and numerous gymnastic skills. Repeated, extreme lumbar hyperextension is associated with increased risk of spondylolysis, a stress fracture of the pars interarticularis region of the spine (7).

Lateral Flexion and Rotation

Movement of the spine away from anatomical position in a lateral direction in the frontal plane is termed lateral flexion. In the lumbar region, the cumulative ROM for lateral flexion is approximately 24°. Spinal rotation capability is small in the lumbar region, with only approximately 2° of motion allowed because of the interlocking of the articular processes there. The lumbosacral joint permits approximately 5° of rotation.

KINETICS OF THE LUMBAR SPINE

As discussed in Chapter 10, forces acting on the spine include body weight, tension in the spinal ligaments and paraspinal muscles, intra-abdominal pressure, and any applied external loads. When the body is in an upright position, the major form of loading on the spine is axial, and the lumbar spine supports the weight of the body segments above it. Although most of the axial compression load on the spine is borne by the vertebral bodies and disks, the facet joints, when the spine is in hyperextension, may bear as much as approximately 30% of the load. Under significant compressive loading, such as during a heavy lifting task, increases in intra-abdominal pressure occur that may help to stiffen the trunk to prevent the spine from buckling (8).

Effect of Body Position

One factor that can dramatically affect the load on the lumbar spine is body position. When the body is in an upright position, the line of gravity passes anterior to the spinal column (Fig. 11.6). As a result, the spine is under a constant, forward bending moment. As the trunk is progressively flexed, the line of gravity shifts farther away from the spine. The farther the line of gravity from the spine, the larger the moment arm for body weight and the greater the bending moment generated. To maintain body position, this moment must be counteracted by tension in the back muscles. The more tension that is required to maintain body position, the greater the compression load on the spine. Lifting with the trunk being erect minimizes the tension requirement for the lumbar muscles, because the moment arm for body weight is minimized. For the same reason, holding the load as close to the trunk as possible during lifting and carrying minimizes the load on the back. In comparison to the load that is present during upright standing, compression on the lumbar spine increases with sitting; increases more with spinal flexion; and increases still further with a slouched sitting position. Box 11.1 lists guidelines for preventing lumbar spinal stress during performance of daily activities.

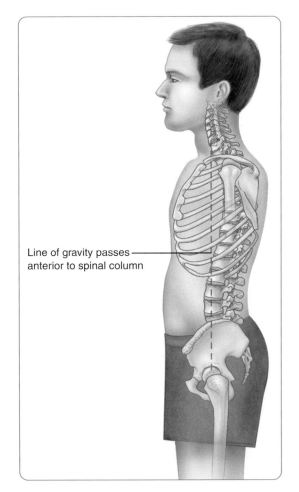

Line of gravity passes anterior to spinal column

■■■ ■ FIGURE 11.6 **Line of gravity.** The line of gravity for the head and trunk passes anterior to the spinal column during upright standing. The moment arm for head/trunk weight at any given vertebral joint is the perpendicular distance between the line of gravity and the spinal column.

Effect of Movement Speed

Another factor that affects loading of the lumbar spine is body movement speed. Executing a lift in a very rapid, jerking fashion dramatically increases compression and shear forces on the lumbar spine as well as tension in the paraspinal muscles (9). This is one reason why isotonic resistance training exercises should be performed in a slow, controlled fashion.

Box 11.1   Preventing Low Back Injuries in Activities of Daily Living

Sitting
- Sit on a firm, straight-backed chair.
- Place the buttocks as far back into the chair as possible to avoid slouching.
- Sit with the feet flat on the floor, not extended and raised on a stool.
- Avoid sitting for long periods of time, particularly with the knees fully extended.

Driving
- Place the seat forward so that the knees are level with the hips and you do not have to reach for the pedals.
- If the left foot is not working the pedals, place it flat on the floor.
- Keep the back of the seat in a nearly upright position to avoid slouching.

Standing
If you must stand in one area for an extended time:
- Shift body weight from one foot to the other.
- Elevate one foot on a piece of furniture to keep the knees flexed.
- Perform toe flexion and extension inside the shoes.
- Hold the chin up, keep the shoulders back, and relax the knees.
- Avoid arching the back

Lifting and Carrying
- Use a lumbosacral belt or have assistance when lifting heavy objects.
- To lift an object:
  - Place the object close to the body.
  - Bend at the knees, not the waist, and keep the back erect.
  - Tighten the abdominal muscles and inhale before lifting the object.
  - Exhale during the lift.
  - Do not twist while lifting.
- To carry a heavy object:
  - Hold the object close to the body at waist level.
  - Carry the object in the middle of the body, not to one side.

Sleeping
- Sleep on a firm mattress. If needed, place a sheet of 3/4-inch plywood under the mattress.
- Sleep on the side, and place pillows between the legs.
- When sleeping supine, place pillows under the knees. Avoid sleeping in the prone position.
- Avoid sleeping with the arms extended overhead.

ANATOMICAL VARIATIONS PREDISPOSING INDIVIDUALS TO SPINAL CONDITIONS

Mechanical stress derived from lateral spinal muscle imbalances or from sustaining repeated impact forces can cause back pain and/or injury. Excessive spinal curvatures can be congenital or acquired through weight training or sport participation. Defects in the pars interarticularis of the neural arch can be caused by mechanical stress, also placing an individual at risk for serious spinal injury.

Lordosis

Abnormal exaggeration of the lumbar curve, or **lordosis**, often is associated with weakened abdominal muscles in combination with tight muscles, especially the hip flexors, tensor fasciae latae, and deep lumbar extensors. Normally, the pelvic angle is approximately 30°. With excessive lordosis, this angle can increase to 40° and be accompanied by a mobile spine and anterior pelvic tilt (Fig. 11.7A). Other causes of lordosis include congenital spinal deformity, such as bilateral congenital hip dislocation, spondylolisthesis, compensatory action resulting from another deformity (e.g., kyphosis), hip flexion contractures, poor postural habits, and overtraining in sports requiring repeated lumbar hyperextension (e.g., gymnastics, figure skating, football linemen, javelin throwing, or swimming the butterfly stroke). Because lordosis places added compressive stress on the posterior elements of the spine, low back pain is a common symptom predisposing many individuals to low back injuries.

Sway Back

An individual with a sway back deformity presents with an increased lordotic curve and kyphosis (Fig. 11.7B). This condition often results from weakness in the lower abdominals, lower thoracic extensors, hip flexors, compensatory tight hip extensors, lower lumbar extensors, and upper abdominals. The deformity results as the spine bends back sharply at the lumbosacral angle. Subsequently, the entire pelvis shifts anteriorly, causing the hips to move into extension. For the center of gravity to remain in its normal position, the thoracic spine flexes on the lumbar spine, increasing the lumbar and thoracic curves.

A. Exaggerated lordosis   B. Swayback   C. Flat back

■■■■ FIGURE 11.7 **Lumbar anomalies. A,** Lordosis.
B, Sway back. **C,** Flat back.

Flat Back Syndrome

The term flat back refers to a relative decrease in lumbar lordosis (20°), which shifts the center of gravity anterior to the lumbar spine and hips (Fig. 11.7C). The condition may result from the use of Harrington rods in the treatment of scoliosis, degenerative disk disease involving multiple levels of the spine, ankylosing spondylitis, and postlaminectomy syndrome compression fractures, most commonly caused by osteoporosis.

The most common clinical sign is the tendency to lean forward when walking or standing. In an effort to bring the body into better alignment, the low back, buttock, and posterior thigh muscles are recruited to tilt the pelvis. This action causes these muscles to fatigue more quickly, leading to aching and pain. The body also may compensate by exhibiting increased hip and knee flexion. If hip flexion is accentuated, however, a hip flexion contracture may occur. Treatment involves strengthening the gluteal, low back, abdominal, and hamstring musculature.

Pars Interarticularis Fractures

The pars interarticularis is the weakest bony portion of the vertebral neural arch, the region between the superior and inferior articular facets. Fracture in this region are termed **spondylolysis** and **spondylolisthesis** (Fig. 11.8). Although some pars defects may be congenital, they also may be caused by mechanical stress from axial loading of the lumbar spine during repeated weight-loading in flexion, hyperextension (i.e., back-arching), and rotation. These repetitive movements cause a shearing stress to the vertebrae, resulting in a stress fracture.

Fractures of the pars interarticularis may range from hairline to complete separation of the bone. A bony defect in spondylolysis tends to occur at an earlier age, typically before 8 years of age, yet often does not produce symptoms until 10 to 15 years of age. The fracture may heal with less periosteal callus and tends to form a fibrous union more often than fractures at other sites.

A bilateral separation in the pars interarticularis, called **spondylolisthesis**, results in the anterior displacement of a vertebra with respect to the vertebra below it (Fig. 11.9). The most common site for this injury is the lumbosacral joint (L_5–S_1), with 90% of the slips occurring at this level. Spondylolisthesis often is diagnosed in children between the ages of 10 and 15 years and is more common in boys than in girls. High-degree slips, however, are seen more commonly in females than in males. (10). Unlike most stress fractures, spondylolysis and spondylolisthesis do not typically heal with time but, rather, tend to persist, particularly in cases with no interruption in participation in sport and physical activity. Those who are particularly susceptible to this condition include female gymnasts, interior football linemen, weight lifters, volleyball players, pole vaulters, wrestlers, and rowers.

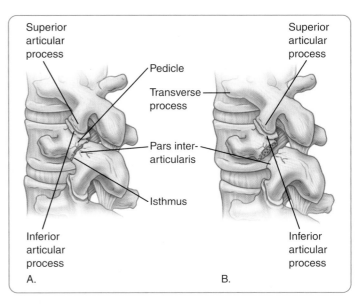

FIGURE 11.8 Spondylolysis and Spondylolisthesis. **A**, Spondylolysis is a stress fracture of the pars interarticularis. **B**, Spondylolisthesis is a bilateral fracture of the pars interarticularis accompanied by anterior slippage of the involved vertebra.

Although most spondylitic conditions are asymptomatic, low back pain and associated neurologic symptoms, when the underlying cause is repeated mechanical stress, are likely to occur. The individual may complain of unilateral, dull backache aggravated by activity, usually hyperextension and rotation. Standing on one leg and hyperextending the back aggravates the condition.

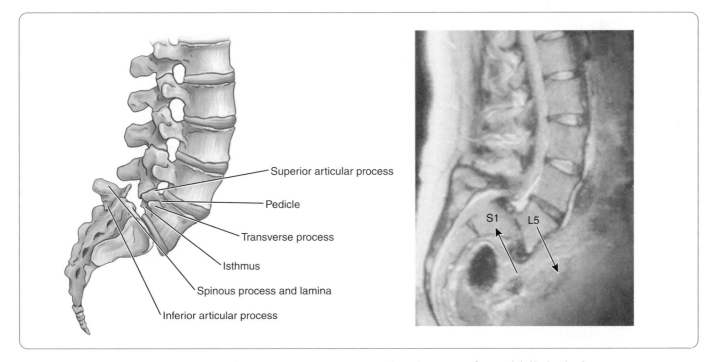

FIGURE 11.9 Spondylolisthesis. This magnetic resonance imaging scan of spondylolisthesis demonstrates an anterior shift of the L_5 vertebra.

Demonstrable muscle spasm occurs in the erector spinae muscles or hamstrings, leading to flattening of the lumbosacral curve, but no sciatic nerve symptoms usually are present. Pain may radiate into the buttock region or down the sciatic nerve if the L_5 nerve root is compressed. This individual should be referred to a physician.

Slippage is measured by dividing the distance the superior vertebral body has displaced forward onto the inferior by the anteroposterior dimensions of the inferior vertebral body. In mild cases (i.e., slippage of 0–25%), modifications in training and technique can permit the individual to continue to participate in physical activity. In moderate cases (i.e., slippage from 25–50%), however, most physicians do not begin active rehabilitation until the individual has been asymptomatic for 4 weeks. Following that period, the focus of rehabilitation is the development of flexibility in the hamstrings and gluteal muscles, combined with strengthening the abdomen and back extensors. If the slip is greater than 50%, the individual presents with flat buttocks, tight hamstrings, and alterations in gait, and a palpable step-off deformity may be present at the level of the defect. This individual should be excluded from participation in contact sports unless the condition is asymptomatic and absence of continued slippage has been documented.

PREVENTION OF SPINAL CONDITIONS

Although most of the load on the spine is borne by the vertebral bodies and disks, the facet joints assist with some load bearing. Protective equipment can prevent some injuries to the spinal region; however, physical conditioning plays a more important role in preventing injuries to this area. In addition, because the low back is subjected to a variety of stresses as part of normal daily activities, an awareness of proper posture is essential in minimizing the risk of injury.

Protective Equipment

Weight-training belts, abdominal binders, and other similar lumbar/sacral supportive devices support the abdominal contents, stabilize the trunk, and potentially, can assist in preventing spinal deformity and damage. These devices place the low back in a more vertical lifting posture, decrease lumbar lordosis, limit pelvic torsion, and lessen axial loading on the spine by increasing intra-abdominal pressure, which in turn reduces compressive forces in the vertebral bodies. Many of these protective devices are discussed in Chapter 3.

Physical Conditioning

Strengthening of the back muscles is imperative to stabilize the spinal column. Exercises to strengthen the low back area should involve back extension, lateral flexion, and rotation. In addition, it is important to strengthen the abdominal muscles to maintain appropriate postural alignment.

Normal range of motion (ROM) also is essential in stabilizing the spine and preventing injury. If warranted, stretching exercises should be used to promote and maintain normal ROM. In particular, it is advantageous to ensure maximal motion in lateral flexion, forward flexion, and rotation.

Proper Skill Technique

Poor posture during walking, sitting, standing, lying down, and running may lead to chronic low back strain or sprains. Cases of postural deformity should be assessed to determine the cause, and an appropriate exercise program should be developed to address the deficits.

Lifting technique also can affect spinal loading. Executing a lift in a very rapid, jerking fashion dramatically increases compression and shear forces on the spine as well as tension in the paraspinal muscles. For this reason, isotonic resistance exercises should always be performed in a slow, controlled fashion. Breathing technique should be emphasized as well. Specifically, it is desirable to inhale deeply as a lift is initiated and exhale forcefully and smoothly at the end of the lift. Use of a supportive weight-training belt and a spotter also can potentially reduce the chance of injury to the lumbar region during heavy weight lifting.

CONDITIONS OF THE LUMBAR SPINE

 What criteria should be used to determine whether an individual who reports low back pain should be referred to a physician?

The lumbar spine must support the weight of the head, trunk, and arms as well as any load held in the hands. In addition, the two lower lumbar motion segments (i.e., L_4–L_5 and L_5–S_1) provide a large ROM in flexion-extension. As such, it is not surprising that mechanical abuse often results in episodes of low back pain or that the lower lumbar disks are injured more frequently than any others in the spine.

Lumbar Contusions, Strains, and Sprains

An estimated 75 to 80% of the population experiences low back pain stemming from mechanical injury to muscles, ligaments, or connective tissue (Box 11.2). Although low back pain typically strikes adults, nearly 30% of children experience low back pain up to the age of 16 years (1). Several known pathologies may cause low back pain, but reduced spinal flexibility, repeated stress, and activities that require maximal extension of the lumbar spine are most associated with chronic low back pain.

Muscle strains may result from a sudden extension action with trunk rotation on an overtaxed, unprepared, or underdeveloped spine. Chronic strains may stem from improper posture, excessive lumbar lordosis, flat back, or scoliosis.

Signs and Symptoms

Pain and discomfort can range from diffuse to localized. Pain does not radiate into the buttocks or posterior thigh, and no signs of neural involvement, such as muscle weakness, sensory changes, or reflex inhibition, are seen. If a muscle strain is present, pain will increase with passive flexion and with active or resisted extension.

Management

Acute protocol is followed to control pain and hemorrhage. Following cold treatment, passive stretching of the low back can help to relieve muscle spasm. A corset-type brace can be worn to compress the area (see Fig. 3.5). Following the acute stage, a graduated stretching and strengthening program can be initiated. In moderate to severe cases, the individual should be referred to a physician. Prescription muscle relaxants or nonsteroidal anti-inflammatory drugs (NSAIDs) may be appropriate.

Low Back Pain in Runners

Many runners develop muscle tightness in the hip flexors and hamstrings. Tight hip flexors tend to produce a forward body lean, which leads to anterior pelvic tilt and hyperlordosis of the lumbar spine. Because the lumbar muscles develop tension to counteract the forward bending moment of the entire trunk when the trunk is in flexion, these muscles are particularly susceptible to strain. Coupled with tight hamstrings, a shorter stride often emerges.

Box 11.2   Causes of Low Back Pain

- Muscle strains and sprains
- Sciatica
- Protruded or herniated disk
- Pathologic fracture
- Disk space infections
- Spinal infections (e.g., tuberculosis)
- Neoplastic tumor (i.e., primary or metastatic)
- Ankylosing spondylitis (arthritis of the spine)
- Benign space-occupying lesions
- Abdominal aortic aneurysm

Box 11.3 Reducing Low Back Pain in Runners

- Wear properly fitted shoes that control heel motion and provide maximum shock absorption.
- Increase flexibility at the hip, knee, ankle plantar flexors, and trunk extensors.
- Increase strength in the abdominal and trunk extensor muscles.
- Avoid excessive body weight.
- Warm up before and after running.
- Run with an upright stance rather than with a forward lean.
- Avoid excessive side-to-side sway.
- Run on even terrain, and limit hill work. Avoid running on concrete.
- Avoid overstriding to increase speed, because this increases leg shock.
- Gradually increase distance, intensity, and duration. Do not increase any parameter more than 10% in 1 week.
- If orthotics are worn and pain persists, check for wear and rigidity.
- Consider alternatives to running, such as cycling, rowing, or swimming.

Signs and Symptoms

Symptoms include localized pain that increases with active and resisted back extension, but radiating pain and neurologic deficits are not present. Anterior pelvic tilt and hyperlordosis of the lumbar spine also may be present.

Management

Treatment focuses on avoiding excessive flexion activities and a sedentary posture (Box 11.3). Flexion causes the mobile nucleus pulposus to shift posteriorly and press against the annulus fibrosus at its thinnest, least-buttressed place. In most cases, this just leads to pain, but in others, it may lead to a herniated disk. In addition, physical activity is necessary to pump fluid through the spinal disks to keep them properly hydrated; by interfering with this process, immobility can prolong pain.

Ice, NSAIDs, muscle relaxants, transcutaneous electrical nerve stimulation (TENS), and electrical muscle stimulation may be used to reduce pain and inflammation. Lumbar stabilization exercises can be combined with extension exercises, progressive activity, and early mobilization. Aerobic exercise, such as walking, swimming, or biking, should be included in all programs. If symptoms do not improve within a week, the individual should be referred to a physician to rule out a more serious underlying condition. In an effort to decrease the incidence of low back pain, training techniques should allow adequate progression of distance and intensity and include extensive flexibility exercises for the hip and thigh region.

Myofascial Pain

Myofascial pain is referred pain that emanates from a myofascial trigger point, a hypersensitive, localized nodule within a taut band of muscle tissue and its surrounding fascia. When compressed or palpated, pain is produced in a predictable distribution of referred pain. In the lumbar area, the piriformis muscle and quadratus lumborum are common trigger point sites associated with extended sitting, standing, running and walking activities. The piriformis in particular can impact the sciatic nerve as it courses through, above, or below the muscle on its path into the posterior leg. Individuals who slip unexpectedly and catch themselves also can irritate the trigger points.

Signs and Symptoms

Aggravation of the piriformis can lead to referred pain in the SI area, posterior hip, and upper two-thirds of the posterior thigh. Aching and deep pain increases with activity or with prolonged sitting with the hip adducted, flexed, and internally rotated. If the sciatic nerve is impinged, pain and possible changes in sensation may extend into the leg.

Referred pain from the quadratus lumborum often gives a false sign of a disk syndrome and often is overlooked as a source of low back pain. The superficial fibers can refer a sharp, aching pain to the low back, iliac crest, or greater trochanter or can extend it to the abdominal wall. The deep fibers may refer pain to the SI joint or lower buttock region. Pain increases during lateral bending toward the involved side, while standing for long periods of time, and during coughing or sneezing.

Management

Trigger point treatment involves stretching the involved muscle back to its normal resting length as a way to relieve the irritation that led to the initial pain. The patient should be placed in a comfortable position on the uninvolved side if the piriformis is involved or prone if the quadratus lumborum is involved. Three potential techniques can be used. One technique involves application of pressure slowly and progressively over the trigger point. Pressure is maintained until the tenderness is gone. Another technique involves ice massage applied over the length of the muscle and then over the referred pain pattern. The ice is applied in longitudinal, parallel strokes in only one direction while a passive stretch is applied progressively to the involved muscle. The third technique involves a deep-stroking massage over the length of the muscle, moving in a distal to proximal direction. As the massage continues, the taut band should relax, the tender nodules soften, and the pain ease.

Facet Joint Pathology

Throughout the longitudinal axis of the spine, three distinct anatomical columns can be defined at any spinal motion segment—namely, the anterior, middle, and posterior columns. The posterior column contains the pars interarticularis, facet joints, and spinous processes and is supported by the ligamentum flavum and interspinous ligaments. The facet joint is a synovial joint richly innervated via the medial branch of the posterior primary rami of at least two adjacent spinal nerves. The facet joint capsules act as passive restraints against excessive lumbar rotation and flexion and serve as a protective mechanism for the intervertebral disk.

Lumbar facet pathology may involve subluxation or dislocation of the facet, facet joint syndrome (i.e., inflammation), or degeneration of the facet itself (i.e., arthritis). The exact pathophysiology is unclear. Theories include possible mechanical irritation of the nearby nerve root, chemical irritation arising from the inflammatory process (e.g., capsular and synovial inflammation), meniscoid entrapment, synovial impingement, joint subluxation, chondromalacia facette, mechanical injury to the joint's capsule, and restriction to normal articular motion from soft or articular causes.

Signs and Symptoms

Signs and symptoms can include nonspecific low back, hip, and buttock pain with a deep and achy quality. The pain may radiate into the posterior thigh, but it does not radiate below the knee. Some patients describe their pain as being worse in the morning, aggravated by rest and hyperextension, and relieved by repeated motion. Flattening of lumbar lordosis may be visible. Point tenderness may be elicited to a unilateral or bilateral paravertebral area. Pain often is exacerbated by trunk rotation, stretching into full extension, lateral bending toward the involved side, and with torsion. Sensory alternations usually are absent unless the nerve root is secondarily involved.

Limited flexibility of the pelvic musculature can directly impact the mechanics of the lumbosacral spine. If facet joint pathology is present, an abnormal pelvic tilt and rotation of the hip secondary to tight hamstrings, hip rotators, and quadratus may be evident. Typically, manual muscle testing is normal; however, a subtle weakness in the erector spinae and hamstring muscles may contribute to pelvic tilt abnormalities. This subtle weakness may be appreciated with trunk, pelvic, and lower extremity extension asymmetry. If facet hypertrophy narrows the neural foramen, causing nerve root impingement, a straight leg raising test may elicit a positive response. Typically, this maneuver is normal.

Management

A definitive diagnosis is made using radiographs or magnetic resonance imaging or by a physician injecting the facet with an anesthetic and noting any change in the symptoms. Initial treatment should focus on education, relative rest, pain relief, and maintenance of positions that provide comfort, exercises, and some modalities. Therapeutic exercises should include instruction regarding proper posture and body mechanics in activities of daily living that protect the injured joints, reduce symptoms, and prevent further injury. Positions that cause pain should be avoided. Modalities such as superficial heat and cryotherapy may help to relax the muscles and reduce pain. In addition, medications such as NSAIDs can be advantageous. Spinal manipulation and mobilization also can be used to reduce pain. Once the painful symptoms are controlled during the acute phase of treatment, stretching and strengthening exercises of the lumbar spine and associated muscles can be initiated.

Sciatica

Sciatica, an inflammatory condition of the sciatic nerve, is classified in terms of four levels of severity, each with its own management strategy (Box 11.4). The condition can be caused by a herniated disk, annular tear, myogenic or muscle-related disease, spinal stenosis, facet joint arthropathy, or compression of the nerve between the piriformis muscle.

Signs and Symptoms

If related to a herniated disk, radiating leg pain is greater than back pain and increases with sitting and leaning forward, coughing, sneezing, and straining. Pain is reproduced during an ipsilateral straight leg raising test (see Fig. 11.18).

In an annular tear, back pain is more prevalent and is exacerbated with straight leg raising. Morning pain and muscular stiffness that worsens if chilled or when the weather changes (arthritic-like symptoms) are characteristic of myogenic or muscle-related disease. Pain typically radiates into the buttock and thigh region.

See *Signs and Symptoms of Sciatic*, available on the companion website at thePoint, for the common signs and symptoms that accompany the various etiologies of sciatica.

If lumbar spinal stenosis is present, back and leg pain develop after the individual walks a limited distance and concomitantly increase as the distance increases. Pain is not reproduced with a straight leg raising test, but it can be reproduced with prolonged spine extension, which is relieved with spine flexion. If a facet joint is involved, pain is localized over the joint on spinal extension and is exacerbated with ipsilateral lateral flexion. If the sciatic nerve is compressed by the piriformis muscle, pain increases during internal rotation of the thigh.

Management

Referral to a physician is necessary to check for a potentially serious underlying condition. Under normal circumstances, bed rest usually is not indicated, although side-lying with the knees flexed may relieve symptoms. Lifting, bending, twisting, and prolonged sitting and standing aggravate the condition and, therefore, should be avoided. When asymptomatic, abdominal and extensor muscle strengthening exercises can begin, with gradual return to activity. If symptoms resume, however, activity should cease, and the individual should be referred back to the physician. Occasionally,

Box 11.4   Classification and Management of Sciatica

- **Sciatica only:** No sensory or muscle weakness. Modify activity appropriately, and develop rehabilitation and prevention program. Any increased pain requires immediate re-evaluation.
- **Sciatica with soft signs:** Some sensory changes, mild or no reflex change, normal muscle strength, and normal bowel and bladder function. Remove from sport participation for 6 to 12 weeks.
- **Sciatica with hard signs:** Sensory and reflex changes, and muscle weakness caused by repeated, chronic, or acute condition. Normal bowel and bladder function. Remove from participation for 12 to 24 weeks.
- **Sciatica with severe signs:** Sensory and reflex changes, muscle weakness, and altered bladder function. Consider immediate surgical decompression.

extended rest is needed for symptoms to resolve totally, and if a significant disk protrusion is present, surgery may be indicated.

Conditions of the Lumbar Disk

Prolonged mechanical loading of the spine can lead to microruptures in the annulus fibrosus, resulting in degeneration of the disk (Fig. 11.10). Bulging or protruded disks refer to some eccentric accumulation of the nucleus with slight deformity of the annulus. When the eccentric nucleus produces a definite deformity as it works its way through the fibers of the annulus, it is called a **prolapsed disk**. It is called an **extruded disk** when the material moves into the spinal canal, where it runs the risk of impinging on adjacent nerve roots. Finally, with a **sequestrated disk**, the nuclear material has separated from the disk itself and, potentially, can migrate. The most commonly herniated disks are the lower two lumbar disks at L_4-L_5 and L_5-S_1, followed by the two lower cervical disks. Most ruptures move in a posterior or posterolateral direction as a result of torsion and compression, not just compression.

Signs and Symptoms

Because the intervertebral disks are not innervated, the sensation of pain does not occur until the surrounding soft-tissue structures are impinged. When compression is placed on a spinal nerve of the sciatic nerve complex (L_4–S_3), sensory and motor deficits are reflected in the myotome and dermatome patterns associated with the nerve root (Fig. 11.11). In addition, alteration in tendon reflexes is apparent. A disk need not be completely herniated to give symptoms, which include sharp pain and muscle spasms at the site of herniation that often shoot down the sciatic nerve into the lower extremity. The individual may walk in a slightly crouched position, leaning away from the side of the lesion. Forward trunk

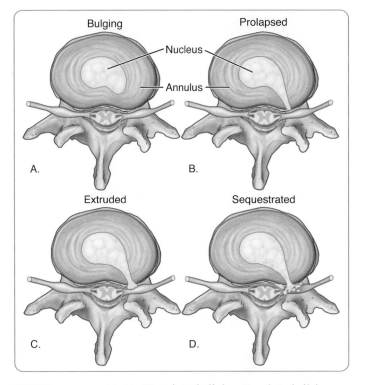

FIGURE 11.10 Herniated disks. Herniated disks are categorized by severity as an eccentrically loaded nucleus progressively moves from **(A)** protruded through, **(B)** prolapsed, and **(C)** extruded, culminating in **(D)** sequestrated when the nuclear material moves into the canal to impinge on the adjacent spinal nerves.

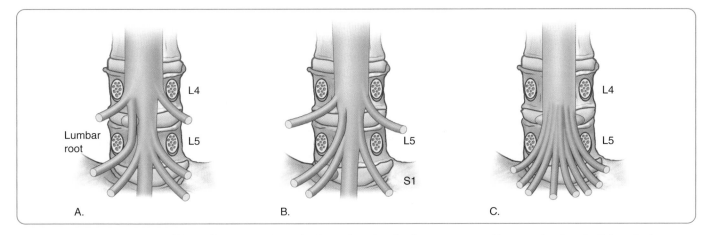

FIGURE 11.11 Possible effects on the spinal cord and spinal nerves according to the level of herniation. **A,** Herniation between L_4 and L_5 compresses the L_5 nerve root. **B,** Herniation between L_5 and S_1 can compress the nerve root crossing the disk (S_1) and the nerve root emerging through the intervertebral foramina (L_5). **C,** A posterior herniation at the L_4–L_5 level can compress the dura mater of the entire cauda equina, leading to bowel and bladder paralysis.

TABLE 11.1 Physical Findings Associated with a Herniated Disk

SIGNS AND SYMPTOMS	L₃–L₄ (L₄ ROOT)	L₄–L₅ (L₅ ROOT)	L₅–S₁ (S₁ ROOT)
Pain	Lumbar region and buttocks	Lumbar region, groin, and sacroiliac area	Lumbar region, groin, and sacroiliac area
Dermatome and sensory loss	Anterior midthigh over patella and medial lower leg to great toe	Lateral thigh, anterior leg, top of foot, and middle three toes	Posterior lateral thigh and lower leg to lateral foot and fifth toe
Myotome weakness	Ankle dorsiflexion	Toe extension (extensor hallux)	Ankle plantar flexion (gastrocnemius)
Reduced deep tendon reflex	Quadriceps	Medial hamstrings	Achilles tendon
Straight leg raising test	Normal	Reduced	Reduced

flexion or a straight leg raising test (see Fig. 11.18) may exacerbate pain and increase distal symptoms. Significant signs indicating the need for immediate referral to a physician include muscle weakness, sensory changes, diminished reflexes in the lower extremity, and abnormal bladder or bowel function. Table 11.1 outlines physical findings associated with disk herniation in the low back region.

Management

In mild cases, treatment consists of minimizing load on the spine by avoiding activities that involve impact, lifting, bending, twisting, and prolonged sitting and standing. Painful muscle spasms can be eliminated with ice and/or heat, administration of prescribed NSAIDs and/or muscle relaxants, ultrasound, TENS, passive exercise, and gentle stretching. Following resolution of spasm and acute pain, rehabilitation should include spine and hamstring flexibility, spinal strength and stabilization exercises, and functional stabilization control in sport and daily activities.

Lumbar Fractures and Dislocations

Transverse or spinous process fractures are caused by extreme tension from the attached muscles or from a direct blow to the low back during participation in contact sports, such as football, rugby, soccer, basketball, hockey, and lacrosse. These fractures often lead to additional injury of surrounding soft tissues but are not as serious as compression fractures. Compression fractures more commonly involve the L_1 vertebra at the thoracolumbar junction.

Hyperflexion, or jack-knifing of the trunk, crushes the anterior aspect of the vertebral body. The primary danger with this injury is the possibility of bony fragments moving into the spinal canal and damaging the spinal cord or spinal nerves. Because of the facet joint orientation in the lumbar region, dislocations occur only when a fracture is present. Fracture-dislocations resulting from sport participation are rare.

Signs and Symptoms

Symptoms include localized, palpable pain that may radiate down the nerve root if a bony fragment compresses a spinal nerve. Because the spinal cord ends at approximately the L_1 or L_2 level, fractures of the lumbar vertebrae below this point do not pose a serious threat but, rather, should be handled with care to minimize potential nerve damage to the cauda equina. Confirmation of a possible fracture is made with a radiograph or computed tomographic scan.

 EMS If a fracture or dislocation is suspected, the emergency plan, including summoning emergency medical services (EMS) for transport to the nearest medical facility, should be activated.

Management

Conservative treatment consists of initial bed rest, cryotherapy, and minimizing mechanical loads on the low back until symptoms subside, which may take 3 to 6 weeks.

If assessment of a low back injury reveals signs of nerve root involvement (i.e., sensory or motor deficits and diminished reflexes) or disk injury, physician referral is warranted.

SACRUM AND COCCYX CONDITIONS

 A 40-year-old man initiated a training program to improve his cardiovascular fitness. His workout for the past month has consisted of running on a treadmill. Over the past week, he began to develop pain in the sacral region during his workout. The pain has now become so persistent and chronic that it hurts to sit for an extended period of time. What injury may be present, and what recommendations can be made to this person relative to caring for the injury?

Because the sacrum and coccyx are essentially immobile, the potential for mechanical injury to these regions is dramatically reduced. In many cases, injuries result from direct blows and stress on the SI joint.

Sacroiliac Joint Sprain

Sprains of the SI joint may result from a single traumatic episode that involves bending and/or twisting, repetitive stress from lifting, a fall on the buttocks, excessive side-to-side or up-and-down motion during running and jogging, running on uneven terrain, suddenly slipping or stumbling forward, or wearing new shoes or orthoses. The injury may irritate or stretch the sacrotuberous or sacrospinous ligament, or it may lead to an anterior or posterior rotation of one side of the pelvis relative to the other. Hypermobility results from rotation of the pelvis. During healing, the joint on the injured side may become hypermobile, allowing the joint to subluxate in either an anterior- or posterior-rotated position.

Signs and Symptoms

Symptoms may involve unilateral, dull pain in the sacral area that extends into the buttock and posterior thigh. On observation, the ASIS or posterior superior iliac spine (PSIS) may appear to be asymmetrical when compared bilaterally. A leg-length discrepancy may be present, but muscle spasm is not often seen. Standing on one leg and climbing stairs may increase the pain. Forward bending reveals a block to normal movement, with the PSIS on the injured side moving sooner than on the uninjured side. Lateral flexion toward the injured side increases pain, as do straight leg raises beyond 45°.

Management

Treatment for SI sprains includes cryotherapy, prescribed NSAIDs, and gentle stretching to alleviate stiffness. As the conditions improves, flexibility, pelvic stabilization exercises, mobilization of the affected joint, and strengthening exercises for the low back should be initiated.

Coccygeal Conditions

Direct blows to the region can produce contusions and fractures of the coccyx. Pain resulting from a fracture may last for several months. Prolonged or chronic pain in the region also may result from irritation of the coccygeal nerve plexus. This condition is termed coccygodynia. Treatment for coccygeal pain includes analgesics, use of padding for protection, and a ring seat to alleviate compression during sitting.

 This individual has probably irritated the SI joint from repeated stress while running on the treadmill. This individual should ice the region to control inflammation and pain and should stretch the low back and buttock region. A detailed assessment (including a gait analysis while running) should be performed to determine the potential cause of the injury so that a proper rehabilitation program and, subsequently, an appropriate cardiovascular conditioning regimen can be developed.

ASSESSMENT OF SPINAL CONDITIONS

> **Q** *A 17-year-old cheerleader reports to the athletic training room complaining of aching pain during trunk flexion and aggravated with resisted hyperextension that produces sharp, shooting pains into the low back and down the posterior leg. How should the assessment of this injury progress to determine the extent and severity of injury?*

Injury assessment of the lumbar spine is difficult and complex. In the event of an acute injury with possible nerve involvement, immobilization and immediate transportation to the nearest medical facility is warranted, regardless of whether a total assessment is completed. Box 11.5 identifies several "Red Flags" that warrant immobilization and immediate referral to a physician.

When the individual walks into the examination room and complains of low back pain, it is relatively safe to assume that a serious spinal injury is not present. Most of the examination will involve differentiating symptoms, including distinguishing the presence of radicular symptoms into the leg from a space-occupying lesion or herniated disk, from other conditions, such as a strain, sprain, or facet problem more likely to cause localized low back pain. Even after a detailed and methodical assessment, a definitive determination of the source of pain may not be obvious. As such, referral to a physician for advanced testing and assessment may be necessary.

 See *Field Strategy: Lumbar Spinal Injury Evaluation*, available on the companion website at thePoint, for a summary of the assessment procedure.

The assessments that follows focuses on a lumbar assessment for a conscious individual. Specific information related to an acute injury is included where appropriate.

HISTORY

> **Q** *The injury assessment of the cheerleader should begin with a history. What questions need to be asked to identify the cause and extent of injury?*

A history of the injury should include information regarding the primary complaint, mechanism of injury, characteristics of the symptoms, disability resulting from the injury, previous injuries to the area, and family history that may have some bearing on this specific condition. In cases of lumbar spinal injury, questions should be asked about the location of pain (i.e., localized or radiating), type of pain (i.e., dull, aching, sharp, burning, or radiating), presence of sensory changes (i.e., numbness, tingling, or absence of sensation), and possible muscle weakness or paralysis. It also is important to determine the length of time the problem has been present. Acute back pain usually lasts 3 to 4 days. Subacute back pain lasts up to 12 weeks, however, and chronic back pain can extend longer than 3 months.

See *Field Strategy: Developing a History for a Spinal Injury*, available on the companion website at thePoint, for general questions related to a lumbar spinal injury.

Box 11.5   Red Flags That Warrant Immobilization and Immediate Referral to a Physician

- Severe pain, point tenderness, or deformity along the vertebral column
- Loss or change in sensation anywhere in the body
- Paralysis or inability to move a body part
- Diminished or absent reflexes
- Muscle weakness in a myotome

- Pain radiating into the extremities
- Trunk or abdominal pain that may be referred from the visceral organs
- Any injury in which uncertainty exists regarding the severity or nature

The cheerleader should be asked questions that would assist in determining the cause and extent of injury. Questions should address the primary complaint (i.e., what, when, and how questions), mechanism of injury, location of pain (i.e., localized or radiating), type of pain (i.e., dull, aching, sharp, burning, or radiating), presence of sensory changes (i.e., numbness, tingling, or absence of sensation) and possible muscle weakness, unusual sensations (i.e., sound or feelings), onset of symptoms, related medical history, and past injuries/treatment.

OBSERVATION AND INSPECTION

The 17-year-old cheerleader has been participating in cheerleading for 5 years. The primary complaint is an aching pain during trunk flexion and aggravated with resisted hyperextension that produces sharp shooting pains into the low back and down the posterior aspect of the right leg. The cheerleader reports the condition has been present for 2 weeks, and she cannot recall a traumatic episode that may have caused the condition. Would it be appropriate to do a scan examination to rule out other painful areas, and what specific factors should be observed to identify the injury?

The observation component of an assessment should be initiated as soon as the examiner sees the patient. Body language can signal pain, disability, and muscle weakness. It is important to note the individual's willingness or ability to move, general posture, ease in motion, and general attitude. Clothing and protective equipment may prevent visual observation of abnormalities in the spinal alignment. As such, the individual should be suitably dressed so that the back is as exposed as possible; for girls and women, a bra, halter top, or swimsuit can be worn. Observation should begin with a postural assessment, progress through a scan examination and gait analysis, and end with an inspection of the injury site.

Posture

Posture assessment can detect congenital or functional problems that may contribute to the injury. A patient with acute back pain usually exhibits some degree of antalgic (painful) posturing. This may present as a decrease in lumbar lordosis with a concomitant lateral shift or scoliosis because of muscle spasm. The individual should be observed from an anterior, lateral, and posterior view, paying particular attention to pelvic tilt. It is important to determine if the pelvis is maintained in a neutral position (i.e., normal lordotic curve with ASIS slightly lower than the PSIS).

The head and neck posture should be observed as well. In particular, it is important to determine:

- If the nose is in alignment with the manubrium, sternum, and umbilicus

- If any abnormal spinal curvatures are present

- If the shoulders and clavicles are level (although the dominant side may be slightly lower)

- If the individual leans to one side and, if so, if it appears to be caused by muscle spasm, scoliosis, or leg length discrepancy

- If the height and position of the ASIS, iliac crests, patella, and malleoli are the same bilaterally

The individual should be instructed to lean forward and touch the toes while keeping the knees straight (Adam's position). The vertebrae and contour of the back should be observed (see Fig. 10.18). The presence of a hump or raised scapula on one side (convex side of curve) and of a hollow (concave side of curve) on the other indicates scoliosis. From the side, the presence of flexed posturing at the hips from tight hip flexors should be noted; this results in a compensatory increase in the lumbar and cervical lordoses. It also is appropriate to determine if the trunk is rotated so that one shoulder is forward. Finally, the presence of prominent ribs on one side should be noted.

From a posterior view, the level of the shoulders, inferior angles of the scapula, and waist angles should be assessed. The PSIS should be level. The gluteal folds and knee joints should be at the same height. The presence of any dark areas of skin

See *Field Strategy: Postural Assessment of the Low Back Region,* available on the companion website at thePoint, for specific postural factors to observe in the head and spinal region.

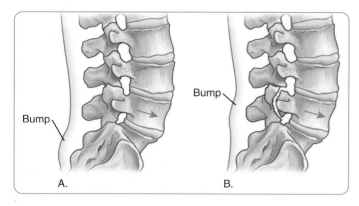

FIGURE 11.12 Step deformity in the lumbar spine. A step deformity occurs when the spinous process of one vertebra is more prominent than the vertebra below or above it. **A,** Spondylitis. **B,** Spondylolisthesis.

pigmentation, such as café-au-lait spots, should be noted, because this could indicate a possible collagen disease or abnormal growth of neural tissues (neurofibromatosis). The lower lumbar spine and sacrum should be observed for tufts of hair (Faun's beard), indicating possible **spina bifida occulta**.

Gait Assessment

The individual should be asked to walk several yards while the examiner observes normal body movement. The examiner should stand behind, in front of, and to the side of the individual to observe from all angles. Subtle posture abnormalities, such as kyphosis, scoliosis, lordosis, or pelvic tilt, should be noted. A low back injury may produce a forward lean, a lean to one side, or a noticeable limp.

Inspection of the Injury Site

Local inspection of the injury site should include observation for deformity, swelling, discoloration, muscle spasm, atrophy, hypertrophy, scars that might indicate previous surgery, and general skin condition. A step deformity in the lumbar spine may indicate a spondylolisthesis (Fig. 11.12).

Gross Neuromuscular Assessment

During an acute on-site injury assessment, a posture and scan may not be possible. It is beneficial, however, to perform a neuromuscular assessment prior to palpation to detect any motor and/or sensory deficits. This can be done without moving the individual by having the person perform a submaximal, bilateral hand-squeeze and ankle dorsiflexion. These two actions assess the cervical and lumbar spinal nerves, respectively. Muscle weakness and/or diminished sensation over the hands and feet indicate a serious injury. If any deficits are noted, the emergency care plan, including summoning EMS, should be activated. If no deficits are noted, it does not rule out possible neurologic involvement or fracture. Therefore, palpation should be done with the individual maintained in the position found.

 What specific factors should be observed and inspected in the on-going assessment of the cheerleader? Is it appropriate to perform a scan examination?

PALPATION

During a scan examination, trunk flexion and extension produced a dull pain in the low back. Lateral flexion to the right caused sharp pain to radiate into the right buttock and posterior leg. Gait analysis showed a shortened stride on the right side. Visual inspection showed no abnormalities. The injury is confined to the low back region. What specific structures need to be palpated to determine if the injury is of bony or soft-tissue origin, and can neural involvement be ruled out during palpation?

Bony and soft-tissue structures are palpated to detect temperature, swelling, point tenderness, deformity, crepitus, muscle spasm, and cutaneous sensation. In injuries that do not involve neural damage, fracture, or dislocation, palpation can proceed with the patient in a supine position. The umbilicus lies at the level of the L_3–L_4 disk space and is the center point for the intersection of the abdominal quadrants. Using careful deep palpation, the examiner may be able to palpate the anterior aspects of the L_4, L_5, and S_1 vertebrae, disks, and accompanying anterior longitudinal ligament. The abdomen also should be palpated for pain and muscle spasm that may be responsible for referred pain into the lumbar region from internal organs. The inguinal area, iliac crest, and symphysis pubis also can be palpated for signs of infection (e.g., enlarged lymph nodes), hip pointers, apophysitis, or osteitis pubis.

When moving into the prone position, a pillow or blanket should be placed under the hip region to tilt the pelvis back and relax the lumbar curvature. Muscle spasm in the lower erector spinae, lower trapezius, serratus posterior, quadratus lumborum, latissimus dorsi, or gluteus maximus can indicate dysfunction of the thoracic or lumbar spine. The following surface landmarks in the lumbar region can facilitate palpation:

- L_4—top of iliac crest
- L_5—demarcated by bilateral dimples
- S_2—level of PSIS

In palpating the spinous processes of the lumbar spine, particular attention should be noted at the L_4, L_5, and S_1 level. A visible or palpable dip or protrusion can indicate spondylolisthesis. If the fingers are moved laterally 2 to 3 cm (0.8–1.2 inches), the facet joints can be palpated for signs of pathology. Because of their depth, it may be difficult to palpate the joints; however, spasm in the overlying paraspinal muscles can be palpated. The spinous processes of the sacrum also can be palpated. Because no interposing soft-tissue spaces are between them, they may be harder to distinguish. The S_2 spinous process is at the level of a line drawn between the two PSIS ("posterior dimples"). In moving to the PSIS, the examiner can palpate the iliac crest for signs of injury and then palpate the gluteal muscles for pain, spasm, or possible nodules. Having the patient flex the hip at 90° allows easier palpation of the ischial tuberosity, greater trochanter, and sciatic nerve, which is located midway between the ischial tuberosity and greater trochanter. Finally, the piriformis muscle should be palpated deep to the gluteal muscles for pathology. The following structures should be palpated:

Anterior Aspect

1. **Umbilicus and abdominal area.** Note any abnormal tenderness or masses indicating internal pathology that is referring pain to the spinal region.

2. **Inguinal area.** Palpate for possible hernia, infection (enlarged lymph nodes), or other pathology.

3. **Iliac crest, ASIS, and symphysis pubis.** Palpate for pain, tenderness, or defect indicating pathology (e.g., avulsion fracture, hip pointer, apophysitis, or osteitis pubis).

Posterior Aspect

1. **Spinous processes of the lumbar vertebrae.** Note any tenderness, crepitus, or presence of a step-off deformity (i.e., one vertebra is more anterior than the one below it). This indicates spondylolisthesis, which most commonly is seen between the L_4 and L_5 or the L_5 and S_1 vertebrae. Pain and tenderness without positive findings on muscle movement may indicate that the problem is not musculoskeletal in origin.

2. **Facet joints.** The facet articulations are approximately a thumb's breadth to either side of the spinous process. Point tenderness at these sites, especially with extension and rotation to the same side, suggests facet joint pain.

3. **Interspinous and supraspinous ligaments, paraspinal muscles, and quadratus lumborum.** Trigger points within specific muscles may refer pain to a more distal area. Tender points that increase with muscular contraction indicate a localized muscle strain. An area that is tender to palpation but is not painful during muscle contraction may indicate referred pain from another area.

4. **Iliac crest, PSIS, and sacrum.** The interspace between L_4 and L_5 lies at the same level as the top of the iliac crest. The S_2 spinous process lies in the middle of a line drawn between the PSIS. Palpate for pain, tenderness, and other pathology (e.g., hip pointer or apophysitis).

5. **Ischial tuberosity, sciatic nerve, and greater trochanter.** Flex the hip to 90° for easier palpation of these structures. The sciatic nerve is located midway between the ischial tuberosity and greater trochanter (Fig. 11.13).

■■■■ **FIGURE 11.13 Sciatic nerve.** To palpate the sciatic nerve, flex the hip, and locate the ischial tuberosity and greater trochanter. The sciatic nerve may be palpated at the midpoint. It is designated here by the white dot.

A   *The palpation component of the assessment of the cheerleader should include bony and soft tissues of the lumbar region (i.e., spinous processes of the lumbar vertebrae; facet joints; interspinous and supraspinous ligaments, paraspinal muscles, and quadratus lumborum; iliac crest, PSIS, and sacrum; and ischial tuberosity, sciatic nerve, and greater trochanter). Palpation also should include anterior structures (i.e., umbilicus and abdominal area, iliac crest, and ASIS).*

Because the cheerleader is younger than 18 years, palpation can only be performed with permission from the parent or guardian. It also is important to recognize that the cheerleader may feel uncomfortable being touched by a health care provider of the opposite gender. If a same-gender clinician is not available, the evaluation should be observed by a third party (e.g., another clinician, parent, or guardian).

PHYSICAL EXAMINATION TESTS

Q   *In the palpation component of the assessment of the cheerleader, point tenderness was elicited in the low back region between the L_3 and S_1 vertebrae, with increased pain in the L_4–L_5 region. Muscle spasm was present on either side of the lumbar region. Pain also was elicited with palpation midway between the ischial tuberosity and greater trochanter. Based on the information obtained through the history, observation, and palpation, what tests should be performed to determine nerve root impingement, and what tests should be conducted as part of a neurologic assessment of the cheerleader's condition.*

It is imperative to work slowly through the tests that are used to assess low back conditions, because injuries to the lumbar region can be very complex. If, at any time, movement leads to increased acute pain or change in sensation, or if the individual resists moving the spine, a significant injury should be assumed and the emergency plan activated.

Functional Tests

Goniometry measurements of the spine are not typically taken because of the difficulty of measuring individual regional motions. Completion of gross movement patterns in a standing position is adequate to determine normal ROM. Further assessment can be conducted if motion is limited or the patient is unwilling to do the movements.

Active Movement

If active movement of the spine was conducted during the scan examination, it need not be repeated. The individual's willingness to perform the movement should be noted. It is important to note if movement is fluid and complete or if pain, spasm, or stiffness block the full ROM. The presence of a painful arc, particularly a lightning-like pain, present during forward flexion and extension should be noted as well. This often indicates a space-occupying lesion (e.g., herniated disk), but it also may be caused by instability. Movements to the left and right should be compared bilaterally. The ROM listed usually is the summation of the entire lumbar spine, not just that at one level, along with hip movement. Basic active movements of the lumbar spine (Fig. 11.14) include:

1. Forward trunk flexion (40–60°)

2. Trunk extension (20–35°)

3. Lateral trunk flexion (left and right; 15–20°)

4. Trunk rotation done in a standing and sitting position (3–18°).

Because spinal injuries seldom occur during a single motion, combined motions of the spine should be included in the examination. These movements include lateral flexion in flexion, lateral flexion in extension, flexion and rotation, and extension and rotation (Fig. 11.15). These movements may lead to signs and symptoms different from the basic motions and are indicated if these motions reproduce the patient's symptoms. For example, extension and rotation are more likely to reproduce symptoms in a facet syndrome compared with only extension or only rotation.

FIGURE 11.14 Active movements of the lumbar spine. A and **B,** Measuring forward flexion with a tape measure. **C,** Extension. **D** and **E,** Lateral flexion. **F,** Rotation (standing). **G,** Rotation (sitting).

■■■■ FIGURE 11.15 **Combined active movements. A,** Lateral flexion in flexion. **B,** Lateral flexion in extension. **C,** Rotation and flexion. **D,** Rotation and extension.

Passive Range of Motion

Passive movements are difficult to perform in the lumbar region. If active movements are full and pain-free, gentle overpressure may be applied as the patient reaches the full range of active motion. Extreme care must be exercised in applying the overpressure, because the upper body weight is already being applied to the lumbar joints by virtue of gravity (i.e., compressive forces) and their position (i.e., shear forces). While sustaining the position at the end of the ROM for 10 to 20 seconds, the patient should be asked if their symptoms increase. Likewise, if symptoms increased during the active combined movements, these movements should be repeated, but only after the patient has completed the basic movements. The normal end feels for the lumbar movements are tissue stretch.

Resisted Muscle Testing

Resisted movement is initially performed in a neutral position with the patient seated to stabilize the hip. The individual is instructed to not allow the examiner to move the body part being tested by applying a maximal isometric contraction in flexion, extension, lateral flexion, and rotation. By

■■■■ FIGURE 11.16 **Resisted isometric movements of the lumbar spine.**
A, Flexion, extension, and lateral flexion. **B**, Rotation to the right.

repetitively loading the patient's resisting muscle with rapid, consecutive impulses, more subtle weakness can be detected. Lumbar movements to be tested are shown in Fig. 11.16.

Stress and Functional Tests

Several stress tests can be used in spinal assessment. Only those deemed to be relevant should be performed. Because many of these tests are designed to put stress on neurologic tissue, they often cause pain or discomfort, which may be bilateral. For a test to be positive, however, the patient's symptoms must be reproduced; otherwise, the test is considered to be negative. Tests are grouped on the basis of patient position.

Lumbar Tests in a Seated Position

SLUMP TEST. This test is designed to assess potential lumbar nerve root compression. While in a seated position on an examining table, the patient is instructed to "slump" so that the spine flexes and the shoulders sag forward. Initially, the examiner maintains the position of the patient's head in a neutral position (Fig. 11.17A). The presence of any symptoms that are produced by the slump should be noted. If no symptoms are present, the patient flexes the neck, and the examiner places pressure on the shoulders of the patient (Fig. 11.17B). If no symptoms are produced, slight overpressure of neck flexion is applied by the examiner (Fig. 11.17C). If no symptoms are elicited, one of the patient's knees is passively extended, and the foot of the same leg is passively dorsiflexed, to see if any symptoms occur (Fig. 11.17D). If no symptoms are reported, the patient is asked to extend the neck, and the presence or lack of symptoms should be noted (Fig. 11.17E). This process is repeated with the opposite leg. A test is positive if symptoms of sciatic pain are reproduced, indicating impingement of the dura and spinal cord or nerve roots. The pain usually is produced at the site of the lesion.

Lumbar Tests in a Supine Position

STRAIGHT LEG RAISING TEST. Also known as Laségue's test, this examination is used to assess SI joint pain, irritation of the sciatic nerve, or tight hamstrings. The individual is placed in a relaxed, supine position with the hip medially rotated and the knee extended. The examiner should grasp the individual's heel with one hand and place the other on top of the patella to prevent the knee from flexing. The leg is slowly raised until the individual complains of pain or tightness. The leg is then

■ ■ ■ FIGURE 11.17 **Slump test.** The test is performed in several stages. **A,** While sitting on a table, the examiner asks the person to "slump" so that the spine flexes and the shoulders sag forward while the examiner holds the head in a neutral position. **B,** If no symptoms are present, the examiner applies light pressure, pushing down on the shoulders while the patient holds the head in a neutral position. **C,** If no symptoms are produced, overpressure is applied to the cervical spine. **D,** If no symptoms occur, the examiner passively extends one of the patient's knees and dorsiflexes the ankle of the same leg. **E,** The patient is instructed to extend the head. The test is considered to be positive if symptoms of sciatic pain are reproduced, indicating impingement of the dura and spinal cord or nerve roots.

lowered until the pain is relieved. Next, the individual is asked to flex the neck onto the chest, to dorsiflex the foot, or to do both actions simultaneously (Fig. 11.18).

The neck flexion movement is called **Hyndman's sign** or **Brudzinski's sign.** Pain that increases with neck flexion or dorsiflexion indicates stretching of the dura mater of the spinal cord. Pain that does not increase with neck flexion or dorsiflexion indicates tight hamstrings. The sciatic nerve is fully stretched at approximately 70° of flexion. As such, pain after 70° usually indicates pain from the lumbar area (facet joints) or SI joints. Pain that occurs opposite the leg that is lifted indicates a space-occupying lesion (e.g., herniated disk).

■■ ■■ FIGURE 11.18 **Straight leg raising test.** The examiner passively flexes the individual's hip while keeping the knee extended until pain or tension is felt in the hamstrings. Next, the leg is lowered slowly until the pain or tension disappears. Next, the examiner dorsiflexes the ankle, has the individual flex the neck, or perform both simultaneously. If pain does not increase with dorsiflexion of the ankle or flexion of the neck, it indicates tight hamstrings.

WELL STRAIGHT LEG RAISING TEST. The well straight leg raising test differs from the previous test in that the unaffected leg is raised. A positive sign is pain on the side opposite the leg being raised, indicating a space-occupying lesion (e.g., a herniated intervertebral disk.)

BOWSTRING TEST (TENSION OR POPLITEAL PRESSURE SIGN). A positive straight leg raising test can then be followed by the tension, or bowstring, test. This test is designed to assess tension or pressure on the sciatic nerve and is a modification of the straight leg raising test. The examiner maintains the leg in the same position, then flexes the knee slightly (20°), reducing the symptoms. Thumb or finger pressure is then exerted over the tibial portion of the sciatic nerve as it passes through the popliteal space to re-establish the painful radiating symptoms (Fig. 11.19). An alternative method is to flex both the hip and the knee at 90°. The examiner then slowly extends the knee as far as possible while applying pressure in the popliteal space. Replication of tenderness or radiating pain is a positive sign for sciatic nerve irritation.

BRUDZINSKI'S TEST. This test is similar to the straight leg raising test, but the movements are actively performed by the patient. The individual is supine, with the hands cupped behind the head (Fig. 11.20A). The test is positive if the individual complains of neck and low back discomfort and attempts to relieve the meningeal irritation by involuntarily flexing the knees and hips.

KERNIG'S TEST. This test can aid in identifying the presence of a bulging disk, nerve root impingement, inflammation of the dural sheath, or irritation of the meninges. In Kernig's position, the individual lies supine, with the hip flexed and the knee extended (Fig. 11.20B). Pain in the head, neck, or lower back suggests meningeal irritation. If the pain is relieved when the individual flexes the knee, it is considered to be a positive test, indicating meningeal irritation, nerve root involvement, or dural irritation. The Brudzinski's and Kernig's tests may be done either separately or together.

BILATERAL STRAIGHT LEG RAISING TEST. This test is used to assess the presence of lesions at the SI joint and in the lumbar spine. The examiner can test both legs simultaneously (bilateral straight leg raising). This must be performed carefully, because the examiner is lifting the weight of both lower limbs, thereby placing a large stress on their own lumbar spine. If the test causes pain before 70° of hip flexion, the lesion is probably in the SI joints; if it causes pain after 70° of hip flexion, the lesion is probably in the lumbar spine.

VALSALVA'S TEST. Valsalva's maneuver is used to determine the presence of space-occupying lesions (e.g., herniated disk, tumor, or osteophytes). While

■■ ■■ FIGURE 11.19 **Bowstring test.** After pain results in a straight leg raising test, the clinician flexes the knee slightly (20°) to reduce the symptoms. Thumb pressure is then exerted in the popliteal area to reproduce the painful radicular symptoms.

Involuntary flexion of knee

A.

Flexion relieves pain

B.   Head and neck   Lower back

▩▩▩▩ FIGURE 11.20 **Brudzinski's and Kernig's tests. A,** In Brudzinski's test, the individual lays supine and dorsiflexes the neck. **B,** In Kernig's test, the individual actively flexes the hip, with the knee extended. The test is considered to be positive if knee extension leads to head, neck, or low back pain that is relieved with knee flexion.

▩▩▩▩ FIGURE 11.21 **Milgram test.** The patient is instructed to raise both legs 2 to 6 inches and hold the position for 30 seconds. The test is considered to be positive if the affected limb or limbs cannot be held for 30 seconds or if symptoms are reproduced in the affected limb.

supine, the individual is asked to take a deep breath and hold it while bearing down, as if moving the bowels. It is important for the examiner to exercise caution with this test, because the maneuver increases intrathecal pressure, which can slow the pulse, decrease venous return, and increase venous pressure, each of which actions may cause fainting. A positive test is indicated by increased pain.

MILGRAM TEST. This test attempts to increase intrathecal pressure, resulting in an increased bulge of the nucleus pulposus, primarily in the lumbar spine. The individual lies supine, simultaneously lifts both legs off the table by 2 to 6 inches, and holds this position for 30 seconds (Fig. 11.21). The test is considered to be positive if the affected limb or limbs cannot be held for 30 seconds or if symptoms are reproduced in the affected limb. This test should be performed with caution, because it places a high stress load on the lumbar spine.

■■■ FIGURE 11.22 **Piriformis muscle stretch test.** With the knees crossed and the involved extremity on top of the involved extremity, the patient pulls the top knee toward the chest in the direction of the opposite shoulder.

■■■ FIGURE 11.23 **Prone knee bending test.** With the patient prone, the examiner passively flexes the knee as far as possible toward the buttocks. Unilateral pain in the lumbar area, buttock, and/or posterior thigh may indicate an L_2 or L_3 nerve root lesion.

PIRIFORMIS MUSCLE STRETCH TEST. This test stretches the piriformis muscle and lateral rotators, a common source of low back pain. The patient lies supine, with the knees flexed and the feet flat on the table. The affected leg is crossed on top of the other, and both knees are brought to the chest. The patient grasps the uninvolved knee and pulls both knees to the chest (Fig. 11.22). The uninvolved knee should be directed toward the opposite shoulder as the knees are brought toward the chest. The test is positive if symptoms are reproduced. This test also can be used to stretch the muscle during rehabilitative exercises.

Lumbar Tests in a Prone Position

PRONE KNEE BENDING TEST. This test can be used to assess nerve root lesion. The individual is placed prone, and the knee is passively flexed until the foot rests against the buttock, making sure the hip is not rotated. This position is maintained for 45 to 60 seconds (Fig. 11.23). If the knee cannot be flexed beyond 90° because of a pathologic condition, passive extension of the hip, with the knee flexed as much as possible, is performed. Unilateral pain in the lumbar region indicates an L_2 or L_3 nerve root lesion. Pain in the anterior thigh indicates tight quadriceps or stretching of the femoral nerve.

SPRING TEST FOR FACET JOINT MOBILITY. Hypomobility of the vertebrae, especially at the facet joint, may be assessed with the spring test (Fig. 11.24). With the patient prone, the examiner stands over the patient with the thumbs placed over the spinous process to be tested. The examiner carefully pushes the spinous process anteriorly, feeling for a springing of the vertebrae. The test is considered to be positive if pain is elicited or the vertebra does not move ("spring").

FARFAN TORSION TEST. This test stresses the facet joints, joint capsule, supraspinous and interspinous ligaments, neural arch, longitudinal ligaments, and lumbar disks. With the patient prone, the clinician stabilizes the ribs and spine with one hand at approximately T_{12} and places the other hand under the anterior aspect of the ilium. The ilium is then pulled backward, causing rotation of the spine on the opposite side to produce torque on the opposite side (Fig. 11.25). The test is considered to be positive if some or all of the patient's symptoms are reproduced.

■■■ FIGURE 11.24 **Facet joint spring test.** While placing the thumbs directly over the spinous process, the examiner carefully pushes the spinous process anteriorly, feeling for the springing of the vertebrae. If pain is elicited or the vertebra is hypomobile, facet joint pathology is present.

TRUNK EXTENSION TEST (PRESS-UPS). This test compresses the lumbar vertebrae. In a prone position, the patient is asked to extend the trunk

▓▓▓■ FIGURE 11.25 **Farfan torsion test.** The examiner stabilizes the patient's ribs and spine at approximately T$_{12}$ with one hand. The other hand lifts the anterior aspect of the ilium backward, causing the spine to rotate to the opposite side. The test is positive if symptoms are reproduced.

▓▓▓■ FIGURE 11.26 **Trunk extension test.** The patient extends the spine by pressing up onto the elbows. If pain radiates into the buttocks or thigh, it may indicate a space-occupying lesion (e.g., herniated disk).

(press-up) and rest the body weight on the elbows (Fig. 11.26). If pain is localized, it may indicate a herniated disk. Generalized lumbar pain may indicate a more serious condition.

Lumbar Tests in a Side-Lying Position

FEMORAL NERVE TRACTION TEST. In applying a stretch to the femoral nerve, the patient is instructed to lie on the unaffected side, with the neck slightly flexed and the unaffected limb flexed at the hip and knee (Fig. 11.27). It is important to make certain that the patient's back is straight and not hyperextended. Next, the examiner grasps the affected limb and slowly extends the knee while gently extending the hip approximately 15°. The patient's knee is then flexed on the affected side to further stretch the femoral nerve. The test is considered to be positive if pain radiates down the anterior thigh.

QUADRATUS LUMBORUM STRETCH TEST. In applying a stretch to the quadratus lumborum, the patient lies on the uninvolved side at the edge of the table, and a pillow is placed under their waist to facilitate slight lateral bending of the lumbar spine. The patient drops the involved leg off the table while the clinician adds a slight overpressure to the distal thigh (Fig. 11.28). The test is considered to be positive if symptoms, such as pain, discomfort, or tightness, are reproduced.

▓▓▓■ FIGURE 11.27 **Femoral nerve traction test.** The examiner extends the knee while extending the hip approximately 15°. The knee is then flexed to further stretch the femoral nerve.

▓▓▓■ FIGURE 11.28 **Quadratus lumborum stretch test.** While lying on the unaffected side, the patient slowly drops the affected leg off the table. The test is considered to be positive if pain or tightness is evident.

Lumbar Tests in a Standing Position

SINGLE-LEG STANCE TEST. This test can aid in the assessment of spondylolysis, spondylolisthesis, and SI joint irritation. The individual stands on one leg and extends the spine while balancing on the single leg (stork position) (Fig. 11.29). The test is then repeated with the opposite leg. If pain is elicited when the opposite leg is lifted, a unilateral lesion to the pars interarticularis should be suspected; if pain is elicited when either leg is lifted, a bilateral pars interarticularis fracture should be suspected. If rotation is combined with extension and pain results, possible facet joint pathology is indicated on the side to which rotation occurs.

QUADRANT TEST. This test can be used to assess dural irritation, facet joint compression, and SI joint dysfunction. The examiner stands behind the patient. The patient extends the spine while the examiner controls the movement by stabilizing the patient's shoulders. If needed, the examiner may use his or her shoulder to support the weight of the patient's head. Overpressure is applied in extension while the patient laterally flexes and rotates toward the painful side. This movement pattern causes maximum narrowing of the intervertebral foramen and stresses the facet joints on the side where rotation occurs. The presence of radicular pain suggests impingement of the lumbar nerve roots. In comparison, localized pain is indicative of facet joint pathology; SI joint dysfunction would be suggested if pain is specific to the area of the PSIS (Fig. 11.30).

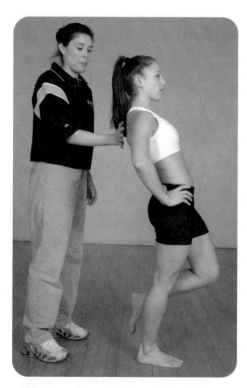

■■■■ FIGURE 11.29 **Single-leg stance test.** The examiner needs to stand behind the patient to support the shoulder region as the patient balances on one leg and then hyperextends the spine. A test is positive when pain is evoked in the back when the opposite leg is raised, indicating a pars interarticularis stress fracture. Bilateral pars fractures result in pain when either leg is lifted.

■■■■ FIGURE 11.30 **Quadrant test.** The patient extends the spine while the clinician controls the movement by holding the shoulders. The examiner applies overpressure in extension while the patient laterally flexes and rotates toward the painful side. This movement is continued until symptoms are reproduced or the end of the range of motion is reached.

■■■■ FIGURE 11.31 **Hoover test. A,** Under normal conditions, when an individual tries to elevate one leg, the action is accompanied by downward pressure on the opposite leg. **B,** When the individual attempts to elevate the "weak" leg but the opposite (asymptomatic) leg does not "help," at least some of the weakness probably is feigned.

Lumbar Tests for Malingering

HOOVER TEST. Because the assessment of lumbopelvic disorders is difficult to perform objectively, the Hoover test is used to determine if the patient is a malingerer. The examiner's hands cup each heel of the supine patient while the legs remain relaxed on the examining table (Fig. 11.31). The individual is then asked to lift one leg off the table while keeping the knees straight, as in an active straight leg raising test. If the individual does not lift the leg or the examiner does not feel pressure under the opposite heel, the patient may not be trying to lift the leg or may be a malingerer. Pressure under the normal heel increases, however, if the lifted limb is weaker because of the increased effort to lift the weak leg. A bilateral comparison then is made to determine any differences.

BURNS TEST. This test also can be used to assess malingering. The patient is asked to kneel on a chair and then bend forward, touching the floor with the fingers (Fig. 11.32). If the patient overbalances or is unable to perform this test, the result is considered to be positive for malingering.

■■■■ FIGURE 11.32 **Burns test.** While kneeling on a chair, the patient is asked to bend forward and touch the floor with his or her fingers. Inability to perform the action suggests malingering.

Sacroiliac Dysfunction

A variety of tests can be used to assess SI pathology. In an effort to improve reliability, it is essential that the examiner incorporate the results of several tests in making decisions regarding to injury status.

SACROILIAC COMPRESSION (TRANSVERSE ANTERIOR STRESS) AND DISTRACTION TEST. The examiner applies a cross-arm pressure both downward and outward to the ASIS of the patient who is lying supine (Fig. 11.33). This action is repeated, with pressure applied downward through the anterior portion of the ilium, spreading the SI joint. Unilateral gluteal or posterior leg pain may indicate a sprain to the anterior SI ligaments. Sharp pain elsewhere along the pelvic ring with outward pressure, or with bilateral compression of the iliac crests, may indicate a pelvic fracture.

APPROXIMATION (TRANSVERSE POSTERIOR STRESS) TEST. With the patient in a side-lying position, a downward force is applied over the iliac crest (Fig. 11.34). The movement causes forward pressure on the sacrum. A positive test produces pain or a feeling of pressure on the SI joints, indicating a sprain of the posterior SI ligaments, a SI lesion, or both. Sharp pain along the pelvic ring may indicate a fracture.

▇▇▇ FIGURE 11.33 **Sacroiliac compression and distraction test.** The examiner applies a cross-arm pressure both downward and outward to the anterior superior iliac spines. Pressure may then be applied down through the anterior portion of the ilium, spreading the sacroiliac (SI) joint. Unilateral pain or posterior leg pain may indicate a sprain to the anterior SI ligaments. Sharp pain elsewhere may indicate a pelvic fracture.

▇▇▇ FIGURE 11.34 **Approximation test.** The examiner applies a downward force over the iliac crest of the side-lying patient. Increased pain or a feeling of pressure on the sacroiliac (SI) joints indicates a possible joint sprain. Pain or pressure in the SI joints indicates a possible SI lesion, sprain of the posterior SI ligaments, or both. Sharp pain may indicate a possible pelvic fracture.

"SQUISH" TEST. The examiner applies pressure both downward and inward at a 45° angle to both of the ASIS of the supine patient. This action stresses the posterior SI ligaments and is considered to be positive if pain is present.

FABER (PATRICK OR FIGURE-FOUR) TEST. In a supine position, the foot and ankle of the involved leg are rested on the contralateral knee. The examiner places one hand on the opposite ASIS and the other on the medial aspect of the flexed knee. The flexed leg is allowed to rest into full external rotation, followed by the examiner applying overpressure at the knee and ASIS (Fig. 11.35). The final position of *f*lexion, *ab*duction, and *e*xternal *r*otation (Faber) at the hip should place the involved leg on the table or at least near a horizontal position with the opposite leg. Overpressure on the knee of the involved leg and the contralateral iliac crest may produce pain in the SI joint on the side of the involved leg, denoting possible SI pathology.

▇▇▇ FIGURE 11.35 **Patrick's (Faber) test.** Also called the figure-four test, the foot and ankle of the involved leg are rested on the contralateral knee. The examiner applies an overpressure on the knee of the involved leg and the contralateral iliac crest. A positive test produces pain in the sacroiliac joint on the side of the involved leg, indicating pathology.

GAENSLEN'S TEST. Gaenslen's test is used to place a rotatory stress on the SI joint by forcing one hip into hyperextension. The patient is positioned so that the hip extends beyond the edge of the table. Both legs are drawn onto the chest, and then one leg is slowly lowered into extension (Fig. 11.36). While stabilizing the patient, the examiner applies overpressure to the near leg, forcing it into hyperextension. The other leg is tested in a similar fashion for comparison. A positive test is indicated with pain in the SI joints. An alternative position is with the patient in a side-lying position,

■■■■ **FIGURE 11.36 Gaenslen's sign. A,** The patient is positioned so that the involved hip extends beyond the edge of the table. **B,** Both legs are drawn onto the chest, and then one is slowly lowered into extension. Increased pain signals an ipsilateral sacroiliac joint lesion, hip pathology, or an L_4 nerve root lesion.

with the upper leg (test leg) hyperextended at the hip. The lower leg is flexed against the chest. The pelvis is stabilized while extending the hip of the uppermost leg. Increased pain may be caused by an ipsilateral SI joint lesion, hip pathology, or a L_4 nerve root lesion.

LONG SITTING TEST. The patient is asked to lie supine, with the legs straight. The examiner places the thumbs over the medial malleoli, ensuring that the malleoli are level. The patient is then asked to sit up while the examiner observes whether one leg moves from a long to a short position (moves proximally). If one leg moves up farther than the other, a functional leg length difference exists, resulting from pelvic dysfunction caused, in turn, by pelvic torsion or rotation. For example, if the right leg moves proximally, it indicates anterior rotation of the right ilium on the sacrum. If the reverse occurs (i.e., the right leg moves from a short position to a longer position), it indicates posterior rotation of the right ilium on the sacrum.

Neurologic Tests

Injury to the lumbar region and spinal cord can be reflected in **hyperreflexia,** muscle weakness, loss of sensation, and ataxia. Several tests should be performed to assess lower motor neuron lesions. Lower-quarter neurologic screening tests the L_1–S_2 nerve roots. Neurologic integrity can be assessed through special tests, myotomes, reflexes, segmental dermatomes, and peripheral nerve cutaneous patterns.

Babinski Test

The individual should be supine with the eyes closed and the leg held in a slightly elevated and flexed position. A pointed object is stroked along the plantar aspect of the foot (see Fig. 9.11). A normal sign is for the toes to curl downward in flexion and adduction. A positive sign suggests an upper motor neuron lesion and is demonstrated by extension of the big toe and abduction (splaying) of the other toes.

Oppenheim Test

The individual should be supine. Using the edge of their fingernail, the examiner strokes the crest of the anteromedial tibia (see Fig. 10.27). A positive sign suggests an upper motor neuron lesion

TABLE 11.2 Myotomes Used to Test Selected Nerves

NERVE ROOT SEGMENT	ACTION TESTED
L_1–L_2	Hip flexion
L_3	Knee extension
L_4	Ankle dorsiflexion
L_5	Toe extension
S_1	Plantar flexion of the ankle, foot eversion, and hip extension
S_2	Knee flexion

and is demonstrated by extension of the big toe and abduction (splaying) of the other toes or hypersensitivity to the test.

Myotomes

Isometric muscle testing is performed in the upper and lower extremities to test specific myotomes (Table 11.2). These were originally discussed in Chapter 5. The ankle movements should be performed with the knee flexed approximately 30°, especially if the patient is complaining of sciatic pain, because full dorsiflexion is considered to be a provocative maneuver for stretching neurologic tissue. Similarly, a fully extended knee increases the stretch on the sciatic nerve and may result in false signs, such as weakness that results from pain rather than from pressure on the nerve root.

Reflexes

Repetitive tapping of the reflexes may show a gradual decline in the reflex response not otherwise noted in a singe tap. Absent or decreased reflexes are not necessarily pathologic, especially in individuals who have well-developed muscles. Upper limb reflexes can be increased by having the individual perform an isometric contraction, such as squeezing the knees together during the test. In the lower extremity, the two major reflexes are the patella (L_3–L_4) and Achilles tendon (S_1) (Table 11.3). Asymmetry between sides should raise suspicion of an abnormality.

Cutaneous Patterns

The wide variation of dermatomal innervation and the subjectivity of the test make it less useful than motor or reflex testing. The segmental nerve dermatome patterns and peripheral nerve cutaneous patterns are demonstrated in Figure 5.8. Testing should be performed bilaterally.

Referred Pain

Pain can be referred to the thoracic spine from various abdominal organs. Figure 5.1 demonstrates the area that the pain is commonly referred to the torso.

TABLE 11.3 Deep Tendon Reflexes In The Lower Extremity

REFLEX	SEGMENTAL LEVELS
Patellar	L_2, L_3, and L_4
Posterior tibial	L_4 and L_5
Medial hamstring	L_5 and S_1
Lateral hamstring	S_1 and S_2
Achilles	S_1 and S_2

Activity-Specific Functional Testing

Before return to play, the individual must have a normal neurologic exam, with pain-free ROM and normal bilateral muscle strength, cutaneous sensation, and reflexes. If pain is present, the individual should not return to competition. Sport-specific functional tests that should be performed include walking, bending, lifting, jogging, running, figure-eight running, karioka running, and sport-specific skills. All must be performed pain-free and with unlimited movement.

> **A** *In assessing the cheerleader, the special tests that are used to determine nerve root impingement should include Valsalva's test, Milgram test, Hoover test, slump test, straight leg raising test, well straight leg raising test, bilateral straight leg raising test, Brudzinski's test, Kernig's test, tension (bowstring) test, femoral nerve stretch test, and single-leg stance test. Neurologic testing for the cheerleader should include Babinski, Oppenheim, myotomes, reflexes, and dermatomes.*

REHABILITATION

> **Q** *The findings from the special tests and neurologic testing revealed increased pain in the right lumbar region on resisted trunk extension, lateral flexion, and rotation to the right; diminished quadriceps reflex on the right side; muscle weakness apparent with knee extension and ankle dorsiflexion; and pain elicited down the right leg during a straight leg raising test. These signs and symptoms suggest the possibility of sciatica resulting from an extruded disk at the L_4 level.*
>
> *The cheerleader was seen by a physician who prescribed NSAIDs, muscle relaxants, and rest until the symptoms subside. When the individual begins rehabilitation, what exercises should be included in the general program?*

Rehabilitation programs must be developed on an individual basis and address the specific needs of the patient. Exercises to relieve pain related to postural problems may not address sciatic pain. Therefore, a variety of exercises are listed in this section to allow selection of those that are appropriate for the patient. The program should relieve pain and muscle tension; restore motion and balance; develop strength, endurance, and power; and maintain cardiovascular fitness. Patient education also is critical in teaching the skills and techniques that are needed to prevent recurrence.

Relief of Pain and Muscle Tension

Maintaining a prolonged posture can lead to discomfort. This can be avoided by doing active ROM exercises to relieve stress on supporting structures, promote circulation, and maintain flexibility. For example, in the lower thoracic and lumbar region, exercises such as back extension, side bending in each direction, spinal flexion (avoiding hip flexion), trunk rotation, and walking a short distance may relieve discomfort in the lumbar region. With nerve root compression injuries, however, extension exercises may increase discomfort and may be contraindicated. In some cases, conscious relaxation training can relax an individual who generally is tense or release tension in specific muscle groups. In addition, grade I and II mobilization exercises can be initiated early in the program to relieve pain and stretch tight structures to restore accessory movements to the joints.

Restoration of Motion

Once pain and muscle guarding are relieved, grade III and IV mobilization exercises can begin. In addition to mobilization exercises, flexibility and ROM exercises also can be initiated. Flexion exercises stretch the lumbar fascia and back extensors, open the intervertebral foramen and facet joints to reduce nerve compression, relieve tension on lumbar vertebrae caused by tight hip flexors, and increase intra-abdominal pressure by strengthening the abdominals. Examples of flexion exercises (Field Strategy 11.1) include the single- and double-knee to the chest stretches, hamstring stretch, hip flexor stretch, lateral rotator stretch, crunch curl-ups, and diagonal crunch curl-ups. Exercises to stretch the upper thoracic and pectoral region, trunk rotators and lateral flexors, and hip adductors, abductors, extensors, and medial and lateral rotators also should be added to improve flexibility. Other exercises include bringing both knees to the chest and gently rocking back and forth in a cranial/caudal direction and, in a standing position, shifting the hips from one side to another, lateral trunk flexion, and rotation exercises. Flexion-based exercises should be avoided if hypermobility or instability is suspected or if the maneuvers increase low back pain.

Extension exercises improve spinal mobility, reduce load on the intervertebral disks, strengthen the back extensors, and allow self-mobilization of the motion segments. Back extension exercises described in Field Strategy 11.1 include prone extension exercises, beginning with raising to the elbows and then to the hands, the alternate arm and leg lift, double-arm and -leg lift, and alternate arm and leg extension on all fours. Other extension exercises may include prone single-leg hip extension and double-leg hip extension while holding onto a table, beginning with the knee or knees flexed and then with the knee or knees extended.

Pelvic and abdominal stabilizing exercises are used to teach an individual to place the hip in a neutral position to maintain the spine in the most comfortable position and control the forces that are exerted during repetitive microtrauma. During each exercise, the individual concentrates on maintaining the hip in a neutral position by contracting and relaxing the abdominal muscles. During functional activities, the individual can initiate stabilization contractions before starting any movement. This presets the posture and can reduce stress on the back. Many of these exercises are demonstrated in Field Strategy 11.2. Pelvic tilt maneuvers can help to reduce the degree of lumbar lordosis and, initially, can be performed with bent-knees standing, straight leg standing, and sitting.

Restoration of Proprioception and Balance

Proprioception and balance are regained through lower extremity closed chain exercises. For example, squats, leg presses, lunges, or exercises on a StairMaster, Pro-Fitter, or slide board can restore proprioception and balance in the hip and lower extremity. Stabilization exercises on "all fours" and use of surgical tubing through functional patterns also can restore proprioception and balance. These exercises should be performed in front of a mirror or videotaped, if possible, so that the individual can observe proper posture and mechanics. In addition, constant verbal reinforcement from the supervising clinician can maximize feedback.

Muscular Strength, Endurance, and Power

Abdominal strengthening exercises, such as those described in Field Strategy 11.2, should begin with pelvic tilts and progress to crunch curl-ups and diagonal crunch curl-ups to reduce functional lordosis. Progressive prone extension exercises and resisted back extension exercises can increase strength in the erector spinae.

Cardiovascular Fitness

Aquatic exercises are very beneficial, because buoyancy can relieve load on sensitive structures. Deep water allows the individual to exercise all muscle groups through a full ROM without the pain associated with gravity. Performing sport-specific skills against water resistance can apply an equal and uniform force to the muscles, similar to that in isokinetic strengthening. With low back pain, an upper body ergometer, stationary bicycle, StairMaster, or slide board may be incorporated as tolerated. Jogging can begin after all symptoms have subsided.

 As acute symptoms subside, pain and muscle tension should be relieved. The following exercises should be included in the rehabilitation program for the cheerleader: Stretching of the piriformis, gluteals, and hamstrings, which should be combined with extension exercises

FIELD STRATEGY 11.1

Flexibility and Strength Exercises for the Lumbar Region

Flexibility Exercises

1. **Sacroiliac angle knee-to-chest stretch.** In a supine position, pull one knee toward the chest with the hands. Keep the back flat. Switch to the opposite leg and repeat.

2. **Double-knee-to-chest stretch.** In a supine position, pull both knees to the chest with the hands. Keep the back flat.

3. **Hamstring stretch, seated position.** Place the leg to be stretched straight out, with the opposite foot tucked toward the groin. Reach toward the toes until a stretch is felt.

4. **Hip flexor stretch (lunge).** Extend the leg to be stretched behind you. Place the contralateral leg in front of you. While keeping the back straight, shift your body weight forward.

5. **Lateral rotator stretch, seated position.** Cross one leg over the thigh, and place the elbow on the outside of the knee. Gently stretch the buttock muscles by pushing the bent knee across the body while keeping the pelvis on the floor.

6. **Lower trunk rotation stretch.** In a supine position, rotate the flexed knees to one side, keeping the back flat and the feet together.

7. **Angry cat stretch (posterior pelvic tilt).** Kneel on all fours, with the knees a hip-width apart. Tighten the buttocks, and arch the back upward while lowering the chin and tilting the pelvis backward. Relax the buttocks, and allow the pelvis to drop downward and forward.

Strengthening Exercises

1. **Crunch curl-up.** In a supine position with the knees flexed, flatten the back, and curl up to elevate the head and shoulders from the floor. Alternate exercises include diagonal crunch curl-ups and hip crunches.

2. **Prone extension.** In a prone position, rise up on the elbows. Progress to rising up onto the hands.

3. **Alternate arm and leg lift.** In a fully extended prone position, lift one arm and the opposite leg off the surface at least 3 inches. Repeat with the opposite arm and leg.

4. **Double-arm and -leg lift.** In a fully extended prone position, lift both arms and legs off the surface at least 3 inches. Hold and return to starting position.

5. **Alternate arm and leg extension on all fours.** Kneel on all fours; raise one leg behind the body while raising the opposite arm in front of the body. Ankle and wrist weights may be added for additional resistance.

6. **Back extension.** Use a back extension machine, or have another individual stabilize the feet and legs. Raise the trunk into a slightly hyperextended position.

FIELD STRATEGY 11.2

Pelvic Stabilization and Abdominal Strengthening Exercises

1. **Stabilization in a neutral position.** With the back in a neutral position, slowly shift forward over the arms, adjusting pelvic position as you move. A tendency exists to "sag" the back; therefore, progressively tighten and relax the abdominal muscles during forward movement and backward movement, respectively.

2. **Stabilization in "two point" position.** Balance on the right leg and left arm. Slowly move forward and back without losing a neutral position. Switch to the opposite arm and leg.

3. **Leg exercise.** Without arching the back, lift one leg out behind you. Do not lift the foot more than a few inches from the floor. A variation is to move a flexed knee sideways, away from the body, and then back to the original position.

4. **Half-knee to stand (lunges).** Move to a standing position while maintaining a neutral hip position. Push evenly with both legs. Repeat several times, and then switch the forward leg.

5. **Pelvic tilt.** With the hips and knees bent and the feet on the floor, do an isometric contraction of the abdominal muscles (posterior pelvic tilt) and hold. Using the phrase "tuck the stomach in" may convey the correct motion. Then, arch the back by doing an anterior pelvic tilt. Alternate between the two motions until the individual can control pelvic motion.

6. **Bridging.** Keeping the back in a neutral position, and raise the hips and back off the floor (contract the abdominal muscles to hold the position). Hold for 5 to 10 seconds, drop down, and relax. Repeat. Variations include adding pelvic tilt exercises, lifting one leg off the floor (keeping the back in neutral position), and combining pelvic tilts and one-leg lift with bridging.

to strengthen the back extensors, stretch the abdominals, and reduce pressure on the intervertebral disks; and stabilization exercises, abdominal strengthening, and strengthening of the medial rotators of the hip through proprioceptive neuromuscular facilitation and Thera-Band exercises. As strength is regained, functional activities can be incorporated, with gradual return to full activity.

SUMMARY

1. Anatomical variations in the low back region that can predispose an individual to spinal injuries include lordosis, sway back, flat back, and par interarticularis fractures, which can lead to spondylolysis or spondylolisthesis.

2. Runners are particularly prone to low back pain resulting from tight hip flexors and hamstrings. Symptoms include localized pain that increases with active and resisted back extension, but radiating pain and neurologic deficits are not present. Anterior pelvic tilt and hyperlordosis of the lumbar spine also may be present.

3. Sciatica may be caused by a herniated disk, annular tear, myogenic or muscle-related disease, spinal stenosis, facet joint arthropathy, or compression of the nerve between the piriformis muscle.

4. The most commonly herniated disks are the lower two lumbar disks at L_4–L_5 and L_5–S_1, followed by the two lower cervical disks. Most ruptures move in a posterior or posterolateral direction as a result of torsion and compression.

5. The assessment of a spinal injury should begin with a thorough history of the injury and include neurologic tests to determine possible nerve involvement. The severity of pain and the presence or absence of neurologic symptoms, spasm, and tenderness can indicate when a backboard and stabilization are needed.

6. If, at any time, an individual complains of acute pain in the spine, change in sensation anywhere on the body, or resists moving the spine, a significant injury should be assumed and EMS summoned.

7. A rehabilitation program should focus on reduction of pain and spasm; restoration of motion and balance; development of strength, endurance, and power; and maintenance of cardiovascular fitness.

REFERENCES

1. Duggleby T, Kumar S. Epidemiology of juvenile low back pain: a review. Disabil Rehabil 1997;19(12):505–512.
2. Burton AK. Low back pain in children and adolescents: to treat or not? Bull Hosp Joint Dis 1996;55(3):127–129.
3. Newcomer K, Sinaki M. Low back pain and its relationship to back strength and physical activity in children. Acta Paediatr 1996;85(12):1433–1439.
4. Bono CM. Low-back pain in athletes. J Bone Joint Surg Am 2004;86:382–396.
5. Anderson MW. Lumbar discography: an update. Semin Roentgenol 2004;39:52–67.
6. Nordin M, Weiner SS. Biomechanics of the lumbar spine. In: Nordin M, Frankel VH, eds. Basic Biomechanics of the Musculoskeletal System, 3rd Ed. Philadelphia: Lippincott Williams & Wilkins, 2001.
7. Soler T, Calderon C. The prevalence of spondylolysis in the Spanish elite athlete. Am J Sports Med 2000;28(1):57–62.
8. Cholewicki J, Juluru K, McGill SM. Intra-abdominal pressure mechanism for stabilizing the lumbar spine. J Biomech 1999;32:13–17.
9. Hall SJ, Evans GG. Biomechanics. In: Mohnsen B, ed. Comprehensive Physical Education: What Every Student Needs to Know, 2nd Ed. Reston, VA: NASPE, 2003.
10. Wilhite JM. Thoracic and lumbosacral spine. In: Mellion MB, Walsh WM, Madden C, Putukian M, Shelton GL, eds. The Team Physician's Handbook. Philadelphia: Hanley & Belfus, 2002.

STUDENT OUTCOMES

1. Identify the important bony and soft-tissue structures of the throat, thorax, and viscera.

2. List the primary and accessory organs in the female and male reproductive systems.

3. Explain the effects of hormones on the human body.

4. Describe measures to prevent injuries to the throat, thorax, and viscera.

5. Describe the signs and symptoms of superficial injuries of the throat, chest wall, and abdominal wall, and explain the management of these injuries.

6. Describe internal complications of the thoracic area, occurring spontaneously or as a result of direct trauma, that can lead to a life-threatening situation.

7. Describe the signs and symptoms of sternal and rib fractures, and explain the management of these injuries.

8. Describe the signs and symptoms of intra-abdominal injuries, and explain the management of these injuries.

9. Identify injuries and conditions of the genitalia related to participation in sport and physical activity.

10. Describe the assessment of the throat, thorax, and visceral regions.

ROLE DELINEATION COMPETENCIES

The following Performance Domains and Tasks defined in the National Athletic Trainers' Association Board of Certification *Role Delineation Study*, 5th Edition are addressed in this chapter:

BOC COMPETENCIES

II. Clinical Evaluation and Diagnosis

    A. Obtain a history through observation, interview, and/or review of relevant records to assess current or potential injury, illness, or condition.

    B. Inspect the involved area(s) visually to assess the injury, illness, or health-related condition.

    C. Palpate the involved area(s) using standard techniques to assess the injury, illness, or health-related condition.

    D. Perform specific tests in accordance with accepted procedures to assess the injury, illness, or health-related condition.

    E. Formulate a clinical impression by interpreting the signs, symptoms, and predisposing factors of the injury, illness, or condition to determine the appropriate course of action.

III. Immediate Care

    A. Employ life-saving techniques through the use of standard emergency procedures in order to reduce morbidity and the incidence of mortality.

    B. Prevent exacerbation of non–life-threatening condition(s) through the use of standard procedures in order to reduce morbidity.

    C. Facilitate the timely transfer of care for conditions beyond the scope of practice of the athletic trainer by implementing appropriate referral strategies to stabilize and/or prevent exacerbation of the condition(s).

IV. Treatment, Rehabilitation, and Reconditioning

    E. Reassess the status of injuries, illnesses, and/or conditions using standard techniques and documentation strategies in order to determine appropriate treatment, rehabilitation, and/or reconditioning and to evaluate readiness to return to a desired level of activity.

    F. Educate the appropriate individual(s) in the treatment, rehabilitation, and reconditioning of injuries, illnesses, and/or conditions using applicable methods and materials to facilitate recovery, function, and/or performance.

Torso injuries occur in nearly every sport, particularly those involving sudden deceleration and impact. Injuries to the reproductive organs, however, are rare, particularly in females. Although protective equipment and padding are available to protect the anterior throat, thorax, and viscera, only football, men's lacrosse, ice hockey, fencing, catchers in baseball and softball, and goalies in lacrosse and field hockey require specific safety equipment for this vital region. Approximately 2% of all athletic injuries affect the abdomen, with the most commonly injured abdominal organs being the spleen, liver, and kidney (1). Most injuries are superficial and are easily recognized and managed. Some injuries, however, may involve the respiratory and circulatory system, leading to a life-threatening situation.

    This chapter begins with a review of the anatomy of the anterior throat, thorax, and viscera, followed by a brief discussion on prevention of injuries. Common injuries are then presented, followed by internal complications that result from trauma or spontaneous rupture. Finally, a step-by-step assessment of injury is presented to help determine the extent and seriousness of injury. Because rehabilitation of the region usually is included with other body regions, specific exercises for the thorax and visceral region are not discussed.

ANATOMY OF THE THROAT

The throat includes the pharynx, larynx, trachea, esophagus, a number of glands, and several major blood vessels (Fig. 12.1). Injuries to the throat are of particular concern because of the life-sustaining functions of the trachea and carotid arteries.

Pharynx, Larynx, and Esophagus

The pharynx, commonly known as the throat, connects the nasal cavity and mouth to the larynx and esophagus. The pharynx lies between the base of the skull and the sixth cervical vertebra. The laryngeal prominence on the thyroid cartilage that shields the front of the larynx is known as the "Adam's apple." A specialized, spoon-shaped cartilage, called the epiglottis, covers the superior opening of the larynx during swallowing to prevent food and liquids from entering. If a foreign body does slip past the epiglottis, the cough reflex is initiated, and the foreign body normally is ejected back into the pharynx. The larynx also contains the vocal cords, which are two bands of elastic connective tissue surrounded by mucosal folds. When expired air from the lungs passes over the vocal cords, sound is able to be produced.

The hyoid bone, the only bone of the body that does not articulate directly with any other bone, lies just inferior to the mandible in the anterior neck. It is anchored by the narrow stylohyoid ligaments to the styloid processes of the temporal bones, and it serves as an attachment point for neck muscles that raise and lower the larynx during swallowing and speech.

The esophagus carries food and liquids from the throat to the stomach. It is a muscle-walled tube that originates from the pharynx in the mid-neck and follows the anterior side of the spine. The body of the esophagus is divided into cervical, thoracic, and abdominal regions. The esophagus is pinched together at both the upper and lower ends by muscles referred to as sphincters. The coordinated action of the esophageal walls propels food into the stomach. The esophageal sphincters maintain a barrier against reverse movement of the esophageal contents into the pharynx and gastric fluids into the esophagus. When the esophagus is empty, the tube is collapsed.

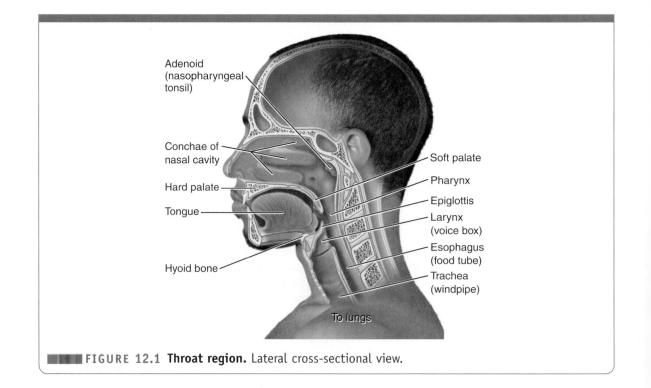

■■■ FIGURE 12.1 Throat region. Lateral cross-sectional view.

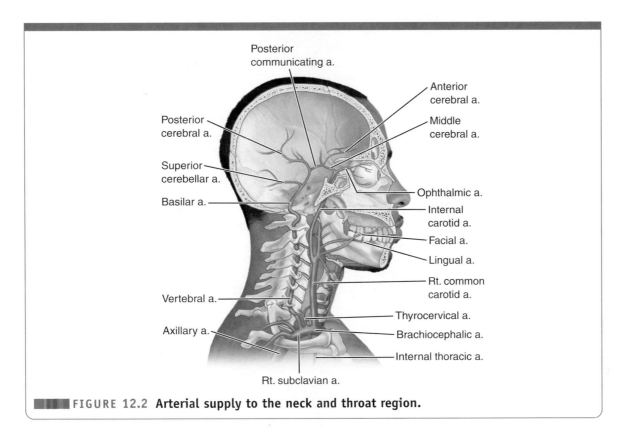

FIGURE 12.2 Arterial supply to the neck and throat region.

Trachea

The trachea extends inferiorly from the larynx through the neck into the midthorax, where it divides into the two right and left bronchial tubes. The tracheal tube is formed by C-shaped rings of hyaline cartilage that are joined by fibroelastic connective tissue. Smooth muscle fibers of the trachealis muscle form the open side of the "C" and allow expansion of the posteriorly adjacent esophagus as swallowed food passes. Contraction of the trachealis muscle during coughing can dramatically reduce the size of the airway and, in doing so, increases the pressure inside the trachea to promote expulsion of mucus.

Blood Vessels of the Throat

The largest blood vessels coursing through the neck are the common carotid arteries (Fig. 12.2). The common carotid arteries, which provide the major blood supply to the brain, head, and face, divide into external and internal carotid arteries at the level of the Adam's apple. Branches from the carotid arteries include the superior thyroid arteries, facial artery, and lingual artery; these arteries supply the thyroid and larynx, the face and sinuses, and the mouth and tongue, respectively. Several arteries branch from the left and right subclavian arteries and course upward through the posterior side of the neck, including the costocervical trunk, thyrocervical trunk, and vertebral artery.

ANATOMY OF THE THORAX

The thoracic cavity, or chest cavity, lies anterior to the spinal column and extends from the level of the clavicle down to the diaphragm. The major organs of the thorax are the heart and lungs. Although these organs are not commonly injured, internal complications caused by direct trauma or spontaneous damage can necessitate emergency action.

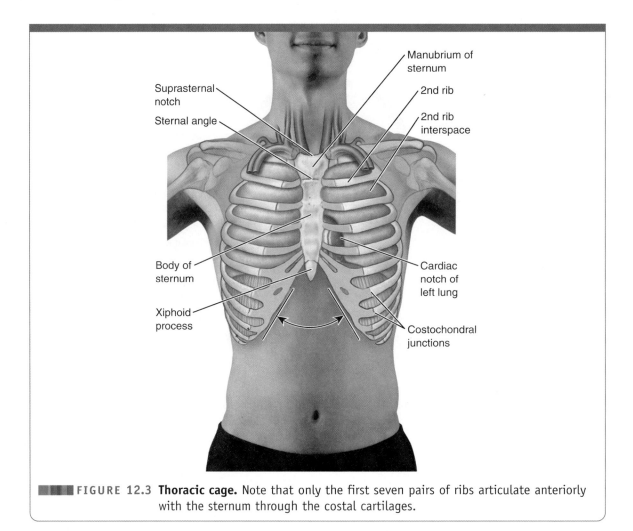

FIGURE 12.3 Thoracic cage. Note that only the first seven pairs of ribs articulate anteriorly with the sternum through the costal cartilages.

Thoracic Cage and Pleura

The thorax includes the sternum, ribs, costal cartilages, and thoracic vertebrae. These structures form a protective cage around the heart and lungs (Fig. 12.3). The sternum consists of the manubrium, which articulates with the first and second ribs; the body, which articulates with the second through seventh ribs; and the xiphoid process, a trapezoidal projection composed of hyaline cartilage that ossifies around 40 years of age. The costal cartilages of the first seven pairs of ribs attach directly to the sternum. The costal cartilages of ribs 8 through 10 attach to the costal cartilages of the immediately superior ribs. The last two rib pairs are known as floating ribs, because they do not attach anteriorly to any other structure.

The thoracic cavity is lined with a thin, double-layered membrane called the pleura. The pleural cavity is a narrow space between the pleural membranes that is filled with pleural fluid secreted by the membranes, which enables the lungs to move against the thoracic wall with minimal friction during breathing. Further discussion on the anatomy of the lungs is provided in Chapter 21.

See *Muscles of the Thorax*, found on the companion website at thePoint, for a summary of the muscles of the thoracic region and the muscles of respiration, including their attachments, primary actions, and nerve innervation.

Muscles of the Thorax

The muscles of the thoracic region and the muscles of respiration are shown in Figures 12.4 and 12.5. The major respiratory muscle is the diaphragm, a powerful sheet of muscle that completely separates the thoracic and abdominal cavities. During relaxation, the diaphragm is dome-shaped. During contraction, it flattens,

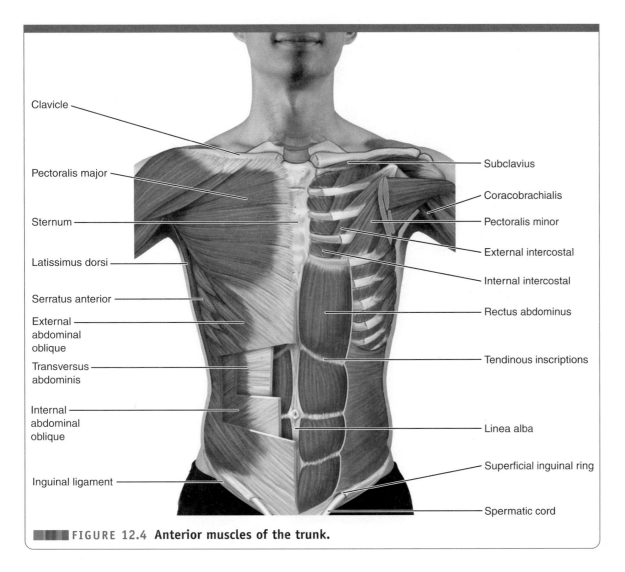

Clavicle

Pectoralis major

Sternum

Latissimus dorsi

Serratus anterior

External
abdominal
oblique

Transversus
abdominis

Internal
abdominal
oblique

Inguinal ligament

Subclavius

Coracobrachialis

Pectoralis minor

External intercostal

Internal intercostal

Rectus abdominus

Tendinous inscriptions

Linea alba

Superficial inguinal ring

Spermatic cord

FIGURE 12.4 Anterior muscles of the trunk.

increasing the size of the thoracic cavity. In turn, this increase in cavity volume causes a decrease in intrathoracic pressure, resulting in inhalation of air into the lungs.

ANATOMY OF THE VISCERAL REGION

The visceral region includes the organs and vessels between the diaphragm and the pelvic floor (Fig. 12.6). The peritoneal space includes the diaphragm, liver, spleen, stomach, and transverse colon. A portion of the cavity is covered by the bony thorax. The retroperitoneal space, which is the region behind the peritoneum and pelvis, includes the aorta, vena cava, pancreas, kidneys, ureters, and portions of the duodenum and colon. The pelvic organs and vessels include the rectum, bladder, uterus, and iliac vessels. The abdomen contains both solid and hollow organs. The solid organs include the spleen, liver, pancreas, kidneys, and adrenal glands. The hollow organs include the stomach, gallbladder, small and large intestines, bladder, and ureters. The pelvic girdle protects the lower abdominal organs.

Pelvic Girdle and Abdominal Cavity

The pelvic girdle, or pelvis, consists of the sacrum, ilium, ischium, and pubis. The joints between these bones are fused in adults, and as such, no movement is allowed. The pelvis forms a protective basin

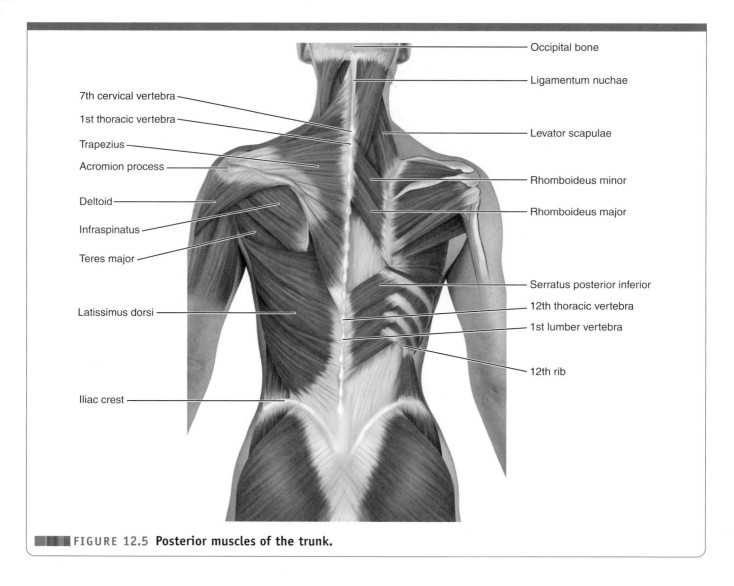

7th cervical vertebra

1st thoracic vertebra

Trapezius

Acromion process

Deltoid

Infraspinatus

Teres major

Latissimus dorsi

Iliac crest

Occipital bone

Ligamentum nuchae

Levator scapulae

Rhomboideus minor

Rhomboideus major

Serratus posterior inferior

12th thoracic vertebra

1st lumber vertebra

12th rib

█████FIGURE 12.5 Posterior muscles of the trunk.

around the internal organs of the abdomen, and it transfers loads between the spine and lower extremity through the hip joint. The pelvis also provides a mechanical link between the upper and lower extremities. Its primary role is to stabilize the lower trunk while motion occurs in the extremities.

Visceral Organs

The stomach is a J-shaped bag positioned between the esophagus and small intestine. Food is stored in the stomach for approximately 4 hours, during which time hydrochloric acid secreted in the stomach breaks it down into a paste-like substance known as **chyme**. The chyme then moves into the small intestine, where it is progressively absorbed. A few substances, including water, electrolytes, aspirin, and alcohol, are absorbed into the bloodstream across the stomach lining without full digestion.

The small intestine is approximately 2 m (6 feet) in length and is responsible for most of the digestion and absorption of food as it is propelled through the organ by waves of alternate circular contraction and relaxation by a process called **peristalsis**. This process takes approximately 3 to 6 hours. During the next 12 to 24 hours, water and electrolytes are further absorbed from the stored material in the large intestine, or colon. Mass peristaltic movements pass through the intestines several times per day to move the feces to the rectum.

The vermiform appendix protrudes from the large intestine in the right lower quadrant of the abdomen. It can become a protected environment for the accumulation of bacteria, leading to inflammation of the appendix, or appendicitis.

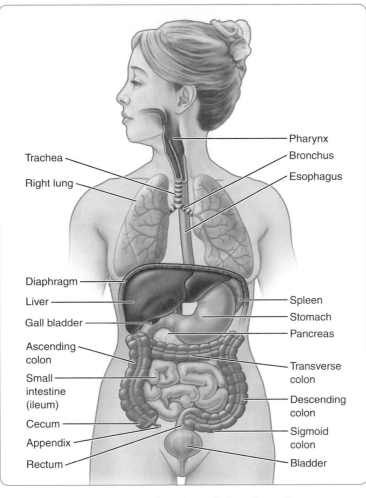

Trachea
Right lung
Diaphragm
Liver
Gall bladder
Ascending colon
Small intestine (ileum)
Cecum
Appendix
Rectum

Pharynx
Bronchus
Esophagus
Spleen
Stomach
Pancreas
Transverse colon
Descending colon
Sigmoid colon
Bladder

FIGURE 12.6 Anterior view of the visceral organs.

The liver, which is located in the upper right quadrant under the diaphragm, produces bile, a greenish liquid that helps to break down fat in the small intestine. The liver also absorbs excess glucose from the bloodstream and stores it, in the form of glycogen, for later use. Additional functions of the liver include processing fats and amino acids, manufacturing blood proteins, and detoxifying certain poisons and drugs. These functions can be severely impaired by alcohol abuse, which can result in cirrhosis of the liver. **Hepatitis** is inflammation of the liver caused by a viral infection that also can reduce the liver's efficiency. The gallbladder functions as an accessory to the liver by storing concentrated bile on its way to the small intestine.

The spleen, which is the largest of the lymphoid organs, performs four vital functions:

1. Cleansing the blood of foreign matter, bacteria, viruses, and toxins

2. Storing excess red blood cells for later reuse, and releasing others into the blood for processing by the liver

3. Producing red blood cells in the fetus

4. Storing blood platelets

The pancreas secretes most of the digestive enzymes that break down food in the small intestine. It also secretes the hormones insulin and glucagon, which lower and elevate blood sugar levels, respectively.

The kidneys filter and cleanse the blood. They are vital for filtering out toxins, metabolic wastes, drugs, and excess ions and excreting them from the body in urine. The kidneys also return

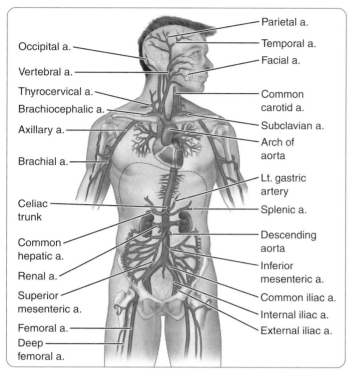

Occipital a.
Vertebral a.
Thyrocervical a.
Brachiocephalic a.
Axillary a.
Brachial a.
Celiac trunk
Common hepatic a.
Renal a.
Superior mesenteric a.
Femoral a.
Deep femoral a.

Parietal a.
Temporal a.
Facial a.
Common carotid a.
Subclavian a.
Arch of aorta
Lt. gastric artery
Splenic a.
Descending aorta
Inferior mesenteric a.
Common iliac a.
Internal iliac a.
External iliac a.

■ ■ ■ ■ **FIGURE 12.7 Arterial system of the trunk.**

needed substances, such as water and electrolytes, to the blood. The ureters connect the kidneys to the urinary bladder, which is an expandable sac that stores urine.

Blood Vessels of the Trunk

The major blood vessel of the trunk is the aorta, with its numerous branches (Fig. 12.7). The left and right coronary arteries branch from the ascending aorta to supply the heart muscle. The first arterial branch from the aortic arch is the brachiocephalic artery, which splits into the right common carotid artery and right subclavian artery. The second and third branches from the aortic arch are the left common carotid artery and the left subclavian artery, respectively. The thoracic aorta yields 10 pairs of intercostal arteries to supply the muscles of the thorax, the bronchial arteries to the lungs, the esophageal artery to the esophagus, and the phrenic arteries to the diaphragm. The distal portion of the descending aorta becomes the abdominal aorta. The first branch of the abdominal aorta is the celiac trunk, which forms the left gastric artery to the stomach, the splenic artery to the spleen, and the common hepatic artery to the liver. Other branches of the abdominal aorta include the superior and inferior mesenteric arteries to the small intestine and the first half of the large intestine, the renal arteries to the kidneys, the ovarian arteries in females, and the testicular arteries in males. The distal portion of the abdominal aorta divides into the common iliac arteries, which further divide into the internal iliac artery to supply the organs of the pelvis, and the external iliac artery, which enters the thigh to become the femoral artery.

See *Muscles of the Pelvic Girdle,* found on the companion website at thePoint, for a summary of the locations, primary functions, and innervations of the major muscles of the pelvic girdle.

Muscles of the Pelvic Girdle

As is the case throughout the neck and trunk, muscles in the pelvic region are named in pairs, with one located on the left and the other on the right side of the body. These muscles cause lateral flexion or rotation when they contract unilaterally, but they contribute to spinal flexion or extension when bilateral contractions occur.

ANATOMY OF THE GENITALIA

The reproductive organs of the female and male include the primary and accessory sex organs. The primary sex organs, the ovaries and testes, produce gametes (specifically, ovum and sperm, respectively) that, when joined together, develop into a fetus. Important sex hormones influence sexual differentiation and development of secondary sex characteristics and, in the female, regulate the reproductive cycle. The sex hormones predominantly are produced by the primary sex organs and belong to the general family known as **steroids**. In the female, estrogen and progesterone are produced by the ovaries. In the male, the adrenal cortex and testes produce hormones collectively known as **androgens**, the most active being testosterone. The accessory sex organs transport, protect, and nourish the gametes after they leave the ovaries and testes. In females, the accessory sex organs include the fallopian tubes, uterus, vagina, and vulva. In males, the accessory sex organs include the epididymis, ductus deferens, seminal vesicles, prostate gland, bulbourethral glands, scrotum, and penis.

Female Reproductive System

The female reproductive system includes the ovaries, which produce ova (female eggs); the fallopian tubes, which transport, protect, and nourish the ova; the uterus, which provides an environment for development of the fertilized embryo; and the vagina, which serves as the receptacle for the sperm (Fig. 12.8). These structures are protected by the pelvic girdle and seldom are injured during participation in sport and physical activity.

The ovarian cycle begins at puberty with the release of an ovum, or egg, from the ovary. The ovum, released at ovulation, travels through a fallopian tube to the uterus, where it embeds itself in the uterine wall. The menstrual cycle lasts anywhere from 28 to 40 days, involves a repeated series of changes within the lining of the uterus, and is controlled by the ovarian cycle. Menses, or menstrual flow, is a phase in the menstrual cycle that lasts 3 to 6 days; during this time, the thickened vascular walls of the uterus, the unfertilized ovum, and the blood from the damaged vessels of the endometrium are discharged.

The hormones estrogen and progesterone are produced by the ovaries. **Estrogens** help to regulate the menstrual cycle and influence the development of female physical sex characteristics, such as the appearance of breasts, pubic and axillary hair, increased subcutaneous fat (particularly in the hips and breasts), and widening of the pelvis. Estrogens also are responsible for the rapid growth spurt seen in girls between the ages of 10 and 13 years. This growth is short-lived, however, because increased levels of estrogen cause early closure of the epiphyses of long bones, in turn causing females to reach their full height between the ages of 15 to 18 years. In contrast, males may continue to grow until the age of 19 to 21 years. **Progesterones** are responsible for regulating the menstrual cycle and stimulating development of the uterine lining in preparation for pregnancy.

The external genital organs of the female are known as the vulva, or pudendum. The outer rounded folds, referred to as the labia majora, protect the vestibule into which the vagina and urethra open.

Male Reproductive System

The male reproductive system includes the testes, which produce spermatozoa; a number of ducts that store, transport, and nourish the spermatozoa; several accessory glands that contribute to the formation of semen; and the penis, through which urine and semen pass (Fig. 12.9). **Testosterone**, which is the primary androgen produced by the testes, stimulates the growth and maturation of the internal and external genitalia at puberty and is responsible for sexual motivation. Secondary sex characteristics that are testosterone-dependent include the appearance of pubic, axillary, and facial hair; enhanced hair growth on the chest or back; and a deepening of the voice as the larynx enlarges. Androgens also increase bone growth, bone density, and skeletal muscle size and mass.

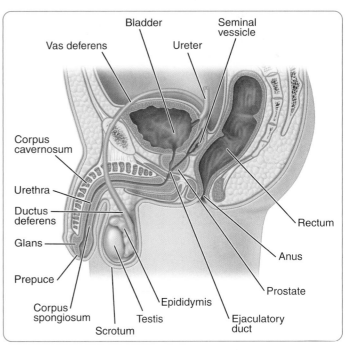

FIGURE 12.8 Median section of the female pelvis.

FIGURE 12.9 Median section of the male pelvis.

PREVENTION OF INJURIES TO THE THROAT, THORAX, AND VISCERA

> **Q** *The throat, thorax, and viscera are vulnerable to direct impact injuries. This region is such a critical area that injuries can be life-threatening. What measures can be taken to prevent injuries to this region?*

Injuries to the throat, thorax, and abdomen occur in nearly every sport, yet few sports require protective equipment for all players. In sports where high-velocity projectiles are present, throat and chest protectors are required only for specific player positions (i.e., catcher or goalie). As with other body regions, protective equipment, in combination with a well-rounded physical conditioning program, can reduce the risk of injury. Although proper skill technique can prevent some injuries, this is not a major factor in this region.

Protective Equipment

Face masks with throat protectors are required for fencing participants, baseball/softball catchers, and field hockey, ice hockey, and lacrosse goalies. Many of these athletes wear an extended pad attached to the mask to protect the throat region.

Many participants in collision and contact sports wear full chest and abdominal protection. In young baseball and softball players (younger than 12 years), it has been suggested that all infield players wear chest protectors. Adolescent rib cages are less rigid, placing the heart at greater risk from a direct impact. In this age group, more baseball and softball deaths occur from impacts to the chest than to the head.

Shoulder pads can protect the upper thoracic region, and rib protectors can provide protection against rib, upper abdominal, or low back contusions. Body suits made of mesh with pockets can hold rib and hip pads to protect the sides and back.

The male genitalia are more susceptible to injury than the female genitalia. Protective cups can protect the penis and scrotum from injury. Sport bras can provide added support to reduce excessive vertical and horizontal breast motion during exercise. Protective equipment is illustrated and discussed in Chapter 3.

Physical Conditioning

Flexibility and strengthening of the torso muscles should not be an isolated program; rather, it should include a well-rounded conditioning program for the back, shoulder, abdomen, and hip regions. Range-of-motion (ROM) and strengthening exercises should include both open and closed kinetic chain activities. Exercises for the thorax and abdominal region are included in the chapters on the hip, shoulder, and spine.

> **A** *Injuries to the throat, thorax, and viscera can be prevented by wearing appropriate protective equipment. Physical conditioning should include a well-rounded flexibility and strengthening program for the shoulder, back, abdominal, and hip region.*

THROAT CONDITIONS

> **Q** *During a rebound attempt, a basketball player is struck in the anterior neck with an elbow. The player is coughing and having difficulty swallowing. What injury should be suspected? How should the situation be managed?*

Neck Lacerations

Although uncommon, lacerations to the neck can occur. If the trauma is sufficiently deep, it can damage the jugular vein or carotid artery on the lateral side of the neck. Immediate control of hemorrhage is imperative. In addition to blood loss, air may be sucked into the vein and carried to the heart as an air embolism. Such an embolism can be fatal.

Management

Activation of the emergency plan, including summoning emergency medical services (EMS), is warranted. While waiting for EMS to arrive, the examiner should apply firm, direct pressure over the wound. The examiner also should maintain the airway, assess vital signs, and treat for shock as necessary.

Contusions and Fractures

Contusions and fractures to the trachea, larynx, and hyoid bone can occur during hyperextension of the neck. In this position, the thyroid cartilage (Adam's apple) becomes prominent and vulnerable to direct impact forces. In rare instances, these injuries can be fatal as a result of the extravasation of blood into the laryngeal tissues, leading to airway edema and asphyxia resulting from obstruction.

Signs and Symptoms

Immediate symptoms include hoarseness, dyspnea (difficulty breathing), coughing, difficulty swallowing, laryngeal tenderness, and an inability to make high-pitched "e" sounds. Significant trauma to the region can result in severe pain, **laryngospasm**, and acute respiratory distress (Box 12.1). Laryngospasm occurs when the adductor muscles of the vocal cords pull together in a shutter-like fashion and the upper surface of the vocal cords closes over the top, causing complete obstruction. The individual may recover on-site, leave the area, and return home, only to have increasing respiratory problems en route. As the internal hemorrhage and swelling increases, the occlusion becomes more complete, and the individual's breathing becomes more difficult. Panic and anxiety can increase respiration and, in doing so, compound the problem. Swelling usually is maximal within 6 hours but may occur as late as 24 to 48 hours after injury. Cyanosis and loss of consciousness may occur with complete occlusion.

Management

In an effort to diminish panic and anxiety resulting from the sudden inability to breathe, the examiner should immediately reassure the individual. The examiner should help the individual to focus on their breathing rate.

With significant trauma, activation of the emergency plan, including summoning EMS, is warranted. In these cases, it is important to consider an associated injury to the cervical spine. The examiner also should maintain the airway, assess vital signs, and treat for shock as necessary.

 If the individual recovers on-site, observation should continue throughout the day to note the presence of any delayed respiratory problems. Field Strategy 12.1 explains the management of tracheal and laryngeal injuries.

 The basketball player struck in the anterior neck could have a contusion or fracture to the trachea, larynx, or hyoid bone. In an effort to diminish panic and anxiety because of the sudden inability to breathe, the examiner should immediately reassure the individual. An open

---

Box 12.1   Signs and Symptoms Indicating Tracheal and Laryngeal Injuries

- Mild bruising and redness
- Shortness of breath
- Pain and point tenderness
- Subcutaneous crepitation
- Difficulty swallowing or coughing
- Spasmodic coughing

- Hoarseness or loss of voice[a]
- Laryngospasm[a]
- Presence of hemorrhage with blood-tinged sputum[a]
- Loss of contour of the Adam's apple (thyroid cartilage)[a]
- Cyanosis or respiratory distress

[a]A "red flag" that necessitates activation of emergency medical services.

FIELD STRATEGY 12.1

Management Algorithm for Tracheal and Laryngeal Injuries

If severe anterior throat trauma has occurred:
Assume a possible spinal injury, and treat accordingly.

 EMS Activate the emergency medical plan, including summoning emergency medical services.

Ensure an open airway:

- If needed, use the jaw-thrust maneuver to achieve a chin-up position.
- Apply ice to control swelling, if appropriate.

If an obvious deformity is present in the pharynx:
Manually straighten the airway.

If a major laceration is present:

- Control hemorrhage with firm, manual pressure.
- Maintain pressure during assessment.
- Loosen any restrictive clothing.
- To reduce panic or anxiety, talk calmly to the individual, providing assurance that you are there to help.
- Treat for shock and monitor vital signs until emergency medical services arrives.

---

airway should be maintained, and the individual should be asked to focus on the breathing rate. In cases involving severe anterior neck trauma or spasm, it is important to consider an associated injury to the cervical spine. If breathing does not return to normal in a few minutes, activation of the emergency medical plan, including summoning EMS, is warranted.

THORACIC CONDITIONS

> **Q** *In an effort to improve his cardiovascular fitness, a healthy, 35-year-old man began a supervised running program. He has been running for 3 weeks and occasionally experiences a stitch in the side while running. A physician has advised him that the condition is not serious and has suggested that he attempt to run though the pain. What techniques can be used to alleviate the pain while running?*

Thoracic injuries frequently are caused by sudden deceleration and impact, which can lead to compression and subsequent deformation of the rib cage. The extent of damage depends on the direction, magnitude of force, and point of impact. For example, a glancing blow may contuse the chest wall, whereas a baseball that strikes the ribs directly may fracture a rib and drive the bony fragments internally, causing subsequent lung or cardiac damage. Box 12.2 identifies signs and symptoms that indicate a serious thoracic condition.

Stitch in the Side

A "stitch in the side" refers to a sharp pain or spasm in the chest wall, usually on the lower right side, during exertion. Potential causes include trapped colonic gas bubbles, localized diaphragmatic hypoxia with spasm, liver congestion with stretching of the liver capsule, and poor conditioning.

Box 12.2   Red Flags Indicating a Serious Thoracic Condition

- Shortness of breath or difficulty breathing
- Deviated trachea or trachea that moves during breathing
- Anxiety, fear, confusion, or restlessness
- Distended neck veins
- Bulging or bloodshot eyes
- Suspected rib or sternal fracture
- Severe chest pain aggravated by deep inspiration

- Abnormal chest movement on affected side
- Coughing up bright red or frothy blood
- Abnormal or absent breath sounds
- Rapid, weak pulse
- Low blood pressure
- Cyanosis

Management

The frequency of a stitch usually diminishes as an individual's level of aerobic conditioning improves. Attempts can be made to run through the pain by:

- Forcibly exhaling through pursed lips
- Breathing deeply and regularly
- Leaning away from the affected side
- Stretching the arm on the affected side over the head as high as possible

Breast Conditions

Excessive breast motion during activity can lead to soreness, contusions, and nipple irritation. Although breast conditions usually are associated with women, men also may have conditions associated with the breast or nipples.

Contusions

Contusions to the breast may produce fat necrosis or hematoma formation, both of which are painful and may result in formation of a localized breast mass. The appearance of these lesions on a mammogram may be indistinguishable from that of a malignant tumor. Direct trauma should be recorded on a woman's permanent medical record to avoid any erroneous conclusions when reading a future mammogram.

MANAGEMENT. Immediate management of a breast contusion includes the application of ice and external support to the area.

Nipple Irritation

Nipple irritation commonly is seen in distance runners. Two commonly seen conditions are called runner's nipples and cyclist's nipples.

SIGNS AND SYMPTOMS. Runner's nipples are associated with friction over the nipple area. As the shirt rubs over the nipples, this friction can lead to abrasions, blisters, or bleeding.

Cyclist's nipples are caused by the combined effects of perspiration and windchill. The nipples become cold and painful, and the condition can persist for several days.

MANAGEMENT. Initial treatment of runner's nipples involves cleansing the wound, applying an antibiotic ointment, and covering the wound with a nonadhering, sterile gauze pad. Infection secondary to the injury may involve the entire nipple region or extend into the breast tissue and may necessitate referral to a physician. This condition can be prevented by applying petroleum-based products and adhesive bandages over the nipples. Initial treatment for cyclist's nipples is to warm the nipples after completion of the event to prevent the irritation. This condition can be prevented by wearing a windproof jacket.

Gynecomastia

Gynecomastia is an excessive development of the mammary glands. The condition usually is bilateral and more prevalent in the adolescent males, particularly those taking anabolic steroids. Other causes include testicular, pituitary, and adrenal pathology.

SIGN AND SYMPTOMS. Symptoms associated with the condition include nipple soreness, tenderness to pressure, and increased susceptibility to irritation through friction from a shirt.

MANAGEMENT. Typically, the condition is physiologic and resolves spontaneously in 6 to 12 months. Occasionally, surgical removal of extra breast tissue may be indicated for cosmetic reasons or as a biopsy specimen to rule out malignancy.

Strain of the Pectoralis Major Muscle

Strains of the pectoralis major muscle can occur in a variety of activities, including power lifting (particularly while bench pressing), boxing, and wrestling. The mechanism of injury usually is indirect, resulting from extreme muscle tension. A rupture results when the actively contracting muscle is overburdened by a load or extrinsic force that exceeds tissue tolerance. A strain of the pectoralis major also can result from direct trauma involving a sudden deceleration maneuver, such as when punching in boxing or blocking with an extended arm in football.

Ruptures are seen almost exclusively in men between 20 and 40 years of age (2). A higher incidence of this injury is seen with anabolic steroid abuse (3,4). Steroid use causes muscle hypertrophy and an increase in power secondary to rapid strength gain not accompanied by a concomitant increase in tendon size.

Signs and Symptoms

An audible pop, snap, or tearing sensation usually is accompanied by immediate, marked pain and weakness. The pain often is described as an aching or fatigue-like pain rather than a sharp pain. If the proximal attachment ruptures, the muscle retracts toward the axillary fold, causing it to appear enlarged. Swelling and ecchymosis are limited to the anterior chest wall. If the distal attachment is ruptured, the muscle bulges medially into the chest region, causing the axillary fold to appear thin. Swelling and ecchymosis occur on the anterior chest wall and upper arm. Shoulder motion is limited by pain. Horizontal adduction and internal rotation of the shoulder are weak and accentuate the deformity.

Management

Treatment depends on the extent of damage and follows standard protocol for muscle strains. If the strain is mild or moderate, subsequent treatment should focus on control of inflammation, protected ROM exercises, and gradual strengthening. When ROM has been achieved, the individual's strength, endurance, and power can be restored.

Rupture of the muscle can require surgical intervention. Surgical treatment has been performed successfully following delays of as long as 5 years after injury; however, the best results are achieved with prompt recognition and surgery (3).

Costochondral Injury

Costochondritis and costochondral sprains may occur during a collision with another object or as a result of a severe twisting motion of the thorax, such as during the sweep motion in rowing (5). This action can sprain or separate the costal cartilage where it attaches to the sternum or where the anterior margin of the rib attaches to the anterior end of the costal cartilage, putting pressure on the intercostal nerve lying between it and the rib above (Fig. 12.10). "Slipping rib syndrome," as it sometimes is called, more frequently involves the tenth rib, followed by the ninth or eighth rib. The onset of symptoms may be insidious, occurring long after the initial trauma.

Signs and Symptoms

The individual may hear or feel a pop. The initial localized sharp pain may be followed by intermittent stabbing pain for several days. Pain may slowly decrease in intensity, but sharp clicks may occur during bending maneuvers as the displaced cartilage overrides the bone. A visible deformity and localized pain can be palpated at the involved joint. The pain can be reproduced either by hooking the fingers under the anterior costal margin and pulling the rib cage anteriorly or by adducting the arm on the affected side coupled with rotation of the head toward the affected side (5). More severe sprains produce pain during deep inhalation and can refer the pain to the epigastric region or the spine.

FIGURE 12.10 Undisplaced costochondral separation. The costal cartilage separates from the site at which the anterior margin of the rib attaches to the anterior end of the costal cartilage.

Management

Standard acute protocol should be followed to reduce pain and inflammation. The individual should be referred to a physician for further assessment.

The discomfort usually resolves itself with 3 or 4 weeks of rest and anti-inflammatory medication, but it may persist for 9 to 12 weeks. Occasionally, a physician may choose to inject the site with steroid medication to relieve chronic pain.

Sternal Fractures

The sternum rarely is fractured in sports, but such an injury may occur as a result of rapid deceleration and high impact into an object or acute flexion that causes the upper fragment to displace anteriorly over the lower fragment. The fracture itself is not significant; however, the incidence of an associated intrathoracic injury is high.

Signs and Symptoms

The injury causes an immediate loss of breath. Localized pain is present, with pressure over the sternum, and is aggravated by deep inspiration if the fracture is incomplete. If the fracture is complete, a palpable defect is present, and pain occurs during normal respiration. Because of the anatomical location, any suspected fracture should be assessed for underlying injury, such as cardiac contusion, injury of internal mammary vessels, retrosternal and mediastinal hematoma, and pulmonary laceration or contusion (4).

Management

If a sternal fracture is suspected, the emergency plan, including summoning EMS, should be activated. Observation in the hospital with a cardiac monitor often is necessary because of the high incidence of associated intrathoracic trauma. While waiting for EMS to arrive, the examiner should maintain the airway, assess vital signs, and treat for shock as necessary.

Rib Fractures

Stress fractures to the ribs can result from an indirect force, such as a violent muscle contraction. They typically occur at the rib's weakest point (i.e., where it changes direction or has the smallest diameter). Opposing contractions of the scalene muscles and upper digitations of the serratus anterior may fracture the first rib at its thinnest segment, where the subclavian artery crosses, as is seen in weight lifting or baseball pitching. Anterolateral stress fractures of the fourth and fifth ribs have been reported in golfers and rowers because of excessive action of the serratus anterior muscle (4,5). Violent muscle contractions also are known to cause fractures to the floating ribs or avulsion fractures to the lower three ribs. In particular, the external oblique muscles often are involved.

Rib fractures are the most common thoracic injury as a result of blunt trauma (6). The force usually is applied in the anteroposterior plane, leading to fractures at the posterior angles of the

■■■■ FIGURE 12.11 **Undisplaced fractured rib.** The arrow is pointing to the fracture site.

fifth through ninth ribs. Nondisplaced fractures are more common than displaced. If the fracture is displaced, the examiner should conduct an internal injury assessment. If a fracture occurs to the lower two ribs, there may be associated damage to the kidneys, liver, or spleen. Splenic trauma has been reported in up to 20% of left lower rib fractures and liver trauma in up to 10% of right lower rib fractures (6).

Signs and Symptoms

Intense localized pain over the fracture site is aggravated by deep inspiration, coughing, or chest movement (Fig. 12.11). In many cases, the individual takes shallow breaths and leans toward the fracture site, stabilizing the area with a hand to prevent excessive movement of the chest to ease the pain. A visible contusion and palpable crepitus may be present at the impact site. Coughing up blood, especially bright red or frothy blood, should be noted. A stethoscope should be used to listen for abnormal or absent breath sounds in the lungs, and the rate and depth of respirations should be recorded. Manual compression of the rib cage in an anteroposterior direction and lateral compression produces pain over the fracture site (see Fig. 12.18). If any signs of respiratory distress, cyanosis, or shock appear, a thorough assessment for an underlying visceral injury should be conducted. Box 12.3 identifies other signs and symptoms indicating a possible sternal or rib fracture.

Management

Treatment involves standard acute protocol. A 6-inch elastic bandage can be wrapped around the thorax with circular motions distal to the injury site, or a sling and swathe may be used to immobilize the chest if pain is intense or multiple fractures are suspected. If one or two ribs are fractured, the individual should be referred to a physician immediately.

Box 12.3 Signs and Symptoms Indicating a Possible Sternal or Rib Fracture

- History of direct blow, compression of the chest, or violent muscle contraction
- Individual may lean toward the fractured side, stabilizing the area with a hand to prevent movement of the chest
- Localized discoloration or swelling over the fracture site
- Visible, slight step deformity
- Palpable pain and crepitus at fracture site
- Increased pain on deep inspiration
- Increased pain on trunk rotation and lateral flexion away from the fracture site
- Increased pain on manual compression of the rib cage in an anteroposterior direction or with lateral compression
- Shallow breathing
- Cyanosis
- Rapid, weak pulse and low blood pressure with multiple fractures; with a fracture that has damaged intercostals, vessels, and nerves; or if the lung or pleural sac has been penetrated

Pain tends to be most severe during the first 3 to 5 days following injury and ultimately disappears after 3 to 6 weeks. Depending on the fracture site, the presence of a displaced or nondisplaced fracture, and the number of ribs involved, it may be necessary to refrain from participation in sport and physical activity until healing is complete. Strapping or taping to reduce chest movement is not recommended, because it may aggravate the condition. With a simple fracture, a flak jacket or rib vest can be worn to protect the area from reinjury.

> If three or more ribs are fractured or signs and symptoms suggesting internal injury are present, the emergency plan, including summoning EMS, should be activated. While waiting for EMS to arrive, the examiner should maintain the airway, assess vital signs, and treat for shock as necessary.

 The male runner could attempt the following: exhaling forcibly through pursed lips, breathing deeply and regularly, leaning away from the affected side, or stretching the arm on the affected side over the head as high as possible.

INTERNAL COMPLICATIONS

Q *During preseason volleyball practice, a player experiences hyperventilation while sprinting. What is the management of this condition?*

Several conditions can alter breathing and cardiac function. Hyperventilation is associated with an inability to catch one's breath and, in most instances, is not a serious problem. Direct trauma to the thorax can lead to serious underlying problems, although these conditions are rare in sport participation. Among the more serious complications are pulmonary contusion, pneumothorax, tension pneumothorax, hemothorax, and heart contusions.

Hyperventilation

Hyperventilation often is linked to pain, stress, or trauma in sport participation. The respiratory rate increases during activity. Rapid, deep inhalations draw more oxygen into the lungs. Conversely, long exhalations result in too much carbon dioxide being exhaled.

Signs and Symptoms

Signs and symptoms include an inability to catch one's breath, numbness in the lips and hands, spasm of the hands, chest pain, dry mouth, dizziness, and occasionally, fainting.

Management

It is important to calm the individual, because panic and anxiety can complicate the condition. Treatment involves concentrating on slow inhalations through the nose and exhalations through the mouth until the symptoms have stopped. Although breathing into a paper bag has proved to be quite successful in restoring the oxygen–carbon dioxide balance, many individuals find it to be embarrassing. Breathing into a paper bag is not needed except in severe cases.

Pulmonary Contusion

Pulmonary contusion usually results from nonpenetrating chest trauma and is rare in sport participation. Force transmitted through the thorax, as in landing on a football or a body slam onto the hard ground, causes blood and protein to leak into the alveoli and interstitial spaces, leading to pulmonary collapse.

Signs and Symptoms

Chest pain, rapid breathing, shortness of breath, rales, and coughing are common signs and symptoms. Breathing may be compromised, and hypoxia may appear 2 to 4 hours after trauma. The condition may go undetected until the individual coughs up blood or has other problems, such as pneumothorax, rib fractures, or **subcutaneous emphysema**.

Management

EMS · If a pulmonary contusion is suspected, the emergency plan, including summoning EMS, should be activated. While waiting for EMS to arrive, the examiner should maintain the airway, assess vital signs, and treat for shock as necessary.

Mild contusions (i.e., no abnormal findings) heal within days. The individual may return to full participation in as few as 10 days. A flak jacket may be worn to protect the region. In more severe cases, hospitalization is required. Ventilatory support may be necessary.

Pneumothorax

Pneumothorax is a condition whereby air is trapped in the pleural space, causing a portion of a lung to collapse. Although the etiology of a pneumothorax can vary, the two most common types are spontaneous and nonspontaneous.

Spontaneous pneumothorax occurs unexpectedly, with or without underlying disease. The condition is believed to result from rupture of a subpleural bleb (a blister-like formation). A precipitating cause usually is not identifiable. In fact, most episodes occur at rest. Risk factors include male gender, cigarette smoking, and an astenic physiognomy [7]. In particular, 20- to 30-year-old males who are tall, lean, and have a long and narrow chest appear to be at increased risk. Other pulmonary conditions that may lead to a spontaneous pneumothorax include asthma, cystic fibrosis, emphysema, and pneumonia [8].

Nonspontaneous, or traumatic, pneumothorax ranks second only to rib fractures as the most common sign of chest injury and can be seen in 40 to 50% of patients with chest trauma [7]. The injury may be caused by a penetrating wound to the chest (e.g., a stab wound), a fractured rib, or severe chest trauma that results in a laceration of lung tissue. Air is allowed to escape into the pleural cavity with each inhalation, preventing the lung from expanding fully (Fig. 12.12A).

Signs and Symptoms

The most common symptoms of a traumatic pneumothorax are **dyspnea**, cyanosis, severe chest pain on the affected side, deviation of the trachea, and decreased or absent breath sounds over the affected area with hyper-resonance to percussion [9] (Box 12.4). Other symptoms may include asymmetric chest expansion, confusion, fatigue, anxiety, restlessness, and decrease in blood pressure. Pain may be referred to the shoulder tip, across the chest, or over the abdomen. If not recognized and treated promptly, the condition can develop into tension pneumothorax.

In a spontaneous pneumothorax, pain can stop abruptly after onset, leading to a delay in treatment. Dyspnea and chest discomfort gradually increase until the individual finally seeks medical care. In some cases, symptoms may flare up suddenly, producing acute pain localized to the side of the pneumothorax and difficulty in breathing.

Management

The individual should be kept calm, quiet, and seated while focusing on controlled breathing. If diminished or absent breath sounds are present over the affected lung, the individual should be

Box 12.4   Signs and Symptoms Indicating Possible Pneumothorax

- Sudden onset or sharp chest pain
- Shortness of breath
- Difficulty breathing
- Referred pain to the tip of the shoulder, across the chest, or over the abdomen
- Light-headedness
- Tightness in chest
- Decreased or absent breath sounds over the collapsed lung
- Asymmetric chest movements on the affected side
- Decrease in blood pressure
- Tachycardia

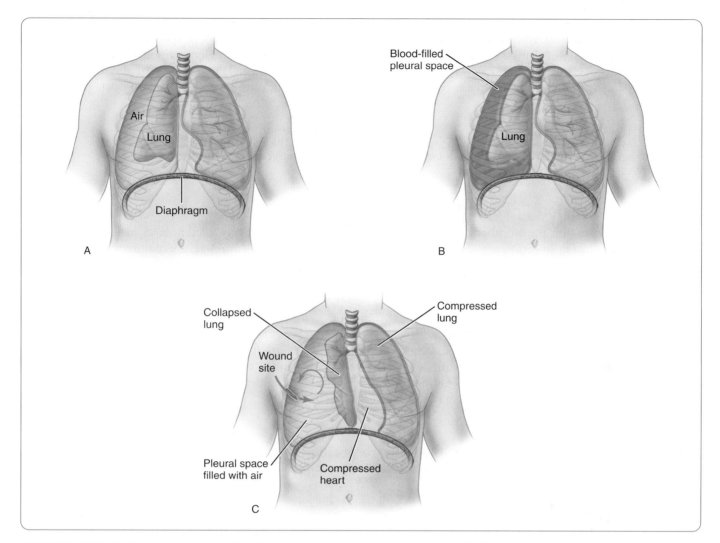

■■■■ FIGURE 12.12 **Internal complication to the lungs. A,** Pneumothorax. **B,** Hemothorax. **C,** Tension pneumothorax. Each condition can become life-threatening if the lung collapses.

transported to the nearest medical facility and should not be given any fluids. Because of the risk of recurrence of spontaneous pneumothorax, individuals treated with conservative measures should be counseled to participate only in nonstrenuous activities. If treatment included a thoracotomy or other invasive procedures, activity usually can resume after 2 to 4 weeks (10). These individuals should be counseled, however, about the increased risk of recurrence, especially on the contralateral side. If pneumothorax recurs, the individual should be advised to discontinue collision and contact sports.

> Activation of the emergency plan, including summoning EMS, is warranted. While waiting for EMS to arrive, the examiner should maintain the airway, assess vital signs, and treat for shock as necessary.

Hemothorax

Hemothorax involves the loss of blood, rather than air, into the pleural cavity (Fig. 12.12B). Fractured ribs may tear lung tissue and blood vessels in the chest or chest cavity.

Signs and Symptoms

The individual usually presents with severe pain, hypoxia, decreased breath sounds unilaterally or bilaterally, dyspnea, tachypnea, and dullness to percussion over the affected side (9). The individual may cough up frothy blood. As the condition deteriorates, the signs and symptoms of shock appear, including hypotension, decreased venous return, and cyanosis. The neck veins may be flat, secondary to hypovolemia, or distended because of the mechanical effects of intrathoracic pressure. Tracheal deviation and/or mediastinal shift are classic signs caused by the contents of the thoracic cavity shifting away from the accumulation of blood as a result of the increased intrathoracic pressure (9).

Management

 Activation of the emergency plan, including summoning EMS, is warranted. The individual should be treated for shock. While waiting for EMS to arrive, the examiner should maintain the airway, assess vital signs, and treat for shock as necessary.

Tension Pneumothorax

Tension pneumothorax occurs when air or blood progressively accumulates in the pleural space during inspiration and cannot escape on expiration. The pleural space expands with each breath, displacing the mediastinum to the opposite side. This displacement compresses the heart, uninjured lung, thoracic aorta, and vena cava, causing a decrease in blood return to the right side of the heart, thereby decreasing cardiac output (Fig. 12.12C).

Signs and Symptoms

Signs and symptoms include chest pain, tracheal deviation away from the tension pneumothorax, respiratory distress, unilateral absence of breath sounds on the affected side, hypotension, and circulatory compromise leading to cyanosis and possibly death (6,9). Asymmetric chest wall movement may be visible, as may distended neck veins.

Management

 Activation of the emergency plan, including summoning EMS, is warranted. While waiting for EMS to arrive, the examiner should maintain the airway, assess vital signs, and treat for shock as necessary.

Traumatic Asphyxia

Traumatic asphyxia results from direct, massive trauma to the thorax.

Signs and Symptoms

Classic symptoms include a bluish tinge over the neck and facial regions, subconjunctival hemorrhage, ecchymosis, and minute hemorrhagic spots on the face. Loss of vision also has been reported as a result of retinal edema, but such loss may improve within hours or days.

Management

Activation of the emergency plan, including summoning EMS, is warranted. While waiting for EMS to arrive, the examiner should maintain the airway, assess vital signs, and treat for shock as necessary.

Heart Injuries

Blunt chest trauma can compress the heart between the sternum and spine, leading to blunt cardiac injury (formally called myocardial contusion). Because it lies directly posterior to the sternum, the right ventricle often is injured. Red blood cells and fluid leak into the surrounding tissues and, in doing so, decreases circulation to the heart muscle. This action leads to localized cellular damage and necrosis of the heart tissue. Decreased cardiac output secondary to arrhythmias, or irregular heart beats, are of major concern.

Blunt trauma also may lead to **cardiac tamponade**. It is the leading cause of traumatic death in youth baseball, and it has been reported in softball, ice hockey, and lacrosse. Massive blunt trauma ruptures the myocardium or lacerates a coronary artery, which leads to an increased volume of blood or edematous exudate into the pericardial sac. As a result, the tension limits venous inflow and diastolic filling, and cardiac output is diminished. The heart is unable to fill and/or pump effectively, and without early recognition and treatment, cardiac arrest occurs.

Signs and Symptoms

Classic signs of cardiac tamponade include jugular venous distention as a result of increased venous pressure or lack of cardiac filling. Beck's triad also is a classic tool for identifying cardiac tamponade. It includes venous pressure elevation that is apparent through distended neck veins, decreased arterial pressure (i.e., hypotension), and muffled heart tones. Another prominent sign is pulsus paradoxus, which is a fall in blood pressure that exceeds 10 mm Hg on inspiration. Pulsus paradoxus is caused by a decrease in cardiac output that results from increased negative intrathoracic pressure during inhalation (9). In nearly all cases, the individual collapses within seconds and goes into respiratory arrest.

Management

In many cases, resuscitation is unsuccessful even if given immediately after injury. This may result from structural cardiac disruption caused by the trauma.

> Activation of the emergency plan, including summoning EMS, is warranted. While waiting for EMS to arrive, the examiner should maintain the airway and, if necessary, initiate breathing and chest compressions.

Sudden Death in Athletes

Sudden death is defined as an event that is nontraumatic, is unexpected, and occurs either instantaneously or within minutes of an abrupt change in an individual's previous clinical state. For individuals younger than 35 years, the most common cause is **hypertrophic cardiomyopathy**, with a higher frequency seen in male athletes as compared with females (11). Other causes of sudden death include abnormalities in the coronary arteries, aortic rupture associated with Marfan's syndrome, and mitral valve prolapse. In individuals older than 35 years, the most common cause is ischemic coronary artery disease. Because of the complexity of sudden death, it is discussed in greater detail in Chapter 19.

Athletic Heart Syndrome

Athletic heart syndrome is a benign condition associated with physiologic alterations in the heart muscle brought on by repetitive, intensive physical training. These changes may produce abnormalities on electrocardiograms, but they are not a contraindication to exercise. Individuals with athletic heart syndrome must be evaluated fully by a physician to rule out serious underlying cardiovascular disorders that may place them at risk.

 Because hyperventilation can produce panic and anxiety, the examiner should initially attempt to calm the individual. Next, the examiner should encourage the individual to concentrate on their breathing. Specifically, the individual should be instructed to inhale slowly through the nose and exhale through the mouth until breathing returns to normal. Breathing into a paper bag has proven to be quite successful in restoring the oxygen–carbon dioxide balance associated with hyperventilation, but this technique can be embarrassing for the individual and is not necessary except in severe cases.

ABDOMINAL WALL CONDITIONS

> *Following a blow to the abdomen, a high-school ice hockey player experiences dyspnea. A solar plexus contusion is suspected. How should the condition be managed?*

The muscles of the abdominal wall are strong and powerful yet also flexible enough to absorb impact. Consequently, injuries to the abdominal wall usually are minor; however, other conditions, such as a contusion to the solar plexus and hernias, can affect sport participation.

Skin Wounds

 If an individual has penetrating trauma, activation of the emergency plan to ensure immediate transportation to the nearest medical facility is warranted. Because further examination is necessary to rule out intra-abdominal injuries, ointments or creams should not be placed on the wound. Instead, the wound should be irrigated with sterile water and covered with an absorbent pad to control hemorrhage.

A superficial skin wound to the abdominal region should be managed in the same manner as any other skin wound.

Management

A superficial skin wound should be cleansed to prevent contamination and covered with a sterile, nonstick dressing. If the wound penetrates the abdominal wall muscles, trauma to internal organs should be suspected.

Skin Contusions

Blunt trauma can result in a minor contusion or damage to internal organs.

Signs and Symptoms

Simple contusions to the abdominal wall are evident by tenderness over the area of impact, pain during active contraction of the abdominal muscles, and the absence of referred pain. Any case involving blunt trauma requires assessment to rule out internal injury. Information specific to intra-abdominal conditions is provided later in this chapter.

If internal injury is suspected, activation of the emergency plan, including summoning EMS, is warranted. While waiting for EMS to arrive, the examiner should maintain the airway, assess vital signs, and treat for shock as necessary.

Management

The management of a simple contusion includes application of ice and compression to limit hemorrhage. A pressure dressing may be applied if a large hematoma forms.

Muscle Strains

Muscle strains are caused by direct trauma, sudden twisting, or sudden hyperextension of the spine. The rectus abdominis is the most commonly injured muscle. Complications arise when the epigastric artery or intramuscular vessels are damaged, leading to a rectus sheath hematoma. Nearly 80% of hematomas occur below the umbilicus.

Signs and Symptoms

Sudden abdominal pain, nausea, vomiting, marked tenderness, swelling, and muscle guarding may be present. Straight leg raising or hyperextension of the back increases the pain. A palpable mass may or may not be present; if a mass is present, it becomes fixed with contraction of the muscle. Other signs include a bluish discoloration around the periumbilical region 72 hours after injury (Cullen's sign) and pain with resisted trunk or hip flexion (4).

Management

Treatment consists of ice, rest, and use of nonsteroidal anti-inflammatory drugs for the first 36 to 48 hours. Local heat and whirlpools can be used after 48 to 72 hours with activity modification until the hematoma and soreness resolve. Activities such as twisting, turning, trunk flexion, or sudden stretching should be avoided until painful symptoms subside.

Solar Plexus Contusion ("Wind Knocked Out")

A blow to the abdomen with the muscles relaxed is referred to as a "solar plexus punch." Although the true cause of the breathing difficulty is unknown, it is thought to be caused by diaphragmatic spasm and transient contusion to the sympathetic **celiac plexus**.

Signs and Symptoms

The blow results in an immediate inability to catch one's breath (dyspnea). Fear and anxiety may complicate the condition.

Management

Assessment should include a thorough airway analysis. Any mouth guard or partial dental plates should be removed. Any restrictive equipment and clothing around the abdomen should be loosened and the individual instructed to flex his or her knees toward the chest. Although it may seem paradoxic, the individual should be instructed to take a deep breath and hold it. This action should be repeated until normal breathing is restored. Another method for restoring normal breathing is to instruct the individual to whistle. This action forces the diaphragm to relax. Because a severe blow may lead to an intra-abdominal injury, assessment should be performed to rule out internal injury.

Hernias

A **hernia,** which is a protrusion of the abdominal viscera through a weakened portion of the abdominal wall, can be either congenital or acquired. Congenital hernias are present at birth and may be related to family history. Acquired hernias occur after birth and may be aggravated by a direct blow, strain, or abnormal intra-abdominal pressure, such as that exerted during heavy weight lifting. The three most common hernias are indirect, direct, and femoral (Fig. 12.13).

An indirect inguinal hernia is the most common type of hernia in young athletes. A weakness in the peritoneum around the deep inguinal ring allows the abdominal viscera to protrude through the ring into the inguinal canal and, occasionally, even extend into the scrotum. This weakness in the peritoneum typically is not present in women. Large indirect hernias may reduce spontaneously, because they cannot extend easily into the inguinal canal. Direct hernias, which tend to be more common in men older than 40 years, result from a weakness in an area of fascia bounded by the rectus abdominis muscle, inguinal ligament, and epigastric vessels. Femoral hernias, more commonly seen in women, allow the abdominal viscera to protrude through the femoral ring into the femoral canal, compressing the lymph vessels, connective tissue, and femoral artery and vein. The herniation presents as a mass that is inferolateral to the pubic tubercle and medial to the femoral artery and vein.

The danger of a hernia lies in continued trauma to the weakened area during falls, blows, or increased intra-abdominal pressure exerted during activity. The hernia can twist on itself and produce a strangulated hernia, which can become gangrenous.

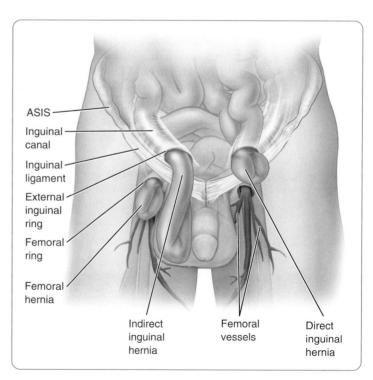

Signs and Symptoms

Symptoms vary, but in most cases, the first sign of a hernia is a visible, tender swelling and an aching feeling in the groin. Some hernias are asymptomatic until the preparticipation examination, when the physician palpates the protrusion by invaginating the scrotum with a finger. Protrusion of the hernia increases with coughing.

Management

Most hernias require surgical repair. Individuals with an indirect hernia repair can begin walking, mild upper extremity exercises, and bicycling within 6 weeks of surgery. Return to noncontact sport participation can occur in 7 weeks and return to contact sports within 8 to 10 weeks.

Repair of direct inguinal and femoral hernias is more extensive. Strenuous activities are prohibited for 3 weeks postsurgery. Return to noncontact sports can occur in 8 weeks and return to contact sports in 12 weeks. Activities that stretch or pull the abdominal

■■■■ FIGURE 12.13 Hernias. A hernia may be classified as **(A)** indirect, in which the small intestine extends into the scrotum; **(B)** direct, in which the small intestine extends through a weakening in the internal inguinal ring; or **(C)** femoral, in which the small intestine protrudes posterior to the inguinal ligament and medial to the femoral artery.

muscles should be avoided. Recommended activities include swimming, biking, and weight training for the upper extremities.

In some situations, an individual with a hernia that has not been repaired can participate in noncontact sports. Surgical repair is recommended to prevent recurrent, irreducible hernias, however, which can lead to small bowel obstruction.

> *The ice hockey player experiencing dyspnea following a blow to the abdomen is believed to have sustained a solar plexus contusion. The management of this condition includes assessing the airway for obstruction, removing any mouth guard or dental apparatus, loosening restrictive equipment around the abdomen, and having the individual flex his knees toward his chest. If breathing does not return to normal within a few minutes, the emergency plan, including summoning EMS, should be activated.*

INTRA-ABDOMINAL CONDITIONS

> *A 22-year-old lacrosse player was struck in the abdomen with an opponent's stick. She experienced a sudden onset of abdominal pain in the upper right quadrant. She also reported pain to the inferior angle of the right scapula. What injury should be suspected, and how should this condition be managed?*

Trauma to the abdomen can lead to severe internal hemorrhage if organs or major blood vessels are lacerated or ruptured. Injuries can be open or closed, with closed injuries typically caused by blunt trauma. If damaged, hollow viscera can leak their contents into the abdominal cavity, causing severe hemorrhage, **peritonitis,** and shock. Many signs and symptoms indicating an intra-abdominal injury, regardless of the organ involved, are similar in nature (Box 12.5). Variations arise in the area of palpable pain and the site of referred pain.

Acute management of suspected intra-abdominal injuries also is very similar, regardless of the injured organ. Initially, the examiner should keep the individual relaxed while assessing airway, breathing, and circulation. If necessary, the emergency medical plan, including summoning EMS, should be activated. While waiting for EMS to arrive, the individual should be placed in a supine position with the knees flexed to relax the low back and abdominal muscles. The vital signs should be monitored regularly and the individual treated for shock. Field Strategy 12.2 summarizes the acute management of intra-abdominal injuries.

Splenic Rupture

Although the spleen rarely is injured in sport participation, certain systemic disorders, such as infectious mononucleosis, can enlarge this organ, making it vulnerable to injury. The spleen is the most commonly injured abdominal organ and is the most frequent cause of death from abdominal blunt trauma in sport (4). Subsequent to trauma, the spleen can lose blood very rapidly because of

Box 12.5   Signs and Symptoms Indicating the Need for Lung Auscultation

- Shortness of breath or dyspnea (could indicate conditions such as pneumonia, pneumothorax, asthma, or heart failure)
- Cough with or without a bloody sputum (could indicate pneumonitis, bronchitis, fibrotic lung disease, or bronchial carcinoma)
- Pleuritic pain (could indicate acute inflammation of the pleural surface, herpes zoster involving the intercostal nerves, or rib fracture)
- A resting respiratory rate of greater than 22 breaths per minute
- Cyanosis or finger clubbing (could indicate several pulmonary diseases, including chronic suppurative disease or pulmonary carcinoma)

FIELD STRATEGY 12.2

Management Algorithm for Suspected Intra-Abdominal Injuries

In case of vomiting:
Roll the person on the side to allow drainage.
Make certain the airway remains open.
Control any external hemorrhage with pressure and a sterile dressing.
Lay the individual supine:
- Keep the knees flexed to relax the abdominal muscles.
- Do not extend the legs or elevate the feet.

Record vital signs:
- Respiratory rate and depth (rapid, shallow breathing indicates shock).
- Pulse rate and strength (rapid, weak pulse indicates shock).
- Blood pressure (a marked drop in both readings indicates shock).
- Pupillary response to light (lackluster, dilated pupils indicates shock).

Do not give anything by mouth to the individual.
Treat for shock, and monitor vital signs until emergency medical services arrives.

> Activate the emergency medical plan, including summoning emergency medical services. EMS

its vascularity; however, the spleen can splint itself and stop hemorrhaging. This may appear to be advantageous but actually is problematic, because the splinting is not sufficient and delayed hemorrhage can be produced days, weeks, or even months later after a seemingly minor jarring motion.

An individual who has infectious mononucleosis should be disqualified from contact and strenuous noncontact sports and physical activity for at least 3 weeks. After 3 weeks, return to strenuous noncontact sports and physical activity is acceptable if the individual feels up to the activity, the spleen is nonpalpable, and the liver function tests are normal. If the spleen remains palpable or the liver function tests are abnormal, contact sports and activities are contraindicated for an additional week or longer (12).

Signs and Symptoms

Indications of a splenic rupture include a history of blunt trauma to the left upper quadrant and a persistent, dull pain in the upper left quadrant, left lower chest, and left shoulder, which is referred to as **Kehr's sign**. This referred pain, which is seen in nearly 60% of patients with a splenic injury, is caused by irritation of the diaphragm innervated by the phrenic nerves, which arise from the ventral rami of segments C3 to C5 (13). The free blood also can irritate the right side of the diaphragm, in which case pain is referred to the dermatome patterns in the right shoulder. Symptoms at the time of injury include nausea, cold and clammy skin, and signs of shock.

Management

Treatment usually involves nonoperative intravenous therapy, strict bed rest, and intensive monitoring of vital signs. Because the spleen is essential to the body's immune system function, it is important to protect the individual by administering additional immunizations and considering the needs of an immunocompromised system. Physical activities should be restricted for at least 2 weeks. Return to vigorous physical activity is not recommended until 2 to 3 months after injury. If surgical repair is indicated, a minimum period of 3 months is needed for the abdominal musculature to heal and regain adequate strength before return to vigorous activity. Most physicians recommend a 6-month interval after a splenectomy before an individual returns to contact sports.

> If splenic injury is suspected, activation of the emergency plan, including summoning EMS, is warranted. While waiting for EMS to arrive, the examiner should maintain the airway, assess vital signs, and treat for shock as necessary. Refer to Field Strategy 12.2 for further management procedures. EMS

Liver Contusion and Rupture

A direct blow to the upper right quadrant can contuse the liver.

Signs and Symptoms

Significant palpable pain, point tenderness, hypotension, and shock are indicative of liver trauma. In addition, pain may be referred to the inferior angle of the right scapula. As with the spleen, systemic diseases, such as hepatitis, can enlarge the liver, making it more susceptible to injury. An individual with an enlarged liver (i.e., hepatomegaly) should avoid contact sports until the liver has returned to its normal size or is nonpalpable. If lacerated, the liver is capable of massive bleeding; however, the bleeding typically stops by the time the wound is exposed during surgery. For this reason, there has been an increasing trend toward nonoperative management (14).

Management

 If a splenic injury is suspected, activation of the emergency plan, including summoning EMS, is warranted. While waiting for EMS to arrive, the examiner should maintain the airway, assess vital signs, and treat for shock as necessary. Refer to Field Strategy 12.2 for further management procedures.

Appendicitis

The vermiform appendix is a pouch extending from the cecum (see Fig. 12.6). If it becomes obstructed (e.g., with hardened fecal material), venous circulation can become impaired, leading to increased bacterial growth and the formation of pus. The resulting inflamed appendix, a condition called **appendicitis,** can lead to ischemia and gangrene. If the appendix ruptures, feces and bacteria are sprayed over the abdominal contents, causing peritonitis.

Signs and Symptoms

Signs and symptoms include acute abdominal pain in the lower right quadrant, loss of appetite, nausea, vomiting, and low-grade fever. Rebound pain can be elicited at **McBurney's point,** which is one-third the distance between the anterior superior iliac spine and the umbilicus.

Management

 Activation of the emergency plan, including summoning EMS, is warranted. While waiting for EMS to arrive, the examiner should maintain the airway, assess vital signs, and treat for shock as necessary. Refer to Field Strategy 12.2 for further management procedures.

Renal and Genitourinary Conditions

The kidneys are located in the retroperitoneal upper lumbar area of the abdomen. The upper third of the right kidney and upper half of the left kidney are located under the twelfth rib. Posteriorly, the organs are protected by the psoas, paravertebral, and latissimus dorsi muscles and are encased in pericapsular fat. Despite this protection, the kidneys can be injured when the body is extended and the abdominal muscles are relaxed, such as when a receiver leaps to catch a pass. The ureters run along the posterior peritoneal wall and are at risk for injury where they cross the bony rim of the pelvis. The bladder lies with the pelvis and is more vulnerable to injury when full. Several chronic and acute conditions can affect these organs.

Kidney Contusion

The kidney may be injured as a result of a direct blow or a contrecoup injury from a high-speed collision. Because the kidney normally is distended by blood, an external force can cause abnormal extension of the engorged kidney. The degree of renal injury depends on the extent of the distention and on the angle and magnitude of the blow.

SIGNS AND SYMPTOMS. The individual may complain of pain, tenderness, and **hematuria.** Pain can be referred posteriorly to the low back region, to the sides of the buttocks, and anteriorly to the lower abdomen. Hypovolemic shock may result from extensive bleeding.

MANAGEMENT. Treatment involves applying ice to control inflammation and pain, treating for shock, and if needed, transporting the individual to the nearest medical facility. A radiograph or computed tomographic scan may be used to determine the extent of injury. Most injuries are handled conservatively, with rest and fluid management. Spontaneous healing and return of normal renal function can be expected. Individuals who have a solitary kidney, especially when the kidney is pelvic, iliac, polycystic, or anatomically abnormal, should be counseled about the increased risk of injury. Although contact sports place the remaining kidney at very little risk, participation in contact or collision sports should be individually assessed. Use of a flak jacket or other customized padding may reduce the incidence of injury during contact or impact sports.

Kidney Stones

Some substances filtered by the kidneys (especially calcium, oxalate, uric acid, and cystine) have a tendency to form crystals. Other substances (e.g., citrate and magnesium) help to prevent crystal formation. When these substances are not in balance, the urine becomes too concentrated, acidic, or alkaline, and crystals can form. Risk factors for this condition include a family history of kidney stones, being a white male between 20 and 40 years of age, certain diseases (e.g., gout, chronic urinary tract infections (UTIs), cystic kidney disease, hyperparathyroidism, renal tubular acidosis, and cystinuria), certain medications (e.g., diuretics), having only one kidney, eating a diet high in protein and low in fiber, lack of adequate water intake, and living a sedentary lifestyle. In some cases, however, the exact cause of kidney stones may be unknown (i.e., idiopathic nephrolithiasis).

There are four main types of kidney stones, each stemming from a different cause:

- **Calcium stones.** Most kidney stones are formed from calcium (85% in men, and 65% in women) (15). These stones may result from large amounts of vitamin D, which may cause the body to absorb too much calcium; drugs, such as thyroid hormones and some diuretics; certain cancers; overactive parathyroid glands; and some kidney conditions.

- **Uric acid stones.** As the name suggests, these stones are formed from uric acid, a byproduct of protein metabolism. A diet high in meat may cause excess amounts of uric acid in the urine. These stones also have been attributed to chemotherapy treatment.

- **Struvite stones.** Found mainly in women, struvite stones almost always are the result of chronic UTIs caused by bacteria that secrete specific enzymes. These enzymes increase the amount of ammonia in the urine, which makes up the crystals in struvite stones. These stones often are large and have a characteristic stag's-horn shape, which can cause serious damage to the kidneys.

- **Cystine stones.** These stones represent approximately 1% of kidney stones. They form in people with a hereditary disorder that causes the kidneys to excrete excessive amounts of certain amino acids (cystinuria).

Over time these crystals may combine to form a small, hard mass. In some cases, this mass or stone breaks off and passes into the ureter, eventually traveling to the bladder for expulsion.

SIGNS AND SYMPTOMS. Individuals may be asymptomatic until the kidney stone is large enough (>7 mm) to cause a blockage or infection. Then, an intense, colicky pain begins suddenly and intensifies over 15 to 30 minutes. The pain usually starts in the back or flank, just below the edge of the ribs, and moves anteriorly toward the groin as the stone moves down the ureter toward the bladder. If the stone stops moving, the pain may stop. Other signs and symptoms may include bloody, cloudy, or foul-smelling urine; nausea; vomiting; persistent urge to urinate; and if an infection is present, fever and chills.

MANAGEMENT. Treatment varies depending on the type of stone and on the cause. Individuals may be able to move the stone through the urinary tract simply by drinking as much as 2 to 3 quarts of water per day and by staying physically active. If the stones are too large to pass on their own or cause bleeding, kidney damage, or an ongoing UTI, surgical intervention with extracorporeal shock wave lithotripsy may be necessary. Extracorporeal shock wave lithotripsy uses shock waves to break the stones into small crystals, which can then be passed in the urine. Following treatment, it may take several months for all the stone fragments to pass.

Urinary Tract Infections

A "urinary tract infection" describes any infection that begins in the urinary system. Although many cases are simply painful and annoying, the condition can become a serious health problem if the infection spreads to the kidneys. Although any structure in the genitourinary system can be infected, most infections occur in the lower tract.

Cystitis (inflammation of the bladder) and **urethritis** (inflammation of the urethra) are the most common UTIs. Most cases are caused by *Escherichia coli*, which ascends the urinary tract from the opening in the urethra. The bacteria also may be introduced during urinary tract catheterization. In addition, urethritis can be caused by sexually transmitted organisms, such as *Chlamydia trachomatis* and *Neisseria gonorrhoeae*, which are the agents of chlamydia and gonorrhea, respectively. Women are 10-fold more likely than men to have ascending UTIs, except when compared to men older than 50 years, largely because women have a shorter urethra. Sexually active women also are more susceptible to cystitis, because sexual intercourse enhances bacterial transfer from the urethra into the bladder.

SIGNS AND SYMPTOMS. Signs and symptoms may not be indicative regarding the severity of the condition. Some individuals may present with very few symptoms yet have significant **bacteriuria**. An individual with cystitis may complain of pain during urination (i.e., **dysuria**), urinary frequency and urgency, and pain superior to the pubic region. Cloudy, bloody, or foul-smelling urine also may be noted. An individual with urethritis may present similar symptoms, with the exception that the quality of the urine often is not affected. Other symptoms, such as high fever, shaking chills, nausea, vomiting, and low back pain, may indicate a simultaneous upper UTI of the kidney (i.e., **acute pyelonephritis**).

MANAGEMENT. Referral to a physician is necessary as a urine culture is required to identify the organism responsible for the infection. Subsequently, medication in the form of antibiotics and sulfa drugs is prescribed to treat the infection. Symptoms usually will clear within a few days of treatment, but it is critical to take the entire course of medication to ensure that the infection is completely eradicated. A longer course of antibiotic treatment may be recommended with recurrent UTIs. In addition, increased clear fluid intake may be recommended to promote urinary outflow. Analgesics, urinary antiseptics, and antispasmodics also may be prescribed for relief of pain and bladder spasms.

Hematuria

Blood in the urine (i.e., **hematuria**) can be macroscopic, gross, or microscopic. The condition may be caused by a direct kidney injury, bladder contusion, UTI, drug or medication use, "march" or foot-strike hemolysis, infection, sickle cell disease, rhabdomyolysis or preexisting pathology. Nontraumatic renal hematuria, referred to as athletic pseudonephritis, is characterized by decreased renal blood flow that leads to ischemia in the kidney and subsequent passage of red blood cells. Traumatic renal hematuria involves obvious direct contact or indirect trauma from repetitive jarring during running or jumping. Traumatic bladder hematuria is believed to result from repetitive contact of the posterior bladder wall against the base of the bladder. Most participants in sport and physical activity void before activity. Running with an empty bladder increases the risk of gross hematuria (i.e., visible blood in the urine), because no fluid cushion exists between the posterior wall and the base of the bladder. This condition commonly is seen in long-distance runners, hence the name "runner's bladder." Hematuria caused by running resolves within 24 to 48 hours of rest.

SIGNS AND SYMPTOMS. Massive external trauma associated with pelvic fractures can seriously damage the bladder, leading to lower abdominal pain and tenderness. Bruising in the lower abdominal region may be visible. Palpation may reveal abdominal tenderness, muscle guarding, or rigidity. An individual with a bladder contusion is able to void, and gross or microscopic hematuria is present. An individual with a bladder rupture usually is unable to void, and a specimen obtained by catheter reveals blood in the pelvic cavity.

MANAGEMENT. Physically active individuals with benign hematuria secondary to exercise may continue to be active but should be encouraged to drink quantities of clear fluids before, during, and after exercise to avoid dehydration. Small amounts of urine should be maintained in the bladder during exercise to cushion against repetitive trauma. If gross or microscopic hematuria persists, referral to a physician is necessary. Additional tests may be necessary to rule out serious underlying conditions, such as renal disease, sickle cell anemia, and urine cytology.

Proteinuria

In the kidney, blood filtration occurs primarily in the glomeruli, which are microscopic, raspberry-shaped tangles of blood vessels. The glomeruli permit small molecules, such as waste products, to escape from the bloodstream into the urine for removal from the body while keeping larger molecules, such as useful proteins, in circulation. Normal protein excretion is 30 to 45 mg/day. Elevated levels of protein, primarily albumin, are thought to occur in as many as 70% of competitive athletes after exertion (15). Other conditions that may lead to elevated protein levels include dehydration, heat-related illness, fever, emotional stress, inflammatory conditions, some acute illnesses (e.g., diabetes, hypertension, and some kidney diseases), orthostatic (postural) disorder, pregnancy, and regular high protein diets.

Excessive protein in the urine (≥150 mg/day) may indicate early signs of renal disease. In the United States, diabetes is the leading cause of end-stage renal disease. In both type 1 and type 2 diabetes, the first sign of deteriorating kidney function is minute amounts of albumin in the urine, a condition called **microalbuminuria**. As kidney function declines, levels of albumin in the urine increase, and microalbuminuria becomes full-fledged proteinuria.

Hypertension is the second leading cause of end-stage renal disease and, if not controlled, can progress to renal failure. African Americans in the age range of 20 to 49 years are 20-fold more likely than their white counterparts to develop hypertension-related kidney failure. Other groups at risk for proteinuria are American Indians, Hispanic Americans, Pacific Islander Americans, older people, and overweight people (16). People with a family history of kidney disease should have their urine tested regularly.

SIGNS AND SYMPTOMS. Albumin functions to retain fluid in the blood by acting like a sponge to soak up fluid from body tissues. Because the protein has been excreted, blood can no longer soak up enough fluid, leading to noticeable swelling in the hands, feet, abdomen, or face. Large amounts of protein in the urine may cause it to look foamy in the toilet. More commonly, however, no signs or symptoms are noticeable.

MANAGEMENT. Testing a urine sample with a chemically treated dipstick is the only way to determine the amount of protein in the urine. In the absence of protein, the dipstick panel is yellow; proteins in solution interfere with the dye-buffer combination, causing the panel to turn green. Exertional proteinuria usually reads 2+ to 3+ by dipstick measurement within 30 minutes of exercise but clears in 24 to 48 hours. Evidence suggests a direct relationship between the intensity of exercise and the amount of proteinuria (15). False-positive results can occur under the following conditions:

- Alkaline urine (pH >7.5)
- Dipstick immersed too long
- Highly concentrated urine
- Gross hematuria
- Presence of penicillin, sulfonamides, or tolbutamide
- Presence of pus, semen, or vaginal secretions

False-negative results can occur with dilute urine and when the urinary proteins are nonalbumin or of low molecular weight (16,17). Because results of urine dipstick analysis are a crude estimate for the urine protein concentration, individuals with positive findings should be referred to a physician for more complete evaluation. More sensitive tests for protein or albumin in the urine are recommended for individuals at risk of kidney disease, especially those with diabetes. If a laboratory test shows high levels of protein, the test should be repeated 1 to 2 weeks later. If the second test also shows high levels, additional tests should be conducted to evaluate kidney function.

A physician may prescribe an angiotensin-converting enzyme inhibitor or an angiotensin-receptor blocker for an individual with diabetes or hypertension. These drugs have been found to protect kidney function even more than other drugs that provide the same level of blood pressure control. Restriction of dietary salt and protein intake also may be recommended (16).

> **A** ▶ *The lacrosse player had a history of direct trauma to the upper right quadrant of the abdomen. In addition to pain at the site of the trauma, she reported pain to the inferior border of the right scapula. This history suggests a possible liver contusion or rupture. This condition warrants activation of the emergency medical plan, including summoning EMS.*

INJURIES AND CONDITIONS OF THE GENITALIA

> **Q** ▶ *While attempting to tag a sliding base runner, a baseball player was struck in the groin by an opponent's foot. He immediately fell to the ground and drew his knees to the chest while grasping the genital region. What possible conditions can occur as a result of direct trauma to the genitalia? What signs and symptoms indicate that immediate referral to a physician is warranted?*

The male genitalia are more susceptible to injury than female genitalia because several structures are external to the body and, as such, are exposed to direct trauma. Protective cups can protect the penis and scrotum from injury. Direct trauma can damage the penis, urethra, and scrotum, which holds the testes. In addition, congenital variations in testicular suspension make certain individuals susceptible to torsion of the testicle.

Male Genital Injuries

Direct trauma to the groin can cause severe pain and dysfunction to the testes and penis. Lacerations are rare, but swelling and hemorrhage inside the scrotal sac can occur. As part of the follow-up management of an injury to the male genital organs, the individual should be instructed to perform periodic self-assessment for pain and swelling and be provided with guidelines on seeking further medical care if necessary.

Penile Injuries

Superficial wounds to the penis may involve a contusion, abrasion, laceration, avulsion, or penetrating wound. In addition, the urethra can be damaged. Most injuries resolve without specific treatment. Superficial bleeding should be controlled by applying a cold compress. Referral to a physician is only necessary if hemorrhage persists or if swelling impairs the function of the urethra, leading to an inability to void.

Cyclists may develop transient paresthesia of the penis as a result of pressure on the pudendal nerve. Adjusting the saddle height, tilt, and number of cycling bouts usually resolves the condition. Rising up on the pedals also can relieve pressure temporarily.

■■■ ■ FIGURE 12.14 **Relieving testicular spasm.** The individual should lie on his back and flex the knees toward the chest until pain is relieved.

Scrotal Injuries

Blunt scrotal trauma can cause a contusion, hematoma, torsion, dislocation, or rupture of a testicle. If the tunica vaginalis ruptures, the vascular and tubercle components of the testes can be seriously damaged. Direct trauma to the groin can compress the testicles against the pelvis, leading to a nauseating, painful condition. Immediate internal hemorrhage, effusion, and muscle spasm occur. Testicular spasm can be relieved by placing the individual on his back and flexing his knees toward the chest (Fig. 12.14). Another method to reduce testicular spasm involves lifting the individual a few inches off the ground and then dropping him to the ground. As the pain subsides, a cold compress should be placed on the scrotum to reduce swelling and hemorrhage.

Occasionally, blunt trauma leads to swelling in the tunica vaginalis, which results in a traumatic **hydrocele** (Fig. 12.15A). In 9 to 19% of men, the plexus of veins on the posterior testicle can become engorged, constituting a **varicocele**. These lesions may be described as "a bag of worms" adjacent to the testicle and cord (Fig. 12.15B). If the plexus ruptures in response to blunt trauma, blood rapidly accumulates in the scrotum, leading to a **hematocele**. In nearly 50% of patients with traumatic hematocele, testicular rupture also is present.

Pain is not a good indicator of which structure is damaged. Swelling and hemorrhage inside the scrotal sac can enlarge the sac to the size of a tennis ball or grapefruit. Each condition can lead to irreparable testicular damage if evaluation and treatment by a physician is delayed. Treatment for swelling inside the scrotal sac involves aspiration of fluid and injection of a solution to toughen the involved tissues. Symptoms disappear in 85 to 90% of the cases with this treatment.

An individual with torsion of a testicle may or may not have a history of trauma. Congenital variations in the testicular suspension can cause rotational twisting of the vascular pedicle and spermatic cord, producing varying degrees of circulatory compromise (Fig. 12.15C). This condition typically is seen at or around puberty, manifesting itself after physical activity. Groin pain may develop gradually or rapidly, and it sometimes occurs with associated nausea and vomiting. Immediate referral to a physician is necessary if correction of the condition is to be successful. High-resolution ultrasound is used to determine if the blood supply is absent to the testicle as well as the extent and severity of injury. Recovery is nearly 100% if corrected within 6 to 8 hours.

A scrotal mass also can be indicative of testicular cancer, which is the most common malignancy in males from 16 to 35 years of age. Males who have an undescended or partially descended testicle are at higher risk than others for developing testicular cancer. The first sign of a mass is a slightly enlarged testicle that has a change in its consistency. The mass is separate from the cord and epididymis. In many cases, a dull ache or sensation of dragging and heaviness is present in the lower abdomen or groin. The diagnosis is established using ultrasound or transillumination with a bright light. Early detection and surgical treatment yields an excellent survival rate.

Female Genital Injuries

Injuries to the vulva usually are caused by trauma associated with a fall, straddling, or penetration resulting in forced perineal stretching because of sudden leg abduction. These injuries have occurred in a variety of activities, including gymnastics, water-skiing, snowmobiling, motorcycling, bicycling, sledding, cross-country skiing, and horseback riding. Nearly all injuries are easily treated by application of ice, mild compression, and bed rest. Occasionally, high-speed water-skiing injuries result in water being forced under high pressure into the vulva and vagina, leading to rupture of the vaginal walls. The water also can be forced through the uterus and fallopian tubes, leading to localized pelvic peritonitis. These injuries are easily preventable by wearing a neoprene wetsuit or nylon-reinforced suit.

 Direct trauma to the groin can lead to a laceration, scrotal contusion, hematoma, torsion, dislocation, or rupture of the testicles. If persistent pain or swelling of the testicles occurs, the individual should seek immediate medical attention.

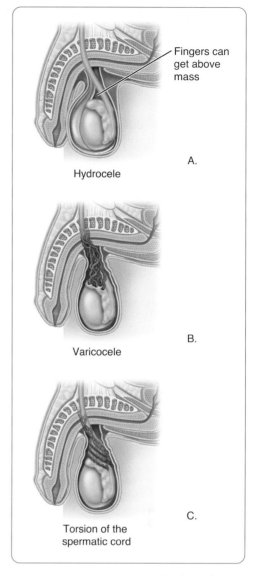

Fingers can get above mass

Hydrocele

A.

Varicocele

B.

Torsion of the spermatic cord

C.

▮▮▮ FIGURE 12.15 **Testicular injury. A,** Hydrocele. **B,** Varicocele. **C,** Spermatic cord torsion around the tunica vaginalis.

ASSESSMENT OF THROAT, THORAX, AND VISCERAL CONDITIONS

Q *During practice, a 20-year-old football player was struck in the abdomen with a helmet and experienced a sudden onset of abdominal pain in the upper left quadrant. How should the assessment of this injury progress to determine the extent and severity of injury?*

Injury assessment for thoracic and visceral injuries should focus on vital signs and the history of the injury. Chest or abdominal trauma, although initially appearing to be superficial and minor, can mask internal hemorrhage and swelling that can seriously compromise the function of vital organs. Such an individual's condition can slowly deteriorate and become a life-threatening condition. Although general observation and palpation can confirm the possibility of a serious underlying condition, an understanding of the history of the injury and constant monitoring of vital signs strengthen the assessment.

The examiner should assess consciousness, respiration, and circulation. If the individual is having difficulty breathing, anxiety and panic may make the task more difficult. If a spinal injury has been ruled out, the individual should be placed in a supine position, with the knees flexed, to facilitate breathing. The airway should be open and clear of any blood or vomitus. The trachea should be in the middle of the throat and should not move during respirations. If breathing does not return to normal within a minute or two, the emergency medical plan, including summoning EMS, should be activated. It is always better to have EMS en route during the assessment than to wait and see if the condition gets better. Several conditions can intensify in severity with time, thereby seriously compromising the health of the injured party. The examiner should record vital signs so that a baseline of information is established. As is the case with an acute abdominal injury, water and food should not be given to the individual. Not only can the condition be aggravated, any food or fluid in the gastrointestinal tract will make the surgery, if necessary, more dangerous. While waiting for EMS to arrive, the vital signs should be monitored frequently and the individual treated for shock.

See *Field Strategy: Thorax and Visceral Region Evaluation*, available on the companion website at thePoint, for a summary of the assessment of the thorax and visceral regions.

HISTORY

Q *The assessment of the football player's injury should begin with a history. The mechanism of injury and the site of the trauma have already been identified. What additional questions need to be asked as part of the on-field assessment of this injury?*

Because few special tests are available for the region, the examiner must rely heavily on information provided in the history. Injuries to the ribs, costal cartilage, or abdominal muscles usually produce tenderness at the site of injury. Abdominal pain may indicate a serious abdominal injury, but it also can be a symptom in conditions as minor as precompetition anxiety. The issue is not to draw a distinction between acute and nonacute pain but, rather, between possible surgical and nonsurgical conditions. Because pain tolerance can vary, every complaint of thoracic or abdominal pain must be assessed.

The examiner should gather information regarding the primary complaint, mechanism of injury, and characteristics of the symptoms (18). Pain that is sudden in onset, severe or explosive, progressive, continuous, and lasts more than 6 hours generally indicates a serious internal problem that necessitates surgical intervention. Persistent pain that awakens the person or that occurs during relative inactivity also is a red flag. Pain that is gradual, mild to moderate, intermittent, recurrent, occurs after exercise or eating, or resolves partially or completely in less than 6 hours indicates a less serious condition that favors a nonsurgical diagnosis (19). Table 12.1 identifies some common nonmusculoskeletal sources of abdominal pain and the typical signs and symptoms that are associated with each condition.

The examiner should ask questions about previous injuries to the area that may have some bearing on this specific condition. It is important to remember that some conditions, such as a ruptured spleen, can delay hemorrhage for hours, days, or even weeks after the initial trauma. Other injuries with an acute onset may have signs and symptoms that subside only to recur later. Questions should be asked about activities that aggravate the pain. Coughing, sneezing, rapid movements, and walking, especially down stairs, can cause peritoneal irritation. Musculoskeletal pain often is relieved by changing position.

TABLE 12.1 Common Nonmusculoskeletal Sources of Abdominal Pain	
CONDITION	**SIGNS AND SYMPTOMS**
Appendicitis (acute)	Inflammation of the appendix resulting in constant pain; progresses in severity; begins in the outer umbilical region; moves to the right lower quadrant; nausea, vomiting, and loss of appetite; low-grade fever.
Cholecystitis (acute)	Inflammation of the gallbladder, resulting in constant pain in the right upper quadrant; onset often follows a meal; nausea and vomiting; tenderness in the right upper quadrant and right shoulder; splinting on the right side.
Perforated peptic ulcer	Perforated stomach ulcer resulting in a sudden onset of pain in the midepigastric region that spreads and is aggravated by movement; individual is reluctant to move and appears acutely ill; rigid abdomen; grunting respiration; absent bowel sounds.
Ectopic pregnancy	Pregnancy in the fallopian tube, which results in a tubal rupture causing a sudden, severe, and persistent pain, generally following a missed or abnormal period; typically epigastric; often associated with hypotension and tachycardia.
Ovarian cyst	An abnormal cystic tumor of the ovary that usually is benign; constant pain with a sharp, sudden onset; usually in the ipsilateral lower area of the abdomen below the umbilicus; may have nausea and vomiting following the pain.
Pelvic inflammatory disease	Chronic inflammation of the pelvis caused by multiple infections, including chlamydia and gonorrhea, resulting in pain at the end of or shortly after a normal menstrual period; bilateral lower quadrant pain aggravated by manipulation of the cervix; rarely, nausea and vomiting; possible cervical discharge; fever.
Urinary calculus	Pain location changes with the movement of the urinary stone and may radiate to the testicle or groin of the involved side; pain is very severe; individual cannot get comfortable.

In younger athletes who are sexually active, females experience abdominal pain twice as often as males of the same age. Males, however, tend to have a higher incidence of conditions necessitating surgical intervention. Pain that is sudden in onset and follows an abnormal menstrual period might stem from an ectopic pregnancy, which would constitute a medical emergency. Pain that occurs shortly after a normal menstrual period, is bilateral, and is accompanied by fever and abdominal pain but not nausea and vomiting suggests pelvic inflammatory disease.

See *Field Strategy: Developing a History for a Thoracic or Abdominal Injury*, found on the companion website at thePoint, for specific questions that can be asked for chest and abdominal injuries.

A ▶ *During the on-field assessment of the football player, the mechanism of injury and the location of trauma have been identified. The examiner should ask questions related to the location and type of pain (including pain in areas other than the injured site) and the presence of any dizziness, nausea, weakness, numbness, or other unusual feelings.*

OBSERVATION AND INSPECTION

Q ▶ *During the history, the individual reports pain in his upper chest and left shoulder. He also complains of feeling weak and light-headed. What factors should be observed and inspected as part of the ongoing on-field assessment of this injury?*

Observation of body position can give an indication regarding the site, nature, and severity of injury. For example, in an acute thoracic injury, the individual may lean toward the injured side, using an arm or a hand to stabilize the region. In an acute abdominal injury, the individual typically lies on the injured side and brings the knees toward the chest to relax the abdominal muscles. Facial expressions can confirm the individual's hesitation to perform any movement because of severe pain. Chest expansion can reveal the rate and depth of respirations.

Inspection

The individual should be sufficiently undressed so that the site of injury can be observed. Inspection should include the neck, back, chest, abdomen, and groin, with any deformity, edema, bruising, ecchymosis, and skin color being noted. Deformity may indicate a sternal or rib fracture, costochondral separation, or muscle rupture. An abrasion or localized bruising on the chest wall could suggest a possible rib fracture or internal complication. Diffuse bruising in the axilla and chest wall may indicate a ruptured pectoralis major. A bruise or ecchymosis in the umbilical area (i.e., Cullen's sign) indicates intraperitoneal bleeding. Distention in the abdomen may indicate internal hemorrhage. Pale, cold, and clammy skin is associated with shock. Cyanosis, or a bluish tinge to the skin, indicates a lack of oxygen resulting from internal pulmonary or cardiac problems. Coughing up bright red or frothy blood indicates a severe lung injury. Vomitus containing blood that looks like used coffee grounds indicates that blood has been swallowed and partially digested.

See *Field Strategy: Observation and Inspection of the Thorax and Viscera,* found on the companion website at thePoint, for specific observations that can help to determine the extent and severity of thoracic or abdominal injuries.

The rate and depth of respirations should be noted, particularly if the individual has any difficulty catching his or her breath. If the condition is only transitory (e.g., the "wind has been knocked out"), breathing and color should quickly return to normal. An individual with an internal injury tends to use rapid and shallow breaths, because deep breathing increases pain. The examiner should observe the symmetric rise and fall of the chest; any abnormal motion may indicate a fractured rib or pneumothorax. If breathing does not quickly return to normal or the individual's condition rapidly deteriorates, the injury should be considered significant, and the emergency medical plan, including summoning EMS, should be activated.

Auscultation and Percussion

If auscultation or percussion is used in the assessment, both should be completed before palpation. Because the visceral organs are interconnected by connective tissue, any palpation in the abdomen moves the internal organs and, as such, can produce inaccurate or false sounds.

Auscultation is used to listen for the presence or absence of sounds in the body and should precede any physical contact with the individual to prevent alteration of peristalsis by physical stimulation. A stethoscope usually has two heads: the bell, and the diaphragm. The bell is used to detect low-pitched sounds, whereas the diaphragm is better at detecting higher-pitched sounds. When using the bell of the stethoscope, light pressure should be applied to maintain contact with the skin surface. Firm pressure is applied when using the diaphragm to keep it pressed tightly to the skin. Because the bell or diaphragm must always be in contact with the skin, listening through clothing is never acceptable. It may take 2 to 3 minutes in each area to adequately evaluate the nature and character of the underlying conditions, particularly with bowel sounds.

Auscultation of the Lungs

In the thorax, the flow of air should be heard throughout the various regions of each lung (Fig. 12.16). Because most breath sounds are high pitched, the diaphragm is used to evaluate lung sounds. Individuals who should be evaluated include those with the following signs and symptoms (see Box 12.5) (20):

- Shortness of breath or dyspnea

- Cough with or without a bloody sputum

- Pleuritic pain

- A resting respiratory rate greater than 22 breaths per minute

- Cyanosis or finger clubbing

The patient should be instructed to breathe deeply through an open mouth. The examiner should listen for at least one full breath at each site, moving from one side to the other and comparing symmetric areas of the lungs. The intensity of breath sounds should be noted. Breath sounds usually are louder in the lower posterior lung fields and may vary from area to area. Characteristics of

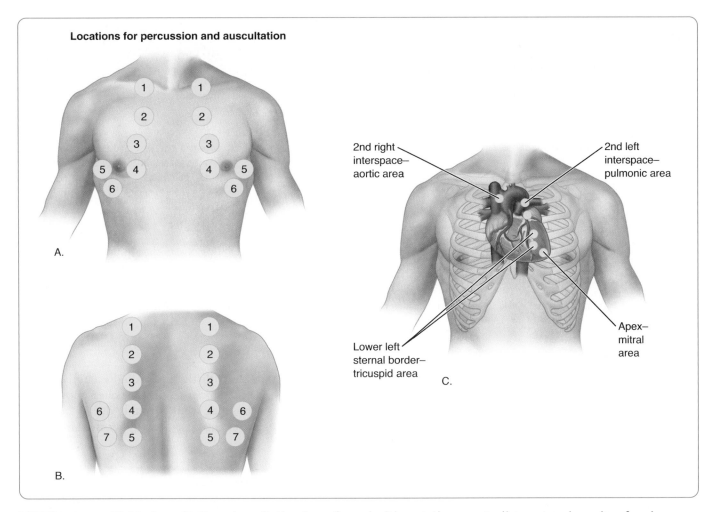

Locations for percussion and auscultation

A.

B.

2nd right interspace—aortic area

2nd left interspace—pulmonic area

Lower left sternal border—tricuspid area

Apex—mitral area

C.

▮▮▮▮ **FIGURE 12.16 Auscultation.** Auscultation is performed with a stethoscope to listen at various sites for air exchange in the lobes of the lungs. **A,** Anterior view. **B,** Posterior view. **C,** Cardiac sounds also can be auscultated over four specific sites.

normal breath sounds in the lungs are summarized in Table 12.2 (21). Abnormal sounds are summarized in Table 12.3 (21).

Auscultation of the Heart

A normal cardiac cycle consists of two sounds, often called "lubb-dubb," which is caused by the blood flowing against the valves as they close. Individuals who should have the heart evaluated include those listed in Box 12.6 (18).

An abnormal sound is called a murmur and is produced by turbulent energy in the walls of the heart and blood vessels. Obstruction to flow, or flow from a narrow to a larger-diameter vessel, produces the turbulence, which sets up motion currents that strike the walls and produce vibrations that can be heard with a stethoscope. Murmurs also can be produced when a large volume of blood is flowing through a normal opening. Murmurs may be described as "blowing," "rumbling," or "harsh." If abnormal sounds, such as a click, snap, or a murmur, are present, the individual should be referred to a physician.

The diaphragm of the stethoscope is more effective in detecting the relatively high-pitched sounds of S_1 (i.e., first sound) and S_2 (i.e., second sound), the murmurs of aortic and mitral regurgitation, and pericardial friction rubs. The bell of the stethoscope is more sensitive to the low-pitched sounds of S_3 and S_4 and the murmur of mitral stenosis.

TABLE 12.2 Characteristics of Normal Breath Sounds

	DURATION OF SOUNDS	INTENSITY OF EXPIRATORY SOUND	PITCH OF EXPIRATORY SOUND	LOCATIONS WHERE NORMALLY HEARD
Vesicular	Inspiratory sounds last longer than expiratory ones	Soft	Relatively low-pitched	Over most of both lungs
Bronchovesicular	Inspiratory and expiratory sounds are about equal	Intermediate	Intermediate-pitched	Often in the first and second interspaces anteriorly and between the scapulae
Bronchial	Expiratory sounds last longer than inspiratory ones	Loud	Relatively high-pitched	Over the manubrium, if heard at all
Tracheal	Inspiratory and expiratory sounds are about equal	Very loud	Relatively high-pitched	Over the trachea in the neck

From Bickley LS, Szilagyi PG. Bates' Guide to Physical Examination and History Taking. Philadelphia: Lippincott Williams & Wilkins, 2003:227; with permission.

The examiner should be on the right side of the patient with the individual recumbent and the head and chest elevated to 45°. This position allows the examiner to observe chest movements associated with cardiac function as well as to place the stethoscope head correctly during auscultation. Some clinicians begin at the apex; others prefer to start at the base (i.e., upper margins of the heart). Either pattern is satisfactory.

TABLE 12.3 Abnormal Breath Sounds

SOUND	CHARACTERISTICS
Crackles	May result from abnormalities of the lungs (e.g., pneumonia, fibrosis, or early congestive heart failure) or the airways (e.g., bronchitis or bronchiectasis).
Fine crackles	Soft, high-pitched, and very brief (5–10 msec). They sometimes are compared to rubbing dry strands of hair together between the thumb and finger close to the ear.
Coarse crackles	Somewhat louder than fine crackles, lower in pitch, and not quite so brief (20–30 msec).
Wheezes	Relatively high-pitched (~400 Hz or higher) and has a hissing or shrill quality. Wheezing suggests narrowed airways, as in asthma, bronchitis, chronic obstructive pulmonary disease, and congestive heart failure.
Rhonchi	Relatively low-pitched (~200 Hz or lower) and have a rumbling or snoring quality. They usually are caused by the passage of air through bronchi obstructed by thick mucus.
Stridor	A wheeze that is entirely or predominantly inspiratory. It often is louder in the neck than over the chest wall, and it indicates partial obstruction of the larynx or trachea.
Pleural rub	Inflamed or roughened pleural surfaces momentarily grate against each other and are delayed by friction, producing creaking sounds known as a pleural rub or pleural friction rub. Pleural rubs resemble crackles acoustically but usually are confined to a relatively small area of the chest wall and typically are heard in both phases of respiration.
Mediastinal crunch (Hamman's sign)	A series of precordial crackles synchronous with heart beat, not with respiration. They are best heard in the left lateral position and are caused by mediastinal emphysema.
Absence of sounds	May be caused by pleural effusion, pneumothorax, tension pneumothorax, hemothorax, or traumatic asphyxia.

Box 12.6   Signs and Symptoms Indicating the Need for Heart Auscultation

- Cyanosis of the skin and mucous membranes accompanied by clubbing of the nails (indicates congenital heart disease)
- Any signs of Marfan's syndrome
- Palpitations or a history of syncope, angina, and fatigue
- Rapid pulse (tachycardia) of more than 100 beats per minute at rest
- Slow pulse (bradycardia) of less than 40 beats per minute at rest
- Unusual and severe dyspnea after routine exercise
- Sustained arterial hypertension
- Retrosternal pain brought on by exertion but relieved with rest
- Traumatic chest injuries that could cause cardiac injury

Four classic sites are used to determine cardiac sounds (see Fig. 12.16):

1. Aortic (second intercostal space, right sternal border)

2. Pulmonic (second intercostal space, left sternal border)

3. Tricuspid (left lower sternal border)

4. Mitral (cardiac apex)

After listening to each site, the examiner should instruct the patient to roll partly onto the left side, which positions the left ventricle closer to the chest wall. In this position, the examiner should place the bell lightly on the apical impulse. Finally, the patient should be instructed to sit up, lean forward, exhale completely, and stop breathing in expiration; this position accentuates aortic murmurs that otherwise might go undetected.

Auscultation of the Abdomen

In the abdomen, auscultation can determine bowel motility. It is important to listen to the abdomen before performing percussion or palpation, because these maneuvers may alter the frequency of bowel sounds.

The diaphragm of the stethoscope should be placed gently on the abdomen. Bowel sounds should be noted relative to their frequency and character. Normal bowel sounds consist of clicks and gurgles, occurring at an estimated frequency of 5 to 34 per minute (20). Because bowel sounds are widely transmitted throughout the abdomen, listening to one area, such as the right lower quadrant, usually is sufficient. Hyperperistalsis with rushes, cramps, and diarrhea suggests gastroenteritis.

Hypoperistalsis, or a silent abdomen, could indicate a serious underlying problem, such as an obstruction or internal hemorrhage. Immediate referral to the nearest medical facility is warranted. Activation of the emergency plan, including summoning EMS, is warranted. While waiting for EMS to arrive, the examiner should maintain the airway, assess vital signs, and treat for shock as necessary.

Percussion

Percussion typically is used over a bony structure to determine a possible fracture, but it also can be used in the chest and abdominal region to indicate internal complications. The examiner should place their nondominant hand on the individual's abdomen over the various internal organs. This is followed by the examiner using the second and third finger of the dominant hand to tap on the distal interphalangeal joint of the middle finger of the nondominant hand. The tapping should be performed as a quick rapid motion (Fig. 12.17). The tone indicates if the organ is hollow (tympanic) or solid (full).

FIGURE 12.17 Percussion. Percussion is used in the abdominal region to indicate internal complications and should be performed before palpation.

In the chest, the same sites used during auscultation are percussed and bilaterally compared. Dullness replaces resonance when fluid or solid tissue replaces air-containing lung tissue. Because pleural fluid usually sinks to the inferior pleural space (i.e., posteriorly in a supine patient), only a very large effusion can be detected anteriorly. The heart normally produces an area of dullness to the left of the sternum from the third to fifth interspace.

In the abdomen, the four quadrants are tested to assess the distribution of tympany and dullness. Tympany usually predominates because of gas in the gastrointestinal tract, but fluid and feces may produce normal, scattered areas of dullness. It is important to note any large, dull areas that may indicate an enlarged organ and any facial expressions to indicate any discomfort.

> **A** *Note the football player's willingness or ability to move, ease in motion, and general attitude. Inspection should include viewing the chest and abdomen, with any deformity, edema, bruising, ecchymosis, and skin color being noted.*

PALPATION

> **Q** *The general attitude of the football player indicates that he is uncomfortable and in pain. No abnormal findings are apparent by inspection. As part of the ongoing on-field assessment of this injury, what areas should be palpated?*

It is important to begin palpation away from the painful area so that pain will not be carried over into other areas. Palpation begins with gentle circular motions, feeling for deformity, crepitus, swelling, rigidity, muscle guarding, or tenderness. The patient should be in a supine position with the knees flexed for more comfort.

The trachea should be palpated during breathing to ensure that it does not move, because movement may indicate tension pneumothorax. The examiner should palpate the clavicle, sternum, costochondral cartilage, and ribs, moving in an anterior-to-posterior direction and noting any pain, deformity, or crepitus. The left anterior rib cage should be palpated for an enlarged spleen. The spleen may be more prominent if the patient raises his or her arms above the head. While palpating the posterior rib cage, the examiner should locate the approximate position of the kidneys. The left kidney is well protected by the posterolateral rib cage; the right kidney rests more inferior.

Possible rib fractures and costochondral separations are assessed with gentle pressure applied to the sternum and vertebrae in an anteroposterior direction (Fig. 12.18A). This action causes the rib cage to bow out laterally. Lateral compression on the sides of the rib cage causes strain on the costochondral junctions (Fig. 12.18B). Compression should begin superiorly and move down, in an inferior direction, until the entire area is covered. Pain at a specific site indicates a positive sign.

The fingernails can be blanched to determine normal capillary refill. Certain cardiac or pulmonary conditions may result in cyanosis of the nail beds, fingers, and toes.

Examination of the abdomen begins by gently stroking the area. Underlying peritoneal irritation causes a light touch to be perceived as a disagreeable sensation, referred to as **dysesthesia**, and

■■■ FIGURE 12.18 **Compression of the rib cage in a supine position. A,** Anteroposterior compression for rib fracture. **B,** Lateral compression for costochondral separation.

suggests a serious underlying condition. Palpation should be performed using the flat part of several fingers, with both hands moving in small, circular motions (Fig. 12.19). It is important to avoid poking or making sudden moves, because this may cause the individual to jerk and tighten the muscles. Palpation should begin away from the injured site and move across the abdomen in a straight line. Any muscle guarding or rigidity should be noted. Muscle guarding that cannot be voluntarily relaxed may indicate internal peritoneal hemorrhage. It is important to palpate for tenderness, muscle resistance, and superficial masses or deficits in the continuity of the abdominal wall. Deeper palpation can detect rigidity, swelling, or masses. Rebound tenderness at McBurney's point is indicative of appendicitis. The rebounding pain is caused when the inflamed appendix is impacted by the viscera returning to the normal position. This phenomenon, however, also can occur with peritonitis.

■■■■■ FIGURE 12.19 **Palpation of the abdomen.** The examiner should use the flat part of several fingers and move both hands in small, circular motions.

> **A** ▶ *The focus of the palpation of the injury to the football player should be the upper left quadrant, but it is important to palpate the entire abdomen. The palpation should assess point tenderness, swelling, deformity, rebound pain, spasms, and rigidity.*

PHYSICAL EXAMINATION TESTS

> **Q** ▶ *Palpation reveals rigidity over the upper left quadrant. Assessment of vital signs indicates the following: Blood pressure is 96/70 mm Hg; pulse is weak at 96 beats per minute; and the skin is cool and clammy. What injury should be suspected, and how should this condition be managed?*

Very few special tests are available for the thorax and visceral area. Most of the information must be gathered during the history, observation, and palpation phase of the assessment. If the condition is not serious and a muscular strain is suspected, active, passive, and resisted muscle testing can be performed. Neck and trunk motion include flexion, extension, lateral flexion, and rotation. The examiner should note the individual's willingness to perform the motion, ease of motion, and bilateral comparison of motions when applicable.

Vital Signs

It is important to note pulse rate and rhythm, blood pressure, temperature, and respiratory rate and characteristics. The pulse usually is taken at the carotid artery; however, a pulse also can be taken at the radial, femoral, or brachial arteries. A normal pulse rate for a physically active individual ranges between 60 and 100 beats per minute, depending on when the pulse is taken. The pulse rate is higher, for example, if taken immediately after exercise. Highly conditioned individuals tend to have lower pulse rates.

Respirations should range between 12 and 20 breaths per minute, with highly conditioned individuals falling into the lower range. Rapid, shallow breaths may indicate internal injury or shock. Deep, quick breaths may indicate asthma or pulmonary obstruction. Noisy, raspy breaths may indicate a partial airway obstruction.

Any sputum should be checked for the presence of blood. Pink or bloody sputum indicates internal bleeding and should be treated as a serious condition.

Painful abdominal conditions frequently are reflected in the vital signs as tachycardia, tachypnea, and elevated temperature. With conditions that involve the upper abdomen or lower lobes of the lung, respiration may be rapid, shallow, painful (grunting), or splinted. Hypotension may result from gastrointestinal bleeding, dehydration, or vagal stimulation.

Urinalysis

Urinalysis is a common test that uses chemically treated dipsticks to provide fast, general results for such information as specific gravity, pH, and levels of leukocytes, nitrate, protein, glucose, ketones, urobilinogen, bilirubin, and blood in the urine. In conducting a urinalysis, the patient should be instructed to clean and rinse the external urethra. In collecting the specimen, the patient should be told to direct the initial flow of urine into the toilet bowl before directing it into a clean specimen cup. One to two ounces of urine should be collected. The examiner should insert the dipstick into the fluid following the manufacturer's recommended immersion times, and the color produced on the dipstick is then matched to the values provided by the manufacturer.

Neurologic Test

Neurologic tests in the thorax and abdomen are somewhat limited. Dermatomes vary and often overlap. Although the dermatomes tend to follow the ribs, the absence of only one dermatome may not lead to a loss in sensation. Sites for referred pain can indicate the origin of injury and are illustrated in Figure 5.1. Myotome testing includes finger abduction and adduction (T1) and hip flexion (L1–L2). No other myotome testing exists for the axial region. In addition, no deep tendon reflexes exist for the region, although it always is appropriate to test the deep tendon lumbar and sacral reflexes (i.e., patellar reflex and Achilles reflex).

Based on the on-field assessment of the football player, a splenic injury should be suspected. As such, activation of the emergency plan, including summoning EMS, is warranted. While waiting for EMS to arrive, the examiner should maintain the airway, assess vital signs, and treat for shock as necessary.

SUMMARY

1. Severe blunt trauma to the anterior neck region, thorax, and viscera can have devastating effects that lead to serious ventilatory and circulatory compromise.

2. Blows to the throat may result in severe pain, laryngospasm, and acute respiratory distress.

3. A "stitch in the side" is a sharp pain or spasm in the chest wall, usually on the lower right side. Several strategies can be used to enable the affected individual to run through the pain.

4. Severe blunt trauma to the breast should be documented on a woman's permanent medical record to avoid misreading a mammogram.

5. A strain of the pectoralis major muscle involves an actively contracting muscle that is overburdened by a load or extrinsic force that exceeds tissue tolerance. If muscle fibers have been ruptured, resisted horizontal adduction and internal rotation of the shoulder are weak and accentuate the deformity.

6. Signs and symptoms indicating a possible internal thoracic condition include:

    ▪ Shortness of breath or difficulty breathing

    ▪ Severe chest pain aggravated by deep inspiration

    ▪ Abnormal chest movement

    ▪ Abnormal or absent breath sounds

7. A hernia is a protrusion of abdominal viscera through a weakened portion of the abdominal wall and can be either congenital or acquired. An indirect inguinal hernia is the most common hernia in young athletes.

8. Signs and symptoms indicating a possible intra-abdominal condition include:

    ▪ Severe abdominal pain

    ▪ Nausea or vomiting

- Distended abdomen
- Tenderness, rigidity, or muscle spasm
- Rebound pain
- Absence of bowel sounds
- Blood in the urine or stool

9. Certain injuries may not develop until hours, days, or even weeks later. As such, the presumption of possible intrathoracic or intra-abdominal injuries with any blunt trauma necessitates a complete assessment.

10. Assessment of injury to the thorax and visceral region should focus on the vital signs and history of the injury.

11. Observation, palpation, and sites of referred pain can confirm suspicions of an existing internal injury.

12. If at any time signs and symptoms indicate an intrathoracic or intra-abdominal injury, the emergency medical plan, including summoning EMS, should be activated. The vital signs should be monitored every 5 to 7 minutes to determine if the individual's condition is improving or deteriorating.

13. If on-site recovery occurs, the individual should still be provided with information identifying the signs and symptoms that could develop later and indicate that the condition is getting worse. The individual also should be provided with instructions for seeking medical assistance.

REFERENCES

1. Finch CF. The risk of abdominal injury to women during sport. J Sci Med Sport 2002;5(1):46–54.
2. Beloosesky Y, Grinblat J, Hendell D, Sommer R. Pectoralis major rupture in a 97-year-old woman. J Am Geriatr Soc 2002;50(8):1465–1468.
3. Dodds SD, Wolfe SW. Injuries to the pectoralis major. Sports Med 2002;32(14):945–952.
4. Chang CJ, Graves DW. Athletic injuries of the thorax and abdomen. In: Mellion MB, Walsh WM, Madden C, Putukian M, Shelton GL, eds. The Team Physician's Handbook. Philadelphia: Hanley & Belfus, 2002.
5. Rumball JS, Lebrun CM, DiCiacca SR, Orland K. Rowing injuries. Sports Med 2005;35(6):537–555.
6. Golden PA. Thoracic trauma. Ortho Nurs 2000;19(5):37–46.
7. Baumann MH, Noppen M. Pneumothorax. Respirology 2004;9(1):157–164.
8. Roman M, Weinstein A, Macaluso S. Primary spontaneous pneumothorax. Medsurg Nurs 2003;12(3):161–169.
9. Yamamoto L, Schroeder C, Beliveau K. Thoracic trauma: the deadly dozen. Crit Care Nurs 2005;28(1):22–40.
10. Moeller JL. Contraindications to athletic participation: cardiac, respiratory, and central nervous system conditions. Phys Sportsmed 1996;24(8):47–58.
11. Van Camp SP, Bloor CM, Mueller FO, et al. Nontraumatic sports death in high school and college athletes. Med Sci Sports Exerc 1995;27(5):641–647.
12. Moeller JL. Contraindications to athletic participation. Spinal, systemic, dermatologic, paired-organ, and other issues. Phys Sportsmed 1996;24(9):57–70.
13. Eckert KL. Penetrating and blunt abdominal trauma. Crit Care Nurs Q 2005;28(1):41–59.
14. Ray T, Lemire JE. Liver laceration in an intercollegiate football player. J Ath Train 1995;30(4):324–326.
15. Burroughs KE, Hilts MJ. Renal and genitourinary problems. In: Mellion MB, Walsh WM, Madden C, Putukian M, Shelton GL, eds. The Team Physician's Handbook. Philadelphia: Hanley & Belfus, 2002.
16. Carroll MF, Temte JL. Proteinuria in adults: a diagnostic approach. Am Fam Physician 2000;62(6):1333–1340.
17. Wilson LA. Urinalysis. Nurs Standard 2005;19(35):51–54.
18. Leung AKC, Sigalet DL. Acute abdominal pain in children. Am Fam Physician 2003;67(11):2321–2326.
19. Bergman RT. Assessing acute abdominal pain: a team physician's challenge. Phys Sportsmed 1996;24(4):72–82.
20. McChesney JA, McChesney JW. Auscultation of the chest and abdomen by athletic trainers. J Ath Train 2002;36(2):190–196.
21. Bickley LS, Szilagyi PG. Bates' Guide to Physical Examination and History Taking. Philadelphia: Lippincott Williams & Wilkins, 2003.

PART

Upper Extremity

4

STUDENT OUTCOMES

1. Identify the major bony and soft-tissue structures of the shoulder.

2. List the major motions at the shoulder and the muscles that produce them.

3. Describe the phases of the throwing motion, and list the common injuries sustained during each phase.

4. Explain the general principles used to prevent injuries to the shoulder.

5. List the common mechanisms of injury that can lead to instability in the sternoclavicular, acromioclavicular, and glenohumeral joints.

6. Describe the common acute injuries and conditions sustained in the shoulder region by physically active individuals.

7. Describe the soft-tissue pathology in the shoulder region that results from overuse.

8. Explain the management strategies for common injuries and conditions of the shoulder.

9. Describe a thorough assessment of the shoulder region.

10. Explain general principles and techniques used in developing a rehabilitation exercise program for the shoulder complex.

ROLE DELINEATION COMPETENCIES

The following Performance Domains and Tasks defined in the National Athletic Trainers' Association Board of Certification *Role Delineation Study*, 5th Edition are addressed in this chapter:

BOC COMPETENCIES

I. Prevention

G. Monitor participants and environmental conditions by following accepted guidelines to promote safe participation.

II. Clinical Evaluation and Diagnosis

A. Obtain a history through observation, interview, and/or review of relevant records to assess current or potential injury, illness, or condition.

B. Inspect the involved area(s) visually to assess the injury, illness, or health-related condition.

C. Palpate the involved area(s) using standard techniques to assess the injury, illness, or health-related condition.

D. Perform specific tests in accordance with accepted procedures to assess the injury, illness, or health-related condition.

E. Formulate a clinical impression by interpreting the signs, symptoms, and predisposing factors of the injury, illness, or condition to determine the appropriate course of action.

III. Immediate Care

A. Employ life-saving techniques through the use of standard emergency procedures in order to reduce morbidity and the incidence of mortality.

B. Prevent exacerbation of non–life threatening condition(s) through the use of standard procedures in order to reduce morbidity.

C. Facilitate the timely transfer of care for conditions beyond the scope of practice of the athletic trainer by implementing appropriate referral strategies to stabilize and/or prevent exacerbation of the condition(s).

V. Treatment, Rehabilitation, and Reconditioning

E. Reassess the status of injuries, illnesses, and/or conditions using standard techniques and documentation strategies in order to determine appropriate treatment, rehabilitation, and/or reconditioning and to evaluate readiness to return to a desired level of activity.

F. Educate the appropriate individual(s) in the treatment, rehabilitation, and reconditioning of injuries, illnesses, and/or conditions using applicable methods and materials to facilitate recovery, function, and/or performance.

The loose structure of the shoulder complex enables extreme mobility but provides little stability. As a result, the shoulder is much more prone to injury compared to the hip. Common shoulder injuries include dislocations, clavicular fractures, muscle and tendon strains, rotator cuff tears, acromioclavicular (AC) sprains, bursitis, bicipital tendonitis, and impingement syndrome (1,2). Shoulder injuries commonly occur during activities involving an overhead motion, such as baseball, swimming, tennis, volleyball, and weight lifting. In fact, shoulder pain is the most common musculoskeletal complaint among competitive swimmers, with 40 to 70% reporting a history of shoulder pain (3). Dislocations of the shoulder articulations are not uncommon in contact sports, such as wrestling and football (4).

This chapter begins with a review of the anatomy of the shoulder region, followed by a synopsis of the kinematics and kinetics of the shoulder joints. A discussion regarding prevention of injuries is followed by an overview of common injuries to the shoulder complex. Management of specific injuries, the assessment process, and examples of rehabilitation exercises then conclude the chapter.

ANATOMY OF THE SHOULDER

The arm articulates with the trunk at the shoulder, or pectoral girdle, which comprises the scapula and clavicle (Figs. 13.1 and 13.2). The shoulder region has five separate articulations:

1. The sternoclavicular (SC) joint

2. The AC joint

3. The coracoclavicular joint

4. The glenohumeral (GH) joint

5. The scapulothoracic joint

The articulation referred to specifically as the shoulder joint is the GH joint; the remaining articulations are collectively referred to as the shoulder girdle. The SC and AC joints enhance motion of the clavicle and scapula, enabling the GH joint to provide a greater range of motion (ROM).

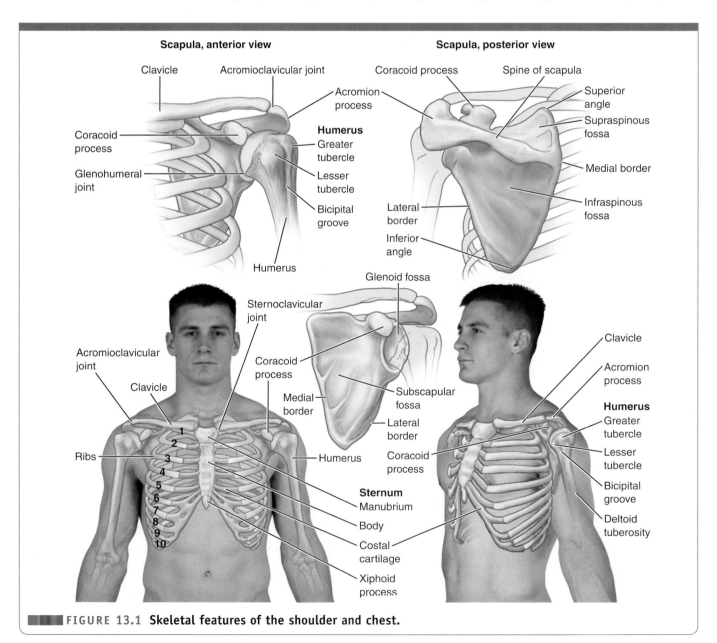

FIGURE 13.1 Skeletal features of the shoulder and chest.

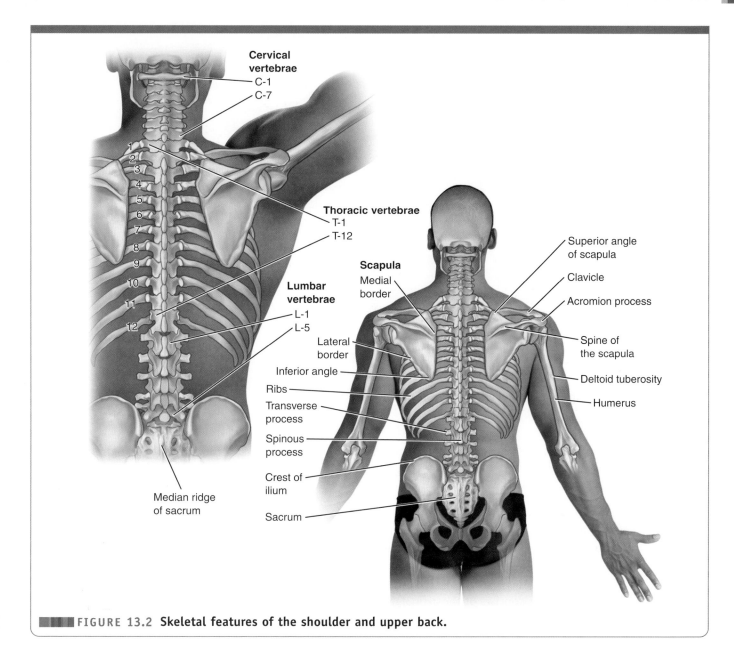

FIGURE 13.2 Skeletal features of the shoulder and upper back.

Sternoclavicular Joint

As the name suggests, the SC joint consists of the articulation of the superior sternum, or manubrium, with the proximal clavicle. The SC joint is surrounded by a joint capsule that is thickened anteriorly and posteriorly by four ligaments, including the interclavicular, costoclavicular, and anterior and posterior SC ligaments (Fig. 13.3). The anterior SC ligament is a broad band supporting the anterior capsule, whereas the posterior SC ligament is smaller and weaker, providing support to the posterior capsule. The costoclavicular ligament runs from the clavicle to the first rib and its adjacent cartilage. The interclavicular ligament provides minimal support to the joint, runs between the two SC joints, and attaches to the manubrium. A substantial fibrocartilaginous disk is found between the manubrium and clavicle, which divides the joint almost completely in half. Because of its attachments, the disk adds significant strength to the joint and, in doing so, prevents medial displacement of the clavicle.

The SC joint enables rotation of the clavicle with respect to the sternum. The joint allows motion of the distal clavicle in superior, inferior, anterior, and posterior directions, along with some forward

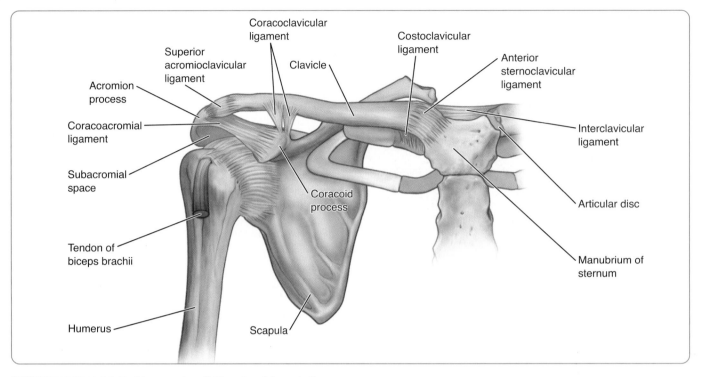

FIGURE 13.3 Ligaments of the shoulder girdle.

and backward rotation of the clavicle. As such, rotation occurs at the SC joint during motions such as shrugging the shoulders, reaching above the head, and most throwing-type activities. Because the first rib is joined by its cartilage to the manubrium just inferior to the joint, motion of the clavicle in the inferior direction is restricted.

The close-packed position for the SC joint occurs with maximal shoulder elevation. Although SC joint dislocations are uncommon, rapid diagnosis and treatment of posterior SC joint dislocations are important because of the proximity of the displaced medial clavicle to the great vessels (5).

Acromioclavicular Joint

The AC joint consists of the articulation of the medial facet of the acromion process of the scapula with the distal clavicle (see Fig. 13.3). As an irregular, diarthrodial joint, limited motion is permitted in all three planes. Highly variable in structure, as many as five different morphological types of AC joint have been identified (6). The joint is enclosed by a capsule, although the capsule is thinner than that of the SC joint. The strong superior and inferior AC ligaments cross the joint, providing stability. The coracoacromial ligament, which sometimes is referred to as the "arch" ligament, also attaches to the inferior lip of the AC joint to serve as a buffer between the rotator cuff muscles and the bony acromion process.

The close-packed position of the AC joint occurs when the humerus is abducted at 90°. Injuries to the AC joint are common among athletes involved in throwing and other overhead activities (7).

Coracoclavicular Joint

The coracoclavicular joint is a syndesmosis in which the coracoid process of the scapula and the inferior surface of the clavicle are joined by the coracoclavicular ligament (see Fig. 13.3). The coracoclavicular ligament, with its conoid and trapezoid branches, resists independent upward movement of the clavicle, downward movement of the scapula, and anteroposterior movement of the clavicle or scapula. Minimal movement is permitted at this joint. The coracoclavicular ligaments frequently are ruptured during contact sports, such as football, hockey, and rugby (8).

Glenohumeral Joint

The GH joint is the articulation between the glenoid fossa of the scapula and the head of the humerus. Although the joint enables a greater total ROM than any other joint in the human body, it lacks bony stability. This partially results from the hemispheric head of the humerus, which has three- to fourfold the surface area as compared to the shallow glenoid fossa. Because the glenoid fossa also is less curved than the humeral head, the humerus not only rotates, it also moves linearly across the surface of the glenoid fossa when humeral motion occurs. Humeral head translation is limited by muscle tension, which also limits rotation, during active positioning of the arm. The largest translations take place during passive movement of the arm at the extremes of the ROM.

The glenoid fossa is somewhat deepened around its perimeter by the glenoid labrum, a narrow rim of fibrocartilage around the edge of the fossa. The GH joint capsule is joined by the superior, middle, and inferior GH ligaments on the anterior side and by the coracohumeral ligament on the superior side (Fig. 13.4). Although joint displacements can occur in anterior, posterior, and inferior directions, the strong coracohumeral ligament protects against superior dislocations. The inferior GH ligament is the thickest of the ligaments and reinforces the inferior capsule. It is the main static stabilizer in the abducted arm.

The tendons of four muscles, including the supraspinatus, infraspinatus, teres minor, and subscapularis, also join the joint capsule. These muscles, which are referred to as the SITS muscles, after the first letter of each muscle's name, also are known as the rotator cuff muscles, both because they act to rotate the humerus and because their tendons merge to form a collagenous cuff around the joint. Tension in the rotator cuff muscles helps to hold the head of the humerus against the glenoid fossa, further contributing to joint stability. The joint is most stable in its close-packed position when the humerus is abducted and laterally rotated.

Scapulothoracic Joint

Because a muscle attaching to the scapula permits its motion with respect to the trunk or thorax, this region sometimes is described as the scapulothoracic joint. Muscles attaching to the scapula include the levator scapula, rhomboids, serratus anterior, pectoralis minor, subclavius, deltoid, subscapularis, supraspinatus, infraspinatus, teres major, teres minor, coracobrachialis, short head of the biceps brachii, long head of the triceps brachii, and the trapezius.

The scapular muscles perform two functions. The first is stabilization of the shoulder region. For example, when a barbell is lifted from the floor, the levator scapula, trapezius, and rhomboids develop tension to support the scapula and, in turn, the entire shoulder through the AC joint. The second is to facilitate movement of the upper extremity through appropriate positioning of the GH joint. For example, during an overhand throw, the rhomboids contract to move the entire shoulder

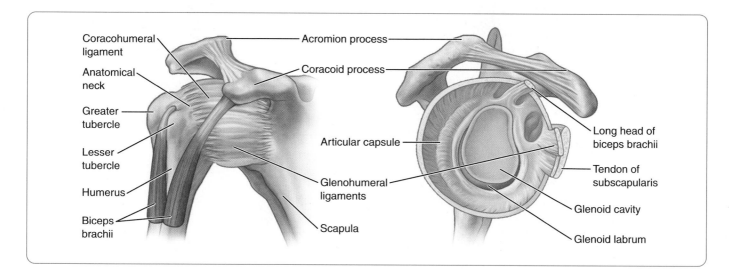

■■■■ FIGURE 13.4 **Ligaments of the glenohumeral joint.**

posteriorly as the arm and hand move backward during the preparatory phase. As the arm and hand then move forward to execute the throw, tension in the rhomboids is released to permit forward movement of the shoulder, enabling medial rotation of the humerus. Abduction of the arm at the GH joint is facilitated by rotation of the scapula (9).

Muscles of the Shoulder

> A detailed table providing the muscles of the shoulder, including each muscle's proximal attachment, distal attachment, primary actions, and nerve innervation, is available on the companion website at thePoint.

A large number of muscles cross the GH joint (Figs. 13.5 and 13.6). Because of the large ROM at the shoulder, however, the action produced by contraction of a given muscle can change with the orientation of the humerus, which complicates the process of identifying the actions of these muscles.

Bursae

The shoulder is surrounded by several bursae, including the subcoracoid, the subscapularis, and the most important, the subacromial. The subacromial bursa lies in the subacromial space, where it is surrounded by the acromion process of the scapula and the coracoacromial ligament above and the GH joint below (see Fig. 13.5). The bursa cushions the rotator cuff muscles, particularly the supraspinatus, from the overlying bony acromion, and it provides the major component of the subacromial gliding mechanism. This bursa is supplied with free nerve endings, Ruffini endings, and pacinian corpuscles and can become irritated when repeatedly compressed during overhead arm action.

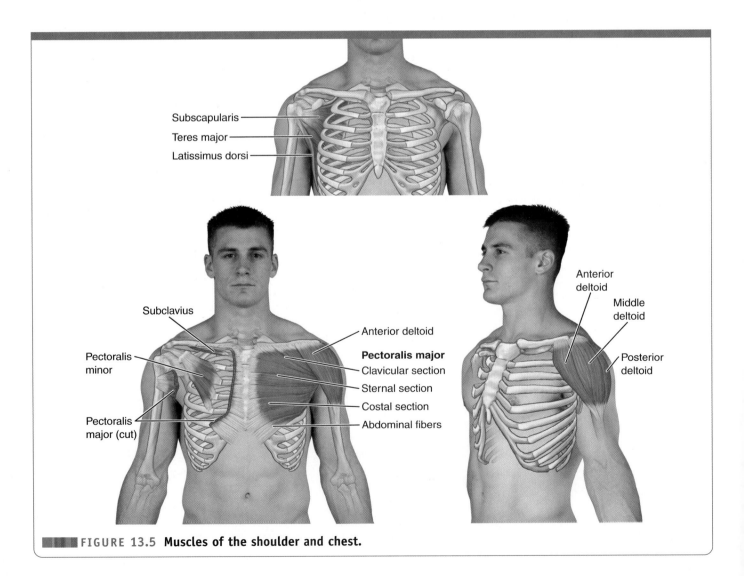

FIGURE 13.5 Muscles of the shoulder and chest.

FIGURE 13.6 Muscles of the shoulder and upper back.

Nerves of the Shoulder

Innervation of the upper extremity arises from the brachial plexus, branching primarily from the lower four cervical (C_5–C_8) and first thoracic (T_1) spinal nerves (see Fig. 10.9). The brachial plexus is positioned between the anterior scalene and middle scalene muscles in approximately 60% of individuals, with the C_5 and/or C_6 nerves coursing through or lying anterior to the anterior scalene in others. The ventral rami of these nerves divide into upper, middle, and lower trunks, which in turn separate into anterior and posterior divisions and then divide into lateral, medial, and posterior cords (see Chapter 10). This network of nerves passes between the clavicle and first

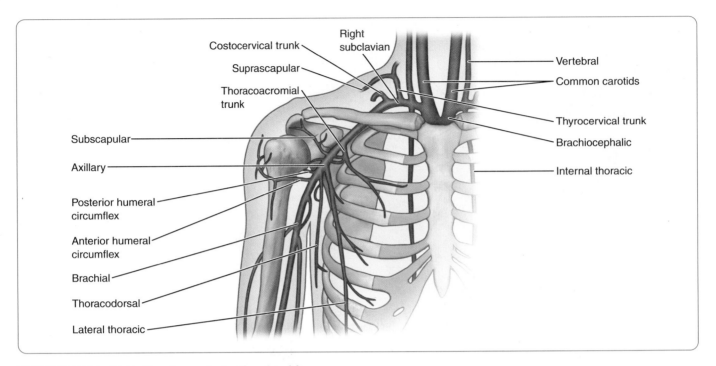

FIGURE 13.7 **Blood supply to the shoulder.**

rib at a distance approximately one-third of the length of the clavicle proximal to the GH joint. Injuries to the clavicle in this region can damage the brachial plexus. Major nerves arising from the brachial plexus that supply the shoulder region are the axillary (C_5, C_6), musculocutaneous (C_5–C_7), dorsal scapular (C_5), subscapular (C_5, C_6), suprascapular (C_5, C_6), and pectoral nerves (C_5–T_1).

Blood Vessels of the Shoulder

The subclavian artery passes beneath the clavicle to become the axillary artery, which provides the major blood supply to the shoulder (Fig. 13.7). Branches of the axillary artery include the thoracoacromial trunk, lateral thoracic artery, subscapular artery, and thoracodorsal artery as well as the anterior and posterior humeral circumflex arteries that supply the head of the humerus.

KINEMATICS AND MAJOR MUSCLE ACTIONS OF THE SHOULDER COMPLEX

The shoulder is the most freely movable joint in the body, with motion capability in all three planes (Fig. 13.8). Sagittal plane movements at the shoulder include flexion (i.e., elevation of the arm in an anterior direction), extension (i.e., return of the arm from a position of flexion to the side of the body), and hyperextension (i.e., elevation of the arm in a posterior direction). Frontal plane movements include abduction (i.e., elevation of the arm in a lateral direction) and adduction (i.e., return of the arm from a position of abduction to the side of the body). Transverse plane movements include horizontal adduction (i.e., a horizontally extended arm is moved medially) and horizontal abduction (i.e., a horizontally extended arm is moved laterally). The humerus also can rotate medially (i.e., the anterior face of the humerus is moved medially) and laterally (i.e., the anterior face of the humerus is moved laterally). Elevation of the humerus in all planes is accompanied by approximately 55° of external rotation (10).

Throwing

Throwing and related motions can produce a variety of both acute and chronic injuries to the shoulder. Throwing styles vary from individual to individual, even across overarm, sidearm, and underarm styles of the throw. Further complicating matters, some sport skills—casually referred to as throwing—actually involve more of a pushing motion than a throwing motion. An example is putting the shot. Nevertheless, overarm throwing can be described in distinct phases (Table 13.1).

Although skillful throwing involves the coordinated action of the entire body, this description focuses on the phases in which potential injury to the shoulder girdle and GH joint may occur. In the preparatory or cocking phase, the arm and hand are drawn behind the body through approximately 90° of abduction and 15° of horizontal abduction at the shoulder, accompanied by maximal external rotation of the humerus (170–180°). The combined motion causes heavy eccentric loading of the horizontal adductors and internal rotators of the shoulder. In particular, the subscapularis has its peak eccentric activity during the late cocking phase and serves to protect the anterior joint, which is under extreme tension. The pectoralis major and latissimus dorsi work eccentrically with the subscapularis to further protect the joint. This arm motion is facilitated by the action of the rhomboids contracting concentrically to pull the scapula and GH joint posteriorly, whereas the serratus anterior provides additional scapular stabilization. As the shoulder proceeds into horizontal abduction and external rotation,

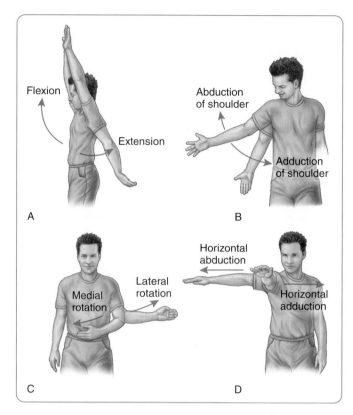

■■■■ FIGURE 13.8 **Movements of the arm at the shoulder. A,** Flexion and extension. **B,** Abduction and adduction. **C,** Internal and external rotation. **D,** Horizontal abduction and adduction.

the humeral head tends to sublux, first posteriorly and then anteriorly, against the anterior capsule; consequently, tendinitis of the anterior muscle tendons is quite common (11,12). Elbow extension begins just before maximal shoulder external rotation. This is immediately followed by the onset of humeral internal rotation.

During the acceleration or delivery phase, the ball is brought forward and released. Humeral horizontal adduction, elbow extension, and rapid internal rotation of the humerus at velocities that can exceed 7,000° per second; are produced by the pectoralis major, latissimus dorsi, and subscapularis; and are coupled with relaxation of the rhomboids to enable anterior movement of the GH joint (12). If the internal rotators are weak, however, the reduced ability to provide forceful arm depression can lead to increased external rotation, superior humeral migration, and impaired scapular rotation, which can cause or aggravate an impingement syndrome. During ball release, the elbow is almost fully extended and positioned slightly anterior to the trunk. Because throwing can involve a whip-like action of the arm, large stresses can be placed on the tendons, ligaments, and epiphyses of the throwing arm during delivery (11).

Arm deceleration occurs after ball release and continues until maximal shoulder internal rotation occurs, and consists primarily of a snap-like flexion of the wrist and pronation of the forearm. Large eccentric loads at the elbow and shoulder decelerate the arm. The infraspinatus, supraspinatus, teres major and minor, latissimus dorsi, and posterior deltoid play major roles in resisting shoulder distraction and anterior subluxation forces. If the rotator cuff muscles are weak, fatigued, or injured, the humeral head distracts and translates in an anterior direction, leading to stress on the posterior capsule. The serratus anterior contracts either concentrically or isometrically to decelerate scapular protraction, and it is assisted by the middle trapezius and rhomboids. Injuries common to the specific phases of throwing are listed in Table 13.1.

TABLE 13.1 Phases and Injuries of the Throwing Motion

PHASE	DESCRIPTION	COMMON INJURIES
Wind-Up Phase	From the first movement until the hands separate. The arms begin with downward swing, then are raised overhead (gathered position). The shoulders and hips rotate as the arms go overhead; the body shifts from facing the target to being perpendicular to the line of throw. Balance is maintained on the "stance leg" as the lead leg or "stride leg" lifts up; the hip and knee flex at about the chest-high level.	—
Stride Phase	From hand separation until the lead foot contacts the ground.	—
Cocking Phase	From foot contact until maximum shoulder external rotation.	Anterior glenohumeral instability or subluxation Anteroinferior glenoid labral tears Acromioclavicular joint pathology Subacromial bursitis Strain to the medial rotators (i.e., pectoralis major and latissimus dorsi), biceps brachii, and triceps brachii Thoracic outlet syndrome
Acceleration Phase	From maximum shoulder external rotation until ball release.	Anterior subluxation Rotator cuff tendinitis or partial tears Subacromial bursitis Proximal humeral apophysitis Glenoid labral pathology Strain to the anterior deltoid, pectoralis major, subscapularis, or latissimus dorsi Bicipital tendinitis or biceps tendon subluxation
Deceleration and Follow-Through Phase	From ball release until maximum shoulder internal rotation and balanced position is achieved.	Rotator cuff tendinitis or partial tears Triceps tendinitis Biceps tendinitis or rupture Teres minor strain Posterior glenohumeral subluxation Posterior capsulitis Glenoid labral pathology Acromioclavicular joint pathology

Coordination of Shoulder Movements

The extensive ROM afforded by the shoulder results in part from the loose structure of the GH joint and in part from the proximity of the other shoulder articulations and the movement capabilities they provide. Movement at the shoulder typically involves some rotation at the SC, AC, and GH joints. For example, as the arm is elevated past 30° of abduction, or the first 45 to 60° of flexion, the scapula also rotates, contributing approximately one-third of the total rotational movement of the humerus. This important coordination of scapular and humeral movements, known as **scapulohumeral rhythm,** enables a much greater ROM at the shoulder than would occur if the scapula were fixed (Fig. 13.9). Also contributing to the first 90° of humeral elevation is the elevation of the clavicle through approximately 35 to 45° of motion at the SC joint. The AC joint contributes to overall movement capability as well, with rotation occurring during the first 30° of humeral elevation and then again as the arm is moved past 135° (13).

Glenohumeral Flexion

The muscles that cross the GH joint anteriorly are positioned to contribute to flexion (see Figs. 13.5 and 13.6). The anterior deltoid and clavicular pectoralis major are the primary shoulder flexors; the coracobrachialis and short head of the biceps brachii provide assistance. Because the biceps brachii also crosses the elbow joint, it is capable of exerting more force at the shoulder when the elbow is in full extension.

■■■ **FIGURE 13.9 Scapulohumeral rhythm.** The coordinated movement of the scapula needed to facilitate motion of the humerus is known as scapulohumeral rhythm. The arrows indicate the direction the scapulae must rotate to raise the arms.

Glenohumeral Extension

When extension is not resisted, the action is caused by gravity. Eccentric contraction of the flexor muscles serves as a controlling or braking mechanism. When resistance to extension is offered, the posterior GH muscles, including the sternocostal pectoralis, latissimus dorsi, and teres major, act with assistance from the posterior deltoid and long head of the triceps brachii (see Fig.s 13.5 and 13.6).

Glenohumeral Abduction

The muscles superior to the GH joint produce abduction and include the middle deltoid and supraspinatus (see Fig. 13.5). During the contribution of the middle deltoid, from approximately 90 through 180° of abduction, the infraspinatus, subscapularis, and teres minor produce inferiorly directed force to neutralize the superiorly directed, dislocating force produced by the middle deltoid. This action serves an important function in preventing impingement of the supraspinatus and subacromial bursa. The long head of the biceps brachii provides GH stability during abduction.

Glenohumeral Adduction

As with extension, adduction in the absence of resistance results from gravitational force, with the abductors controlling the speed of motion. When resistance is present, adduction is accomplished through the action of the muscles positioned on the inferior side of the GH joint, including the latissimus dorsi, teres major, and sternocostal pectoralis (see Fig. 13.5). The short head of the biceps and long head of the triceps contribute minor assistance. When the arm is elevated above 90°, the coracobrachialis and subscapularis also assist.

Lateral and Medial Rotation of the Humerus

Lateral rotators of the humerus lie on the posterior aspect of the humerus, including the infraspinatus and teres minor; the posterior deltoid provides assistance. Muscles on the anterior side of the humerus contribute to medial rotation; these include the subscapularis and teres major, with assistance from the pectoralis major, anterior deltoid, latissimus dorsi, and short head of the biceps (see Fig. 13.5). Table 13.2 summarizes the primary muscles that act on the arm.

TABLE 13.2 Primary Muscles Producing Movement at the Glenohumeral Joint					
FLEXION	**EXTENSION**	**ABDUCTION**	**ADDUCTION**	**MEDIAL ROTATION**	**LATERAL ROTATION**
Anterior deltoid	Latissimus dorsi	Middle deltoid	Latissimus dorsi	Subscapularis	Infraspinatus
Pectoralis major (clavicular)	Pectoralis major (sternal)	Supraspinatus	Pectoralis major (sternal)	Teres major	Teres major
	Teres major		Teres major		

KINETICS OF THE SHOULDER

Although the articulations of the shoulder girdle are interconnected, the GH joint sustains much greater loads compared to the other shoulder joints, primarily because the GH joint provides mechanical support for the entire arm. Although the weight of the arm is only approximately 9% of body weight, the length of the horizontally extended arm creates large torques that must be countered by the shoulder muscles. When these muscles contract to support the extended arm, large compression forces are generated inside the joint. The compression force acting on the articulating surfaces of the GH joint when the arm is abducted to 90° has been estimated to reach 50% of body weight (13). This load is reduced by approximately half when the elbow is maximally flexed, but because of the shortened moment arm, the shoulder is considered to be a major load-bearing joint.

During the throwing motion, two critical instances increase the potential for shoulder injury. The first is during the cocking phase, when the arm has not quite reached maximum lateral rotation and a large internal rotation torque develops at the shoulder, heightening the possibility of a glenoid labral tear. The second occurs just after ball release, when both a large compression force and a large horizontal abduction torque are generated at the shoulder, creating the potential for rotator cuff tension failure and subacromial impingement (11).

Muscles that attach to the humerus at small angles with respect to the glenoid fossa contribute more to shear than to compression at the joint. These muscles stabilize the humerus in the fossa when the contractions of the powerful muscles that move the humerus might otherwise dislocate the joint. Maximum shear force has been found to be present at the GH joint when the arm is elevated approximately 60° (13).

PREVENTION OF SHOULDER CONDITIONS

Acute and chronic injuries to the shoulder complex are common in sport participation. Many contact and collision sports require some protective equipment, but in most cases, flexibility, physical conditioning, and proper technique are the primary factors that can reduce the risk of injury to this vulnerable area.

Protective Equipment

Contact and collision sports, such as football, lacrosse, and ice hockey, require shoulder pads to protect exposed bony protuberances from impact (see Chapter 3). Although shoulder pads do prevent some soft-tissue injuries in this region, they do not protect the GH joint from excessive motion. Several other commercial pads and braces that are used to protect the region are illustrated in Chapter 3.

Physical Conditioning

Lack of flexibility can predispose an individual to joint sprains and muscular strains. Warm-up exercises should focus on general joint flexibility and may be performed either alone or with a partner using proprioceptive neuromuscular facilitation (PNF) stretching techniques. Individuals using the throwing motion in their sport should increase ROM in external rotation, because this has been shown to increase the velocity of the throwing arm and to decrease shearing forces on the GH joint. Several flexibility exercises for the shoulder complex are demonstrated in Field Strategy 13.1.

FIELD STRATEGY 13.1

Flexibility Exercises for the Shoulder Region

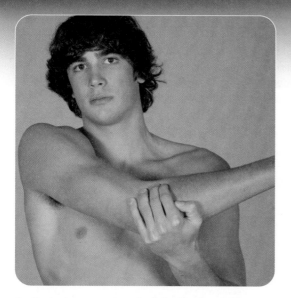

1. Posterior capsular stretch. Horizontally adduct the arm across the chest while the opposite hand assists the stretch.

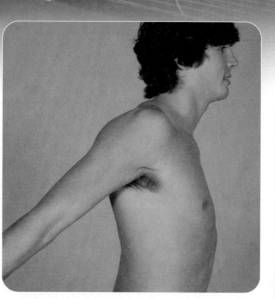

3. Anterior and posterior capsular stretch. Hold onto both sides of a doorway with the hands behind the back. Straighten the arms while leaning forward. Repeat with the hands in front while leaning backward.

2. Inferior capsular stretch. Hold the involved arm over the head with the elbow flexed. Use the opposite hand to assist in the stretching. Add a side stretch.

4. Medial and lateral rotators. Using a towel, bat, or racquet, pull the arm to stretch it into lateral rotation. Repeat in medial rotation.

FIELD STRATEGY 13.2

Strengthening Exercises for the Shoulder Complex

1. Shoulder shrugs. Elevate the shoulders toward the ears and hold. Pull the shoulders back, pinch the shoulder blades together, and hold. Relax, and repeat.
2. Scapular abduction (protraction). Lift the weight directly upward while also lifting the posterior shoulder from the table. Relax and repeat.
3. Scapular adduction (retraction). Perform bent-over rowing while flexing the elbows. When the end of the motion is reached, pinch the shoulder blades together, and hold.
4. Bench press or incline press. Place the hands a shoulder's width apart, and push the barbell directly above the shoulder joint. This exercise should be performed with a spotter.
5. Bent arm lateral flies, supine position. Keeping the elbows slightly flexed, lift the dumbbells directly over the shoulders. Lower the dumbbells until they are parallel to the floor, and then repeat. An alternative method is to move the dumbbells in a diagonal pattern. In the prone position, the exercise strengthens the trapezius.
6. Lateral pull-downs. In a seated position, grasp the handle, and pull the bar behind the head. An alternative method is to pull the bar in front of the body.
7. Surgical tubing. Secure the tubing, and then work in diagonal functional patterns similar to those skills experienced in a specific sport/activity.

Strengthening programs should focus on muscles acting on both the GH and scapulothoracic regions. Strength in the infraspinatus, teres minor, and posterior shoulder musculature is necessary to:

- Begin the cocking phase of throwing.

- Fix the shoulder girdle during the acceleration phase.

- Provide adequate muscle tension, with eccentric contractions, for smooth deceleration through the follow-through phase.

A weakened supraspinatus is present in many chronic shoulder problems, particularly among throwers. Concentric and eccentric contractions with light resistance during the first 30° of abduction can strengthen this muscle. Strengthening the scapular stabilizers can be accomplished by doing push-ups or moving the arm through a resisted, diagonal pattern of external rotation and horizontal abduction. Other strengthening exercises are demonstrated in Field Strategy 13.2.

Proper Skill Technique

Coordinated muscle contractions are necessary for the smooth execution of the throwing motion. Any disruption in the sequencing of integrated movements can lead to additional stress on the GH joint and surrounding soft-tissue structures. High-speed photography, often used to record the mechanics of the throwing motion, can lead to early detection of improper technique. In addition to proper throwing technique, participants in contact and collision sports should be taught the shoulder-roll method of falling rather than falling on an outstretched arm. This technique reduces direct compression of the articular joints and disperses the force over a wider area.

SPRAINS TO THE SHOULDER COMPLEX

 A soccer player fell on an outstretched arm. A physician diagnosed a type II AC sprain. What are the signs and symptoms of a type II AC sprain?

Ligamentous injuries to the SC, AC, and GH joints can result from compression, tension, and shearing forces occurring in a single episode or from repetitive overload. A common method of injury is a fall or direct hit on the lateral aspect of the acromion. The force is transmitted first to the site of impact, then to the AC joint and the clavicle, and finally, to the SC joint. Failure can occur at any one of these sites. Acute sprains are common in hockey, rugby, football, soccer, equestrian sports, and the martial arts.

Sternoclavicular Joint Sprain

The SC joint is the main axis of rotation for movements of the clavicle and scapula. The majority of injuries result from compression related to a direct blow, as when another participant lands on a supine individual or, more commonly, by indirect forces transmitted from a blow to the shoulder or a fall on an outstretched arm. The disruption typically drives the proximal clavicle superior, medial, and anterior, disrupting the costoclavicular and SC ligaments and leading to anterior displacement.

Signs and Symptoms

Grade I (first-degree) injuries are characterized by point tenderness and mild pain over the SC joint, with no visible deformity. Grade II (second-degree) injuries involve a joint subluxation that leads to bruising, swelling, and pain. The individual is unable to horizontally adduct the arm without considerable pain and may hold the arm forward and close to the body, supporting it across the chest, which indicates disruption of the stabilizing ligaments. In addition, scapular protraction and retraction can reproduce pain associated with ligamentous or disk damage. Grade III (third-degree) sprains involve a prominent displacement of the sternal end of the clavicle and may involve a fracture. The individual has a complete rupture of the SC and costoclavicular ligaments. Pain is severe when the shoulders are brought together by a lateral force.

Although rare, posterior, or retrosternal, displacement is more serious because of the potential injury to the esophagus, trachea, internal thoracic artery and vein, and brachiocephalic and subclavian artery and vein. The most common mechanism of injury is a blow to the posterolateral aspect of the shoulder with the arm adducted and flexed, such as a fall on the shoulder that displaces the distal clavicle anteriorly (14). This action may occur during a piling-on injury in football; less commonly, the injury may be caused by a direct blow to the anteromedial end of the clavicle. The individual has a palpable depression between the sternal end of the clavicle and manubrium, is unable to perform shoulder protraction, and may have difficulty swallowing and breathing. The patient also may complain of numbness and weakness of the upper extremity secondary to the compression of structures in the thoracic inlet. If the venous vascular vessels are impinged, the patient may have venous congestion or engorgement in the ipsilateral arm and a diminished radial pulse (14).

Management

Grade I sprains of the SC joint are treated with rest, ice, and anti-inflammatory drugs. The arm may be immobilized with a sling for 1 to 2 weeks, followed by early ROM exercises. Grade II sprains may require longer immobilization (3–6 weeks) in a sling or a soft figure-eight brace, followed by ROM exercises. Grade III sprains require immediate reduction of the dislocation by a physician. Immobilization usually is maintained by a Velpeau bandage, soft figure-eight brace, clavicle strap harness, or bulky pressure pad over the medial clavicle for 4 to 6 weeks. Scar tissue may form, but typically, no function is lost. There remains, however, a high incidence of recurrent SC sprains. When immobilization is discontinued, the arm motion should still be protected for an additional 2 weeks. Elbow exercises and shoulder ROM can be started at 3 weeks (15). Surgical intervention may be necessary in the treatment of recurrent anterior SC joint or trauma that results in significant cosmetic issues. Table 13.3 summarizes the signs and symptoms as well as the management of anterior SC sprains.

Posterior displacement can become life-threatening, and the emergency plan, including summoning emergency medical services, should be activated.

EMS

Acromioclavicular Joint Sprain

The AC joint is weak and easily injured by a direct blow, fall on the point of the shoulder (called a shoulder pointer), or force transmitted up the long axis of the humerus during a fall with the humerus in an adducted position (16). In these cases, the acromion is driven away from the clavicle, or vice versa. Although often referred to as a "separated shoulder," ruptures of the AC and/or coracoclavicular ligaments can result in an AC dislocation; therefore, they are more correctly referred to as "sprains."

TABLE 13.3 Management of a Sternoclavicular Sprain

SIGNS AND SYMPTOMS	FIRST DEGREE	SECOND DEGREE	THIRD DEGREE
Deformity	None	Slight prominence of medial end of the clavicle	Gross prominence of medial end of the clavicle
Swelling	Slight	Moderate	Severe
Palpable pain	Mild	Moderate	Severe
Movement	Usually unlimited, but may have discomfort with movement	Unable to abduct the arm or horizontally adduct the arm across the chest without noticeable pain	Limited as in second degree, but pain is more severe
Treatment	Ice, rest, and immobilization with sling/swathe	Ice, rest, immobilization with figure-eight or clavicular strap with a sling, for 3–4 weeks. Initiate strengthening program after 3–4 weeks.	Apply a figure-eight immobilizer with scapulas retracted. Immediately refer to a physician. Check radial pulse, respiration, and ability to swallow. If significant findings are present, activate the emergency action plan.

Classification of Injury

Like other joint injuries, AC sprains may be classified as first degree (i.e., mild), second degree (i.e., moderate), or third degree (i.e., severe). Because of the complexity of the joint, however, AC sprains often are classified as types I to VI based on the extent of ligamentous damage, degree of instability, and direction in which the clavicle displaces relative to the acromion and coracoid process (Table 13.4).

Signs and Symptoms

Type I injuries have no disruption of the AC or coracoclavicular ligaments. Minimal swelling and pain are present over the joint line and increase with abduction past 90°. The injury is inherently stable, and pain is self-limiting.

Type II injuries result from a more severe blow to the shoulder. The AC ligaments are torn, but the coracoclavicular ligament, only minimally sprained, is intact. Vertical stability is maintained, but sagittal plane stability is compromised. The clavicle rides above the level of the acromion, and a minor step or gap is present at the joint line. Pain increases when the distal clavicle is depressed or moved in an anterior-posterior direction and during passive horizontal adduction.

Type III injuries have complete disruption of the AC and coracoclavicular ligaments, resulting in visible prominence of the distal clavicle. The individual will have obvious swelling and bruising and, more significantly, depression or drooping of the shoulder girdle.

Higher-grade injuries (types IV–VI) are caused by more violent forces. Extensive mobility and pain in the area may signify tearing of the deltoid and trapezius muscle attachments at the distal clavicle. These rare injuries must be carefully evaluated for associated neurologic injuries.

TABLE 13.4 Classification of Acromioclavicular (AC) Joint Sprains

GRADE	DEGREE	INJURED STRUCTURES
Type I	First	Stretch or partial damage of the AC ligament and capsule
Type II	Second	Rupture of AC ligament, and partial strain of coracoclavicular ligament
Type III	Second	Rupture of AC ligament and coracoclavicular ligament
Type IV to VI	Third	Rupture of AC ligament and coracoclavicular ligament, and tearing of deltoid and trapezius fascia

Management

Type I and II injuries are treated with rest, ice, and nonsteroidal anti-inflammatory drugs (NSAIDs), followed by ROM exercises as tolerated. Immobilization in a sling for one to three weeks is only necessary if pain is present. The individual may return to activity when pain and strength permit normal use of the extremity, but the area should be padded to protect it from further insult. The majority of type I and II injuries heal without complications. Occasionally, however, persistent limiting pain may necessitate a cortisone injection to diminish inflammation. Rehabilitation involves regaining ROM and, once ROM is bilaterally equal, beginning a progressive resistance exercise program.

The management of type III injuries is controversial, because they are managed both operatively and nonoperatively. Most type III injuries are treated conservatively, with 90 to 100% having satisfactory results. Nonsurgical treatment involves immobilization in a sling for 2 to 4 weeks, followed by pendulum exercises, elbow ROM exercises, isometrics in all planes, and rope-and-pulley exercises for shoulder flexion and abduction as tolerated. If treatment includes surgery, pendulum and isometric exercises in all planes are encouraged during the initial stages of rehabilitation, although abduction and flexion to 90° are limited for approximately 3 to 4 weeks. Rehabilitation should focus on strengthening the rotator cuff and scapula stabilizers and on restoring neuromuscular control and arthrokinematics. Return to activity may take as long as 10 to 12 weeks, depending on the restoration of full, pain-free ROM and the stability of the joint. Participation in contact sports usually is permitted 3 to 5 months after the injury, depending on functional recovery.

In severe cases (types IV–VI) involving total disruption of the supporting ligaments, intra-articular disk damage, or an intra-articular fracture, open or arthroscopic intervention may be necessary. Immobilization may be necessary for as long as 4 to 6 weeks. The individual is permitted to use the arm for most activities of daily living but is restricted from active forward elevation or abduction. Pushing, pulling, or carrying more than 5 pounds also is prohibited. In approximately 6 weeks, a progressive ROM and strengthening regimen begins. Complete sport and physical activity participation usually is not permitted until isokinetic testing shows results equal to those of the contralateral side, which occurs approximately 6 months after surgery. Table 13.5 summarizes the signs and symptoms as well as the management of AC sprains.

TABLE 13.5 Management of an Acromioclavicular (AC) Sprain			
SIGNS & SYMPTOMS	**TYPE I**	**TYPE II**	**TYPE III**
Deformity	None; ligaments are still intact	Slight elevation of lateral clavicle; AC ligaments are disrupted, but coracoclavicular is still intact	Prominent elevation of clavicle; AC ligaments and coracoclavicular ligaments are disrupted
Swelling	Slight	Moderate	Severe
Palpable pain	Mild over joint line	Moderate with downward pressure on distal clavicle; palpable gap or minor step present; snapping may be felt on horizontal adduction	Severe on palpation and depression of acromion process; definite palpable step deformity present
Movement	Usually unlimited, but may have some discomfort on abduction greater than 90°	Unable to abduct the arm or horizontally adduct the arm across the chest without noticeable pain	Limited as in type II, but pain is more severe
Stability	No instability	Some instability	Demonstrable instability
Treatment	Ice, NSAIDs, regain full ROM and strength; return to activity as tolerated, with protection	Ice, NSAIDs, immobilize with sling; TENS, interferential EMS for pain relief; ultrasound; strengthening and stability exercises; return to activity with protection	Ice, immobilize, and immediately refer to physician; if treated conservatively, deformity remains, but function should be within normal limits

EMS, electrical muscle stimulation; *NSAIDs*, nonsteroidal anti-inflammatory drugs; *ROM*, range of motion; *TENS*, transcutaneous electrical nerve stimulation.

Glenohumeral Joint Sprain

Damage to the GH joint can occur when the arm is forcefully abducted (e.g., when making an arm tackle in football), but such damage more commonly is caused by excessive shoulder external rotation and extension (i.e., arm in the overhead position). When the arm rotates externally, the anterior capsule and GH ligaments are stretched or torn, causing the humeral head to slip out of the glenoid fossa in an anterior-inferior direction (Fig. 13.10). A direct blow or forceful movement that pushes the humerus posteriorly also can result in damage to the joint capsule.

Signs and Symptoms

In a first-degree injury, the anterior shoulder is particularly painful to palpation and movement, especially when the mechanism of injury is reproduced. Active ROM may be slightly limited, but pain does not occur on adduction or internal rotation, in contrast to a muscular strain. A second-degree sprain produces some joint laxity. In addition, pain, swelling, and bruising usually are significant, and ROM, particularly abduction, is limited.

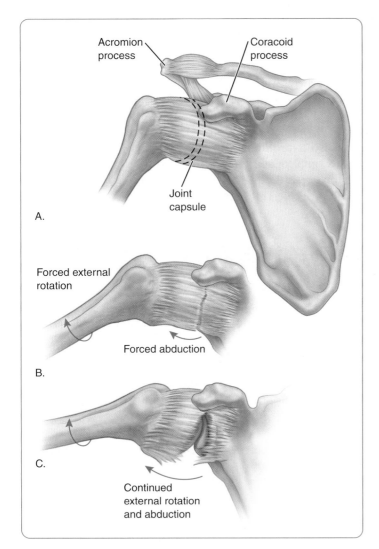

Management

Treatment includes cryotherapy, rest, NSAIDs, and immobilization with a sling during the initial 12 to 24 hours. Early emphasis is placed on pain-free ROM exercises, elastic-band strengthening, and PNF exercises. Exercises to regain full external rotation and abduction should be delayed for at least 3 weeks to allow capsular healing. A more extensive resistance program can be started as tolerated.

Glenohumeral Instability

Glenohumeral instability is based on joint play movements, or the relative displacement of the humeral head in the glenoid fossa, and may be classified as anterior, posterior, inferior, or multidirectional instability. Instability can range from a vague sense of shoulder dysfunction (atraumatic instability) to traumatic dislocation. Although GH instability can occur in any direction, most acute dislocations are anterior, with posterior dislocations being the second most frequent.

Anterior Instability

Anterior instability may result from a blow to the posterolateral aspect of the shoulder, but it more commonly is caused by excessive indirect forces that push the arm into abduction, external rotation, and extension. Failure of the capsule ligamentous complex, particularly the middle and inferior GH ligaments, causes the head of the humerus to lodge under the anteroinferior portion of the glenoid fossa adjacent to the coracoid process. As the humerus slides forward, the inferior GH ligament may be avulsed from the anterior lip of the labrum or in combination with a portion of the labrum. This condition is referred to as a **Bankart lesion**.

Posterior Instability

Posterior instability most often occurs when the humerus is flexed and internally rotated and a posterior

FIGURE 13.10 Glenohumeral sprains. A, Normal abduction with some stretching of the fibers. **B,** Forced external rotation and abduction with minimal tears to the joint capsule, leading to a moderate or second-degree sprain. **C,** Continuation of the forced movement causes a third-degree sprain or shoulder dislocation.

force is directed along the long axis of the humerus. This action often is associated with blocking in football. Although a single traumatic episode may lead to posterior instability, the condition more commonly results from a series of accumulated microtraumatic episodes.

Inferior Instability

Inferior instability is rare. The primary restraint against inferior translation is the superior GH ligament. When the arm is abducted 45° in neutral rotation, the anterior portion of the inferior GH ligament is the primary restraint; when the arm is at 90° of abduction, the entire GH ligament, particularly the posterior band, is responsible for restricting inferior displacement. Superior translation is limited by the coracoacromial arch and acromion process.

Multidirectional Instability

Multidirectional instability of the shoulder occurs when damage takes place in more than one plane. Acutely, most, if not all, anterior and posterior dislocations are associated with some preexisting, inferior laxity or laxity in the opposite direction. Pain and/or clicking can occur during simple tasks, such as picking up a box or backpack. It is essential that a shoulder evaluation differentiate between unidirectional and multidirectional instability. Failure to identify multidirectional instability, and, subsequently, provision of treatment only for a unidirectional instability can significantly alter joint mechanics and predispose the individual to continued instability in one or more planes.

Treatment is initially conservative, with 50 to 70% of patients responding favorably to rehabilitation and activity modification. Surgical repair is indicated for individuals who do not respond to conservative measures.

Glenohumeral Dislocations and Subluxations

The GH joint is the most frequently dislocated major joint in the body. Ninety percent of shoulder dislocations are anterior; posterior dislocations rank second in occurrence. Inferior dislocations are rare and often are accompanied by neurovascular injury and fracture (15). Dislocations can be acute or chronic.

Acute Dislocations

Many acute dislocations have an associated fracture or nerve damage. Therefore, this injury is considered to be serious, and it necessitates immediate transportation to the nearest medical facility for reduction.

SIGNS AND SYMPTOMS. An initial dislocation presents with intense pain. Recurrent dislocations may be less painful. Tingling and numbness may extend down the arm into the hand. In a first-time anterior dislocation, the injured arm often is held in slight abduction (20–30°) and external rotation and is stabilized against the body by the opposite hand. Visually, a sharp contour on the affected shoulder, with a prominent acromion process, can be seen when compared with the smooth deltoid outline on the unaffected shoulder. The humeral head may be palpated in the axilla anterior to the acromion and resting adjacent to the coracoid process. The individual will not allow the arm to be brought across the chest. It is important to assess the axillary nerve and artery, because both structures can be damaged in a dislocation. A pulse may be taken on the medial proximal humerus over the brachial artery, and the axillary nerve can be assessed by stroking the skin on the upper lateral arm to assess sensation. Because the deltoid is not only a key shoulder abductor but also contributes to shoulder flexion and extension, damage to this nerve can be devastating.

Occasionally, posterior dislocations occur from a fall on or a blow to the anterior surface of the shoulder which drives the head of the humerus posteriorly. If dislocated, the arm is carried tightly against the chest and across the front of the trunk in rigid adduction and internal rotation. The anterior shoulder appears to be flat, the coracoid process is prominent, and a corresponding bulge may be seen posteriorly (if not masked by a heavy deltoid musculature). Any attempt to move the arm into external rotation and abduction produces severe pain. Because the biceps brachii is unable to function in this position, the individual is unable to supinate the forearm with the shoulder flexed.

MANAGEMENT. Muscle spasm sets in very quickly following dislocation and makes reduction more difficult. Management of a first-time dislocation requires immediate referral to a physician. As such, in some settings, it may be necessary to activate the emergency action plan. The injury should be treated as a fracture and the arm immobilized in a comfortable position. To prevent unnecessary movement of the humerus, a rolled towel or thin pillow can be placed between the thoracic wall and humerus before applying a sling. Ice should be applied to control hemorrhage and muscle spasm.

Following reduction, the shoulder is immobilized in a sling and swathe. Traditionally, immobilization for 4 weeks followed by rehabilitation is recommended, but this protocol has not been proved to diminish the risk of recurrent dislocations. A 67 to 97% chance of sustaining another dislocation exists, particularly in patients younger than 30 years (15). When the individual is able to tolerate movement, ROM exercises can begin, but it is important to avoid an aggressive flexibility program in extension, abduction, and external rotation. Resisted isometric and stretching exercises can begin immediately after the acute phase has ended. Elastic band exercises below 90° of abduction can be incorporated early during the program to maintain and improve strength. Interferential current stimulation can be used to reduce inflammation, stimulate muscle re-education, promote deep tissue circulation, and minimize fibrotic infiltration. Strength development of the lateral rotators can reduce strain on the anterior structures of the joint by pulling the humeral head posteriorly during lateral rotation of the shoulder, thus reducing anterior instability. Strong scapula stabilizers (e.g., trapezius, rhomboids, and serratus anterior) also are believed to improve anterior stability by placing the glenoid in the optimal position to perform the skill techniques required. Isokinetic internal rotation and adduction can begin within 3 to 4 weeks and advance as tolerated. More aggressive shoulder rehabilitation exercises are not typically initiated until 5 to 6 weeks after removal of the immobilization device and subsequent to achieving full ROM.

A common finding after an anterior dislocation is a Hill-Sachs lesion (Fig. 13.11). The lesion is a small defect in the articular cartilage of the humeral head caused by the impact of the humeral head on the glenoid fossa as the humerus dislocates. The lesion usually is located on the posterior

■■■■ FIGURE 13.11 **Hill-Sachs lesions. A,** In this radiograph of a reduced anterior dislocation with the humeral head held in internal rotation, Hill-Sachs compression fracture is evident. Note the posterolateral humeral head defect with a sharp, dense spine of bone running downward from the top of the humeral head toward the center of the humeral head. This line of condensation of bone is the result of an impaction fracture caused by the anterior glenoid rim. **B,** This radiograph demonstrates a subacromial posterior dislocation of the right shoulder with a large, anteromedial compression fracture defect of the humeral head, the so-called reverse Hill-Sachs sign (arrow).

aspect of the humeral head, but it may be found on the anterior portion of the humeral head following a posterior dislocation, in which it is called a reverse Hill-Sachs lesion. The lesion is used as a diagnostic tool in determining the severity of the dislocation. In individuals reporting that the shoulder dislocated but spontaneously reduced, the lesion may be visible on radiographs. Although the lesion rarely is symptomatic, the condition may lead to early degeneration of the GH joint.

Chronic Dislocations

Recurrent dislocations, or "trick shoulders," tend to be anterior dislocations that are intracapsular. The mechanism of injury is the same as that for acute dislocations. As the number of occurrences increase, however, the forces that are needed to produce the injury decrease, as do the associated muscle spasm, pain, and swelling. The individual is aware of the shoulder displacing, because the arm gives the sensation of "going dead," which is referred to as the **dead arm syndrome**. Activities in which recurrent posterior subluxations are common include the follow-through of a throwing motion or a racquet swing, the ascent phase of a push-up or a bench press, the recoil following a block in football, and certain swimming strokes.

SIGNS AND SYMPTOMS. Pain is the major complaint, with crepitation and/or clicking after the arm shifts back into the appropriate position. Many individuals voluntarily reduce the injury by positioning the arm in flexion, adduction, and internal rotation.

MANAGEMENT. If the injury does not reduce, the individual should be placed in a sling and swathe, or the arm may be stabilized next to the body with an elastic wrap. Ice should be applied to control pain and inflammation. The individual should be referred immediately to a physician for reduction of the injury and further care. Following reduction, conservative treatment involves rest and immobilization, restoration of shoulder motion, and strengthening of the rotator cuff muscles. Surgery may be indicated if persistent instability occurs.

Glenoid Labrum Tears

The glenoid labrum is a fibrocartilaginous rim that lines the glenoid fossa to better receive the humeral head. The capsule and inferior GH ligament are contiguous with the labrum at their attachment to the glenoid. Tearing of the labrum and inferior GH ligament is referred to as a **Bankart lesion.** The lesion is associated with recurrent anterior shoulder instability. Tears of the labrum also may result from degeneration or trauma. In many instances, the tears are asymptomatic and incidental. Longitudinal or flap tears may occur in the anterior or posterior labrum, with or without associated GH instability.

An injury to the superior labrum may begin posteriorly and extend anteriorly, disrupting the attachment of the long head of the biceps tendon to the superior glenoid tubercle (**SLAP lesion**). Fig. 13.12 demonstrates both a Bankart lesion and a SLAP lesion.

Signs and Symptoms

The individual may complain of pain, catching, or weakness, usually when the arm is overhead in an abducted and externally rotated position. The pain often is associated with clicking or popping within the joint. If a tear is the result of a dislocation or subluxation, symptoms of instability also may be present. Superior tears may be symptomatic and can be reproduced with ROM and translation testing, particularly with use of the clunk test and compression rotation test. Speed's test and Yergason's test may be positive as well. Axial loading of the joint with forced internal and external rotation and the arm elevated 160° in the scapular plane with the elbow flexed (e.g., anterior impingement "crank" test) also may reproduce symptoms (17).

Management

Treatment is based on the tear pattern and the presence or absence of GH instability. Initial conservative treatment may involve rest, anti-inflammatory drugs, and if applicable, rehabilitation exercises. For those individuals who do not respond well to conservative measures, arthroscopic debridement may be necessary.

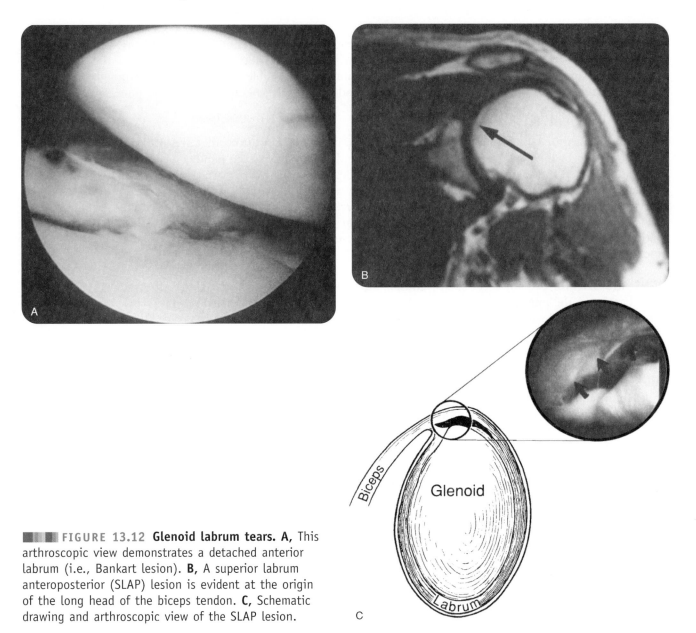

FIGURE 13.12 Glenoid labrum tears. A, This arthroscopic view demonstrates a detached anterior labrum (i.e., Bankart lesion). **B,** A superior labrum anteroposterior (SLAP) lesion is evident at the origin of the long head of the biceps tendon. **C,** Schematic drawing and arthroscopic view of the SLAP lesion.

The soccer player with the type II AC sprain experienced the following signs and symptoms: slight elevation of the lateral clavicle; moderate swelling over the joint; moderate, palpable pain with downward pressure on distal clavicle; palpable gap at the joint; inability to abduct the arm or horizontally adduct the arm across the chest without noticeable pain; and compromised sagittal plane stability.

OVERUSE CONDITIONS

Why is impingement syndrome a problem for swimmers in particular?

Individuals who perform repetitive overhead activities often develop anterior shoulder pain. The GH capsular ligaments are the prime stabilizers of the shoulder, especially the anteroinferior GH ligament. As muscles contract to move the arm, they create compressive and shear forces within the joint. The compression force produced by muscles acting perpendicular to the glenoid fossa stabilizes the humeral head, and the muscles acting more parallel to the glenoid produce a translational shear force. The resultant force derived from the sum of the compressive and shear forces determine the vector direction of the total joint force. A larger superior shear force produces impingement, and a larger compression force centers the humeral head in the glenoid, reducing rotator cuff impingement under the acromion.

During abduction, the strong deltoid and supraspinatus muscles pull the humeral head superiorly relative to the glenoid fossa. The remaining rotator cuff muscles must counteract this migration by producing an inferior shear force to resist the pull from the supraspinatus and deltoid muscles. If the rotator cuff tendons are weak or fatigued, they are incapable of depressing the humeral head in the glenoid fossa during overhead motions. In addition, fatigue of the infraspinatus and teres minor that resist anterior joint translation also may lead to intracapsular impingement and GH instability. The resulting compression can lead to impingement of the supraspinatus tendon and subacromial bursa between the acromion, the coracoacromial ligament, and the greater tubercle of the humerus, resulting in rotator cuff strain, impingement syndrome, bursitis, or bicipital tendinitis.

Rotator Cuff and Impingement Injuries

Chronic rotator cuff tears to the SITS muscles result from repetitive microtraumatic episodes that primarily impinge on the supraspinatus tendon just proximal to the greater tubercle of the humerus (Fig. 13.13). Partial tears usually are seen in young individuals, with total tears typically seen in adults older than 30 years. In older age groups, chronic tears can lead to cuff thinning, degeneration, and total rupture of the supraspinatus tendon.

Impingement syndrome implies an actual, mechanical abutment of the rotator cuff and the subacromial bursa against the coracoacromial ligament and acromion. This injury is caused from the force overload to the rotator cuff and bursa that occurs during the abduction, forward flexion, and medial rotation cycle of shoulder movements. Along with injury to the supraspinatus tendon and subacromial bursa, the glenoid labrum and long head of the biceps brachii also may be injured. Impingement syndrome sometimes is called "painful arc" syndrome or "swimmer's shoulder." Box 13.1 lists several factors that can increase the risk for an impingement syndrome.

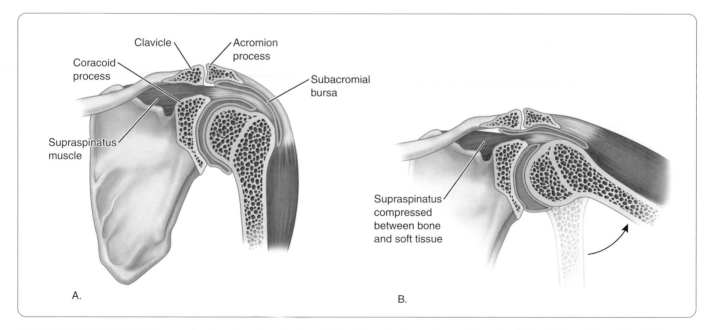

■■ ■ FIGURE 13.13 **Supraspinatus tendon during abduction. A,** Normal position. **B,** Abducted position. Repetitive overhead motions can impinge the muscle or tendon between the acromion process and coracoacromial ligament, resulting in a chronic rotator cuff injury.

Box 13.1   Factors Contributing to Impingement Syndrome

- Excessive amount of overhead movement (i.e., overuse)
- Limited subacromial space under the coracoacromial arch, and limited flexibility of the coracoacromial ligament
- Thickness of the supraspinatus and biceps brachii tendon
- Lack of flexibility and strength of the supraspinatus and biceps brachii
- Weakness of the posterior cuff muscles (e.g., infraspinatus or teres minor)
- Tightness of the posterior cuff muscles
- Hypermobility of the shoulder joints
- Imbalance in muscle strength, coordination, and endurance of the scapular muscles (e.g., serratus anterior or rhomboids)
- Shape of the acromion
- Training devices (e.g., use of hand paddles or tubing)

Signs and Symptoms

Initially, pain is described as being deep in the shoulder and present at night. Activity increases the pain, but only in the impingement position. As repetitive trauma continues, pain becomes progressively worse, particularly between 70 and 120° (i.e., "painful arc") of active and resisted abduction. Because forced scapular protraction leads to further impingement and pain, the individual may be unable to sleep on the involved side. Pain can be palpated in the subacromial space. If a full-thickness tear has been sustained, atrophy may be apparent in the supraspinatus or infraspinatus fossa. Depending on the extent of the injury (Box 13.2), positive results may be elicited in the drop

Box 13.2   Stages of Impingement Syndrome

Stage 1
- Condition typically is seen in individuals younger than 25 years and is reversible.
- Localized hemorrhage and edema are present in the supraspinatus tendon.
- Minimal pain is felt with activity, but no restriction or weakness of motion occurs.
- Atrophy of the rotator cuff muscles may be present.

Stage 2
- Condition typically is seen in individuals between 25 and 40 years of age.
- Marked reactive tendinitis is present, with significant pain felt between 70 and 120° abduction.
- Inflammation may affect the biceps brachii tendon and subacromial bursa, leading to thickening and fibrotic changes in the structures.
- Limited range of motion is found in external rotation and abduction.
- Possible clicking sounds are heard on resisted adduction and internal rotation.

Stage 3
- The individual has a history of chronic, long-term shoulder pain with significant weakness.
- Rotator cuff tear usually is less than 1 cm.
- Prominent capsular laxity with multidirectional instability is seen.
- Noticeable atrophy of the supraspinatus and infraspinatus muscles occurs.
- Arthroscopy may show a damaged labrum.

Stage 4
- Rotator cuff tear is greater than 1 cm.

arm test, empty can test, Neer shoulder impingement test, and anterior impingement test (Hawkins-Kennedy test).

Management

Initially, conservative treatment involves restricting motion below 90° of abduction, cryotherapy, NSAIDs, pain-relieving medication, 1 to 2 weeks of rest, activity modification, and occasionally, steroid injection. Ultrasound, electrical muscle stimulation, interferential therapy, and heat can supplement treatment. Overall, NSAIDs and subacromial steroid injections are effective in the short-term treatment of shoulder pain (18). Concern exists, however, that delaying repair of a supraspinatus tear makes the eventual repair harder or even impossible; initial surgical repair generally has a good outcome (19).

Mobility should be maintained with mild stretching exercises, particularly in external rotation at 90, 135, and 180° of abduction. Pendulum exercises with abduction and forward flexion up to 90°, rope-and-pulley exercises in flexion, and T-bar exercises in flexion and external rotation should be initiated early during the rehabilitation process. In addition, muscles of the rotator cuff as well as muscles that perform scapular retraction, depression, and rotation should be strengthened. In terms of strength about the shoulder, adduction should be the strongest, followed by extension, flexion, abduction, internal rotation, and external rotation. Exercises such as pull-ups or push-ups should be avoided during the early stages of rehabilitation, because they can impinge on the rotator cuff and complicate the condition. Field Strategy 13.3 outlines the management of an impingement syndrome.

Swimmers present a special problem, because many strokes use adduction and internal rotation with excessive propulsion forces. Because of fatigue and lack of coordination in the scapular muscles, this motion may allow subclinical anterior subluxations to occur, resulting in damage to the glenoid labrum. This anterior lesion may be frayed but not detached, resulting in a roughened leading edge that may mechanically catch during overhead motions. As such, swimmers may feel a snapping sensation, clicking, or sense that the shoulder is "going out" when moving through the pull phase of the stroke. Occasionally, a defect or crepitus in the supraspinatus tendon may be palpated just anterior to the acromion process when the arm is extended at the GH joint. Pain also can be palpated anteriorly over the coracoacromial ligament, laterally at the insertion of the supraspinatus, posteriorly at the insertion of the infraspinatus and teres minor, or over the long head of the biceps

FIELD STRATEGY 13.3

Management of an Impingement Injury

- Use cryotherapy initially; later, replace with moist heat therapy twice a day.
- Electrical muscle stimulation, interferential current, and transcutaneous electrical nerve stimulation may be helpful for pain management.
- Use ultrasound and nonsteroidal anti-inflammatory drugs to reduce inflammation.
- Use selective rest. Concentrate on motions that do not cause pain for 4 to 6 weeks. Avoid abduction above 90°.
- Evaluate skill technique, and correct movements that produce shoulder stress.
- Eliminate partner stretching, overhead training, and for swimmers, use of hand paddles.
- Wand and T-bar exercises can improve sport-specific mobility but should not encourage hypermobility.
- Perform pain-free isometric and elastic band exercises at least two to three times daily to maintain muscle tone. Use low weights and high repetitions.
- Strengthen the lateral rotators (i.e., infraspinatus and teres minor) to control superior displacement of the humeral head.
- After 4 to 6 weeks, incorporate isokinetic exercises at high speeds and elastic band exercises in diagonal patterns.
- Begin a gradual return to activity, as long as the symptoms do not recur.

tendon. Atrophy of the shoulder muscles with subsequent weakness in the supraspinatus and biceps brachii may be present as well. Because rest translates into detraining, other steps may need to be taken to allow continued activity. The intensity and quantity of training need to be reduced and paddle work eliminated. Stroke mechanics should be assessed to determine if changes are needed to reduce shoulder stress.

Bursitis

Bursitis is not generally an isolated condition; rather, it is associated with other injuries, such as an impingement syndrome and preexisting degenerative changes in the rotator cuff. The large subacromial bursa is a common site of injury in swimmers and in baseball, softball, and tennis players. Located between the coracoacromial ligament and the underlying supraspinatus muscle, this bursa provides the shoulder with some inherent gliding ability. During an overhead throwing motion, this bursa can become impinged in the subacromial space.

Signs and Symptoms

Frequently, sudden shoulder pain is reported during initiation and acceleration of the throwing motion. Point tenderness can be elicited on the anterior and lateral edges of the acromion process. A painful arc exists between 70 and 120° of passive abduction. Inability to sleep, especially on the affected side, occurs because of forced scapular protraction that leads to further impingement of the bursa. Pain often is referred to the distal deltoid attachment.

Management

Standard acute protocol is followed by referral to a physician. A physician may inject a corticosteroid solution into the subacromial space to relieve the symptoms. In addition, other underlying conditions, such as a rotator cuff tear, impingement syndrome, or bicipital tendinitis, must be ruled out. Treatment is symptomatic and is the same as for a rotator cuff strain or impingement syndrome.

Bicipital Tendinitis

Injury to the biceps brachii tendon often occurs from repetitive overuse during rapid overhead movements involving excessive elbow flexion and supination activities, such as those performed by racquet-sport players, shot-putters, baseball/softball pitchers, football quarterbacks, swimmers, and javelin throwers. Irritation of the tendon occurs as it passes back and forth in the intertubercular (bicipital) groove of the humerus. The tendon may partially sublux because of laxity of the traverse humeral ligament, a poorly developed lesser tubercle, or both. A direct blow to the tendon or tendon sheath can lead to bicipital tenosynovitis. Anterior impingement syndrome associated with overhead rotational activity also may damage the tendon.

Signs and Symptoms

Pain and tenderness is present over the bicipital groove when the shoulder is internally and externally rotated. In internal rotation, the pain stays medial; in external rotation, the pain is located in the midline or just lateral to the groove. Pain also may be elicited when the tendon is passively stretched in extreme shoulder extension with the elbow extended and the forearm pronated. Resisted supination of a flexed elbow while externally rotating the shoulder (e.g., Yergason's test) increases pain, as does forward shoulder flexion of the extended, supinated elbow (e.g., Speed's test).

Management

Treatment involves restriction of rotational activities that exacerbate symptoms. Because of potential vascular impingement of the biceps tendon when the shoulder is at the side, the arm should be propped or wedged into slight abduction if immobilized in a sling. During the early stages of the condition, cryotherapy, NSAIDs, ultrasound, electrical muscle stimulation, or interferential therapy can control inflammation. Icing before and after activity should be combined with a gradual program of stretching and strengthening as soon as pain subsides. Patients experiencing bicipital tendinitis secondary to impingement should avoid horizontal abduction exercises, which can aggravate symptoms (20).

Biceps Tendon Rupture

Prolonged tendinitis can make the tendon vulnerable to forceful rupture during repetitive overhead motions, as commonly are seen in swimmers, or during forceful flexion activities against excessive resistance, as are seen in weight lifters or gymnasts. The rupture occurs as a result of the avascular portion of the proximal long head of the biceps tendon constantly passing over the head of the humerus during arm motion. This condition often is seen in degenerative tendons in older individuals and in individuals who have had corticosteroid injections into the tendon.

Signs and Symptoms

The individual often hears and feels a snapping sensation and experiences intense pain. Ecchymosis and a visible, palpable defect can be seen in the muscle belly when the individual flexes the biceps. If the muscle mass moves distally as a result of a proximal long head rupture, a "Popeye" appearance clearly is visible. Partial ruptures may produce only slight muscular deformity but are still associated with pain and weakness in elbow flexion and supination. Distal biceps rupture results in marked weakness with flexion and supination of the forearm.

Management

Standard acute care protocol is followed by immediate referral to a physician. Surgical repair usually is not suggested for noncompetitive individuals or older patients, because return to normal physical activity can occur after completing an appropriate rehabilitation program. Surgical repair and fixation is indicated, however, for competitive individuals to restore elbow flexion and forearm supination strength needed for participation in competitive sports.

Thoracic Outlet Compression Syndrome

Thoracic outlet compression syndrome is a condition in which nerves and/or vessels become compressed in the proximal neck or axilla (Fig. 13.14). This condition has two clearly defined forms. One is a neurologic syndrome, accounting for approximately 90% of all cases, that involves the lower trunk of the brachial plexus and is caused by abnormal nerve stretch or compression. Another is a vascular form that involves the subclavian artery and vein and is more common in men than in women (21). Thoracic outlet compression syndrome often is aggravated in activities that require overhead rotational stresses while muscles are loaded, such as weight lifting and swimming. Disorders associated with thoracic outlet syndrome include:

- Compression of the medial cord of the brachial plexus
- Compression of the subclavian artery and vein
- Cervical rib syndrome
- Scalenus anterior syndrome
- Hyperabduction syndrome
- Costoclavicular space syndrome
- Poor posture with drooping shoulders

Signs and Symptoms

If a nerve is compressed, an aching pain, pins-and-needles sensation, or numbness in the side or back of the neck extends across the shoulder down the medial arm to the ulnar aspect of the hand. Weakness in grasp and atrophy of the hand muscles also may be present. If arterial or venous vessels are compressed, signs and symptoms vary depending on the specific structure being obstructed. Blockage of the subclavian vein, for example, produces edema, stiffness (especially in the hand), and venous engorgement of the arm with cyanosis (Fig. 13.15). If untreated, this may result in thrombophlebitis. The individual may present these signs and symptoms several hours after a bout of intense exercise. Occlusion of the subclavian artery results in a rapid onset of coolness, numbness in the entire arm, and fatigue after exertional overhead activity. The radial pulse may be obliterated

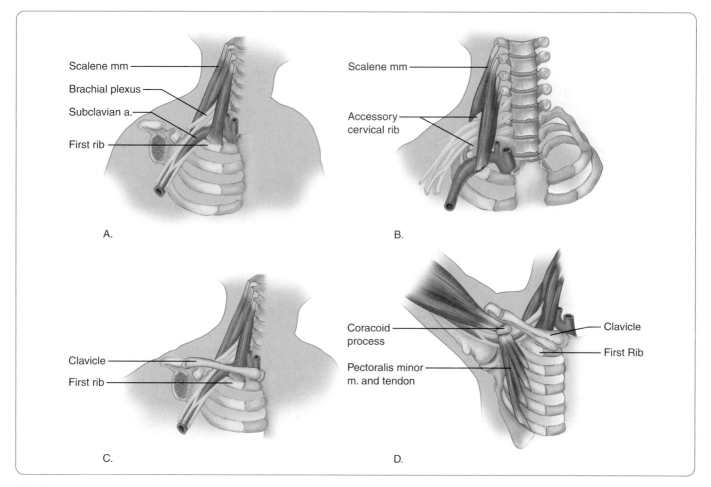

FIGURE 13.14 Location and etiology of thoracic outlet syndrome. A, Scalenus anterior syndrome. **B,** Cervical rib syndrome. **C,** Costoclavicular space syndrome. **D,** Hyperabduction syndrome.

FIGURE 13.15 Thoracic outlet syndrome. This 20-year-old pitcher presented with "burning" pain, swelling, and erythema of the right arm. His right arm has distended veins, which stemmed from right subclavian vein thrombosis.

while performing the Adson test, Allen test, or costoclavicular syndrome (military brace) test. A detailed history is needed, and it is essential to evaluate the cervical spine, shoulder, elbow, and hand for evidence of neural compression. Instability of the shoulder also should be ruled out. In addition, a postural assessment should be conducted.

Management

Immediate referral to a physician is necessary for more extensive assessment to rule out serious vascular involvement. Conservative treatment involves assessing muscle strength and posture. Noted deficits should lead to an appropriate retraining program to develop strength and muscle balance in the shoulder girdle and facilitate maintenance of a corrected posture. If the condition was precipitated by a sudden increase in activity, treatment involves anti-inflammatory drugs, activity modification, and reassessment of the training program. Return to full activity may occur after ROM and strength in the shoulder musculature have been regained.

A ▶ *Swimmers present a special problem with regard to impingement, because many strokes use adduction and internal rotation with excessive propulsion forces. Because of fatigue and lack of coordination in the scapular muscles, this motion may allow subclinical anterior subluxations to occur, resulting in damage to the glenoid labrum. This anterior lesion may be frayed but not detached, resulting in a roughened leading edge that may mechanically catch during overhead motions.*

FRACTURES

Q ▶ *How can atraumatic osteolysis of the distal clavicle occur?*

Most fractures to the shoulder region result from a fall on the point of the shoulder, from rolling over onto the top of the shoulder, or from indirect forces caused by falling on an outstretched arm. Clavicular fractures are more common than fractures to the scapula and proximal humerus, with nearly 80% occurring in the midclavicular region.

Clavicular Fractures

Because of the S-shaped configuration of the clavicle, it is highly susceptible to compression forces caused by a blow or fall on the point of the shoulder, a direct blow to the bone by an opponent or object, or a fall on an outstretched arm. Activities that have a high incidence of clavicular injury include ice hockey, football, the martial arts, lacrosse, gymnastics, weight lifting, wrestling, racquetball, squash, and bicycling.

Osteolysis of the Distal Clavicle

Atraumatic osteolysis of the distal clavicle is an overuse injury resulting from repetitive microtrauma. It also has been described as a sequelae following traumatic injury to the distal clavicle or AC joint. The condition is seen most often in weight lifting, but it also has been seen in sports where cross-training is popular and in younger individuals who weight train year-round for higher-level sports (22). During repetitive activity, subsequent bone resorption causes cystic and erosive changes, and bone remodeling cannot occur because of the continual stress to the area.

SIGNS AND SYMPTOMS. Individuals usually complain of a dull ache over the AC joint, which often is worse at the beginning of an exercise period. Pain and a sense of weakness during abduction and flexion of the arm also are noted. This pain and weakness may occur from weeks to years after the actual injury (23). Palpable pain, crepitus, and swelling is present over the distal clavicle. Increased pain is experienced with horizontal adduction of the arm; any abduction of the arm greater than 90° is extremely painful. Radiographs tend to show osteopenia and lucency in the distal clavicle.

MANAGEMENT. The treatment of choice is conservative but requires patient compliance. Rest, particularly from weight training, and anti-inflammatory drugs are recommended. Surgical resection of the distal clavicle may be necessary depending on the patient's functional demands and symptoms (22,23).

Traumatic Clavicular Fractures

Nearly 80% of traumatic fractures occur in the middle third of the clavicle (15). The sternocleidomastoid muscle pulls the proximal bone fragment upward, allowing the distal shoulder to collapse downward and medially from the force of gravity and the pull of the pectoralis major muscle.

SIGNS AND SYMPTOMS. Swelling, ecchymosis, and a deformity may be visible and palpable at the fracture site. Greenstick fractures, which typically are seen in adolescents, also produce a noticeable deformity. Pain occurs with any shoulder motion and may radiate into the trapezius area. In older adults, fractures of the distal clavicle may involve tears of the coracoclavicular ligament, producing an increased deformity. Although rare, complications may arise if bony fragments penetrate local arteries or nerves.

FIGURE 13.16 Figure-eight clavicular straps. A, Anterior view. **B,** Posterior view.

MANAGEMENT. Immediate treatment involves immobilization in a sling and swathe. Following assessment by the physician, a figure-eight brace or strapping often is used to pull the shoulder backward and upward for 4 to 6 weeks in young adults and for 6 or more weeks in older adults (Fig. 13.16). Although this immobilization prevents movement in nearly all planes, it does not prevent scapular elevation. As a result, healing may be delayed, and excessive callus formation may occur at the fracture site. This bump tends to remodel, to some degree, over a period of years but may never completely disappear. Following immobilization, gentle isometric and mobilization exercises should begin with gradual return to activity.

Scapular Fractures

Scapular fractures may involve the body of the scapula, spine of the scapula, acromion process, coracoid process, or GH joint. Avulsion fractures to the coracoid process result from direct trauma or from forceful contraction of the pectoralis minor or short head of the biceps brachii. Fractures to the glenoid area are associated with shoulder subluxations and dislocations. In this case, treatment is dictated by the shoulder dislocation rather than by the fracture and often requires open reduction and internal fixation or shoulder reconstruction.

Signs and Symptoms

Most fractures result in minimal displacement and exhibit localized hemorrhage, pain, and tenderness. The individual is reluctant to move the injured arm and prefers to maintain it in adduction. Arm abduction is painful. It is critical to note any signs or symptoms that would suggest an underlying pulmonary injury (e.g., pneumothorax or hemothorax).

Management

The arm should be immobilized immediately in a sling and swathe, and ice should be applied to minimize hematoma formation. The individual should be referred to a physician. Complications may arise from scarring and adhesions in the muscles overlying the scapula. Subsequently, the muscles in the region must compensate for the limited scapular motion, leading to overuse injuries. The development of adhesions in the area can be reduced with an early program of passive and active stretching exercises, usually within 2 weeks. Early mobilization also is important to avoid loss of ROM, which could lead to a frozen shoulder.

Epiphyseal and Avulsion Fractures

Epiphyseal centers around the shoulder region remain unfused for a longer span of time than typically is seen at other epiphyseal sites. For example, the medial clavicular growth plate does not close until approximately 25 years of age, and this situation often is misdiagnosed as a SC subluxation/dislocation. The proximal humeral epiphysis does not close until 18 to 21 years of age. An epiphyseal fracture at this site, called **little league shoulder**, often is caused by repetitive medial rotation and adduction traction forces placed on the shoulder during pitching (Fig. 13.17). Catchers also may sustain this fracture, because they throw the ball as hard and as often as pitchers, but with less of a windup. The injury usually occurs during the deceleration and follow-through phases of throwing or pitching.

Avulsion fractures to the coracoid process can be seen in a young individual when forceful, repetitive throwing places too much stress on the growth plate. Fractures of the greater and lesser tubercle often are associated with anterior and posterior GH dislocations, respectively. When the tubercle cannot be maintained in a stable position, open reduction and internal fixation often are required.

Signs and Symptoms

In an epiphyseal fracture, the individual complains of acute shoulder pain when attempting to throw hard, which if ignored may result in an acute displacement of the weakened physis. Pain may be elicited by deep palpation in the axilla. In an avulsion fracture, pain can be elicited by deep palpation over the specific bony landmark.

Management

The arm should be immobilized in a sling and swathe, and ice should be applied to control pain and swelling. Immediate referral to a physician for further care is warranted. Radiographs are necessary to view the widened epiphyseal line and demineralization. Treatment is conservative, with symptoms disappearing after 3 to 4 weeks of rest. The condition may recur if activity is resumed too quickly.

■■■ **FIGURE 13.17 Epiphyseal fracture to the proximal humeral growth center.**

Humeral Fractures

Humeral fractures result from violent compression forces from a direct blow, a fall on the upper arm, or a fall on an outstretched hand with the elbow extended. The surgical neck is the most common site for proximal humeral fractures and may display an appearance similar to that of a dislocation (Fig. 13.18).

Signs and Symptoms

Pain, swelling, hemorrhage, discoloration, inability to move the arm, inability to supinate the forearm, and possible paralysis may be present. The arm often is held splinted against the body.

Management

The arm should be immobilized in a sling and swathe, and ice should be applied to control pain and swelling. Immediate referral to a physician for further care is warranted. In some settings, this injury may warrant activation of the emergency action plan.

Up to 85% of proximal humeral fractures can be treated nonoperatively (15). For cases in which the fracture is impacted, closed reduction allows early mobilization after 3 to 4 weeks of immobilization. Early complications of a fracture to the proximal humerus include brachial plexus injury and/or vascular injury. Late complications include shoulder stiffness, malunion, nonunion, avascular necrosis, and myositis ossificans.

■■■ **FIGURE 13.18 Fracture to the surgical neck of the humerus.**

(A) *A traumatic osteolysis of the distal clavicle is an overuse injury resulting from repetitive microtrauma. It also has been described as a sequelae following traumatic injury to the distal clavicle or AC joint. During repetitive activity, subsequent bone resorption causes cystic and erosive changes, and bone remodeling cannot occur because of the continual stress imposed on the point.*

ASSESSMENT OF SHOULDER CONDITIONS

(Q) *A collegiate swimmer reports to the athletic training room with anterior pain in the right shoulder. How should the assessment of this injury progress to determine the extent and severity of injury?*

 See *Field Strategy: Shoulder Evaluation,* available on the companion website at thePoint.

The shoulder complex is a complicated region to assess because of the number of important structures that are located in such a small area. Furthermore, the biomechanical demands on each structure during overhead motion are not fully understood, so identification of all injured structures is difficult. As a result, each joint must be methodically assessed to determine any limitation of function. Improper biomechanical skill technique is a leading cause of many acute and overuse injuries at the shoulder. Assessment of the individual's activity-specific techniques may determine if improper technique contributed to the injury. By correcting minor mechanical flaws in technique and identifying deficits in flexibility and strength, many shoulder injuries can be prevented. It also is important to remember pain may be referred to the shoulder from the cervical region, heart, spleen, lungs, and other internal organs.

HISTORY

(Q) *The injury assessment of the swimmer should begin with a history. What questions need to be asked to identify the cause and extent of this injury?*

See *Field Strategy: Developing a History of the Injury,* available on the companion website at thePoint, for specific questions related to the shoulder region.

Questions about a shoulder injury should focus on the current primary complaint, past injuries to the region, and other factors that may have contributed to the current problem (e.g., referred pain, alterations in posture, change in technique, or overuse). Many conditions may be related to family history, age, improper biomechanical execution of skills, and recent changes in training programs. Because the shoulder and upper arm are common sites for referred pain from orthopaedic or visceral origins, a complete examination of the cervical spine, thorax, and abdomen may be indicated, particularly when the individual presents a vague history of injury to the shoulder girdle.

(A) *The swimmer should be asked questions that address type of pain, changes in training regimen, strokes that are most painful, previous injuries and their treatment, and any medications being taken for the current injury.*

OBSERVATION AND INSPECTION

(Q) *The history reveals a chronic injury. The swimmer reports a feeling of subluxation during the power phase of the crawl and butterfly stroke. The swimmer also complains of an inability to sleep on the right side of the body. Explain the observation component in the ongoing assessment of the swimmer.*

On-site (e.g., field or court) assessment may be somewhat limited, because uniforms and protective equipment may obscure the region from observation and assessment. The examiner may need to slide their hands under the protective pads to palpate the region and determine the presence of a possible fracture or major ligament damage. If necessary, the pads could be cut and gently removed to expose the area more fully. Following the initial examination, the individual may need to be removed from the on-site location to complete a more comprehensive assessment in the examination room.

A postural examination, looking for faulty posture or congenital abnormalities that could place additional strain on the anatomical structures, should be completed. The individual should be viewed from the anterior, lateral, and posterior views. The entire shoulder and arm should be as exposed as possible during the examination.

From an anterior view, the position of the head should be noted. A head that is tilted or rotated may suggest a muscle spasm, pressure on a cervical nerve root, or stretching of the cervical nerves. Shoulder height should be observed. A painful shoulder often is held in an elevated position. The height and symmetry of the SC joints, clavicle, and AC joints also should be observed. An elevated distal clavicle at the AC joint (step deformity) indicates an AC sprain. It is important to note the symmetry of the deltoid musculature; if the deltoid musculature on one side appears to be flattened, the individual may have a dislocated GH joint.

The musculature on the posterior chest wall should be inspected for symmetry. Superficial muscles usually are easily identifiable. Atrophy of the supraspinatus or infraspinatus muscles results in the spine of the scapulae being more pronounced. The position of the scapulae on the chest wall should then be noted. The base of the spine of the scapula should be at the T_4 level, and the inferior pole of the scapula should be at the T_7 level. An undescended scapula (i.e., Sprengel's deformity) is a congenital deformity that may affect one or both scapulae. The medial borders should be an equal distance from the vertebral spinous processes. The presence of medial elevation off the chest wall should be noted. In a chronic or acutely weakened serratus anterior muscle, the affected side usually is depressed (i.e., lower on the chest wall), protracted (i.e., further from the vertebral spinous processes), and elevated (i.e., winged) off the chest wall, each reflecting a weakened muscle in spasm or one with decreased flexibility.

From a lateral view, it is important to examine for possible thoracic kyphosis or the shoulders being slumped forward, indicating weakness of the erector spinae muscles and tightness in the pectoral muscles. The presence of scoliosis or lordosis also should be noted.

The position of the arm should be observed, and it is important to note possible splinting of the arm alongside the body or the arm hanging limp at the side. The shape and contour of the biceps brachii should be inspected as well. A ruptured tendon is characterized by the muscle belly bulging away from the involved structure.

Inspection should be performed at the specific injury site, looking for obvious deformity, swelling, discoloration, symmetry, hypertrophy, muscle atrophy, or previous surgical incisions. The affected limb should always be compared to the unaffected limb.

> See *Field Strategy: Postural Assessment of the Shoulder Region,* available on the companion website at thePoint, for specific areas in which to focus for this region.

A ▶ *Observation of the swimmer should include a postural assessment of the upper body. In addition, the injury site should be inspected for swelling, discoloration, deformity, muscle hypertrophy or atrophy, and other signs of existing or previous trauma.*

PALPATION

Q ▶ *Observation of the swimmer reveals slight kyphosis. Otherwise, the individual has no abnormal findings. Explain the palpation for this injury.*

Bilateral palpation can determine temperature, swelling, point tenderness, crepitus, deformity, muscle spasm, and cutaneous sensation. Increased skin temperature could indicate inflammation or infection; decreased skin temperature could indicate a reduction in circulation. Swelling should be differentiated between localized, extra-articular swelling and joint effusion. In the shoulder, intra-articular swelling prevents full adduction of the arm against the body. Crepitus may indicate an inflamed subacromial bursa, bicipital tenosynovitis, or irregular articular surface. Vascular pulses can be taken at the radial and ulnar arteries in the wrist, the brachial artery on the medial arm, or the axillary artery in the armpit.

Fractures can be assessed through palpation of pain at the fracture site, compression of the humeral head against the glenoid fossa, compression along the long axis of the humerus, percussion on a specific bony landmark, or use of a tuning fork. If a fracture or dislocation is suspected, circulatory and neural integrity distal to the site should be assessed immediately.

In general, when palpating the shoulder region, the examiner should stand behind the individual to begin bilateral palpation, which should move from proximal to distal. The areas that are anticipated to be most painful should be palpated last. The following structures should be palpated:

Anterior

1. Sternocleidomastoid muscle.

2. Sternoclavicular joint, interclavicular ligament, SC ligament, and sternal end of the clavicle.

3. Clavicle and costoclavicular ligament.

4. Acromioclavicular joint, acromion process, and AC ligament.

5. Coracoid process, pectoralis minor, short head of the biceps brachii, and coracoacromial ligament.

6. Pectoralis major and anterior deltoid muscle.

7. Greater tuberosity and the distal attachments of the supraspinatus, infraspinatus, and teres minor.

8. Biceps brachii muscle and tendon. The bicipital groove should be palpated with the arm in external rotation. The lesser tubercle is medial to the groove where the subscapularis is attached.

9. Subacromial bursa and supraspinatus tendon. The arm should be in a position of extension.

Lateral

1. Middle deltoid muscle and greater tubercle.

2. Glenohumeral capsule.

Posterior

1. Posterior deltoid and trapezius muscles.

2. Spine of the scapula, medial and lateral borders, and inferior angle.

3. Rhomboid muscles, latissimus dorsi, serratus anterior, levator scapulae, and scaleni.

 Bilateral palpation includes bony and soft-tissue structures of the shoulder for point tenderness, swelling deformity, crepitus, sensation, and other signs of trauma.

PHYSICAL EXAMINATION TESTS

Palpation reveals tenderness along the anterior and posterior GH joint. A click is felt during active shoulder abduction and external rotation. What anatomical structures could be involved with this injury, and what injury should be suspected?

The individual should be placed in a comfortable position for the physical examination. Depending on the history, some tests are compulsory, whereas others may be used to confirm or exclude suspected injury or pathology. Caution should be used while moving through the assessment, and bilateral comparison should always be performed.

Functional Tests

The arm and shoulder may act as an open kinetic chain when the hand is free to move or as a closed kinetic chain when the hand is fixed to a relatively immovable object. Depending on the activity-specific skills performed by the individual and when the pain occurs, the components of the kinetic chain can have different effects on the shoulder. The first movements to be performed are active movements.

Active Movements

Active movements may be performed in a seated or prone position. The movements that are expected to be most painful should be performed last. Because pain frequently is referred from the cervical region into the shoulder, active ROM should be performed initially at the neck. Neck flexion, extension, rotation, and lateral flexion should be assessed for fluid motion and presence of pain. If pain is elicited on active motion at the neck, a full neck evaluation should be completed.

If findings are significant, the neck should be immobilized in a cervical collar, and the emergency action plan, including summoning emergency medical services, should be activated.

If no problems are noted during neck movement, the shoulder evaluation should continue. The individual should perform gross movement patterns at the shoulder, and the arms should be viewed from an anterior and a posterior view. When the examiner is standing behind the individual, it is important to note if the scapula and humerus move together in a freely coordinated motion. The scapula should not move until the humerus is elevated to at least 30°.

To facilitate active movement, Apley's scratch test can be used to measure gross movement patterns at the shoulder and arm (Fig. 13.19). The advantage of these simple tests is that they quickly assess bilateral symmetry in gross motor movements. Any deficit can be easily seen and investigated in further detail.

The motions that should be assessed and the normal ROM for each are as follows:

- Shoulder abduction (170–180°)

- Shoulder flexion (160–180°)

- Shoulder extension (50–60°)

- Lateral or external rotation (80–90°)

- Medial or internal rotation (60–100°)

- Adduction (50–70°)

- Horizontal abduction/adduction (130°)

- Upward/downward rotation of the scapula

Goniometry measurements for the GH joint are illustrated in Fig. 13.20.

■■■■ FIGURE 13.19 **Apley's scratch test. A,** Medial rotation and adduction. The individual reaches in front of the head to touch the opposite shoulder. **B,** Medial rotation, extension, and adduction. The individual reaches behind the back to touch the inferior angle of the opposite scapula. **C,** Abduction, flexion, and lateral rotation. The individual reaches behind the head to touch the superior angle of the opposite scapula.

■■ ■ FIGURE 13.20 **Goniometry measurements. A,** Shoulder flexion. Align the proximal arm with the midaxillary line of the thorax with the fulcrum close to the acromion process. Align the distal arm along the humerus in line with the lateral epicondyle of the humerus. **B,** Shoulder extension. Use the same landmarks as for shoulder flexion. **C,** Shoulder abduction. The proximal arm is parallel to the midline of the sternum with the fulcrum close to the acromion process. Align the distal arm with the humerus using the medial epicondyle for reference. **D,** Lateral rotation. Flex the elbow at 90° with the fulcrum centered over the olecranon process. The proximal arm is placed perpendicular to the floor, with the distal arm aligned with the olecranon process and ulnar styloid process. **E,** Medial rotation. Use the same landmarks as for lateral rotation.

Passive Range of Motion

If the individual is able to perform full ROM during active movements, gentle pressure should be applied at the extremes of motion to determine end feel. The normal end feels are as follows:

- **Tissue stretch**—shoulder flexion, extension, lateral rotation, medial rotation, abduction, and horizontal abduction

- **Tissue approximation**—shoulder adduction

- **Tissue stretch or approximation**—horizontal adduction of the shoulder

- **Bone-to-bone or tissue stretch**—abduction of the shoulder

Resisted Muscle Testing

The hip and trunk should be stabilized during muscle testing to prevent any muscle substitution. The testing begins with the examiner placing the muscle on a stretch. In moving through the various motions, the examiner should apply gentle resistance throughout the full ROM. Motion should be assessed several times to note any weakness or fatigue. A painful arc is a common finding at the shoulder. As such, it is important to assess full ROM and to note if movement through an isolated ROM is particularly painful. Any sudden or jarring motions should be avoided, because this may lead to undue pain. Any lag or muscle weakness should be noted. Muscle actions that may cause extreme pain should be delayed until the final phase of muscle testing. Figure 13.21 demonstrates

FIGURE 13.21 Manual muscle testing for the scapula. Myotomes are listed in parentheses. **A,** Elevation (C₄). **B,** Depression. **C,** Protraction. **D,** Retraction. Arrows indicate the direction the individual moves the scapula against applied resistance.

resisted scapular motions to be tested, and Figure 13.22 demonstrates GH and elbow motions to be tested.

Stress Tests

By this point in the assessment, the history, observation, palpation, and functional testing should have established a strong suspicion regarding the structures that may be damaged. In using stress tests, only those tests that are absolutely necessary should be performed (Table 13.6). In moving through the various tests, the examiner should begin with gentle stress and apply it several times to note any weakness or instability.

Test for Sternoclavicular Instability

The individual should be in a seated position while the examiner applies pressure to the medial clavicular head to force the clavicle downward, upward, anteriorly, and posteriorly to determine any instability or increased pain. Pain that is present in all movements may stem from a SC sprain, damage to the SC joint disk, or complete disruption of the joint capsule, which would indicate a possible dislocation or subluxation of the joint.

Tests for Acromioclavicular Joint Instability

ACROMIOCLAVICULAR INSTABILITY TEST. The examiner grasps the distal clavicle and applies pressure in all four directions to determine stability and any increase in pain. This is followed by compression of the AC joint, which is accomplished by applying pressure to the tip of the shoulder, to determine the presence of increased pain.

FIGURE 13.22 Manual muscle testing for the glenohumeral and elbow.
Myotomes are listed in parentheses. **A,** Flexion. **B,** Extension. **C,** Abduction (C_5).
D, Adduction. **E,** External or lateral rotation. **F,** Internal or medial rotation. **G,** Elbow
flexion (C_6). **H,** Elbow extension (C_7). Arrows indicate the direction the individual moves
against applied resistance.

TABLE 13.6 Common Stress and Special Tests Performed at the Shoulder

JOINT	TEST
Sternoclavicular joint	Sternoclavicular instability test
Acromioclavicular joint	Acromioclavicular instability test
	Piano key test
	Acromioclavicular distraction/ compression test
Glenohumeral instability, anterior	Apprehension test ("crank test")
	Relocation test
	Anterior load and shift test
Glenohumeral instability, posterior	Posterior load and shift test
	Posterior apprehension test
Glenohumeral instability, inferior	Sulcus sign
Labral lesions	Clunk test
	Compression rotation test
Impingement tests	Neer shoulder impingement test
	Anterior impingement test (Hawkins-Kennedy test)
Muscle tendon pathology	Serratus anterior weakness test
	Pectoralis major contracture test
	Lift-off test for subscapularis
	Drop arm test
	Empty can (Centinela) supraspinatus test
	Transverse humeral ligament test
	Yergason's test
	Speed's test
	Ludington test
Thoracic outlet syndrome	Adson's test
	Allen test
	Costoclavicular syndrome (military brace) test

PIANO KEY SIGN. If a step deformity is noted at the AC joint, the examiner should apply a downward pressure on the distal end of the clavicle. The pressure may produce a bobbing motion, which indicates damage to the coracoclavicular ligament.

ACROMIOCLAVICULAR DISTRACTION-COMPRESSION. If the AC joint is unstable, downward traction on the upper extremity leads to downward movement of the acromion process away from the clavicle. Assessment involves grasping the arm in one hand and applying steady downward traction while palpating the joint with the other hand (Fig. 13.23A). A positive test produces pain and/or joint movement. Horizontal adduction of the humerus across the chest compresses the AC joint and also leads to increased pain if the joint is injured (Fig. 13.23B).

FIGURE 13.23 Acromioclavicular testing. A, Acromioclavicular traction. **B,** Acromioclavicular compression. Arrows indicate the direction the examiner moves the arm.

Tests for Glenohumeral Joint Instability

APPREHENSION TEST ("CRANK TEST") FOR ANTERIOR INSTABILITY. This test involves positioning the individual in a supine position and then slowly abducting and externally rotating the individual's humerus (Fig. 13.24A). If the individual does not allow passive movement to the extremes of motion or shows apprehension in his or her facial expression, the test is considered to be positive for chronic anterior subluxation or dislocation of the GH joint. This motion should always be done slowly to prevent recurrence of a dislocation.

RELOCATION TEST FOR ANTERIOR INSTABILITY. Position for this test is identical to the apprehension test. If the individual demonstrates a positive apprehension test, the examiner slowly applies a posterior stress to the arm (Fig. 13.24B). The individual's apprehension and pain should diminish. In addition, further lateral rotation of the GH joint may be possible before the apprehension returns. This test is considered to be positive if pain decreases during the maneuver, even if the individual showed no apprehension. If the arm is released in the newly acquired range, any pain and forward translation of the humeral head indicates a positive sign. The resulting pain from this release procedure may be caused by anterior shoulder instability, labral lesion (i.e., Bankart or SLAP lesion), or bicipital tendinitis. The release should be performed slowly, because it may dislocate the joint, leading to distrust on the part of the patient. Lateral rotation should be released before the posterior stress is released.

ANTERIOR LOAD AND SHIFT TEST. While the individual is seated and the test arm is resting on the thigh, the examiner stands or sits slightly behind the individual and stabilizes the shoulder with one

FIGURE 13.24 Glenohumeral anterior instability. A, Apprehension or "crank" test. The examiner should apply gentle pressure in an abducted and laterally rotated position. **B,** Relocation test. The examiner applies abduction and lateral rotation combined with posterior translation of the humerus.

hand over the clavicle and scapula. The head of the humerus is grasped with the examiner's other hand, placing the thumb over the posterior humeral head and the fingers over the anterior humeral head (Fig. 13.25). The examiner then gently pushes the humerus into the glenoid to "seat" it properly in the glenoid fossa. This is the "load" portion of the test, and it is necessary for true translation to occur. If the load is not applied, movement is greater, and the "feel" is altered. While pushing the humeral head anteriorly (i.e., assessing anterior instability) or posteriorly (i.e., assessing posterior instability), the amount of translation should be noted. This is the "shift" portion of the test. Normally, the head translates 0 to 25% of the diameter of the humeral head. The test is considered to be positive if translation is between 25 and 50% and the head feels as if it is riding over the glenoid rim but spontaneously reduces.

FIGURE 13.25 Load and shift test. The humerus is compressed into the glenoid to "load" the humeral head. Subsequently, the examiner pushes the humeral head anteriorly or posteriorly, noting the amount of "shift" or translation.

POSTERIOR LOAD AND SHIFT TEST. In a posterior load and shift test, posterior translation of 50% of the humeral head is considered to be normal. Differences between the normal and injured sides should be bilaterally compared for the amount of translation and the ease with which that translation occurs. This comparison, along with the individual's symptoms, is considered to be more important than the amount of movement that occurs. If multidirectional instability is present, both anterior and posterior translation may be excessive on the affected side as compared to the normal side. The test also may be done in a supine position.

POSTERIOR APPREHENSION TEST. While the individual is supine, the arm is moved into forward flexion and internal rotation as a steady downward force is applied on the elbow to drive the humeral head posteriorly on the glenoid fossa (Fig. 13.26). While applying the axial load, the examiner horizontally adducts and medially rotates the arm. A positive test is indicated by apprehension, resistance to further motion, or reproduction of symptoms. Reproducing pain is more likely than apprehension to occur. A positive sign indicates a possible posterior dislocation.

SULCUS SIGN. The examiner applies traction to the humerus to determine the integrity of the supportive structures. If the space widens between the acromion process and humeral head, producing an indentation or "sulcus," the test is considered to be positive for inferior instability. In the sulcus test, only the humerus is distracted away from both the clavicle and scapula. In comparison, the AC distraction test involves distraction of both the humerus and scapula away from the clavicle.

Special Tests

A variety of special tests can be used for detecting shoulder injury or related pathology (e.g., labral lesions, impingement, muscle-tendon trauma, or thoracic outlet syndrome) (Table 13.6). In general, special tests occur across planes and are not graded.

Tests for Labral Lesions

CLUNK TEST. While the individual is supine, the examiner places one hand on the posterior aspect of the shoulder under the humeral head. Next, the humerus is grasped above the elbow, and the arm is fully abducted over the individual's head. The hand over the humeral head applies a slow push in an anterior direction while the other hand moves the humerus into lateral rotation (Fig. 13.27A). A positive test results in a clunk or grinding sound, indicating a tear of the labrum. This test also may cause apprehension if anterior instability is present.

FIGURE 13.26 Posterior apprehension test. The examiner applies a steady downward force on the elbow to displace the humeral head posteriorly on the glenoid fossa.

FIGURE 13.27 Glenoid labral pathology. A, Clunk test. Using the hand placed under the humeral head, the examiner applies an anterior force while the other hand rotates the humerus into lateral rotation. **B,** Compression rotation test. With the arm slightly abducted and the elbow flexed, the examiner applies a compression force along the long axis of the humerus while the other hand rotates the humerus medially and laterally.

COMPRESSION ROTATION TEST. The individual is supine, with the arm positioned at approximately 20° of abduction and the elbow flexed. The humerus is slowly compressed into the glenoid fossa by pushing on the elbow with one hand while the other hand rotates the humerus medially and laterally (Fig. 13.27B). If a snapping or catching sensation is present as the humeral head is felt, the test is considered to be positive for a labral tear (i.e., Bankart or SLAP lesion).

Tests for Shoulder Impingement

NEER SHOULDER IMPINGEMENT TEST. The individual is seated, and the arm is placed in anatomical position. First, the examiner stabilizes the posterior shoulder. Next, the examiner grasps the individual's arm at the elbow joint and passively moves the arm through forward flexion (Fig. 13.28A). The test is considered to be positive if pain occurs with motion, particularly near the end of the ROM. A positive test indicates impingement of the supraspinatus or the long head of the biceps tendon between the greater tuberosity of the humerus and acromion process or cora-coacromial arch.

FIGURE 13.28 Anterior impingement tests. A, Neer shoulder impingement test. The arm is internally rotated and forcibly flexed forward to jam the greater tuberosity against the anteroinferior surface of the acromion. **B,** Anterior impingement test. An alternative method is to forcibly, medially rotate the proximal humerus when the arm is forward flexed to 90°. (This also is known as the Hawkins-Kennedy impingement test.)

FIGURE 13.29 Pectoralis major contracture test. The individual begins by clasping both hands behind the head. The elbows are then slowly lowered to the table. A positive test, indicating a tight pectoralis major muscle, occurs if the elbows do not reach the table.

ANTERIOR IMPINGEMENT TEST (HAWKINS-KENNEDY TEST). This test involves internally rotating and abducting the humerus through shoulder flexion while depressing the scapula. This action forces the greater tubercle underneath the anteroinferior border of the acromion process. The arm is returned to 90° of abduction (with the elbow flexed at 90°) and then is horizontally adducted across the chest while maintaining internal rotation of the humerus (Fig. 13.28B). Pain or apprehension may indicate an overuse injury to the supraspinatus or biceps brachii tendon. This test also is called the Hawkins-Kennedy impingement test.

Tests for Muscle Tendon Pathology

SERRATUS ANTERIOR WEAKNESS. Weakness of the serratus anterior, often called winging of the scapula, is determined by having the individual perform a push-up against the wall. If the muscle is weak or the long thoracic nerve is injured, the medial border of the scapula pulls away from the chest wall.

PECTORALIS MAJOR CONTRACTURE TEST. The individual lies supine, with the hands clasped together behind the head. The individual is instructed to lower the arms until the elbows touch the examination table (Fig. 13.29). A positive test occurs if the elbows do not reach the table, indicating a tight pectoralis major muscle.

LIFT-OFF TEST FOR SUBSCAPULARIS. The individual stands with the dorsum of the hand on the lumbar region of the back. The individual is instructed to lift the hand away from the back (Fig. 13.30). An inability to perform this action indicates a lesion of the subscapularis muscle. Abnormal motion of the scapula during the test indicates scapular instability. If the medial border of the scapula wings during the test, the rhomboids also may be affected.

DROP ARM TEST. This test assesses the integrity of the supraspinatus muscle and tendon. The individual is positioned with the shoulder abducted to 90° with no humeral rotation. The individual is instructed to slowly lower the arm to the side. The test is positive if the arm does not lower smoothly or increased pain is felt during the motion.

An alternative test is to abduct the arm to 90° with no rotation. The individual is instructed to hold that position while the examiner applies downward resistance to the distal end of the humerus (Fig. 13.31A). A positive test is indicated if the individual is unable to maintain the arm in the abducted position.

FIGURE 13.30 Lift-off test. Failure to lift the hand away from the small of the back indicates a weakened subscapularis muscle, scapular instability, or weak rhomboids.

FIGURE 13.31 Supraspinatus testing. A, Drop arm test. The examiner instructs the patient to abduct the humerus to 90° and subsequently applies mild, downward pressure on the distal humerus. **B,** Empty can test. The patient horizontally adducts the arm approximately 30 to 60° with the humerus internally rotated. The examiner applies mild, downward pressure on the distal humerus.

EMPTY CAN (CENTINELA) TEST FOR SUPRASPINATUS PATHOLOGY. Both arms are positioned at 90° of abduction. The arms are then horizontally adducted approximately 30 to 60°, and the humerus is internally rotated, with the thumbs pointing downward ("empty can position") (Fig. 13.31B). The examiner applies a downward pressure proximal to the elbow. Pain and/or weakness should be assessed. The arms should rebound to the 90° abducted position. A positive test indicates a tear to the supraspinatus muscle or tendon.

TRANSVERSE HUMERAL LIGAMENT TEST. The individual is positioned with the shoulder in 90° of abduction and external rotation and the elbow flexed at 90°. The examiner places the fingers over the bicipital groove. A torn transverse humeral ligament is indicated by an audible and/or palpable snap, which may be accompanied by pain, as the arm is moved into internal rotation (Fig. 13.32).

YERGASON'S TEST FOR BICIPITAL TENDINITIS. The individual should be positioned with the arm stabilized against the body, the elbow flexed at 90°, and the forearm pronated. The examiner instructs the individual to supinate the forearm, flex the elbow, and externally rotate the humerus. Simultaneously, the examiner resists the motion with one hand while applying downward traction on the elbow with the other hand (Fig. 13.33A). The test is considered to be positive if pain is elicited over the bicipital groove or if the tendon snaps out of the groove.

SPEED'S TEST FOR BICIPITAL TENDINITIS. In this test, the tendon moves over the bone during movement rather than simply having tension applied to it. As such, it provides a more effective, accurate result than Yergason's test. The arm is supinated, with the elbow fully extended. The examiner places one hand over the bicipital groove and resists forward flexion of the arm with the other hand. A positive test results in tenderness over the groove (Fig. 13.33B).

LUDINGTON'S TEST FOR BICEPS BRACHII PATHOLOGY. The individual may sit or stand during this test. The individual's hands are placed on top of the head with the fingers interlocked. The examiner should stand behind the patient while palpating the long head of the biceps brachii tendon in the bicipital groove. The patient alternately contracts and relaxes the biceps brachii muscles

FIGURE 13.32 Transverse humeral ligament test. The patient is instructed to place the extended arm in 90° of abduction and external rotation. The examiner places his or her fingers over the bicipital groove and moves the arm into internal rotation. In a positive test, an audible or palpable snap, which may be accompanied by pain, occurs during internal rotation.

FIGURE 13.33 Bicipital tendinitis. A, Yergason's test. The examiner stabilizes the flexed arm against the body, with the forearm pronated. The patient is asked to supinate the forearm, flex the elbow, and externally rotate the humerus. The examiner applies resistance throughout the range of motion and, with the other hand, simultaneously applies downward traction on the elbow. **B,** Speed's test. The patient is instructed to supinate the hand, with the elbow fully extended. The examiner places one hand over the bicipital groove and resists forward flexion of the arm.

(Fig. 13.34). If no contraction or tension is palpated on one side, a rupture of the long head of the biceps brachii likely is present.

Tests for Thoracic Outlet Syndrome

ADSON'S TEST. This test begins by having the examiner palpate the radial pulse. Next, the individual is instructed to turn the head toward the affected shoulder and extend the head. The examiner then slowly extends and laterally rotates the humerus (Fig. 13.35A). The individual is instructed to take a deep breath and hold it. A diminished or absent pulse indicates a positive test, verifying occlusion of the subclavian artery between the anterior and middle scalene muscles. This test sometimes is referred to as the anterior scalene syndrome test.

ALLEN TEST. Similar to Adson's test, the examiner palpates the radial pulse while the individual abducts the shoulder, flexes the elbow to 90°, and looks toward the opposite shoulder (Fig. 13.35B). Next, the examiner instructs the individual to take a deep breath and hold it. A diminished or absent pulse indicates a positive test, suggesting that the pectoralis minor muscle is compressing the neurovascular bundle. It is important to note, however, that this test often produces false-positive results.

An alternative position, called the Halstead maneuver, is performed with the arm extended and the neck hyperextended and rotated to the opposite side. While palpating the radial pulse, the examiner applies a downward traction to the arm. An absent or diminished pulse indicates a positive test for thoracic outlet syndrome.

COSTOCLAVICULAR SYNDROME (MILITARY BRACE) TEST. The individual stands in a relaxed position. The examiner stands behind the individual and palpates the radial pulse. Next, the individual retracts the shoulders as if coming to military attention. The examiner then extends and abducts the arm to 30° while the individual hyperextends the neck

FIGURE 13.34 Ludington's test for biceps brachii pathology. The examiner stands behind the patient and palpates the long head of the biceps brachii while the patient contracts the biceps by applying force to the top of the head. The test is positive for rupture of the long head of the biceps brachii tendon if decreased or no tension is felt under the involved tendon.

FIGURE 13.35 Thoracic outlet compression syndrome. A, Adson's maneuver. The examiner extends and externally rotates the humerus while the individual extends the head. **B,** Allen test. The examiner abducts the shoulder and flexes the elbow while the individual looks toward the opposite shoulder. An alternative position is to extend the elbow and apply downward traction while the individual hyperextends the neck and rotates the head to the opposite side (Halstead maneuver).

(Fig. 13.36). If the radial pulse diminishes or disappears, it indicates that the subclavian artery is being blocked by the costoclavicular structures of the shoulder.

Neurologic Tests

Neurologic integrity can be assessed with the use of myotomes, reflexes, and cutaneous patterns that include both the segmental dermatomes and peripheral nerve patterns.

Myotomes

Isometric muscle testing should be performed in the following motions to test specific myotomes in the upper extremity:

FIGURE 13.36 Costoclavicular syndrome test. The individual retracts the shoulders as if coming to military attention. The arm is extended and abducted approximately 30° while the head and neck are hyperextended. If the radial pulse disappears, it indicates the subclavian artery is blocked by the costoclavicular structures in the shoulder.

- Scapular elevation (C_4)
- Shoulder abduction (C_5)
- Elbow flexion and/or wrist extension (C_6)
- Elbow extension and/or wrist flexion (C_7)
- Thumb extension and/or ulnar deviation (C_8)
- Abduction and/or adduction of the hand intrinsics (T_1)

These tests are demonstrated in Figures 13.21, 13.22, and 14.12.

Reflexes

Reflexes in the upper extremity include the biceps (C_5–C_6) and triceps (C_7). The biceps reflex is tested with the individual's arm flexed and supported by the examiner's forearm. The examiner's thumb is placed over the biceps tendon, and the thumb is struck with the reflex hammer using a quick, downward thrust (Fig. 13.37A). A normal response is slight elbow flexion.

The triceps reflex is tested with the individual's arm abducted and extended with the elbow flexed. The triceps tendon is placed on a slight stretch, and the triceps tendon is then tapped with the reflex hammer (Fig. 13.37B). A normal response is slight elbow extension.

FIGURE 13.37 **Reflex testing. A,** Biceps reflex (C_5, C_6). **B,** Triceps reflex (C_7).

Cutaneous Patterns

The segmental nerve dermatome patterns for the shoulder region are illustrated in Figure 13.38. The peripheral nerve cutaneous patterns are illustrated in Figure 13.39. Bilateral testing should be performed for altered sensation with sharp and dull touch by running the open hand and fingernails over the neck, shoulder, anterior and posterior chest walls, and both sides of the arms.

Activity-Specific Functional Tests

Occasionally, activity-specific functional movements are the only activities that reproduce signs and symptoms. Throwing a ball, performing a swimming stroke, doing the arm part of jumping jacks, or performing an overhead serve or spike may replicate the painful pattern. The examiner should look for smooth, coupled motion of the scapulothoracic and GH joints. Disharmony constitutes

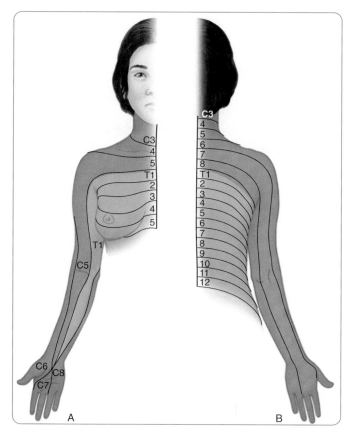

FIGURE 13.38 Dermatome patterns for the shoulder region. A, Anterior view. **B,** Posterior view.

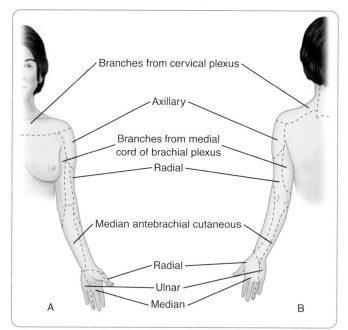

FIGURE 13.39 Cutaneous patterns for the peripheral nerves. A, Anterior view. **B,** Posterior view.

scapulothoracic dyskinesia, which is an inability to perform fluid, voluntary movements. Based on knowledge of the mechanics of the motion, it may be possible to narrow down the few definitive results of the assessment to determine the actual injury. These movements also commonly are used to determine when the individual can return to participation in activity. All functional patterns should be fluid and pain-free.

 The assessment of the swimmer suggests that the humerus, glenoid fossa, glenoid labrum, rotator cuff muscles, and anterior GH ligament could be involved with this injury. The swimmer should be suspected of having recurrent GH dislocations or subluxations.

REHABILITATION

The swimmer has a painful shoulder as a result of recurrent subluxations. What areas should be the focus of a rehabilitation program for this condition?

Rehabilitation program of the shoulder must address the specific needs of the individual. The program should relieve pain and muscle tension; restore motion and balance; develop strength, endurance, and power; and maintain cardiovascular fitness. Progress within any program is dictated by the type and severity of injury, amount of immobilization, and the supervising physician's treatment plan.

Restoration of Motion

Gentle ROM exercises, such as Codman's circumduction and pendulum swings, often are used immediately after injury. The exercise is performed by making small circles and a pendulum motion in the actions of flexion and extension, and horizontal abduction and adduction. The extent of ROM should increase as pain-free motion is regained. Exercises can progress to active, assistive T-bar exercises in the supine position (Field Strategy 13.4). In throwing activities, the ROM needed to

FIELD STRATEGY 13.4

Range of Motion Exercises for the Glenohumeral Joint

Wand and T-bar exercises. Hold the stretch for 5 to 10 seconds, and repeat 10 to 20 times per session. Initially, range of motion exercises can be performed two to three times daily.

1. **Supine shoulder flexion.** Grasp the wand with both hands palm-down at waist height. Raise the wand directly overhead, leading with the uninvolved arm until a stretch is felt in the involved shoulder. If an impingement syndrome is present, this exercise can be performed palm-up.
2. **Shoulder abduction.** Hold the wand with the involved arm palm-up and the uninvolved arm palm-down. With the uninvolved arm, push the wand sideward and upward toward the involved side until a stretch is felt in the involved shoulder.
3. **Shoulder·adduction/horizontal adduction.** Reverse the hand positions from Exercise 2. Pull the wand toward the uninvolved side until a stretch is felt in the involved shoulder.
4. **Shoulder internal/external rotation.** Keeping both palms down, abduct the shoulders, and flex the elbows. Move the wand upward toward the head, and then return to waist level.
5. **Shoulder horizontal abduction/adduction.** Keeping both palms down, push the wand across the body with the uninvolved arm, and then pull back across the body. Do not allow the trunk to twist.
6. **Supine external rotation.** Abduct the shoulder, and flex the elbow to 90°. Grip the T-bar in the hand on the involved arm. Use the opposite arm to push the involved arm into external rotation. Perform external rotation with the arm abducted at 135° and 180°.
7. **Supine internal rotation.** With the arms in the same position as in Exercise 6, use the uninvolved arm to push the involved arm into internal rotation.

adequately complete the cocking phase exceeds 90° of external rotation when the arm is abducted 90°. Special attention should be focused on regaining this additional ROM, but not to the point of hypermobility. A rope-and-pulley system can augment active, assistive GH flexion and abduction. Shoulder shrugs performed in three directions (i.e., superior, anterior, and posterior) can increase scapular ROM.

Restoration of Proprioception and Balance

Closed chain exercises can be performed after acute inflammation has been controlled. Shifting body weight from one hand to the other may be performed on a wall, tabletop, or unstable surface, such as a foam mat or biomechanical ankle platform system (BAPS) board. Push-ups and exercises in a frontal and sagittal plane can be performed on a ProFitter or slide board. Step-ups can be completed on a box, stool, or StairMaster. This activity can progress to stepping up and down on boxes of differing heights arranged so that the exercise is performed in diagonal patterns, circles, figure-eights, or any other pattern.

Use of free weights can develop balance, coordination, and skill in moving through diagonal patterns; however, it is imperative to include transference of proprioceptive training to the actual motions. For example, pertaining to the throwing motion, this training could involve a slow, deliberate rehearsal of the throwing motion that incorporates visual feedback through the use of mirrors or videotape. As the motion is performed, biomechanical errors are corrected. Once motion has been perfected, speed of movement and distance of throw are gradually increased.

Muscular Strength, Endurance, and Power

Gentle, resisted isometric exercises often can begin immediately after injury or surgery, even while the arm is immobilized. The exercises are initiated with the GH joint in a resting position. This is followed by application of a slow, mild overload in each of the various directions of shoulder movement. A disadvantage of isometric exercise is that strength gains are relatively specific to the joint angle at which the exercise is performed; therefore, isometric contractions must be performed at multiple positions to strengthen the joint. As the individual improves, a more moderate isometric overload is applied. Finally, a higher, rapid, unexpected resistance is provided at various positions, including the end of the ROM.

When ROM approximates normal for the individual, open chain kinetic exercises can be performed in a prone, side-lying, supine, or standing position to add gravity as resistance (Field Strategy 13.5). A sandbag or dumbbell can be used for added resistance. The individual should complete 50 to 100 repetitions with a 1-pound weight and should not progress in resistance until 100 repetitions are achieved. Resistance should be limited to 5 pounds, because this decreases the chance of rotator cuff inflammation during the strengthening program. Careful attention should be directed to a potential painful arc of motion during concentric and eccentric contractions, because pain can further aggravate the injury. As such, the individual should work within a pain-free arc of motion with light resistance to the point of fatigue.

Muscular strength and endurance can be developed through PNF-resisted exercises in diagonal patterns to mimic functional skills or through surgical tubing used through a functional pattern. As strength improves, free-weight or machine-weight exercises for the upper body are incorporated. Many of these exercises are demonstrated in Field Strategy 13.2.

Plyometric exercises may involve catching a weighted ball using a quick, eccentric stretch of the muscle to facilitate a concentric contraction in throwing the ball. The exercise can progress through various one- and two-arm chest passes and overhead passes. A minitramp also can be used to do plyometric bounding push-ups.

Cardiovascular Fitness

Cardiovascular conditioning should be maintained throughout the rehabilitation program (see Chapter 8).

 Management of the swimmer's condition likely will involve rest and immobilization. As such, rehabilitation should focus on restoring shoulder motion, but it is important to avoid an

FIELD STRATEGY 13.5

Rehabilitation Exercises for the Shoulder Complex

Progressive exercises should begin when pain subsides.

Exercises should be controlled and focus on the line of movement.

Resistance should progress from gravity to light dumbbells or sandbags. The exercises listed in Field Strategy 13.2 should be progressively incorporated as tolerated.

1. **Side-lying medial and lateral rotation.** Maintaining the elbow in a flexed position, perform lateral and medial rotation.

2. **Prone horizontal abduction (90°).** Positioned with the arm hanging over the table and the hand rotated outward, raise the arm, and laterally rotate the humerus until it is parallel to the floor.

3. **Prone horizontal abduction (100°).** Positioned with the arm abducted at 100°, raise the arm, and laterally rotate the humerus.

4. **Prone flexion and extension.** With the hand rotated outward as far as possible, raise the arm forward into flexion. Repeat, moving the arm into extension.

5. **Prone medial and lateral rotation.** With the shoulder abducted 90° and the elbow flexed, perform lateral and medial rotation. Repeat in the supine position.

6. **Prone rows (scapular adduction).** With the shoulder abducted 90° and the elbow flexed, raise the arm off the table as if pinching the shoulder blades together. Do not raise the chest off the table.

7. **Wall push-ups and press-ups.**

aggressive flexibility program in extension, abduction, and external rotation. Strengthening exercises should progress from resisted isometric exercises to elastic band exercises below 90° of abduction. In particular, developing the strength of the lateral rotators can reduce strain on the anterior structures of the joint by pulling the humeral head posteriorly during lateral rotation of the shoulder. Strong scapula stabilizers (e.g., trapezius, rhomboids, and serratus anterior) also are believed to improve anterior stability by placing the glenoid in the optimal position to perform the required skill techniques. Isokinetic internal rotation and adduction should begin as tolerated. More aggressive shoulder rehabilitation exercises eventually should be introduced on a gradual and progressive basis.

SUMMARY

1. The shoulder complex does not function in an isolated fashion; rather, a series of joints work together in a coordinated manner to allow complicated patterns of motion. Subsequently, injury to one structure can affect other structures.

2. The throwing motion occurs in several distinct phases: wind-up, stride, cocking, acceleration, deceleration, and follow-through.

3. Scapulohumeral rhythm is the combined scapular and GH movement that allows coordinated shoulder motion.

4. A moderate SC sprain is characterized by pain and swelling over the joint and an inability to horizontally adduct the arm without increased pain. The arm typically is held forward and close to the body.

5. A moderate AC sprain is characterized by an elevated distal clavicle, indicating that the coracoclavicular ligament and the AC ligaments have been torn. The individual typically has a depressed or drooping shoulder.

6. Glenohumeral instability may be classified as anterior, posterior, inferior, or multidirectional. Anterior instability indicates injury to the middle and inferior GH ligaments and may have an associated Bankart lesion. Multidirectional instability often is associated with pain and/or clicking during simple tasks.

7. Anterior GH dislocations are more common than posterior dislocations. The injured arm often is stabilized against the body as it is held in slight abduction and external rotation.

8. A Hill-Sachs lesion may occur with an anterior dislocation; a reverse Hill-Sachs lesion may occur with a posterior dislocation. A SLAP lesion is a superior labral tear that may disrupt the attachment of the long head of the biceps tendon and may occur with or without associated GH instability.

9. Impingement syndromes involve an abutment of the supraspinatus tendon and subacromial bursa under the coracoacromial ligament and acromion process. The glenoid labrum and long head of the biceps brachii also may be injured.

10. Thoracic outlet compression syndrome may involve compression of the lower trunk of the brachial plexus or the subclavian artery and vein. If a nerve is compressed, an aching pain or numbness may extend across the shoulder to the ulnar aspect of the hand. If arterial or venous vessels are compressed, then coolness, numbness in the entire arm, and fatigue occur after exertional, overhead activity.

11. The surgical neck is the most common site for proximal humeral fractures in adults. Adolescents, however, have a high degree of proximal humeral epiphyseal fractures because of repetitive medial rotation and adduction traction forces that are placed on the shoulder during pitching motions.

12. Pain may be referred to the shoulder from other areas of the body, particularly the heart, lungs, visceral organs, and cervical spine region.

13. Injuries that should be immediately referred to a physician include:

   ▪ Obvious deformity suggesting a suspected fracture, separation, or dislocation

   ▪ Significant loss of motion or weakness in the myotomes

   ▪ Joint instability

   ▪ Abnormal sensations in either the segmental dermatomes or peripheral cutaneous patterns

   ▪ Absent or weak pulse distal to the injury

   ▪ Any significant, unexplained pain

14. Subsequent to the history, observation, and palpation components of an assessment, the examiner should have established a strong suspicion regarding which structures may be damaged. As such, during the physical examination component, some tests will be compulsory, whereas others will be used to confirm or exclude suspected injury or pathology. Only those tests that are absolutely necessary should be performed.

15. A rehabilitation program should focus on reduction of pain and spasm; restoration of motion and balance; development of strength, endurance, and power; and maintenance of cardiovascular fitness. The individual should have bilateral strength, flexibility, and muscular endurance, as well as an appropriate cardiovascular level, before returning to participation in sport and physical activity. Whenever possible, protective equipment or padding should be used to prevent reinjury.

REFERENCES

1. Nadler SF, Sherman AL, Malanga GA. Sport-specific shoulder injuries. Phys Med Rehabil Clin North Am 2004;15(vi):607–626.
2. Quillen DM, Wuchner M, Hatch RL. Acute shoulder injuries. Am Fam Physician 2004;70:1947–1954.
3. Yanai T, Hay JG, Miller GF. Shoulder impingement in front-crawl swimming: I. A method to identify impingement. Med Sci Sports Exer 2000;32(1):21–29.
4. Kelly BT, Barnes RP, Powell JW, Warren RF. Shoulder injuries to quarterbacks in the national football league. Am J Sports Med 2004;32:328–331.
5. Bicos J, Nicholson GP: Treatment and results of sternoclavicular joint injuries. Clin Sports Med 2003;22:359–370.
6. Poncelet E, Demondion X, Lapegue F, et al. Anatomic and biometric study of the acromioclavicular joint by ultrasound. Surg Radiol Anat 2003;25:439–445.
7. Buss DD, Watts JD. Acromioclavicular injuries in the throwing athlete. Clin Sports Med 2003;22(vii):327–341.
8. Costic RS, Vangura A Jr, Fenwick JA, et al. Viscoelastic behavior and structural properties of the coracoclavicular ligaments. Scand J Med Sci Sports 2003;13:305–310.
9. Hallaceli H, Manisali M, Gunal I. Does scapular elevation accompany glenohumeral abduction in healthy subjects? Arch Orthop Trauma Surg 2004;124:378–381.
10. Stokdijk M, Eilers PH, Nagels J, Rozing PM. External rotation in the glenohumeral joint during elevation of the arm. Clin Biomech (Bristol, Avon) 2003;18:296–302.
11. Fleisig GS, Escamilla RF, Andrews JR. Biomechanics of throwing. In: Zachazewski JE, Magee DJ, Quillen WS, eds. Athletic Injuries and Rehabilitation. Philadelphia: WB Saunders, 1996.
12. Meister K. Injuries to the shoulder in the throwing individual. Part one: biomechanics/pathophysiology/classification of injury. Am J Sports Med 2000;28(2):265–275.
13. Hall SJ. Basic Biomechanics. Dubuque, IA: McGraw-Hill, 2003.
14. Asplund C. Posterior sternoclavicular joint dislocation in a wrestler. Mil Med 2004;169(2):134–136.
15. Bicos J, Nicholson GP. Treatment and results of sternoclavicular joint injuries. Clin Sports Med 2003;22(2):359–370.
16. Quillen DM, Wuchner M, Hatch RL. Acute shoulder injuries. Am Fam Phys 2004;70(10):1947–1955.
17. Wang DH. New exam for glenoid labral tears. Phys Sportsmed 1997;25(2):15.
18. Trojian T, Stevenson JH, Agrawal N. What can we expect from nonoperative treatment options for shoulder pain? J Fam Pract 2005;54(3):216–223.
19. Boileau P, Brassart N, Watkinson DJ, et al. Arthroscopic repair of full-thickness tears of the supraspinatus: does the tendon really heal? J Bone Joint Surg Am 2005;87(96):1229–1240.
20. Patton WC, McCluskey GM. Biceps tendinitis and subluxation. Clin Sports Med 2001;20(3):505–529.
21. Samarasam In, Sadhu D, Agarwal S, Nayak S. Surgical management of thoracic outlet syndrome: a 10-year experience. Aust N Z J Surg 2004;74(6):450–454.
22. Kocher MS, Waters PM, Micheli LJ. Upper extremity injuries in the pediatric athlete. Sports Med 2000;30(2):117–135.
23. Ryan RS, Munk PL. Radiology for the surgeon: musculoskeletal case 33. Can J Surg 2004;47(5):373–374.

Upper Arm, Elbow, and Forearm Conditions

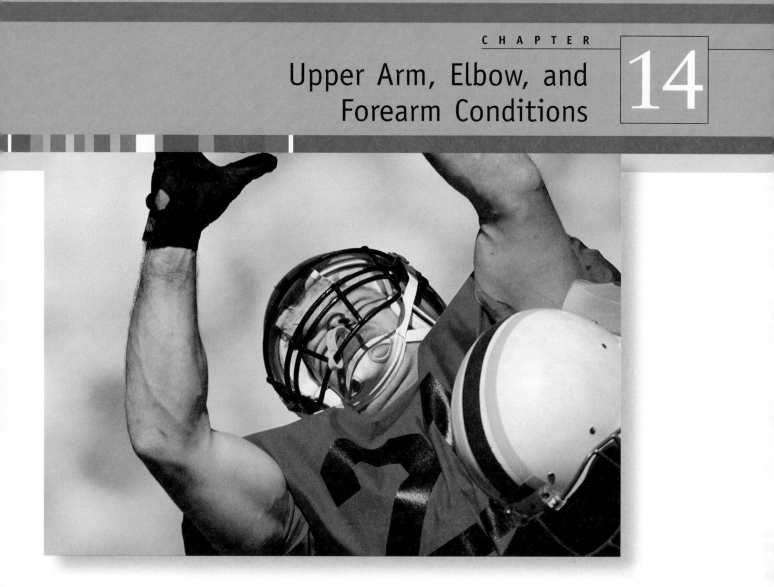

STUDENT OUTCOMES

1. Identify the important bony and soft-tissue structures in the upper arm, elbow, and forearm.

2. Describe the major motions at the elbow, and list the muscles that produce them.

3. Explain the general principles used to prevent injuries to the shoulder.

4. Describe the forces that produce the loading patterns responsible for common injuries to the upper arm, elbow, and forearm.

5. List the common acute injuries and conditions sustained in the upper arm, elbow, and forearm regions by physically active individuals.

6. Describe the soft-tissue pathology in the upper arm, elbow, and forearm regions resulting from overuse.

7. Explain the management strategies for common injuries and conditions of the upper arm, elbow, and forearm.

8. Describe the various types of fractures found at the elbow, and explain their management.

9. Describe a thorough assessment of the elbow region.

10. Explain the general principles and techniques used in developing a rehabilitation exercise program for the shoulder complex.

ROLE DELINEATION COMPETENCIES

The following Performance Domains and Tasks defined in the National Athletic Trainers' Association Board of Certification *Role Delineation Study*, 5th Edition are addressed in this chapter:

BOC COMPETENCIES

I. Prevention

   G. Monitor participants and environmental conditions by following accepted guidelines to promote safe participation.

II. Clinical Evaluation and Diagnosis

   A. Obtain a history through observation, interview, and/or review of relevant records to assess current or potential injury, illness, or condition.
   B. Inspect the involved area(s) visually to assess the injury, illness, or health-related condition.
   C. Palpate the involved area(s) using standard techniques to assess the injury, illness, or health-related condition.
   D. Perform specific tests in accordance with accepted procedures to assess the injury, illness, or health-related condition.
   E. Formulate a clinical impression by interpreting the signs, symptoms, and predisposing factors of the injury, illness, or condition to determine the appropriate course of action.

III. Immediate Care

   A. Employ life-saving techniques through the use of standard emergency procedures in order to reduce morbidity and the incidence of mortality.
   B. Prevent exacerbation of non–life threatening condition(s) through the use of standard procedures in order to reduce morbidity.
   C. Facilitate the timely transfer of care for conditions beyond the scope of practice of the athletic trainer by implementing appropriate referral strategies to stabilize and/or prevent exacerbation of the condition(s).

IV. Treatment, Rehabilitation, and Reconditioning

   E. Reassess the status of injuries, illnesses, and/or conditions using standard techniques and documentation strategies in order to determine appropriate treatment, rehabilitation, and/or reconditioning and to evaluate readiness to return to a desired level of activity.
   F. Educate the appropriate individual(s) in the treatment, rehabilitation, and reconditioning of injuries, illnesses, and/or conditions using applicable methods and materials to facilitate recovery, function, and/or performance.

The arms perform lifting and carrying tasks, cushion the body during collisions, and lessen body momentum during falls. In many sports, performance is contingent on the ability of the arms to effectively swing a racquet or club or the hands to position for throwing and catching. Common sports-related injuries to the elbow region include supracondylar fracture, lateral condyle fracture, radial head/neck fracture, elbow dislocation, ulnar collateral ligament tears, ulnar neuritis, osteochondritis dissecans of the capitellum, medial epicondyle avulsion, medial **epicondylitis** ("little league elbow"), and lateral epicondylitis ("tennis elbow") (1,2).

This chapter begins with a review of anatomy and an overview of the kinematics and kinetics of the upper arm, elbow, and forearm. A discussion concerning prevention of injury is followed by information regarding common injuries to the upper arm, elbow, and forearm. Finally, the injury assessment process is presented, followed by examples of rehabilitation exercises.

ANATOMY OF THE ELBOW

Although the elbow generally may be thought of as a simple hinge joint, the elbow actually is categorized as a trochoginglymus joint that encompasses three articulations: the humeroulnar, humeroradial, and proximal radioulnar joints (3). The bony structure of the elbow and forearm are displayed in Figure 14.1. Several strong ligaments bind these articulations together, and a single joint capsule surrounds all three. Twenty-three muscles associated with the elbow provide dynamic stability (3).

Humeroulnar Joint

The hinge joint at the elbow is the humeroulnar joint. It is the articulation of the trochlea of the humerus with the reciprocally shaped trochlear fossa of the ulna. Motion capabilities primarily are flexion and extension. In some individuals, particularly women, however, a small amount (i.e., 5–15°) of overextension is allowed. The joint is most stable in the close-packed position of extension.

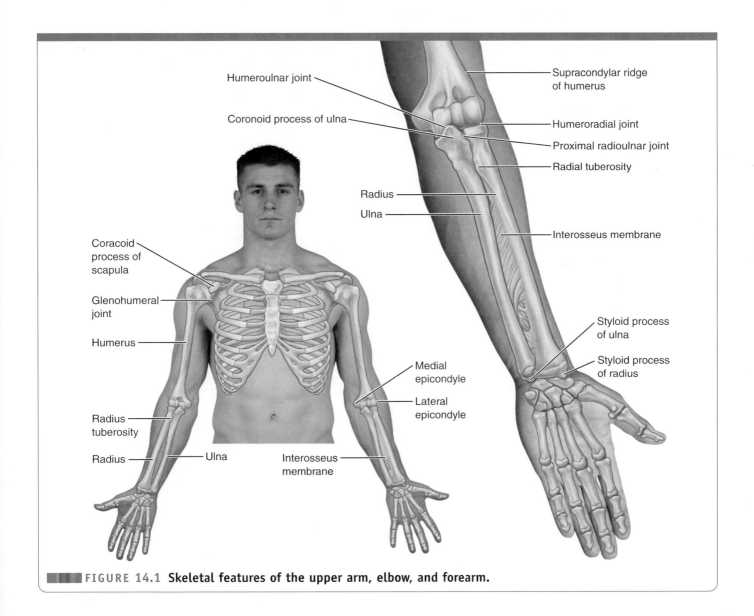

FIGURE 14.1 Skeletal features of the upper arm, elbow, and forearm.

Humeroradial Joint

The humeroradial joint, which is lateral to the humeroulnar joint, is formed between the spherical capitellum of the humerus and the proximal radius. It is a gliding joint, with motion restricted to the sagittal plane by the adjacent humeroulnar joint. The close-packed position is with the elbow flexed at 90°, and the forearm is supinated approximately 5°.

Proximal Radioulnar Joint

The annular ligament binds the head of the radius to the radial notch of the ulna, forming the proximal radioulnar joint. It is a pivot joint that permits forearm pronation and supination occurring as the radius rolls medially and laterally over the ulna (Fig. 14.2). The close-packed position is at 5° of forearm supination.

Carrying Angle

The angle between the longitudinal axes of the humerus and the ulna when the arm is in anatomical position is known as the carrying angle. The angle is so-named because it causes the forearm to angle away from the body when a load is carried in the hand. Given, however, that loads typically are carried with the forearm in a neutral rather than a fully supinated position, the functional significance of the carrying angle is questionable. Nevertheless, the size of the carrying angle at the elbow is one of the skeletal differences between females and males and is attributed to differences in the shape of the trochlea. When the elbow is fully extended and the forearm fully supinated, the carrying angle ranges from approximately 10 to 15° in adults and generally is greater in females

A

B

■■■■■ FIGURE 14.2 **Forearm movements. A,** Supination occurs when the radius and ulna are parallel to each other. **B,** Pronation involves the rotation of the radius over the ulna.

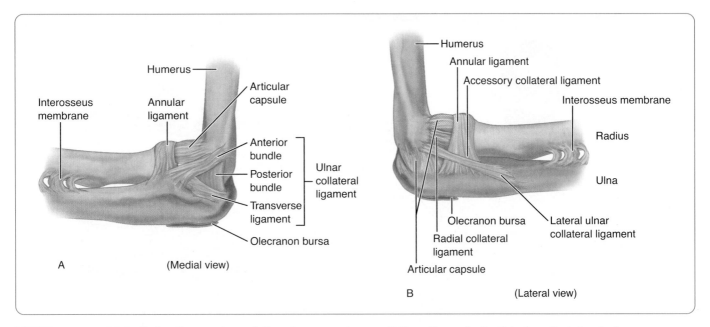

FIGURE 14.3 Major ligaments and the olecranon bursa of the elbow. A, Medial view. **B,** Lateral view.

than in males. The carrying angle changes with skeletal growth and maturity and is always greater on the side of the dominant hand (4).

Ligaments of the Elbow

The elbow is reinforced by capsuloligamentous structures that are thickenings of the capsule. These form the medial and lateral ligamentous complexes (Fig. 14.3). The medial (ulnar) collateral ligament, the most important ligament for stability of the elbow joint, is divided into three oblique bands denoted by their anatomical location—namely, anterior, transverse, and posterior. The anterior oblique band is taut throughout the elbow's full range of motion (ROM) and is the primary restraint against valgus forces. The transverse oblique band provides little, if any, support to the medial elbow. The posterior oblique band is a fan-shaped, capsular thickening that generally is taut when the elbow is flexed beyond 90°.

The lateral (radial) collateral ligament complex consists of four components: the lateral ulnar collateral, radial collateral, annular, and accessory ligaments. The radial collateral ligament, which runs from the lateral epicondyle of the humerus and terminates at the annular ligament, resists varus forces. The posterior portion of this ligament, which is referred to as the lateral ulnar collateral ligament, extends distally to the lateral ulna.

The annular ligament fits tightly around the radial head and upper portion of the neck. It permits pronation and supination of the forearm as the radius rotates, internally and externally, on the ulna. Superior and inferior oblique bands of the annular ligament attach proximally and distally to the ulna (5). During extreme supination, the anterior fibers of the annular ligament are taut; during extreme pronation, the posterior fibers are taut. The accessory lateral collateral ligament is a superficial layer of fibers that blends with the annular ligament to insert onto the supinator tubercle of the ulna.

Bursae of the Elbow

Although the elbow has several small bursae, the most clinically relevant is the subcutaneous olecranon bursa located between the olecranon and the skin surface. The lubricating function of the bursa facilitates smooth gliding of the skin over the olecranon process during elbow flexion and extension.

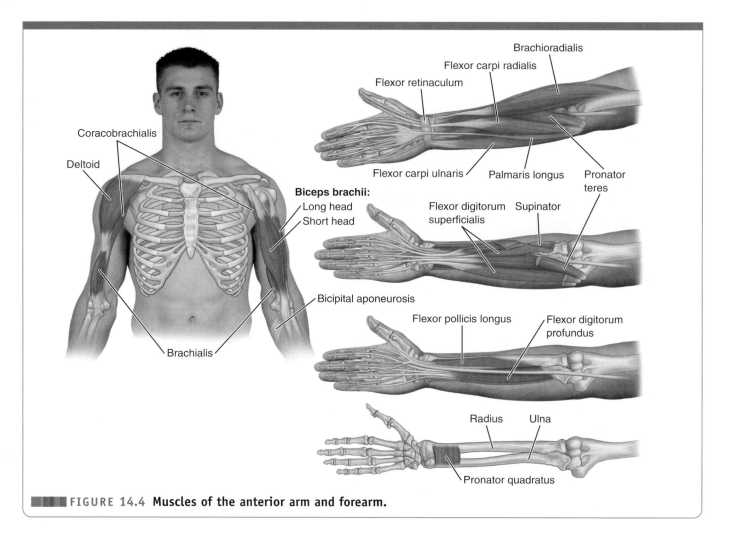

FIGURE 14.4 Muscles of the anterior arm and forearm.

See Muscles of the Elbow, available on the companion website at thePoint, for a summary of these muscles, including attachments, primary actions, and innervation.

Muscles of the Elbow

A large number of muscles cross the elbow (Figs. 14.4 and 14.5). Identifying the actions of these muscles is complicated by the fact that several muscles are two-joint muscles, which extend into the shoulder or the hand and fingers.

Nerves of the Elbow

The major nerves of the elbow and forearm descend from the brachial plexus and include the musculocutaneous (C5–C7), median (C5–T1), ulnar (C8–T1), and radial nerves (C5–T1) (Fig. 14.6). The musculocutaneous nerve provides motor supply to the flexor muscles of the anterior arm and sensory innervation to the skin of the lateral forearm. The median nerve supplies most of the flexor muscles of the anterior forearm and the skin on the palmar aspect of the hand, including the thumb, index finger, and middle finger, and the lateral half of the ring finger. The ulnar nerve provides innervation to the flexor carpi ulnaris and the medial half of the flexor digitorum profundus and to the skin on the medial border of the hand, including the little finger and the medial half of the ring finger. The radial nerve, which is the largest branch of the brachial plexus, passes anteriorly to the lateral epicondyle at the elbow, then divides into superficial and deep branches to continue along the posterolateral aspect of the forearm. The radial nerve supplies the arm and forearm extensor muscles and the skin on the posterior aspect of the arm and forearm.

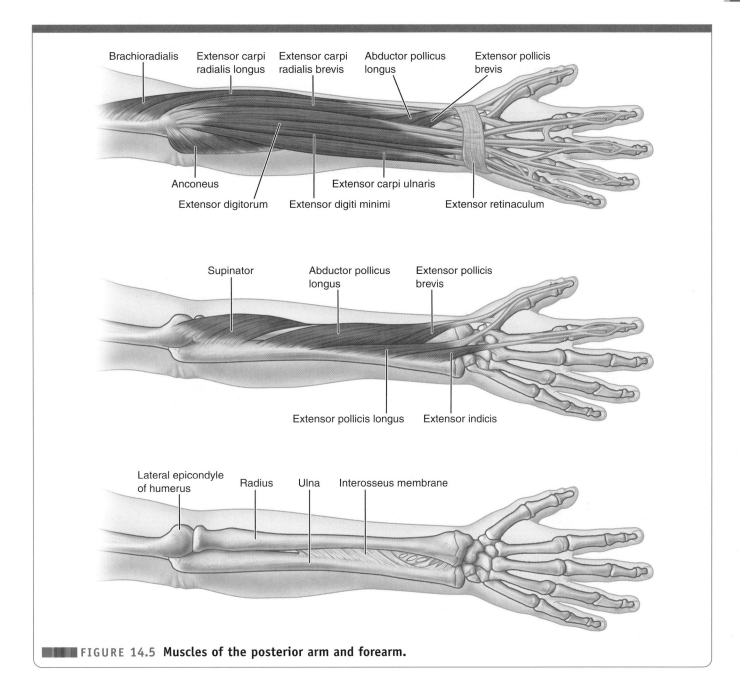

FIGURE 14.5 Muscles of the posterior arm and forearm.

Blood Vessels of the Elbow

The major arteries of the elbow and forearm region are the brachial, ulnar, and radial arteries (Fig. 14.7). The brachial artery courses down the medial side of the arm, providing blood supply to the flexor muscles of the arm. The deep brachial artery branches off to supply the triceps brachii. In the elbow, the brachial artery forms an **anastomosis**, or a network of communicating blood vessels, to supply the elbow joint. The main branch of the brachial artery crosses the anterior aspect of the elbow, where the brachial pulse can be readily palpated.

Distal to the elbow, the brachial artery splits into the ulnar and radial arteries. The ulnar artery supplies the medial forearm and, via one of its branches, the common interosseous artery, supplies the deep flexors and extensors of the forearm. The radial artery, which courses along the anterior aspect of the radius, supplies the lateral forearm muscles. Pulses can be taken for both arteries on the anterior aspect of the wrist (see Fig. 5.3).

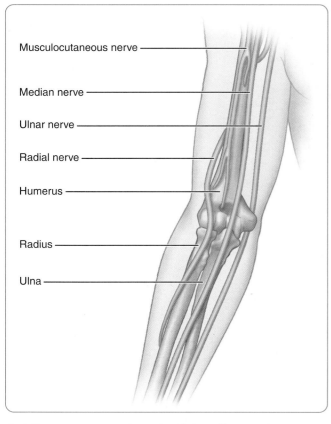

Musculocutaneous nerve

Median nerve

Ulnar nerve

Radial nerve

Humerus

Radius

Ulna

■■■■■ FIGURE 14.6 **Nerves of the elbow region.**

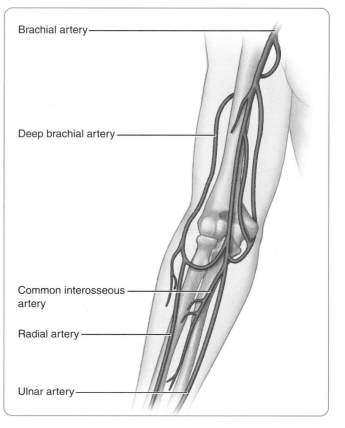

Brachial artery

Deep brachial artery

Common interosseous artery

Radial artery

Ulnar artery

■■■■■ FIGURE 14.7 **Arteries of the elbow region.**

KINEMATICS AND MAJOR MUSCLE ACTIONS OF THE ELBOW

The three associated joints at the elbow allow motion in two planes. Flexion and extension are sagittal plane movements that occur at the humeroulnar and humeroradial joints; pronation and supination are longitudinal rotational movements that take place at the proximal radioulnar joint.

Flexion and Extension

The elbow flexors include those muscles that cross the anterior side of the joint. The primary elbow flexor is the brachialis. Because the distal attachment of the brachialis is the coronoid process of the ulna, the muscle is equally effective when the forearm is in supination or in pronation. Another elbow flexor, the biceps brachii, has both long and short heads attached to the radial tuberosity via a single common tendon. When the forearm is supinated, the biceps contributes effectively to flexion, because it is slightly stretched. When the forearm is pronated, the muscle is less taut and, consequently, less effective. The brachioradialis, which also is an elbow flexor, is most effective when the forearm is in a neutral position (i.e., midway between full pronation and full supination). Other flexor muscles that cross the elbow are important dynamic stabilizers of the joint. In particular, the flexor carpi ulnaris and flexor digitorum superficialis provide significant stability to the medial elbow during a variety of activities, including throwing.

The triceps is the major elbow extensor. Although the three heads have separate origins, they attach to the olecranon process of the ulna through a common distal tendon. The small anconeus muscle also assists with extension at the elbow.

Pronation and Supination

Pronation and supination of the forearm occur when the radius rotates around the ulna. Three radioulnar articulations exist: the proximal, middle, and distal radioulnar joints. The proximal and distal joints are pivot joints. The middle radioulnar joint is a syndesmosis, with an elastic, interconnecting membrane that permits supination and pronation but prevents longitudinal displacement of one bone with respect to the other. The primary pronator muscle is the pronator quadratus, which attaches to the distal ulna and radius. The pronator teres, which crosses the proximal radioulnar joint, assists with pronation. As the name suggests, the supinator is the muscle primarily responsible for supination. During resistance or elbow flexion, the biceps also participates in supination.

KINETICS OF THE ELBOW

Although the elbow is not considered to be a weight-bearing joint, it sustains significant loads during daily activities. For example, it has been estimated that the compressive load at the elbow reaches 300 Newtons (N) (67 lb) during activities such as dressing and eating, 1,700 N (382 lb) when the body is supported by the arms when rising from a chair, and 1,900 N (427 lb) when pulling a table across the floor (6). During performance of a one-handed push-up, compression at the elbow ranges around 65% of body weight (7). Extremely large forces are generated by muscles crossing the elbow during forceful pitching and throwing motions as well as during weight lifting and many resistance training exercises. In fact, during an activity such as pitching, valgus stress at the elbow during the late cocking and acceleration phases of the throw can exceed the strength of the ulnar collateral ligament, resulting in microscopic tears within it (8,9). The triceps, wrist flexor-pronator muscles, and anconeus must develop tension to assist the ulnar collateral ligament in resisting the valgus load. During the execution of many skills in gymnastics and wrestling, the elbow functions as a weight-bearing joint.

Because the attachment of the elbow extensors to the ulna is closer to the joint center than the attachments of the elbow flexors on the radius and ulna, the extensor moment arm is shorter than the flexor moment arm. This means that the elbow extensors must generate more force than the elbow flexors to produce the same amount of joint torque. This translates to greater joint compression forces during extension than during flexion, when movements with comparable speed and force requirements are executed.

PREVENTION OF ELBOW CONDITIONS

The elbow often is subjected to compressive forces when the arm is placed in a position to cushion a fall or lessen the body's impact with another object. In addition, microtraumatic forces caused by repetitive valgus and varus stresses can lead to overuse injuries, many of which are related to poor skill technique. Few sports require protective equipment at the elbow; therefore, physical conditioning and proper skill technique are major factors in preventing injury to this region.

Protective Equipment

A variety of equipment types can be advantageous in preventing injury to the elbow. Because standard shoulder pads may not extend far enough to protect the upper arm, many football players attach an additional biceps pad to the shoulder pads to protect this vulnerable area. Special pads are available to protect the elbow during falls and collisions. Padded elbow sleeves or neoprene sleeves are worn in many sports to protect the olecranon from direct trauma and abrasions, particularly when playing on artificial turf. Counterforce braces, which commonly are used by participants in racquet sports, are intended to reduce muscle tensile forces that can lead to medial or lateral epicondylitis. Finally, hinged braces can add compression and support to the elbow to reduce excessive varus and valgus forces.

Physical Conditioning

Many of the muscles that move the elbow also move the shoulder and wrist. Therefore, flexibility and strengthening exercises must focus on the entire arm. General flexibility exercises for the shoulder can be used in conjunction with warm-up exercises that mimic specific sport skills. For example, a tennis player may begin the warm-up session with slow, controlled forehand and backhand strokes that gradually increase in intensity. A pitcher or outfielder may begin with short, controlled throws, increasing the distance and intensity as the arm is warmed up. Strengthening exercises for the shoulder can be combined with those listed in Field Strategy 14.1. These exercises are designed to improve general strength in elbow flexion and extension, forearm pronation and supination, wrist flexion and extension, and radial and ulnar deviation. Physical conditioning programs should begin with light resistance and progress to a heavier resistance.

Proper Skill Technique

Nearly all overuse injuries are directly related to repetitive, throwing-type motions that produce microtraumatic tensile forces on the surrounding soft-tissue structures. Children who use a sidearm throwing motion are threefold more likely to develop problems compared with those who use a more traditional overhead technique. Movement analysis can detect improper technique in the acceleration and follow-through phase that contribute to these excessive tensile forces. High-speed photography may aid in this analysis.

Teaching sport participants the shoulder-roll method of falling is another preventive measure. Falling on an extended hand or flexed elbow is the most common mechanism for acute injuries in the upper extremity. Excessive compressive forces can be transmitted along the long axis of the bones, leading to a fracture or dislocation.

CONTUSIONS

> *Following practice, a lacrosse player is complaining of pain in his right arm after being struck by another player's stick. He reports receiving several blows to the area over the past week. Palpation reveals a hardened mass of soft tissue over the distal anterior arm that is very tender and sore. Bilateral strength is good. What potentially serious condition might develop, and how should this condition be managed?*

Direct blows to the arm and forearm frequently are associated with contact and collision sports. Contusions result from a compressive force sustained from a direct blow. Such injuries vary in severity according to the area and depth over which blood vessels are ruptured. Contusions occur more frequently over bony prominences.

Signs and Symptoms

Ecchymosis may be present if the hemorrhage is superficial. Significant trauma can lead to internal hemorrhage, rapid swelling, and hematoma formation that can limit ROM. Chronic blows to the anterior arm can result in the development of ectopic bone in either the belly of the muscle (i.e., **myositis ossificans**) or as a bony outgrowth (i.e., **exostosis**) of the underlying bone. The belly of the deltoid and brachialis muscles is the common site for the development of myositis ossificans after trauma. A particularly vulnerable site is just proximal to the deltoid's insertion on the lateral aspect of the humerus, where the bone is least padded by muscle tissue. Standard shoulder pads do not extend far enough to protect the area, and the edge of the pad itself may contribute to the injury. The developing mass can become painful and disabling if the radial nerve is contused, leading to transitory paralysis of the extensor forearm muscles.

"Tackler's exostosis," also known as blocker's spur and commonly seen in football linemen, is not a true myositis ossificans, because the ectopic formation is not infiltrated into the muscle but, rather, is an irritative exostosis arising from the bone. A painful bony mass, usually in the form of a spur with a sharp edge, can be palpated on the anterolateral aspect of the humerus.

Management

Treatment involves standard acute care with ice, compression, and protected rest. Activity modification, nonsteroidal anti-inflammatory drugs (NSAIDs), and a gradual, active ROM and strengthening exercise program should be initiated as tolerated. Aggressive stretching and strengthening exercises should be avoided to prevent further injury to muscle tissue.

If conservative measures do not alleviate the condition, the individual should be referred to a physician for further care, because a more serious condition may have developed. Visible radiograph

FIELD STRATEGY 14.1

Exercises to Prevent Injury to the Elbow Region

Begin all exercises with light resistance using dumbbells or surgical tubing.

1. Biceps curl. Support the involved arm on the leg, and fully flex the elbow. This also can be performed bilaterally in a standing position with a barbell.

2. Triceps curl. Raise the involved arm over the head, and extend the involved arm at the elbow. This also can be performed bilaterally in a supine or standing position with a barbell.

3. Wrist flexion. Support the involved forearm on a table or your leg with the hand off the edge. With the palm facing up, slowly do a full wrist curl, and then return to the starting position.

4. Wrist extension. Support the involved forearm on a table or your leg with the hand off the edge. With the palm facing down, slowly do a full reverse wrist curl, and then return to the starting position.

5. Forearm pronation-supination. Support the involved forearm on a table or your leg with the hand off the edge. With surgical tubing or a hand dumbbell, roll the forearm into pronation, and then return to supination. Adjust the surgical tubing, and reverse the exercise, stressing the supinators. The elbow should remain stationary.

6. Ulnar-radial deviation. Support the involved forearm on a table or your leg with the hand off the edge. With surgical tubing or a hand dumbbell, perform ulnar deviation. Reverse directions, and perform radial deviation. An alternate method is to stand with the arm at the side while holding a hammer or a weighted bar. Raise the wrist in ulnar deviation. Repeat in radial deviation.

7. Wrist curl-ups. Exercising the wrist extensors is performed by gripping the bar with both palms facing down. Slowly wind the cord onto the bar until the weight reaches the top, and then slowly unwind the cord. Reverse the hand position to work the wrist flexors.

changes in the muscle can be noted after 2 to 3 weeks. As the condition progresses and becomes chronic, a painful **periostitis** and **fibrositis** may develop. Surgical excision of the calcification is seldom necessary, because function usually is not impaired. If function is adversely affected, however, surgery should be delayed until the calcification is mature (usually 12–18 months), because it may redevelop. The area should be protected with a special pad during participation.

> **A** *The lacrosse player may be developing myositis ossificans in the brachialis muscle. Standard acute care should be followed, with referral to a physician for further assessment and possible radiography.*

OLECRANON BURSITIS

> **Q** *A football player has acute swelling of approximately 1 inch in diameter on the proximal posterior ulna. His history reveals constant friction to the area, attributed to contact with artificial turf. What condition might be suspected, what anatomical structures are involved, and how should this condition be managed?*

The subcutaneous olecranon bursa is the largest bursa in the elbow region. The superficial location predisposes the bursa to either direct macrotrauma or cumulative microtrauma by repetitive elbow flexion and extension. The bursitis can be acute or chronic, aseptic or septic. Common mechanisms of olecranon bursa injury include:

- A fall on a flexed elbow
- Constantly leaning on one's elbow ("student's elbow")
- Repetitive pressure and friction
- Repetitive flexion and extension
- Infection

Acute and Chronic Bursitis

A fall on a flexed elbow can lead to an acutely inflamed bursa. Constantly leaning on one's elbow, repetitive pressure, and friction can lead to a chronic inflamed bursa.

Signs and Symptoms

The acutely inflamed bursa presents with an immediate, tender, swollen area of redness in the posterior elbow. The swelling is relatively painless. If the bursa ruptures, a discrete, sharply demarcated goose egg is visible directly over the olecranon process. Approximately half of the patients with olecranon bursitis have a history of an abrupt onset of pain and swelling; the other half have a more insidious onset over several weeks, leading to chronic inflammation. Motion is limited at the extreme of flexion as tension increases over the bursa.

Management

Acute management involves ice, rest, and a compressive wrap applied for the first 24 hours. Significant distention may necessitate aspiration followed by a compressive dressing for several days.

Chronic bursitis is managed with cryotherapy, NSAIDs, and use of elbow cushions to protect the area from further insult. In long-term cases of chronic bursitis, the bursa may be aspirated or totally excised, although a risk of poor wound healing over the olecranon process exists. Corticosteroid injections also may be performed.

Septic and Nonseptic Bursitis

Occasionally, a bursa can become infected in the absence of trauma to the area. Septic bursitis sometimes is related to seeding from an infection at a distant site, such as **paronychia**, cellulitis of the hand, or forearm infection.

Nonseptic bursitis can be caused by crystalline deposition disease or rheumatoid involvement. It has been associated with atopic dermatitis.

Signs and Symptoms

Individuals with septic bursitis are more likely to show traditional signs of infection, including malaise (lethargy), fever, pain, localized heat, restricted motion, tenderness, and swelling at the elbow. These signs and symptoms usually present within 1 week of developing symptoms. Approximately 50% of patients present with a skin lesion overlying the bursa, 92 to 100% have bursal tenderness, and 40 to 100% have peribursal cellulitis. In contrast, nonseptic bursitis is associated with an overlying skin lesion in 5% of the cases, bursal tenderness in 45% of the cases, and cellulitis in 23 to 25% (10).

Management

An individual with an infected bursa should be referred to a physician. The physician generally aspirates the bursa and takes a sample of the fluid for culture to determine the presence of septic bursitis. Following aspiration, the elbow is immobilized in a sling, and continuous hot packs and appropriate antibiotics typically are prescribed. If an infected bursa is suspected, corticosteroids should not be injected.

 The football player has acute olecranon bursitis. Standard acute care should resolve the condition; however, the player should be closely observed for signs and symptoms of infection. Applying a pad to the area can help to prevent recurrence.

SPRAINS

A gymnast misses the vault, falls to the mat on an outstretched arm, and sustains a visible posterior dislocation of the elbow. The athlete is unwilling to move the elbow and is in extreme pain. Explain the circulatory and neurologic assessment for this injury.

Collateral Ligament Sprain

Acute tears to ligamentous and joint structures at the elbow are rare, but such injuries may occur during a fall on an extended hand, resulting in elbow hyperextension, or through a valgus/varus tensile force. More commonly, however, repetitive tensile forces irritate and tear the ligaments, particularly the ulnar collateral ligament. If the ulnar collateral ligament is damaged, the ulnar nerve also may be affected.

Signs and Symptoms

A history of pain localized to the medial aspect of the elbow during the late cocking and acceleration phases of throwing is common. Examination reveals point tenderness on the joint line as well as increased pain and instability with the valgus stress test applied to the elbow at 15 to 20° of flexion.

Management

Treatment involves standard acute care with ice, compression, and protected rest. A brief immobilization may be necessary in acute cases. This is followed by early, protected ROM exercises to stretch the forearm flexor-pronator group and the forearm extensors.

Anterior Capsulitis

Anterior joint pain caused by hyperextension usually is attributed to acute anterior capsulitis rather than chronic, repetitive throwing. Microtears in the capsule usually are not sufficient to cause dislocation.

Signs and Symptoms

Diffuse, anterior elbow pain presents after a traumatic episode. It is accompanied by deep tenderness on palpation, particularly on the anteromedial side. A strain to the pronator teres should be ruled out, as should entrapment of the median nerve as it courses through the pronator teres. With nerve entrapment, tingling or numbness of the thumb and index finger usually are noted.

Management

Treatment involves standard acute care with ice, compression, and protected rest. The condition is managed with immobilization for 3 to 5 days, after which active ROM exercises can begin as pain allows. Flexion contracture may result from fibrosis caused by repeated injury to the capsule.

Dislocations

In adolescents, the most common traumatic injury to the elbow is subluxation or dislocation of the proximal radial head, often associated with an immature annular ligament. Referred to as "nurse-maid's elbow" or "pulled-elbow syndrome," this condition results from longitudinal traction of an extended and pronated upper extremity, such as when a young child is swung by the arms. A small tear in the annular ligament allows the radial head to migrate out from under the annular ligament. If an individual is unable to pronate and supinate the forearm without pain, immediate referral to a physician is warranted.

Most ulnar dislocations occur in individuals younger than 20 years, with a peak incidence during the teenage years (1). The mechanism of injury usually is hyperextension or a sudden, violent unidirectional valgus force that drives the ulna posteriorly or posterolaterally. Approximately 60% of patients have associated fractures of the medial epicondyle, radial head, coronoid process, or olecranon process (11). When the dislocation is associated with both radial head and coronoid fractures, it has been termed the "terrible triad of the elbow" because of the difficulties that are inherent in treatment and the consistently poor reported outcomes as compared to a simple elbow dislocation (12). The injury also may involve disruption of the anterior capsule, tearing of the brachialis muscle, injury to the ulnar collateral ligament, and rarely, brachial artery compromise or nerve injury to the median or ulnar nerves (1).

Signs and Symptoms

A snapping or cracking sensation is experienced on impact, followed by severe pain, rapid swelling, total loss of function, and an obvious deformity (Fig. 14.8). The anterior capsule, brachialis muscle,

▮▮▮▮ **FIGURE 14.8 Elbow dislocation. A,** Clinical view of a posterior dislocation. **B,** Radiograph of a typical posterior dislocation. Note that the coronoid process is adjacent to the olecranon fossa.

Box 14.1   Signs and Symptoms of a Posterior Elbow Dislocation

- Snapping or cracking sensation
- Immediate, severe pain with rapid swelling, primarily on the medial aspect of the elbow
- Total loss of function

- Obvious deformity as the olecranon is pushed posteriorly
- A slightly flexed elbow is supported, if possible, by the uninjured arm
- Pain is predominantly localized over the medial aspect of the elbow
- Crepitation may be palpated if an associated fracture is present

and flexor and extensor muscle masses also may be disrupted. The arm frequently is held in flexion, with the forearm appearing shortened. The olecranon and radial head are palpable posteriorly, and a slight indentation in the triceps is visible just proximal to the olecranon. Signs and symptoms of a posterior elbow dislocation are listed in Box 14.1.

Nerve palsies are common, making pre- and postreduction neurovascular examination critical. Ulnar nerve dysfunction usually is transient. If damaged, numbness will extend into the little finger. The median nerve, however, may become trapped within the joint, trapped within a healing medial epicondylar fracture, or looped anteriorly into the joint. Persistent, unexplained pain and median nerve dysfunction (e.g., finger flexor weakness or numbness in the palm of the hand) necessitate immediate re-evaluation by a physician.

Management

Reduction usually is performed under general or regional anesthesia. Early reduction minimizes the amount of muscle spasm. For cases in which the forearm flexors, extensors, and annular ligament have maintained their integrity with no associated fracture, limited immobilization, early ROM exercises, and proprioceptive neuromuscular facilitation exer-

Activation of the emergency action plan, including summoning emergency medical services (EMS), is warranted. Because of the risk of neurovascular injury, on-site reduction is not indicated. Additional guidelines for management of an elbow dislocation are discussed in Field Strategy 14.2.

cises have proved to be quite successful. Although rare, recurrent dislocations often are related to laxity in the lateral ulnar collateral ligament of the elbow, leading to posterolateral rotary subluxation.

FIELD STRATEGY 14.2

Management Algorithm for Posterior Elbow Dislocation

1. Apply ice to reduce swelling and inflammation.
2. To rule out circulatory impairment, assess:
   - Radial pulse
   - Skin color
   - Blanching of the nails
3. To rule out nerve impairment, assess motor and sensory function:
   - Have the patient (if able) flex, extend, abduct, and adduct the fingers with the person looking away:
   - Stroke the palm and dorsum of the hand in several different locations with a blunt and sharp object
   - Ask the individual to identify where you are touching and whether the object is sharp or dull

4. Immobilize the area with a vacuum splint or other appropriate splint.
5. Take vital signs, recheck pulse and sensory functions, and treat for shock.

This injury should be considered a medical emergency. The emergency action plan, including summoning emergency medical services, should be activated.

A recurrent dislocation in the first 6 months after initial injury is more often attributed to a missed osteochondral fracture. Elbow dislocations involving fractures of the radial head and capitellar fracture dislocations are more complex and require internal fixation.

> **A** *In assessing the dislocation sustained by the gymnast, circulatory assessment should include checking for a distal pulse, assessing skin color and temperature, and assessing capillary refill. Neurologic assessment includes checking for sensation distal to the injury.*

STRAINS

> **Q** *After receiving a severe blow to the right forearm, an offensive lineman is having problems flexing his wrist and fingers. The lineman has rapid swelling, discoloration, and diminished pulse. Passive stretching of the wrist flexors increases pain. What condition should be suspected, what structures are involved, and how should this injury be managed?*

Muscular strains commonly result from inadequate warm-up, excessive training past the point of fatigue, and inadequate rehabilitation of previous muscular injuries. A less common cause of strains in this area is a single, massive contraction or sudden overstretching. Field Strategy 14.3 summarizes the management of isolated muscular strains.

Flexor and Extensor Strains

Repetitive tensile stresses to the elbow flexors (i.e., brachialis, biceps brachii, and brachioradialis) and pronator teres can lead to a self-limiting muscle strain, especially after an inadequate warm-up or fatigue. In rowing, excessive wrist motion during the feathering action can lead to chronic forearm tendinitis and tenosynovitis (13). In a triceps strain, the mechanism generally is a decelerating-type injury. It has been reported in tennis and baseball players as well as in weight lifters with a history of anabolic steroid use or local steroid injections (14).

FIELD STRATEGY 14.3

Management Algorithm for Muscular Strains

1. Control inflammation, swelling, and pain. Use ice, compression, elevation, nonsteroidal anti-inflammatory drugs, and rest if necessary.
2. Use ice, ultrasound, electrical muscle stimulation, interferential current, or thermotherapy to precede therapeutic exercise.
3. Restore range of motion. (Assess flexibility at the shoulder region, because limitations may increase stress at the elbow.)
4. Perform isometric exercises throughout a pain-free range of motion.
5. Progress to isotonic exercises with light resistance, building from 1 to 5 pounds, throughout a pain-free range.
6. Improve neuromuscular control with closed kinetic chain exercises, such as shifting a weighted ball in the hand, press-ups, or walking on the hands in a push-up position between boxes of varying heights.
7. Add surgical tubing exercises as tolerated.
8. When pain-free, ensure adequate warm-up and gradual return to functional exercises.
9. Recommend activity modification, biomechanical analysis of skill performance, or equipment modifications.

If involved in a throwing activity:

1. Begin functional throwing with a light toss over a distance of 20 to 30 feet for 5 minutes, then progressing to between 15 and 20 minutes.
2. When the individual can throw for 15 to 20 minutes, gradually increase the distance to 150 feet.
3. When proper throwing mechanics are present, gradually increase velocity.
4. Continue a strengthening and stretching program as return to activity is initiated.

Signs and Symptoms

Palpable pain can be elicited over the involved muscle mass. Pain increases with active and resisted motion.

Management

Treatment involves standard acute care with ice, compression, and protected rest. A brief immobilization may be necessary in acute cases. Activity modification, NSAIDs, and a program of gradual active ROM and strengthening exercises should be initiated as tolerated. In rowing, special attention should be paid to improper technique, wrongly sized grips, poor rigging, and limiting rowing during wet or rough conditions, which can cause the rower to use excessive wrist motion (13).

Rupture of the Biceps Brachii

Approximately 97% of all biceps brachii ruptures are proximal; only 3% involve the distal attachment (11,15). In many cases, preexisting degenerative changes in the distal tendon make it vulnerable to rupture following a sudden eccentric load (e.g., during weight lifting or trying to catch oneself during a fall). Individuals at increased risk for this injury tend to be men under 30 years of age with a history of using steroid medication (11).

Signs and Symptoms

Tenderness, swelling, and ecchymosis are visible in the antecubital fossa. The biceps tendon is not palpable, because the belly muscle retracts proximally. The individual is still able to flex the elbow and supinate the forearm, but these movements are weak when resisted.

Management

Treatment for a rupture may involve a nonoperative approach or surgical repair. Some studies have found a significant loss of elbow flexion (30%) and supination (40%) strength with a nonoperative approach (16). Although this decreased level of function may suffice for daily activities, the distal biceps tends to scar to the brachialis muscle, illuminating the normal contour of the muscle.

Surgical repair to reattach the avulsed distal biceps tendon to the radial tuberosity provides the greatest likelihood of maximal functional results and return to physical activity. Following repair, the elbow is immobilized at 90° of flexion with moderate forearm supination for 8 weeks, followed by gradual active ROM and strengthening (11,15).

Rupture of the Triceps Brachii

Occasionally, a direct blow to the posterior elbow or an uncoordinated triceps contraction during a fall results in an acute rupture of the tendon. In addition to the tendon rupture, 80% of all injuries involve an olecranon avulsion fracture (11). Spontaneous ruptures of the tendon can occur, but these are rare and usually associated with systemic diseases or steroid use.

Signs and Symptoms

Pain and swelling are present over the distal attachment of the extensor mechanism on the olecranon process. A palpable defect in the triceps tendon or a step-off deformity of the olecranon also may be present. Active extension of the elbow may be weak (if a partial tear is present) or nonexistent (with a total rupture).

Management

Treatment involves standard acute care with ice, compression, and immobilization in a sling followed by immediate referral to a physician. Partial tears are treated conservatively. Surgical reattachment of the tendon onto the olecranon process is necessary in a total rupture. If an avulsion fracture of the olecranon is present, open reduction and internal fixation of the fragment are necessary. Subsequently, the elbow is immobilized in 45° of flexion for 4 weeks, followed by allowing 0 to 45° of flexion for 4 weeks and then gradual incorporation of active ROM and strengthening exercises.

Compartment Syndrome

The deep fascia of the forearm encloses the wrist and finger flexor and extensor muscle groups in a common sheath. The two groups are separated into compartments by an interosseous membrane between the radius and ulna. The wrist and finger flexors are in the anterior compartment; the wrist and finger extensors are in the posterior compartment.

A compartment often is secondary to an elbow fracture or dislocation, crushing injury, forearm fracture, postischemic edema, or excessive muscular exertion, as in weight lifting. Hemorrhage or edema causes increased pressure within the compartment, leading to excessive pressure on neurovascular structures and tissues within the space.

Signs and Symptoms

Onset of symptoms usually is rapid, including swelling, discoloration, absent or diminished distal pulse, and subsequent onset of sensory changes and paralysis. Severe pain at rest, aggravated by passive stretching of the muscles in the compartment, signals a potential problem.

Management

Treatment involves immobilization of the forearm and wrist as well as application of ice and elevation above the heart to limit pain and swelling. External compression should not be applied to the area, because the neurovascular structures already are compressed by the swelling. Immediate referral to a physician is necessary, because a fasciotomy may be needed to decompress the area.

 The football player most likely has a compartment syndrome. Injury usually involves the wrist flexors, finger flexors, and median nerve. The condition warrants immediate referral to a physician.

OVERUSE CONDITIONS

The athletic trainer for a summer tennis camp has been asked to provide suggestions to decrease the risk of lateral epicondylitis. What recommendations should be made?

The throwing mechanism discussed in Chapter 14 also can lead to overuse injuries at the elbow. During the initial acceleration phase, the body is brought forward rapidly, but the elbow and hand lag behind the upper arm. This results in a tremendous tensile valgus stress being placed on the medial aspect of the elbow, particularly the ulnar collateral ligament and adjacent tissues. As acceleration continues, the elbow extensors and wrist flexors contract to add velocity to the throw. This whipping action produces significant valgus stress on the medial elbow and concomitant lateral compressive stress in the radiocapitellar joint (Fig. 14.9). Before release of the ball, the elbow is almost fully extended and is positioned slightly anterior to the trunk. During release, the elbow is flexed approximately 20 to 30°. As these forces decrease, however, the extreme pronation of the forearm places the lateral ligaments under tension. During the deceleration phase, eccentric contractions of the long head of the biceps brachii, supinator, and extensor muscles decelerate the forearm in pronation. Additional stress occurs on structures around the olecranon as pronation and extension jam the olecranon into its fossa. Impingement can occur during this jamming.

Epicondylitis is a common, chronic condition seen in activities involving pronation and supination, such as in tennis, javelin throwing, pitching, volleyball, and golf. This condition sometimes is referred to as a **tendinosis,** because degeneration rather than an inflammatory condition exists. A pattern of poor technique, fatigue, and overuse often is associated with this condition.

Medial Epicondylitis

Medial epicondylitis is caused by repeated, medial tension/lateral compression (valgus) forces placed on the arm during the acceleration phase of the throwing motion (17). The medial humeral apophyseal growth plate in the pediatric athlete is particularly vulnerable to injury and, if affected, is called little league elbow. In a recent study of 9- to 12-year-old pitchers, medial elbow pain was found in

26% (18). Efforts have been imposed in leagues and recreational programs to limit the number of innings pitched per game (to three or four per game) and/or the number of pitches per week (to less than 200) in an attempt to decrease the incidence of medial epicondylitis in adolescents (17).

Injury occurs when valgus forces produce a combined flexor muscle strain, ulnar collateral ligament sprain, and ulnar neuritis. The two most commonly involved tendons are the pronator teres and the flexor carpi radialis. Simultaneously, lateral compressive and shearing forces generated in the olecranon fossa can damage the lateral condyle of the humerus and radial head, leading to capitellar osteochondral injuries. Posterior stresses may lead to triceps strain, synovial impingement, olecranon fractures, or loose bodies and degenerative joint changes.

Signs and Symptoms

Assessment reveals swelling, ecchymosis, and point tenderness over the humeroulnar joint or the flexor/pronator origin, slightly distal and lateral to the medial epicondyle. Pain usually is severe over the medial epicondyle, extending distally 1 to 2 cm along the track of the flexor carpi radialis and pronator teres. Pain is aggravated by resisted wrist flexion and pronation and by a valgus stress applied at 20 to 30° of elbow flexion. There will be a negative Tinel's sign at the cubital tunnel for ulnar neuritis. If the ulnar nerve is involved, tingling and numbness may radiate into the forearm and hand, particularly the fourth and fifth fingers.

■■■■■ FIGURE 14.9 **Traction-compression mechanism.** An excessive valgus force can lead to both medial tensile stress and lateral compression stress, causing injury to both sides of the joint.

Management

Most conditions can be managed with ice, NSAIDs, and immobilization in a sling, with the wrist in slight flexion, for 2 to 3 weeks. In cases involving apophysitis, the resting period may extend from 4 to 6 weeks with limitation or elimination of throwing (19). Transcutaneous electric nerve stimulation (TENS), high-voltage galvanic stimulation, ultrasound, and interferential current are used to decrease pain and inflammation. Early ROM exercises and gentle, resisted isometric exercises should progress to isotonic strengthening and use of surgical tubing. Activity should not resume until the individual can complete all functional tests without pain. A functional brace may limit valgus stress and allow early resumption of strenuous activities. In moderate injuries, throwing or overhead motions should be avoided for up to 6 to 12 weeks (11).

With intra-articular injuries, ulnar nerve problems, or moderate to severe cases of pain or instability, referral to a physician is indicated. Field Strategy 14.4 describes management of medial epicondylitis.

Common Extensor Tendinitis (Lateral Epicondylitis)

Pain over the lateral epicondyle denotes extensor tendon overload and is the most common overuse injury in the adult elbow. The condition typically is caused by eccentric loading of the extensor muscles, predominantly the extensor carpi radialis brevis, during the deceleration phase of the throwing motion or tennis stroke. Faulty mechanics (e.g., "leading" with the elbow and off-center hits in racquet sports), poorly fitted equipment (e.g., improper grip size and improper racquet string tension), and age (i.e., 30–50 years of age) contribute to this condition (11).

Signs and Symptoms

Pain is anterior or just distal to the lateral epicondyle and may radiate into the forearm extensors during and after activity. Pain initially subsides but then becomes more severe with repetition and increases with resisted wrist extension, the "coffee cup" test (i.e., pain increases while picking up a full cup of coffee), and the tennis elbow test.

FIELD STRATEGY 14.4

Management Algorithm for Medial Epicondylitis

1. Limit pain and inflammation with ice, compression, nonsteroidal anti-inflammatory drugs, and rest.
2. Avoid all activities that lead to pain; immobilization may be necessary if simple daily activities cause pain.
3. Other therapies also may supplement the treatment plan, such as ice massage, contrast baths, ultrasound therapy, electrical muscle stimulation, interferential current, and friction massage over the flexor tendons.
4. Maintain range of motion and strength at the wrist and shoulder.
5. Stretching exercises, within pain-free motions, should include wrist flexion-extension, forearm pronation-supination, and radial and ulnar deviation.
6. Begin with fast contractions using light resistance:
   - Perform tennis ball squeezes and other strengthening exercises within pain-free ranges.
   - Add surgical tubing as tolerated.
   - Work up to three to five sets of 10 repetitions per session before moving on to heavier resistance.

7. Incorporate early, closed chain exercises, such as press-ups, wall push-ups, or walking on the hands.
8. Add strengthening exercises for all shoulder, elbow, and wrist motions.
9. Perform a biomechanical analysis of the throwing motion to determine proper technique, and make adjustments as necessary.

After return to protected activity:

1. Continue stretching exercises before and after practice
2. Continue ice after practice to control any inflammation
3. Return to full activity as tolerated

In the adolescent, if an apophyseal fracture or an avulsion fracture of the medial epicondyle is suspected, immediate referral to a physician is warranted. In some settings, this may require activation of the emergency action plan.

FIGURE 14.10 **Ulnar nerve.** As the ulnar nerve passes through the cubital tunnel between the ulnar collateral ligament and the olecranon fossa, it passes under the two heads of the flexor carpi ulnaris. This tendon is slack during extension, but it becomes taut during flexion, contributing to ulnar nerve compression.

Management

Initial treatment should include ice, compression, NSAIDs, and rest. Grasping an object with the forearm pronated is highly discouraged until acute symptoms resolve. Rehabilitation should focus on increasing the strength, endurance, and flexibility of the extensor muscle group. If appropriate, evaluation of mechanics and equipment should be conducted. A counterforce strap placed 2 to 3 inches distal to the elbow joint can limit excessive muscular tension placed on the epicondyle and usually is sufficient to eliminate symptoms. Field Strategy 14.5 describes management of common extensor tendinitis.

Neural Entrapment Injuries

The ulnar nerve passes behind the medial epicondyle of the humerus through the cubital tunnel to rest against the posterior portion of the ulnar collateral ligament (Fig. 14.10). The nerve is vulnerable to compression and tensile stress, which may be caused by trauma (i.e., acute or chronic), cubital valgus deformity, irregularities within the ulnar groove, or subluxation as a result of a lax ulnar collateral ligament. The condition often is referred to as **cubital tunnel syndrome.** The individual complains of a shocking sensation along the medial aspect of the elbow, radiating as if "hitting the crazy bone." Palpation or percussion in the ulnar groove generally produces tingling

FIELD STRATEGY 14.5

Management of Common Extensor Tendinitis

1. Use ice, compression, elevation, nonsteroidal anti-inflammatory drugs, and rest to limit pain and inflammation.
2. Immobilize the wrist in slight extension to allow functional use of the hand.
3. Use cryotherapy, ultrasound, thermotherapy, electrical muscle stimulation, interferential current, and/or friction massage over the extensor tendons to reduce pain and inflammation.
4. Avoid strong gripping activities and any activities that aggravate symptoms.
5. Perform stretching exercises within pain-free motion, including wrist flexion-extension, forearm pronation-supination, and radial and ulnar deviation.

6. Perform isotonic strengthening exercises, and add surgical tubing exercises as tolerated. Begin with fast contractions using light resistance.
7. Work up to three to five sets of 10 repetitions per session before moving on to heavier resistance.
8. Continue active range of motion and strengthening exercises for all shoulder, elbow, and wrist motions.
9. Incorporate closed chain exercises, such as press-ups, wall push-ups, or walking on the hands.
10. Perform a biomechanical analysis of the skills to determine if improper technique may have contributed to the problem, and make appropriate changes.
11. Return to full activity as tolerated, but continue stretching exercises before and after practice. Apply ice after practice to control any inflammation.

and numbness down the medial aspect of the forearm into the ring and little finger (Tinel's sign). Observation may reveal the disappearance of the concavity of the ulnar nerve sulcus. Because the ulnar nerve innervates several intrinsic muscles of the hand, the patient may develop gradual hand weakness, hypotrophy of the first dorsal interosseous muscle, and reduced strength of the deep fifth digit flexor and flexor carpi ulnaris, all of which result in grip and pinch weakness (20).

The median nerve travels across the cubital fossa, passing between the two heads of the pronator teres and the two heads of the flexor digitorum superficialis, to give off its largest branch, the anterior interosseous nerve. Compression may be caused by hypertrophied muscles, particularly the pronator teres, or by compression from fibrous arches near the flexor digitorum superficialis muscle, bicipital aponeurosis, or supracondylar process. It can lead to a condition called **"pronator syndrome,"** in which pain is felt in the anterior proximal forearm and is aggravated with pronation activities. Numbness may occur in the anterior forearm or in the middle and index fingers and thumb.

The radial nerve may be damaged during a midshaft humeral fracture. Less frequently, direct trauma or entrapment occurs at the elbow as the nerve passes anterior to the cubital fossa, pierces the supinator muscle, and runs posterior, again, into the forearm. The condition is referred to as **radial tunnel syndrome**. The terminal branch, the posterior interosseous nerve, supplies the deeper-lying extensor muscles of the forearm. Symptoms of injury often mimic those of lateral epicondylitis. An aching lateral elbow pain may radiate down the posterior forearm. Significant point tenderness can be elicited over the supinator muscle, and resisted supination generally is more painful than wrist extension. Extensor weakness of the wrist, called **wrist drop**, is seen in extreme cases, but no sensory loss tends to be present.

Management

The individual should be referred to a physician immediately. Treatment for neural entrapment depends on the frequency, duration, intensity, magnitude, and cause of the problem. If recognized early, complete rest and NSAIDs can help in acute cases. If the injury is secondary to direct blows, a pad can protect the area. Occasionally, chronic nerve damage may require surgery to release any pressure or constriction on the nerve.

 The following recommendations may help to decrease the risk of lateral epicondylitis: use of a well-fitted racquet with appropriate grip size and string tension, limiting the number of single backhand strokes, increasing the strength of the wrist extensors and supinators, and performing wrist flexibility exercises.

FRACTURES

 A forearm fracture is suspected in a hockey player who was hit by an opposing player's stick. What tests can be used to determine whether a fracture is, in fact present?

Displaced and undisplaced fractures to the humerus, radius, and ulna usually result from violent compressive forces caused by direct trauma, such as an impact with a helmet or implement, a fall on a flexed elbow or outstretched hand with or without a valgus/varus stress, or tensile forces associated with throwing. Because major nerves and vessels run along the bones, serious neurovascular injury can result from the jagged bone fragments. Fractures to the growth plates also are common in javelin throwers, gymnasts, water polo and tennis players, and adolescent baseball and softball pitchers, whereas stress fractures have been reported in gymnasts, volleyball players, and weight lifters.

Epiphyseal and Avulsion Fractures

Because the closing growth plate of the medial epicondyle in adolescents is sensitive to tension stress, a repetitive or sudden contraction of the flexor-pronator muscle group may result in a partial or complete avulsion fracture of the medial epicondyle of the humerus. Referred to as little league elbow, the tension stress is related to throwing curve balls and other breaking pitches that require forceful pronation. Use of this term, however, negates the fact that other individuals, such as golfers, gymnasts, javelin throwers, tennis players, bowlers, squash and racquetball players, wrestlers, and weight lifters, also are susceptible to the condition. Fracture to the secondary growth center of the lateral epicondyle is similar to a medial epicondyle fracture and is treated in a similar manner.

Signs and Symptoms

In the initial phase of the injury, the individual complains of aching during performance, but no limitations in performance and no residual pain are present. As the condition progresses, however, an aching pain during activity limits performance, and a mild postexercise ache is present. Some localized tenderness can be elicited directly over the epicondyle. In severe cases, pain can be intense, with point tenderness, swelling, and ecchymosis directly on the epicondyle.

Management

Standard acute protocol, with activity modification, is followed during the initial stages of injury. If performance is limited because of pain and if postexercise pain is present, the individual should be referred to a physician. The fracture is managed conservatively, with rest and immobilization in a sling for as little as 2 to 3 weeks. Usually, however, throwing is not allowed for 6 to 12 weeks. Surgery is only necessary if a valgus instability is present, the medial epicondyle is incarcerated within the elbow joint, or ulnar nerve symptoms are present.

Stress Fractures

Stress fractures to the diaphysis of the ulna can occur during intensive weight lifting. Bilateral distal radial and ulnar fractures have been found in young individuals who lift heavy weights or lose control of the barbells, resulting in added shear stress. For this reason, adolescents in a weight-lifting program should be properly instructed and supervised.

Osteochondritis Dissecans

An unusual complication of repetitive stress to the skeletally immature elbow is osteochondritis dissecans. The mechanism is attributed to lateral compressive forces exerted during the throwing motion, which can damage the radial head, capitellum, or both. It is the leading cause of permanent elbow disability in adolescent athletes (19). In adolescents with open growth plates (age, 12–15 years), a focal lesion can lead to destruction of the overlying articular cartilage, with fragmentation and softening of the underlying subchondral bone. A microfracture (i.e., loose bodies) and eventual avascular necrosis lead to further joint degeneration.

An associated osteochondrosis condition, called Panner's disease, is the most common cause of chronic lateral elbow pain, encompassing the entire capitellum in young athletes under 10 years of age (19). Pain is present over the lateral and anterior elbow. The pain increases with deep palpation or pronation-supination, but it quickly resolves with decreased activity. Elbow extension may be limited by 20° or more secondary to synovitis and a deformed capitellar congruity. Loose body formation is much less likely to occur in Panner's disease.

Signs and Symptoms

Signs and symptoms of osteochondritis dissecans mirror little league elbow. An insidious onset of dull, activity-related, and poorly localized pain may precede other, more severe symptoms, such as locking, decreased motion, and flexion contractures of more than 15° (19). Swelling and tenderness is centralized over the radiocapitellar joint, and grating may be present during passive pronation and supination. The ability to fully extend the elbow may be limited.

Management

Management involves referral to a physician. Treatment usually is conservative, with rest for 6 to 18 months. If no loose body is present, no further treatment may be needed. If a fragment is displaced, surgery may be necessary to reattach a large articular fragment or to excise a small fragment.

Displaced and Undisplaced Fractures

Supracondylar fractures, which are caused by falling on an outstretched hand, occur largely in children, with the peak incidence occurring between 4 and 8 years of age (21). A catastrophic complication from this fracture is ischemic necrosis of the forearm muscles, known as **Volkmann's contracture.** The brachial artery or median nerve can be damaged by the fractured bone ends, leading to major circulatory or neural impairment of the forearm and hand. As a result, the hand is cold, white, and numb. The presence of a radial or ulnar pulse does not automatically indicate adequate circulation to the forearm muscles. Severe pain in the forearm is aggravated by passive extension of the fingers. These symptoms indicate a serious problem.

> The arm should be immobilized in a vacuum splint. The emergency action plan should be activated to ensure immediate transport of the individual to the nearest medical facility. EMS

Fracture of the olecranon process of the ulna results from direct trauma, such as being struck with an implement or falling on a flexed elbow. The tension of the triceps pulls the bone fragment superiorly. Because this fracture is intra-articular, it does not respond to conservative treatment and requires surgical intervention.

The head of the radius may be fractured as a result of a valgus stress that tears the ulnar collateral ligament, leading to traumatic compressive and shearing stress on the radial head. The fracture may be nondisplaced (type I), displaced (type II), or comminuted (type III). Tenderness can be elicited on palpation of the radial head, and swelling can be seen lateral to the olecranon. Flexion and extension may or may not be limited. In contrast, passive pronation and supination is both painful and restricted. There also may be an associated valgus instability of the elbow or axial instability of the forearm. A nondisplaced fracture is treated nonoperatively, with early ROM exercises to prevent joint stiffness. With more than one-third of the articular surface involved, more than 30° of angulation, or more than 3 mm of fracture gap, open reduction is recommended (11).

The **"nightstick fracture,"** which is seen in football and hockey players, is caused by a direct blow to the forearm that fractures the ulna. Following closed reduction, splinting or casting for 7 to 10 days is needed to allow the initial swelling and discomfort to subside. If a radial head dislocation or a distal radial ulnar joint subluxation is present, open reduction and internal fixation are necessary.

In gymnastics, a unique forearm fracture occurs as a result of wearing leather grips with enclosed dowels. The dowels help to grip the horizontal bar. Problems arise, however, when the leather grip "catches" or grabs onto the bar and holds the hand in position, preventing the individual from continuing during a giant swing maneuver. This action causes the forearm to "wrap around" and sustain multiple fractures. Severe pain and disability with this fracture require immediate immobilization in a vacuum splint and transport to the nearest medical facility.

Fracture Management

Fractures should be suspected in all elbow and forearm injuries. Palpation, compression, traction, and percussion, which can assist in determining possible fractures, are explained in Field Strategy 14.6. In addition, a neurologic and circulatory assessment should be conducted. If the radial nerve is damaged, forearm supination and extension at the elbow, wrist, or fingers will be weak, and sensory changes may occur on the dorsum of the hand. If the median nerve is damaged, active wrist and finger flexion will be weak, and sensory changes may occur on the palm of the hand.

If the ulnar nerve is damaged, ulnar deviation and finger abduction and adduction will be weak, and sensory changes may occur on the ulnar border of the hand. The examiner should take a pulse

FIELD STRATEGY 14.6

Determining a Possible Fracture in the Upper Arm and Forearm

1. **Compression.** Palpate the region for any pain, deformity, crepitus, or loose bodies. Ask if the individual heard any cracking sounds that might indicate a possible fracture. Apply gentle compression along the long axis of the bone. Then, encircle the distal ulna and radius with your hand, and give mild compression. This will produce some distraction at the proximal end of the ulna and radius. Increased pain in either position indicates a possible fracture.
2. **Distraction.** Slowly distract the bones. If pain eases, this may indicate a possible fracture. If pain increases, it indicates soft-tissue damage.
3. **Percussion.** Gently tap the superficial bony landmarks. Vibrations travel along the bone and cause

increased pain at the fracture site. For example, tap the following sites:

- **Humerus**—medial and lateral epicondyles
- **Ulna**—olecranon process and distal styloid process
- **Radius**—distal styloid process

4. **Tuning fork.** Tap a tuning fork, and place the base on the superficial bone sites mentioned in the preceding. Increased pain indicates a possible fracture.

Any positive signs indicate a possible fracture. Immobilize the limb in a vacuum splint or other appropriate splint or sling, and transport the individual to the nearest medical facility.

at the wrist or the ulnar and radial arteries, or the examiner should blanch the fingernails and note capillary refill. A vacuum splint should be applied and the individual transported immediately to the nearest medical facility.

The tests to determine a possible forearm fracture include applying gentle compression along the long axis of the bone and noting any pain; encircling the distal ulna and radius with the hand, applying mild compression, and noting any pain; and performing percussion over superficial bony landmarks or using a tuning fork over the bony prominences and noting any increase in pain at the fracture site.

ASSESSMENT OF ELBOW CONDITIONS

A little league baseball player is complaining of pain on the medial elbow during pitching. How should the assessment of this injury progress to determine the extent and severity of injury?

The elbow's primary role is to place the forearm and hand in the most appropriate position to perform efficient motion. Biomechanical errors in throwing technique at the shoulder can place additional stress at the elbow. Because use of equipment often is associated with overuse problems, it is important to determine if the individual uses a bat, racquet, field hockey or lacrosse stick, or other implement. Assessment of skill technique to rule out possible contributing factors also is advisable.

> See *Field Strategy: Elbow Evaluation,* available on the companion website at thePoint, for a summary of the assessment of the upper arm, elbow, and forearm.

    Because of the severity of the trauma, recognizing possible fractures and dislocations early in an assessment is essential. It also is important to understand that pain may be referred from the cervical region, shoulder, or wrist to the arm. As in any assessment, both arms should be fully visible to allow bilateral comparison.

HISTORY

The injury assessment of the little league baseball player should begin with a history. What questions need to be asked to identify the cause and extent of this injury?

The onset and location of symptoms are two of the most critical facts surrounding elbow trauma. This information forms the basis for determining the cause-and-effect relationship between the mechanism and the onset of injury. In gathering information about the primary complaint, questions should focus on the individual's perception of pain, weakness, or sensory changes. It also is important to note if the nature of the injury is acute or overuse. Specific questions should be asked related to equipment, technique, and recent changes in training intensity, frequency, or duration.

> See *Field Strategy: Developing a History of the Injury,* available on the companion website at thePoint, for specific questions that should be included in an elbow evaluation.

The little league baseball player should be asked questions that address the following: when, where, and how; throwing technique and training regimen; phase of throwing motion in which pain occurs; intensity, location, and type of pain; actions that relieve pain; and any previous injury, treatment, and medication.

OBSERVATION AND INSPECTION

The history of the little league player reveals an aching pain has been present for 2 to 3 days. The pain intensifies during the acceleration phase of throwing and has started to affect his performance. Explain the observation component in the ongoing assessment of the little league player.

If the history has indicated an insidious onset of elbow trauma, the individual's full-body posture, especially of the neck and shoulder area, should be observed. In an acute injury, if the individual is in great pain or is unable or unwilling to move the elbow, the assessment should be completed in the position that is most comfortable for the individual.

Initially, the arm should be observed from an anterior position for any noticeable deformity and possible holding of the arm. If swelling is present in the joint, the individual may be unable to fully extend the elbow, resulting in a slightly flexed position. This **resting position** allows the joint to have maximal volume to accommodate intra-articular swelling. The carrying angle of the arms should be noted. A normal angle is slight valgus, with the forearm fully supinated and the elbow extended. Angles of greater than 20° are referred to as **cubital valgus**; angles of less than 10° are referred to as **cubital varus**. Baseball pitchers may exhibit cubital valgus in the throwing arm as an adaptation to repeated valgus loading during the throwing motion. The alignment of the forearm and humerus normally is fully extended, although extension beyond 0° (**cubital recurvatum**) is common, especially in females.

In the next portion of the observation, the elbow should be observed in the position of function, namely 90° of flexion, with the hand being held halfway between supination and pronation. The entire region should be assessed for symmetry and any abnormal deformity, muscle atrophy, hypertrophy, swelling, discoloration, or previous surgical incisions. In particular, the cubital fossa, which is a triangular area bounded laterally by the brachioradialis muscle and medially by the pronator teres muscle, should be inspected. The biceps brachii tendon, median nerve, and brachial artery pass through the fossa. The presence of swelling in the fossa can place pressure on the neurovascular structures as they pass through the area.

Next, the medial aspect of the arm should be inspected. The medial epicondyle of the humerus should be prominent rather than obscured by excessive swelling. The wrist flexor muscle mass should appear bilaterally equal in terms of muscle tone and mass. Atrophy of the mass may result from disuse associated with long-term tendinitis or prolonged immobilization.

Observation should then move to the lateral aspect of the arm. The wrist extensor muscle mass on the lateral aspect of the elbow also should appear bilaterally equal in terms of muscle tone and mass. Atrophy of the mass may result from disuse associated with long-term tendinitis, prolonged immobilization, or radial nerve pathology.

Finally, the arm should be observed from a posterior position. It is important to note the position of the olecranon relative to the epicondyles of the humerus. In a flexed position, the olecranon process and epicondyles should form an isosceles triangle; in an extended position, the olecranon process and epicondyles should form a straight line. The olecranon process should be clearly visible rather than obscured by excessive swelling.

(A) Observation of the little league player should include the following: full-body posture, carrying angle and position of function, and inspection at the site for swelling, discoloration, deformity, muscle hypertrophy, atrophy, and other signs of trauma.

PALPATION

(Q) Observation of the little league player reveals minor swelling over the medial epicondyle. No other visible signs are apparent. Explain palpation specific to the injury sustained by the player.

The injured arm should be supported during palpation. Bilateral palpation should determine temperature, swelling, point tenderness, crepitus, deformity, muscle spasm, and cutaneous sensation. In general, palpation should move from proximal to distal, leaving the areas that are anticipated to be the most painful for last. Pulses can be taken at the radial and ulnar arteries at the wrist and at the brachial artery in the cubital fossa. The following structures should be palpated:

Anterior Palpation

1. Cubital fossa, biceps brachii tendon, median nerve, and brachial artery

2. Coracoid process and head of radius

Lateral Palpation

1. Lateral supracondylar ridge and brachioradialis muscle

2. Lateral epicondyle, common wrist extensors, and supinator muscle

3. Radial collateral ligament

4. Annular ligament and head of the radius (this is facilitated by supination and pronation of the forearm)

Posterior Palpation

1. Triceps muscle

2. Olecranon process and olecranon fossa (this is facilitated by positioning the elbow in 45° of flexion to relax the triceps)

3. Olecranon bursa (the skin overlying the olecranon process should be grasped, which permits palpation to note any thickening or presence of loose bodies)

4. Ulnar nerve in the cubital tunnel

5. Ulnar border distal to the styloid process at the wrist

Medial Palpation

1. Medial supracondylar ridge

2. Medial epicondyle and common wrist flexor-pronator tendons and muscles

3. Ulnar collateral ligament

During the assessment of the little league player, the following structures should be palpated for point tenderness, swelling, deformity, skin temperature, sensation, and other signs of trauma: medial supracondylar ridge, medial epicondyle, proximal attachment of wrist flexors and pronators, ulnar collateral ligament, ulna, olecranon, and ulnar nerve.

PHYSICAL EXAMINATION TESTS

Palpation of the little league player revealed point tenderness and swelling directly on the medial epicondyle. Based on the information obtained through the history, observation, and palpation, what tests should be performed as part of the physical examination of the little league player?

If a fracture or dislocation is suspected, testing should not be performed. Instead, the arm should be immobilized in an appropriate splint, and the emergency action plan should be activated. In some settings, summoning EMS may be warranted. Only those tests that are necessary to assess the current injury should be performed.

Functional Tests

The available ROM in elbow flexion-extension, forearm pronation-supination, and wrist flexion-extension should be determined. If trauma to the ulnar, median, or radial nerves is suspected, ROM testing of the thumb and fingers also should be performed.

Active Movements

The examiner should stabilize the upper arm against the body to prevent muscle substitution. As with previous assessments, bilateral comparison with the uninvolved arm is necessary. Active movements that are anticipated to be painful should be performed last to prevent painful symptoms from overflowing into the next movement.

The motions that should be assessed and the normal ROM for each are as follows:

- Flexion at the elbow (140–150°)
- Extension at the elbow (0–10°)
- Supination of the forearm (90°)
- Pronation of the forearm (90°)
- Flexion of the wrist (80–90°)
- Extension of the wrist (70–90°)

During elbow extension, it is important to recognize that some females can extend as much as 5 to 15° below the straight line. Bilateral comparison verifies whether this extra motion is normal for the individual. In performing active pronation and supination, the individual should be instructed to flex the elbow to 90° and then secure the elbow next to the body to avoid any glenohumeral motion. Goniometry measurements are demonstrated in Figure 14.11.

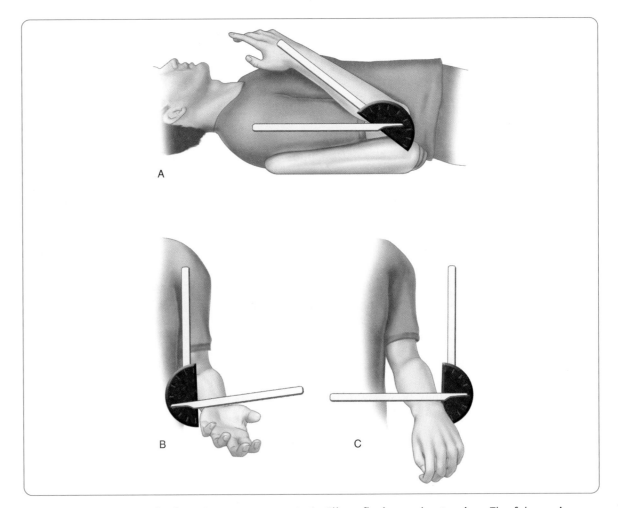

■■ ■■ FIGURE 14.11 **Goniometry measurement. A,** Elbow flexion and extension. The fulcrum is centered over the lateral epicondyle of the humerus. The proximal arm is aligned along the humerus, using the acromion process for reference. The distal arm is aligned along the radius, using the styloid process for reference. **B,** Forearm supination. The fulcrum is centered medial to the ulnar styloid process. The proximal arm is parallel to the midline of the humerus, and the distal arm is placed across the palmar aspect of the forearm just proximal to the styloid processes of the radius and ulna. **C,** Forearm pronation. The fulcrum is centered lateral to the ulnar styloid process. The arms are placed in the same position but on the dorsal aspect of the forearm.

Passive Movements

If the individual is able to perform full ROM during active movements, gentle pressure should be applied at the extremes of motion to determine end feel. The normal end feels are as follows:

- **Tissue stretch**—elbow flexion; supination; pronation
- **Tissue approximation**—shoulder adduction
- **Bone to bone**—elbow extension

Resisted Muscle Testing

The elbow should be stabilized against the body during muscle testing to prevent any muscle substitution. The testing begins with the examiner placing the muscle on a stretch. When performing the various motions, the examiner should apply gentle resistance proximal to the wrist throughout the full ROM. To avoid allowing finger flexors or extensors to assist during movement, instruct the individual to keep the thumb and fingers relaxed. Motion should be assessed several times to note any weakness or fatigue. Any sudden or jarring motions should be avoided, because this may lead to undue pain. Any lag or muscle weakness should be noted. Muscle actions that may cause extreme pain should be delayed until the final phase of muscle testing. Figure 14.12 demonstrates motions that should be tested.

Stress Tests

In using stress tests, only those tests that are absolutely necessary should be performed. In moving through the tests, the examiner should begin by applying gentle stress. The force should be applied several times with increasing overpressure. The presence of pain or joint laxity should be noted.

■■■■■ FIGURE 14.12 **Resisted manual muscle testing for the elbow.** The myotomes for each motion are listed in parentheses. **A,** Elbow flexion (C$_6$). **B,** Elbow extension (C$_7$). **C,** Forearm supination. **D,** Forearm pronation. **E,** Wrist flexion (C$_7$). **F,** Wrist extension (C$_6$).

FIGURE 14.13 Ligamentous instability tests. A, The ulnar collateral ligament: a valgus force at multiple angles. **B,** The radial collateral ligament: a varus force at multiple angles. Arrows indicate the direction in which the examiner applies stress.

Ulnar Collateral Ligament Stress Test

Because of the amount of rotation that occurs at the shoulder, it is difficult to get an accurate valgus or varus stress at the elbow. As such, tests should be performed at multiple angles, from full extension to 20 to 30° of flexion. When the olecranon is "unlocked" from the olecranon fossa, the ligamentous structures are isolated. While the individual is seated, the arm should be stabilized and a valgus or abduction force applied to the distal forearm to stress the ulnar collateral ligament (Fig. 14.13A).

Radial Collateral Ligament Stress Test

Following the same procedures as used for testing the ulnar collateral ligament, a varus or adduction force should be applied at the forearm in the various angles to stress the radial collateral ligament (Fig. 14.13B).

Special Tests

Several special tests can be used for detecting injury or related pathology (e.g., epicondylitis and neuritis).

Common Extensor Tendinitis Test (Lateral Epicondylitis or Tennis Elbow Tests)

The examiner stabilizes the individual's flexed elbow and palpates the lateral epicondyle. The individual is instructed to make a fist and pronate the forearm. Next, the individual attempts to radially deviate and extend the wrist while the examiner applies resistance (Fig. 14.14A). A positive sign is indicated if severe pain is present over the lateral epicondyle of the humerus. The same results can be elicited through passively stretching the extensor muscles by simultaneously pronating the forearm, flexing the wrist, and extending the elbow (Fig. 14.14B). In some cases, discomfort also can

FIGURE 14.14 Tests for common extensor tendinitis. A, Resisted extension and radial deviation of the wrist. **B,** Passive stretching of the wrist extensors. **C,** Resisted extension of the extensor digitorum communis in the middle finger with the wrist extended. Arrows indicate the direction in which the individual moves the joint.

be produced by testing the extensor digitorum communis of the third digit through the application of resistance distal to the proximal interphalangeal joint with the wrist extended (Fig. 14.14C).

Medial Epicondylitis Tests

Initially, the flexed elbow is stabilized against the body, and the forearm is supinated. The examiner palpates the medial epicondyle. Next, the examiner extends the wrist and elbow while the individual resists the movement. A positive sign is indicated by pain over the medial epicondyle of the humerus.

Tinel's Sign for Ulnar Neuritis

The cubital tunnel is tapped on the posteromedial side of the elbow. A positive sign is indicated by a tingling sensation that runs down the ulnar aspect of the forearm into the medial half of the fourth finger and all of the fifth finger (Fig. 14.15).

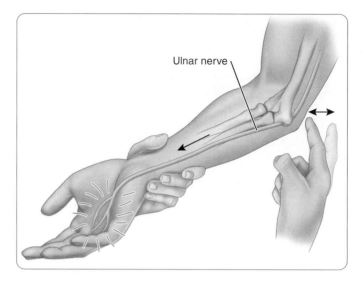

■■ ■ FIGURE 14.15 Tinel's sign. Tapping over the cubital tunnel produces a tingling sensation down the ulnar nerve into the forearm and hand. A positive Tinel's sign indicates ulnar nerve entrapment.

Elbow Flexion Test for Ulnar Neuritis

This test determines whether the ulnar nerve is entrapped in the cubital tunnel. The individual is instructed to flex the elbow completely and hold it in that position for 5 minutes. A positive test is indicated by tingling or numbness in the ulnar nerve distribution pattern of the forearm and hand.

Test for Pronator Teres Syndrome

The individual sits with the elbow flexed at 90°. The examiner strongly resists forearm pronation while the elbow is extended. A positive test is indicated by tingling or paresthesia in the median nerve distribution of the forearm and hand.

Pinch Grip Test

The individual is instructed to pinch the tip of the index finger and thumb together (Fig. 14.16). Normally, there should be a tip-to-tip pinch. If an abnormal pulp-to-pulp pinch is performed, the anterior interosseous nerve, which is an extension of the median nerve, may be entrapped at the elbow as it passes between the two heads of the pronator teres.

■■ ■ FIGURE 14.16 Pinch grip test. The individual is instructed to make an "0" with the thumb and forefinger. **A,** Normal tip-to-tip. **B,** Abnormal pulp-to-pulp, which signifies entrapment of the interior interosseous nerve.

■■■■ FIGURE 14.17 Reflex testing.
Brachioradialis reflex.

Neurologic Tests

Neurologic integrity can be assessed with the use of myotomes, reflexes, and cutaneous patterns, which include both segmental dermatomes and peripheral nerve patterns.

Myotomes

Isometric muscle testing should be performed in the following motions to test specific myotomes in the upper extremity:

- Scapular elevation (C_4)
- Shoulder abduction (C_5)
- Elbow flexion and/or wrist extension (C_6)
- Elbow extension and/or wrist flexion (C_7)
- Thumb extension and/or ulnar deviation (C_8)
- Abduction and/or adduction of the hand intrinsics (T_1)

Reflexes

Reflexes in the upper extremity include the biceps (C_5–C_6), brachioradialis (C_6), and triceps (C_7). The individual should be relaxed, with the elbow flexed. The biceps and triceps reflex testing is explained in Figure 13.37.

The brachioradialis reflex is tested in a similar manner. The elbow is flexed and supported by the examiner's forearm, with the wrist in slight ulnar deviation. A reflex hammer is used to strike the brachioradialis tendon at the distal end of the radius (Fig. 14.17). In some individuals, the tap may need to be applied 2 to 3 inches proximal to the wrist. A slight jerk in elbow flexion is a normal sign.

Cutaneous Patterns

The segmental nerve dermatome patterns for the elbow region are demonstrated in Fig. 14.18. The peripheral nerve cutaneous patterns are demonstrated in Fig. 14.19. Testing is performed bilaterally for altered sensation with sharp and dull touch by running the open hand and fingernails over the neck, shoulder, and anterior and posterior chest walls as well as down both sides of the arms and hands.

■■■ FIGURE 14.18 Dermatome patterns for the elbow region. A, Anterior view. **B,** Posterior view.

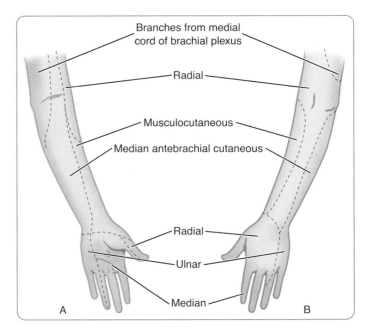

■■■ FIGURE 14.19 Cutaneous patterns for the peripheral nerves. A, Anterior view. **B,** Posterior view.

Box 14.2   Signs and Symptoms That Necessitate Immediate Referral to a Physician

- Possible epiphyseal or apophyseal injuries
- Tingling or numbness in the forearm or hand
- Obvious deformity suggesting a dislocation or fracture
- Excessive joint swelling
- Significantly limited range of motion

- Weakness in a myotome
- Gross joint instability
- Abnormal or absent reflexes
- Absent or weak pulse
- Any unexplained pain

Activity-Specific Functional Tests

The elbow is in the middle of the upper extremity kinetic chain. Therefore, it must function properly to position the hand so that daily activities can be performed smoothly and efficiently. Activities such as combing the hair, throwing a ball, lifting an object, or pushing an object should be performed without pain. The individual should be instructed to perform the skills that are needed to complete activities of daily living and sport-specific tasks. Each movement should be pain-free and fluid. If any of the conditions listed in Box 14.2 are present, the individual should be referred to a physician.

A *Bilateral testing of the little league player should include AROM, PROM, and RROM for elbow flexion, elbow extension, pronation, supination, wrist flexion, and wrist extension; medial epicondylitis test; Tinel's sign for ulnar neuritis; elbow flexion test for ulnar neuritis; pronator teres syndrome test; grip strength; and varus stress.*

REHABILITATION

Q *The little league baseball player is diagnosed with little league elbow. The fracture was managed conservatively with a sling for 3 weeks. When the individual begins rehabilitation, what exercises should be included in the general program?*

Rehabilitation of the upper arm, elbow, and forearm must involve exercises for the entire kinetic chain, because muscles in the upper arm cross the shoulder and elbow and muscles in the forearm cross the elbow and wrist. Traumatic injuries to the elbow often require immobilization. Although the elbow is immobilized, early ROM and strengthening exercises can be conducted at the wrist, hand, and shoulder.

The management of some injuries will not require immobilization, but pain may be exacerbated by certain motions. The exercise program should focus on early mobilization in the available pain-free motions and expand to the other motions once the pain has subsided. Individuals who are involved in throwing-type activities also should include scapular stabilization exercises along with strengthening exercises for the shoulder.

The reader should refer to Chapter 13 for appropriate shoulder exercises. This section focuses only on those exercises specific to the upper arm, elbow, and forearm.

Restoration of Motion

Range-of-motion exercises should focus on elbow flexion and extension, forearm pronation and supination, wrist flexion and extension, and wrist radial and ulnar deviation. The individual can use the opposite hand to apply a low-load, prolonged stretch in the various motions to minimize joint trauma and increase flexibility (Fig. 14.20). The upper body ergometer also is an effective ROM tool.

FIGURE 14.20 Range-of-motion exercises can be facilitated by using the opposite hand to apply a sustained stretch.

Restoration of Proprioception and Balance

Closed chain exercises may be performed immediately after the acute phase of injury. Shifting body weight from one hand to the other may be performed on a wall, table top, or unstable surface, such as a foam mat or a biomechanical ankle platform system board. Push-ups and exercises in a frontal and sagittal plane can be performed on a ProFitter or slide board, if available. Step-ups can be completed on a box, stool, or StairMaster. This activity can progress to stepping up and down on boxes of differing heights, arranged so that the exercise is performed in diagonal patterns, circles, or figure-eights.

As with the shoulder injury, the throwing motion should be rehearsed using mirrors or videotape. As the motion is performed, biomechanical errors at the elbow are corrected. When motion is perfected, speed of movement and distance of throw are increased gradually.

Muscular Strength, Endurance, and Power

Gentle, resisted isometric exercises can begin immediately after injury or after surgery while the arm is still immobilized. As the individual improves, more overload is applied. When normal ROM is achieved, open kinetic chain exercises can be performed in the various motions using lightweight dumbbells; many of these exercises were demonstrated in Field Strategy 14.1. The individual should complete 30 to 50 repetitions using a 1-pound weight and should not progress in resistance until 50 repetitions are achieved. Wrist curls, reverse wrist curls, pronation, and supination should be performed with the forearm supported on a table. A weighted bar or hammer can be used for both radial and ulnar deviation and for pronation and supination. Another common exercise is the wrist curl-up. Using a broomstick with a light weight suspended on a 3- to 4-foot rope, the individual slowly winds the rope up around the stick and then slowly unwinds the rope. Proprioceptive neuromuscular facilitation, resisted exercises, and surgical tubing are used for concentric and eccentric loading.

Plyometric exercises may involve catching a weighted ball and using a quick, eccentric stretch of the muscle to facilitate a concentric contraction in throwing the ball. The exercise can progress through various one- and two-arm chest passes and overhead passes. A minitramp can also be used to perform plyometric bounding push-ups.

Cardiovascular Fitness

Cardiovascular conditioning should be maintained throughout the rehabilitation program. Several examples of such programs are provided in Field Strategy: Cardiovascular-Conditioning Exercises located on thePoint website.

The little league baseball player should focus on restoring ROM in elbow flexion-extension, forearm pronation-supination, wrist flexion-extension, and radial and ulnar deviation. Isometric strengthening exercises should begin immediately in pain-free motions, with active exercises beginning as soon as normal ROM is achieved. The program also should include general body conditioning and strengthening exercises for the shoulder, elbow, and wrist.

SUMMARY

1. The elbow encompasses three articulations: the humeroulnar, humeroradial, and proximal radioulnar joints.

2. The medial collateral ligament is the most important ligament for stability of the elbow joint. It is divided into the anterior, transverse, and posterior oblique bands.

3. The major nerves of the elbow and forearm include the musculocutaneous, median, ulnar, and radial nerves.

4. Chronic blows to the arm can result in the development of ectopic bone, either in the belly of the muscle (myositis ossificans) or as an outgrowth (exostosis) of the underlying bone.

5. The subcutaneous olecranon bursa is the largest bursa in the elbow region. Bursitis may be acute or chronic, aseptic or septic.

6. In adolescents, the most common traumatic injury to the elbow is subluxation or dislocation of the radial head, referred to as "nursemaid's elbow" or "pulled-elbow syndrome."

7. Most ulnar dislocations occur in individuals younger than 20 years, with a peak incidence during early adolescence. The mechanism usually is hyperextension or a sudden, violent, unidirectional valgus force that drives the ulna posterior or posterolateral. Because 60% of elbow dislocations have an associated fracture, the limb should be immobilized in a vacuum splint and the individual transported immediately to the nearest medical facility.

8. Chronic injuries can result from inadequate warm-up, excessive training past the point of fatigue, inadequate rehabilitation of previous injuries, or neglect of seemingly minor conditions that progress to major complications.

9. Repetitive throwing motions place a tremendous tensile stress on the medial joint structures (i.e., medial collateral ligament, ulnar nerve, and common flexor tendons) and concomitant lateral compressive stress in the radiocapitellar joint.

10. Medial epicondylitis produces severe pain on resisted wrist flexion and pronation and with a valgus stress applied at 15 to 20° of elbow flexion.

11. Common extensor tendinitis produces severe pain on resisted wrist extension and supination and with a varus stress applied at 15 to 20° of elbow flexion.

12. Lateral compressive forces on the radiocapitellar joint can lead to osteochondritis dissecans of the skeletally immature elbow.

13. If a decision is made to refer an individual to a physician for care, the limb should be appropriately immobilized to protect the area.

14. Subsequent to the history, observation, and palpation components of an assessment, the examiner should have established a strong suspicion of the structures that may be damaged. As such, during the physical examination component, some tests will be compulsory, whereas others are used to confirm or exclude suspected injury or pathology. Only those tests that are absolutely necessary should be performed.

15. A rehabilitation program should focus on the following: reduction of pain and spasm; restoration of motion and balance; development of strength, endurance, and power; and maintenance of cardiovascular fitness. The individual should have bilateral strength, flexibility, and muscular endurance as well as an appropriate cardiovascular level before returning to participation in sport and physical activity. Whenever possible, protective equipment or padding should be used to prevent reinjury.

REFERENCES

1. Kocker MS, Waters PM, Micheli LJ. Upper extremity injuries in the pediatric athlete. Sports Med 2000;30(2): 117–135.

2. Cain EL Jr, Dugas JR, Wolf RS, Andrews JR. Elbow injuries in throwing athletes: a current concepts review. Am J Sports Med 2003;31:621–635.

3. Alcid JG, Ahmad CS, Lee TQ. Elbow anatomy and structural biomechanics. Clin Sports Med 2004;23:503–517.

4. Paraskevas G, Papadopoulos A, Papaziogas B, et al. Study of the carrying angle of the human elbow joint in full extension: a morphometric analysis. Surg Radiol Anat 2004;26:19–23.

5. Bozkurt M, Acar HI, Apaydin N, et al. The annular ligament: an anatomical study. Am J Sports Med 2005;33: 114–118.

6. Rettig AC, Patel DV. Epidemiology of elbow, forearm, and wrist injuries in the athlete. Clin Sport Med 1995;14(2): 289–297.

7. Chou PH, Lin CJ, Chou YL, et al. Elbow load with various forearm positions during one-handed push-up exercise. Int J Sports Med 2002;23(6):457–462.

8. Chen FS, Rokito AS, Jobe FW. Medial elbow problems in the overhead-throwing athlete. J Am Acad Orthop Surg 2001;9(2):99–113.

9. Rettig AC, Sherrill C, Snead DS, et al. Nonoperative treatment of ulnar collateral ligament injuries in throwing athletes. Am J Sports Med 2001;29(1):15–17.

10. Salzman KL, Lillegard WA, Butcher JD. Upper extremity bursitis. Am Fam Physician 1997;56(7):1797–1806.

11. Mehlhoff TL, Bennett JB. Elbow injuries. In: Mellion MB,

Walsh WM, Madden C, Putukian M, Shelton GL, eds. The Team Physician's Handbook. Philadelphia: Hanley & Belfus, 2002.

12. Pugh DM, Wild LM, Schemitsch EH, et al. Standard surgical protocol to treat elbow dislocations with radial head and coronoid fractures. J Bone Joint Surg Am 2004;86(6): 1122–1130.

13. Rumball JS, Lebrun CM, DiCiacca SR, Orland K. Rowing injuries. Sports Med 2005;35(6):537–555.

14. Caldwell GL Jr, Safran MR. Elbow problems in the athlete. Orthop Clin North Am 1995;26(3):465–485.

15. Özyürekölu T, Tsai TM. Ruptures of the distal biceps tendon: results of three surgical techniques. Hand Surg 2003;8(1):65–73.

16. Pearl ML, Bessos K, Wong K. Strength deficits related to distal biceps tendon rupture and repair. Am J Sports Med 1998;26(2):295–296.

17. Adirim TA, Cheng TL. Overview of injuries in the young athlete. Sports Med 2003;33(1):75–81.

18. Lyman S, Fleisig GS, Roseman JM, et al. Longitudinal study of elbow and shoulder pain in youth baseball pitchers. Med Sci Sports Exerc 2001;33(11):1803–1810.

19. Klingele KE, Kocher MS. Little league elbow: valgus overload injury in the pediatric athlete. Sports Med 2002; 32(15):1005–1015.

20. Matev B. Cubital tunnel syndrome. Hand Surg 2003;8(1): 127–131.

21. Platt B. Supracondylar fracture of the humerus. Emerg Nurse 2004;12(2)22–29.

Wrist and Hand Conditions

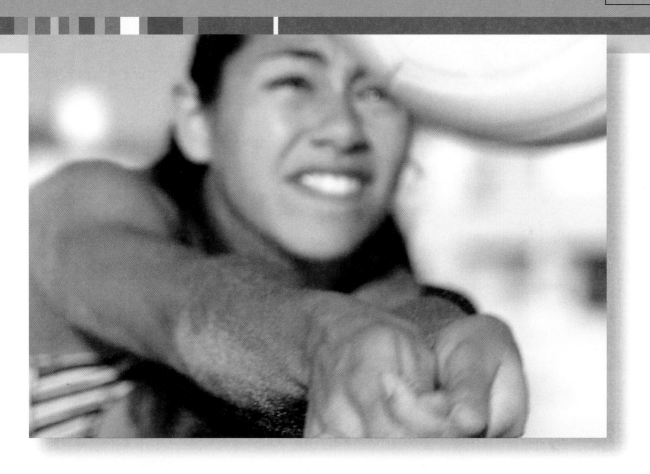

STUDENT OUTCOMES

1. Identify the major bony and soft-tissue structures of the wrist and hand.

2. Describe the pathways of the median, ulnar, and radial nerves, and identify the motor and sensory components of each nerve.

3. Describe the motions of the wrist and hand, and identify the muscles that produce them.

4. Describe the forces that produce the loading patterns responsible for common injuries of the wrist and hand.

5. Explain the general principles used to prevent injuries to the wrist and hand.

6. List the common injuries and conditions sustained to the wrist and hand by physically active individuals (including sprains, dislocations, strains, tendinopathies, and nerve entrapment syndromes).

7. Describe the various types of fractures that can occur in the wrist and hand, and explain their management.

8. Explain management strategies for common injuries and conditions of the wrist and hand.

9. Describe a thorough assessment of the wrist and hand.

10. Explain general principles and techniques used in developing a rehabilitation exercise program for the wrist and hand.

ROLE DELINEATION COMPETENCIES

The following Performance Domains and Tasks defined in the National Athletic Trainers' Association Board of Certification *Role Delineation Study*, 5th Edition are addressed in this chapter:

BOC COMPETENCIES

I.   Prevention

    G. Monitor participants and environmental conditions by following accepted guidelines to promote safe participation.

II.   Clinical Evaluation and Diagnosis

    A. Obtain a history through observation, interview, and/or review of relevant records to assess current or potential injury, illness, or condition.
    B. Inspect the involved area(s) visually to assess the injury, illness, or health-related condition.
    C. Palpate the involved area(s) using standard techniques to assess the injury, illness, or health-related condition.
    D. Perform specific tests in accordance with accepted procedures to assess the injury, illness, or health-related condition.
    E. Formulate a clinical impression by interpreting the signs, symptoms, and predisposing factors of the injury, illness, or condition to determine the appropriate course of action.

III. Immediate Care

    A. Employ life-saving techniques through the use of standard emergency procedures in order to reduce morbidity and the incidence of mortality.
    B. Prevent exacerbation of non–life threatening condition(s) through the use of standard procedures in order to reduce morbidity.
    C. Facilitate the timely transfer of care for conditions beyond the scope of practice of the athletic trainer by implementing appropriate referral strategies to stabilize and/or prevent exacerbation of the condition(s).

IV. Treatment, Rehabilitation, and Reconditioning

    E. Reassess the status of injuries, illnesses, and/or conditions using standard techniques and documentation strategies in order to determine appropriate treatment, rehabilitation, and/or reconditioning and to evaluate readiness to return to a desired level of activity.
    F. Educate the appropriate individual(s) in the treatment, rehabilitation, and reconditioning of injuries, illnesses, and/or conditions using applicable methods and materials to facilitate recovery, function, and/or performance.

The wrist and hand are used extensively during activities of daily living and in nearly all sport skills. Injuries to the region often result from the natural tendency to sustain the force of a fall on the hyperextended wrist. Many hand and wrist injuries also are directly related to specific sports. For example, in wrestling, football, hockey, and skiing, forced abduction of the thumb can damage the ulnar collateral ligament of the thumb, leading to an injury called a gamekeeper's thumb. Receivers in football and catchers in baseball and softball are subject to "mallet" deformity of the finger, which is caused when a ball hits the end of the finger and avulses an extensor tendon from its distal attachment. Carpal tunnel syndrome also has been reported among the physically active population in badminton, baseball, cycling, gymnastics, field hockey, racquetball, rowing, skiing, squash, tennis, and rock climbing (1).

This chapter begins with a review of the anatomy, kinematics, and kinetics of the wrist and hand. Measures to prevent injury are followed by information regarding common injuries to the wrist and hand and their management. Finally, assessment techniques and rehabilitation exercises are presented.

ANATOMY OF THE WRIST AND HAND

The wrist and hand are composed of numerous small bones and articulations. These function effectively to enable the dexterous movements performed by the hands during both daily living and sport activities.

Wrist Articulations

The wrist consists of a series of radiocarpal and intercarpal articulations (Fig. 15.1). Most wrist motion occurs at the radiocarpal joint. It is a condyloid joint that includes the articulation of the radius with the scaphoid, lunate, and triquetrum. The joint allows sagittal plane motions (i.e., flexion, extension, and hyperextension) and frontal plane motions (i.e., radial deviation and ulnar deviation) as well as circumduction.

During wrist motions, the scaphoid, lunate, capitate, triquetrum, and pisiform exhibit significant nonplanar motions, with the axis of rotation for each bone shifting with the direction of the wrist movement (2–5). The individual motions and interactions among these proximal carpal bones become particularly complex during the combined wrist motions, such as extension and pronation (6). Alternately, the bones of the distal carpal row function as a single unit and are separated by gliding joints that contribute little to wrist motion. The distal carpal bones are directly linked to the motion of the third metacarpal (7).

The distal radioulnar joint is immediately adjacent to the radiocarpal joint. The triangular fibrocartilage (TFC) is a cartilaginous disk overlying the distal ulnar head. This disk binds the end of the ulna and the radius together (i.e., head of the ulna and ulnar notch of the radius) and the distal end of the ulna and the carpal bones (i.e., lunate and triquetral bones). It makes up a portion of the TFC complex (TFCC), which acts as a stabilizer of the distal radioulnar joint. The TFCC also is the ulnar continuation of the radius, providing an articular surface for the carpal condyle. Although the ulna and radius share the articular disk, they have separate joint capsules. The volar radiocarpal, dorsal radiocarpal, radial collateral, and ulnar collateral

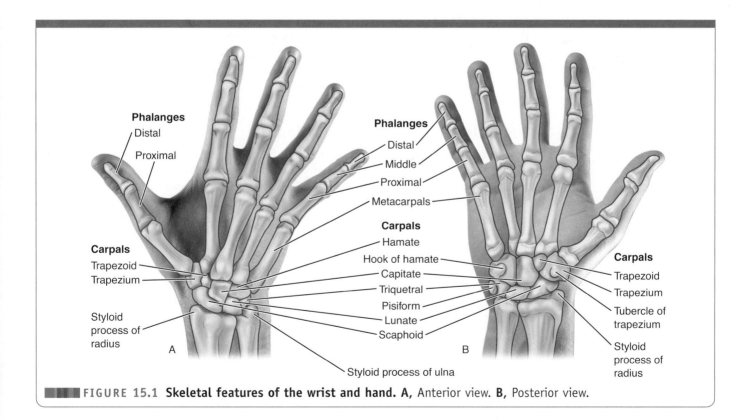

FIGURE 15.1 Skeletal features of the wrist and hand. A, Anterior view. **B,** Posterior view.

ligaments reinforce the radiocarpal joint capsule. Its close-packed position is in extension with radial deviation.

Hand Articulations

A large number of joints are required to provide the extensive motion capabilities of the hand. Included are the carpometacarpal (CM), intermetacarpal, metacarpophalangeal (MP), and interphalangeal (IP) joints. The fingers are numbered as digits 1 through 5, with the first digit being the thumb.

Carpometacarpal and Intermetacarpal Joints

The CM joint of the thumb is a classic saddle joint. A capsule surrounding the joint serves to restrict motion. The flexion-extension axis and abduction-adduction axis at the joint are not perpendicular to each other or to the bones, and they do not intersect (8). The articulating trapezium and metacarpal bones at the joint appear to have greater congruence, or better fit, in males than in females, which may predispose the female joint to osteoarthritis (9).

The CM joints of the four fingers are essentially gliding joints, although some anatomists have described them as modified saddle joints. The CM and intermetacarpal joints of the fingers are mutually surrounded by joint capsules that are reinforced by the dorsal, volar, and two interosseous CM ligaments. Among these, the V-shaped interosseous ligaments are the strongest, providing very strong interconnections between the bases of the adjacent metacarpals.

Metacarpophalangeal Joints

The knuckles of the hand are formed by the MP joints. These are condyloid joints formed by the articulation of the rounded, distal heads of the metacarpals with the concave, proximal ends of the phalanges. The MP joints are each enclosed in a capsule that is reinforced by strong collateral ligaments. A dorsal ligament also merges with the MP joint of the thumb. Close-packed positions of the MP joints in the fingers and thumb are full flexion and opposition, respectively.

Interphalangeal Joints

The proximal IP (PIP) and distal IP (DIP) joints of the fingers, and the single IP joint of the thumb, are hinge joints. Subtle differences in the geometry of the articulating bone surfaces and soft-tissue restraints govern the motion capabilities at the PIP joints. An articular capsule joined by volar and collateral ligaments surrounds each IP joint. These joints are most stable in the close-packed position of full extension.

See *Major Muscles of the Hand and Fingers*, available on the companion website at thePoint, for a summary of the muscles, including their attachments, primary actions, and nerve innervation.

Muscles of the Wrist and Hand

Given the numerous, highly controlled, precision movements of which the hand and fingers are capable, it is no surprise that a relatively large number of muscles are responsible. Nine extrinsic muscles cross the wrist, and 10 intrinsic muscles have both of their attachments distal to the wrist. The muscles of the wrist and hand are shown in Figures 15.2 (anterior) and Figure 15.3 (posterior).

Retinacula of the Wrist

The fascial tissue surrounding the wrist is thickened into strong, fibrous bands called retinacula. They form protective passageways through which tendons, nerves, and blood vessels pass. The flexor retinaculum protects the extrinsic flexor tendons and the median nerve as they pass into the hand through the carpal tunnel on the palmar side of the wrist. Within the tunnel, the tendons are enclosed in bursal tissue and tenosyniovioma. The extensor retinaculum provides a passageway for the extrinsic extensor tendons on the palmar side of the wrist.

Tendon Sheaths

The level of the metacarpal heads is the point where the flexor tendons enter a flexor tendon sheath, which is a double-walled, hollow tube sealed at both ends (Fig. 15.4). Filled with synovial fluid, the

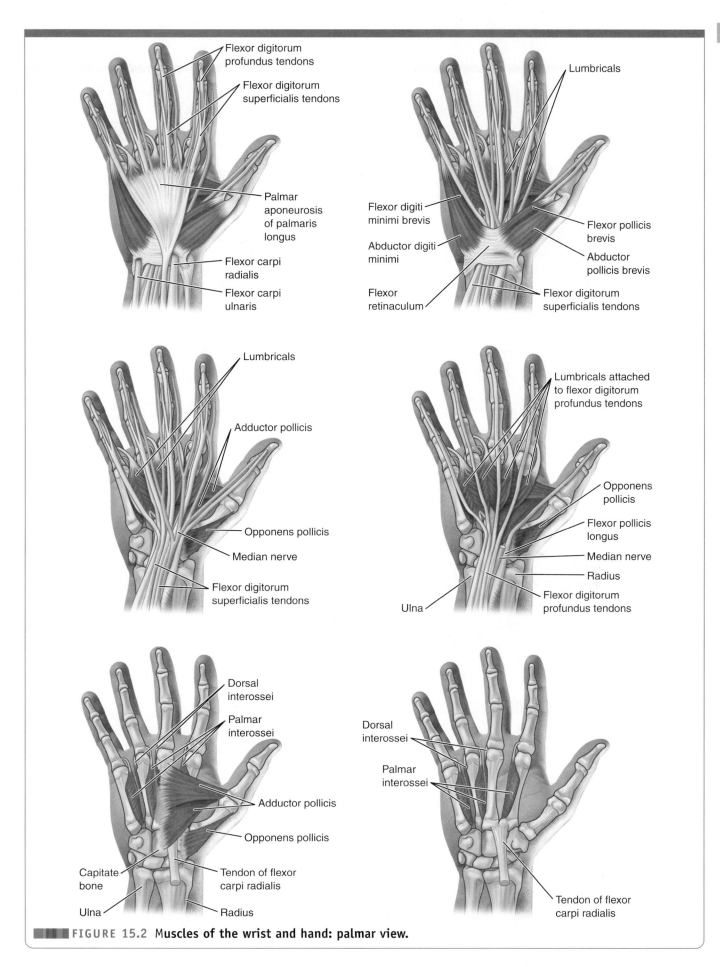

Flexor digitorum profundus tendons

Flexor digitorum superficialis tendons

Palmar aponeurosis of palmaris longus

Flexor carpi radialis

Flexor carpi ulnaris

Lumbricals

Flexor digiti minimi brevis

Abductor digiti minimi

Flexor retinaculum

Flexor pollicis brevis

Abductor pollicis brevis

Flexor digitorum superficialis tendons

Lumbricals

Adductor pollicis

Opponens pollicis

Median nerve

Flexor digitorum superficialis tendons

Lumbricals attached to flexor digitorum profundus tendons

Opponens pollicis

Flexor pollicis longus

Median nerve

Radius

Ulna

Flexor digitorum profundus tendons

Dorsal interossei

Palmar interossei

Adductor pollicis

Opponens pollicis

Tendon of flexor carpi radialis

Capitate bone

Ulna

Radius

Dorsal interossei

Palmar interossei

Tendon of flexor carpi radialis

FIGURE 15.2 Muscles of the wrist and hand: palmar view.

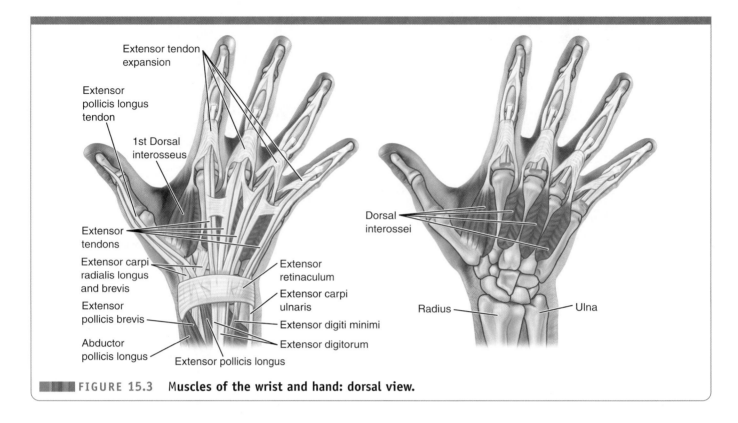

FIGURE 15.3 **Muscles of the wrist and hand: dorsal view.**

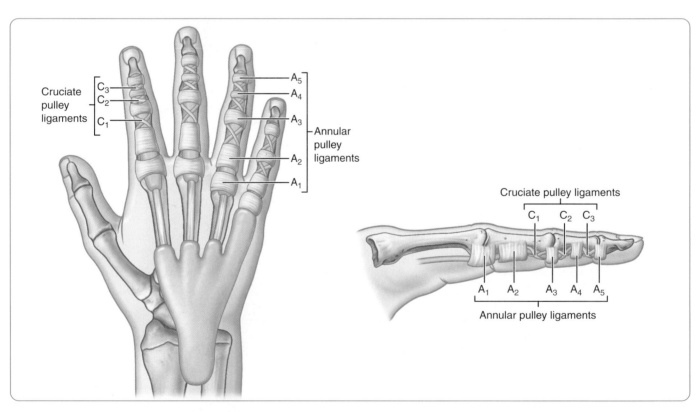

FIGURE 15.4 **Flexor tendons, sheath, and pulley system.** The tendons from the finger flexors pass through strong annular pulleys (A1 through A5), which keep the tendons and their encircling sheath closely applied to the phalanges. The thin, pliable cruciate pulleys (C1 through C3) collapse to allow full digital flexion.

sheath provides low-friction gliding and nutrition for the flexor tendons. The sheath is supported by a series of retinacular thickenings called annular pulleys or cruciform pulleys, depending on their configuration. The pulleys prevent tendon bowstringing with flexion. The second (A2) and fourth (A4) annular pulleys, which are located at the proximal and middle phalanges, respectively, are the most important for preventing tendon bowstringing during active flexion.

Nerves of the Wrist and Hand

The median, ulnar, and radial nerves are major terminal branches of the brachial plexus that provide motor and sensory innervation to the wrist and hand (Fig. 15.5). The median nerve supplies the majority of the flexor muscles of the wrist and hand, as well as the intrinsic flexor muscles on the radial side of the palm, and cutaneous sensation to the skin on the lateral two-thirds of the palm and the dorsum of the second and third fingers. The ulnar nerve innervates the flexor carpi ulnaris, the ulnar portion of the flexor digitorum profundus, and most of the intrinsic muscles of the hand. It also provides cutaneous sensation to the fifth finger and half of the fourth finger on both the dorsal and palmar sides. The radial nerve divides into superficial and deep branches distal to the lateral epicondyle of the elbow. The superficial branch supplies the skin on the dorsum of the hand, and the deep branch innervates most of the extensor muscles of the forearm.

Blood Vessels of the Wrist and Hand

The major vessels supplying the muscles of the wrist and hand are the radial and ulnar arteries (Fig. 15.6). The radial artery supplies the muscles on the radial side of the forearm as well as the

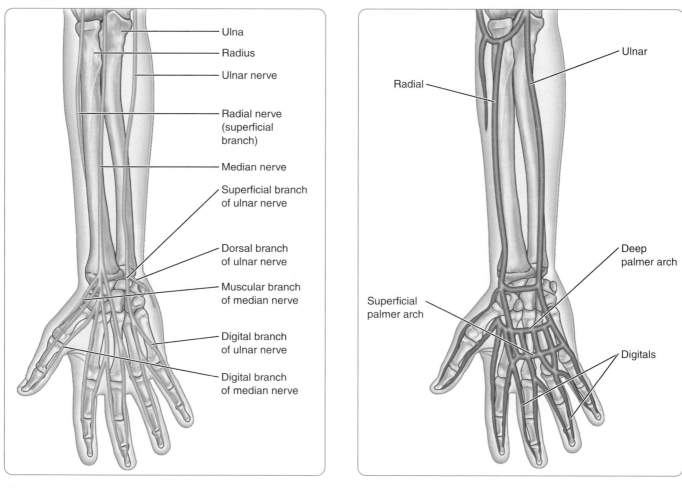

■■■ FIGURE 15.5 **Peripheral nerve supply to the wrist and hand.**

■■■ FIGURE 15.6 **Blood supply to the wrist and hand.**

thumb and index finger. The ulnar artery divides into anterior and posterior interosseous arteries to supply the deep flexor muscles and extensor muscles, respectively, of the forearm. In the palm, the radial and ulnar arteries merge to form the superficial and deep palmar arches. Another connecting branch from these arteries forms the carpal arch on the dorsal side of the wrist. Digital arteries branch from the palmar arches to supply the fingers, and branches from the carpal arch run distally along the metacarpal bones. The radial artery is superficial on the anterior aspect of the wrist. The pulse is readily palpable at this site.

KINEMATICS AND MAJOR MUSCLE ACTIONS OF THE WRIST AND HAND

The wrist is capable of both sagittal and frontal plane movements (Fig. 15.7). Flexion occurs when the palmar surface of the hand is moved toward the anterior forearm. Extension involves the return of the hand to anatomical position from a position of flexion, and hyperextension occurs when the dorsal surface of the hand is brought toward the posterior forearm. Movement of the hand toward the radial side of the arm is known as radial deviation; movement in the opposite direction is known as ulnar deviation. Movement of the hand through all four directions is termed circumduction.

Flexion

The major flexor muscles of the wrist are the flexor carpi radialis and flexor carpi ulnaris (see Fig. 15.2). The palmaris longus, which often is absent in one or both forearms, contributes to flexion. The flexor digitorum superficialis and flexor digitorum profundus assist with flexion at the wrist when the fingers are completely extended, but when the fingers are in flexion, these muscles cannot develop sufficient tension to assist.

Extension and Hyperextension

The extensor carpi radialis longus, extensor carpi radialis brevis, and extensor carpi ulnaris produce extension and hyperextension at the wrist. The other posterior wrist muscles also may assist with extension movements, particularly when the fingers are in flexion. Included are the extensor pollicis longus, extensor indicis, extensor digiti minimi, and extensor digitorum (see Fig. 15.3). When the

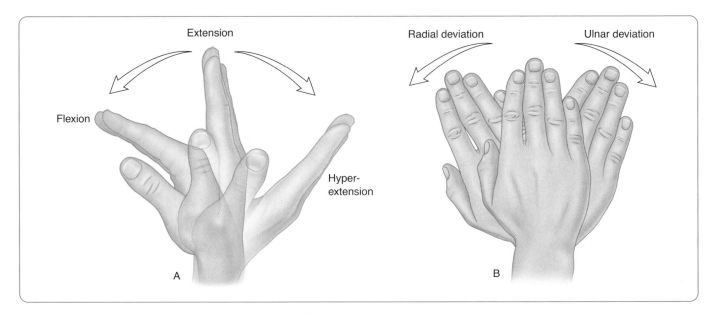

■■■ FIGURE 15.7 **Directional movement capabilities at the wrist. A,** Sagittal plane movements. **B,** Frontal plane movements.

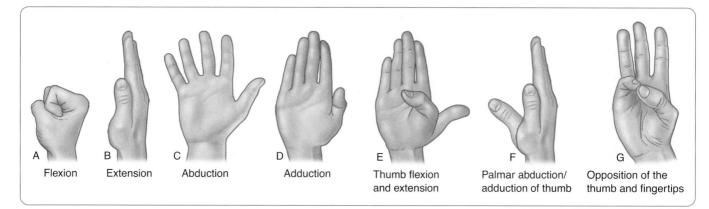

FIGURE 15.8 Directional movement capabilities at the fingers and thumb. A, Flexion. **B,** Extension. **C,** Abduction. **D,** Adduction. **E,** Thumb flexion and extension. **F,** Palmar abduction/adduction of the thumb. **G,** Opposition of the thumb and fingertips.

wrist moves from full flexion to full extension, the passive tension in the extrinsic muscles causes the DIP joints to go from approximately 12 to 31° of flexion and the PIP joints from approximately 19 to 70° of flexion (10).

Radial and Ulnar Deviation

The flexor and extensor muscles of the wrist cooperatively develop tension to produce radial and ulnar deviation of the hand at the wrist. The flexor carpi radialis and extensor carpi radialis act to produce radial deviation, and the flexor carpi ulnaris and extensor carpi ulnaris cause ulnar deviation.

Carpometacarpal Joint Motion

The CM joint of the thumb allows a large range of movement, comparable to that of a ball-and-socket joint. The fifth CM joint permits significantly less range of motion, however, and only a very small amount of motion is allowed at the second through fourth CM joints because of the presence of restrictive ligaments.

Metacarpophalangeal Joint Motion

The MP joints of the fingers allow flexion, extension, abduction, adduction, and circumduction (Fig. 15.8). Among the fingers, abduction is defined as movement away from the middle finger and adduction as movement toward the middle finger. The MP joint of the thumb, however, functions more as a hinge joint, with the primary movements being flexion and extension.

Interphalangeal Joint Motion

The IP joints permit flexion and extension and, in some individuals, slight hyperextension. These joints are classic hinge joints.

KINETICS OF THE WRIST AND HAND

The extrinsic flexor muscles of the hand are more than twice as strong as the extrinsic extensor muscles. This should come as little surprise given that the flexor muscles of the hand are used extensively in everyday activities involving gripping, grasping, or pinching movements, whereas the extensor muscles rarely exert much force.

Three types of hand grips are predominantly used in sport activities (Fig. 15.9). The power grip, as typified by the baseball bat grip, is one in which the fingers and thumb are used to clamp the grip of the bat against the palm of the hand. The wrist is held in a position of ulnar deviation and slight hyperextension to increase the tension in the flexor tendons. In contrast to the power grip,

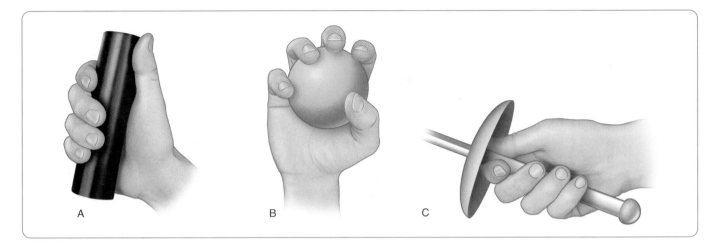

▪▪▪▪ FIGURE 15.9 **Hand grips.** Muscles of the hand contract to provide several grips. **A,** **P**ower grip. **B,** **P**recision grip. **C,** Fencing grip.

the precision grip, as exemplified by the baseball grip, involves use of the semiflexed fingers and thumb to pinch the ball against the palm, with the wrist in slight hyperextension. A third grip, which is intermediate to the two previously described, is referred to as the fencing grip. Fencing requires both power and precision. The grip on the foil is essentially a power grip; however, because the thumb is aligned along the long axis of the foil handle, it enables precise control over the direction of force application.

PREVENTION OF WRIST AND HAND CONDITIONS

The very nature of many contact and collision sports places the wrist and hand in an extremely vulnerable position for injury. The hands almost always are the first point of contact to cushion the body during collisions, deflect flying objects, or lessen body impact during a fall. Falling on an out-stretched hand is the leading cause of fractures and dislocations at the distal forearm, wrist, and hand. Although several pads and gloves are available, few sports require protective padding for the region.

Protective Equipment

Goalies, baseball and softball catchers, and field players in sports such as ice hockey and lacrosse are required to wear wrist and hand protection. Padded gloves prevent direct compression from a stick, puck, or ball. Several other gloves have extra padding placed at high-impact areas, aid in gripping, and protect the hand from abrasions, particularly when playing on artificial turf or a base-ball or softball field. Whenever possible, protective pads and gloves should be worn during sport participation to lessen the risk of injury.

Physical Conditioning

Several muscles that move the wrist and hand cross the elbow. As such, range-of-motion and strengthening exercises for the wrist and hand also must include exercises for the elbow (see Field Strategy 14.1). The exercises include elbow flexion and extension, forearm pronation and supination, wrist flexion and extension, and radial and ulnar deviation. Other exercises, such as squeezing a tennis ball or a spring-loaded grip device, can be used to strengthen the finger flexors.

Proper Skill Technique

Unlike the shoulder and elbow, which is subjected to excessive stress during a throwing-type motion, the majority of wrist and hand injuries result from direct trauma. Although analysis of specific movements may detect improper technique, the analysis in many cases is incidental. An important skill technique that can prevent injury of the wrist and hand is proper instruction on the shoulder-roll method of falling. In this technique, the force of impact is dispersed over a wider area, lessening the risk for injury from direct axial loading on the extended wrist.

CONTUSIONS AND SKIN WOUNDS

In attempting to catch a pass, a football player fell and slid on the artificial turf field. He sustained an abrasion on the palmar side of one hand. What are the immediate and long-term concerns associated with cleaning this superficial wound?

Direct impact to the back of the hand can produce a soft, painful, bluish discoloration. Although many contusions are minor, it is always important to be alert for an underlying fracture. Initial treatment involves ice, compression, elevation, and rest. Symptoms usually disappear in 2 to 3 days. If not, the individual should be referred to a physician for follow-up care.

Skin wounds on the hand may involve abrasions, lacerations, and puncture wounds. Each must be thoroughly cleansed of any foreign matter. With an abrasion, a 10-minute wash using surgical soap, a water-soluble iodine solution, and a brush can remove imbedded foreign matter. When the wound has been cleansed, an antiseptic should be applied and the wound covered with a nonocclusive dressing. The dressing should be changed daily and the wound inspected for signs of infection. If the wound appears red, swollen, or purulent or is hot and tender, immediate referral to a physician is warranted.

Completely lacerated digital vessels tend to retract, constrict, and clot, whereas partial transactions may continue to hemorrhage and may result in a traumatic aneurysm (11). Direct pressure applied to the wound for 10 to 15 minutes with a sterile, semicompressible material should be followed by elevation of the limb above the heart and immediate transportation to the nearest medical facility. A puncture wound is characterized by sharp, localized pain on palpation. The wound should be irrigated with normal saline to flush as much of the foreign material as possible from the wound. After covering the wound with a sterile dressing, the individual should be transported to a physician for further evaluation to ensure that all foreign matter has been eliminated from the wound. Although infection is the most common complication with any open wound, particularly puncture wounds, the use of prophylactic antibiotics remains controversial; however, tetanus prophylaxis is warranted when these injuries are sustained (11).

The abrasion sustained by the football player should be cleansed thoroughly. Next, an antiseptic and a nonocclusive dressing should be applied. The wound should be inspected daily for signs of infection.

SPRAINS

Following the completion of a floor routine, a gymnast reports pain in the right wrist. What signs and symptoms would suggest that the injury is a wrist sprain?

Ligamentous sprains in the wrist and hand are the result either of a single episode of trauma or of repetitive stress. When caused by a single episode of trauma, the severity of injury is dependent on:

- Characteristics of the injury force (i.e., point of application, magnitude, rate, and direction)

- Position of the hand at impact

- Relative strength of the carpal bones and ligaments

Most injuries to the region result from a compressive load that is applied while the hand is in some degree of extension, although hyperflexion or rotation also may lead to injury. Unfortunately, because of the need to perform simple daily activities, most individuals do not allow ample time for healing. Consequently, many sprains are neglected, leading to chronic instability.

Wrist Sprains

Axial loading on the proximal palm during a fall on an outstretched hand is the leading cause of wrist sprains (12). The most common ligamentous instability at the wrist occurs between the scaphoid and the lunate (13). Gymnasts have a high incidence of dorsal wrist pain when excessive forces are exerted on the wrist, producing combined hyperextension, ulnar deviation, and intercarpal supination. These excessive forces occur during vaulting, floor exercise, and pommel horse routines. Divers who enter the water with the hands in extension, as well as skaters and wrestlers who fall on an extended hand, are prone to this injury.

Signs and Symptoms

Assessment reveals point tenderness on the dorsum of the radiocarpal joint. A high degree of pain is palpable between the distal radius and the scaphoid and lunate. Pain increases with active or passive extension.

Management

Immediate treatment involves immobilization, application of ice to reduce swelling and inflammation, and immediate referral to a physician to rule out a fracture or carpal dislocation. Subsequent management includes decreasing intensity of training, cryotherapy before and after physical activity, nonsteroidal anti-inflammatory drugs (NSAIDs), and use of an appropriate bandage, taping technique, or splint to prevent excessive hyperextension. As pain decreases, range-of-motion exercises as well as wrist- and hand-strengthening exercises can be initiated (see Field Strategy 14.1).

Gamekeeper's Thumb

The thumb is exposed to more force than the fingers by virtue of its position on the hand. Integrity of the ulnar collateral ligament at the MP joint is critical for normal hand function, because it stabilizes the joint as the thumb is pushed against the index and middle fingers while performing many pinching, grasping, and gripping motions. **Gamekeeper's thumb** is common in football, baseball/softball, and hockey, as well as in skiing when the individual falls on the ski pole (skier's thumb). Tearing of the ulnar collateral ligament at the MP joint occurs when the MP joint is near full extension and the thumb is forcefully abducted away from the hand.

Signs and Symptoms

The palmar aspect of the joint is painful and swollen, and it may have visible bruising. Instability is detected by replicating the mechanism of injury or by stressing the thumb in flexion. In partial tears, only moderate laxity is present, as is a definite end feel. In more severe cases, laxity of greater than 35° and the absence of an end feel indicate total rupture of the ulnar collateral ligament. Bilateral comparison (as well as assessment of laxity at other major joints) helps to determine normal joint laxity for the individual.

Management

Initial treatment includes ice, compression, elevation, and referral to a physician for further care. If no instability is present, treatment involves early mobilization accompanied by cryotherapy, contrast baths, ultrasound, and NSAIDs. Strapping or taping the thumb can prevent reinjury. If joint instability is present, a thumb spica cast should be applied for 3 to 6 weeks, followed by further taping for another 3 to 6 weeks during risk activities. Severe cases require surgical repair.

Interphalangeal Collateral Ligament Sprains

Excessive varus/valgus stress and hyperextension can damage the collateral ligaments of the fingers. Ligament failure usually occurs at its attachment to the proximal phalanx or, less frequently, in the midportion. Hyperextension of the proximal phalanx can stretch or rupture the volar plate on the palmar side of the joint (Fig. 15.10).

Signs and Symptoms

An obvious deformity may not be present unless there is a fracture or total rupture of the supporting tissues, causing a dorsal dislocation. Rapid swelling makes assessment difficult. A radiograph is needed to rule out an associated dislocation or fracture.

Management

Following standard acute care, a mild sprain can be treated by taping the injured finger to an adjacent finger (e.g., buddy taping). This provides some support and mobility, but such taping should not be used on an acutely swollen, painful finger because of possible constriction to the vascular flow. If more support is needed, the involved joint can be splinted in extension with a molded polypropylene splint to avoid flexion contractures.

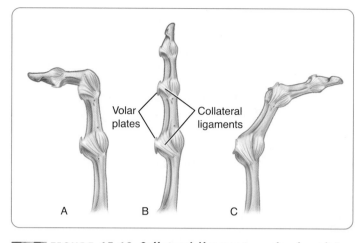

■■ ■ FIGURE 15.10 **Collateral ligaments and volar plate of the fingers can be damaged in hyperextension injuries. A**, Flexion. **B**, Extension. **C**, Hyperextension.

Dislocations

Similar to many other wrist and hand injuries, dislocations often are caused by a fall on the outstretched hand or by traumatic hyperflexion, hyperextension, or rotary movement.

Distal Radioulnar Joint Injury

An acute dislocation and subluxation of the distal radioulnar joint (DRUJ) can be an isolated injury or may occur in conjunction with a fracture of the radius. The mechanism of injury almost always involves hyperextension. If an ulnar dorsal dislocation of the joint occurs, hyperpronation also is present, whereas an ulnar volar dislocation occurs in conjunction with hypersupination. Because the TFCC functions as a sling to support the ulnar border of the wrist and connects the distal ulna to the ulnar side of the radius, dislocation of the DRUJ can result in damage to some portion of this complex or its attachments.

SIGNS AND SYMPTOMS. The clinical appearance of a DRUJ dislocation can vary significantly, depending on the presence or absence of an associated fracture. Generally, following dislocation or subluxation, the joint is deformed, swollen, and very painful. In fact, swelling may be so extensive that it obscures the prominence of the ulnar head. In a dorsal dislocation, the ulnar head is more prominent dorsally. In volar dislocations, the wrist typically appears to be narrow as a result of an overlap of the distal parts of the radius and ulna. If soft-tissue swelling is not excessive, a depression may be noted near the sigmoid notch of the radius, where the ulnar head normally is located. Flexion and extension of the elbow are normal unless there is an associated fracture, but pronation and supination of the forearm is limited.

MANAGEMENT. Immediate action involves immobilization of the limb in a vacuum splint and immediate transportation of the individual to a physician. The prognosis and rehabilitation program depend on the extent of tissue damage and instability. Simple DRUJ dislocations may be stabilized after the internal fixation of associated fractures and immobilized in an above-the-elbow cast. Range-of-motion exercises should be started 6 weeks after fixation.

Perilunate and Lunate Dislocation

Because of the shape of the lunate and its position between the large capitate and lower end of the radius, it is particularly prone to dislocation during axial loading that causes displacement in a volar direction (Fig. 15.11). As force initially impacts the carpals, the distal row is displaced away from the lunate, resulting in the lunate resting dorsally relative to the other carpals (i.e., **perilunate dislocation**). If the force continues to extend the wrist, however, the dorsal ligaments rupture, relocating

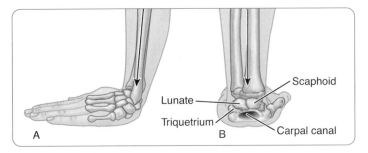

FIGURE 15.11 Lunate dislocation. A, The lunate can dislocate during a fall on an outstretched hand when the load from the radius compresses the lunate in a volar direction. **B,** If the bone moves into the carpal tunnel, the median nerve can become compressed, leading to sensory changes in the first and second fingers.

the carpals and rotating the lunate. The lunate then rests in a volar position relative to the other carpals (i.e., **lunate dislocation**).

SIGNS AND SYMPTOMS. The dorsum of the hand is point tender, and a thickened area on the palm can be palpated just distal to the end of the radius (proximal to the third metacarpal) if not obscured by swelling. Passive and active motion may not be painful. If the bone moves into the carpal tunnel, compression of the median nerve leads to pain, numbness, and tingling in the first and second fingers.

MANAGEMENT. Immediate action involves immobilization of the wrist in a vacuum splint and immediate transportation of the individual to a physician. Following reduction, the wrist is immobilized in moderate flexion with a silicone cast for 3 to 4 weeks. The wrist is then placed into a neutral position and protected from any wrist extension, particularly during sport participation. This condition often is overlooked until complications, such as flexor tendon contractures and median nerve palsies, arise from chronic dislocations. Repeated trauma to the lunate can lead to vascular compromise, resulting in degeneration or osteochondritis of the lunate (**Kienböck's disease**).

Dislocation of the Metacarpals and Phalanges

Metacarpophalangeal joint dislocations are rare but readily recognizable as a serious injury. Hyperextension or a shearing force causes the anterior capsule to tear, allowing the proximal phalanx to move backward over the metacarpal and stand at a 90° angle to the metacarpal (Fig. 15.12).

The most common dislocation in the body occurs at the PIP joint (Fig. 15.13). Because digital nerves and vessels run along the sides of the fingers and thumb, these dislocations are potentially serious. The mechanism of injury usually is hyperextension and axial compression, such as when a ball hits the end of the finger and forces it into hyperextension.

Distal interphalangeal dislocations usually occur dorsally and may be associated with an open wound. These individuals often reduce the injury on their own. As with MP joint dislocations, injuries to the collateral ligaments at the PIP and DIP joints can involve ruptures of the volar plate.

SIGNS AND SYMPTOMS. A swollen, painful finger is the most frequent initial complaint. Pain is present at the joint line and increases when the mechanism of injury is reproduced. With an MP dislocation, the proximal phalanx may stand at a 90° angle to the metacarpal. When the stability of an injured collateral ligament of the PIP joint exceeds 20° or has no end point on manual stress, it is considered to be a complete rupture (14). Because of the probability of entrapping the volar plate in an IP joint, which can lead to permanent dysfunction of the finger, no attempt should be made by an untrained individual to reduce a finger dislocation.

FIGURE 15.12 Metacarpophalangeal dislocation. The volar plates protect the anterior joint capsules of the fingers. During hyperextension, the anterior capsule and supporting ligaments can rupture, dislocating the phalanx. The resulting deformity signals a serious dislocation.

MANAGEMENT. Immediate treatment for all dislocations involves immobilization in a wrist or finger splint, application of ice to reduce swelling and inflammation, and immediate referral to a physician for reduction of the dislocation.

■■ ■ ■ FIGURE 15.13 **Dislocation variants of the proximal interphalangeal joint.** The most common are (**A**) dorsal, followed by (**B**) pure volar with a central slip rupture. The least common is (**C**) rotatory subluxation.

If the MP joint is stable, protection with buddy taping for 2 to 3 weeks usually is sufficient. Early active range-of-motion exercises are encouraged. In an uncomplicated dislocation of the PIP joint, the finger may be splinted in approximately 30° of flexion, with active motion being started at 10 to 14 days. Volar-displaced PIP dislocations with suspected central slip injury should have the PIP joint splinted in complete extension for 6 full weeks. During this time, active exercises of the DIP joint are imperative to maintain muscle integrity and strength of the flexor digitorum profundus and extensor mechanism. If inadequately managed, however, dislocations at the PIP joint can result in a painful, stiff finger with a fixed flexion deformity called a **"coach's finger."** If the volar plate is trapped in the joint, the deformity may result in the PIP joint being held in flexion and the DIP joint in hyperextension (a pseudo-boutonniere deformity). Immobilization for a DIP joint dislocation involves splinting the DIP joint with a volar splint for approximately 3 weeks. The PIP joint can be left free so that motion can continue at this joint. Protective splinting is continued for at least 3 weeks until the finger is pain free.

A *The signs and symptoms that would suggest the gymnast has sustained a wrist sprain include excessive forces producing a hyperextension mechanism; point tenderness on the dorsum of the radiocarpal joint; point tenderness between the distal radius, scaphoid, and lunate; and pain that increases with active or passive extension.*

STRAINS

Q *While holding an opponent's jersey tightly, a basketball player felt a sharp pain in the distal phalanx of the ring finger. After releasing the jersey, the player was unable to flex the DIP joint of the ring finger. What injury should be suspected?*

Muscular strains occur as a result of excessive overload against resistance or stretching the tendon beyond its normal range. In mild or moderate strains, pain and restricted motion may not be a major factor. In many injuries, muscular strains occur simultaneously with a joint sprain. The joint sprain takes precedence in priority of care, especially with an associated dislocation; as a result, tendon damage may go unrecognized and untreated.

Jersey Finger (Profundus Tendon Rupture)

This injury typically occurs when an individual grips an opponent's jersey while the opponent simultaneously twists and turns to get away. This jerking motion may force the individual's fingers to rapidly extend, rupturing the flexor digitorum profundus tendon from its attachment on the distal phalanx. The ring finger is most commonly involved, because this finger assumes a position of slight extension relative to the other fingers, which are more flexed during the grip.

Signs and Symptoms

Flexor tendon disruption is indicated by one finger lying in complete extension while others are in slight (10°) flexion at the IP joints (11). If avulsed, the tendon can be palpated at the proximal aspect of the involved finger; it typically has a hematoma formation along the entire flexor tendon sheath. If a portion of bone also is avulsed, it may become trapped distal to the A4 pulley over the middle phalanx, or distal to the A2 pulley, or it may retract all the way into the palm. Because of the avulsion, the individual is unable to flex the DIP joint against resistance.

Management

Following standard acute care, the individual should be referred to a physician for further treatment. For cases in which the tendon has retracted into the palm, surgical reattachment of the tendon must be performed within 7 to 10 days (before permanent contracture occurs).

Mallet Finger

Mallet finger, or baseball finger, occurs when an object hits the end of the finger while the extensor tendon is taut, such as when catching a ball. The resulting forceful flexion can avulse the lateral bands of the extensor mechanism from its distal attachment, or the tendon may remain attached to an avulsed piece of bone or fracture fragment, leaving a characteristic mallet deformity (Fig. 15.14).

Signs and Symptoms

Unlike the jersey finger, in which the flexor tendon retracts into the proximal aspect of the finger, isolated rupture of the extensor tendon usually does not retract. Examination reveals pain, swelling, and a variable lack of active extension at the DIP joint.

FIGURE 15.14 Mallet finger. This individual was asked to straighten the middle finger but was unable to extend the distal interphalangeal joint, suggesting that the extensor tendon is avulsed from the attachment on the distal phalanx. The tendon also may avulse a small piece of bone, leading to an avulsion fracture.

Management

Following standard acute care, the individual should be referred to a physician for further treatment, which usually involves splinting the DIP joint in complete extension for 6 to 8 weeks. Motion at the PIP and MP joints, however, is highly encouraged. An additional 6 to 8 weeks of splinting should be employed during athletic participation. Soft-tissue irritation or ulceration on the dorsum of the DIP may occur secondary to splinting; this can be avoided by keeping the splint dry and alternating its position between the dorsal and palmar aspects of the finger. Extreme hyperextension of the distal phalanx also may impair vascular supply to the tip of the finger, leading to further skin damage. If large fracture fragments are present, surgical repair may be necessary.

Boutonniere Deformity

A boutonniere deformity is caused by blunt trauma to the dorsal aspect of the PIP joint or by rapid, forceful flexion of the joint against resistance. The central slip of the extensor tendon ruptures at the middle phalanx, leaving no active extensor mechanism intact over the PIP joint. An injury to the volar plate also can lead to a flexion deformity of the PIP joint that resembles a boutonniere deformity; however, the central slip of the extensor tendon is not involved. This condition is called a **pseudo-boutonniere deformity**.

Signs and Symptoms

The deformity is not usually present immediately; rather, it develops over 2 to 3 weeks, as the lateral slips move in a palmar direction and cause hyperextension at the MP joint, flexion at the PIP joint, and hyperextension at the DIP joint (Fig. 15.15). Because the head of the proximal phalanx protrudes through the split in the extensor hood, this condition sometimes is referred to as a "buttonhole rupture." The PIP joint is swollen and lacks full extension.

Management

Any injury that limits PIP extension to 30° or less and produces dorsal tenderness over the base of the middle phalanx should be treated as an acute tendon rupture and immediately referred to a physician. Initial treatment involves splinting the PIP joint in complete extension for 5 to 6 weeks. To avoid the development of adhesions, the DIP joint should not be immobilized.

■■■■ FIGURE 15.15 **Boutonniere deformity.** In a boutonniere deformity, the proximal joint flexes while the distal joint hyperextends.

Tendinopathies

Individuals who are involved in strenuous and repetitive training often inflame tendons and tendon sheaths in the wrist and hand. Tendon injury can be acute or chronic in nature, but tendons are most at risk for injury when tension is rapidly applied at an oblique angle. Tendons that are already under tension and muscles that are maximally innervated or stretched are risk factors for rupture. Overuse can lead to derangement of both the mechanical and physiological components of the normal tendon. This condition is referred to clinically as tendinitis. In comparison, when the tendon sheath is inflamed as a result of trauma, overuse, or infection, it is called tenosynovitis (Fig. 15.16).

Trigger Finger

Snapping flexor tendons, or trigger finger, may be present in individuals who have multiple, severe traumas to the palmar aspect of the hand or in individuals who perform repeated movement and clenching of the fingers. It most commonly occurs in the middle or ring finger, but it also may occur in the thumb and other fingers. Repeated trauma and inflammation results in a thickening of the tendon sheath as it passes over the proximal phalanx. A nodule can form and grow within the thickened, synovium-lined tendon sheath that eventually prevents the tendon from sliding within the annular ligaments of the finger. The finger becomes locked in flexion when the nodule becomes too thick, or the sheath too constricted, to allow the finger to be actively re-extended (Fig. 15.17).

SIGNS AND SYMPTOMS. The locking action usually occurs when the individual first wakes from sleep. A painful popping sensation often is perceived when the flexed PIP joint is passively returned to extension. Additional palpable crepitus may indicate an underlying systemic disease (e.g., systemic sclerosis, rheumatoid arthritis, or granulomatous infection).

MANAGEMENT. Treatment includes NSAIDs, resting the finger, splinting when necessary, and possible cortisone injections into the sheath. For those individuals who do not respond to a steroid injection or who prefer quick, more definitive relief, an

■■■■ FIGURE 15.16 **Tenosynovitis.** This 13-year-old boy complained of pain in the finger for 3 days after a paronychia had been drained. Note the swelling and erythema of the distal phalanx.

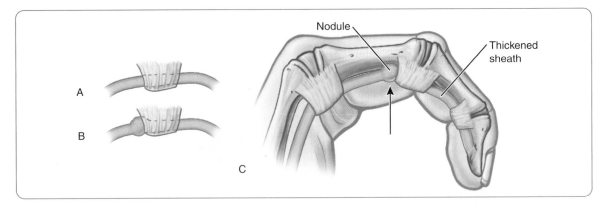

■■ ■ FIGURE 15.17 **Trigger finger. A,** Under normal conditions, the flexor tendons slide within the synovial sheaths under the annular ligaments at the proximal and middle phalanx. **B,** Repeated trauma can cause a nodule to form in the tendon sheath, or the sheath may become thickened. **C,** Flexion occurs, and the finger becomes locked in flexion when the nodule becomes too thick or the sheath too constricted. The finger is then unable to re-extend.

incision proximal to the palpable nodule may be necessary to cut the annular ligament and allow the tendon to slide freely (15).

De Quervain's Tenosynovitis

Individuals who must use a forceful grasp, combined with repetitive use of the thumb and ulnar deviation, are particularly at risk for de Quervain's tenosynovitis. Sports such as tennis, golf, fly fishing, and javelin and discus throwing place a high demand on the abductor pollicis longus (APL) and extensor pollicis brevis (EPB). These two tendons share a single synovial tendon sheath that travels through a bony groove over the radiostyloid process, then turns sharply (as much as 105°) to enter the thumb when the wrist is in radial deviation. Tenosynovitis results from friction among the tendons, stenosing sheath, and bony process (Fig. 15.18). The tendons slide within the sheath not only during movements of the thumb but also during movements of the wrist with the thumb fixed, as in bowling and throwing.

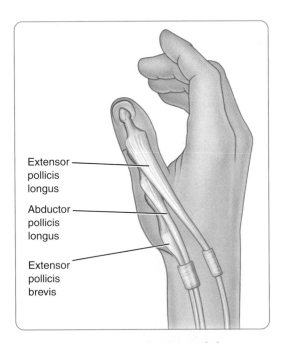

SIGNS AND SYMPTOMS. The individual complains of pain over the radial styloid process that increases with thumb and wrist motion. Palpation reveals point tenderness over the tendons, either at or just proximal to the radial styloid, and occasionally crepitation. Movements of the thumb are painful, and snapping of the tendons may be present with some activities. Pain is reproduced in two ways: (1) by abducting the thumb against resistance, and (2) by flexing the thumb and cupping it under the fingers, then flexing the wrist in ulnar deviation to stretch the thumb tendons (see Fig. 15.32). Swelling may be present in the first dorsal compartment.

Extensor pollicis longus

Abductor pollicis longus

Extensor pollicis brevis

■■ ■ FIGURE 15.18 **De Quervain's tenosynovitis.** The abductor pollicis longus and extensor pollicis brevis share the same synovial sheath. Excessive friction among the tendons, sheath, and bony process leads to tenosynovitis of the tendons.

MANAGEMENT. Treatment is conservative, with ice, rest, and NSAIDs. If symptoms are not relieved, steroid injections, immobilization with a thumb spica for 3 weeks, or both may be indicated. In severe cases, surgical decompression may be necessary.

Intersection Syndrome

Intersection syndrome is a tendinitis or friction tendinitis in the first and second dorsal compartments. It has been described in rowers, indoor raquet players, canoeists, and weight lifters who overuse the radial extensors of the wrist by excessive curling (16). The muscle and tendons of these two compartments traverse each other at a 60° angle at a site approximately two to three finger breadths proximal to the wrist joint on the dorsal aspect (i.e., 4–6 cm proximal to Lister's tubercle). The condition also has been described as a stenosing tenosynovitis of the sheath of the second compartment (i.e., the radial extensors) at the area where it traverses the muscle bellies of the first compartment (i.e., APL and EPB).

SIGNS AND SYMPTOMS. Examination reveals point tenderness on the dorsum of the forearm, two to three finger breadths proximal to the wrist joint. Crepitation or squeaking is noted with passive or active motion. Visible swelling is present along the course of the affected tendons.

MANAGEMENT. Treatment consists of ice massage, rest, NSAIDs, splinting, and avoidance of exacerbating activities. A corticosteroid injection may be necessary to relieve acute symptoms. Rehabilitation should consist of range-of-motion exercises and wrist extensor strengthening. A tenosynovectomy and a fasciotomy of the APL muscle may be necessary if conservative treatment is not effective.

Dupuytren's Contracture

For unknown reasons, nodules can develop in the palmar aponeurosis. These nodules limit finger extension and, eventually, cause a flexion deformity. The condition, known as Dupuytren's contracture, is rare but can impact normal function of the fingers.

SIGNS AND SYMPTOMS. A fixed flexion deformity is visible, occurring more frequently on the ring or little finger. The finger cannot be extended.

MANAGEMENT. Because normal finger function cannot occur with the flexion deformity, the nodule causing the contracture must be surgically removed.

Gymnast's Wrist

The distal radial epiphyseal plate is the classic location for the stress injury commonly called "gymnast's wrist." In contrast to other growth-plate overuse syndromes in adolescents, this fracture is caused by compression. Repetitive performances on the pommel horse and uneven bars cause excessive wrist loading, leading to pain over the dorsum of the wrists. Pain increases as the wrist is carried into maximum dorsiflexion, such as occurs in vaulting, tumbling, and beam work.

SIGNS AND SYMPTOMS. Diffuse tenderness typically is present over the dorsum of the midcarpal area. Pain increases with the extremes of wrist motion. Edema, discoloration, and clinical instability generally are not present. The distal ulnar epiphysis also may be involved.

MANAGEMENT. Treatment involves splinting, NSAIDs, and avoidance of the offending exercises until the individual is asymptomatic. Complete resolution of symptoms may require 3 to 6 months or longer. A dorsal block splint may be beneficial for practice and competition to avoid extremes of wrist extension.

Ganglion Cysts

Ganglion cysts are benign tumor masses typically seen on the dorsal aspect of the wrist, although they may occur on the volar aspect. Associated with tissue sheath degeneration, the cyst itself contains a jelly-like, colorless fluid of mucin and is freely mobile and palpable. Occurring spontaneously, cysts seldom cause any pain or loss of motion. Discomfort from the pressure may occur as the ganglion increases in size. Treatment is symptomatic: Aspiration, injection, and rupture of the cyst have not proved to be successful, because the condition may recur. Surgical excision remains the treatment of choice.

The mechanism of injury and the symptoms suggest that the basketball player has sustained a rupture of the profundus tendon (i.e., jersey finger). Avulsion of the tendon from the distal phalanx results in an inability to flex the DIP.

FINGERTIP INJURIES

 A high school cheerleader has a mild case of paronychia. Are antibiotics required in the management of this condition?

Direct trauma to the nail bed, such as that caused when the finger is impacted by a ball, jammed into an object, or crushed when stepped on, can lead to a subungual hematoma. Infections also can occur in the nail fold, leading to a condition called paronychia.

Subungual Hematomas

Direct trauma to the nail bed can result in blood forming under the fingernail, which is called a subungual hematoma. Increasing pressure can lead to throbbing pain. After ruling out an underlying fracture, the finger should be soaked in ice water for 10 to 15 minutes to numb the area and reduce the bleeding under the nail bed. If the pain diminishes, it may not be necessary to drain the hematoma. This is preferable, because draining the hematoma opens an avenue for infection. If discomfort interferes with the ability to perform physical activities, however, the hematoma should be drained under the direction of a physician. This is performed by cutting a hole through the nail with a rotary drill or a number-11 surgical blade or by melting a hole through the nail with the end of a paper clip heated to a bright red color (Fig. 15.19). Field Strategy 15.1 explains the proper care

FIELD STRATEGY 15.1

Management Algorithm for Subungual Hematoma[a]

To numb the area and reduce hemorrhage:

1. Soak the finger in ice water for 10–15 minutes.
2. Clean your hands thoroughly with antiseptic soap and water, and apply latex gloves.
3. Cleanse the finger thoroughly with:

   - Antiseptic soap, or
   - An antibacterial solution

4. Make a hole through the nail. Either:
5. Cut the hole, using: **OR:** Melt the hole with the end of a paper clip
                                              heated to bright red.
   - A sterile, number-11 surgical blade, or
   - A rotary drill, cleaned and disinfected
     with iodine solution

6. Have the individual exert mild pressure on the distal pulp of the finger to drive excess blood through the hole.
7. Watch carefully for signs of shock, and treat accordingly by:

   - Placing the individual in a supine position, and
   - Elevating the feet above the level of the heart

8. Soak the finger in an iodine solution for 10 minutes.
9. Cover the phalanx with a sterile dressing, and apply a protective splint.

Follow up:

1. Do not apply heat for 48 hours.
2. Check the finger daily for signs of infection; if any appear, immediately refer the individual to a physician.

[a]Because of the nature of opening a wound and the potential for subsequent infection, this procedure should be discussed with the supervising physician and documented as a standing order.

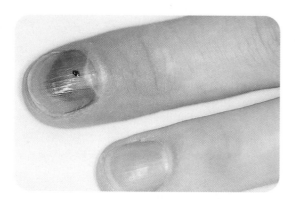

■■■ FIGURE 15.19 **Subungual hematoma.** Note the hole that was made to drain the excess blood and relieve pain.

■■■ FIGURE 15.20 **Paronychia of the right middle finger.** The infection is clearly localized to the dorsal surface, although the pulp is slightly swollen because of edema.

for a subungual hematoma. After the blood has been drained, the area must be checked daily for signs of infection; if signs of infection are present, immediate referral to a physician is warranted.

Paronychia

Paronychia is an infection along the nail fold. It commonly is seen with a hangnail and in individuals whose hands are frequently immersed in water. The nail fold becomes red, swollen, and painful, and it can produce purulent drainage (Fig. 15.20). The condition is treated with warm-water soaks and germicide. In more severe cases, the physician may recommend systemic antibiotics and drainage of localized pus or may perform a partial-nail resection.

A *Treatment of the cheerleader's paronychia should include warm-water soaks and germicide. An antibiotic is only necessary in severe cases.*

NERVE ENTRAPMENT SYNDROMES

Q *An ice-hockey goalie complains of numbness in the little finger. He is unable to grasp a piece of paper between the thumb and index finger and has a weakness in grip strength. Inspection reveals atrophy of the hypothenar mass. What condition should be suspected, and how should this condition be managed?*

Nerve entrapment syndromes, or compressive neuropathies, can be subtle and often are overlooked. They occur in activities such as bowling, cycling, karate, rowing, baseball/softball, field hockey, lacrosse, rugby, weight lifting, handball, and wheelchair athletics. Mechanisms of injuries most commonly involve repetitive compression, contusion, or traction. A compressive neuropathy also may be caused by anatomical structures such as anomalous muscles or vessels, fibrous bands, osteofibrous tunnels, or muscle hypertrophy. Pathologic structures, such as ganglia, lipomas, osteophytes, aneurysms, and localized inflammation, also can compress a nerve. This discussion of compressive neuropathies is limited to those found in the distal forearm, wrist, and hand (Box 15.1).

Median Nerve Entrapment

The median nerve lies medial to the brachial artery in the cubital fossa and passes distally between the two heads of the pronator teres. The nerve divides at the distal margin to form the anterior interosseous nerve to supply the flexor pollicis longus, flexor digitorum superficialis to the index and middle digits, and pronator quadratus. The main trunk of the median nerve continues distally beneath the fibrous arch of the flexor digitorum superficialis. The palmar cutaneous branch supplies sensation to the volar wrist, thenar eminence, and palm. The median nerve continues through the

Box 15.1   Nerve Entrapment Syndromes

Median Nerve	**Ulnar Nerve**	**Radial Nerve**
▪ Anterior interosseous syndrome	▪ Ulnar tunnel syndrome	▪ Distal posterior interosseous nerve syndrome
▪ Carpal tunnel syndrome	▪ Cyclist's palsy	▪ Superficial radial nerve entrapment
	▪ Bowler's thumb	

carpal tunnel beneath the flexor retinaculum to supply sensation to the palm and the radial three and one-half digits. The deep motor branch supplies the abductor pollicis brevis, opponens pollicis, superficial head of the flexor pollicis brevis, and two lateral lumbricales.

Anterior Interosseous Nerve Syndrome

Seen sporadically, anterior interosseous nerve syndrome can occur after a set of strenuous or repetitive elbow motion exercises. Structurally, there may be compression of the nerve by fibrous bands from the deep head of the pronator teres or flexor digitorum superficialis, affecting any or all of the muscles innervated by the nerve. Because the nerve has no sensory cutaneous portion, however, no sensory changes occur.

SIGNS AND SYMPTOMS. The individual presents in one of two ways:

1. **Acute onset:** The individual suddenly loses use of the flexor pollicis longus and index finger profundus tendons.

2. **Slow, insidious onset:** Gradual weakening of these muscles becomes apparent, with weakness during heavy activity.

Examination reveals weakness or loss of flexion of the IP joint of the thumb and DIP joint of the index finger. The individual characteristically is unable to make a circle with the index finger and thumb (i.e., pinch grip test).

MANAGEMENT. Initial treatment involves splinting the extremity and avoiding heavy activity. If no return of function is noted after 6 months, surgical intervention and decompression of the nerve may be necessary.

Carpal Tunnel Syndrome

The floor of the carpal tunnel is formed by the volar wrist capsule, with the roof formed by the transverse retinacular ligament traveling from the hook of the hamate and pisiform on the lateral side to the volar tubercle of the trapezium and tuberosity of the scaphoid on the medial side. This unyielding tunnel accommodates the median nerve, finger flexors in a common sheath, and flexor pollicis longus in an independent sheath (Fig. 15.21). Any irritation of the synovial sheath covering these tendons can produce swelling or edema that puts pressure on the median nerve.

Carpal tunnel syndrome (CTS) is the most common compression syndrome of the wrist and hand, although it is not commonly seen in the physically active population. Movement of tendons and nerves during prolonged, repetitive hand movements may contribute to the development of CTS (17). In addition, CTS may be caused by direct trauma or anatomical anomalies. It typically is seen in the dominant extremity. Sporting activities that predispose an individual to CTS include those that involve repetitive or continuous flexion and extension of the wrist, such as cycling, throwing sports, racquet sports, archery, and gymnastics. Etiologies for CTS other than traumatic causes include infectious origins (e.g., diphtheria, mumps, influenza, pneumonia, meningitis, malaria, syphilis, typhoid, dysentery, tuberculosis, and gonococcus) and metabolic causes (e.g., hypothyroidism, diabetes, rheumatoid arthritis, gout, vitamin deficiency, heavy metals poisoning, and carbon monoxide poisoning) (18).

SIGNS AND SYMPTOMS. A common sign is pain that awakens the individual in the middle of the night but that often is relieved by "shaking out the hands" (known as a positive "flick"). Pain, numbness, tingling, or a burning sensation may be felt only in the fingertips on the palmar aspect of the thumb, index, and middle finger. Generally, only one extremity is affected. Grip and pinch strength may be limited. A common complaint is difficulty manipulating coins. Symptoms are reproduced when direct compression is applied over the median nerve in the carpal tunnel for approximately 30 seconds. Although a positive Phalen's maneuver and Tinel's sign are classic clinical signs of the syndrome, diminished sensitivity to pain and weak thumb abduction are more predictive of abnormal nerve conduction (19).

MANAGEMENT. Individuals with suspected CTS should be referred to a physician for care. Immobilization in slight wrist extension with a dorsal splint is used to rest the wrist for up to 3 to 5 weeks, particularly at night when symptoms occur. Cold, NSAIDs, or in some situations, diuretics can initially reduce swelling and pain in the area caused by tenosynovitis. Use of a compression wrap should be avoided, however, because this adds additional compression on the already impinged structures. More than half of the individuals with this condition respond

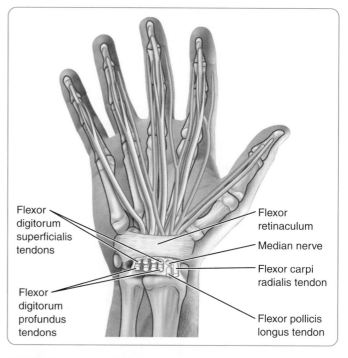

Flexor digitorum superficialis tendons

Flexor digitorum profundus tendons

Flexor retinaculum

Median nerve

Flexor carpi radialis tendon

Flexor pollicis longus tendon

■■ ■ FIGURE 15.21 Carpal tunnel. The flexor tendons of the fingers pass through the carpal tunnel in a single synovial sheath.

well to conservative treatment, although symptoms may recur, necessitating a corticosteroid injection into the canal. Long-term benefits from corticosteroid injections, however, may not include symptomatic relief as compared to a properly applied splint (20). In cases that do not respond well to conservative treatment, surgical decompression or carpal tunnel release can be necessary.

Ulnar Nerve Entrapment

The ulnar nerve passes through the ulnar groove posterior to the medial epicondyle to enter the cubital tunnel formed by the aponeurosis and two heads of the flexor carpi ulnaris. The nerve continues distally between the flexor digitorum profundus dorsally and the flexor carpi ulnaris palmarly. The palmar cutaneous nerve arises in the midforearm to supply the proximal hypothenar eminence. The dorsal cutaneous nerve arises 5 to 8 cm proximal to the ulnar styloid and supplies the dorsum of the ulnar side of the hand. In the wrist, the nerve courses between the hook of the hamate and pisiform, then passes through Guyon's canal to move distally into the fingers (Fig. 15.22). The superficial branch supplies the overlying palmaris brevis, then becomes entirely sensory to supply the hypothenar eminence and the ring and small fingers. The deep branch curves around the hook of the hamate to supply the ulnar intrinsics, ending its terminal branch in the first dorsal interossei.

Ulnar Tunnel Syndrome

Compression of the ulnar nerve may occur as the nerve enters the ulnar tunnel or as the deep branch curves around the hook of the hamate and traverses the palm. This condition frequently is seen in cycling and racquet sports and in baseball/softball catchers, hockey goalies, and handball players who experience repetitive compressive trauma to the palmar aspect of the hand. Distal ulnar nerve palsy also may be seen as push-up palsy, following fractures of the hook of the hamate, or as a result of a missed golf shot or baseball swing.

SIGNS AND SYMPTOMS. The lesion may present with motor, sensory, or mixed symptoms. Coincident involvement of the median nerve is common. The individual complains of numbness in the ulnar

Transverse carpal
ligament (Flexor retinaculum)

Deep branch of ulnar nerve

Volar carpal ligament

Guyon's canal

Ulnar artery

Ulnar nerve

■■■■■■ FIGURE 15.22 **Impingement of the ulnar nerve.**
The ulnar nerve can become impinged in the tunnel of
Guyon as it runs under the ligament between the hamate
and pisiform.

nerve distribution, particularly in the little finger, and is unable to grasp a piece of paper between the thumb and index finger (see Fig. 15.37). Slight weakness in grip strength and atrophy of the hypothenar mass also may be present. Tapping just distal to the pisiform bone produces a tingling sensation that radiates into the little finger and ulnar aspect of the ring finger (i.e., positive Tinel's sign).

MANAGEMENT. Treatment involves splinting, NSAIDs, and avoidance of any precipitating activity. If symptoms do not disappear within 6 months of conservative treatment, surgical decompression of Guyon's canal may be necessary.

Cyclist's Palsy

Cyclist's palsy, which also is linked to ulnar nerve entrapment, occurs when a biker leans on the handlebar for an extended period of time, leading to swelling in the hypothenar area. Symptoms mimic those of the more serious ulnar nerve entrapment syndrome, but they usually disappear rapidly after completion of the ride. Properly padding the handlebars, wearing padded gloves, varying hand position, and properly fitting the bike to the rider can greatly reduce the incidence of this condition.

Bowler's Thumb

Bowler's thumb involves compression of the ulnar digital sensory nerve, on the medial aspect of the thumb in the web space, while gripping the ball. Constant pressure on this spot can lead to scarring in the area. The radial digital nerve of the index finger is similarly at risk in racquet sports.

SIGNS AND SYMPTOMS. Numbness, tingling, or pain may develop on the medial aspect of the thumb. The individual may have swelling or thickening over the medial palmar aspect at the base of the thumb. Although no true motor involvement is present, grip strength may be decreased secondary to pain. Athletic trainers develop similar symptoms from excessive use of dull scissors or from added pressure on the thumb as one cuts through thick tape jobs or pads.

MANAGEMENT. Treatment depends on the stage of injury. Because the predominant cause is inflammatory in nature, treatment is directed at reducing inflammation. Cryotherapy, immobilization with a molded plastic thumb guard, NSAIDs, and if necessary, a corticosteroid injection usually are successful in relieving symptoms.

Radial Nerve Entrapment

The radial nerve bifurcates near the radiocapitellar joint to become the posterior interosseous and superficial radial nerves. The posterior interosseous nerve travels between the two heads of the supinator, around the proximal radius, and under the forearm extensors to supply the terminal articular branches to the wrist. The superficial radial nerve travels underneath the brachioradialis to become subcutaneous in the distal forearm and supply sensation to the dorsoradial portion of the hand, including the first web space and the proximal phalanges of the first three digits. The most common compressive neuropathy of the radial nerve, which occurs at the radial tunnel, is discussed in Chapter 14.

Distal Posterior Interosseous Nerve Syndrome

Compression of the distal posterior interosseous nerve occurs as it passes dorsally over the distal radius and enters the wrist capsule. Gymnasts are particularly prone to this injury because of repetitive and forceful wrist dorsiflexion.

SIGNS AND SYMPTOMS. The individual usually complains of a deep, dull ache in the wrist that is reproduced with forceful wrist extension or deep palpation of the forearm with the wrist in flexion. Because the condition often can be confused with carpal instability, ganglions, and wrist sprains, the examiner should perform several tests for carpal stability.

MANAGEMENT. If the condition does not improve following standard acute care and activity modification, referral to a physician for further treatment is warranted.

Superficial Radial Nerve Entrapment

The superficial branch of the radial nerve can be compressed at the wrist as it pierces the deep fascia to become subcutaneous between the tendons of the extensor carpi radialis longus and brachioradialis. This constriction is made worse by sports that require repeated pronation and supination, such as batting, throwing, and rowing; by gloves that are strapped too tight; or by the use of tight wrist bands.

SIGNS AND SYMPTOMS. The individual complains of burning pain, sensory changes, and night pain over the dorsoradial aspect of the wrist, hand, dorsal thumb, and index finger. Typically, the Finkelstein's test is negative, but Tinel's sign over the wrist is positive. The absence of pain with wrist motions can rule out a tendinitis-, arthritis-, or impingement-type syndrome.

MANAGEMENT. If the condition does not improve following standard acute care and activity modification, referral to a physician is warranted.

 The ice-hockey goalie may have ulnar tunnel syndrome. Treatment involves splinting, NSAIDs, and avoidance of any precipitating activity. If symptoms do not disappear within 6 months of conservative treatment, surgical decompression of Guyon's canal may be necessary.

FRACTURES OF THE WRIST AND HAND

 A volleyball player appears to have sustained a boxer's fracture. What is the immediate management of this injury?

Fractures of the distal ulna and radius and of the carpal bones usually are caused by axial loading when an individual falls on an outstretched hand. The majority are simple and nondisplaced. Subsequent to the advent of external orthoses, many fractures can be immobilized adequately to allow individuals to continue with regular sport participation. Specific rules governing special protective equipment, however, require that braces, casts, or any unyielding substances on the elbow, forearm, wrist, or hand be padded on all sides so as not to endanger other players. When the fracture has reached a stage at which external support is no longer necessary during daily activities, it may be advantageous to wear a splint during sport participation.

Distal Radial and Ulnar Fractures

Fractures to the distal radius and ulna present a special problem. In adolescents, epiphyseal and metaphyseal fractures are common. These fractures usually heal without residual disability. In older

■■■ **FIGURE 15.23 Clinical view of a Colles'
fracture.**

individuals, one or both bones may be fractured, or one bone may be fractured with the other bone dislocated at the elbow or wrist joint. A Colles' fracture occurs within 1½ inches of the wrist joint and results in a "dinner-fork" deformity when the distal segment displaces in a dorsal and radial direction (Fig. 15.23). A reverse of this fracture is the Smith's fracture, which tends to move toward the palmar aspect (volar). A Monteggia fracture is characterized by a fracture of the proximal third of the ulna accompanied by a dislocation of the radial head. In a Galeazzi fracture, the distal radioulnar dislocation is secondary to the marked shortening of the radius caused by the severe ulnar displacement and dorsal angulation of the distal radial fragment. Figure 15.24 demonstrates the four common fractures of the forearm.

Signs and Symptoms

In adolescents, fractures of the growth plate may present with the distal fragment being dorsally displaced. Other signs and symptoms associated with traumatic fractures include intense pain, swelling, deformity, and a false joint. Swelling and hemorrhage may lead to circulatory impairment, or the median nerve may be damaged as it passes through the forearm.

■■■ **FIGURE 15.24 Forearm fractures. A,** Colles' fracture. The extra-articular distal radial fracture is associated with a fracture of the base of the ulnar styloid. **B,** Smith's fracture. This type of fracture is characterized by a transverse fracture of the distal radius, with volar and proximal displacement of the distal radial fragment **C,** Monteggia fracture. This type of fracture is characterized by a fracture of the proximal third of the ulna, accompanied by a dislocation of the radial head. **D,** Galeazzi fracture. The distal radioulnar dislocation is secondary to the marked shortening of the radius caused by the severe ulnar displacement and dorsal angulation of the distal radial fragment.

Management

Immediate immobilization in a vacuum splint and a careful neurovascular evaluation of the hand should be followed by immediate referral to a physician. In many instances, open reduction and internal fixation with rigid plates and screws are necessary to restore function.

Carpal Fractures

The small bones of the wrist greatly enhance the mobility of the hand. Of the eight bones, only the scaphoid and lunate articulate with the radius; therefore, these two bones transmit the entire force of a fall on an outstretched hand to the forearm.

Scaphoid Fractures

Scaphoid fractures account for more than 70% of all carpal bone injuries in the general population and are the most common wrist bone fracture in physically active individuals (21). Peak incidence is between 12 and 15 years of age (22). In many cases, the individual falls on the wrist, has normal radiographs, and is discharged with the diagnosis of a wrist sprain and without further care. Several months later, however, the individual continues to experience persistent wrist pain. Radiographs at this time may reveal an established nonunion fracture of the scaphoid (Fig. 15.25A). Because of a poor blood supply to the area, aseptic necrosis (death of the tissue) is a common complication with this fracture.

SIGNS AND SYMPTOMS. Assessment reveals a history of falling on an outstretched hand. Pain is present during palpation of the anatomical snuff box (Fig. 15.25B), which lies directly over the scaphoid, or with inward pressure along the long axis of the first metacarpal bone. Pain increases during wrist extension and radial deviation.

MANAGEMENT. Treatment involves ice, compression, immobilization in an appropriate splint, and immediate referral to a physician. Nondisplaced scaphoid fractures can be immobilized in a thumb spica cast, with the wrist in slight radial deviation. The cast is changed at 2-week intervals to ensure proper molding around the forearm until union occurs (22). Follow-up radiographs are obtained at 3- to 4-week intervals to monitor healing and detect signs of delayed union, nonunion, malunion, or avascular necrosis. Some fractures may take several weeks or months to heal; during this time, the individual may participate with a padded, short-arm thumb cast or silicone cast. Displaced scaphoid fractures are secured with internal fixation.

■■■■ FIGURE 15.25 **Scaphoid fracture. A,** Radiograph of a scaphoid fracture. Nonunion fractures occur when the area has a poor blood supply. **B,** The scaphoid forms the floor of the anatomical snuff box. It is bounded by the extensor pollicis brevis medially and by the extensor pollicis longus laterally. Increased pain during palpation in this region indicates a possible fracture to the scaphoid bone.

Lunate Fracture/Keinböck's Disease

Of the carpal bones, the lunate has the largest area, proportionately, of cartilage surface; however, a true lunate fracture is rare in sports. These fractures are difficult to identify and diagnose; therefore, some may be overlooked. Because a large portion of the lunate is cartilage and cancellous bone, the amount of pain associated with a fracture to this area is minimal. Avascular necrosis of the lunate, however, which also is known as **Keinböck's disease**, is common if the vascular pathway is disrupted. Its cause has yet to be determined, but it is thought to arise from repetitive trauma or an unrecognized lunate fracture.

SIGNS AND SYMPTOMS. A history of trauma may or may not be present. The individual usually complains of dorsal wrist pain, swelling, and weakness of the wrist associated with use. If left untreated, Keinböck's disease can result in chronic tenderness, pain, and swelling over the lunate as well as in decreased grip strength and weakness during wrist extension. Pain during passive extension of the third finger is a common characteristic with this condition.

MANAGEMENT. Treatment involves ice, compression, immobilization in an appropriate splint, and immediate referral to a physician. Early radiographs are needed to ascertain the correct diagnosis. The preferred treatment is early surgical intervention.

Hamate Fracture

Direct impact to the hamate may lead to a nonunion fracture. This typically occurs when an individual strikes a stationary object with a racquet or club in full swing. Once fractured, the ligamentous insertions of the transverse carpal ligament, pisohamate ligament, short flexor, and opponens digiti minimi act to displace the fragment and prevent union.

SIGNS AND SYMPTOMS. Physical examination reveals tenderness over the hypothenar muscle mass. Painful abduction of the small finger against resistance is present, as is decreased grip strength.

MANAGEMENT. Treatment involves ice, compression, immobilization in an appropriate splint, and immediate referral to a physician. Radiographs and tomograms using a carpal tunnel view with the wrist in extension confirm the diagnosis. Care usually is symptomatic, with a protective orthoses worn for 4 to 6 weeks (until tenderness subsides). It may be 2 to 3 months before a racquet or bat will feel comfortable in the hand again.

Triquetrum Fractures

Fractures of the triquetrum are fairly common. An avulsion fracture is believed to be caused by sudden wrist flexion or sudden, forceful impingement of the ulnar styloid into the dorsum of the triquetrum. The ulna tends to shear a portion of bone away from the triquetrum. This type of fracture occurs when pressure is put on the wrist during a fall and the wrist is hyperextended and deviated to the ulnar side.

SIGNS AND SYMPTOMS. The individual usually reports a history of acute wrist dorsiflexion injury or direct trauma to the wrist area. Pain in the dorsal wrist is present over the triquetrum.

MANAGEMENT. Treatment involves ice, compression, immobilization in an appropriate splint, and immediate referral to a physician. Immobilization in a short-arm cast with mild extension of the wrist for 4 to 6 weeks is the treatment of choice. Some fractures may become nonunion and require surgical excision.

Metacarpal Fractures

Uncomplicated fractures of the metacarpals result in severe pain, swelling, and deformity. Unique fractures at the base of the first metacarpal may involve a simple intra-articular fracture (i.e., Bennett's fracture) or a comminuted fracture (i.e., Rolando fracture). A unique fracture involving the

FIELD STRATEGY 15.2

Determining a Possible Fracture to a Metacarpal

1. Palpate for pain along the shaft of the bone.
2. Apply compression along the long axis of the bone. A positive sign occurs if pain is felt at the injury site.
3. Apply percussion or vibration at the end of the bone. A positive sign occurs if pain is felt at the injury site.
4. Apply distraction at the end of the bone. A positive sign occurs if pain is decreased; increased pain may indicate a ligamentous injury.

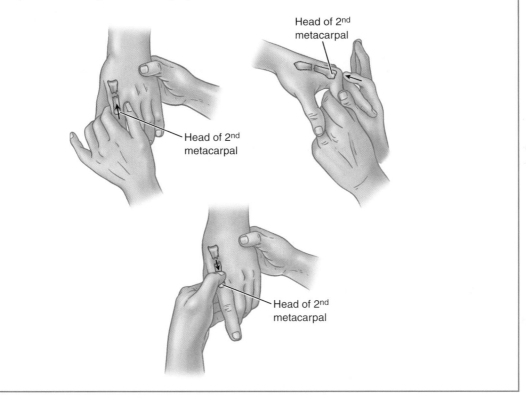

neck of the fourth or fifth metacarpal is called a boxer's fracture, and it occurs when an individual punches an object with a closed fist, leading to rotation of the head of the metacarpal over the neck.

Uncomplicated Fractures

Axial compression on the hand can lead to a fracture-dislocation of the proximal end of the metacarpal. This often goes undetected, however, because edema obscures the extent of injury. Fractures of the shaft of the metacarpal are more easily recognized.

SIGNS AND SYMPTOMS. Increased pain and a palpable deformity are present in the palm of the hand directly over the involved metacarpal. Gentle percussion and compression along the long axis of the bone increase pain at the fracture site (Field Strategy 15.2). These same techniques can be used to detect possible fractures in the carpals and phalanges.

MANAGEMENT. Fractures should be immobilized in the position of function, with the palm face down and the fingers slightly flexed. Ice should be applied to reduce hemorrhage and swelling; an elastic compression bandage should not be applied to a swollen hand, because it may lead to increased

■■ ■■ FIGURE 15.26 **Bennett's fracture.** A Bennett's fracture usually is associated with a dislocation of the metacarpophalangeal joint of the thumb. An avulsion fracture, however, occurs when a segment of the metacarpal is held in place by the deep volar ligament.

distal swelling in the fingers. The fingernails must remain uncovered so that circulation can be periodically assessed. The individual should be referred immediately to a physician for further assessment.

Bennett's Fracture

A Bennett's fracture is an articular fracture of the proximal end of the first metacarpal and usually is associated with a dislocation. It typically is caused by axial compression, as occurs when a punch is thrown with a closed fist or the individual falls on a closed fist. The pull of the APL tendon at the base of the metacarpal displaces the shaft proximally. A small medial fragment, however, is held in place by the deep volar ligament, leading to a fracture-dislocation (Fig. 15.26).

SIGNS AND SYMPTOMS. Pain and swelling are localized over the proximal end of the first metacarpal, but deformity may or may not be present. Inward pressure exerted along the long axis of the first metacarpal elicits increased pain at the fracture site.

MANAGEMENT. Acute care consists of ice, compression, immobilization in a wrist splint, and immediate referral to a physician. The preferred treatment for this fracture is closed reduction and percutaneous pinning for less than 3 mm of fracture displacement and open reduction and fixation for greater displacements.

Rolando Fracture

Similar to a Bennett's fracture, a Rolando fracture involves only an intra-articular fracture of the first metacarpal, with no dislocation. The potential for serious complications is significantly increased, however, because it tends to be more comminuted.

SIGNS AND SYMPTOMS. Pain and swelling are localized over the proximal end of the first metacarpal. Deformity is more apparent than with a Bennett's fracture. Inward pressure exerted along the long axis of the first metacarpal elicits increased pain at the fracture site.

MANAGEMENT. Acute care consists of ice, compression, immobilization in a wrist splint, and immediate referral to a physician. Open reduction and internal fixation with multiple Kirschner wires may be necessary for excellent results. When the fracture is accurately reduced and fixated, complete healing leads to excellent joint range of motion; however, because the joint surface was involved in the fracture, arthritic symptoms may eventually develop.

Boxer's Fracture

Fractures involving the distal metaphysis or neck of the fourth or fifth metacarpals are commonly seen in young males involved in punching activities, hence the name boxer's fracture (although the fracture rarely occurs in boxers) (Fig. 15.27). The fracture typically has an apex dorsal angulation and is inherently unstable secondary to the deforming muscle forces and the frequent volar comminution.

SIGNS AND SYMPTOMS. Sudden pain, inability to grip objects, rapid swelling, and possible deformity are present. Palpation reveals tenderness and pain over the fracture site as well as possible crepitus and bony deviation. Delayed ecchymosis is common. Pain increases with axial compression of the involved metacarpal and percussion.

■■ ■■ FIGURE 15.27 **Boxer's fracture.** These fractures usually involve the fourth and fifth metacarpals.

MANAGEMENT. Acute care consists of ice, compression, immobilization in a wrist splint, and immediate referral to a physician. Closed reduction is followed by immobilization in a splint for 4 to 6 weeks, followed by early range-of-motion exercises.

Phalangeal Fractures

Fractures of the phalanges are very common in sport participation, and these fractures can be difficult to manage. They may be caused by having the fingers stepped on or impinged between two hard objects, such as a football helmet and the ground, or by hyperextension that may lead to a fracture-dislocation (Figure 15.28).

FIGURE 15.28 Phalangeal fracture. This fracture demonstrates a shearing pattern in the diaphysis.

SIGNS AND SYMPTOMS. Increased pain is present with circulative compression around the involved phalanx. Gentle percussion and compression along the long axis of the bone increase pain at the fracture site. Particular attention should be given to a possible fracture of the middle and proximal phalanges. These fractures tend to have marked deformity because of the strong pull of the flexor and extensor tendons. The four fingers move as a unit. Failure to maintain the longitudinal and rotational alignments of the fingers can lead to long-term disability in grasping or manipulating small objects in the palm of the hand. This deformity often results in one finger overlapping another when a fist is made.

MANAGEMENT. Acute care involves ice to reduce pain and swelling. While the hand is immobilized in a full-wrist splint, gauze pads or a gauze roll are placed under the fingers to produce approximately 30° of finger flexion and reduce the pull of the flexor tendons. The individual should be referred immediately to a physician. Immobilization depends on the type of fracture and its location and may vary from 2 to 4 weeks.

 Immediate management for the suspected boxer's fracture includes ice, compression, immobilization in a wrist splint, and immediate referral to a physician.

ASSESSMENT OF WRIST AND HAND CONDITIONS

 A cheerleader is complaining of pain over the right anatomical snuff box. How should the assessment of this injury progress to determine the extent and severity of injury?

The wrist and hand can be difficult to evaluate because of the number of anatomical structures providing motor and sensory function to the region. A thorough examination in this area often takes longer than with other joints of the body because of the multiple structures and joints that are involved. When assessing this region, two major objectives must be kept in mind. First, the injury or condition must be evaluated as accurately as possible to ensure adequate treatment. Second, the examiner must ascertain the remaining function to determine whether the individual has any incapacity in performing sport-specific skills and activities of daily living.

The examiner also must keep in mind that if the mechanism of injury involves axial loading at the wrist, additional assessment may be necessary at the elbow or shoulder. Although uncommon, pain at the wrist and hand may be referred from the cervical spine, shoulder, and elbow. As such, it may be necessary to evaluate these joints before assessing the wrist and hand.

See *Field Strategy: Wrist and Hand Evaluation,* available on the companion website at thePoint.

HISTORY

The injury assessment of the cheerleader should begin with a history. What questions need to be asked to identify the cause and extent of this injury?

Questions about a wrist injury should focus on the primary complaint, past injuries, and other factors that may have contributed to the current problem (e.g., demands of the sport, changes in technique, overuse, occupational requirements, or referred pain). Questions should be asked to determine how the injury occurred, because it is important to determine if the region has been subjected to repetitive trauma, such as constant impact from a ball, racquet, bat, or stick. Current symptoms and their progression must be determined. Questions also must be asked regarding the pain (i.e., localized, general, radiating, or activities that increase or decrease pain), as should questions concerning the presence of sounds and unusual feelings. Recent changes, if any, in the training program should be noted.

See *Field Strategy: Developing a History of the Injury,* available on the companion website at thePoint, for specific questions regarding the wrist and hand region.

The cheerleader should be asked questions that address the following: when, where, and how the injury occurred; current symptoms and their progression; pain (i.e., localized, general, or radiating); activities that cannot be performed because of the pain; actions or motions that replicate the pain; and previous injury, treatment, and medication.

OBSERVATION AND INSPECTION

The history reveals falling on an outstretched hand approximately 1 month ago. The cheerleader reports pain is more pronounced during activities that involve wrist extension. Explain the observation component in the ongoing assessment of the cheerleader.

The entire arm should be exposed for observation and inspection. Although the individual may have a wrist injury, the elbow and shoulder region also may need to be evaluated, depending on the mechanism of injury. First, the examiner should observe the position of the wrist, hand, and fingers, noting any noticeable deformity and general presentation. If swelling is present in a specific joint, the individual may be unable to fully extend that joint and may be supporting it in a slightly flexed position. If a fracture or dislocation is not present, the individual's willingness and ability to place the hand in the various positions that are requested should be observed. The functional position of the wrist, sometimes called the position of rest, is with the wrist in 20 to 35° of extension and 10 to 15° of ulnar deviation. This position allows the greatest amount of flexion of the fingers; inability to assume this position may suggest a tendon or nerve disruption (13). The palm of the hand should be inspected for palmar creases; swelling in one or more of the hand compartments may obliterate these lines. In a bilateral comparison, the dominant hand tends to be slightly larger than the nondominant hand. The specific site of injury should be inspected for obvious abrasions, deformity, swelling, discoloration, symmetry, hypertrophy, muscle atrophy, or previous surgical incisions. Subtle skin changes may be indicative of a possible nerve injury. For example, the hand normally has moisture on it, and the absence of moisture on the distal phalanx may indicate a digital nerve injury (13).

See *Field Strategy: Observation and Inspection of the Wrist and Hand,* available on the companion website at thePoint, for a summary of the observations at the wrist and hand from the dorsal and palmar views.

During the assessment of the cheerleader's injury, a general observation regarding the presentation of the hand and wrist as well as of the elbow and shoulder should be performed. In addition, the injury site should be inspected for swelling, discoloration, deformity, muscle hypertrophy or atrophy, and other signs of existing or previous trauma.

PALPATION

A bilateral comparison of the cheerleader's wrist and hand reveals no abnormal findings. Explain palpation for this injury.

If the individual is in great pain and is unable or unwilling to move the wrist or hand, the possibility of a fracture or dislocation should be determined before moving the wrist or hand. Fracture tests, including compression, percussion, vibration, and traction, should be performed. If a fracture is suspected, it should be treated accordingly. Acute care consists of ice, immobilization, and immediate referral to a physician.

The wrist and hand should be palpated in a direction from proximal to distal. While supporting the individual's hand throughout palpation, the examiner should begin on the dorsal aspect and move to the palmar aspect. Bilateral palpation can determine temperature, swelling, point tenderness, crepitus, deformity, muscle spasm, and cutaneous sensation. Temperature changes may indicate inflammation, infection, or reduction in circulation. Crepitus may indicate tenosynovitis, an irregular articular surface, or possible fracture. Circulation can be assessed by blanching the fingernails; this is performed by squeezing the nail and observing the changes in color. Initially, the nails should turn white, but color should return within 2 seconds of release. Pulses also can be taken at the radial and ulnar arteries in the wrist. The following structures should be palpated:

Dorsal Aspect

1. Radial styloid process and tubercle of the radius

2. Styloid process of the ulna

3. Finger and thumb extensors and thumb abductor

4. The carpal bones on the dorsal and palmar aspect (should be palpated at the same time):

   - *Scaphoid*—Lies distal to the radial styloid process and forms the floor of the anatomical snuff box.
   - *Lunate*—Lies just distal to the radial tubercle and is easily palpated during wrist flexion.
   - *Triquetrum*—Lies one finger's breadth distal to the ulnar styloid process.
   - *Pisiform*—Palpable on the medial palmar side when the wrist is slightly flexed.
   - *Trapezium*—Lies distal to the anatomical snuff box.
   - *Trapezoid*—Lies medial to the trapezium.
   - *Capitate*—Lies distal to the lunate and a slight indentation before the metacarpal.
   - *Hamate*—Lies distal to the triquetrum; the hook of the hamate is more easily palpated on the palmar aspect.

5. Metacarpal bones and phalanges

Palmar Aspect

1. Flexor tendons

2. Carpal transverse arch that forms the carpal tunnel, and the longitudinal arch comprised of the carpal bones, metacarpals, and phalanges

3. Palmar fascia and intrinsic muscles within the thenar and hypothenar muscle masses

 During the assessment of the cheerleader, the bony and soft tissue structures of the distal radius/ulna, wrist, and hand should be palpated for point tenderness, swelling, deformity, skin temperature, sensation, and other signs of trauma.

PHYSICAL EXAMINATION TESTS

Palpation reveals pain over the anatomical snuff box, and the physical examination of the injury reveals pain at the end range of PROM with wrist extension and ulnar deviation. Pain also is elicited during RROM of those motions. What injury should be suspected, and what is the immediate management for that injury?

The wrist or hand should not be forced through any sudden motions, and caution should be used in proceeding through the physical examination. Only those tests that are necessary to assess the current injury should be performed. Tests should be performed bilaterally.

Functional Tests

The examiner should determine the available range of motion in forearm pronation-supination, wrist flexion-extension, radial/ulnar deviation, finger flexion-extension, finger abduction-adduction, thumb flexion-extension, thumb abduction-adduction, and opposition of the thumb and little finger. As always, bilateral comparison is critical to distinguish normal from abnormal movement.

Active Movements

In determining active movements at the wrist and hand, the movements that are anticipated to be most painful should be performed last. Finger active motion usually is done in a continuous pattern of flexion and extension. The examiner should ask the individual to:

1. Make a tight fist (flexion).
2. Straighten the fingers (extension).
3. Spread the fingers (abduction).
4. Bring the fingers together (adduction).

It is important to note the fluidness as each digit moves throughout the range of motion. If one finger does not move through the full range of motion, that finger can be evaluated separately. The motions that should be assessed and the normal ranges of motions for each are as follows:

- Pronation/supination of the forearm (85–90°)
- Wrist flexion (80–90°)
- Wrist extension (70–90°)
- Radial deviation (15°)
- Ulnar deviation (30–45°)
- Finger flexion and extension
- Finger abduction and adduction
- Thumb flexion, extension, abduction, and adduction
- Opposition of the thumb and little finger (tip to tip)

The techniques for taking goniometry measurements of wrist flexion and extension, and of radial and ulnar deviation, are shown in Figure 15.29.

■■■■ FIGURE 15.29 Goniometry measurement. A, Wrist flexion and extension. The fulcrum is centered over the lateral aspect of the wrist close to the triquetrum. Align the proximal arm along the lateral aspect of the ulna using the olecranon process as a reference. Then, align the distal arm along the midline of the fifth metacarpal. **B,** Radial and ulnar deviation. Center the fulcrum over the middle of the dorsum of the wrist close to the capitate. Align the proximal arm with the midline of the forearm using the lateral epicondyle as a reference. Then, align the distal arm along the midline of the third metacarpal.

Passive Movements

If the individual is unable to perform active movements in all ranges, the individual's passive movements should be assessed. Slight overpressure at the end of each motion can test the end feel of each joint. The normal end feels are as follows:

- **Tissue Stretch**—movements of the wrist and finger joints
- **Bone to bone**—pronation

Resisted Muscle Testing

Active movements are tested using resisted movements throughout the full range of motion. The individual can be standing or seated. The proximal joint is stabilized, and a mild resistance is applied to the distal joint. Figure 15.30 demonstrates motions that should be tested.

Stress Tests

Stress tests are performed when in those individuals with a clear indication of the damaged structures. Only those tests deemed to be relevant should be used, and results should be compared bilaterally.

Ligamentous Instability Test for the Wrist

The elbow flexed at 90° and the forearm pronated, the examiner grips the distal forearm with one hand and the metacarpals with the other. A varus (i.e., ulnar deviation) and valgus (i.e., radial

■■■■ FIGURE 15.30 **Resisted manual muscle testing. A,** Forearm supination and pronation. **B,** Wrist flexion and extension. **C,** Ulnar and radial deviation. **D,** Finger flexion and extension. **E,** Finger abduction and adduction. **F,** Thumb flexion and extension. **G,** Thumb abduction and adduction. **H,** Opposition.

■■■ FIGURE 15.31 **Ligament instability test.** To stress the ligamentous structures around the joints, the examiner applies varus and valgus forces at the specific joint.

■■■ FIGURE 15.32 **Finkelstein's test.** The examiner should instruct the individual to make a fist with the thumb inside the fingers. The examiner then flexes the wrist in an ulnar direction. A positive Finkelstein's test produces pain over the APL and EPB tendons.

deviation) stress is applied to the wrist joint. Pain or laxity indicates damage to the ulnar collateral or radial collateral ligaments, respectively. This test may elicit signs of trauma to the TFC.

Ligamentous Instability Test for the Fingers

The examiner stabilizes the thumb or finger with one hand proximal to the joint being tested. This is followed by applying valgus and varus stresses to the joint to test the integrity of the collateral ligaments (Fig. 15.31) and anteroposterior glide to stress the joint capsule. This test is used for gamekeeper's thumb and joint sprains of the fingers.

■■■ FIGURE 15.33 **Carpal tunnel compression test.** Compression over the carpal tunnel may lead to tingling into the palmar aspect of the thumb, index finger, and middle finger and indicates a carpal tunnel syndrome.

Special Tests

A variety of special tests can be used for detecting injury or related pathology (e.g. muscle/tendon injury, nerve entrapment, or fracture).

Finkelstein's Test

While the individual makes a fist with the thumb inside the fingers (Fig. 15.32), the examiner stabilizes the forearm and flexes the wrist in an ulnar direction. A positive Finkelstein's test, indicating de Quervain's tenosynovitis, produces pain over the APL and EPB tendons at the wrist. Because the test may be uncomfortable even for a healthy individual, all positive test results should be compared bilaterally to the uninvolved wrist.

Carpal Tunnel Compression Test

The examiner exerts even pressure with both thumbs directly over the carpal tunnel and holds it for at least 30 seconds (Fig. 15.33). A positive test produces numbness or tingling into the palmar aspect of the thumb, index finger, and middle finger.

Phalen's (Wrist Flexion) Test

The examiner instructs the individual to place the dorsum of the hands together to maximally flex the wrists and hold this position for 1 minute by gently pushing the wrists together (Fig. 15.34). It is important to ensure that the individual does not shrug the shoulders during the test, because this causes compression of the median branch of the brachial plexus as it passes through the thoracic outlet. An alternative position is to have the examiner

FIGURE 15.34 Phalen's test. Phalen's (wrist flexion) test indicates that the median or ulnar nerve is compressed if numbness or tingling occur in the specific nerve distribution pattern.

FIGURE 15.35 Tinel's sign. Tinel's sign at the wrist also is used to indicate median nerve compression.

apply overpressure during passive wrist flexion and hold the position for 1 minute. A positive test, indicating either median or ulnar nerve compression, produces numbness or tingling into the specific nerve distribution pattern: If the median nerve is compressed, sensory changes are evident in the thumb, index finger, third finger, and lateral half of the ring finger; if the ulnar nerve is compressed, sensory changes occur in the fifth finger and medial half of the ring finger.

Tinel's Sign

Testing for median nerve compression involves tapping over the carpal tunnel at the wrist (Fig. 15.35). A positive test produces numbness or tingling in the median nerve distribution. This test also can be adapted for ulnar nerve compression in the hypothenar mass and for radial nerve compression on the dorsoradial aspect of the wrist.

Pinch Grip Test for Entrapment of the Anterior Interosseous Nerve

The examiner instructs the individual to pinch the tip of the index finger and thumb together (Fig. 15.36). If an abnormal pulp-to-pulp pinch is performed, the anterior interosseous nerve, which is an extension of the median nerve, may be entrapped at the elbow as it passes between the two heads of the pronator teres.

FIGURE 15.36 Pinch grip test. The examiner instructs the individual to make an "O" with the thumb and forefinger. **A,** Normal tip-to-tip. **B,** Abnormal pulp-to-pulp, which signifies entrapment of the interior interosseous nerve.

FIGURE 15.37
Froment's sign. The Froment's test is positive if the individual flexes the distal phalanx of the thumb to prevent a piece of paper from being pulled away, which indicates paralysis of the adductor pollicis muscle resulting from possible ulnar nerve damage.

Froment's Sign for Ulnar Nerve Paralysis

The patient grasps a piece of paper between the thumb and forefinger (Fig. 15.37), and the examiner attempts to pull the paper away. If the distal phalanx of the thumb flexes to hold the paper, it indicates paralysis of the adductor pollicis muscle, which is indicative of ulnar nerve damage.

Allen Test for Circulation

The examiner instructs the individual to quickly open and close the hand several times and then squeeze the hand tightly. This is followed by the examiner placing his or her thumb and index finger over the radial and ulnar arteries to compress them. The individual then opens the hand while pressure is maintained over the arteries. Each artery is tested by releasing the pressure over that artery to see if the hand flushes. Bilateral comparison can determine the effectiveness of the two arteries and which artery provides the major blood supply to the hand.

Neurologic Tests

Neurologic integrity can be assessed with the use of myotomes, reflexes, and segmental dermatomes as well as peripheral nerve cutaneous patterns.

Myotomes

Isometric muscle testing to assess the myotomes should be performed in the loose-packed position and include scapular elevation (C_4), shoulder abduction (C_5), elbow flexion and/or wrist extension (C_6), elbow extension and/or wrist flexion (C_7), thumb extension and/or ulnar deviation (C_8), and abduction and/or adduction of the hand intrinsics (T_1).

Reflexes

Reflexes in the upper extremity include the biceps (C_5–C_6), brachioradialis (C_6), and triceps (C_7). These are discussed and demonstrated in Chapters 13 and 14.

Cutaneous Patterns

The segmental nerve dermatome patterns for the wrist and hand region are demonstrated in Figure 15.38. The peripheral nerve cutaneous patterns are demonstrated in Figure 15.39. Bilateral testing

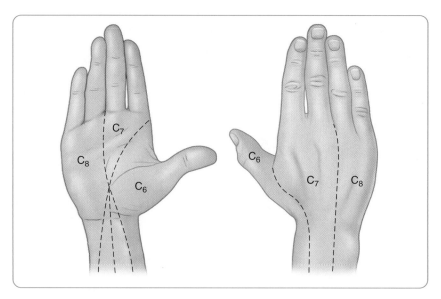

FIGURE 15.38 Segmental dermatomes for the wrist and hand.

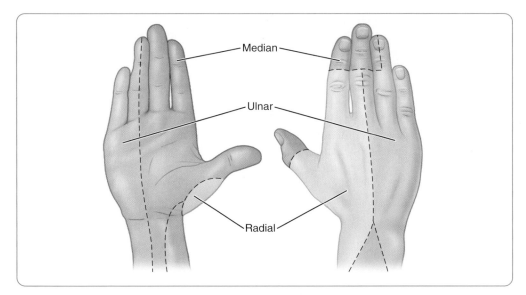

FIGURE 15.39 Cutaneous nerve distribution patterns for the wrist and hand.

for altered sensation should be performed using sharp and dull touch by running the open hand and fingernails over the shoulder and down both sides of the arms and hands.

Activity-Specific Functional Tests

Because the wrist, hand, and fingers are vital in performing activities of daily living, individuals should be assessed for manual dexterity and coordination. It is important to assess the abilities to hook, pinch, and grasp an object as well as activities such as combing the hair, holding a fork, brushing the teeth, or picking up a backpack. Before return to activity, the individual should be able to perform these simple functional skills in addition to having bilateral range of motion and strength in the wrist and fingers. Conditions that warrant immediate referral to a physician include:

- Suspected fracture or dislocation
- Significant pain and/or excessive swelling in soft tissues or around joints
- Joint instability
- Loss or impairment of motion or function
- Presence of any sensory or circulatory changes

 The assessment of the cheerleader suggests a fracture of the scaphoid. Immediate management involves ice, compression, immobilization in an appropriate splint, and immediate referral to a physician.

REHABILITATION

 A scaphoid fracture can take several weeks or months to heal. What exercises could be included during this period to help the cheerleader maintain her fitness?

Injuries to the wrist and hand often require immobilization; however, early range-of-motion and strengthening exercises should be conducted at the elbow and shoulder. Many of the exercises for the wrist and hand are discussed and demonstrated in Chapter 14, because they often are combined with rehabilitation of the elbow.

Restoration of Motion

Immobilization typically results in joint contractures and stiffness in the fingers. Therefore, active range-of-motion exercises should begin as soon as possible. In the acute phase, exercises can be performed using cryokinetic techniques. Ice immersion is alternated with active range-of-motion exercises. The individual can use the opposite hand to apply a low-load, prolonged stretch in the various motions to minimize joint trauma and increase flexibility. As inflammation decreases, a warm whirlpool or paraffin bath may be used to facilitate motion.

Restoration of Proprioception and Balance

Closed chain exercises may involve shifting body weight from one hand to the other on a wall, tabletop, or unstable surface, such as a foam mat or BAPS (biomechanical ankle platform system) Board®. Push-ups and step-ups on a box, stool, or StairMaster also can be used. Precision techniques to restore dexterity can be performed by picking up and manipulating the following objects:

1. Coins of different thickness

2. Playing cards

3. Small objects of differing shapes

4. Large, light objects

5. Large, heavy objects

In addition, the individual can tear tape, use scissors to cut paper, or juggle balls of different sizes.

Muscular Strength, Endurance, and Power

Once the range of motion approximates what is normal for the individual, open chain kinetic exercises are performed in the various motions using lightweight dumbbells. Many of these exercises are listed and explained in Field Strategy 14.1. The individual should complete 30 to 50 repetitions with a 1-pound weight and should not progress in resistance until 50 repetitions have been achieved. Using a table to support the forearm, wrist curls, reverse wrist curls, pronation, and supination can be performed. Wrist curl-ups using a light weight suspended from a broomstick on a 3- to 4-foot rope can be used to increase strength in the wrist flexors and extensors. A weighted bar or hammer can be used for radial and ulnar deviation and for pronation and supination. PNF-resisted exercises, surgical tubing, or strong rubber bands can be used in all motions for concentric and eccentric loading. Gripping exercises using a tennis ball or putty can be combined with pinching small and large objects. Plyometric exercises may involve catching a weighted ball in a single hand and throwing it straight up and down or using a minitramp to do bounding push-ups.

Cardiovascular Fitness

Cardiovascular conditioning should be maintained throughout the rehabilitation program. Several examples of such programs are provided on thePoint (Chapter 8).

 The cheerleader should engage in general body conditioning and strengthening exercises. Only those exercises that aggravate the condition are contraindicated.

SUMMARY

1. Most wrist motion occurs at the radiocarpal joint. The TFC is the cartilaginous disk that acts as a stabilizer of the DRUJ and serves as the ulnar continuation of the radius.

2. The CM joint of the thumb is a classic saddle joint, which allows it to have more motion than the CM joints of the other four digits.

3. Retinacular tissue is found throughout the hand and forms protective passageways through which tendons, nerves, and blood vessels pass.

4. Most injuries to the wrist are a result of axial loading on the proximal palm during a fall on an outstretched hand.

5. Excessive varus/valgus stress and hyperextension can damage the collateral ligaments of the fingers. Failure of a ligament usually occurs at its attachment to the proximal phalanx or, less frequently, in the midportion.

6. The most common dislocation in the body occurs at the PIP joint. Because digital nerves and vessels run along the sides of the fingers and thumb, dislocation can be serious if it is reduced by an untrained individual.

7. Muscular strains occur as a result of excessive overload against resistance or stretching the tendon beyond its normal range. Ruptures of a muscle tendon may cause the tendon to retract, necessitating surgical reattachment of the tendon in its proper position.

8. Chronic overuse of a tendon can lead to a tendinitis or friction tendinitis in one or more of the dorsal tunnels. Treatment usually consists of ice, rest, NSAIDs, splinting, and avoidance of exacerbating activities.

9. Carpal tunnel syndrome is the most common compression syndrome of the wrist and hand. It is characterized by pain and numbness that wakes the individual in the middle of the night and that often is relieved by shaking the hands.

10. Compression of the ulnar nerve leads to weakness in grip strength, atrophy of the hypothenar mass, and loss of sensation over the little finger.

11. If pain is present during palpation of the anatomical snuff box or with inward pressure along the long axis of the first metacarpal bone, a fracture of the scaphoid should be suspected.

12. Any injury that impairs the function of the hand or fingers should be referred to a physician. The area should be immobilized to prevent further damage, ice applied to control hemorrhage and swelling, and the individual transported in an appropriate manner.

REFERENCES

1. Dimeff RJ. Entrapment neuropathies of the upper extremity. Curr Sports Med Rep 2003;2(5):255–261.

2. Moojen TM, Snel JG, Ritt MJ, et al. Pisiform kinematics in vivo. J Hand Surg Am 2001;26(5):901–907.

3. Moojen TM, Snel JG, Ritt MJ, et al. Three-dimensional carpal kinematics in vivo. Clin Biomech 2002;17(7): 506–514.

4. New CP, Crisco JJ, Wolfe SW. In vivo kinematic behavior of the radiocapitate joint during wrist flexion-extension and radioulnar deviation. J Biomech 2001;34(11):1429–1438.

5. Wolfe SW, New C, Crisco JJ. In vivo scaphoid, lunate, and capitate kinematics in flexion and in extension. J Hand Surg Am 2000;25(5):860–869.

6. Upal MA. Carpal bone kinematics in combined wrist joint motions may differ from the bone kinematics during simple wrist motions. Biomed Sci Instrum 2003;39: 272–277.

7. Kobayashi M, Berger RA, Linscheid R, An KN. Intercarpal kinematics during wrist motion. Hand Clin 1997; 13(1):143–149.

8. Hollister A, Buford WL, Myers LM, et al. The axes of rotation of the thumb carpometacarpal joint. J Orthop Res 1992;10(3):454–460.

9. Ateshian GA, Rosenwasser MP, Mow VC. Curvature characteristics and congruence of the thumb carpometacarpal joint: differences between female and male joints. J Biomech 1992;25(6):591–607.

10. Su F-C, Chou YL, Yang CS, Lin GT, An KN. Movement of finger joints induced by synergistic wrist motion. Clin Biomech 2005;20(5):491–497.

11. Daniels JM II, Zook EG, Lynch JM. Hand and wrist injuries: Part II. Emergent evaluation. Am Fam Physician 2004;69(8):1949–1956.

12. Tiedeman JJ, Ferlic TP. Hand and wrist injuries. In: Mellion MB, Walsh WM, Madden C, Putukian M, Shelton GL, eds. The Team Physician's Handbook. Philadelphia: Hanley & Belfus, 2002.

13. Daniels JM II, Zook EG, Lynch JM. Hand and wrist injuries: Part I. Nonemergent evaluation. Am Fam Physician 2004;69(8):1941–1948.

14. Kato N, Nemoto K, Nakajima H, Motosuneya T, Fujikawa K. Primary repair of the collateral ligament of the proximal interphalangeal joint using a suture anchor. Scand J Plast Reconstr Surg Hand Surg 2003;37(2): 117–120.

15. Finsen V, Hagen S. Surgery for trigger finger. Hand Surg 2003;8(2):201–203.

16. Servi JT. Wrist pain from overuse: detecting and relieving intersection syndrome. Phys Sports Med 1997;25(12):41–44.

17. Ugbolue UC, Hsu W-H, Goitz RJ, Li Z-M. Tendon and nerve displacement at the wrist during finger movements. Clin Biomech 2005;20(1):50–56.

18. Holm G, Moody LE. Carpal tunnel syndrome: current

theory, treatment, and the use of B_6. Clin Pract 2003; 15(1):18–22.

19. Viera AJ. Management of carpal tunnel syndrome. Am Fam Physician 2003;68(2):265–272.

20. Sevim S, Dogu O, Camdeviren H, et al. Long-term effectiveness of steroid injections and splinting in mild and moderate carpal tunnel syndrome. Neurol Sci 2004; 25(2):48–52.

21. McNally C, Gillespie M. Scaphoid fractures. Emergency Nurse 2004;12(1):21–25.

22. Kocher MS, Water PM, Micheli LJ. Upper extremity injuries in the pediatric athlete. Sports Med 2000; 30(2):117–135.

23. Daniels JM, Zook EG, Lynch JM. Hand and wrist injuries: Part I. Nonemergent evaluation. Am Fam Physician 2004; 69(8):1941–1948.

Lower Extremity

5

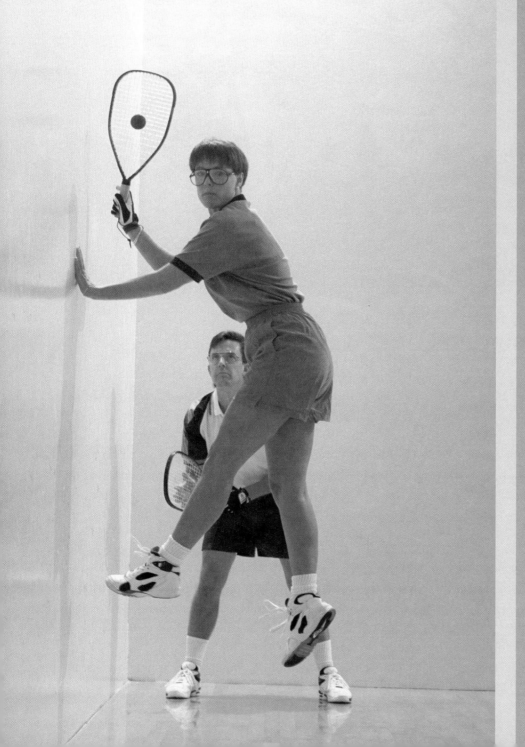

Chapter 16
Pelvic, Hip, and Thigh
Conditions

Chapter 17
Knee Conditions

Chapter 18
Lower Leg, Ankle, and
Foot Conditions

16

Pelvic, Hip, and Thigh Conditions

STUDENT OUTCOMES

1. Identify the major bony and soft-tissue structures of the pelvis, hip, and thigh.

2. Describe the functions of the various soft-tissue structures that support the sacroiliac joint, sacrococcygeal joint, and hip joint.

3. Describe the motions of the hip, and identify the muscles that produce them.

4. List the major nerves and blood vessels that course through the pelvic and proximal femoral region.

5. Describe the forces that produce loading patterns responsible for common injuries of the pelvis, hip, and thigh.

6. Explain general principles used to prevent injuries to the pelvis, hip, and thigh.

7. Identify the common injuries and conditions sustained in the pelvis, hip, and thigh by physically active individuals (including sprains, dislocations, contusions, strains, bursitis, and vascular and neural disorders).

8. Explain the management strategies for common injuries and conditions of the wrist and hand.

9. Describe the various types of fractures that can occur in the wrist and hand, and explain their management.

10. Describe a thorough assessment of the pelvis, hip, and thigh.

11. Explain the general principles and techniques used in developing a rehabilitation exercise program for pelvis, hip, and thigh.

ROLE DELINEATION COMPETENCIES

The following Performance Domains and Tasks defined in the National Athletic Trainers' Association Board of Certification *Role Delineation Study*, 5th Edition are addressed in this chapter:

BOC COMPETENCIES

I.   Prevention

G. Monitor participants and environmental conditions by following accepted guidelines to promote safe participation.

II.   Clinical Evaluation and Diagnosis

A. Obtain a history through observation, interview, and/or review of relevant records to assess current or potential injury, illness, or condition.
B. Inspect the involved area(s) visually to assess the injury, illness, or health-related condition.
C. Palpate the involved area(s) using standard techniques to assess the injury, illness, or health-related condition.
D. Perform specific tests in accordance with accepted procedures to assess the injury, illness, or health-related condition.
E. Formulate a clinical impression by interpreting the signs, symptoms, and predisposing factors of the injury, illness, or condition to determine the appropriate course of action.

III.   Immediate Care

A. Employ life-saving techniques through the use of standard emergency procedures in order to reduce morbidity and the incidence of mortality.
B. Prevent exacerbation of non–life threatening condition(s) through the use of standard procedures in order to reduce morbidity.
C. Facilitate the timely transfer of care for conditions beyond the scope of practice of the athletic trainer by implementing appropriate referral strategies to stabilize and/or prevent exacerbation of the condition(s).

IV.   Treatment, Rehabilitation, and Reconditioning

E. Reassess the status of injuries, illnesses, and/or conditions using standard techniques and documentation strategies in order to determine appropriate treatment, rehabilitation, and/or reconditioning and to evaluate readiness to return to a desired level of activity.
F. Educate the appropriate individual(s) in the treatment, rehabilitation, and reconditioning of injuries, illnesses, and/or conditions using applicable methods and materials to facilitate recovery, function, and/or performance.

Although the pelvis, hip, and thigh have a sturdy anatomical composition, this region can be subjected to large, potentially injurious forces when individuals engage in sports or exercise. For example, the soft tissues of the anterior thigh often sustain compressive forces, particularly during contact sports. Although the resulting contusions are not usually serious, mismanagement of these injuries can lead to more serious problems. Daily activities, such as sitting, walking, and climbing stairs, rarely involve stretching of the hamstrings. A lack of hamstring flexibility combined with an imbalance of strength between the hamstrings and the quadriceps, place the physically active individual at higher risk for sustaining a hamstring strain.

Because of their strong bony stability, the hip and pelvis are seldom injured. Because the hip sustains repetitive forces of four- to sevenfold the body weight during walking and running, however, the joint is subject to stress-related injuries.

This chapter begins with a review of the anatomy, kinematics, and kinetics of the pelvis, hip, and thigh. Next, preventative measures are discussed, followed by information regarding basic injuries to the region. A step-by-step process of injury assessment is then followed by examples of rehabilitation exercises for the region.

ANATOMY OF THE PELVIS, HIP, AND THIGH

The pelvis, hip, and thigh have an extremely stable bony structure that is further reinforced by a number of large, strong ligaments and muscles. This region is well-suited anatomically for withstanding the large forces to which it is subjected during daily activities.

The Pelvis

The pelvis, or pelvic girdle, consists of a protective bony ring formed by four fused bones—namely, the two innominate bones, the sacrum, and the coccyx (Fig. 16.1). The innominate bones articulate with each other anteriorly at the pubic symphysis and with the sacrum posteriorly at the sacroiliac (SI) joints. Each innominate bone consists of three fused bones—namely, the ilium, the ischium, and the pubis. Among these, the ilium forms the major portion of the innominate bone, including the prominent iliac crests. The anterior superior iliac spine (ASIS) is a readily palpable landmark on the iliac crest; the posterior superior iliac spine (PSIS) typically is marked by an indentation in the soft

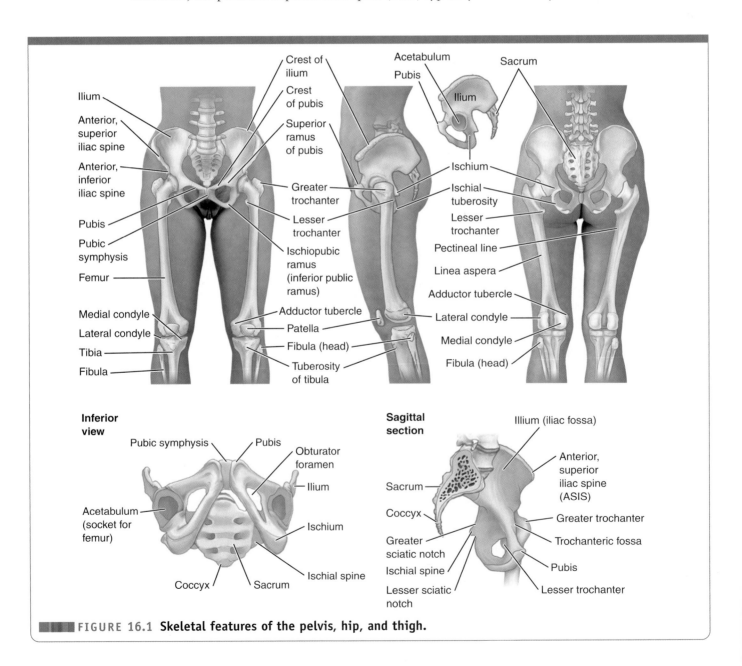

FIGURE 16.1 **Skeletal features of the pelvis, hip, and thigh.**

tissues just lateral to the sacrum. The pelvis protects the enclosed inner organs, transmits loads between the trunk and lower extremity, and provides a site for a number of major muscle attachments.

Sacroiliac Joints

The SI joints form the critical link between the two pelvic bones. Working with the pubic symphysis, they help to transfer the weight of the torso and skull to the lower limbs, provide elasticity to the pelvic ring, and conversely, act as a buffer to decrease impact forces from the foot as they are transmitted to the spine and upper body.

The SI joints are synovial as well as syndesmosis joints. The synovial portion of the joint is C-shaped, with the convex iliac surface of the "C" facing an anterior and inferior direction. The articular surface of the ilium is covered with fibrocartilage; the articular surface of the sacrum is covered with hyaline cartilage and is threefold thicker than that of the ilium. The size, shape, and texture of the articular surfaces vary across the life span. In children, the surfaces are smooth. In adults, irregular depressions and elevations are formed that fit into one another. As a result, the articulation is very strong and has a limited range of motion (ROM). In older individuals, portions of the joint surfaces may be obliterated by adhesions.

The strong fibers of the interosseous SI ligaments bind the anterior portion of the ilium and the posterior portion of the sacrum, filling the void behind the articular surfaces of these bones (Fig. 16.2). The joint also is strengthened anteriorly and posteriorly by the dorsal and ventral SI ligaments. The dorsal SI ligament runs transversely to bind the posterior ilium to the upper portion of the sacrum, and vertical fibers connect the lower sacrum to the PSIS. The ventral SI ligament lines the anterior portion of the pelvic cavity, attaching onto the anterior portion of the sacrum. These SI ligaments, particularly the ventral bond, play a significant role in restricting movement at the SI joints (1,2). Two accessory ligaments also assist in maintaining the stability of the SI joint. The sacrotuberous

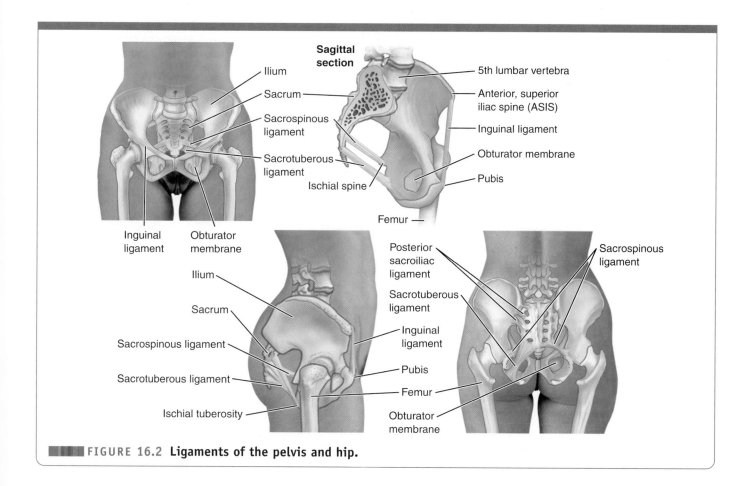

FIGURE 16.2 Ligaments of the pelvis and hip.

ligament arises from the ischium to merge with the inferior fibers of the dorsal SI ligaments. The sacrospinous ligament, indirectly supporting the sacrum, runs from the ischial spine and attaches to the coccyx.

Sacrococcygeal Joint

The sacrococcygeal joint usually is a fused line (i.e., symphysis) that is united by a fibrocartilaginous disk. Occasionally, the joint is freely movable and synovial, but with advanced age, the joint may fuse and be obliterated.

Pubic Symphysis

The pubic symphysis is a cartilaginous joint with a disk of fibrocartilage, called the interpubic disk, that is located between the two joint surfaces. A small degree of spreading, compression, and rotation occurs between the two halves of the pelvic girdle at this joint.

Bony Structure of the Thigh

The femur, a major weight-bearing bone, is the longest, largest, and strongest bone in the body (see Fig. 16.1). Its weakest component is the femoral neck, which is smaller in diameter than the rest of the bone and is weak internally, because it is composed primarily of cancellous bone. The head of the femur is angled at approximately 125° in the frontal plane, although it can vary from 90 to 135°. This relationship, known as the **angle of inclination** (Fig. 16.3), allows the femur to angle medially downward from the hip during the support phase of walking and running, producing single-leg support beneath the body's center of gravity. Because women have a wider pelvis, this angulation tends to be more pronounced than the angulation in men. Angles of inclination greater than 125° are termed **coxa valga**, and angles less than 125° are referred to as **coxa vara**.

In the transverse plane, the relationship between the femoral head and the femoral shaft is called the **angle of torsion**, which is approximately 12° (Fig. 16.4). A decreased angle between the femoral condyles and femoral head is called **retroversion**; an increased angle is called **anteversion**. Retroversion causes a tendency for external rotation of the leg during the swing phase of gait, and

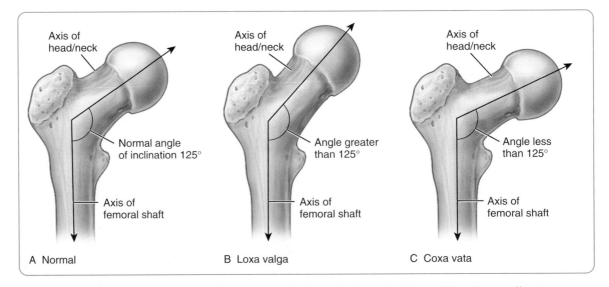

FIGURE 16.3 Angle of inclination. In the frontal plane, the femoral head normally assumes a 125° angle with the long axis of the femur **(A)**. This angle allows the femur to angle medially downward from the hip during the support phase of walking and running, producing single-leg support beneath the body's center of gravity. Because women have a wider pelvis, this angulation tends to be slightly increased, which is called coxa valga **(B)**; a decrease is called coxa vara **(C)**.

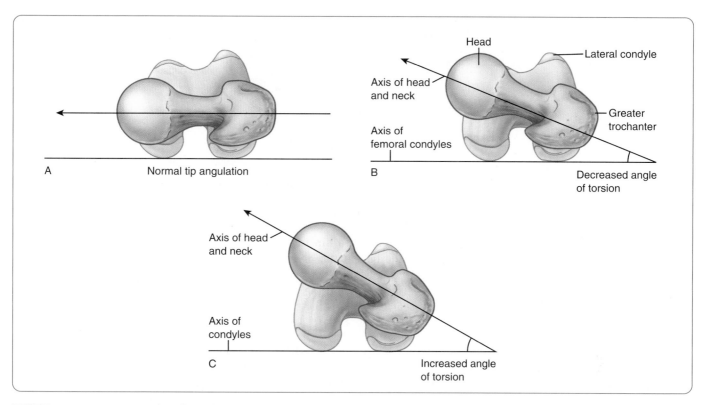

FIGURE 16.4 Angle of torsion. A, In the transverse plane, deviations may occur from the norm. **B,** A decreased angle between the femoral condyles and femoral head is called retroversion. **C,** An increased angle is called anteversion.

anteversion causes the opposite tendency (i.e., toward internal rotation). Both are relatively common in children but tend to normalize with maturity (3).

The Hip Joint

The hip is the articulation between the concave acetabulum of the pelvis and the head of the femur. It functions as a classic ball-and-socket joint (Fig. 16.5). The acetabulum angles obliquely in an inferior, anterior, and lateral direction. Because the socket is deep, it provides considerable bony stability to the joint. Both articulating surfaces are covered with friction-reducing joint cartilage. The cartilage on the acetabulum is thickened around the periphery, where it merges with the U-shaped fibrocartilaginous acetabular labrum, which further contributes to stability of the joint.

Hip Joint Capsule

The joint capsule of the hip, the coxofemoral joint, is large and loose. It completely surrounds the joint, attaching to the labrum of the acetabular socket. The labrum forms a seal around the joint, with increased fluid pressure within the labrum contributing to lubrication of the joint (4). The joint capsule also passes over a fat pad internally to join to the distal aspect of the femoral neck. Because the capsular fibers attaching to the femoral neck are arranged in a circular fashion, they are known as the zona orbicularis and are an important contributor to hip stability.

Ligaments of the Hip Joint

Several large, strong ligaments support the hip (see Fig. 16.2). The anterior aspect of the hip includes the extremely strong, Y-shaped iliofemoral ligament, sometimes referred to as the Y-ligament of Bigelow. It extends from the anterior inferior iliac spine (AIIS) to the intertrochanteric line on the femur, enabling it to limit hip hyperextension. The pubofemoral ligament, which also is located

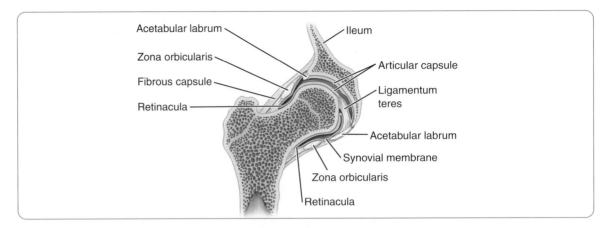

anteriorly, connects the pubic ramus to the intertrochanteric line, limiting abduction and hyperextension of the hip. The ischiofemoral ligament reinforces the hip posteriorly, extending from the posterior acetabular rim of the ischium in a superior, lateral direction and attaching to the inner surface of the greater trochanter of the femur. The spiraling nature of this ligament causes it to limit extension of the hip. Tension in these major ligaments twists the head of the femur into the acetabulum on hip extension, as occurs when a person rises from a seated position.

Within the joint, the ligamentum teres serves as a conduit for the medial and lateral circumflex arteries but provides little support to the hip joint. The inguinal ligament, which runs from the ASIS and inserts at the pubic symphysis, contains the soft tissues as they course anteriorly from the trunk to the lower extremity. The structure demarcates the superior border of the femoral triangle.

Femoral Triangle

The femoral triangle is formed by the inguinal ligament superiorly, the sartorius laterally, and the adductor longus medially (Fig. 16.6). This region is significant in that the femoral nerve, artery, and vein are located within the area. The femoral pulse can be palpated as it crosses the crease between the thigh and the abdomen. In addition, with an infection of or active inflammation in the lower extremity, enlarged lymph nodes may be palpated in this region.

Bursae

Four primary bursae are present in the hip and pelvic region. The iliopsoas bursa is positioned between the iliopsoas and articular capsule, serving to reduce the friction between these structures. The deep trochanteric bursa provides a cushion between the greater trochanter of the femur and the gluteus maximus at its attachment to the iliotibial tract. The gluteofemoral bursa separates the gluteus maximus from the origin of the vastus lateralis. Finally, the ischial bursa serves as a weight-bearing structure when an individual is seated, cushioning the ischial tuberosity where it passes over the gluteus maximus.

Q-Angle

The **Q-angle** is defined as the angle between the line of resultant force produced by the quadriceps muscles and the line of the patellar tendon (see Fig. 17.3). One line is drawn from the middle of

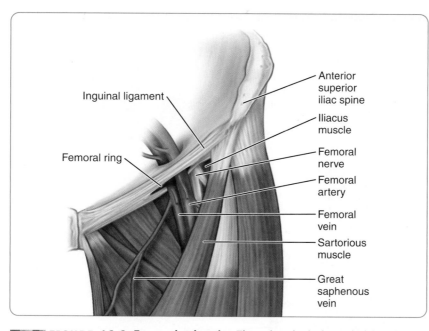

Inguinal ligament

Femoral ring

Anterior superior iliac spine

Iliacus muscle

Femoral nerve

Femoral artery

Femoral vein

Sartorious muscle

Great saphenous vein

■■ ■ FIGURE 16.6 Femoral triangle. The triangle is bounded by the inguinal ligament superiorly, the adductor longus medially, and the sartorius laterally. The femoral artery, vein, and nerve pass through this area to enter the thigh.

the patella to the ASIS of the ilium, and a second line is drawn from the tibial tubercle through the center of the patella. When the knee is fully extended, the normal Q-angle ranges from approximately 13° in males to approximately 18° in females (5). This angle can predispose an individual to patellar injuries. The Q-angle is explained in more detail in Chapter 17.

Muscles of the Hip Joint

A large number of muscles cross the hip (Figs. 16.7 to 16.9). Identifying the actions of these muscles is complicated by the fact that several muscles are two-joint muscles.

> See *Muscles of the Hip,* available on the companion website at thePoint, for a summary of these muscles, including their attachments, primary actions, and innervation.

Nerves of the Pelvis, Hip, and Thigh

The major nerve supply to the pelvis, hip, and thigh arises from the lumbar and sacral plexi. The **lumbar plexus** is formed from the first four lumbar spinal nerves (see Fig. 11.4). It innervates portions of the abdominal wall and psoas major, with branches into the thigh region. The largest branch is the femoral nerve (L_2–L_4), which supplies the muscles and skin of the anterior thigh. Another branch, the obturator nerve (L_2–L_4), provides innervation to the hip adductor muscles.

The **sacral plexus** is positioned just anterior to the lumbar plexus and has some intermingling of fibers with the lumbar plexus. The lower spinal nerves, including L_4 through S_4, spawn the sacral plexus (see Fig. 11.5). Twelve nerve branches arise from the sacral plexus. The major nerve is the sciatic nerve (L_4, L_5, and S_1–S_3), which is the largest and longest single nerve in the body. The sciatic nerve passes through the greater sciatic notch of the pelvis, courses through the gluteus maximus muscle, and then innervates the hamstrings and adductor magnus. The tibial and common peroneal nerves that branch from the sciatic nerve in the posterior thigh region are discussed in Chapters 17 and 18.

FIGURE 16.7 Muscles of the pelvis, hip, and thigh. Anterior view.

FIGURE 16.8 **Muscles of the pelvis, hip, and thigh.** Lateral view.

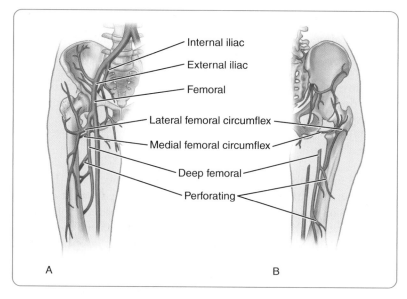

Internal iliac

External iliac

Femoral

Lateral femoral circumflex

Medial femoral circumflex

Deep femoral

Perforating

A   B

FIGURE 16.10 Arterial supply to the hip and thigh region.
A, Anterior view. **B,** Posterior view.

Blood Vessels of the Pelvis, Hip, and Thigh

The external iliac arteries become the femoral arteries at the level of the thighs (Fig. 16.10). The femoral artery gives off several branches in the thigh region, including the deep femoral artery, which serves the posterior and lateral thigh muscles, and the lateral and medial femoral circumflex arteries, which supply the region of the femoral head.

KINEMATICS AND MAJOR MUSCLE ACTIONS OF THE HIP

Because the hip is a ball-and-socket joint, the femur can move in all planes of motion. The massive muscles crossing the hip tend to limit ROM, however, particularly in the posterior direction.

Pelvic Positioning

During many activities, the positioning of the pelvic girdle facilitates motion of the femur at the hip. For example, abduction of the leg during the preparatory phase of a kick in one of the martial arts is made easier by a lateral tilt of the pelvis toward the side opposite the kicking leg. Likewise, flexion at the hip is assisted by posterior pelvic tilt, and extension at the hip is enhanced by anterior pelvic tilt.

Flexion

The major hip flexors are the iliacus and psoas major, which because of their common attachment at the femur are referred to jointly as the iliopsoas. Four other muscles cross the anterior aspect of the hip to contribute to hip flexion—namely, the pectineus, the rectus femoris, the sartorius, and the tensor fascia latae. Because the rectus femoris is a two-joint muscle that is active during both hip flexion and knee extension, it functions more effectively as a hip flexor when the knee is in flexion, as occurs when a person kicks a ball. The sartorius also is a two-joint muscle. Crossing from the ASIS to the medial surface of the proximal tibia just below the tuberosity, the sartorius is the longest muscle in the body.

Extension

The hip extensors are the gluteus maximus and the three hamstrings—namely, the biceps femoris, the semitendinosus, and the semimembranosus. The gluteus maximus usually is active only when the hip is in flexion, as occurs during stair climbing or cycling, or when extension at the hip is resisted. The nickname "hamstrings" derives from the prominent tendons of the three muscles, which are readily palpable on the posterior aspect of the knee. The hamstrings cross both the hip and the knee, contributing to hip extension and knee flexion.

Abduction

The gluteus medius is the major abductor at the hip, with assistance from the gluteus minimus. The hip abductors are active in stabilizing the pelvis during single-leg support of the body and during the support phase of walking and running (see Chapter 18). For example, when body weight is supported by the right foot during walking, the right hip abductors contract isometrically and eccentrically to prevent the left side of the pelvis from being pulled downward by the weight of the swinging left leg. This allows the left leg to move freely through the swing phase without scuffing the toes. If the hip abductors are too weak to perform this function, lateral pelvic tilt occurs with every step.

Adduction

The hip adductors include the adductor longus, adductor brevis, and adductor magnus. These muscles are active during the swing phase of gait, bringing the foot beneath the body's center of gravity for placement during the support phase. The relatively weak gracilis assists with hip adduction. The hip adductors also contribute to flexion and internal rotation at the hip, especially when the femur is externally rotated.

Medial and Lateral Rotation of the Femur

Although several muscles contribute to lateral rotation of the femur, six function solely as lateral rotators. These six muscles are the piriformis, gemellus superior, gemellus inferior, obturator internus, obturator externus, and quadratus femoris. The femur of the swinging leg rotates laterally to accommodate the lateral rotation of the pelvis during the stride.

The major medial rotator of the femur is the gluteus minimus, with assistance from the tensor fascia latae, semitendinosus, semimembranosus, gluteus medius, and the four adductor muscles. The medial rotators are relatively weak; their estimated strength is approximately one-third that of the lateral rotators. Table 16.1 summarizes the muscles responsible for the various motions at the hip joint.

TABLE 16.1 Hip Movements and Involved Muscles

FLEXION	EXTENSION	ABDUCTION	ADDUCTION	MEDIAL ROTATION	LATERAL ROTATION
Iliopsoas	Gluteus maximus	Gluteus medius	Pectineus	Gluteus medius	Piriformis
Rectus femoris	Biceps femoris	Gluteus minimus	Adductor brevis	Gluteus minimus	Obturator internus
Pectineus	Biceps femoris	Gluteus minimus	Adductor magnus	Tensor fasciae latae	Obturator externus
Sartorius	Semitendinosus	Tensor fasciae latae	Adductor longus		Superior gemelli
Tensor fasciae latae	Semimembranosus	Sartorius	Adductor magnus		Inferior gemelli
	Adductor magnus	Piriformis	Gracilis		Quadratus femoris
					Gluteus maximus

KINETICS OF THE HIP

Forces at the Hip During Standing

The hip is a major weight-bearing joint that is subject to extremely high loads during sport participation. During upright standing, with weight evenly distributed on both legs, the weight supported at each hip is half the weight of the body segments above the hip. The total load on each hip in this situation is greater than the weight that is being supported, however, because tension in the large, strong hip muscles further adds to compression at the joint.

Forces at the Hip During Gait

Compression on the hip is approximately the same as body weight during the swing phase of normal walking gait but increases up to three- to sixfold the body weight during the stance phase (3). Body weight, impact forces translated upward through the skeleton from the foot, and muscle tension contribute to this compressive load. Walking or running increases the forces on the hip. Use of a crutch or a cane on the side opposite an injured lower limb serves to more evenly distribute the load between the legs throughout the gait cycle. It is better to use no assistive device than to use a crutch or a cane on the same side as the lower extremity injury, because this actually increases joint forces on the injured side (6).

PREVENTION OF PELVIC, HIP AND THIGH CONDITIONS

The hip joint is well protected within the pelvic girdle and seldom is injured. Several factors, however, such as wearing protective equipment, wearing shoes with adequate cushioning and support, and participating in an extensive physical conditioning program, can further reduce the incidence of acute and chronic injuries to the region.

Protective Equipment

Several collision and contact sports require special pads composed of hard polyethylene covered with layers of specialized foam rubber to protect vulnerable areas, such as the iliac crests, sacrum and coccyx, and genital region. A girdle with special pockets can hold the pads in place. The male genital region is best protected by a protective cup placed in an athletic supporter. Special commercial thigh pads also may be used to prevent contusions to the anterior thigh, and neoprene sleeves can provide uniform compression, therapeutic warmth, and support for a quadriceps or hamstrings strain. Many of these items can be seen in Chapter 3.

Physical Conditioning

Because several of the muscles in the pelvis, hip, and thigh are two-joint muscles, physical conditioning should include ROM and strengthening exercises for both the hip and the knee. Field Strategy 16.1 demonstrates specific exercises for the hip flexors, extensors, adductors, abductors, and medial and lateral rotators. Exercises for the muscles that govern the knee are presented in Chapter 17.

Shoe Selection

Sport and physical activities take place on a variety of terrains and floor surfaces. Shoes should adequately cushion impact forces as well as support and guide the foot during the stance and final push-off phases of running, regardless of the terrain or surface. Inadequate cushioning in the heel region can transmit forces up the leg, leading to inflammation of the hip joint, or stress fractures of the femoral neck or pubis. Therefore, it is important to purchase shoes that provide an adequate heel cushion and a thermoplastic heel counter, which can maintain its shape and firmness even during adverse weather conditions. The soles should be designed for the specific type of playing surface to avoid slipping or sliding.

Exercises to Prevent Injury at the Thigh, Hip, and Pelvis

The following exercises can be performed for motions at the hip. Exercises for the hamstrings, quadriceps, and iliotibial band, which also cross the knee joint, can be seen in Chapter 17.

1. **Hip flexor stretch (lunge).** Place the leg to be stretched in front. Bend the contralateral knee as the hips are moved forward. Keep the back straight. Alternative method: Place the foot on a chair or table, and lean forward until a stretch is felt.

2. **Lateral rotator stretch, seated position.** Cross one leg over the thigh, and place the elbow on the outside of the knee. Gently stretch the buttock muscles by pushing the bent knee across the body while keeping the pelvis on the floor.

3. **Adductor stretch, standing position.** Place the leg to be stretched out to the side. Slowly bend the contralateral knee. Keep the hips in a neutral or extended position.

4. **Elastic tubing exercises.** Secure elastic tubing to a table. Perform hip flexion, extension, abduction, adduction, and medial and lateral rotation in a single plane or in multidirectional patterns.

5. **Full squats.** A weight belt should be worn during this exercise. Place the feet at shoulder width or wider. Keep the back straight by keeping the chest out and the head up at all times. Flex the knees and hips to no greater than 90°. Begin the upward motion by extending the hips first.

6. **Hip extension.** With the trunk stabilized and the back flat, extend the hip while keeping the knee flexed. Alternate legs.

CONTUSIONS

 A volleyball athlete was digging for a ball and fell directly on her left hip. She experienced immediate severe pain and extreme tenderness over the iliac crest. What painful movements would confirm a suspected hip pointer?

Direct impact to soft tissue, such as a kick to the thigh or a fall onto a hard surface, causes a compressive force to crush soft tissue. The condition may be mild and resolve on its own in a matter of days, or the bleeding and swelling may be more extensive, resulting in a large, deep hematoma that takes months to resolve. Contusions may occur anywhere in the hip region but typically are seen on the crest of the ilium or in the quadriceps muscle group.

Hip Pointer

A **hip pointer** generally refers to a contusion of the iliac crest over the tensor fascia latae muscle belly with an associated hematoma, but the term also may be used to identify tearing of the external oblique muscle from the iliac crest, periostitis of the crest, and trochanteric contusions. Most injuries are sustained when a direct blow impacts the iliac crest.

Signs and Symptoms

Deep, rapid bleeding and swelling can be subperiosteal, intramuscular, or subcutaneous. Because so many trunk and abdominal muscles attach to the iliac crest, any movement of the trunk, including coughing, laughing, and even breathing, is painful. Immediate pain, discoloration, spasm, and loss of function prevent the individual from rotating the trunk or laterally flexing the trunk toward the injured side. Extreme tenderness is present over the iliac crest, and abdominal muscle spasm may be present. Within 24 to 48 hours, the swelling is more diffuse, and ecchymosis is evident. In severe injury, the individual may be unable to walk or bear weight, even with crutches, because of the intense pain caused by muscular tension at the injury site. Table 16.2 lists the signs and symptoms of the various grades of hip pointers.

TABLE 16.2 Signs and Symptoms of Hip Pointers	
INJURY GRADE	**SIGNS AND SYMPTOMS**
Grade I	Normal gait and normal posture
	Slight pain on palpation
	Little or no swelling present
	Full trunk range of motion
	Return to activity may take 3–7 days
Grade II	Abnormal gait pattern
	Posture may be slightly flexed toward the side of injury
	Noticeable pain on palpation of iliac crest, with visible swelling
	Active trunk range of motion is painful and limited, especially lateral flexion to the opposite side and trunk rotation
	Return to activity may take 5–14 days
Grade III	Severe pain, swelling, and ecchymosis
	Gait is slow, with short stride length and swing-through
	Posture may have severe tilt to injured side
	Trunk range of motion is painful and limited in all directions
	Return to activity may take 14–21 days

Management

Treatment involves ice, compression, and total rest during the first 2 to 3 days following injury. Mild stretching and electrical stimulation to the muscles during icing may reduce secondary muscle spasm. If intense pain is palpated directly over the iliac crest, the individual should be referred to a physician to rule out a fracture of the iliac crest, because the same mechanism of injury may cause both injuries.

In an uncomplicated hip pointer, the individual can return to activity in 3 to 7 days. To prevent reinjury, however, the area should be protected with a pad.

In a grade II or III injury, crutches should be used for ambulation. Analgesic medications for pain and nonsteroidal anti-inflammatory drugs (NSAIDs) are indicated after 48 hours. Later treatment may include heat therapy, ultrasound, transcutaneous electrical nerve stimulation (TENS), and pain-free ROM exercises as tolerated. As soon as pain-free active ROM exercise can be accomplished, the individual should progress to resistive exercise, including lower extremity and trunk strengthening. Return to activity should be gradual, with the individual possibly wearing a dense foam donut pad fitted into a custom-formed plastic shell or a compression garment to protect the area from further injury.

Quadriceps Contusion

The most common site for a quadriceps contusion is the anterolateral thigh. If the contusion is located adjacent to the intermuscular septum, pain and hemorrhage tend to resolve more rapidly. Contusions within the muscle itself often are associated with greater tearing, hemorrhage, and pain and with a greater tendency toward abnormal pathology. Severity of the injury is almost always underestimated, leading to undertreatment.

Signs and Symptoms

Pain and swelling may be extensive immediately after impact. In a mild (grade 1) contusion, the individual has mild pain and swelling and is able to walk without a limp. Passive flexion beyond 90° may be painful, but resisted knee extension may cause less discomfort. In a moderate (grade II) contusion, the individual can flex the knee between 45 and 90° and walks with a noticeable limp. Swelling prevents the knee from being fully flexed. In a severe (grade III) contusion, little evidence of bruising is seen initially, but within 24 hours, progressive bleeding and swelling occur, preventing knee flexion beyond 45°. There may be a palpable, firm hematoma, resulting in an inability to contract the quadriceps or do a straight leg raise. The individual will require crutches for ambulation.

Management

For the first 24 to 48 hours, treatment involves application of ice and a compressive wrap, applied with the knee in maximal flexion (Fig. 16.11). This position preserves the needed flexion and limits intramuscular bleeding and spasm. After 48 hours, re-evaluation may necessitate continuation of the ice, compression, and flexion for another 12 to 24 hours. Continued swelling despite proper acute care protocol indicates continued hemorrhage. In these cases, immediate referral to a physician is necessary to assess the level of bleeding.

The individual should begin gentle passive and active, pain-free stretching with daily ice treatments and use of NSAIDs. If unable to perform a pain-free gait, the individual should be placed on crutches (non–weight bearing) for 48 hours; as motion capability improves, partial weight bearing should be initiated. Proprioceptive neuromuscular facilitation exercise patterns may be used to strengthen, relax, or gain ROM. Isometric quadriceps strengthening and hamstrings resistive exercises can progress to an active stretching

FIGURE 16.11 Management of a quadriceps contusion. Ice should be applied, with the knee in maximal flexion to place the muscles on stretch.

FIELD STRATEGY 16.2

Management Algorithm for a Quadriceps Contusion

Acute Phase (First 24–48 Hours)

- Ice and compression with knee flexed at 120°
- Crutches with partial or no weight bearing
- Pain-free passive and active ROM
- NSAIDs after 24 hours

Subacute Phase (2–5 Days)

- Cryotherapy and passive stretching exercises
- NSAIDs
- Active ROM and pain-free resisted proprioceptive neuromuscular facilitation relaxation and strengthening exercises
- Continue partial weight bearing until 90° of flexion are attained
- High-voltage galvanic stimulation, hot packs, or hydromassage (when no swelling is present)
- Swimming with gentle kicking exercises

Final Phase

- Discontinue crutches (when no limp is present)
- Cycling, light jogging, or running as tolerated
- High-voltage galvanic stimulation
- Radiography at 3 weeks to rule out myositis ossificans

Return to Play

- Range of motion within 10° of that for the unaffected leg
- Bilaterally equal strength and endurance
- Work on jumping, starts, stops, changing directions, sprinting
- Must pass all functional tests
- Consider protective padding to prevent reinjury

and progressive resistance strengthening program. Pulsed ultrasound or high-voltage galvanic stimulation may be helpful in the early stages to reduce edema. Continuous ultrasound, hydrotherapy, and massage should be avoided during the early stages, because they may irritate the inflammatory process, but may be used during later stages to aid recovery.

When full ROM has been restored, full weight-bearing gait should be resumed, the progressive strengthening program can be expanded, and cycling, jogging, running, and functional activities specific to the sport can be incorporated. Field Strategy 16.2 explains the care of a quadriceps contusion.

Myositis Ossificans

Myositis ossificans is an abnormal ossification involving bone deposition within muscle tissue. It may stem from a single traumatic blow, or from repeated blows, to the quadriceps. Several risk factors following a quadriceps contusion can predispose an individual to this condition, including:

- Innate predisposition to ectopic bone formation
- Continuing to play after injury
- Early massage, hydrotherapy, or thermotherapy during the acute stage
- Passive, forceful stretching
- Too rapid a progression in the rehabilitation program
- Premature return to play
- Reinjury of same area

Common sites are the anterior and lateral thigh. Although the precise mechanism that triggers the bone formation has yet to be established, it is thought that during resolution of the hematoma, within a week after injury, the existing fibroblasts involved in the repair process begin to differentiate into osteoblasts. The evidence of calcification on a radiograph becomes visible after 2 to 4 weeks.

As the calcification continues to progress, a palpable, firm mass can be felt in the deep tissues. After 6 to 7 weeks, the mass generally stops growing, and resorption occurs. Total resorption may not occur, however, leaving a visible, cortical-type bony lesion (Fig. 16.12).

Signs and Symptoms

Examination reveals a warm, firm, swollen thigh nearly 2 to 4 cm larger than the unaffected side. A palpable, painful mass may limit passive knee flexion to 20 to 30°. Active quadriceps contractions and straight leg raises may be impossible.

Management

This individual should be referred to a physician. Treatment includes ice, compression, elevation, crutches, and protected rest. Nonsteroidal anti-inflammatory drugs are only indicated after 48 hours because they inhibit platelet function and promote hemorrhage. Periodic radiographs generally are taken until the abnormal ossification matures, which typically occurs within 6 to 12 months. For cases in which the mass fails to reabsorb completely, many individuals return safely to participation, using adequate protection to prevent injury from subsequent blows. Surgery is only indicated in cases where activity is limited by pain, weakness, and decreased ROM. Excision before the mass matures may result in reformation, with the new mass sometimes being larger than the original mass.

FIGURE 16.12 Myositis ossificans. In myositis ossificans, full resorption of the calcification may not occur, leaving a visible, cortical-type bony lesion.

Acute Compartment Syndrome

A serious complication of a quadriceps contusion is the development of an acute compartment syndrome. Compartment syndrome is defined as increased tissue pressure in a closed facial compartment that compromises circulation to the nerves and muscles within that compartment. The condition often follows severe blunt trauma to the thigh, but it also may occur as a result of a crushing injury or fracture of the femur. It is considered to be a true surgical emergency and requires prompt clinical diagnosis and treatment.

Signs and Symptoms

The individual complains of a progressive, severe pain that occurs with passive motion and isometric contraction of the quadriceps. The individual is unwilling to flex the knee because of thigh pain. As pressure increases within the compartment, decreased femoral sensation and motor weakness may occur, although distal pulse and capillary refill may be normal.

Management

Ice should be applied to reduce swelling, and the individual should be immediately referred to a physician. Because motor function of the femoral nerve is difficult to assess in the presence of a large hematoma, diagnosis is based on measurements of compartment pressure as taken by a physician. Pressure readings of greater than 40 mm Hg usually indicate surgical intervention consisting of an anterior or anterolateral skin incision, fasciotomy, and evacuation of the hematoma. Untreated compartment syndrome can lead to muscle necrosis, fibrosis, scarring, and limb contractures, whereas nerve injury can result from either a direct blow or compartment compression (7).

In the assessment of the volleyball player, the painful movements that would confirm a suspected hip pointer include active trunk motion, especially lateral flexion to the opposite side and trunk rotation. In addition, because so many trunk and abdominal muscles attach to the iliac crest, pain can be elicited from coughing, laughing, and even breathing.

BURSITIS

Q *A 36-year-old woman is complaining of pain while running. Pain is located on the postero-lateral aspect of her hip near the grater trochanter and, occasionally, is accompanied by a snapping sensation. Further assessment suggests the individual has snapping hip syndrome. Describe a rehabilitation program for this condition*

Bursitis is common in runners and joggers and typically affects the greater trochanteric bursa, iliopsoas bursa (iliopectineal), and ischial bursa (Fig. 16.13). The most common mechanism is inflammation secondary to excessive friction or shear forces caused by overuse. A second mechanism is direct trauma, such as galling on the lateral hip.

Greater Trochanteric Bursitis

The greater trochanteric bursa lies between the greater trochanter and the gluteus maximus and tensor fascia latae (iliotibial tract). Inflammation of this bursa is seen more often in females because of their wider pelvis and larger Q-angle. It also is seen in runners who cross their feet over the midline as they run, thereby functionally increasing the Q-angle. Because streets are crowned to allow for runoff, individuals who typically run on streets are at increased susceptibility for irritating the greater trochanteric bursa. The down leg (i.e., the leg closest to the gutter) usually is affected.

Signs and Symptoms

Trochanteric bursitis is characterized by a burning or aching pain over or just posterior to the tip of the greater trochanter that intensifies with walking or exercise. The condition is aggravated by contraction of the hip abductors against resistance or during hip flexion and extension on weight bearing. Referred pain also may move distally into the lateral aspect of the thigh. If accompanied by a sudden, sharp pain that occurs during certain movements, it can be secondary to a snapping hip problem.

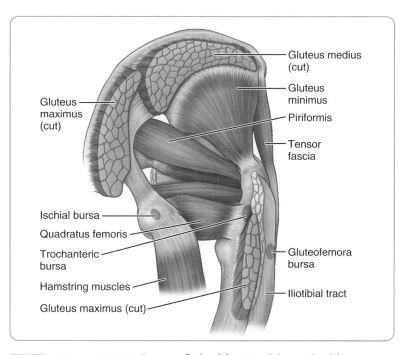

■■ ■■ **FIGURE 16.13 Bursa of the hip.** Bursitis at the hip may involve the trochanteric bursa, iliopsoas bursa, or ischial bursa.

Iliopsoas Bursitis

The iliopsoas bursa, which is the largest bursa in the body, can be irritated when the iliopsoas muscle repeatedly compresses the bursa against either the joint capsule of the hip or the lesser trochanter of the femur. Osteoarthritis of the hip also may lead to the condition.

Signs and Symptoms

Pain is felt more medial and anterior to the joint and cannot be easily palpated. When the knee is supported to relax the muscles, point tenderness may be elicited with the hip and knee flexed and the leg externally rotated. Passive rotary motions at the hip and resisted hip flexion, abduction, and external rotation also may produce increased pain. Iliopsoas bursitis may be associated with symptoms of a snapping hip syndrome as well.

Ischial Bursitis

Direct bruising from a fall can lead to compression of the ischial bursa. Often, however, the individual has a history of prolonged sitting, especially with the legs crossed or on a hard surface—hence the nickname "bench warmer's bursitis." Although it is relatively uncommon, it must be differentiated from a hamstring tear at the tendinous attachment or an epiphyseal fracture.

Signs and Symptoms

Pain is aggravated by prolonged sitting, uphill running, and even carrying a wallet in the back pocket. When the hip is flexed, point tenderness can be palpated directly over the ischial tuberosity. Pain increases with passive and resisted hip extension.

Management of Bursitis

Treatment for bursitis includes cryotherapy, deep friction massage, protected rest, NSAIDs, and a stretching program for the involved muscles. The use of ultrasound or interferential current also may be helpful. A postural examination and biomechanical analysis of the running motion performed by trained professionals can be used to determine if certain factors contributed to the individual's condition. Different shoes, orthotics, or alteration of the running technique may correct the problem and avoid recurrence. If the condition does not improve rapidly, a bone scan should be performed to rule out possible femoral neck stress fractures. Individuals who do not respond to conservative treatment may require local injections with anesthetics and cortisone, or surgery may be necessary.

Snapping Hip Syndrome

Chronic bursitis can lead to **snapping hip syndrome**, a condition very prevalent in dancers, runners, and cheerleaders that may develop secondary to a variety of both intra-articular and extra-articular causes (Box 16.1). The three types of the condition include:

- **External.** The most common cause is the iliotibial band or gluteus maximus snapping over the greater trochanter during hip flexion, leading to trochanteric bursitis.

- **Internal.** The iliopsoas snaps over structures deep to the musculotendinous unit, such as the iliopsoas bursa, pelvic pectineal eminence, femoral head, or lesser trochanter.

- **Intra-articular.** Lesions of the joint, such as a labral tear, can lead to the condition.

Signs and Symptoms

Snapping hip syndrome is characterized by a snapping sensation, rather than pain, that is either heard or felt during certain motions at the hip. It usually occurs when an individual laterally rotates and flexes the hip joint while balancing on one leg. If the iliopsoas bursa is affected, the individual may complain of snapping, chronic pain, or both in the femoral triangle of the medial groin.

Box 16.1   Causes of Snapping Hip Syndrome

Intra-Articular Causes
- Osteocartilaginous nodules occurring in the synovial membrane of the joint (synovial chondromatosis)
- Loose bodies
- Osteocartilaginous exostosis
- Subluxation of the hip
- Negative pressure in the joint capsule

Extra-Articular Causes
- Iliotibial band friction syndrome
- Snapping of the iliopsoas over the iliopectineal eminence on the medial aspect of the inferior ilium
- Snapping of the iliofemoral ligaments over the femoral head
- Snapping of the long head of the biceps femoris over the ischial tuberosity

Management

The condition usually is handled with limitation of hip motion, particularly limitation of extension by use of an elastic wrap. Ice and NSAIDs are used to relieve inflammation and pain. If associated with pain or a sense of hip joint instability, the individual should be referred to a physician. A rehabilitation program should address specific deficits, including muscle tightness, muscle imbalance, poor training techniques, or poor biomechanics of movement.

 A rehabilitation program for the 36-year-old female diagnosed with snapping hip syndrome should address specific deficits: muscle tightness, muscle imbalance, poor training techniques, or poor biomechanics of movement.

SPRAINS AND DISLOCATIONS

A van transporting a collegiate swim team to a meet was involved in a multivehicle accident. The van was struck in the rear and forced into the vehicle in front of it. The assistant coach, sitting in the front seat on the passenger's side, was thrown into the dashboard of the vehicle. He is experiencing severe pain, and the hip is slightly flexed and internally rotated. Explain management for this condition.

Hip joint sprains are rare, both because of the multitude of movements allowed at the ball-and-socket joint and because of the level of protection provided by layers of muscles that add to its stability. Injury can occur in violent, twisting actions or in catastrophic trauma when the knee strikes a stationary object, such as during an automobile accident when the knee is driven into the dashboard. Traumatic hip dislocations in children are rare but more common than femoral neck fractures. This may largely result from the pliable cartilage composition of the acetabulum during the early- to mid-teen years.

Signs and Symptoms

Symptoms of a mild or moderate hip sprain mimic those of synovitis, or stress fractures about the hip, and involve pain on hip rotation. Severe hip sprains and dislocations result in immediate intense pain and an inability to walk or even move the hip. The hip remains in a characteristic flexed and internally rotated position, indicating a posterosuperior dislocation (Fig. 16.14).

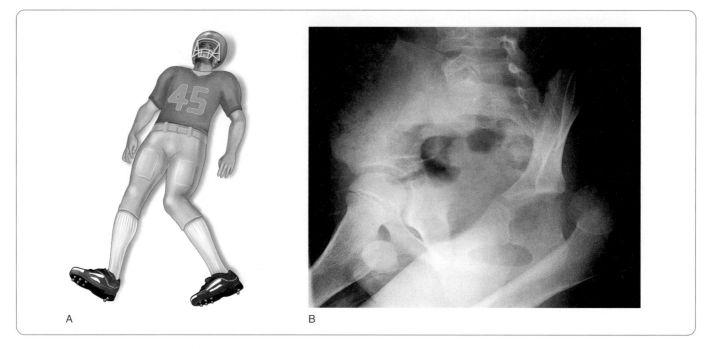

A   B

■■■■ FIGURE 16.14 **Hip dislocation.** Most hip dislocations drive the head of the femur posterior and superior, leaving the leg in a characteristically flexed and internally rotated position.

Management

Treatment for a mild to moderate sprain is symptomatic and may include cryotherapy, NSAIDs, rest, and protected weight bearing on crutches until walking is pain-free. Radiographs or bone scans usually are obtained to rule out degenerative joint disease, slipped femoral capital epiphysis, and femoral stress fractures.

The individual should not be moved until EMS arrives. With a fracture to the posterior rim of the acetabulum or head of the femur, movement could damage the blood supply to the head of the femur and cause avascular necrosis or further damage to surrounding soft-tissue structures. The vital signs should be monitored frequently and the individual treated for shock. Because the sciatic nerve may be damaged, nerve function should be assessed by determining if the individual has full or partial sensation.

EMS A hip dislocation is considered to be a medical emergency. As such, it requires activation of the emergency action plan, including summoning emergency medical services (EMS).

Ⓐ *Management of the hip injury sustained by the assistant coach requires activation of the emergency action plan, including summoning EMS. While waiting for EMS to arrive, the examiner should maintain the airway, assess vital signs, check for nerve and circulatory impairment at the lower leg and ankle, and treat for shock as necessary. The individual should not be moved until EMS arrives.*

STRAINS

Ⓠ *A first-base softball player stretches for an overthrown ball. During the stretch, the athlete feels a twinge in her left inner groin region. What painful movements would suggest an adductor strain?*

Muscular strains of the hip and thigh muscles frequently are seen not only in sport but in many occupations involving repetitive motions. Strains may range from mild to severe, with the severity of symptoms paralleling the amount of disruption to the fibers.

Quadriceps Strain

Quadriceps strains are less common than hamstring strains. An explosive muscular contraction of the rectus femoris can lead to an avulsion fracture at the proximal attachment on the AIIS, but tears more commonly occur in the midsubstance of the muscle belly. Because the rectus femoris is the most superficial muscle of the quadriceps, any disruption in its continuity is easily visible. The vastus lateralis and vastus medialis are more rarely injured, but when an injury does occur, it usually involves the mid to upper third of the muscle belly.

Signs and Symptoms

In a grade I injury, the individual complains of tightness in the anterior thigh, but gait is normal. No swelling or pain can be palpated, although passive knee flexion beyond 90° may be painful. In a grade II injury, the individual reports a snapping or tearing sensation during an explosive jumping, kicking, or running motion, followed by immediate pain and loss of function. The knee may be held in extension as a means for protecting the injured area. Assessment reveals tenderness, swelling, a palpable defect if continuity is disrupted, discoloration, pain on passive knee flexion between 45 and 90°, and pain and weakness during resisted knee extension. Grade III strains are extremely painful, and ambulation is not possible. Palpation reveals an obvious defect in the muscle. Resisted knee extension is not possible, and ROM is severely limited. An isometric contraction may reveal a muscle bulge or defect in the quadriceps muscles, especially the rectus femoris of the thigh. Box 16.2 lists the signs and symptoms of a quadriceps strain.

Hamstrings Strains

During the initial swing phase of gait, the hamstrings act to flex the knee. In the late swing, the hamstrings contract eccentrically to decelerate knee extension and re-extend the hip in preparation for the stance phase. The hamstrings are the most frequently strained muscles in the body, and these strains typically are caused by a rapid contraction of the muscle during a ballistic action or a violent stretch. Several factors can increase the risk of injury, including:

- Poor flexibility
- Poor posture
- Muscle imbalance
- Improper warm-up
- Muscle fatigue
- Lack of neuromuscular control
- Previous injury
- Overuse
- Improper technique

Box 16.2   Signs and Symptoms of a Quadriceps Strain

- Snapping or tearing sensation at the anterior inferior iliac spine or at midthigh during an explosive movement
- Increased pain or weakness elicited during:
  - Passive knee flexion
    - Grade I: >90° is painful
    - Grade II: Limited to 45–90°
    - Grade III: Limited to <45°
  - Active knee extension with a flexed hip
  - Resisted knee extension
- Isolated rectus femoris strain produces increased pain and weakness during:
  - Passive knee flexion and hip extension
  - Active knee extension and hip flexion
  - Resisted hip flexion with the knee flexed at 45°

Box 16.3 Signs and Symptoms of a Hamstrings Strain

- History of poor posture, inflexibility, and muscle imbalance
- Injury often occurs when muscle function suddenly changes from a stabilizing knee flexor to an active hip extensor, as occurs in sprinting, and may occur midstride
- Sharp pain in the posterior thigh
- Increased pain or weakness during:
  - Passive knee extension
  - Passive hip flexion
  - Active knee flexion
  - Active hip extension with an extended knee
  - Resisted knee flexion:
    - Medial hamstrings—tibia internally rotated
    - Lateral hamstrings—tibia externally rotated
  - Resisted hip extension with an extended knee

Signs and Symptoms

In mild strains, the individual complains of tightness and tension in the muscle. Passive stretching of the hamstrings may be painful. In second- and third-degree strains, the individual may report a tearing sensation or feeling a "pop," leading to immediate pain and weakness in knee flexion. In more severe cases, a sharp pain in the posterior thigh may occur during midstride. The individual limps and is unable to do a heel-strike or to fully extend the knee. Pain and muscle weakness are elicited during active knee flexion. If assessed early enough, a noticeable defect in the muscle belly may be palpated. Frequently, profuse swelling and ecchymosis become visible in the popliteal fossa 1 to 2 days after injury. Although rare, total rupture of the ischial origin can result from a sudden, forceful flexion of the hip joint when the knee is extended and the hamstring muscles contract powerfully. Box 16.3 lists the signs and symptoms of a hamstrings strain.

A hamstrings strain has a reputation of being both chronic and recurring. Rehabilitation should focus on regaining flexibility and strengthening the muscles. It is important to maintain an appropriate strength balance between the quadriceps and hamstrings.

Adductor (Groin) Strain

Adductor strains are common in activities that require quick changes of direction as well as explosive propulsion and acceleration. A strength imbalance between the hip abductors and adductors may be a predisposing factor in many of these injuries. The more severe strains typically occur at the proximal attachment of the muscle on the hip, particularly the adductor longus. Milder strains tend to occur more distally, at the musculotendinous junction.

Signs and Symptoms

The individual often experiences an initial "twinge" or "pull" of the groin muscles and is unable to walk because of the intense, sharp pain. As the condition worsens, increased pain, stiffness, and weakness in hip adduction and flexion become apparent. Running straight ahead or backward may be tolerable, but any side-to-side movement leads to more discomfort and pain. Localized tenderness can be palpated on the ischiopubic ramus, lesser trochanter, or musculotendinous junction. Increased pain is felt during passive stretching with the hip extended, abducted, and externally rotated and with resisted hip adduction. Occasionally, a palpable defect may be found, indicating a more serious injury.

Gluteal Muscles

Because of their size and strength, the gluteal muscles rarely are injured except in activities that require muscle overload, such as power weight lifting and rowing. Signs and symptoms are similar to those of other muscular strains and include:

- History of muscle overload or repetitive muscular contractions, as occurs in weight lifting or rowing

- Increased pain or weakness during:
  - Passive hip flexion with the knee flexed
  - Active hip extension with the knee flexed
  - Resisted hip extension with the knee flexed

Piriformis Syndrome

The sciatic nerve passes through the sciatic notch beneath the piriformis muscle to travel into the posterior thigh (see Fig. 16.9). In approximately 10 to 15% of the population, the nerve passes through or above the muscle, subjecting the nerve to compression from trauma, hemorrhage, or spasm of the piriformis muscle. More commonly, the peroneal portion of the nerve is compressed. The incidence of piriformis syndrome has been reported to be sixfold more prevalent in women than in men (8). A history of prolonged sitting, stair climbing, repetitive squatting and rising, recent increase in activity, or buttock trauma may be reported. Resulting symptoms may mimic those of a herniated lumbar disk with nerve root impingement. With a herniated disk, pain usually is increased on coughing, sneezing, or straining during defecation, indicating epidural involvement; such pain is not noted in a piriformis syndrome.

Signs and Symptoms

Low back pain is not usual, although the individual may complain of a dull ache in the midbuttock region; pain that worsens at night. particularly when turning from one side to the other in bed; difficulty walking up stairs or on an incline; and weakness or numbness extending down the back of the leg. Assessment reveals point tenderness in the midbuttock region over the greater sciatic notch. Increased pain and weakness on active hip external rotation, passive hip flexion, adduction, and internal rotation, and resisted hip external rotation are present. The individual may stand with the leg in slight external rotation. Pain can be elicited with the individual supine and the hip flexed, adducted, and internally rotated (i.e., reverse Patrick's test), because this stretches the piriformis muscle. Straight leg raising may be limited.

Management of Strains

Treatment for muscular strains involves immediate ice, compression, elevation, and protected rest. Whenever possible, the injured muscles should be iced in a stretched position. If the individual cannot walk with a normal gait, crutches should be used. With severe strains, a compression wrap may be indicated from the toe to the groin to prevent venous thrombosis and distal edema. Nonsteroidal anti-inflammatory drugs typically are used for the first 7 to 10 days.

   If the condition does not improve within 2 to 5 days, referral to a physician is necessary to rule out other underlying conditions. Nontraumatic diagnostic possibilities can include an avulsion fracture, osteitis pubis, myositis ossificans, hip joint disease, nerve entrapment, hernia-related conditions, urologic disorders, and gynecologic problems.

   When the acute inflammatory phase has progressed to resolution of the hematoma, pain-free gentle stretching and isometric contractions can be initiated in conjunction with cryotherapy and electrical modalities. Compression shorts can provide symptomatic relief and expedite return to activity. If compression shorts are not available, a hip spica wrap or compressive wrap can provide both warmth and support. Active stretching, progressive resistance exercises, soft-tissue mobilization, as well as swimming, cycling, mild jogging, and stair climbing can begin when the region is pain-free and ROM is within 10° of the uninvolved limb. Several stretching and strengthening exercises are discussed in Field Strategy 16.1; other exercises for muscles crossing the knee joint can be seen in Field Strategy 17.1. When jogging is comfortable, skipping and rope jumping may be initiated. Rapid stops, starts, and changes in direction are not allowed until the individual can achieve full, pain-free motion. The individual should not return to activity until normal muscular strength and power are achieved.

The softball player suspected of having an adductor strain would experience pain with the following movements: sliding sideways (no pain with running straight ahead or backward), passive hip abduction, active hip adduction, and resisted hip adduction.

VASCULAR AND NEURAL DISORDERS

A 12-year-old soccer player is seen limping after a game. When asked about a possible injury, he reports that his groin and knee have hurt since the start of the season, nearly 10 weeks ago. When the parents were questioned about the pain, they reported that the pain comes and goes. They have been having the child ice the hip and stretch the groin muscles but have not thought the situation was serious enough to see a physician. What recommendations are appropriate?

Vascular disorders should be suspected in any lower extremity injury caused by a high-velocity, low-mass projectile and in an injury for which no physical findings support the continued discomfort. If an acute circulatory problem exists, the lower leg and foot may appear to be pale or cyanotic, be cool to the touch, or have diminished or totally absent pulse. In these cases, immobilization of the limb and transportation to the nearest medical center is warranted. Other vascular problems are more insidious but can be just as serious. Neural entrapment is very rare in the hip region, particularly as a result of sport participation.

FIGURE 16.15 Osteochondrosis of the left femoral head (Legg-Calvé-Perthes disease). This picture demonstrates the destruction of articular cartilage.

Legg-Calvé-Perthes Disease

Legg-Calvé-Perthes disease, or avascular necrosis of the capital femoral epiphysis, is a noninflammatory, self-limiting disorder of the hip seen in young children, especially males, between the ages of 3 and 8 years (8). It is considered to be an osteochondrosis condition of the femoral head caused by diminished blood supply to the capital region of the femur. This leads to a progressive necrosis of the bone and marrow of the epiphysis of the femoral head (Fig. 16.15). The natural history of the condition occurs in the following stages:

1. Edema develops at the synovial membrane and capsule over 1 to 6 weeks.

2. Necrosis of the femoral epiphysis occurs, lasting from several months to 1 year.

3. Regeneration/resorption lasts 1 to 3 years. Granulation tissue invades necrotic bone, leaving isolated areas of bone sequestered. Connective tissues invade the area, leading to resorption and replacement by new immature bone, which results in a weakened subchondral support system.

4. Repair occurs when new, normal bone replaces dead bone. Outcome is related to the percentage of epiphysis involved, age of the patient, and promptness of diagnosis.

Signs and Symptoms

The most common complaint is a gradual onset of a limp and mild hip or knee pain of several months' duration. The pain most often is referred to the groin region, but up to 15% of patients report knee pain as the primary symptom (8). Pain generally is related to activity, which often contributes to delayed recognition. Examination reveals a decreased ROM in hip abduction, extension, and external rotation caused by muscle spasm in the hip flexors and adductors.

Management

This condition should be suspected in young children when pain in the groin, anterior thigh, or knee region cannot be explained. If pain persists for more than 1 week after initial acute care or the individual continues to limp after activity, immediate referral to a physician is needed to rule out nontraumatic causes of the pain that have similar signs and symptoms. Possibilities include a slipped capital femoral epiphysis, septic arthritis, transient synovitis, juvenile rheumatoid arthritis, or bone tumor. Confirmation of the condition is made through radiographs, bone scans, or magnetic resonance images.

Treatment depends on the extent of the disease and the philosophy of the supervising physician. Nonoperative treatment may involve several different progressive protocols, including:

- Therapy to improve hip ROM
- Non–weight bearing in a brace
- Weight bearing in a brace that limits hip motion
- Weight bearing in a brace that allows free movement

Treatment can be quite extensive, sometimes taking 1 to 2 years. It may involve immobilization, non–weight bearing, and possible surgery to prevent any further deformity of the femoral head caused by the avascular necrosis.

Venous Disorders

A direct blow from a baseball, softball, puck, or helmet may damage a vein, causing thrombophlebitis or phlebothrombosis. **Thrombophlebitis** is an acute inflammation of a vein; **phlebothrombosis** is a thrombosis, or clotting, in a vein without overt inflammatory signs and symptoms. Plebothrombosis is discussed in more detail in Chapter 18. Superficial thrombophlebitis is the preferred term for inflammation of superficial veins, and term deep venous thrombosis (DVT) is preferred term for problems with deep veins. Superficial thrombophlebitis tends to be more painful than DVT and almost always is associated with varicose veins. Other predisposing factors include obesity, smoking, surgery, hospitalization, cancer, and trauma. An increased incidence of complications from the condition are seen among individuals who are older than 60 years, are male, have a history of DVT or prolonged bed rest, have bilateral superficial thrombophlebitis, and have infection in the involved leg (9).

Signs and Symptoms

Superficial thrombophlebitis may present itself as acute, red, hot, palpable, tender cord in the course of a superficial vein. Extension of superficial thrombophlebitis to the deep venous system occurs through the proximal long and short saphenous veins to the common femoral and popliteal veins, respectively, and through the perforating veins. The most reliable signs are chronic swelling and edema in the involved extremity and a positive Homans' sign (see Fig. 18.35).

Management

Treatment may involve a variety of actions, including anticoagulant therapy; external support with compression stockings or elastic bandages; ambulation and lower extremity exercises, particularly with hydrotherapy; periodic elevation of the extremity; and avoidance of long-term sitting or standing in one position.

Toxic Synovitis

An infrequent condition that occurs largely in children is **toxic synovitis** of the hip.

Signs and Symptoms

The transient inflammatory condition is characterized by a painful hip joint accompanied with an antalgic gait and limp.

Management

Early referral to a physician is necessary to rule out septic arthritis of the hip and other more serious conditions that may require surgery to drain the septic joint, relieve pressure, and preserve blood supply to the femoral head. Rest is the key to treatment, along with appropriate medication and traction for prompt resolution.

Obturator Nerve Entrapment

The obturator nerve is derived from the anterior portion of the lumbar plexus (L_2–L_4). It innervates the adductor brevis, longus, and magnus; the obturator externus; and the gracilis as well as provides sensory innervation for the hip joint and the distal, medial thigh. A fascial entrapment of the obturator nerve may occur where it enters the thigh as a result of pelvic tumors, obturator hernias, or pelvic and proximal femoral fractures.

Signs and Symptoms

A characteristic clinical pattern of exercise-induced, medial thigh pain presents from the adductor muscle origin distally along the medial thigh. This pain may be described as vague groin or medial knee pain.

Management

With no abnormal findings during special stress tests for the hip and knee region, an individual who reports vague groin or medial knee pain should be referred to a physician. If the obturator nerve is entrapped, surgical intervention is necessary. Return to activity usually occurs within several weeks of treatment.

The soccer player's symptoms have been present for more than 10 weeks, and icing and stretching of the groin muscles have not improved the injury. Because of the age of the athlete, the vague groin and knee pain, and the length of time for the disability, which has now resulted in a noticeable limp, you should recommend that the child see a physician immediately. He may have Legg-Calvé-Perthes disease or another degenerative condition involving the hip joint.

HIP FRACTURES

A rugby player is down on the field after receiving a severe blow to the anterior right thigh. The thigh is externally rotated and severely angulated, and the involved limb appears to be shorter than the uninvolved limb. The athlete is in severe pain. What injury should be expected? Explain and demonstrate management for this injury.

Major fractures of the pelvic girdle and hip often result from severe direct trauma. In some sports (e.g., football and ice hockey), the pelvic region usually is adequately protected by padding to prevent such injuries. Fractures that may be sustained in this region include avulsion and apophyseal fractures, epiphyseal fractures, and stress fractures.

Avulsion Fractures

Individuals who perform moves involving rapid, sudden acceleration and deceleration are at risk for the following avulsion fractures:

- The ASIS with the displacement of the sartorius
- The AIIS with displacement of the rectus femoris

- The ischial tuberosity with displacement of the hamstrings
- The lesser trochanter with displacement of the iliopsoas

Many of these apophyseal sites do not unite with the bone until 18 to 25 years of age and, as such, continue to be prone to fracture.

Signs and Symptoms

The individual complains of sudden, acute, localized pain that may radiate down the muscle. Examination reveals severe pain, swelling, and discoloration directly over the tendinous attachment on the bony landmark. In a completely displaced avulsion fracture, a gap may be palpated between the tendon's attachment and the bone. Pain increases with passive stretching of the involved muscle, active ROM, and resisted ROM.

Management

Depending on the fracture site, immobilization from an elastic compression spica wrap may limit motion and decrease pain. The individual should be fitted with crutches and referred immediately to a physician for radiography. Ice, rest, modified activity, and protected weight bearing with crutches for 4 to 6 weeks should provide adequate healing for an undisplaced fracture. Range-of-motion exercises should be discouraged until the fracture has healed, but isometric exercises can be performed if pain-free. When healing is complete, restoration of ROM and strength should be initiated, with gradual return to activity. If the individual is returned to vigorous activity too soon, a bony prominence may form at the site of the avulsion.

Slipped Capital Femoral Epiphysis

The capital femoral epiphysis is the growth plate at the femoral head. A fracture to this area, sometimes referred to as adolescent coxa vara, is seen in adolescent boys from 12 to 15 years of age. In particular, the condition commonly is seen in obese adolescents with underdeveloped sexual characteristics and, occasionally, in rapidly growing, slender boys. In a slipped capital femoral epiphysis, the femoral head slips at the epiphyseal plate and displaces inferiorly and posteriorly relative to the femoral neck (Fig. 16.16). As the proximal femoral growth plate deteriorates, the individual begins to develop a painful limp with groin pain. Pain also may be referred to the anterior thigh or knee region. The condition may lead to synovitis of the hip and an accompanying psoas major spasm.

Signs and Symptoms

Early signs and symptoms may go undetected. Frequently, the only complaint is diffuse knee pain. During later stages, the individual feels more comfortable holding the leg in slight flexion. The individual is unable to touch the abdomen with the thigh, because the hip externally rotates with flexion. The individual also is unable to rotate the femur internally or to stand on one leg. If the obturator nerve is damaged during the fracture, an aching pain may be referred to the groin, medial thigh, or knee.

Management

The individual should be fitted with crutches and referred to a physician for further assessment. Radiographs of the hip are necessary to confirm the condition and to rule out other possible conditions, such as tumors, bone cysts, and underlying osteochondromas. Prognosis is good with early detection, although those with more severe slips likely have residual deformity and progressive disability. Surgery is indicated in nearly all cases.

■■■■■ FIGURE 16.16 **Slipped capital femoral epiphysis.** An epiphyseal fracture, seen in adolescents from 12 to 15 years of age, occurs through the growth plate at the femoral head. An individual who sustains this fracture will not be able to rotate the femur internally.

Stress Fractures

Stress fractures of the pubis, femoral neck, and proximal third of the femur are seen in individuals who engage in extensive jogging or aerobic dance activities to the point of muscle fatigue. Several factors can increase the risk of sustaining a stress fracture, including:

- Sudden increase in training (mileage, intensity, or frequency)
- Change in running surface or terrain
- Improper footwear
- Biomechanical abnormalities
- Nutritional and hormonal factors (anorexia, amenorrhea, or osteopenia)

Signs and Symptoms

Signs and symptoms usually involve a diffuse or localized, aching pain in the anterior groin or thigh region during weight-bearing activity that is relieved with rest. Night pain is a frequent complaint. An antalgic gait may be present. Deep palpation in the inguinal area will produce discomfort. Diffuse or localized swelling also may be present. Increased pain on the extremes of hip rotation, an abduction lurch, and an inability to stand on the involved leg (i.e., positive Trendelenburg sign or "one-legged hop" test) may indicate a femoral neck stress fracture.

Management

Referral to a physician is necessary. Bone scans or magnetic resonance images frequently are used for early diagnosis. If the diagnosis is established early enough, rest is indicated for at least 1 to 4 weeks, with no weight-bearing activity until the fracture is completely healed. Stress fractures of the ischium and pubis may require 2 to 3 months of rest. Biking and swimming can help the individual to maintain cardiovascular fitness; however, during swimming, the whip kick and scissors kick should be avoided. Displaced stress fractures of the femoral neck require surgical pin fixation to prevent a complete fracture and avascular necrosis of the femoral head.

Osteitis Pubis

Osteitis pubis is an inflammatory process involving continued stress on the pubic symphysis from repeated overload of the adductor muscles or repetitive running activities.

Signs and Symptoms

The most common complaint is a gradual onset of pain in the adductor musculature, which is aggravated by kicking, running, and pivoting on one leg. Sit-ups and abdominal muscular strengthening exercises will increase pain in the lower abdominal muscles and over the pubic symphysis. Pain also may radiate distally into the groin or medial thigh.

Management

Treatment is symptomatic with ice, protected rest, and NSAIDs until the condition is resolved. Prolonged rest extending over 2 to 3 months, however, may be necessary to alleviate symptoms. Hydrotherapy exercises may help in rehabilitation. Use of a stationary bike and light jogging may be added as tolerated.

Displaced and Nondisplaced Pelvic Fractures

Major fractures of the pelvis seldom occur in sport participation except in activities such as equestrian sports, ice hockey, rugby, skiing, and football. Three distinct mechanisms are involved in traumatic pelvic fractures:

1. Avulsion or traction injury of the bony origin or attachment of muscle
2. Direct compression, with disruption of the pelvic osseous ring
3. Direct blow to the pelvis

Because the pelvis is a closed ring, an injury to one location in the pelvis can cause a countrecoup fracture or sprain on the other side of the pelvic ring. For example, if the superior and inferior pubic rami are fractured on the right side, the left side often has an SI disruption.

Signs and Symptoms

This crushing injury produces severe pain, total loss of function, and in many cases, severe loss of blood, leading to hypovolemic shock. The extent of blood loss is unknown, because hemorrhage within the pelvic cavity is not visible. In addition, possible internal injuries to the genitourinary system, such as rupture of the bladder or laceration of the urethra, also may occur. In dramatic, severe fractures, this internal damage and subsequent shock can lead to death. A fracture to the pelvis can be assessed by applying slight compression to the sides of the ilium and the ASIS. Fractures of the acetabulum can be detected by placing gentle, upward pressure on the femur against the acetabulum.

Management

If a fracture is suspected, the emergency action plan, including summoning EMS, should be activated. While waiting for EMS to arrive, the examiner should assess vital signs and treat for shock as necessary.

Sacral and Coccygeal Fractures

Fractures of the sacrum and coccyx rarely occur in sports. They typically are caused by a direct blow onto the sacrococcygeal area subsequent to a fall on the buttock region.

Signs and Symptoms

Direct impact leads to an extremely painful injury. Subsequent to pain, the individual is unable to sit.

Management

The individual should be referred immediately to a physician. These fractures usually heal within 6 weeks and without any functional impairment, but clinically healed fractures often show evidence of fibrous union. In rare cases, coccygodynia, or persistent severe pain, can occur. This condition is very difficult to treat because of the rich complex of pain nociceptors in the area. Return to activity should only be restricted if pain interferes with the activity.

Femoral Fractures

Fractures of the femoral shaft can be very serious because of potential damage to the neurovascular structures from bony fragments. Femoral shaft fractures are caused by tremendous impact forces, such as shearing or torsion forces when an alpine skier falls, or from direct compressive forces, such as tackles in football, ice hockey, or rugby. Fractures may be open or closed, but in either case, significant bleeding occurs at the fracture site. Signs and symptoms indicating a femoral fracture are listed in Box 16.4.

Management

It is not unusual for significant bleeding in the thigh to lead to hypovolemic shock, similar to that seen in pelvic fractures. Vascular damage may lead to impaired circulation distal to the injury, causing a pale, cold, pulseless foot. Distal neurovascular function should be assessed immediately and monitored frequently; this can be performed by palpating a pulse at the posterior tibial artery and dorsalis pedis artery, looking for pale skin at the foot, and feeling for cool skin temperature. Sensation testing can be performed by stroking the dorsum and plantar aspect of both feet.

If a fracture is suspected, the emergency action plan, including summoning EMS, should be activated. This type of fracture is best immobilized in a traction splint, which should be applied only by trained personnel. While waiting for EMS to arrive, the examiner should assess vital signs and treat for shock as necessary. Any external bleeding should be covered with a dry, sterile dressing to protect the area from further contamination.

Box 16.4   Signs and Symptoms of Femoral Fractures

Displaced Fracture
- Shortened limb deformity
- Severe angulation with the thigh externally rotated
- Swelling into the soft tissues
- Severe pain
- Total loss of function
- Loss of, or change in, distal neurovascular functions

Nondisplaced Fractures
- Extreme pain on palpation
- Crepitation
- Muscle weakness
- Muscle spasm
- Swelling into the soft tissues

Table 16.3 summarizes signs and symptoms of the various fractures seen in the pelvis and thigh region.

> *The rugby player has signs and symptoms that suggest a fracture of the femoral shaft. The emergency action plan, including summoning EMS, should be activated. This fracture is best immobilized in a traction splint, which should be applied by trained personnel. While waiting for EMS to arrive, the examiner should maintain the airway, assess vital signs, check for nerve and circulatory impairment at the lower leg and ankle, and treat for shock as necessary.*

TABLE 16.3   Fractures and Associated Signs and Symptoms

FRACTURE	COMMON SITES	SIGNS AND SYMPTOMS
Avulsion and apophyseal	Anterior superior iliac spines Anterior inferior iliac spine Ischial tuberosity Lesser trochanter	Severe pain and tenderness over bony landmark. Increased pain with active motion of involved muscle
Epiphyseal	Capital femoral epiphysis	Unable to internally rotate the thigh Possible pain in groin, medial thigh, or knee
Stress	Pubis Femoral neck Proximal third of femur	May have point tenderness over fracture site Pain is worse before and after activity and is relieved with rest Possible limp as the fracture progresses
Pelvic girdle	Wing of ilium or acetabulum	Severe pain over fracture site Total loss of function Positive fracture tests Show signs of shock
Femoral	Shaft of femur or femoral neck	Severe angulation with thigh externally rotated Shortened limb; swelling into soft tissue Severe pain and crepitation at fracture site Total loss of function and signs of shock Positive fracture tests Vascular damage may lead to pale, cold, pulseless foot

ASSESSMENT OF PELVIC, HIP, AND THIGH CONDITIONS

Q ► *A high school basketball player reports to the athletic training room complaining of discomfort in the anterior thigh for the past 2 weeks. How should the assessment of this player progress to determine the extent and severity of injury?*

The lower extremity works as a unit to transmit load from the upper body to the ground through a closed kinetic chain. In the closed chain, the foot, ankle, leg, and hip also absorb force from the ground and dissipate the stress throughout the various structures. When excessive loads and stress exceed the yield points of a tissue, an injury occurs. Furthermore, the hip is a common site for referred pain from visceral, low back, and knee conditions. Evaluations therefore must be inclusive, particularly with adolescents who are complaining of groin pain. In the absence of direct trauma to the hip, or when improvement is not seen in 2 to 5 days, always refer the individual to a physician to rule out serious underlying conditions.

See *Field Strategy: Hip Evaluation,* available on the companion website at thePoint.

HISTORY

Q ► *The injury assessment of the basketball player should begin with a history. What questions need to be asked to identify the cause and extent of this injury?*

Many conditions at the hip may be related to family history, age, congenital deformity, improper biomechanical execution of skills, and recent changes in training programs, surfaces, or foot attire. The examiner should gather information regarding the mechanism of injury, associated symptoms, progression of symptoms, any disabilities that may have resulted from the injury, and related medical history. For example, deep groin pain may originate in the hip joint itself or be referred from the lumbar spine or SI joint, and Box 16.5 lists other conditions that can cause groin pain. Sacroiliac pathology almost always manifests itself with pain over the PSIS of the affected side. Trochanteric bursitis usually presents with pain in the posterior aspect of the greater trochanter.

See *Field Strategy: Developing a History of the Injury,* available on the companion website at thePoint, for specific questions related to the pelvis, hip, and thigh region.

A ► *The high school basketball player should be asked questions that address when, where, and how the injury occurred; intensity, location, and type of pain; when the pain begins (e.g., when you get out of bed, while sitting, while walking, during exercise, or at night); how long the condition has been present; how long the pain lasts; if the pain has changed or stayed the same; if the pain is worse before, during, or after activity; activities that aggravate or alleviate the symptoms; as well as previous injury, treatment, and medication.*

Box 16.5 Conditions that Can Cause Groin Pain

- Referred pain from the bowel, bladder, testicle, kidney, abdomen, rectum, hip joint, sacroiliac joint, pubic symphysis, lymph nodes, or rectus abdominis muscle
- Apophysitis, stress fracture, or avulsion fracture
- Osteitis pubis
- Toxic synovitis of the hip
- Testicular torsion or rupture
- Testicular cancer and other neoplasms

- Ovarian cysts
- Pelvic inflammatory disease
- Urinary tract infections
- Avascular necrosis of the femoral head, or slipped capital femoral epiphysis
- Lymphadenopathy
- Hernia
- Osteoarthritis

OBSERVATION AND INSPECTION

Q ▶ *The basketball player reports having sustained a severe blow to the right anterior thigh 2 weeks earlier. He did not report the injury when it occurred. During today's practice, he received a mild blow to the same area. He complains of discomfort after the initial injury that became progressively worse. In particular, he reports pain and weakness during activity. Explain the observation component in the ongoing assessment of the basketball player.*

In the examination room, the individual should wear shorts to allow full view of the lower extremity. This may not be possible during an on-field or on-site examination, however, because protective equipment or the uniform may obstruct the view. In these cases, determination of the condition may rest more heavily on palpation and stress tests. If the individual is nonambulatory, it is important to complete all observations, inspection, and palpation for possible fractures and dislocations before moving the individual.

In general, observation should include a full postural assessment and gait analysis. The individual should be viewed from anterior, lateral, and posterior positions, and the position of the ilium relative to the SI joint should be noted (Fig. 16.17). If contranutation occurs at the SI joint, it indicates anterior torsion of the joint or posterior rotation of the sacrum on the ilium on one side; the limb on that side probably is medially rotated. Contranutation occurs when, on one side, the ASIS is lower and the PSIS is higher. As a result, the iliac bones move apart, and the ischial tuberosities approximate. **Contranutation** is limited by the posterior SI ligaments; **nutation** is the backward rotation of the ilium on the sacrum. If nutation occurs on only one side, the ASIS is higher and the PSIS is lower on that side. The iliac innominate bones move together, and the ischial tuberosities move apart, resulting in an apparent or functional short leg on the same side. Nutation is limited by the anterior SI ligaments, the sacrospinous ligament, and the sacrotuberous ligament. Nutation occurs when a person assumes a pelvic tilt position; contranutation occurs when a person assumes a lordotic or anterior pelvic tilt position.

See *Field Strategy: Postural Assessment of the Hip Region,* found on the companion website at thePoint, for specific areas on which to focus in this region.

The symmetry in the region should be observed, noting any visible congenital deformity, such as excessive femoral torsion, abnormal positioning of the patella, toeing in, or toeing out. An increase in the angle of torsion greater than 15° (i.e., anteversion) is evidence of external femoral rotation characterized by a toe-out gait. When the angle is decreased (i.e., retroversion), the femur internally rotates, causing a toe-in position of the feet. An increase in the angle of inclination (i.e., coxa valga), may be visible through either **genu varum** or laterally positioned patellae. Decreases in this angle (i.e., coxa vara) may be visible with **genu valgum** or medially positioned, "squinting" patellae.

Following the completion of a static examination, the examiner should observe the individual walking. This observation should include an anterior, posterior, and lateral view, noting any abnormalities in gait and determining if any actions cause pain or discomfort. With an abnormal gait, it is important to determine the onset of the limp, if the limp is constant or intermittent, and the activities that make the condition better or worse.

The specific site of injury should be inspected for obvious deformities, discoloration, edema, scars that might indicate previous surgery, and general condition of the skin.

A ▶ *Observation of the basketball player should include a full postural assessment and gait analysis. The specific site of injury should be inspected for obvious deformities, discoloration, edema, scars that might indicate previous surgery, and general condition of the skin.*

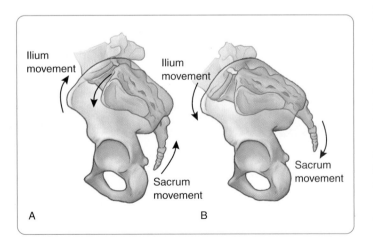

FIGURE 16.17 Abnormal pelvic tilt. Movements of nutation **(A)** and contranutation **(B)** occurring at the sacroiliac joint.

PALPATION

 Observation of the basketball player reveals a swollen thigh (i.e., 3 cm larger than the uninvolved thigh). Explain palpation specific to the injury sustained by the basketball player.

Bilateral palpation can determine temperature, swelling, point tenderness, crepitus, deformity, muscle spasm, and cutaneous sensation. Vascular pulses can be taken at the femoral artery in the groin, popliteal artery in the posterior knee, and posterior tibial artery and dorsalis pedis artery in the foot.

Pain during palpation of bony structures may indicate a displaced avulsion fracture or a femoral shaft fracture. Compression, distraction, percussion, or use of a tuning fork on specific bony landmarks also may be used to determine a possible fracture. For example, to determine a possible fracture to the acetabulum or to the femoral neck or head, a slow, compressive force is applied to the hip through the longitudinal axis of the femur by pushing through the femoral condyles (Fig. 16.18). A possible pelvic fracture can be determined with the SI compression and distraction test (see Fig. 16.21).

■■ ■ FIGURE 16.18 **Axial compression of the femur.** Increased pain with gentle compression along the long axis of the femur indicates a possible fracture of the femur or acetabulum.

During palpation, the individual should be non–weight bearing, preferably on a table. When the individual is prone on the table, a pillow should be placed under the hip and abdominal area to reduce strain on the low back region. Palpation should proceed proximal to distal, but the area anticipated to be the most painful should be palpated last. The following structures should be palpated:

Anterior Palpation

1. Iliac crest, ASIS, tensor fascia latae, and sartorius

2. Inguinal ligament, lymph nodes, pubic symphysis, greater trochanter, trochanteric bursa, and abductors (i.e., gluteus medius and gluteus minimus)

3. Femoral triangle, femoral artery, iliopsoas bursa, and flexor and adductor muscles (i.e., pectineus, adductor brevis, adductor longus, adductor magnus, and gracilis)

4. Quadriceps muscles (i.e., vastus lateralis, rectus femoris, vastus medialis, and vastus intermedius)

Posterior Palpation

1. Iliac crest and PSIS

2. Ischial tuberosity, ischial bursa, hamstring muscles (i.e., biceps femoris is lateral, and semi-tendinosus and semimembranosus are medial), and greater trochanter

3. SI, lumbosacral, and sacrococcygeal joints

 Bilateral palpation should include point tenderness, swelling, muscle spasms, deformity, hardness or a firm mass, and skin temperature.

PHYSICAL EXAMINATION TESTS

Palpation of the basketball player revealed a warm, firm, swollen thigh. A palpable mass was not detected. What physical examination findings would suggest that the individual has myositis ossificans?

The individual should be placed in a comfortable position for the physical examination. Depending on the history, some tests are compulsory, whereas others may be used to confirm or exclude suspected injury or pathology. Caution should be used while moving through the assessment, and bilateral comparison should always be performed.

Functional Tests

The examiner should determine the available ROM in hip flexion-extension, hip abduction-adduction, hip internal/external rotation, and knee flexion-extension. Bilateral comparison is critical to determine normal or abnormal movement.

Active Movements

Active movements can be performed in a seated or prone position. Active movements that are anticipated to be painful should be performed last to prevent painful symptoms from overflowing into the next movement.

The motions that should be assessed, and the normal ROM for each, are as follows:

- Knee extension (0–15°)
- Lateral rotation (40–60°)
- Medial rotation (30–40°)
- Hip flexion (110–120°) with knee flexed
- Abduction (30–50°)
- Adduction (30°)
- Knee flexion (0–135°)
- Hip extension (10–15°)

Measuring ROM at the hip with a goniometer is demonstrated in Fig. 16.19.

Passive Range of Motion

If the individual is able to perform full ROM during active movements, gentle pressure is applied at the extremes of motion to determine end feel. The end feel for hip flexion and adduction is tissue approximation; the end feel for hip extension, abduction, and medial and lateral rotation is tissue stretch. When testing passive movement, the aim is to reproduce the patient's symptoms, not just pain or discomfort.

Resisted Muscle Testing

It is important to stabilize the hip during manual muscle testing to prevent any muscle substitution. The examiner begins with the muscle on stretch and applies resistance throughout the full ROM, noting any muscle weakness compared to the uninvolved limb. Painful motions should be delayed until last. Fig. 16.20 demonstrates the motions that should be tested.

■■■■ FIGURE 16.19 Goniometry measurements for the hip. A, Hip flexion. Center the fulcrum over the greater trochanter of the femur. Align the proximal arm with the lateral margin of the pelvis, and then align the distal arm along the lateral midline of the femur, using the lateral epicondyle as reference. **B,** Hip extension. Alignment is the same as for measuring hip flexion, except that the individual is prone. **C,** Hip abduction and adduction. Center the fulcrum over the anterior superior iliac spine (ASIS) of the extremity being measured. Align the proximal arm along an imaginary horizontal line extending to the other ASIS, and then align the distal arm along the middle of the femur, using the midline of the patella for reference. **D,** Hip medial and lateral rotation. Center the fulcrum over the anterior aspect of the patella. Align the proximal arm perpendicular to the floor, and then align the distal arm, using the crest of the tibia and a point midway between the two malleoli for reference.

FIGURE 16.20 **Resisted manual muscle testing. A,** Knee extension (L_3). **B,** Lateral hip rotation. **C,** Medial hip rotation. **D,** Hip flexion (L_2). **E,** Hip abduction. **F,** Hip adduction. **G,** Knee flexion (S_2). **H,** Hip extension (S_1).

■■■■■ FIGURE 16.21 **Sacroiliac (SI) compression and distraction test.** The examiner applies a cross-arm pressure downward and outward to the anterior superior iliac spine with the thumbs. The action is repeated with pressure applied down through the anterior portion of the ilium, spreading the SI joint. Unilateral pain or posterior leg pain may indicate a sprain to the anterior SI ligaments. Sharp pain elsewhere may indicate a pelvic fracture.

Stress Tests

When using stress tests, only those tests that are absolutely necessary should be performed. While moving through the tests, the examiner should begin by applying gentle stress. The force should be applied several times with increasing overpressure. The presence of pain or joint laxity should be noted.

Sacroiliac Compression (Transverse Anterior Stress) and Distraction Test

The individual is in a supine position. The examiner applies a cross-arm pressure downward and outward to the ASIS with their thumbs (Fig. 16.21). This action is repeated with pressure applied down through the anterior portion of the ilium, spreading the SI joint. Unilateral gluteal or posterior leg pain may indicate a sprain to the anterior SI ligaments. Sharp pain elsewhere along the pelvic ring with outward pressure, or with bilateral compression of the iliac crests, may indicate a pelvic fracture.

"Squish" Test

The individual is in a supine position. The examiner pushes both ASIS downward and inward at a 45° angle. This action stresses the posterior SI ligaments. The test is considered to be positive if pain is present.

Sacroiliac Rocking (Knee-to-Shoulder) Test

This test also is called the sacrotuberous ligament stress test. The individual is in a supine position. The examiner fully flexes the individual's knee and hip toward the opposite shoulder and adducts the hip (Fig. 16.22). The hip and knee must both demonstrate no pathology and have full ROM. The SI joint is rocked by flexion and adduction of the hip. If bringing a single knee to the chest causes pain in the posterolateral thigh, irritation of the sacrotuberous ligament may be indicated. If pain

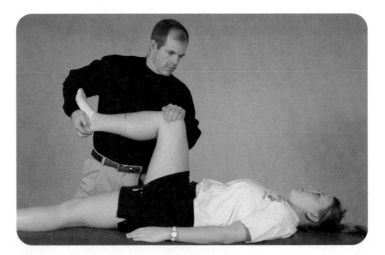

■■■■■ FIGURE 16.22 **Sacroiliac (SI) rocking (knee-to-shoulder) test.** The individual's knee and hip are fully flexed toward the opposite shoulder, and the hip is adducted. The SI joint is rocked by flexion and adduction of the hip. Pain in the posterolateral thigh indicates irritation of the sacrotuberous ligament. Pain in the region of the posterior superior iliac spine when pulling the leg toward the opposite shoulder indicates SI ligament irritation.

is produced in the area around the PSIS when pulling the leg toward the opposite shoulder, SI ligament irritation is indicated.

Approximation (Transverse Posterior Stress) Test

The individual is in a side-lying position. The examiner exerts a downward force over the iliac crest (Fig. 16.23). The movement causes forward pressure on the sacrum. A positive test produces pain or a feeling of pressure on the SI joints, indicating a sprain of the posterior SI ligaments, an SI lesion, or both. Sharp pain along the pelvic ring may indicate a fracture.

Patrick's (Faber) Test

In a supine position, the foot and ankle of the involved leg are rested on the contralateral knee. Then, the flexed leg is slowly lowered into abduction (Fig. 16.24). The final position of *f*lexion, *ab*duction, and *e*xternal *r*otation (Faber) at the hip should place the involved leg on the table, or at least near a horizontal position with the opposite leg. Overpressure on the knee of the involved leg and the contralateral iliac crest may produce pain in the SI joint on the side of the involved leg, denoting possible pathology.

Special Tests

A variety of special tests can be used for detecting injury or related pathology.

Leg Length Measurement

Nutation of the ilium on the sacrum results in decreased leg length, as does contranutation on the opposite side. If the iliac bone on one side is lower, the leg on that side usually is longer. Anatomical discrepancy, or true leg length, is measured in a supine position with the ASIS square, level, and balanced. The legs should be parallel to each other, with the

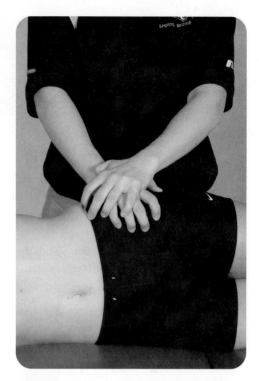

■ ■ ■ **FIGURE 16.23 Approximation test.** In a side-lying position, a downward force is applied over the iliac crest. Increased pain or a feeling of pressure on the sacroiliac (SI) joints indicates a possible joint sprain. Pain or pressure in the SI joints indicates a possible SI lesion, sprain of the posterior SI ligaments, or both. Sharp pain may indicate a possible pelvic fracture.

■ ■ ■ **FIGURE 16.24 Patrick's (Faber) test.** Also called the figure-four test, the foot and ankle of the involved leg is rested on the contralateral knee. Overpressure on the knee of the involved leg and the contralateral iliac crest may produce pain in the sacroiliac joint on the side of the involved leg, indicating pathology.

FIGURE 16.25 Measuring leg length. A, In measuring leg length, the pelvis should be square, level, and balanced. For anatomical discrepancy, or true leg length, the measure is from the anterior superior iliac spines to the distal aspect of the medial malleolus of each ankle. **B,** For apparent leg length discrepancies, the measure is from the umbilicus to the medial malleolus of each ankle.

heels approximately 6 to 8 inches apart. Using a flexible tape measure, the distance from the distal edge of the ASIS to the distal aspect of the medial malleolus of each ankle is measured (Fig. 16.25A). The measurement is repeated on the other side, and the results are then compared. A difference of 1.0 to 1.3 cm (0.5–1.0 inch) is considered to be normal.

Apparent leg length discrepancies as a result of lateral pelvic tilt or flexion or adduction contractures are measured from the umbilicus to the medial malleolus of each ankle (Fig. 16.25B). The test is meaningful only if the result for true leg length discrepancy is negative.

Thomas Test for Flexion Contractures

The individual is lying supine on a table. The examiner should note the presence of lumbar lordosis. If contractures are present, the examiner may be able to slip his or her hand under the low back. Next, the individual is instructed to flex the uninvolved leg to the chest and hold it in that position. This action should flatten the lumbar region. If the test is negative, the straight leg (i.e., the involved leg) remains in contact with the table; if the test is positive, the straight leg rises off the table (Fig. 16.26).

Gaenslen's Test

A modification of the Thomas test, Gaenslen's test is used to place a rotary stress on the SI joint by forcing one hip into hyperextension. The individual is positioned so that the test hip extends beyond

FIGURE 16.26 Thomas test. The individual is instructed to flex the uninvolved leg to the chest and hold it. A positive test occurs when the extended leg moves up off the table, indicating hip flexion contractures.

■■■■ FIGURE 16.27 **Gaenslen's sign. A,** The individual is positioned so that the involved hip extends beyond the edge of the table. **B,** The individual draws both legs onto the chest and then slowly lowers one leg into extension. Increased pain signals an ipsilateral sacroiliac joint lesion, hip pathology, or L_4 nerve root lesion.

the edge of the table. Next, both legs are drawn onto the chest, and then one is slowly lowered into extension (Fig. 16.27). The other leg is tested in a similar fashion for comparison. A positive test is indicated with pain in the SI joints.

An alternative position is with the individual in a side-lying position, with the upper leg (i.e., the test leg) hyperextended at the hip and the lower leg flexed against the chest. Next, the pelvis is stabilized while the hip of the uppermost leg is extended. Increased pain may indicate an ipsilateral SI joint lesion, hip pathology, or a L_4 nerve root lesion.

Kendall Test for Rectus Femoris Contracture

The individual lies supine on the table, with both knees flexed at 90° over the edge of the table. The individual flexes the unaffected knee to the chest and holds it in that position. The other knee should remain flexed at 90°. If the knee slightly extends, a contracture in the rectus femoris may be present in that leg (Fig. 16.28). If the results are positive, the muscle is palpated for tightness to confirm the contracture. With no palpable tightness, the condition may be caused by tight joint structures (i.e., capsular or ligamentous). If the hip abducts during the test, it may result from iliotibial band tightness. Then, Ober's test should be performed bilaterally (see Fig. 16.33).

Patrick's (Faber or Figure-Four) Test

The individual lies supine with the foot and ankle of the involved leg resting on the contralateral knee. The flexed leg is then slowly lowered into abduction (see Fig. 16.24). The final position should place the involved leg on the table or, at least, near a horizontal position with the opposite leg. If the leg is unable to relax to this position and remains above

■■■ FIGURE 16.28 **Kendall test.** The Kendall test is similar to the Thomas test, except that the individual lies supine, with both knees flexed over the edge of the table. The uninvolved leg is flexed to the chest and held. A positive test occurs when the leg flexed over the end of the table extends.

FIGURE 16.29 Hamstring contractures.
The individual flexes one hip against the chest to stabilize the pelvic region. The test is considered to be positive if the individual cannot touch the toes of the extended leg.

the opposite leg, an iliopsoas spasm or hip joint contracture may be indicated.

Hamstring Contracture Test

In a seated position on a table, the individual flexes the hip and brings one leg against the chest to stabilize the pelvic region. Next, the individual is instructed to touch the toes of the extended leg (Fig. 16.29). Inability to do so indicates tight hamstrings on the extended leg.

90°-90° Straight Leg Raising Test

The individual is supine, with the hips flexed to 90° and the knees bent. The examiner grasps behind the knee to stabilize the hip at 90° and extends each knee one at time. Knee extension within 20° of full extension is considered to be normal flexibility for the hamstrings.

In some cases, nerve root symptoms may be produced. The test is similar to the slump test, performed in a supine rather than a sitting position.

Straight Leg Raising (Lasegue's) Test

Although this test typically is used to stretch the dura mater of the spinal cord and assess possible intervertebral disk lesions, it also is used to rule out tight hamstrings. The individual is in a supine position. Maintaining the knee in extension, the examiner flexes the individual's hip until the individual complains of tightness or pain (Fig. 16.30). The examiner then slowly lowers the leg until the pain or tightness disappears. Next, the examiner dorsiflexes the ankle and instructs the individual to flex the neck. Pain that increases with dorsiflexion and neck flexion, or both, indicates stretching of the dura mater of the spinal cord. Pain that does not increase with dorsiflexion or neck flexion usually indicates tight hamstrings. If both legs are passively raised simultaneously and pain occurs before 70° of flexion, SI joint problems are indicated.

FIGURE 16.30 Straight leg raising (Lasègue's) test.
The examiner passively flexes the individual's hip while keeping the knee extended, until pain or tension is felt in the hamstrings. The examiner slowly lowers the leg until the pain or tension disappears. Then, the examiner dorsiflexes the ankle, and the individual flexes the neck. If pain does not increase with dorsiflexion of the ankle or flexion of the neck, it indicates tight hamstrings.

Trendelenburg Test

The individual is asked to stand and balance first on one leg and then on the other (Fig. 16.31). While the individual is balancing, the movement of the pelvis is noted. If the pelvis on the side of the nonstance leg rises, the test is considered to be negative, because the gluteus medius muscle on the opposite (i.e., stance) side is lifting it up as it normally does in a one-legged stance. If the pelvis on the side of the nonstance leg falls, however, the test is considered to be positive, indicating weakness or instability of the hip abductor muscles, primarily the gluteus medius on the stance side. Although the examiner is watching what happens on the nonstance side, the stance side is being tested.

Piriformis Test

The individual is in a side-lying position resting on the uninvolved leg. The involved hip is flexed at 60° with the knee flexed. The examiner stabilizes the involved hip with one hand and applies a downward pressure to the knee (Fig. 16.32). If the piriformis muscle is tight, pain will be elicited in the muscle. If the sciatic nerve is compressed by the piriformis muscle, the patient may experience sciatic-like symptoms. Resisted lateral rotation with the muscle on stretch (i.e., with the hip medially rotated) also may cause the same sciatica.

Long Sitting Test

The individual is asked to lie supine with the legs straight. The examiner places the thumbs over the medial malleoli, ensuring that the malleoli are level. The individual is then asked to sit up while the examiner observes whether one leg moves from a long position to a short position (i.e., moves proximally). If one leg moves up farther than the other, a functional leg length difference exists, resulting from pelvic dysfunction caused by pelvic torsion or rotation. For example, if the right leg moves proximally, it indicates anterior rotation of the right ilium on the sacrum. If the reverse occurs (i.e., the right leg moves from a short position to a longer position), it indicates posterior rotation of the right ilium on the sacrum.

FIGURE 16.31 Trendelenburg test. If an individual is unable to stand on the left leg with the hips level, it indicates weakness in the left hip abductors.

FIGURE 16.32 Piriformis test. The patient lies on the uninvolved side. The involved hip is flexed at 60°, and the knee is flexed. The examiner stabilizes the hip with one hand and applies a downward pressure to the knee. Pain over the piriformis muscle indicates a positive test.

■ ■ ■ FIGURE 16.33 **Ober's test.** The examiner passively abducts and slightly extends the hip. Then, the extended leg is slowly lowered. If the iliotibial band is tight, the leg will remain in the abducted position.

Ober's Test

The individual is side-lying, with the lower leg slightly flexed at the hip and knee for stability. The examiner stabilizes the pelvis with one hand to prevent the pelvis from shifting posteriorly during the test. Next, the examiner abducts and slightly extends the hip so that the iliotibial tract passes over the greater trochanter (Fig. 16.33). Next, the examiner slowly lowers the upper leg. If the tensor fascia latae, or iliotibial band, is tight, the leg remains in the abducted position. Although the original Ober's test called for the knee to be flexed at 90°, the iliotibial tract has a greater stretch if the knee is extended. If the knee is flexed during the test, greater stress is placed on the femoral nerve, which may result in neurologic signs (i.e., pain, tingling, or paresthesia).

Buttock Test

This test determines the presence of pathology in the buttock region, such as a bursitis, tumor, or abscess that may restrict hip flexion. The straight leg raising test is performed as above. If a restriction is reached in hip flexion, the examiner flexes the knee to determine if hip flexion increases (Fig. 16.34). If a problem exists in the lumbar spine, hip flexion increases, denoting a negative buttock test. A positive buttock test is determined when hip flexion does not increase after the knee is flexed.

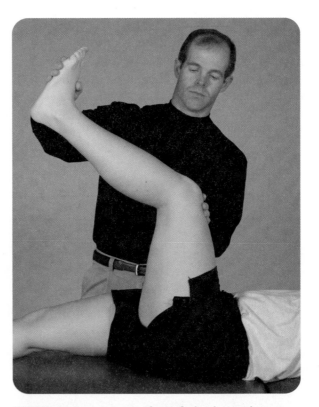

■ ■ ■ FIGURE 16.34 **Sign of the buttock test.** A unilateral straight leg raising test is performed. If a restriction is felt, the examiner flexes the knee. If hip flexion increases, a problem may exist in the lumbar spine. A positive buttock test occurs when hip flexion does not increase.

Neurologic Tests

Neurologic integrity is assessed with the use of myotomes, reflexes, and cutaneous patterns, including segmental dermatomes and peripheral nerve patterns.

Myotomes

Isometric muscle testing in the loose-packed position should be performed in the following motions to test specific segmental myotomes:

- Hip flexion (L_1, L_2)
- Knee extension (L_3)
- Ankle dorsiflexion (L_4)
- Toe extension (L_5)
- Ankle plantar flexion, foot eversion, or hip extension (S_1)
- Knee flexion (S_2)

Testing of these motions is demonstrated in Figures 17.22 and 18.31.

Reflexes

The pelvic or hip area has no specific reflexes to test. Other reflexes in the lower extremity include the patella (L_3, L_4) and Achilles tendon reflexes (S_1) (see Fig. 17.38).

Cutaneous Patterns

The segmental nerve dermatome patterns for the pelvis, hip, and thigh are demonstrated in Fig. 16.35. The peripheral nerve cutaneous patterns are demonstrated in Fig. 16.36.

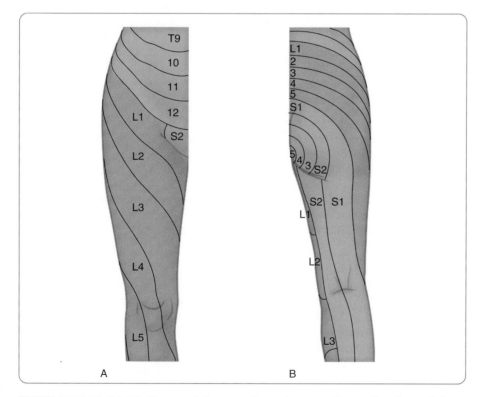

■■■■ FIGURE 16.35 Segmental nerve dermatome patterns for the pelvis, hip, and thigh. A, Anterior view. **B,** Posterior view.

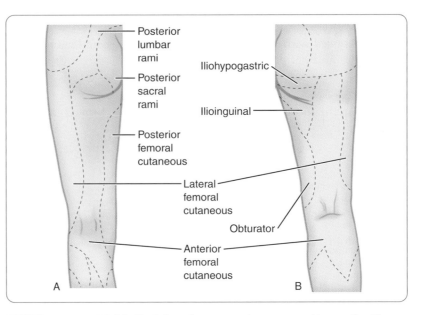

FIGURE 16.36 Peripheral nerve cutaneous patterns for the pelvis, hip, and thigh. A, Anterior view. **B,** Posterior view.

Activity-Specific Functional Tests

Functional tests should be performed before clearing any individual to return to activity. The individual should be able to perform activities pain-free, with no limp or antalgic gait. Examples of functional activities include walking, going up and down stairs, jogging, squatting, jumping, running straight ahead, running sideways, and changing directions while running.

Physical examination findings that would suggest the individual has myositis ossificans include passive knee flexion limited to 20 to 30°, and inability to perform active quadriceps contractions and straight leg raises.

REHABILITATION

The basketball player was referred to the team physician, who recommended treatment including ice, compression, elevation, crutches, and protected rest. Is it advantageous to treat this condition using NSAIDs?

Rehabilitation of the hip area should restore motion and proprioception; improve muscular strength, endurance, and power; and maintain cardiovascular fitness. In addition to focusing on muscles that move the hip, exercises also should involve the muscles that govern the knee.

Restoration of Motion

Range-of-motion exercises for the hip region should focus on the hip flexors, extensors, abductors, adductors, medial and lateral rotators, and quadriceps and hamstrings. Several of the stretching exercises were demonstrated in Field Strategy 16.1; other ROM exercises for muscles crossing the knee joint appear in Field Strategy 17.1. These exercises can be active or passive, and they should include proprioceptive neuromuscular facilitation stretching techniques.

Restoration of Proprioception and Balance

Proprioception and balance are regained in the early stages of exercise, with activities such as shifting one's weight while on crutches, performing straight leg raises while weight bearing on one leg, performing bilateral minisquats, and using a biomechanical ankle platform system (BAPS) board, slide board, or minitramp. Straight leg raises can be further supplemented with ankle weights and elastic tubing. Attaching the tubing to the opposite limb from the one being worked can develop balance in one limb while strengthening the other. Movement patterns can work in a single plane or in multidirectional patterns.

Muscular Strength, Endurance, and Power

Isometric exercises may be used early to strengthen the muscle groups. Open chain exercises, such as straight leg raises, can be completed in a single plane or in multidirectional patterns and can be supplemented with ankle weights or tubing. Closed chain exercises may include minisquats and modified lunges and should progress to full squats and lunges. Resistance may be added with hand-held weights, a weighted bar, or use of a leg-press machine. A variety of commercial isotonic and isokinetic machines are available to strengthen the individual muscle groups using both open and closed chain techniques.

Cardiovascular Fitness

Cardiovascular fitness exercises can include early use of an upper body ergometer or hydrotherapeutic exercise. Running in water and performing sport-specific exercises in deeper water can allow the individual to maintain sport-specific functional skills in a non–weight bearing position. When ROM is adequate, a stationary bike can be used, beginning with a light to moderate load and increasing the load as tolerated. A slide board also may be used. Light jogging can begin with one-quarter speed and progress to half-speed, three-quarter speed, and full sprints. Plyometric exercises, including jumping, skipping, and bounding, can be combined with running, side-to-side running, or cutting and changing directions. Timed sprints, shuttle runs, karioca runs, and hops or vertical jump tests may be used to measure return to full activity. The individual should not be cleared for participation until they have bilaterally equal ROM, balance, muscular strength, endurance, and power as well as an appropriate level of cardiovascular fitness for the specific sport.

Use of NSAIDs can be dependent on the stage of healing. Because the basketball player sustained another blow during today's practice, NSAIDs are not indicated for 48 hours postinjury, because they inhibit platelet function and promote hemorrhage.

SUMMARY

1. The SI joints help to transfer the weight of the torso and skull to the lower limbs, provide elasticity to the pelvic ring, and conversely, act as a buffer to decrease impact forces from the foot as they are transmitted to the spine and upper body.

2. The hip joint is the most stable joint in the body. It is protected by a deep, bony socket called the acetabulum and is stabilized by several strong ligaments, including the iliofemoral, pubofemoral, and ischiofemoral ligaments.

3. Compression on the hip is approximately the same as body weight during the swing phase of normal walking, but compression increases to at least sixfold body weight during the stance phase.

4. Muscle imbalance and dysfunction, congenital abnormalities, and postural deviations can predispose an individual to injury.

5. Contusions typically are seen on the crest of the ilium or in the quadriceps muscle group. Severe quadriceps contusions can lead to myositis ossificans or an acute compartment syndrome.

6. Bursitis can result from inflammation secondary to excessive friction or shear forces or can stem from a direct blow that causes bleeding in the bursa. The greater trochanteric bursa is the most commonly injured bursa.

7. The hamstrings are the most frequently strained muscle group in the body. Injuries typically are caused by a rapid contraction of the muscle during a ballistic action or by a violent stretch.

8. Adductor strains are common in activities that require quick changes of direction and explosive propulsion and acceleration.

9. Piriformis syndrome is sixfold more prevalent in women than in men, and it can mimic the signs and symptoms of a herniated lumbar disk problem with nerve root impingement.

10. In adolescents, any unexplained groin pain associated with a gradual onset of a limp should be referred to a physician to rule out Legg-Calvé-Perthes disease or a slipped capital femoral epiphysis.

11. Avulsion fractures may occur in individuals who perform rapid moves involving sudden acceleration and deceleration, with the following sites being most affected:

   - **ASIS**—proximal sartorius muscle or tensor fascia latae
   - **AIIS**—proximal rectus femoris muscles
   - **Ischial tuberosity**—proximal hamstrings attachment
   - **Lesser trochanter**—distal iliopsoas attachment

12. Physician referral is warranted if any of the following conditions are suspected:

   - Obvious deformity suggesting a dislocation or fracture
   - Significant loss of motion or palpable defect in a muscle
   - Severe joint disability that may be evident by a noticeable limp
   - Excessive soft-tissue swelling, particularly in the quadriceps
   - Any adolescent with groin pain that does not improve within 5 to 7 days or is associated with a gradual onset of a limp
   - Any abnormal or absent reflexes, or weakness in a myotome
   - Abnormal sensations in either the segmental dermatomes or peripheral cutaneous patterns
   - Absent or weak pulse

13. Radiographs, bone scans, or magnetic resonance images can be used to rule out underlying bone cysts, tumors, osteochondromas, or congenital defects that could lead to permanent disability.

REFERENCES

1. Pool-Goudzwaard A, Hoek Van Dijke G, Mulder P, et al. The iliolumbar ligament: its influence on stability of the sacroiliac joint. Clin Biomech 2002;18(2):99–105.
2. Pool-Goudzwaard A, Kleinrensink GJ, Snijders C, et al. The sacroiliac part of the iliolumbar ligament. J Anat 2001;199(Pt 4):457–463.
3. Nordin M, Frankel VH. Basic biomechanics of the hip. In: Nordin M, Frankel V, eds. Basic Biomechanics of the Musculoskeletal System. 3rd Ed. Philadelphia: Lea & Febiger, 2001.
4. Ferguson SJ, Bryant JT, Ganz R, Ito K. An in vitro investigation of the acetabular labral seal in hip joint mechanics. J Biomech 2003:36(2):171–178.
5. Harrington L, Nester C. Q-angle undervalued? The relationship between Q-angle and mediolateral position of the patella. Clin Biomech 2004:19(10):1070–1073.
6. Chan GNY, Smith AW, Kirtley C, Tsang WWN. Changes in knee moments with contralateral versus ipsilateral cane usage in females with knee osteoarthritis. Clin Biomech 2005;20(4):396–404.
7. Newton M, Walker J. Acute quadriceps injury: a case study. Emerg Nurse 2004;12(8):24–29.
8. Esposito PW. Pelvis, hip, and thigh injuries. In: Mellion MB, Walsh WM, Madden C, Putukian M, Shelton GL, eds. The Team Physician's Handbook. Philadelphia: Hanley & Belfus, 2002.
9. Kalodiki E, Nicolaides AN. Superficial thrombophlebitis and low-molecular-weight heparins. Angiology 2002;53(6):659–663.

Knee Conditions

STUDENT OUTCOMES

1. Identify the major bony and soft-tissue structures of the knee region.

2. Identify the primary and secondary ligamentous restraints of the knee.

3. Describe the motions of the knee, and identify the muscles that produce them.

4. Describe the forces that produce the loading patterns responsible for common injuries at the knee.

5. Explain the general principles used to prevent injuries to the knee.

6. Describe the common injuries to and conditions of the knee by physically active individuals (including sprains, dislocations, contusions, strains, bursitis, meniscal tears, and patellofemoral pain).

7. Explain the management strategies for common injuries and conditions of the knee.

8. List the various types of fractures that can occur at the knee, and explain their management

9. Describe a thorough assessment of the knee and patellofemoral joint.

10. Explain the basic principles associated with rehabilitation of the knee.

ROLE DELINEATION COMPETENCIES

The following Performance Domains and Tasks defined in the National Athletic Trainers' Association Board of Certification *Role Delineation Study*, 5th Edition are addressed in this chapter:

BOC COMPETENCIES

I.   Prevention

G. Monitor participants and environmental conditions by following accepted guidelines to promote safe participation.

II.   Clinical Evaluation and Diagnosis

A. Obtain a history through observation, interview, and/or review of relevant records to assess current or potential injury, illness, or condition.
B. Inspect the involved area(s) visually to assess the injury, illness, or health-related condition.
C. Palpate the involved area(s) using standard techniques to assess the injury, illness, or health-related condition.
D. Perform specific tests in accordance with accepted procedures to assess the injury, illness, or health-related condition.
E. Formulate a clinical impression by interpreting the signs, symptoms, and predisposing factors of the injury, illness, or condition to determine the appropriate course of action.

III.   Immediate Care

A. Employ life-saving techniques through the use of standard emergency procedures in order to reduce morbidity and the incidence of mortality.
B. Prevent exacerbation of non–life threatening condition(s) through the use of standard procedures in order to reduce morbidity.
C. Facilitate the timely transfer of care for conditions beyond the scope of practice of the athletic trainer by implementing appropriate referral strategies to stabilize and/or prevent exacerbation of the condition(s).

IV.   Treatment, Rehabilitation, and Reconditioning

E. Reassess the status of injuries, illnesses, and/or conditions using standard techniques and documentation strategies in order to determine appropriate treatment, rehabilitation, and/or reconditioning and to evaluate readiness to return to a desired level of activity.
F. Educate the appropriate individual(s) in the treatment, rehabilitation, and reconditioning of injuries, illnesses, and/or conditions using applicable methods and materials to facilitate recovery, function, and/or performance.

The knee is a complex joint that frequently is injured during participation in physical activity. While walking and running, the knee moves through a considerable range of motion (ROM) while bearing loads equivalent to three- to fourfold body weight. Because the knee is positioned between the two longest bones in the body (i.e., the femur and the tibia), the potential exists for creating large, injurious torques at the joint. These factors, coupled with minimal bony stability, make the knee susceptible to injury. The knee is the predominant site of injury among runners and is one of the most frequently injured joints for sport participants (1).

This chapter begins with a review of the anatomy of the knee and a discussion of the associated kinematics and kinetics. General principles to prevent injuries then are followed by a discussion regarding common injuries to the knee complex. Finally, a step-by-step injury assessment of the region is presented, and examples of rehabilitative exercises are provided.

ANATOMY OF THE KNEE

The knee is a large, synovial joint that includes three articulations within the joint capsule. The weight-bearing joints are the two condylar articulations of the tibiofemoral joint; the third articulation is the patellofemoral joint. The soft-tissue connections of the proximal tibiofibular joint also exert a minor influence on knee motion.

Bony Structure of the Knee

The proximal bone of the knee joint is the femur. The prominent posterior ridge of the femur, the linea aspera, serves as an attachment for many of the muscles that move the hip and knee. The distal portion of the femur broadens to form the medial and lateral epicondyles. The area between the epicondyles on the anterior surface of the femur is the femoral trochlea, through which the patella glides as the knee moves into flexion and extension (Fig. 17.1).

The lateral epicondyle is wider than the medial epicondyle. Arising from the most superior crest of the medial epicondyle is the palpable adductor tubercle. Inferior to each epicondyle are the medial and lateral condyles, with the medial condyle being the longer. Sharing a common anterior surface, these condyles bifurcate posteriorly and are separated by the deep intercondylar notch.

Corresponding to the femoral condyles are the medial and lateral tibial plateaus. To accommodate for the longer medial femoral condyle, the medial tibial plateau is 50% larger than the lateral tibial plateau. Separating the two tibial plateaus are the intercondylar eminences, which are raised areas that match the femur's intercondylar notch. The anterior aspect of the tibia includes the prominent tibial tubercle, which serves as the distal attachment of the infrapatellar ligament.

The patella is a sesamoid bone located in the quadriceps (patellar) tendon. It improves the biomechanical function of the extensor mechanism and protects the anterior portion of the knee. The fibula is not a direct part of the knee joint. The head of the fibula, however, does serve as a site for several soft-tissue attachments that support and stabilize the knee.

Tibiofemoral Joint

The distal femur and proximal tibia articulate to form two side-by-side condyloid joints that collectively are known as the **tibiofemoral joint** (see Fig. 17.1). These joints function together primarily as a modified hinge joint. Because of the restricting ligaments, some lateral and rotational motions are allowed at the knee. The medial and lateral condyles of the femur differ somewhat in size, shape, and orientation. As a result, the tibia rotates laterally on the femur during the last few degrees of extension to produce "locking" of the knee. This phenomenon, known as the **"screwing-home" mechanism**, brings the knee into the close-packed position of full extension.

Menisci

The **menisci**, which also are known as semilunar cartilages because of their half-moon shapes, are disks of fibrocartilage firmly attached to the superior plateaus of the tibia by the coronary ligaments and joint capsule. They provide several functional advantages, including absorption and dissipation of force and significantly improved congruency of the joint surfaces to even the distribution of stress across the joint (Box 17.1). In addition, because 74% of the total weight of the menisci is water, much of the fluid is squeezed out into the joint space when the knee undergoes compression during weight bearing, which provides lubrication to promote gliding of the joint structures (2). The menisci also increase knee stability by serving as soft-tissue restraints that resist anterior tibial displacement.

When viewed in cross-section, the menisci are thicker along the lateral margin and thinner on the medial margin, serving to deepen the concavities of the tibial plateaus. When viewed from above, the medial meniscus is semicircular, whereas the lateral meniscus is somewhat more circular (see Fig. 17.1). The inner edges of both menisci are unattached to the bone, but the two ends of the menisci, known as the anterior and posterior horns, are attached to the intercondylar tubercles. The anterior horns of each meniscus are joined to each other by the transverse ligament and are connected to the infrapatellar tendon via the patellomeniscal ligaments.

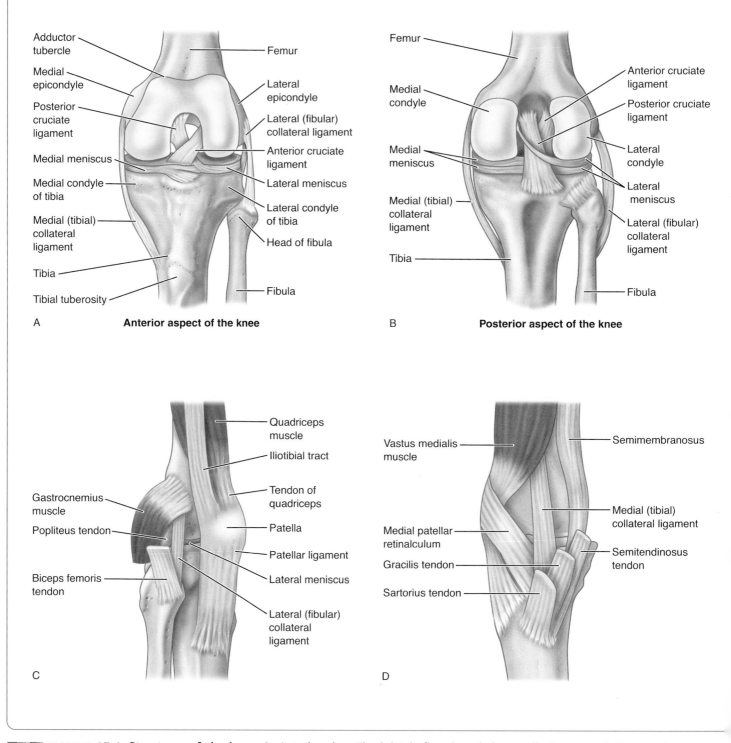

Anterior aspect of the knee

B **Posterior aspect of the knee**

C

D

▪▪▪▪ FIGURE 17.1 **Structures of the knee. A,** Anterior view. The joint is flexed, and the patella is removed. **B,** Posterior view. The knee is in extension. **C,** Lateral view. **D,** Medial view. **E,** Superior surface of the tibia. **F,** Bursae of the knee.

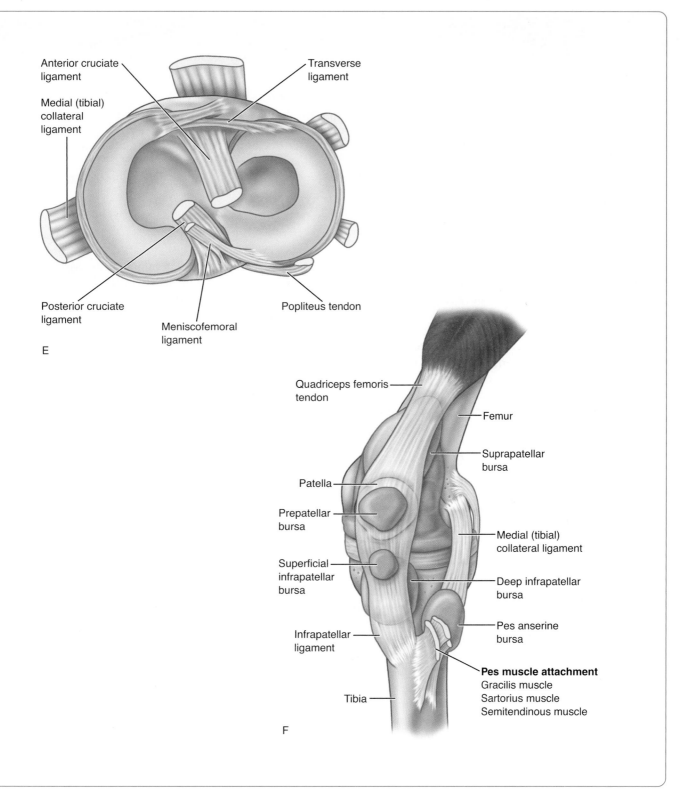

Anterior cruciate ligament

Medial (tibial) collateral ligament

Transverse ligament

Posterior cruciate ligament

Meniscofemoral ligament

Popliteus tendon

E

Quadriceps femoris tendon

Femur

Suprapatellar bursa

Patella

Prepatellar bursa

Medial (tibial) collateral ligament

Superficial infrapatellar bursa

Deep infrapatellar bursa

Pes anserine bursa

Infrapatellar ligament

Pes muscle attachment
Gracilis muscle
Sartorius muscle
Semitendinous muscle

Tibia

F

Box 17.1 Functions of the Menisci

- Deepen the articulation, and fill the gaps that occur during knee motion.
- Aid in lubrication and nutrition of the joint.
- Reduce friction during movement.
- Increase area of contact between the condyles, thus improving weight distribution.
- Provide shock absorption by dissipating stress over the articular cartilage, thus decreasing cartilage deterioration.
- Assist the ligaments and capsule in preventing hyperextension.
- Prevent the joint capsule from entering the joint during the locking mechanism by directing the movement of the femoral articular condyles.

The medial meniscus has an attachment to the deep medial collateral ligament (MCL) and fibers from the semimembranosus muscle. It is injured much more frequently than the lateral meniscus, in part because the medial meniscus is more securely attached to the tibia and, therefore, is less mobile.

In comparison, the lateral meniscus is a smaller and more freely moveable structure. In addition to its attachments to the joint capsule, intercondylar tubercles, and transverse ligament, the lateral meniscus is attached to the posterior cruciate ligament through the meniscofemoral ligament (ligament of Wrisberg) and to the popliteus muscle via the joint capsule and coronary ligament. Contraction of the popliteus serves to retract the lateral meniscus. During flexion and extension of the knee, the medial and lateral menisci move posteriorly and anteriorly, respectively. The outer third of each meniscus is innervated and contains nociceptors that, when a meniscus is injured, send signals of pain to the brain (3).

Joint Capsule and Bursae

The thin articular capsule at the knee is large and lax, encompassing both the tibiofemoral and patellofemoral joints. Anteriorly, it extends approximately 2.5 cm above the patella to attach along the edges of the superior patellar surface. The deep bursa formed by this capsule above the patella, known as the suprapatellar bursa, is the largest in the body (Fig. 17.2). The suprapatellar bursa lies between the femur and quadriceps femoris tendon, and it functions to reduce friction between the two structures.

Posteriorly, two other bursae communicate with the joint capsule—namely, the subpopliteal and semimembranosus bursae. The subpopliteal bursa lies between the lateral condyle of the femur and the popliteal muscle. The semimembranosus bursa lies between the medial head of the gastrocnemius and the semimembranosus tendon.

During flexion and extension, synovial fluid moves throughout the bursal recesses to lubricate the articular surfaces. In extension, the gastrocnemius and subpopliteal bursae are compressed, driving the synovial fluid anteriorly. In flexion, the suprapatellar bursa is compressed, forcing the fluid posteriorly. When the knee is in a semiflexed or open-packed position, the synovial fluid is under the least amount of pressure; this position provides relief of pain caused by swelling in the joint capsule and surrounding bursae.

Four other key bursae are associated with the knee but not contained in the joint capsule—namely, the prepatellar, superficial infrapatellar, deep infrapatellar bursae, and pes anserine bursa. The prepatellar bursa is located between the skin and anterior surface of the patella, allowing free movement of the skin over the patella during flexion and extension. The superficial infrapatellar bursa is located between the skin and patellar tendon. Inflammation of this bursa caused by excessive kneeling sometimes is referred to as "housemaid's knee." The deep infrapatellar bursa is located between the tibial tubercle and the infrapatellar tendon, and it is separated from the joint cavity by the infrapatellar fat pad. This bursa reduces friction between the ligament and the bony tubercle. The pes anserine bursa is located between the MCL and the sartorius, gracilis, and semitendinosus tendons and distal to the joint line, in close proximity and posterior to the MCL.

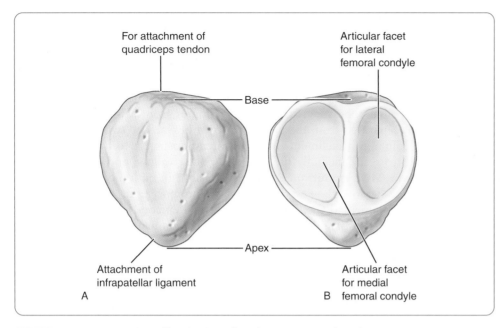

For attachment of
quadriceps tendon

Articular facet
for lateral
femoral condyle

Base

Apex

Attachment of
infrapatellar ligament

A

Articular facet
for medial
femoral condyle

B

FIGURE 17.2 Patella. A, Anterior view. **B,** Posterior view.

Ligaments of the Knee

Because the shallow articular surfaces of the tibiofemoral joint contribute minimally to knee stability, the stabilizing role of the ligaments crossing the knee is of great significance. Two major ligaments of the knee are the anterior and posterior **cruciate ligaments** (see Fig. 17.1). The name cruciate is derived from the fact that the two ligaments cross each other, with anterior and posterior referring to their respective tibial attachments. These ligaments are termed **intracapsular ligaments,** because they are located within the articular capsule, and **extrasynovial ligments,** because they lie outside the synovial cavity.

The anterior cruciate ligament (ACL) stretches from the anterior aspect of the intercondyloid fossa of the tibia just medial and posterior to the anterior tibial spine in a superoposterior direction to the posteromedial surface of the lateral condyle of the femur. The ACL is a critical stabilizer that prevents:

- Anterior translation (movement) of the tibia on a fixed femur

- Posterior translation of the femur on a fixed tibia

- Internal and external rotation of the tibia on the femur

- Hyperextension of the tibia

The ACL has two discrete bands—namely, an anteromedial and a posterolateral bundle. Occasionally, a third, intermediate band also is present. When the knee is fully extended, the femoral attachment of the anteromedial bundle is anterior to the attachment of the posterolateral bundle. When the knee is flexed, the positions are reversed, causing the ACL to wind on itself. The result of this action is that varying portions of the ACL are taut as the knee moves through a normal ROM. When the knee is fully extended, the posterolateral bundle is taut; when the knee is fully flexed, the anteromedial bundle is taut. Generally, loads on the ACL correspond to anteriorly directed shear force at the knee (4). During gait, this force is maximum in early stance and small in late stance. The ACL frequently is subject to deceleration injuries; internal tibial torque is the most dangerous loading mechanism, particularly when combined with an anterior tibial force (5).

The shorter and stronger posterior cruciate ligament (PCL) runs from the posterior aspect of the tibial intercondyloid fossa in a anterosuperior direction to the lateral anteromedial condyle of the femur. It consists of a large anterolateral and a smaller posteromedial bundle. The PCL is considered to be the primary stabilizer of the knee, and it resists posterior displacement of the tibia on a fixed femur. The posterior fibers of the PCL are taut when the knee is fully extended, and the anterior fibers are taut when it is fully flexed.

The medial and lateral **collateral ligaments** also are referred to as the tibial and fibular collateral ligaments, respectively, after their distal attachments. Formed by two layers, the deep fibers of the MCL merge with the joint capsule and medial meniscus to connect the medial epicondyle of the femur to the medial tibia. The superficial layer originates from a broad band just below the adductor tubercle and is separated from the deep layer by a bursa. The two layers insert just below the pes anserinus, the common attachment of the semitendinosus, sartorius, and gracilis, thereby positioning the ligament to resist medially directed shear (i.e., valgus) and rotational forces acting on the knee. As a unit, the MCL is taut in complete extension. In midrange, its posterior fibers are the most taut; in complete flexion, the anterior fibers are the most taut.

The lateral collateral ligament (LCL) connects the lateral epicondyle of the femur to the head of the fibula, contributing to lateral stability of the knee. The ligament is separated from the lateral meniscus by a small fat pad. The LCL is the primary restraint against varus forces when the knee is between full extension and 30° of flexion, and it provides secondary restraint against external rotation of the tibia on the femur.

Other Structures Stabilizing the Knee

Several other structures contribute to knee integrity. Posteriorly, the oblique popliteal ligament forms an extension of the semimembranosus tendon, and the arcuate popliteal ligament connects the lateral condyle of the femur to the head of the fibula. These two ligaments, which are called the **arcuate–popliteal complex**, provide support to the posterior joint capsule. The complex limits anterior displacement of the tibia relative to the femur as well as hyperextension and hyperflexion of the knee. It becomes taut during internal and external tibial rotation and during valgus and varus loading of the knee.

Although the knee is only partially surrounded by a joint capsule, the capsule is reinforced by several tendons, including the expanded tendons of the quadriceps, the tendon of the semimembranosus, and the iliotibial (IT) band. Laterally, the IT band is a broad, thickened band of fascia that extends from the tensor fascia latae over the lateral epicondyle of the femur to Gerdy's tubercle on the lateral tibial plateau. The IT band is well supplied with free nerve endings that transmit signals for pain and proprioception to the brain, enhancing the structure's ability to promote lateral knee stability. The tissue under the IT band is a lateral extension and invagination of the knee joint capsule. Table 17.1 lists the structures providing stability to the knee, including primary and secondary restraints.

Patellofemoral Joint

The patella (i.e., the kneecap) is a triangular bone that rests between the femoral condyles to form the patellofemoral joint (see Fig. 17.2). The posterior surface of the patella is composed of three

TABLE 17.1 Structures Contributing to the Stability of the Knee		
TIBIAL MOTION	**PRIMARY RESTRAINTS**	**SECONDARY RESTRAINTS**
Anterior translation	ACL	MCL, LCL, middle third of the mediolateral capsule, IT band
Posterior translation	PCL	MCL, LCL, posterior third of the mediolateral capsule, popliteus tendon, anterior and posterior meniscofemoral ligaments
Valgus rotation	MCL	ACL, PCL, posterior capsule when the knee is fully extended
Varus rotation	LCL	ACL, PCL, posterior capsule when the knee is fully extended
Lateral rotation	MCL, LCL	Popliteus corner, ACL, PCL
Medial rotation	ACL, PCL	Anteroposterior meniscofemoral ligaments

ACL, anterior cruciate ligament; *LCL,* lateral (fibular) collateral ligament; *MCL,* medial collateral ligament; *PCL,* posterior cruciate ligament.

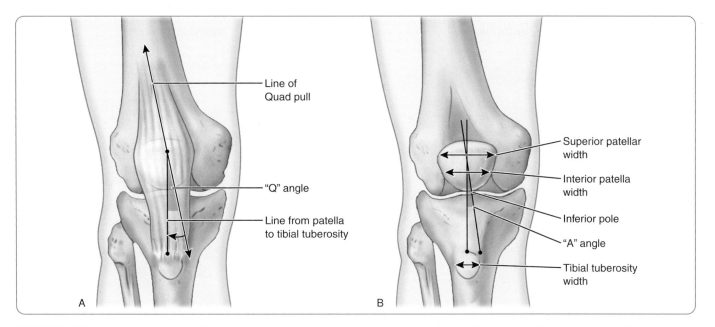

FIGURE 17.3 Angles at the knee. A, The Q-angle is formed between the line of quadriceps pull and the imaginary line connecting the center of the patella to the center of the tibial tubercle. **B,** The A-angle measures the relationship of the patella to the tibial tubercle.

distinct facets, although the number, size, and shape of these facets vary from person to person (6). A central, vertical ridge separates the medial and lateral regions, each having a superior, middle, and inferior articular surfaces. The odd facet, lying medial to the medial facet, has no articular subdivisions. The thickest articular cartilage in the body covers these facets, with the cartilage ranging up to 5 mm in thickness (7).

In the sagittal plane, the patella serves to increase the angle of pull of the patellar tendon on the tibia, thereby improving the mechanical advantage of the quadriceps muscles to produce knee extension. Patellar positioning is both maintained and restrained by the patellar retinaculum. The lateral retinaculum originates from the vastus lateralis and the IT band and inserts on the patella's lateral border. The medial retinaculum originates from the distal portion of the vastus medialis and adductor magnus, and it inserts on the medial border of the patella. The superior portion of the knee's joint capsule thickens and inserts on the patella's superior border, forming the medial and lateral patellofemoral ligaments.

The Q-angle is defined as the angle between the line of resultant force produced by the quadriceps muscles and the line of the patellar tendon (Fig. 17.3A). One line is drawn from the middle of the patella to the anterior superior iliac spine of the ilium, and a second line is drawn from the tibial tubercle through the center of the patella. When the knee is fully extended, the normal Q-angle ranges from approximately 13° in males to approximately 18° in females. A Q-angle of less than 13° or greater than 18° is considered to be abnormal and can predispose individuals to patellar injuries or degeneration. Cadaver studies show that increasing the Q-angle increases lateral patellofemoral contact pressures and could promote lateral patellar dislocation, whereas decreasing the Q-angle could increase the medial tibiofemoral contact pressure (8). Factors that contribute to an increased angle in women include a wider pelvis, increased femoral anteversion, increased knee valgus, external tibial torsion, increased ligamentous laxity, and hyperpronation of the foot (9).

Another measurement, similar to the Q-angle, is the **A-angle**, which measures the relationship of the patella to the tibial tubercle (Fig. 17.3B). This measurement consists of a vertical line that divides the patella in half. A second line is drawn from the tibial tubercle to the apex of the inferior pole of the patella. An A-angle of 35° or greater has been linked to increased patellofemoral pain, although some have questioned the reliability of this measurement because of the difficulty in consistently finding appropriate landmarks.

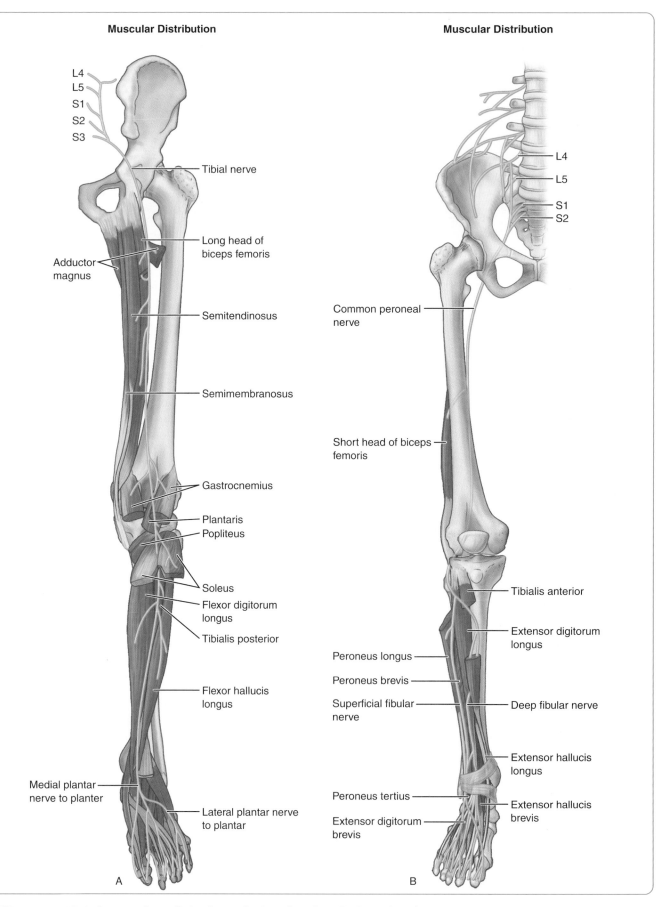

Muscular Distribution

L4
L5
S1
S2
S3

Tibial nerve

Adductor magnus

Long head of biceps femoris

Semitendinosus

Semimembranosus

Gastrocnemius

Plantaris
Popliteus

Soleus
Flexor digitorum longus
Tibialis posterior

Flexor hallucis longus

Medial plantar nerve to planter

Lateral plantar nerve to plantar

A

Muscular Distribution

L4
L5
S1
S2

Common peroneal nerve

Short head of biceps femoris

Tibialis anterior

Extensor digitorum longus

Peroneus longus
Peroneus brevis
Superficial fibular nerve

Deep fibular nerve

Extensor hallucis longus

Peroneus tertius

Extensor hallucis brevis

Extensor digitorum brevis

B

FIGURE 17.4 Innervation of the knee. A, Anterior view. **B,** Posterior view.

Muscles Crossing the Knee

The muscles of the knee develop tension to produce motion at the knee and contribute to the knee's stability.

Nerves of the Knee

The tibial nerve (L_4, L_5, S_1–S_3) is the largest and most medial continuation of the sciatic nerve. It innervates all the muscles in the hamstring group except for the short head of the biceps femoris, and it also supplies all muscles in the calf of the leg (Fig. 17.4).

The common peroneal nerve (L_4, L_5, S_1, S_2) is the lateral branch of the sciatic nerve (see Fig. 17.4). It innervates the short head of the biceps femoris in the thigh, then circles around Gerdy's tubercle, or the lateral tubercle of the proximal tibia, with a radius of approximately 45 mm (10). Proceeding inferiorly, it passes through the popliteal fossa to wind laterally along the subcutaneous surface to just below the proximal head of the fibula, where it can be easily damaged. As it passes between the fibula and the peroneus longus muscle, it subdivides into the superficial and deep peroneal nerves. An articular branch to the knee may arise either from the deep peroneal nerve or from both the deep and superficial peroneal nerves as a terminal branch of the common peroneal nerve.

The femoral nerve (L_2–L_4) courses down the anterior aspect of the thigh adjacent to the femoral artery to supply the quadriceps group. The L_2 and L_3 branches of the femoral nerve also innervate the sartorius.

Blood Vessels of the Knee

Just proximal to the knee, the main branch of the femoral artery becomes the popliteal artery. The popliteal artery courses through the popliteal fossa and then branches, forming the medial and lateral superior genicular, the middle genicular, and the medial and lateral inferior genicular arteries that supply the knee (Fig. 17.5). The superior and inferior genicular arteries intertwine with each other about the knee.

See *Muscles Acting on the Knee*, available on the companion website at the Point, for a summary of these muscles, including their attachments, primary actions, and innervation.

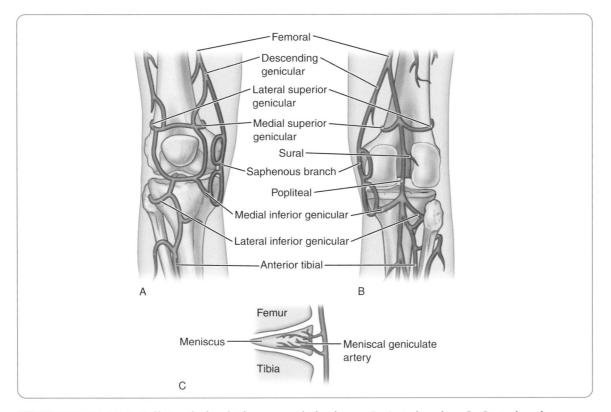

■■■■ FIGURE 17.5 **Collateral circulation around the knee. A,** Anterior view. **B,** Posterior view. **C,** Circulation to meniscus.

KINEMATICS AND MAJOR MUSCLE ACTIONS OF THE KNEE

The knee functions primarily as a hinge joint. The different shapes of the femoral condyles, however, serve to complicate joint function.

Flexion and Extension

The primary motions permitted at the tibiofemoral joint are flexion and extension. Knee flexion is performed primarily by the hamstrings and is assisted by the popliteus, gastrocnemius, gracilis, and sartorius. In addition, the flexor musculature has a secondary responsibility of rotating the tibia. The flexors attaching on the tibia's medial side (i.e., semitendinosus, semimembranosus, gracilis, and sartorius) internally rotate the tibia, whereas those attaching on the lateral side (i.e., biceps femoris) externally rotate the tibia. Knee extension is carried out by the quadriceps femoris muscle group. Although the name implies four muscles, most clinicians describe five—namely, the vastus lateralis, vastus intermedius, vastus medialis, vastus medialis oblique (VMO), and rectus femoris. The VMO is a discrete group of fibers arising from the medial femoral condyle and the fascia of the adductor magnus. Each muscle has a common attachment on the tibial tubercle via the patella and infra-patellar ligament.

In the terminal 20° of knee extension, the tibia externally rotates approximately 15° in what is called the "screw-home" mechanism. In full extension, the joint's close-packed position, maximal bony contact occurs between the femur and tibia, resulting in the joint being anatomically "locked." This rotation occurs because the articulating surface of the medial condyle of the femur is longer than that of the lateral condyle in this locked position, rendering motion almost completely impossible. Initiation of flexion from a position of full extension requires that the knee first be "unlocked." The role of "locksmith" in the closed kinetic chain is provided by the popliteus, which acts to externally rotate the femur with respect to the tibia and, in doing so, frees the joint for motion.

Once the knee is unlocked from full extension, bony contact is diminished, and motion in the transverse and frontal planes becomes freer. In an open kinetic chain, contraction of the popliteus causes internal rotation of the tibia on the femur. As the knee moves into flexion, the medial femoral condyle moves very little anteroposteriorly, but the lateral femoral condyle rolls back and the point of femorotibial contact shifts posteriorly, producing internal rotation of the tibia, with 120° of flexion accompanied by 20° of internal tibial rotation (11). This motion is facilitated by the inferior sloping of the lateral compartment of the tibial plateau. The reverse occurs during extension as the lateral femoral condyle of the femur slides anteriorly on the tibia.

Rotation and Passive Abduction and Adduction

The rotational capability of the tibia with respect to the femur is maximal at approximately 90° of knee flexion. A few degrees of passive abduction and adduction are permitted when the joint is positioned in the vicinity of 30° of flexion.

Knee Motion During Gait

During midstance of normal gait, the knee is flexed to approximately 20°, internally rotated approximately 5°, and slightly abducted. Knee motion during the swing phase includes approximately 70° of flexion, 15° of external rotation, and 5° of adduction. Gait is explained in more detail in Chapter 18.

Patellofemoral Joint Motion

During movements of knee flexion and extension, the patella glides in the trochlear groove, primarily in a vertical direction, with an excursion of as much as 8 cm. When the knee is fully extended, the inferior pole of the patella rests on the distal portion of the femoral shaft, just proximal to the femoral groove. During flexion, the patella makes initial contact with the groove at 10 to 20° of flexion, and it becomes seated within the groove as the knee approaches 20 to 30°. In this position, the lateral border of the trochlea is prominent, forming a barrier against lateral displacement of the patella. The inferior border of the patella tilts upward and medially during knee flexion, with the contact area increasingly shifted superiorly on the medial and lateral facets of the posterior patella (12,13). The patella also undergoes medial and lateral displacement as the tibia is rotated laterally and medially, respectively.

Tracking of the patella against the femur is dependent on the direction of the net force produced by the attached quadriceps. The vastus lateralis tends to pull the patella laterally in the direction of the muscle's action line, parallel to the femoral shaft. The IT band and lateral extensor retinaculum also exert a lateral force on the patella. Although considerable debate exists regarding its role, the VMO seems to oppose the lateral pull of the vastus lateralis and, in doing so, keeps the patella centered in the patellofemoral groove. If the magnitude of the force produced by the vastus lateralis exceeds that produced by the VMO, the patella is pulled laterally out of its groove during tracking. Mistracking of the patella during knee flexion-extension can be extremely painful and lead to several chronic patellofemoral conditions.

KINETICS OF THE KNEE

Because the knee is positioned between the body's two longest bony levers (i.e., the femur and the tibia), the potential for torque and force development at the knee is significant. The key role played by the knee during weight bearing makes the knee subject to large forces during the gait cycle.

Forces at the Tibiofemoral Joints

Both compression and shear forces are created at the tibiofemoral joints during daily activities. Weight bearing and tension development in muscles crossing the knee contribute to these forces, with compression dominating when the knee is fully extended. During knee flexion, the shear component of joint force that is produced by weight bearing increases. Shear at the knee, which causes a tendency for the femur to displace anteriorly on the tibial plateaus, is resisted primarily by the ACL and the PCL. Because of the potential for injury to the cruciate ligaments as well as to the collateral ligaments and menisci, the parallel squat is recommended over the deep squat (14). Individuals with previous knee injuries should restrict quadriceps exercise to the functional 0 to 50° of knee flexion (15).

Compressive force at the tibiofemoral joint can reach an estimated threefold body weight during the stance phase of gait, increasing to around three- to sixfold body weight during stair climbing (16). During sport participation, knee forces undoubtedly are greater, although quantitative estimates are lacking. Tension in the knee extensors also increases lateral stability of the knee, with tension in the knee flexors contributing to medial stability.

The menisci assist with force absorption at the knee, bearing as much as an estimated 45% of the total load (17). The medial two-thirds of each meniscus have an internal structure that is particularly well suited to resisting compression. The menisci also serve to distribute force from the femur over a broader area and, in doing so, reduce the magnitude of joint stress. Tibiofemoral joint stress is an estimated threefold higher during weight bearing when the menisci have been removed. Because the menisci also serve to protect the articulating bone surfaces from wear, knees that have undergone complete or partial meniscectomies still may function adequately, but such knees are more likely to develop degenerative conditions.

Forces at the Patellofemoral Joint

Compressive force at the patellofemoral joint has been found to be half the body weight during normal walking gait, increasing up to eightfold body weight during stair climbing (18). Although the greatest amount of contact with the surface area is reached between 60 and 90° of flexion, the greatest compressive forces are exerted on the patella at 30° of flexion (19).

The squat exercise, which is known for being particularly stressful to the knee complex, produces a patellofemoral joint reaction force more than sevenfold body weight. Given the small contact area between the articulating bone surfaces, the transmitted stress at the patellofemoral joint during such maneuvers is high. The point of application of the resultant contact force moves superiorly as the knee goes through 20 to 90° of flexion.

PREVENTION OF KNEE CONDITIONS

Because many of the muscles that move the knee also move the hip, prevention of knee injuries must focus on a well-rounded physical conditioning program. Although much debate continues as to the effectiveness of prophylactic knee braces (see Chapter 3), recent rule changes and improved shoe design have contributed significantly to a reduction of injuries at the knee.

Physical Conditioning

The development of a well-rounded physical conditioning program is the key to injury prevention. Exercises should include flexibility and muscular strength, endurance, and power as well as speed, agility, balance, and cardiovascular fitness. Lack of flexibility can predispose an individual to muscular strains. Exercises should focus on general flexibility and may be performed either alone or with a partner using proprioceptive neuromuscular facilitation stretching techniques. In particular, stretching exercises should focus on the quadriceps, hamstrings, gastrocnemius, IT band, and adductors. Because many of these muscles contribute to knee stability, strengthening programs also should focus on these muscle groups. Specific exercises to prevent injury to the musculature that moves the knee are provided in Field Strategy 17.1. Additional exercises for muscles that cross the hip region

FIELD STRATEGY 17.1

Exercises to Prevent Injury at the Knee

1. **Hamstrings stretch, seated position.** Place the leg to be stretched straight out, with the opposite foot tucked toward the groin. Reach toward the toes until a stretch is felt.

3. **Iliotibial band stretch, supine position.** With the trunk stabilized, adduct the leg to be stretched over the other leg, and allow gravity to passively stretch the iliotibial band.

2. **Quadriceps stretch, prone position.** Push the heel toward the buttocks, and then raise the knee off the floor until tension is felt.

4. **Iliotibial band stretch, standing position.** Cross the limb to be stretched behind the other, extending and adducting the hip as far as possible.

5. Closed chain exercises:

- Step-ups, step-downs, and lateral step-ups
- Leg press
- Lunges
- Squats (never below 85–90°)

6. Open chain exercises:

- Knee extension (quadriceps)
- Knee flexion (hamstrings)

are demonstrated in Field Strategy 16.1. Many of these exercises can be supplemented with tubing to add resistance to the exercise.

Rule Changes

Rule changes in contact sports, particularly football, have significantly reduced injuries to the knee region. Specifically, modifications in acceptable techniques that prohibit blocking at or below the knee and blocking from behind have reduced traumatic injuries. Proper training methods on correct technique should continue throughout the season to ensure compliance with specific rules designed to prevent injury.

Shoe Design

Shoe design is discussed in Chapter 3. In field sports, shoes may have a flat-sole, long-cleat, short-cleat, or multicleated design. The cleats should be properly positioned under the major weight-bearing joints of the foot and should not be felt through the sole of the shoe. Shoes with longer, irregular cleats placed at the peripheral margin of the sole with a number of smaller, pointed cleats in the middle produce higher torsional resistance and are associated with a significantly higher ACL injury rate compared with shoe models having flat cleats and screw-in cleats or with pivot-disk models (19). In football, a cleated shoe with a higher number of shorter, broader cleats can prevent the foot from becoming fixed to the ground yet allow good traction during running and cutting maneuvers.

CONTUSIONS

A volleyball player fell on the knee and felt an intense pain on the anterior of the joint. Pain is palpable on either side of the patellar tendon but not directly on the tendon. The individual reports a "catching" sensation. Extreme pain is felt with forced knee extension. What condition should be suspected, and how should the injury be managed?

Contusions resulting from compressive forces (i.e., a kick or falling on the knee) are common at the knee. General signs and symptoms include localized tenderness, pain, swelling, and ecchymosis. Other injuries may be obscured if swelling is extensive. For example, being kicked on the medial aspect of the tibia may appear as a contusion when, in fact, the impact may have caused an avulsion fracture of the MCL or an epiphyseal injury in an adolescent. Extreme point tenderness and positive findings on any of the special tests should indicate a more serious injury, and referral to a physician is indicated.

Fat Pad Contusion

The infrapatellar fat pad may become entrapped between the femur and tibia or inflamed during arthroscopy, leading to a tender, puffy, fat pad contusion.

Signs and Symptoms

Signs and symptoms include locking, catching, giving way, palpable pain on either side of the patellar tendon, and extreme pain on forced extension.

Management

Following a full assessment to rule out fracture and major ligament damage, initial treatment includes ice, compression, elevation, rest, and nonsteroidal anti-inflammatory drugs (NSAIDs). Participation in sport and physical activity usually is not limited; however, the area should be protected to prevent further insult.

Peroneal Nerve Contusion

The common peroneal nerve leaves the popliteal space and winds around the fibular neck to supply motor and sensory function to the anterior and lateral compartments of the lower leg (see Fig. 17.4). A kick or blow to the posterolateral aspect of the knee can contuse this nerve, leading to temporary or permanent paralysis. The nerve also may be injured by prolonged compression from a knee brace or elastic wrap, prolonged squatting (e.g., baseball or softball catcher), or traction caused by a varus stress or hyperextension at the knee.

Signs and Symptoms

In a mild acute injury, an immediate "shocking" feeling of pain may radiate down the lateral aspect of the leg and foot. If the actual nerve is not damaged, tingling and numbness may persist for several minutes. In severe cases (i.e., when the nerve is crushed), initial pain is not immediately followed by tingling or numbness. Rather, as swelling increases within the nerve sheath, muscle weakness in dorsiflexion or eversion as well as loss of sensation on the dorsum of the foot, particularly between the great and second toes, may progressively occur days or weeks later.

Management

Treatment involves standard acute care for contusions. If the condition does not rapidly improve, however, it is necessary to monitor any sensory changes or motor weakness as indicated and, at the first sign of change, refer the individual to a physician.

The volleyball player probably contused the infrapatellar fat pad during the fall onto the knee. Standard acute care (i.e., ice, compression, elevation, and protected rest) should be sufficient to address the injury.

BURSITIS

As part of rehabilitation for a shoulder injury, a 30-year-old man is maintaining cardiovascular fitness by using a stationary bike. Following 1 week on the bike, the individual complains of pain on the proximal, medial tibia just distal to the knee joint. The pain is particularly evident after his workout. What structure may be inflamed, and are there any factors that may contribute to this condition?

Bursitis can be caused by direct trauma, overuse, infections, metabolic abnormalities, rheumatic afflictions, and **neoplasms** (tumors). Compressive forces from a direct blow can be associated with a grossly distended, warm bursal sac filled with bloody effusion, called a hemobursa. Repeated insult can lead to the more common chronic bursitis, in which the bursal wall thickens and, when filled with fluid, appears to be distended.

Abrasions or penetrating injuries can lead to infected bursitis caused by bacteria entering broken skin. This condition differs from acute bursitis because of the localized and intense redness, increased pain, enlarged regional lymph nodes, spreading cellulitis, and subsequent fever and malaise. If infection is suspected, immediate referral to a physician is warranted for proper cleansing, irrigation, and closure (often with a drain). The infection can enter the lymph system, causing pyarthrosis, or suppurative arthritis, at the knee.

The suprapatellar bursa rarely is injured by direct trauma, except in the case of a puncture wound. It may, however, become enlarged and inflamed secondary to inflammation in the knee joint capsule.

Because of its location, the prepatellar bursa is injured more frequently by direct blows and shearing forces. Swelling can occur immediately or over a 24-hour period, obscuring the visible outline of the patella. Direct pressure over the bursa and passive flexion of the knee lead to considerable pain. Chronic prepatellar bursitis is more common than an acute episode and usually is the result of repeated episodes of microtrauma. The condition may remain asymptomatic except for mild discomfort when firm pressure is applied directly over the bursa.

Inflammation of the deep infrapatellar bursa usually is caused by overuse and subsequent friction between the patellar tendon and the structures behind it (i.e., fat pad and tibia). Because this bursa lies posterior to the patellar tendon, inflammation of the bursa often is confused with Osgood-Schlatter disease in adolescents and with patellar tendinitis in older individuals. In extension, the fat pad is squeezed between the patellar tendon and tibia and often extends beyond the sides of the tendon. Carefully palpating over the distal patellar tendon and noting the specific area of tenderness will determine which condition is present. In flexion, bursitis is indicated by pain deep to the patellar tendon. In extension, pain palpated on either side of the patellar tendon indicates a fat pad contusion.

Inflammation of the pes anserine bursa typically develops from friction, but it also may occur in direct trauma. It often is seen in runners, cyclists, and swimmers who are subjected to excessive valgus stress at the knee or in individuals who have tight hamstrings. Initial symptoms include point tenderness beneath the pes tendons (usually 2 cm below the joint line), localized swelling, and crepitation. When inflamed, contraction of the hamstring muscles, rotational movements of the tibia, and direct pressure over the bursa produce pain. Inflammation of this bursa more commonly is seen in middle-aged or older, overweight women, many of whom also have osteoarthritis of the knee (20). To avoid recurrence, the individual should begin an extensive flexibility program for the hamstrings and gastrocnemius–soleus complex.

The term Baker's cyst identifies almost any synovial herniation of the posterior joint capsule, or bursitis on the posterior aspect of the knee. With no posterior obstruction, internal derangement injuries (i.e., meniscal problems, cruciate ligament tears, or arthritis) commonly lead to joint effusion that expands into the bursal sac. The semimembranosus bursa most commonly is involved, because it often communicates with the joint capsule. A soft, tumorous mass can be palpated in the medial popliteal space and may or may not be painful. A Baker's cyst does not pose a serious problem, although it may be bothersome during full flexion or extension of the knee.

Signs and Symptoms

Common symptoms of bursitis include swelling and pain in the prepatellar region (i.e., prepatellar bursitis), in the distal patellar tendon region (i.e., deep infrapatellar bursitis), in the proximal medial tibia (i.e., pes anserine bursitis), or over the medial joint line (i.e., tibial collateral ligament bursitis).

Management

Treatment consists of ice therapy, a compressive wrap, NSAIDs, avoiding activities that irritate the condition, or total rest until acute symptoms subside. A protective foam, or doughnut, pad may protect the area from further insult. A risk of infection exists if the skin is broken during the initial injury, in which case the individual should be referred to a physician immediately. The physician may culture any aspirated fluid to detect bacteria and subsequently prescribe medication.

Corticosteroid injections may be administered by the physician in cases of chronic or persistent bursitis when other means of treatment have been ineffective in decreasing inflammation (20). Because these injections can weaken surrounding tendons or ligaments, they should not be injected close to these structures.

(A) *The 30-year-old man using the stationary bike to maintain cardiovascular fitness could have pes anserine bursitis. Tight hamstrings and excessive valgus stress placed on the knee during the pedaling motion can predispose an individual to this injury. In addition to standard acute care, this individual should begin an extensive flexibility program for the hamstrings and gastrocnemius–soleus complex.*

LIGAMENTOUS CONDITIONS

(Q) *A basketball player decelerated, set the left foot, and then forcefully pushed off the left leg to perform a right-handed lay-up shot. The player felt a sudden popping sensation and intense pain, and then the knee collapsed. Initial evaluation revealed point tenderness on the anteromedial joint line. The basketball player has swelling but no signs of deformity. What structures might be involved with this injury?*

Knee joint stability depends on a static, passive system of support from its ligaments and capsular structures. The American Academy of Orthopaedic Surgeons (AAOS) classifies ligamentous injuries at the knee according to the functional disruption of a specific ligament, or amount of laxity (Box

Box 17.2   Signs and Symptoms of Ligament Failure

Minimal Ligament Failure (Distraction, <5 mm)
- Less than one-third of the fibers are torn.
- Mild swelling and pain are localized over the injury site (with the medial collateral ligament, pain is in the proximal 1–2 inches).
- Active and passive range of motion are normal; and muscular strength is normal or slightly decreased.
- No joint laxity is apparent during the stress test.
- Definite end feel is present.

Partial Ligament Failure (Distraction, 5–10 mm)
- One- to two-thirds of the ligament is damaged, with microtears present.
- Localized swelling and joint effusion may result from deep capsular tears, meniscal damage, or cruciate ligament damage.
- Pain is sharp and may be either transient or lasting.
- Individual may complain of instability and an inability to walk with the heel on the ground.
- Range of motion is decreased initially by pain and hamstring muscle spasm and later by soft-tissue swelling or effusion.
- Inability to fully extend the knee actively.
- Visible translation of the tibia during stress tests.

Complete Ligament Failure (Distraction, >10 mm)
- More than two-thirds of the ligament is ruptured.
- Swelling is diffuse, indicating severe capsular tear and damage to intracapsular structures.
- Pain is initially sharp and often disappears within a minute.
- Individual is aware of the feeling of instability or the knee giving way.
- Significant loss of range of motion.
- Visible distraction of greater than 10 mm during stress testing may appear as a subluxation.

17.2), and the direction of laxity. The AAOS identifies four straight instabilities and four rotary instabilities (Table 17.2). Knowing the knee position at impact and the direction the tibia displaces or rotates is beneficial in determining the damaged structures.

Unidirectional Instabilities

A straight plane (i.e., unidirectional) instability implies instability in one of the cardinal planes. Injury to the ACL or PCL produces instability in the sagittal plane, allowing equal anterior or posterior **translation** (i.e., shifting) of the medial and lateral tibial plateaus on the femur. Injury to the MCL and LCL leads to valgus or varus instability in the frontal plane. Although several structures may be damaged, the resulting instability involves a single plane.

Straight Medial Instability

In straight medial instability, or **valgus instability,** lateral forces cause tension on the medial aspect of the knee, potentially damaging the MCL and posteromedial capsular ligaments as well as the PCL (Fig. 17.6A).

SIGNS AND SYMPTOMS A grade I sprain is characterized by mild pain on the medial joint line, little or no joint effusion, full ROM that may include some discomfort, and a stable joint when doing the valgus stress test. A positive valgus test in 30° of flexion with a positive end feel indicates at least a grade II injury to the middle third of the capsular ligament and MCL. The individual may be unable to fully extend the leg and often walks on the ball of the foot, unable to keep the heel flat on the ground. A grade III MCL injury often has no significant intra-articular effusion, but if such effusion is found, injuries to the cruciate ligaments, patella, or meniscus should be assessed.

TABLE 17.2 Classification of Knee Instability and Structures Injured

INSTABILITY	STRESS TEST	POSSIBLE STRUCTURES INJURED IF TEST IS POSITIVE
Straight valgus (medal)	Abduction (valgus) stress with knee in full extension	1. Medial collateral ligament 2. Oblique popliteal ligament 3. Posteromedial capsule 4. Anterior cruciate ligament 5. Posterior cruciate ligament 6. Medial quadriceps expansion 7. Semimembranosus muscle
	Abduction (valgus) stress with knee slightly flexed (20–30°)	1. Medial collateral ligament 2. Oblique popliteal ligament 3. Posterior cruciate ligament
Straight varus (lateral)	Adduction (varus) stress with knee in full extension	1. Lateral collateral ligament 2. Posterolateral capsule 3. Arcuate–popliteus complex 4. Biceps femoris tendon 5. Anterior cruciate ligament 6. Posterior cruciate ligament 7. Lateral gastrocnemius muscle
	Adduction (varus) stress with knee slightly flexed (20–30°) and tibia laterally rotated	1. Lateral collateral ligament 2. Posterolateral capsule 3. Arcuate–popliteus complex 4. Iliotibial band 5. Biceps femoris tendon
Straight anterior	Anterior drawer test (90° knee flexion)	1. Anterior cruciate ligament (anteromedial bundle) 2. Posterolateral and posteromedial capsule 3. Deep medial collateral ligament 4. Iliotibial band 5. Oblique popliteal ligament 6. Arcuate–popliteus complex
	Lachman's test Modified Lachman's test	1. Anterior cruciate ligament (anteromedial bundle) 2. Oblique popliteal ligament 3. Arcuate–popliteus complex
Straight posterior	Posterior sag (gravity) test Posterior drawer sign Reverse Lachman's test	1. Posterior cruciate ligament (anterolateral bundle) 2. Arcuate–popliteus complex 3. Oblique popliteal ligament 4. Anterior cruciate ligament
Anteromedial rotary	Slocum drawer test (tibia internally rotated)	1. Medial collateral ligament 2. Oblique popliteal ligament 3. Posteromedial capsule 4. Anterior cruciate ligament
Anterolateral rotary	Slocum drawer test (tibia externally rotated) Lateral pivot shift test Jerk test Slocum ALRI Crossover test Flexion-rotation drawer test	1. Anterior cruciate ligament 2. Posterolateral capsule 3. Arcuate–popliteus complex 4. Lateral collateral ligament 5. Iliotibial band

TABLE 17.2 CONTINUED		
INSTABILITY	**STRESS TEST**	**POSSIBLE STRUCTURES INJURED IF TEST IS POSITIVE**
Posteromedial rotary	Posteromedial drawer test Posteromedial pivot shift test	1. Posterior cruciate ligament 2. Oblique popliteal ligament 3. Medial collateral ligament 4. Semimembranosus muscle 5. Posteromedial capsule 6. Anterior cruciate ligament
Posterolateral rotary	Posterolateral drawer test External rotation recurvatum test	1. Posterior cruciate ligament 2. Arcuate–popliteus complex 3. Lateral collateral ligament 4. Biceps femoris tendon 5. Posterolateral capsule 6. Anterior cruciate ligament

ALRI, anterolateral rotary instability.

A grade III injury has a positive valgus test with a soft or even absent end point because of a complete tear of the MCL, usually at the femoral attachment.

Straight Lateral Instability

Straight lateral instability, or **varus instability**, results from medial forces that produce tension on the lateral compartment, damaging the LCL, lateral capsular ligaments, PCL, and joint structures (Fig. 17.6B). This isolated injury is rare, because the biceps femoris, IT band, and popliteus provide a strong stabilizing effect. A potential mechanism for this injury can be seen in the sport of wrestling, in which an opponent often is between the individual's legs and is able to deliver an excessive varus force that can lead to injury.

SIGNS AND SYMPTOMS. Damage to the LCL has the same general signs and symptoms that are associated with an MCL sprain. Occasionally, the individual may hear or feel a pop, accompanied by sharp, lateral pain. Swelling is minimal, because the ligament is not attached to the joint capsule. Instability is subtle, because other structures are intact. A positive varus test in 30° of flexion, however, should confirm damage to the ligament. If tenderness is detected on the head of the fibula, an avulsion fracture or peroneal nerve injury may be present, although these injuries usually are associated with more severe knee injuries.

Straight Anterior Instability

In a straight anterior instability, both tibial plateaus sublux anteriorly by an equal amount when an anterior drawer test is performed. This translation is resisted by the ACL. Isolated anterior instability is rare; instead, an anteromedial or anterolateral laxity usually occurs. Damage to the ACL commonly occurs during a cutting or turning maneuver, landing, or sudden deceleration (Fig. 17.6C).

The rate of ACL injuries is higher in women that in men, particularly for those women who are involved with jumping and pivoting sports (21). Several theories have been put forth to explain this phenomenon, and recent research has begun to look at muscle strength imbalance between the hamstrings and quadriceps in both men and women. During a landing/deceleration maneuver, flexion moments are occurring at the hip and knee. Simultaneous eccentric contractions of the quadriceps to stabilize the knee and of the hamstrings to stabilize the hip decelerate the horizontal velocity of the body. The hamstrings also act to neutralize the tendency of the quadriceps to cause ante-

See *Possible Factors Influencing Increased Rate of Anterior Cruciate Ligament Injuries in Women,* available on the companion website at thePoint.

FIGURE 17.6 Knee instability. A, When a valgus force is applied to the knee, the medial collateral ligament and medial capsular ligaments are damaged, leading to valgus laxity. **B,** An isolated varus force damages the lateral collateral ligament, leading to varus laxity. **C,** When changing directions during deceleration, the anterior cruciate ligament can be damaged. **D,** During hyperextension of the knee or when the knee is flexed and the tibia is driven posterior, the posterior cruciate ligament can be damaged.

rior tibial translation. If the muscles are unable to meet the demand of stabilization, inert internal tissues, such as ligaments, cartilage, and bone, are at risk for injury. Therefore, a deficit in eccentric hamstrings strength relative to eccentric quadriceps strength could predispose an individual to an ACL injury. Prophylactic bracing has not been shown to prevent ACL injuries (22,23).

SIGNS AND SYMPTOMS. Pain can range from minimal and transient to severe and lasting. It may be described as being deep in the knee but more often is felt anterior, on either side of the patellar tendon, or laterally, on the joint line. In approximately 80% of ACL injuries, individuals experience a popping, snapping, or tearing sensation, and in a similar percentage of cases, individuals note a rapid onset (i.e., usually within 3 hours) of swelling (hemarthrosis). Weight bearing leads to a feeling of the knee giving way or "just not feeling right." The high incidence of damage to other internal structures necessitates immediate referral to a physician.

Straight Posterior Instability

In straight posterior instability, the medial and lateral tibial plateaus have equal translation posteriorly in a neutral position without rotation. The PCL, along with the arcuate complex and oblique popliteal ligament, provides nearly all resistance to prevent this motion. Hyperextension is the most common mechanism for injury. The PCL, however, also can be damaged during a fall on a flexed knee with the foot plantar flexed, resulting in a blow to the tibial tubercle that drives the tibia posteriorly (Fig. 17.6D).

SIGNS AND SYMPTOMS. In milder cases, intense pain and a sense of stretching are felt in the posterior aspect of the knee. In a total rupture, a characteristic pop or snap is felt and heard, and this may be followed by autonomic symptoms of dizziness, sweating, faintness, or slight nausea (23). A large effusion and hemarthrosis usually occur within the first 2 hours after the acute injury. Knee extension is limited because of the effusion and stretching of the posterior capsule and gastrocnemius. A positive posterior sag (gravity) test or reverse Lachman's test confirms damage to the PCL. When the PCL is torn, the extensor mechanism, including the patella and the patellar tendon, forcefully holds the tibia in a reduced position, which results in increased patellofemoral pressure. Increased patellofemoral loading also is caused by a vector change resulting from posterior tibial displacement. This concept may explain complaints of patellofemoral pain in individuals with PCL-deficient knees.

Multidirectional Instabilities

Whereas unidirectional instability involves damage that results in instability to a single plane, multidirectional instability involves instability in more than one plane. This injury also is called a multiplane or rotary instability.

Anteromedial Rotary Instability

Anteromedial rotary instability results from anterior external rotation of the medial tibia condyle on the femur, leading to damage of the medial compartment ligaments and oblique popliteal ligament (Fig. 17.7). This instability can be accentuated by a tear of the medial meniscus and ACL. Although referred to as the "unhappy triad," the MCL is the primary ligamentous restraint to this motion. In anteromedial rotary instability, valgus stress testing at 0 and 30° of flexion is positive. In addition, increased anterior translation of the medial tibial plateau is noted when a Slocum drawer test or Lachman's test is performed with the tibia externally rotated.

Anterolateral Rotary Instability

Anterolateral rotary instability (ALRI) is characteristic of an anterior internal subluxation of the lateral tibial condyle on the femur. The ACL is the primary structure damaged by this instability, but the IT band and lateral capsule ligaments also can be damaged. The injury typically is caused by a sudden deceleration and cutting maneuver, and it is the most frequent rotary instability at the knee. In anterolateral instability, the Slocum drawer test with the tibia internally rotated, jerk test, Slocum ALRI test, cross-over test, and flexion-rotation drawer test show increased anterior translation of the lateral tibial plateau.

Posteromedial Rotary Instability

In posteromedial rotary instability, the medial tibial plateau shifts posteriorly on the femur and opens medially. This is a severe injury and is indicative of damage to the superficial MCL, posteromedial capsule, oblique popliteal ligament, and both cruciate ligaments. Injury of the posteromedial capsule is suspected if joint space opening and a soft end point are apparent on valgus stress at 0°. The posteromedial drawer test and posteromedial pivot shift test are positive.

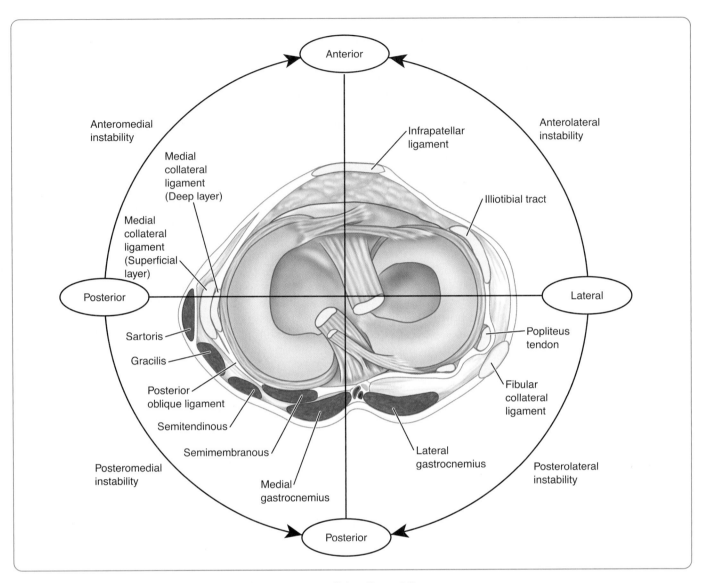

Anterior

Anteromedial
instability

Anterolateral
instability

Infrapatellar
ligament

Medial
collateral
ligament
(Deep layer)

Illiotibial tract

Medial
collateral
ligament
(Superficial
layer)

Posterior

Lateral

Sartoris

Popliteus
tendon

Gracilis

Posterior
oblique ligament

Fibular
collateral
ligament

Semitendinous

Semimembranous

Lateral
gastrocnemius

Posteromedial
instability

Posterolateral
instability

Medial
gastrocnemius

Posterior

■■■■■ FIGURE 17.7 **Instabilities at the knee.** *MCL,* medial collateral ligament.

Posterolateral Rotary Instability

In posterolateral rotary instability, a greater posterior translation of the lateral tibial plateau is noted, as compared to the medial tibial plateau, when a posterior drawer force is applied. This injury often is caused by a sudden anteromedial force that brings the knee joint from near-full extension into hyperextension. This mechanism, when combined with a varus moment, disrupts the posterolateral structures, which include the PCL, arcuate–popliteal complex, posterolateral capsule, and LCL. Other mechanisms may include a combined hyperextension and external rotation force, contact and noncontact hyperextension, severe varus bending moment, and severe tibial external rotation torque (24). Injury of the posterolateral capsule is suspected if joint space opening and a soft end point are apparent on varus stress at 0 and 30°. In addition, the posterolateral drawer and external rotation recurvatum tests are positive.

Knee Dislocations

Knee dislocations and less severe multiligament injuries make up approximately 20% of all grade III knee ligament injuries. Frequent two-ligament injuries include the ACL-MCL (most common), PCL-MCL, ACL-LCL, and ACL-PCL. Damage to only two ligaments does not result in enough translation of the joint to cause neurovascular injury. The exception, however, is injury to the LCL and a cruciate ligament that results in enough lateral opening to damage the peroneal nerve.

A minimum of three ligaments must be torn for the knee to dislocate. Most often, this involves the ACL, PCL, and one collateral ligament. Although dislocations may occur in any direction, the most common is in an anterior or posterior direction. As with any dislocation, additional damage can occur to other joint structures, including the ligaments, capsular structures, menisci, articular surfaces, tendons, and neurovascular structures. Associated injuries include vascular damage in 20 to 40% of knee dislocations and nerve damage in 20 to 30%. Posterior knee dislocations are associated with the highest incidence of damage to the popliteal artery; posterolateral rotary dislocations have the highest incidence of nerve injury.

Signs and Symptoms

The individual may describe a severe injury to the knee and hear a loud pop. Deformity of the knee may be present if the knee has dislocated and remained unreduced. Knee dislocations often reduce spontaneously, however, making identification difficult. Swelling occurs within the first few hours, but swelling may not be large because of an associated capsular injury and extravasation of the hemarthrosis. It is critical to identify the dislocated knee by the ligamentous structures that have been disrupted. If a vascular injury is left untreated or not repaired within 8 hours after injury, the amputation rate is 86%. If surgery is completed within 6 to 8 hours, however, the amputation rate drops to 11%. Associated nerve injury has a poor prognosis regardless of the treatment.

Management of Ligament Conditions

Injuries involving minimal ligament failure are managed conservatively, with ice application, compression, elevation, and protected rest until acute symptoms subside. A compression wrap, consisting of an inverted horseshoe around the patella secured by an elastic wrap, can be used with a knee immobilizer to reduce swelling. Cryotherapy and NSAIDs are used to reduce pain and inflammation. In suspected ACL injuries, radiographs should be obtained to rule out an associated intra-articular fracture. Avulsion fractures of the tibial eminence may occur, particularly in adults older than 35 years who have some associated osteopenia. Magnetic resonance imaging can clarify the diagnosis.

In consultation with a physician, a moderate injury with partial ligament failure is managed with ice, compression, elevation, and protected rest for 24 to 72 hours. Crutches are used until the individual walks without a limp. Progression to partial weight bearing with heel-to-toe gait can begin as tolerated. Rehabilitation should be initiated as soon as acute symptoms subside. Range-of-motion exercises should include assisted knee flexion and knee extension. Isometric exercises of the quadriceps and straight leg raises in all directions should progress to resisted exercises throughout the full ROM. Closed chain strengthening exercises and maintenance of ROM can be supplemented with cardiovascular exercises as tolerated.

The physician may determine that surgical repair is necessary for injuries in which isolated complete ligament failure has occurred or in which more than one major ligament is involved. Surgical reconstruction is based on the degree of laxity, activity-specific demands, hours per week of activity, intensity of activity, frequency of instability, and associated repairable meniscal tear. Reconstruction usually is delayed at least 3 weeks postinjury to allow swelling to decrease and ROM to increase. Field Strategy 17.2 describes the management and rehabilitation of a mild ACL injury.

 The basketball player may have sustained an injury to the medial meniscus, the ACL, or the MCL. Additional assessment is necessary to confirm the involved structure.

MENISCAL CONDITIONS

A 40-year-old golfer complains of mild swelling and tenderness on the medial joint line. Slight joint effusion is present, and pain can be elicited with rotation of the tibia on the femur and during extreme knee flexion. What injury may be present, and what is the management for this injury?

FIELD STRATEGY 17.2

Management of an Anterior Cruciate Injury

Phase 1

1. Protect, restrict activity, ice, compression, elevation, and rest with a knee immobilizer to reduce swelling.
2. Use crutches if the individual cannot bear weight without pain.
3. Range-of-motion exercises within pain-free limits:
   - Heel slides.
   - Prone knee flexion, assisted with the opposite leg.
   - Passive knee extension in a supine or seated position.
4. Strengthening exercises:
   - Bent leg raises in all directions.
   - Multiangle isometric exercises for the quadriceps, hamstrings, and hip adductors.
5. Cardiovascular fitness. Upper body ergometer and unilateral leg cycling.

Phase 2

1. Range of motion. Continue exercises to regain full range of motion.
2. Unilateral balance activities. See Field Strategy 17.1, and progress as tolerated.
3. Strengthening exercises:
   - Perform slow, controlled, eccentric closed chain exercises, such as two-legged squats to 60°, step-ups, step-downs, and lateral step-ups.
   - Calf raises (seated position) can progress to standing position when pain-free.
   - Perform straight leg raises in all directions, with tubing added as tolerated.

Phase 3

1. Range of motion. Maintain full range of motion and flexibility in the lower extremity.
2. Strengthening:
   - Hip leg press and squats.
   - Toe raises with weights.
   - Lunges.
   - Isokinetic open and closed chain exercises.
3. Cardiovascular fitness:
   - Bilateral, minimal tension cycling if 110 to 115° of knee flexion is present. Avoid full knee extension.
   - Pool running, swimming with a flutter kick, jogging in place on a trampoline, and power walking.

Phase 4

1. Balance and proprioception. Continue exercises from the preceding.
2. Functional activities:
   - Running drills, such as circles, figure-eights, crossover steps (kariocas), and jumping with double limb/single limb progressing from standing in place, front to back, to diagonals.
   - Multidirectional, high-speed balance drills are added after the individual can run 2 to 3 miles.
   - Jumping, bounding, and skipping (plyometrics).
   - Slide board.

Menisci, which become stiffer and less resilient with age, are injured in manners similar to the ligamentous structures. In addition to compression and tensile forces, shearing forces caused when the femur rotates on a fixed tibia trap the posterior horns of both menisci, leading to some tearing. Tears are classified according to age, location, or axis of orientation. Medial meniscus damage is more common than lateral meniscus damage because of the lower mobility of the structure.

Longitudinal tears result from a twisting motion when the foot is fixed and the knee is flexed (Fig. 17.8A). This action produces compression and torsion on the posterior peripheral attachment. The tear can be partial, affecting only the peripheral segment of the meniscus, or a complete tearing of the inner substance of the meniscus. A **"bucket-handle"** tear occurs when an entire longitudinal segment is displaced medially toward the center of the tibia (Fig. 17.8B). This tear can lead to locking of the knee at approximately 10° flexion; however, this only occurs in approximately 40% of complete meniscal tears.

Horizontal cleavage tears result from degeneration and often affect the posteromedial portion of the meniscus (Fig. 17.8C). With age, shearing forces from rotational motions tear the inner substance of the meniscus. If detached, momentary locking, associated pain, and instability may occur. A parrot-beak tear is actually two tears that commonly occur in the middle segment of the lateral menisci, leading to the characteristic shape of a parrot's beak. It is seen more frequently in individuals with a history of previous trauma or some cystic pathology that makes the meniscus more fixed at its periphery (Fig. 17.8D).

■■■ FIGURE 17.8 **Meniscal tears. A,** Longitudinal. **B,** Bucket-handle. **C,** Horizontal. **D,** Parrot-beak.

Signs and Symptoms

Meniscal injuries are difficult to assess, both because they are not innervated by nociceptors and because only 10 to 30% of the peripheral medial meniscus border and 10 to 25% of the lateral meniscus border receive direct blood supply. Localized pain and joint-line tenderness near the collateral ligament probably are the most common findings. Anterior joint-line pain rarely reflects meniscal pathology unless a bucket-handle or ruptured bucket-handle tear is present. Because the meniscal periphery is attached to the synovial lining, tensile forces may cause synovial inflammation and slight joint effusion more than 12 hours after the initial injury. Pain occurs on rotation and extreme flexion of the knee (e.g., duck walk or deep knee squats). In the initial assessment, it is important to determine whether the knee lacked full extension from the time of injury (i.e., locked knee from displaced fragment) or lacked full extension the next day (i.e., pseudolocking from a hamstring spasm).

A chronic degenerative meniscal tear often results from multiple episodes of minimal trauma leading to almost no pain, disability, or swelling, although atrophy of the quadriceps may be present. Recurrent locking is typical. Chronic tears in the absence of degeneration have point tenderness only over the site of the lesion. The individual may experience a popping, grinding, or clicking sensation that can lead to the knee buckling or giving way. Special tests used to identify meniscal injuries include McMurray's test, Apley's compression test, and the "bounce home" test.

Management

Initial treatment depends on the extent of damage. Mild cases with no ligamentous instability are managed with standard acute care, including ice, compression, elevation, protected rest, NSAIDs, and use of crutches as needed. Isometric strengthening exercises can be initiated when swelling has subsided. Field Strategy 17.3 summarizes the initial management and suggested rehabilitation exercises for a mild meniscal injury.

If joint effusion is extensive, immediate referral to a physician is warranted. Immediate referral also is necessary if the knee is locked and cannot be spontaneously reduced.

Bucket-handle tear segments can be excised surgically without removing the total meniscus, although regeneration of the centrally displaced portion will not occur. Arthroscopic meniscectomy is performed as an outpatient procedure under local anesthesia, with return to function following partial meniscectomy within 2 to 6 weeks. Total meniscectomy increases rotary instability and can lead to arthritis.

(A) *The golfer has mild joint effusion and pain on the medial joint line that increases with rotation and extreme flexion of the knee. This suggests a possible chronic meniscal tear. This individual should be referred to a physician.*

PATELLAR AND RELATED CONDITIONS

(Q) *A high school wrestler complains of an aching pain on the lateral side of the patella that increases during the workout. Slight effusion is present in the patellofemoral joint, and pain is elicited over the lateral patellar border. Intense pain is felt when the patella is pushed downward into the patellofemoral groove. What factors may contribute to this condition, and what long-term management should be considered after acute symptoms have subsided?*

FIELD STRATEGY 17.3

Management of a Partial Meniscectomy

Phase 1

1. Protect, restrict activity, ice, compression, elevation, and bracing to reduce swelling. Use crutches if needed.
2. Range-of-motion exercises within pain-free limits:

   - Heel slides.
   - Supine wall slides.
   - Prone knee flexion, assisted with the opposite leg.
   - Passive knee extension in a supine or seated position.

Phase 2

1. Range of motion. Continue exercises as tolerated.
2. Unilateral balance activities. See Field Strategy 17.1.
3. Strengthening exercises. Include:

   - Multiangle isometric exercises for the quadriceps, hamstrings, and hip adductors.
   - Straight leg raises in all directions. Add tubing or ankle weights during later stages.
   - Short-arc quadriceps extension exercises. Place a pillow or bolster under the knee to support the knee at 45° of flexion. Extend the knee, and hold for 10 seconds. Add ankle weights to increase resistance.
   - Toe raises from a seated position can progress to standing position when pain-free.
   - Straight leg raises in all directions, with tubing added as tolerated.

4. Cardiovascular fitness:

   - Use upper body ergometer and a stationary cycle with bilateral minimal tension if 115 to 120° of knee flexion is present. Avoid full knee extension.

Phase 3

1. Range of motion. Maintain full range of motion and flexibility in the lower extremity.
2. Strengthening:

   - Hip leg press and squats.
   - Toe raises with weights.
   - Lunges.
   - Isokinetic open and closed chain exercises.

3. Cardiovascular fitness:

   - Pool running, swimming with a flutter kick, jogging on a trampoline, and power walking.

Phase 4 (Return to Activity)

1. Maintain range of motion, flexibility, strength, and balance.
2. Functional activities. See Field Strategy 17.2.

The patellofemoral joint is the region most commonly associated with anterior knee pain. Patellar tracking disorders and instability within the joint, along with obesity, direct trauma, and repetitive motions, all contribute to a variety of injuries. Patellofemoral pain may be classified into mechanical causes (e.g., patellar subluxation or dislocation), inflammatory causes (e.g., prepatellar bursitis or patellar tendinitis), and other causes (e.g., reflex sympathetic dystrophy or tumors).

The main dynamic stabilizer is the quadriceps mechanism. More accurately called the **extensor mechanism**, it is made up of the vastus lateralis, vastus intermedius, vastus medialis, and rectus femoris, each of which is innervated by the femoral nerve. The vastus medialis has two heads, the superior longus head (vastus medialis longus) and the VMO. The VMO fibers approach the patella at a 55° angle. Although the VMO is incapable of producing knee extension, it provides a dynamic restraint to forces that would laterally displace the patella. Atrophy of this muscle nearly always is evident in patellofemoral dysfunction. The pes anserinus muscle group and the biceps femur influence patellar stability, because they control tibial internal and external rotation, which can significantly influence patellar tracking.

The static stabilizers include the anteriorly projected, lateral aspect of the femoral sulcus, the extensor retinaculum, IT band, quadriceps tendon, and patellar tendon. Oblique condensations of the retinacula produce the patellofemoral ligament and the medial and lateral patellotibial ligaments (Fig. 17.9). The structures that resist medial displacement of the patella (i.e., lateral retinaculum and

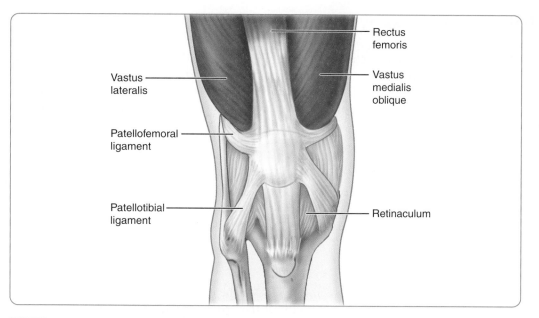

■■■■ FIGURE 17.9 Extensor mechanism. The extensor mechanism is composed of dynamic and static stabilizers. Working together, they combine rolling and gliding motions to place the femur and patella in specific positions to effect the deceleration mechanism of the patellofemoral articulation and provide stability and function at the knee.

IT band) are thicker and stronger than the soft-tissue structures that resist lateral displacement forces (i.e., medial retinaculum and lateral aspect of femoral sulcus). The patellar tendon resists superior displacement forces on the patella, whereas the quadriceps tendon resists inferior displacement of the patella. Both medial and lateral retinacula assist in knee extension even though the patellar tendon may be ruptured.

Deficiencies in stabilization of the extensor mechanism can be caused by several abnormalities of the patellofemoral region (Box 17.3), which can lead to anterior knee pain. Each condition can be counterbalanced in a healthy knee by the triangular shape of the patella, depth of the patellofemoral groove, and limiting action of the static ligamentous structures. Failure of medial structures to restrain the patella in a balanced position, or the presence of bony anomalies, can result in lateral tilting or lateral excursion of the patella, which in turn leads to patellofemoral **arthralgia**, or severe joint pain.

Box 17.3   Causes of Patellofemoral Pain

- Patellar instability caused by:
  - Abnormally shaped medial patellar facet
  - Shallow patellofemoral (trochlear) groove
  - Variable length and width of the patellar tendon
  - Patella alta (high-riding patella)
- Weak vastus medialis oblique (VMO) or VMO dysplasia
- Hypermobility of the patella caused by:
  - Muscle atrophy after an injury
  - Tightness of the lateral retinaculum, iliotibial band, and hamstrings

- Anatomical malalignment caused by:
  - Shallow patellofemoral groove
  - Excessive femoral anteversion or external tibial rotation
  - Genu valgum or genu recurvatum
  - Increased Q-angle
  - Excessive foot pronation
- Plica syndromes and repetitive minor trauma

Patellofemoral Stress Syndrome

Patellofemoral stress syndrome, also called lateral patellar compression syndrome, is pain in the patellofemoral joint without documented instability. The condition often occurs when either the VMO is weak or the lateral retinaculum that holds the patella firmly to the femoral condyle is excessively tight. Pain results when a tense lateral retinaculum passes over the trochlear groove or when increased patellofemoral stresses are transferred from the articular cartilage to pain fibers in the subchondral bone.

Signs and Symptoms

The individual may report a dull, aching pain in the anterior knee that is made worse by squatting, sitting in a tight space with the knee flexed, and descending stairs or slopes. Point tenderness can be located over the lateral facet of the patella, with intense pain and crepitus elicited when the patella is manually compressed into the patellofemoral groove. Synovial inflammation also may be present.

Management

Treatment involves standard acute care and NSAIDs. The entire lower extremity should be assessed for gait characteristics, flexibility, and strength of the proximal and distal portions. It is important to determine the presence of decreased rotation or strength in the lateral rotators of the hip as well as tightness in the hamstrings, quadriceps, and Achilles tendon. The McConnell taping technique uses both passive taping of the patella to correct patellar position and tracking during knee motion. Patellofemoral support devices may be used to prevent lateral displacement of the patella, or orthotics may be employed to correct foot malalignment conditions.

Rehabilitation should focus on recruiting the VMO, normalizing patella mobility, and increasing flexibility and muscle control of the lower extremity. Resisted terminal knee extension exercises, straight leg raises in hip flexion and adduction, and quadriceps isometric, isotonic, and high-speed isokinetic exercises in a 60 to 90° arc may be performed. If the VMO is not monitored using biofeedback devices, proper recruitment is difficult to determine. Closed chain exercises often are preferred because of the decrease in patellofemoral compression forces. Examples of closed kinetic chain exercises include knee flexion of 30 to 70° and lateral steps up of from 1 to 8 inches to allow eccentric and concentric movements. Eccentric quadriceps strengthening is emphasized, because the quadriceps muscle is an important decelerator. Strengthening of the hip muscles to prevent adduction and internal rotation is critical to allow the progression of closed chain exercises. Restoring proprioception also is critical in re-establishing neuromuscular control. Weight-training programs that load the patellofemoral joint, such as bent-knee exercises, should be avoided.

Chondromalacia Patellae

Chondromalacia patellae is a true degeneration in the articular cartilage of the patella, which results when compressive forces exceed the normal physical range or when alterations in patellar excursion produce abnormal shear forces that damage the articular surface. Because articular cartilage does not contain nerve endings, chondromalacia should not be considered as the true source of anterior knee pain. Chondromalacia is a surgical finding that represents areas of hyaline cartilage trauma or aberrant loading; it is not the cause of pain. The medial and lateral patellar facets are most commonly involved. The condition is confirmed when pain results from Clarke's test and Waldron's test. Chondromalacia has four stages, which are detailed in Figure 17.10.

Management

Asymptomatic chondromalacia does not require treatment; if the condition becomes symptomatic, standard acute care is the appropriate protocol. Most individuals respond well to mild anti-inflammatory medication, quadriceps strengthening, and a hamstring flexibility program. All resisted exercises with knee extension from a fully flexed position, crouches, and deep knee bends should be avoided, because these positions may aggravate the condition. A knee sleeve with a patellar cutout may be helpful. If this does not reduce the symptoms, the condition may require surgical intervention, such

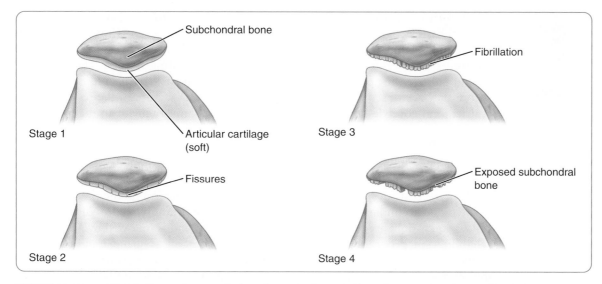

■■ ■ FIGURE 17.10 Four stages of chondromalacia patellae. Stage 1 involves softening or blistering of the cartilage. Stage 2 reveals fissures in the cartilage. Stage 3 is reached when fibrillation of the cartilage occurs, causing a "crabmeat" appearance. Stage 4 reveals cartilage defects with subchondral bone exposed.

as arthroscopic patellar debridement, lateral retinacular release, extensor mechanism realignment, or elevation of the tibial tubercle to relieve patellar compression forces.

Patellar Instability and Dislocations

Patellar instability occurs when the patella has normal or abnormal alignment in the trochlear groove but is displaced by internal or external forces. Displacement can range from microinstability to subluxation or gross dislocation. Factors that may lead to congenital malalignment of the extensor mechanism include VMO dysplasia, vastus lateralis hypertrophy, high and lateral patellar posture, increased Q-angle, and bony deformity.

Signs and Symptoms

In a subluxation, transient partial displacement of the patella from the femoral trochlea may occur acutely, as in a patellar dislocation, or be intermittent, with spontaneous reduction of the displacement. The individual may or may not have a history of complete dislocation or patellofemoral pain but reports a feeling of the patella slipping when cutting, twisting, or pivoting. Joint effusion may develop, but it improves rapidly when the individual resumes activity.

Chronic subluxations produce less swelling, pain, and disability. The condition is verified by observing patellar position during active knee flexion and extension and by a positive patellar apprehension test. An individual with patellofemoral stress syndrome is not apprehensive with this test, whereas one with patellar pain resulting from subluxation resists any attempt to displace the patella laterally.

Acute patellar subluxations and dislocations appear the same and generally occur during deceleration with a cutting maneuver (Fig. 17.11). Distinguishing one from the other depends on patient history. In a dislocation, the individual reports that the patella moved and had to be pushed back into place; with a subluxation, the individual reports that the patella slipped out and then went back into place spontaneously. The majority of the medial muscular and retinacular attachments are torn from the medial aspect of the patella, leading to an audible pop and violent collapse of the knee. Localized tenderness also may occur along the medial extensor retinaculum or at the adductor tubercle, which is the origin of the medial patellofemoral ligament. In addition, there may be localized tenderness along the peripheral edge of the lateral femoral condyle, where impaction from the patella occurs with flexion of the knee.

Typically, a traumatic displacement has acute effusion associated with a hemarthrosis occurring within the first 2 hours. A dislocation without acute effusion should signal chronic laxity; the tissues are so lax that the patella moves in and out of the groove without traumatizing surrounding tissues. The examiner should palpate the area to assess any defects in the medial retinaculum and VMO before they are obscured by swelling. Occasionally, a fracture of the patella or lateral femoral condyle occurs, resulting in a loose, bony fragment in the joint.

Management

Treatment includes ice, elevation, immobilization, and immediate referral to a physician. Following reduction of the dislocation by the physician, aspiration of the hemarthrosis may be indicated for comfort or to determine the presence of fat in the blood secondary to an osteochondral fracture. Immobilization of a first-time dislocation is only needed to control acute symptoms and is followed by an extensive rehabilitation program and functional patellar bracing. During immobilization, isometric quadriceps exercises and straight leg raises can be performed. When immobilization is removed, a full rehabilitative program to strengthen the dynamic stabilizers of the patellofemoral joint, particularly the VMO, and a flexibility program for the hamstrings and IT band should be initiated. A knee sleeve with a lateral pad to restrict lateral excursion and activity modification may be helpful. Most individuals with patellofemoral tracking disorders and instability can improve and return to activity without surgical intervention. An obvious disruption of the VMO insertion into the medial patellar edge, however, or a rupture of the medial patellofemoral ligament from the adductor tubercles responds best with early surgical repair (23).

■■ ■■ FIGURE 17.11 **Dislocated patella.** A dislocated patella often displaces laterally and is accompanied by an audible pop and violent collapse of the knee following deceleration involving a cutting maneuver.

Patella Plica Syndrome

The patella plica shelf is a fold in the synovial lining that projects into the joint cavity. This congenital abnormality is a remnant of the embryologic walls that divide the knee into medial, lateral, and suprapatellar pouches. Typically, it is crescent-shaped and extends from the infrapatellar fat pad medially (medial plica), loops around the femoral condyle, crosses under the quadriceps tendon in the suprapatellar region (suprapatellar plica), then passes laterally over the lateral femoral condyle to the lateral retinaculum (Fig. 17.12). Normally, a synovial plica remains asymptomatic until traumatized by a direct blow to the capsule or becomes inflamed and thickened from overuse, resulting from friction caused as the plica bow-strings across the medial femoral condyle. This bow-stringing results in two reservoirs for synovial fluid—namely, a suprapatellar reservoir and the cavity of the knee joint itself.

Signs and Symptoms

Anterior knee pain comes on gradually and is aggravated by quadriceps exercises. Approximately 25% of cases have a positive "movie-goer's sign" (i.e., pain with prolonged sitting). As the individual stands and begins to walk, a sharp pain is felt for 8 to 10 steps and then disappears. The pain is caused by the plica being maximally stretched and impinged within the patellofemoral joint. As the articularis genus muscle contracts several times, it elevates the plica enough to prevent further impingement. Occasionally, adhesions in the plica lead to a distinctive pop or snap as the individual extends the knee, or pseudolocking may occur over the medial patellofemoral joint, mimicking a torn meniscus. Assessment reveals slight joint effusion, palpable pain, and crepitus in the medial and lateral retinacular regions, particularly along the edge of the medial femoral condyle with the knee flexed at 45°. The test for medial synovial plica and the stutter test are positive.

Management

Treatment is symptomatic, with ice therapy, NSAIDs, activity modification, phonophoresis, and use of an external patellar support device. The condition may improve with hamstring stretching, heel cord stretching, and VMO strengthening exercises, especially if the VMO is dysplastic (abnormally developed). If the condition warrants, the plica shelf can be removed arthroscopically.

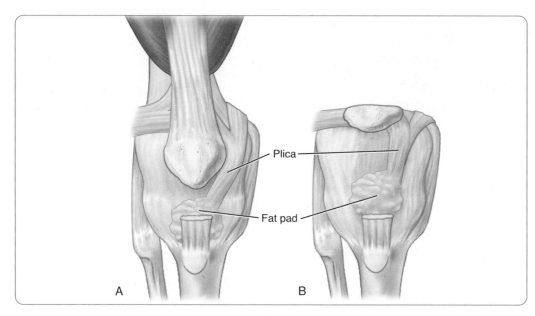

██ ██ ██ FIGURE 17.12 **Patella plica.** The patella plica is a fold in the synovial lining of the knee joint that can become inflamed and thickened by trauma where it extends over the femoral condyle or by microtrauma from overuse. **A,** Fully extended. **B,** Flexion of 90°.

Patellar Tendinitis (Jumper's Knee)

The patellar tendon frequently becomes inflamed and tender from repetitive or eccentric knee extension activities; these occur in running and in sports, such as volleyball and basketball, in which jumping is a critical action, hence the name "jumper's knee." Patellar subluxation, patellofemoral stress syndrome, and other conditions also can overload the patellar tendon, predisposing an individual to this condition. Extrinsic factors that can lead to the condition include frequency of training, years of play, playing surface, type of training, stretching and warm-up practices, and type of shoe that is worn. Some intrinsic factors that may have a role in contributing to the condition include lower extremity malalignment, leg-length discrepancies, muscle imbalance, anthropometric variables, muscle length, and muscle strength (25).

Signs and Symptoms

Most individuals will complain of chronic anterior knee pain of insidious onset, which might be described as a sharp or aching pain. Initially, pain after activity is concentrated on the inferior pole of the patella or the distal attachment of the patellar tendon on the tibial tubercle. As the condition progresses, pain is present at the beginning of activity, subsides during warm-up, then reappears after activity. Increased pain often is reported while ascending and descending stairs or after prolonged sitting. Eventually, pain is present both during and after activity and can become too severe for the individual to participate. Pain can be elicited during passive knee flexion beyond 120° and during resisted knee extension. It also is common to find tightness in the hamstrings, quadriceps, and heel cord, with weakness in the ankle dorsiflexors. Chronic tendinitis occasionally may lead to cystic changes at the distal pole of the patella or ectopic calcification and nodule formation in the tendon.

Management

Immediate treatment involves standard acute care and NSAIDs. Field Strategy 17.4 summarizes the management of patellar tendinitis.

Osgood-Schlatter Disease

Osgood-Schlatter disease is a traction-type injury to the tibial apophysis where the patellar tendon attaches onto the tibial tubercle (Fig. 17.13). Osgood-Schlatter disease typically develops in girls between the ages of 8 and 13 years and in boys between the ages 10 and 15 years at the beginning

FIELD STRATEGY 17.4

Management of Patellar Tendinitis

- Rest for 2 to 3 weeks to allow symptoms to subside.
- Modalities that may be used during the early stages of healing include heat therapy, electrical stimulation, phonophoresis, iontophoresis, and ultrasound.
- Transverse friction massage for 6 to 8 minutes.
- Initiate early flexibility exercises for the gastrocnemius-soleus complex, quadriceps, and hamstrings.
- Aquatic therapy during the early stages can reduce gravitational forces.
- Progressive resistance strengthening exercises may include:
  - Straight leg raises in all directions
  - Short-arc knee extension exercises
  - One-quarter knee squats
- Eccentric strengthening exercises for the quadriceps and dorsiflexors, such as drop squats (i.e., landing from a jump). Focus on the deceleration between the upward and downward phase. Increase deceleration as tolerated by the individual.
- Cardiovascular fitness should be maintained with exercises that do not involve powerful knee extension (i.e., upper body ergometer, swimming, and stationary bike with minimal tension).
- During the later stages, plyometrics may be incorporated (i.e., single-leg hop, double-leg hop, single-leg vertical jump, and bounding).
- A patellofemoral knee sleeve may reduce mobility of the patellar tendon during activity.

■■■■ FIGURE 17.13 **Patellar tendon traction-type injuries.** Patellar tendon traction-type injuries may involve Sinding-Larsen-Johansson disease or Osgood-Schlatter disease. The location of pain typically defines which problem is present.

of their growth spurt. It is estimated that the condition occurs in 21% of adolescent athletes, compared with 4.5% of age-matched nonathletes (26). The condition has been more common in boys, but with girls' increased participation in sports, the ratio may be equalizing.

Signs and Symptoms

Assessment of the condition usually is straightforward. Individuals point to the tibial tubercle as the source of pain, and the tubercle appears to be enlarged and prominent. Individuals report that pain generally occurs during activity and is relieved with rest. Point tenderness can be elicited directly over the tubercle, but ROM is not usually affected. Pain is present at the extremes of knee extension and forced flexion. Severity is rated in three grades, depending on the duration of pain:

- **Grade 1**—Pain after activity that resolves within 24 hours
- **Grade 2**—Pain during and after activity that does not hinder performance and resolves within 24 hours
- **Grade 3**—Continuous pain that limits sport performance and daily activities

Management

Treatment is symptomatic and self-limiting, but it may take 12 to 24 months for the condition to run its course. In most cases, activity is unrestricted unless pain is disabling. Shock-absorbent insoles in shoes may decrease peak stress on the tendon and tubercle. Application of cold for 20 minutes after activity should be beneficial, as should hamstrings and quadriceps stretching. Knee pads may protect the tibial tubercle when kneeling, or a knee strap (e.g., Cho-Pat® straps) may decrease the traction forces on the tibial tubercle. The condition rectifies with closure of the apophysis, but a small percentage of individuals develop a painful ossicle, which can necessitate surgical excision. Others may develop painful kneeling as adults.

Sinding-Larsen-Johansson Disease

A condition similar to Osgood-Schlatter disease is **Sinding-Larsen-Johansson disease**. Pain, swelling, and tenderness result from excessive strain on the inferior patellar pole at the origin of the patellar tendon (see Fig. 17.13). The condition usually is seen in children 8 to 13 years of age.

Signs and Symptoms

The onset of pain over the inferior patellar pole is gradual and seen in children who are involved in running and jumping sports. The condition often is missed unless the clinician palpates the inferior patellar pole with the individual's knee extended and the patellar tendon relaxed. Repeating the examination with the knee flexed at 90° should reveal diminished tenderness as the patellar tendon becomes taut.

Management

Treatment is symptomatic and similar to that for Osgood-Schlatter disease. Symptoms generally resolve quickly with standard acute care, NSAIDs, and activity modification.

Extensor Tendon Rupture

Extensor tendon ruptures can occur at the superior or inferior pole of the patella, the tibial tubercle, or within the patellar tendon itself. Ruptures result from powerful eccentric muscle contractions or in conjunction with severe ligamentous disruption at the knee. The rupture may be partial or total.

Signs and Symptoms

A partial rupture produces pain and muscle weakness in knee extension. If a total rupture occurs distal to the patella, assessment reveals a high-riding patella, a palpable defect over the tendon, and an inability to perform knee extension or perform a straight leg raise. If the quadriceps tendon is ruptured from the superior pole of the patella and the extensor retinaculum is still intact, knee extension is still possible, although it is weak and painful. Individuals with a history of previous corticosteroid injections, anabolic steroid abuse, or use of systemic steroids are at a greater risk for tendon ruptures. Steroid use can cause softening or weakening of collagen fibers in the muscle tendon, predisposing the tendon to premature rupture.

Management

Treatment involves standard acute care, use of a knee immobilizer, fitting the individual for crutches, and immediate referral to a physician. Treatment depends on the location and displacement of any bony fragment. In partial ruptures involving a shredded tendon, wiring through the patella may be necessary to relieve tension on the healing tendon. Surgical repair is necessary in total ruptures. Overall, the results of a delayed repair are less satisfactory than the results with an acute repair, but a delayed repair still provides an extensor mechanism and adequate function (27).

The high school wrestler complains of lateral patellofemoral pain that increases with certain maneuvers during practice. Precipitating factors that increase stress on the patellofemoral region include patellar instability, a weak VMO, hypermobility of the patella, and anatomical malalignment conditions. Following standard acute care, a total assessment of the lower extremity should be conducted to address deficiencies in muscle strength or biomechanical problems that contributed to the condition.

ILIOTIBIAL BAND FRICTION SYNDROME

Q *Following an evening practice session on the third day of preseason, a field-hockey player complains of a sharp ache over the lateral epicondyle of the femur that has gotten progressively worse since the start of the week. A history reveals that the daily double sessions have concentrated on technique drills and conditioning exercises. Observation reveals excessive foot pronation and genu varus. What actions might be taken to reduce the pain and correct the injury?*

A common condition in runners, cyclists, weight lifters, and volleyball players is IT band friction syndrome. The band originates on the lateral iliac crest and continues the line of pull from the tensor fasciae latae and gluteus maximus muscle; the deep fibers are associated with the lateral intermuscular septum. The distal fibers become thicker at their attachment on Gerdy's tubercle adjacent to the tibial tubercle on the lateral proximal tibia. The band drops posteriorly, behind the lateral femoral epicondyle, with knee flexion and then snaps forward over the epicondyle during extension (Fig. 17.14). Weight bearing increases compression and friction forces over the greater trochanter and lateral femoral condyle. Individuals with a malalignment problem are predisposed to this condition; see Box 17.4 for a listing of predisposing factors.

Signs and Symptoms

Initially, pain is present over the lateral aspect of the knee after running a certain mileage, typically late in the run, but does not restrict distance or speed. As the condition progresses, the pain begins to occur earlier and earlier, and it does restrict distance and speed. Pain may occur while running uphill and downhill and while climbing stairs. It is particularly intense on weight bearing from foot strike through midstance. During this part of the gait cycle, the IT band is most compressed between the lateral femoral epicondyle and greater trochanter of the femur. With continued activity, the initial lateral ache progresses into a more painful, sharp, and localized discomfort over the lateral femoral condyle approximately 2 to 3 cm above the lateral joint line and, occasionally, radiates distally to the tibial attachment or proximally up the thigh. Swelling may be noted at the distal IT band and palpation of the affected limb may reveal multiple trigger points in the vastus lateralis, gluteus medius, and biceps femoris (28). Palpation of these trigger points may cause referred pain to the lateral aspect of the affected knee. Flexion and extension of the knee may

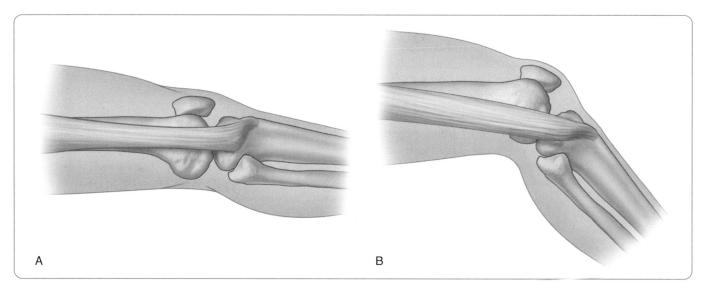

A   B

FIGURE 17.14 Iliotibial band. The iliotibial band drops posteriorly behind the lateral femoral epicondyle during knee flexion, then snaps forward over the epicondyle during extension. Malalignment problems or constant irritation can inflame the iliotibial band or lead to bursitis. **A,** Extension. **B,** Flexion.

Box 17.4 Predisposing Factors for Iliotibial Band Friction Syndrome

- Genu varus
- Excessive pronation in feet
- Leg-length discrepancy
- Prominent greater trochanter of femur
- Preexisting iliotibial band tightness
- Muscle weakness in knee extensors, knee flexors, and hip abductors
- Training errors, such as excessive distance in a single run, increasing mileage too quickly, inadequate warm-up, and running on the same side of a crowned road

produce a creaking sound. Positive Noble's and Ober's compression tests confirm the condition. Magnetic resonance images have shown that the distal band becomes thickened and that the potential space deep to the IT band over the femoral epicondyle becomes inflamed and filled with fluid (28). Eventually, pain restricts all running and becomes continuous during activities of daily living.

Management

The immediate treatment should be focused on alleviating inflammation with standard acute care and NSAIDs. Any activity that requires repeated knee flexion and extension should be limited. Field Strategy 17.5 describes the management of IT band friction syndrome.

The field-hockey player has IT band friction syndrome. The double sessions, coupled with the preexisting genu varus and pronated feet, have added strain to the IT band. Following standard acute care to control inflammation, an extensive flexibility program for the IT band should be initiated.

FIELD STRATEGY 17.5

Management of Iliotibial Band Friction Syndrome

- Ice, compression, elevation, nonsteroidal anti-inflammatory drugs, and rest until acute symptoms subside.
- Stretch hip abductors, flexors, and lateral thigh muscles.
- Foot orthotics may correct some structural problems.
- Non–weight bearing strengthening exercises, such as leg lifts and isometric exercises for knee flexion, extension, hip abduction, and adduction, can be initiated when pain-free, followed by concentric and eccentric strengthening of the hip and thigh muscles.
- Hill running should be avoided until asymptomatic.
- Running or training should be modified to the point of little or minimal pain during activity. Initially, this may necessitate an easy pace on level ground, progressing to increased mileage while maintaining pain-free activity.
- Cardiovascular fitness can be maintained with swimming.
- Ice massage before and after running may be helpful.
- Steroid injections may be used in resistant cases.
- Full return to participation should be gauged on pain-free completion of all functional tests.

FRACTURES AND ASSOCIATED CONDITIONS

> **Q** *A 14-year-old soccer player complains of an aching, diffuse pain in his right knee. The pain increases with strenuous activity and twisting motions. Because of the pain, he tends to walk with the leg externally rotated. What condition should be suspected, and what is the immediate management for this condition?*

Traumatic fractures about the knee area are rare in sports competition, except for high-velocity sports, such as motorcycling and auto racing. These fractures usually are associated with multiple traumas. Other, more common fractures and associated bony conditions can occur with regular participation in sport and physical activity. Displaced and undisplaced fractures of the femoral shaft are discussed in Chapter 16.

Avulsion Fractures

Avulsion fractures are caused by direct trauma, excessive tensile forces from an explosive muscular contraction, repetitive overuse, or a tensile force that pulls a ligament from its bony attachment. For example, getting kicked on the lateral aspect of the knee may avulse a portion of the lateral epicondyle, or the tibial tubercle may be avulsed when the extensor mechanism pulls a fragment away.

Signs and Symptoms

The individual has localized pain and tenderness over the bony site. In some instances, a fragment may be palpated. If a musculotendinous unit is involved, muscle function is limited. When the anterior cruciate is involved, the bony fragment may lodge in the joint, causing the knee to "lock."

Management

Treatment involves standard acute care and application of a knee immobilizer. The individual should be referred immediately to a physician for further care. If necessary, the individual should be fitted for crutches and instructed to use a non–weight bearing gait en route to the physician.

Epiphyseal and Apophyseal Fractures

Adolescents in contact sports are particularly susceptible to epiphyseal fractures in the knee region. A shearing force across the cartilaginous growth plate may lead to disruption of growth and a shortened limb.

Tibial Tubercle Fractures

The tibial tubercle, a common site for apophyseal fractures in boys, may occur as a result of Osgood-Schlatter disease. The typical patient is a muscular, well-developed individual who has almost reached skeletal maturity and who almost always is involved in a jumping sport, most commonly basketball. These fractures usually result from forced flexion of the knee against a straining quadriceps contraction or a violent quadriceps contraction against a fixed foot.

SIGNS AND SYMPTOMS. The individual has pain, ecchymosis, swelling, and tenderness directly over the tubercle. Difficulty going up and down stairs also is reported. When the fracture extends from the tubercle to the tibial epiphysis (type II) or through the secondary epiphysis and into the joint (type III), quadriceps insufficiency makes knee extension both painful and weak. In larger fractures involving extensive retinacular damage, the patella rides high, and knee extension is impossible.

MANAGEMENT. Treatment involves standard acute care and application of a knee immobilizer. The individual should be referred immediately to a physician for further care. If necessary, the individual should be fitted for crutches and instructed to use a non–weight bearing gait en route to the physician. Displaced fractures need open reduction and internal fixation.

Distal Femoral Epiphyseal Fractures

Fractures to the distal femoral epiphysis are 10-fold more common than proximal tibial fractures and are more serious because of possible arterial damage to the growth plate. They may occur at any age but often are seen in boys between 10 and 14 years of age. These fractures occur when a varus or valgus stress is applied on a fixed, weight-bearing foot, as when someone falls on the outer aspect of the knee while the foot is planted.

SIGNS AND SYMPTOMS. The individual complains of pain around the knee and is unable to bear weight on the injured leg.

MANAGEMENT. Treatment involves standard acute care and application of a knee immobilizer or vacuum splint. The individual should be referred immediately to a physician for further care. Undisplaced type I fractures usually are treated with closed reduction and casting and with use of crutches and protective weight bearing for 4 weeks, followed by rehabilitation to restore motion and strength. This fracture has a history of fairly good resolution, although such resolution may take weeks to occur. More serious fractures require internal fixation and may result in angular or leg-length discrepancy.

Stress Fractures

The femoral supracondylar region, medial tibial plateau, and tibia tubercle are common regions for stress fractures. These fractures occur when:

- Load on the bone is increased (e.g., jumping or high-impact activity)
- The number of stresses on the bone increase (e.g., changes in training intensity, duration, frequency, or running surface, or unevenly worn shoes)
- The surface area of the bone that receives the load is decreased (i.e., during the normal process of bone repair, certain portions of the bone remain immature and less able to tolerate stress for a period of time)

Signs and Symptoms

The individual complains of localized pain before and after activity that is relieved with rest and non–weight bearing. In a stress fracture of the medial tibial plateau, pain runs along the anteromedial aspect of the proximal tibia just below the joint line. Localized tenderness and edema are present, but initial radiographs of the stress fracture may be negative. As the condition progresses, pain becomes more persistent. Follow-up radiographs 3 weeks postinjury may show periosteal new bone development. Early bone scans are highly recommended.

Management

Once a stress fracture is identified, treatment involves rest, crutches, and/or casting.

Chondral and Osteochondral Fractures

A chondral fracture is a fracture involving the articular cartilage at a joint. An osteochondral fracture involves the articular cartilage and the underlying bone (Fig. 17.15). These fractures are the result of compression from a direct blow to the knee, causing shearing or forceful rotation. A substantial amount of articular surface on the involved bone can be damaged.

Signs and Symptoms

The individual usually feels a painful "snap" and reports considerable pain and swelling within the first few hours after injury. Displaced fractures can cause locking of the joint and produce crepitation during ROM.

■■■ FIGURE 17.15 **Osteochondral fracture.** This traumatic osteochondral fracture involves the articular cartilage and subchondral bone on the medial epicondyle of the tibia.

Management

Following standard acute care and immobilization in a vacuum splint, the individual should be referred immediately to a physician for further care. Aspiration of the joint often yields bloody fluid containing fat. Magnetic resonance images may be indicated, because some fractures may not appear on standard radiographs. Small fragments can be removed during arthroscopic surgery; internal fixation is necessary with larger fragments. Following surgery, ROM exercises are performed to improve articular cartilage nutrition, limit joint adhesions, and prevent muscular atrophy.

Osteochondritis Dissecans

Osteochondritis dissecans (OCD) occurs when a fragment of bone adjacent to the articular surface of a joint is deprived of its blood supply, leading to avascular necrosis (Fig. 17.16). The avascular bone fragment may be in its normal anatomical location with a smooth articular surface (i.e., stable), or the lesion may displace and form a loose body within the joint space, leaving a defect in the articular cartilage (i.e., unstable). The cartilage remains healthy even if the fragment is loose, because cartilage is nourished by synovial fluid rather than a direct blood supply. Repetitive trauma and loss of mechanical support, however, may cause the cartilage to undergo softening and degenerative changes. Although found in other joints, it more commonly affects the knee joint, particularly in males from 10 to 20 years of age, with the femoral condyles accounting for 75% of all lesions. Of these, the medial femoral condyle accounts for 75 to 85% of all femoral lesions (29). Causes include direct and indirect trauma, skeletal abnormalities associated with endocrine dysfunction, a prominent tibial spine that impacts the medial femoral condyle, and generalized ligamentous laxity.

See *Classification and Prognosis of Osteochondritis Dissecans*, available on the companion website at thePoint.

Signs and Symptoms

The most common symptom is an aching, diffuse pain, or swelling, with activity. Locking or giving way of the knee may develop as the disease progresses. Pain increases with strenuous activity and twisting motions, especially internal rotation of the tibia, which causes the medial tibial spine to strike the lateral aspect of the medial femoral condyle (the site of most OCD lesions). As a result, the individual walks with the affected leg externally rotated. Lesions of the lateral femoral condyle may produce a painful "clunk" with knee flexion and extension. Individuals with OCD of the patella usually present with retropatellar pain and crepitus. Thigh circumference may be diminished because of muscle disuse atrophy.

Management

Following standard acute care and immobilization with a knee immobilizer or vacuum splint, the individual should be referred immediately to a physician for further care. Treatment depends on the age of the individual, the size and location of the lesion, and the radiographic appearance of the fragment and articular cartilage.

Individuals in categories 1 and 2 (those <20 years of age) are treated nonsurgically if the fragment has not separated. A soft knee immobilizer is worn, and activity is restricted for 1 to 2 weeks, with minimal weight bearing to control pain and initiate healing. Activities are then modified for 6 to 12 weeks; younger individuals generally require a shorter period of activity modification compared with older individuals. Rapid or strenuous movement of the lower extremities should be avoided, especially high-impact activities, such as running, cutting, and jumping. Plain radiographs usually reveal evidence of healing between 3 and 6 months after treatment. Full activity may be permitted once the following criteria are met:

- The individual is pain-free.

■■ ■ FIGURE 17.16 **Osteochondritis dissecans.** Osteochondritis dissecans occurs when a fragment of bone adjacent to the articular surface of a joint is deprived of its blood supply, leading to avascular necrosis. In this individual, a portion of the medial epicondyle of the femur is damaged.

- Physical examination is normal, including full ROM, and no joint effusion or tenderness is present.
- Radiographic evidence of healing is present, as noted by disappearance of the radiolucent line that outlined the fragment.

If the individual is older than 20 years, the fragment is unstable (regardless of the individual's age), or a chronic lesion does not respond to conservative measures, internal fixation or removal of the fragment is indicated. Older individuals do not heal as well, because degenerative joint changes may have already developed within the joint. For OCD lesions of the patella, conservative management often is unsuccessful, necessitating early surgical intervention to excise the fragment. For these individuals, brief postsurgical immobilization followed by activity limitations usually brings about gradual healing.

Patellar Fractures

Stress fractures of the patella are rare and typically involve the inferior pole of the patella. Traumatic fractures can be transverse, stellate or comminuted, or longitudinal (Fig. 17.17). Displaced patellar fractures, which generally are associated with disruption of the quadriceps retinaculum, require open reduction and internal fixation. These fractures occur as a result of a fall onto the knee, a direct blow to the knee, or an eccentric contraction of the quadriceps that overloads the intrinsic tensile strength of the bone, as occurs in jumping activities. Patellar fracture also is a rare complication of ACL reconstruction using a bone–patellar tendon–bone **autogenous** (i.e., from within the body) graft. These fractures occur an average of 7 weeks postsurgery and result from external trauma, rapid flexion movement while preventing a fall backward, or a twisting maneuver. A **bipartite** (i.e., having two parts) patella, although not a fracture, is present in 1 to 4% of individuals and is more common in males than in females. It typically is seen on the superolateral corner of the patella and has rounded rather than sharp edges. The individual lacks point tenderness over the area and can maintain knee extension, which differentiates the condition from a true fracture.

■■■■ FIGURE 17.17 **Traumatic patellar fracture.** This radiograph provides a lateral view of a transverse fracture of the patella.

Signs and Symptoms

Generally, 2 mm of articular incongruity signifies a displaced fracture, which produces diffuse extra-articular swelling on and about the knee. A portion of the patella is retracted proximally. A visible and palpable defect lies between the fragments, which are mobile. A straight leg raise is impossible to perform.

Management

Initial treatment involves ice, elevation, immobilization in a knee immobilizer, and immediate referral to a physician. Radiographs are needed for verification. Nondisplaced patellar fractures are treated nonoperatively, with either a long-leg cylinder cast or a knee immobilizer for 4 to 6 weeks. Partial weight bearing is then allowed, and a full rehabilitation program is initiated. Surgery is indicated in a displaced fracture with major disruption to the extensor mechanism.

The 14-year-old soccer player may have OCD. Following standard acute care and immobilization with a knee immobilizer or vacuum splint, the individual should be referred immediately to a physician for further care.

ASSESSING KNEE CONDITIONS

A female high school basketball player is complaining of a deep, aching pain in the knee during activity. How should the assessment of this injury progress to determine the extent and severity of injury?

See *Special Tests for the Knee* and *Field Strategy: Knee Evaluation*, both available on the companion website at thePoint.

The lower extremity works as a unit to provide motion, and the knee plays a major role in supporting the body during dynamic and static activities. Biomechanical problems at the foot and hip can directly affect strain on the knee. As such, assessment of the knee complex must encompass an overview of the entire lower extremity. Refer to Table 17.2 for a summary of the various knee instabilities, the tests used, and the injured structures as indicated by the various positive tests.

HISTORY

Q *The injury assessment of the female high school basketball player should begin with a history. What questions need to be asked to identify the cause and extent of this injury?*

Conditions at the knee can be related to family history, age, congenital deformities, mechanical dysfunction, and recent changes in training programs, surfaces, or foot attire. Assessment should begin by gathering information on the mechanism of injury, associated symptoms, progression of the symptoms, any disabilities that may have resulted from the injury, and related medical history. Injuries seldom occur in an absolute frontal or sagittal plane; instead, most injuries involve a fixed, weight-bearing foot, with the individual trying to change directions or pivot. These acute, noncontact injuries most likely involve a rotational stress on the knee, which may injure several structures.

See *Field Strategy: Developing a History of the Injury*, available on the companion website at thePoint, for specific questions related to the knee.

Sprains of the collateral ligaments usually result in pain directly over the injury site. Injury to the ACL may be described as "deep in the knee" or "under the kneecap," whereas pain associated with a PCL tear is located in the posterior knee near the proximal attachment of the gastrocnemius. Unlike ACL injuries, PCL injuries usually do not cause incapacitating pain but, rather, produce vague symptoms, such as unsteadiness or insecurity of the knee. Individuals with meniscal injuries frequently report knee pain after twisting their leg while the foot is bearing their full weight.

The individual also may describe an associated pop or snap or other unusual sensation at the time of injury. Hearing a "pop" is a classic sign of an ACL tear. Symptoms such as locking of the knee may indicate a meniscal tear; "giving way" may indicate a patellar subluxation or internal derangement of the knee. Pain following extended periods of sitting, the "moviegoer's" or "theater" sign, usually indicates prolonged pressure being placed on one of the patellar facets. Individuals who have symptoms of patellar instability may have had a dislocation or recurrent subluxation.

A *The high school basketball player should be asked questions that address when, where, and how the injury occurred; intensity, location, and type of pain; when the pain begins (e.g., when you get out of bed, while sitting, while walking, during exercise, or at night); how long the condition been has present; how long the pain lasts; if the pain has changed or stayed the same; if the pain is worse before, during, or after activity; activities that aggravate or alleviate the symptoms; changes in training; changes in footwear; and previous injury, treatment, and medication.*

OBSERVATION AND INSPECTION

Q *The female high school basketball player indicates a deep, aching pain in the knee during activity that began 7 to 10 days ago. She reports that practice has been taking place in two facilities. One gym has hardwood floors, and the other gym has composite flooring. She reports that there has been increased focus on cardiovascular conditioning during the past 2 weeks of practice. Explain the observation component in the ongoing assessment of the basketball player.*

Both legs should be clearly visible to check symmetry, any congenital deformity, swelling, discoloration, hypertrophy, muscle atrophy, or previous surgical incisions. The individual should wear running shorts to allow a full view of the entire lower extremity. In addition, the individual should bring the shoes normally worn when pain is present so that they can be inspected for unusual wear, which could be indicative of a biomechanical abnormality.

The injured knee should be placed on a folded towel or pillow at 30° of flexion to relieve any strain on the joint structures. The injury site should be inspected for obvious deformities, discoloration, swelling, or scars that might indicate previous surgery. Swelling proximal to the patella may indicate suprapatellar bursitis or quadriceps involvement. Swelling distal to the patella may indicate patellar tendinitis, fat pad contusion, or internal derangement. Posterior swelling may indicate a Baker's cyst, gastrocnemius strain, or venous thrombosis. Medial swelling over the pes anserine may indicate bursitis or tendinitis. Girth measurements should be taken to determine the presence of swelling. One measurement should be at the joint line; subsequent measurements should be taken at 2-inch increments (1-inch for smaller individuals) above the superior pole of the patella.

Faulty posture or congenital abnormalities can increase stress on any joint. In an ambulatory patient, observation should include a thorough postural examination. It is important to observe the alignment of the femur on the tibia. Normally, the angle between the femoral and tibial shafts ranges from 180 to 195°. An angle of less than 180° is called **genu valgus** (i.e., "knock knee"); an angle of greater than 195° is called **genu varum** (i.e., "bowlegs"). Hyperextension, or posterior bowing of the knee, is called **genu recurvatum**.

The examiner should observe patella alignment for any abnormalities (Box 17.5). A high-riding patella exposes the infrapatellar fat pad, leading to a double hump when viewed from the lateral side (i.e., "camel sign"). Although some misalignments may be observed during a postural examination radiographs often are required to establish a definitive diagnosis.

Tibial torsion should be evaluated. Normally, the patella faces straight ahead while the foot faces slightly lateral (i.e., Fick angle). Medial torsion is associated with genu varum, in which the feet point toward each other, resulting in a "pigeon-toed" foot deformity. Genu valgum is associated with lateral tibial torsion, in which the feet point outward. When standing, most people exhibit a lateral tibial torsion. Femoral torsion, or anteversion (see Chapter 16), can impact the position of the patella relative to the femur and tibia.

While the individual is seated, the examiner should observe whether the tibial tubercles are directly below the patella or are displaced laterally by more than 10°, indicating an increased tubercle sulcus angle. Lateral displacement of the tubercle suggests bony patellofemoral malalignment and predisposition to lateral patellar tracking. The examiner should ask the individual to actively extend and flex the knee and should observe the dynamic tracking of the patella. The patella should be palpated for crepitus during the movement and compared with the contralateral knee. Although asymptomatic crepitus is common in certain individuals, symptomatic crepitus in the injured knee may indicate articular cartilage damage on the patella or trochlea.

Following completion of a static examination, the examiner should observe the individual walking. This observation should include an anterior, posterior, and lateral view, with the examiner noting any abnormalities in gait, favoring of one limb, tibial torsion, increased Q-angle, or inability to perform a fluid motion.

See *Field Strategy: Postural Assessment of the Knee Region,* found on the companion website at thePoint.

Ⓐ *Observation of the basketball player should include a full postural assessment and gait analysis. In particular, it is important to note the presence of pes planus, pes cavus, foot*

Box 17.5 Patellar Abnormalities

Patella alta	High-riding patella caused by a long patellar tendon
Patella baja	Low-riding patella caused by a short patellar tendon
Squinting patella	Medial-riding patella caused by hip anteversion (internal rotation of the femur) or internal tibial rotation
"Frog-eyed" patella	Lateral-riding patella caused by hip retroversion (external rotation of the femur) or external tibial rotation

pronation, foot supination, genu varus, genu valgum, tibial torsion, patella alta, Q-angle, and leg-length discrepancies. The specific injury site should be inspected for obvious deformities, discoloration, edema, scars that might indicate previous surgery, and the general condition of the skin.

PALPATION

Q *Observation of the female basketball player reveals an increased Q-angle, genu valgum, and excessive foot pronation. Explain palpation specific to the injury sustained by the basketball player.*

Bilateral palpation can determine temperature, swelling, point tenderness, crepitus, deformity, muscle spasm, and cutaneous sensation. Vascular pulses can be taken at the popliteal artery in the posterior knee, posterior tibial artery behind the medial malleolus, and dorsalis pedis artery in the dorsum of the foot. Before palpating for tenderness, which may lead to additional pain and apprehension, patella mobility should be evaluated. While the individual is supine, the patellar tilt test should be performed. The examiner grasps the patella, pushing down on the medial edge, and attempts to rotate the patella in the coronal plane to determine if the lateral patellar tilt can be corrected to "neutral" (i.e., when the patella's anterior surface comes parallel to the surface of the examination table). Then, while holding the patella in a corrected or neutral position, the examiner should attempt to displace the patella first medially and then laterally. Medial glide of the patella stresses the lateral patellar retinaculum and the other soft-tissue restraints. Lateral glide stresses the medial patellar retinaculum, the VMO, and the knee's medial joint capsule. The patella should move half its width (one to two quadrants of the size of the patella) in both directions, with an end feel of tissue stretch (Fig. 17.18). If lateral displacement produces apprehension or reproduces symptoms of a subluxation (apprehension test), the test is considered to be positive, indicating patellar instability. Movement of one quadrant or less is called a **hypomobile patella**; movement of three quadrants or more is a **hypermobile patella**, indicating laxity of the restraints. A hypermobile lateral glide may predispose the individual to a laterally subluxating or dislocating patella. Comparing superior and inferior patellar glide sometimes can reveal side-to-side differences, especially in individuals who have undergone surgery. Bilateral comparison should be performed and any asymmetry noted.

Palpation should move proximal to distal, leaving the most painful area until last. The individual should be non–weight bearing, with a pillow placed under the knee to relax the limb. It may be necessary to change knee position to palpate certain structures more effectively. For example, meniscal lesions are best palpated at 45°; the joint line is more prominent at 90°. Externally rotating the knee exposes the anteromedial border of the medial meniscus; internally rotating the knee exposes the lateral meniscus.

Extreme pain or point tenderness during palpation of bony structures may indicate a fracture. Compression, distraction, and percussion also may be used to detect fracture. For example, compression at the distal tibia and fibula causes distraction at the proximal tibiofibular joint. Percussion or tapping on the malleoli, or use of a tuning fork, may produce positive signs at the fracture site as well.

FIGURE 17.18 Patellar glide. Passive lateral glide of the patella demonstrating subluxation to its second quadrant. Hypomobility is manifested by less than one quadrant of displacement; hypermobility is manifested by three or more quadrants (greater than half of patellar width).

Palpation should proceed proximal to distal, but the area anticipated to be the most painful should be left to last. The following structures should be palpated:

Anterior Palpation

1. Quadriceps muscles, adductor muscles, and sartorius.

2. Patellar surface, edges, and retinaculum.

3. Patellar tendon, fat pad, tibial tubercle, medial and lateral tibial plateaus, and bursa. When the knee is extended, the infrapatellar fat pad can be palpated on the medial and lateral sides of the patellar tendon.

4. Patella plica (medial to the patella, with the knee flexed at 45°).

5. Medial femoral condyle and epicondyle and MCL.

6. Pes anserinus.

7. Iliotibial band, lateral femoral condyle and epicondyle, LCL, and head of fibula. The LCL can be palpated further by having the individual place the foot of the affected limb on the knee of the unaffected leg while palpating the lateral joint line.

8. While the knee is flexed at 90°, the tibiofemoral joint line, medial and lateral tibial plateaus, medial and lateral femoral condyles, and adductor muscles should be palpated.

Posterior Palpation with Knee Slightly Flexed

1. Popliteal fossa for Baker's cyst and popliteal artery

2. Popliteus muscle in posterolateral corner

3. Hamstring muscles and gastrocnemius

Palpation for Swelling

Two special tests are used to determine if the swelling is intra-articular or extra-articular. Intra-articular swelling feels heavy and mushy, because blood often is mixed with the synovial fluid. Extra-articular swelling is light and fluid and can easily be moved between the fingers from one side to the other.

Brush or Stroke Test (Milking) for Joint Swelling

This test differentiates between synovial thickening and joint effusion. With effusion, the knee assumes a resting position of 15 to 25° of flexion, which allows the synovial cavity maximum capacity for holding fluid. Beginning below the medial joint line, the examiner strokes two or three times toward the individual's hip, moving proximal to the suprapatellar pouch (Fig. 17.19A). Next, using the opposite hand, the examiner strokes down the lateral side of the patella (Fig. 17.19B). An effusion is present if a wave of fluid passes to the medial side of the joint and bulges just below the medial, distal portion of the patella.

Patellar Tap ("Ballotable Patella") Test

While the knee is relaxed, the examiner pushes the patella downward, into the patellofemoral groove (Fig. 17.20). If swelling is intra-articular, the fluid under the patella causes it to rebound, exhibiting the outlines of

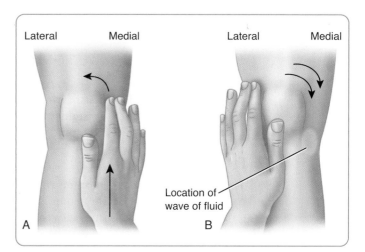

■■ ■ ■ FIGURE 17.19 **Assessment of joint swelling.**
A, To assess joint swelling, the examiner strokes the medial side of the knee several times, toward the hip. **B,** Using the opposite hand, the examiner strokes down the lateral side of the patella and notes any wave of fluid as it moves to the medial side of the joint.

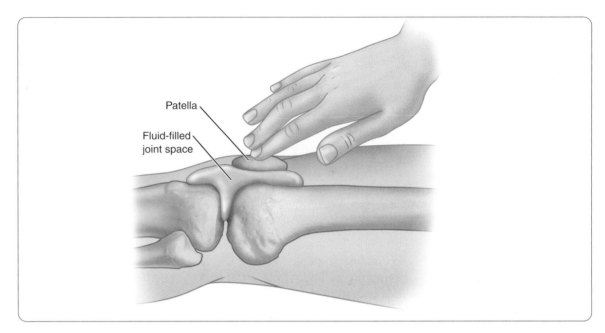

■ ■ ■ FIGURE 17.20 **Patellar tap test.** The leg should be relaxed. The examiner gently pushes the patella downward into the groove. If joint effusion is present, the patella rebounds and floats back up.

the floating patella. If the swelling is extra-articular, a click or definite stopping point is felt when the patella strikes the patellofemoral groove. The outline of the patella usually is obscured by extra-articular swelling, typically seen with a ruptured bursa.

A *Bilateral palpation of the basketball player's knee, with a particular focus on the patella, should include swelling, point tenderness, deformity, crepitus, temperature, other signs of trauma, and patellofemoral joint pain.*

PHYSICAL EXAMINATION TESTS

Q *In palpating the basketball player's patella, point tenderness is elicited over the lateral facet. In addition, pain and crepitus are elicited when the patella is manually compressed into the patellofemoral groove. Explain the physical examination of the basketball player.*

Physical examination tests are performed with the individual in a comfortable position, preferably supine. Pain and muscle spasm can restrict motion and cause an inaccurate result. The limb should not be forced through any sudden motions. It may be necessary to place a rolled towel under the knee to relieve strain on the joint structures.

Functional Tests

The examiner should determine the available ROM in knee flexion-extension and medial-lateral rotation of the tibia on the femur. Bilateral comparison with the noninjured knee is critical to determine normal or abnormal movement.

Active Movements

Active movements can first be performed while the individual is sitting, with the leg flexed over the end of the table, and then repeated in a prone or supine position. The thigh must be stabilized and the most painful movements performed last to prevent painful symptoms from overflowing into the next movement. The motions that should be assessed and the normal ROM for each are as follows:

- Knee flexion (0–135°)
- Knee extension (0–15°)

- Medial rotation of the tibia on the femur (20–30°) with the knee flexed at 90°
- Lateral rotation of the tibia on the femur (30–40°) with the knee flexed at 90°

Measuring ROM at the knee with a goniometer is demonstrated in Figure 17.21.

Passive Range of Motion

If the individual is able to perform full ROM during active movements, the examiner should apply gentle pressure at the extremes of motion to determine end feel. The end feel for flexion is tissue approximation. The end feel for extension is medial rotation, and that for lateral rotation is tissue stretch. Patellar motion should be performed passively, before palpation for point tenderness.

Resisted Muscle Testing

The individual is in a seated position during testing, except for hamstring testing, in which the individual is prone. The examiner must stabilize the hip during testing to prevent muscle substitution. The biceps femoris is isolated by placing the tibia in external rotation and performing knee flexion against resistance. Internal tibial rotation and knee flexion test the medial hamstrings. During knee extension, any abnormal tibial movement or excessive pain from patellar compression should be noted. Figure 17.22 demonstrates motions that should be tested.

■■■■ FIGURE 17.21 **Goniometry measurement for knee flexion and extension.** Center the fulcrum over the lateral epicondyle of the femur. Using the greater trochanter for reference, align the proximal arm along the femur. Align the distal arm in line with the lateral malleolus.

■■■■ FIGURE 17.22 **Resisted manual muscle testing. A,** Knee extension (L_3). **B,** Ankle plantar flexion (S_1). **C,** Ankle dorsiflexion (L_4). **D,** Knee flexion (S_1, S_2). Myotomes are listed in parentheses.

Stress Tests

From information gathered during the history, observation, inspection, and palpation, the examiner determines which tests will assess the condition most effectively. Only those tests deemed to be absolutely necessary should be performed. If ACL damage is suspected, tests for anterior cruciate instability should be performed as soon as possible, before swelling, joint effusion, and muscle spasm occludes the extent of instability. Possible structures injured with the various positive tests for unidirectional and multidirectional instability are listed in Table 17.2 and are not repeated in this section, except when necessary to explain the test.

Straight Anterior Instability

ANTERIOR DRAWER TEST. The individual is supine, with the hip flexed at 45° and the knee flexed at 90°. The examiner stabilizes the foot by placing it under the thigh to prevent any tibial rotation. In this position, the ACL is nearly parallel to the tibial plateau. The examiner places both thumbs on either side of the patellar tendon to palpate the anteromedial and anterolateral joint line and to determine anterior translation as the tibia is drawn forward on the femur. The fingers are placed in the popliteal fossa to ensure that the hamstrings are relaxed. A step-off at the medial tibial plateau should first be palpated to ensure the proper starting position (see *Posterior Drawer Test*). While palpating the joint line, apply an alternating anterior (i.e., anterior drawer) and posterior (i.e., posterior drawer) displacement force on the proximal tibia (Fig. 17.23A). Stability can be visualized from a lateral view or palpated with the thumb at the joint line. The knee is tested with the foot in neutral rotation, external rotation, and finally, internal rotation. The amount of translation and the end point are compared with those for the contralateral knee. The examiner should be aware that the anterior drawer test is not as effective as Lachman's test for a variety of reasons (Box 17.6).

LACHMAN'S TEST. A modification of the drawer test is Lachman's test, which tends to isolate the posterolateral bundle of the ACL. The individual is supine, with the knee joint at 20 to 30° of flexion. When the knee is in slight flexion, the ACL is the primary restraining force that prevents anterior translation, because the secondary restraints are relaxed. The examiner stabilizes the femur with one hand while placing the other hand over the proximal tibia to displace the tibia anteriorly (Fig. 17.23B). If the individual has heavy, muscular legs, or if the examiner has small hands, a small support, such as a pillow or tightly rolled towel, can be placed under the femur. A positive sign results in a "mushy" or soft end feel when the tibia is moved anterior in relation to the femur. When the tibia is in slight internal rotation, anterior displacement indicates additional damage to the IT band and to the anterior and middle lateral capsule. When the tibia is in slight external rotation, anterior displacement indicates damage to the ACL, MCL, and medial meniscus.

■■ ■ FIGURE 17.23 Anterior cruciate ligament tests. A, Drawer test. The knee is flexed, and the examiner applies an anterior and posterior displacement force on the proximal tibia. **B,** Lachman's test. Using one hand to stabilize the femur, the examiner applies firm pressure on the posterior proximal tibia in an attempt to move the tibia anteriorly.

Box 17.6 Limitations of the Anterior Drawer Test

- Gravity also has an effect.
- Guarding by the hamstrings group can mask anterior displacement of the tibia on the femur.
- The triangular shape of the meniscus can form a block against anterior movement of the tibia.
- A displaced "bucket-handle" meniscal tear can block anterior movement.
- Knee flexion at 90° may lead to anterior displacement of tibia, masking further displacement during the test.
- Increased pain is elicited in an acute injury at 90° of flexion, masking the true extent of injury.
- If the posterior cruciate ligament is absent, anterior movement to the neutral position can be misread as abnormal anterior displacement.
- Because the knee is flexed at 90°, only the anteromedial bundle is tested.

MODIFIED (PRONE) LACHMAN'S TEST. This test is used to differentiate abnormal tibiofemoral glide caused by tears of the ACL from glide caused by PCL deficiencies. It often is favored over the traditional Lachman's position when the individual has large thighs or the examiner has small hands, because the weight of the femur is supported by the examination table and the tibia may be supported by the examiner's thigh or forearm (30). The individual is in a prone position, and the knee is flexed at 30°. The examiner supports the tibia with one hand while palpating either side of the joint line. The other hand applies a downward pressure on the proximal portion of the posterior tibia (Fig. 17.24). The examiner notes any anterior tibial displacement. Positive anterior translation found with an anterior drawer, Lachman's test, or modified Lachman's test indicates a tear of the ACL. Positive anterior translation with the anterior drawer test or Lachman's test and a negative modified Lachman's test indicate a tear in the PCL.

■■ ■ **FIGURE 17.24 Modified Lachman's test.** The examiner applies downward pressure on the proximal posterior tibia and notes any anterior translation.

Straight Posterior Instability

POSTERIOR SAG (GRAVITY) TEST. The true posterior sag test is performed in a supine position with the hips flexed at 45° and the knees at 90°. When viewed laterally, a loss of tibial tubercle prominence in a PCL-deficient knee is evident when the tibia falls back or sags on the femur because of gravitational forces. The posterior displacement is more noticeable, however, when the hips and knees are both flexed at 90°. The examiner holds both relaxed legs distally to prevent manual reduction of the tibia. Next, the examiner moves to the side of the individual and looks for the position of the tibia as it sags back on the femur (Fig. 17.25A). This maneuver is called Godfrey's sign. It is important to note the sag, because if the sag goes unnoticed, it may produce a false-positive Lachman's test.

POSTERIOR DRAWER TEST. The individual is positioned in the same pose as described for the anterior drawer test. The examiner initially observes the resting position of the tibial plateau in relation to the femoral condyles. When the knee is flexed to 90°, the medial tibial plateau normally lies approximately 1 cm anterior to the medial femoral condyle. This can be felt by running the thumb or index finger down the medial femoral condyle toward the tibia. In a PCL-deficient knee, this relationship is not present. The examiner then applies a posteriorly directed force to the tibia (see Fig. 17.22A). The knee is tested with the foot in neutral position, external rotation, and finally, internal rotation. Isolated PCL tears often produce only minimal posterior translation when the secondary restraints of the knee, particularly the posterior capsule and the posteromedial and posterolateral structures, are intact.

FIGURE 17.25 Posterior cruciate ligament tests. A, Posterior sag (gravity) test. The hips and knees are flexed, and the examiner looks from the side and compares the anterior contours of both legs. If one leg sags back and the prominence of the tibial tubercle is lost, the posterior cruciate may be damaged (Godfrey's sign). **B,** Reverse Lachman's test. The examiner stabilizes the femur with one hand while the other lifts the tibia up (superiorly). Any posterior translation and the quality of the end feel is noted.

False-negative results can occur with a displaced bucket-handle meniscal tear, hamstring or quadriceps spasm, or hemarthrosis.

REVERSE LACHMAN'S TEST. Positioning of the patient is identical to that in the modified Lachman's test. While the individual is prone and the knee flexed to between 20 and 30°, the examiner holds the distal femur to the table and grasps the proximal tibia (Fig. 17.25B). Using the hand on the femur to stabilize the thigh and ensure that the hamstrings are relaxed, the examiner lifts the proximal tibia posteriorly (up), noting the amount of translation and the quality of end point. A false-positive test may occur if the ACL is torn, allowing gravity to cause an anterior shift of the tibia. The test is not as sensitive for detecting a torn PCL, because the PCL functions more at 90° of knee flexion.

Straight Valgus Instability

ABDUCTION (VALGUS STRESS) TEST. The individual is supine, with the leg extended. The examiner places the heel of one hand on the lateral joint line, and the other hand stabilizes the distal lower leg. Next, a lateral force is applied at the joint line with the lower leg stabilized in slight lateral rotation (Fig. 17.26A). If positive (i.e., the tibia abducts), primary damage involves the structures of the medial

FIGURE 17.26 Valgus and varus stress tests. A, Valgus stress test. The knee is flexed at 30° to isolate the medial collateral ligament. The examiner applies a gentle valgus stress at the knee joint while moving the lower leg laterally. The test is repeated with the knee fully extended. **B,** Varus stress test. The knee is flexed at 30° to isolate the lateral collateral ligament. The examiner applies a varus stress at the knee joint while moving the lower leg medially. The test is repeated with the knee fully extended.

FIGURE 17.27 Slocum drawer test. A, An anterior drawer force is applied for anteromedial rotary instability with the tibia externally rotated 15°. **B,** Anterolateral rotary instability is tested with the tibia internally rotated 25 to 30°.

joint capsule. The tibial collateral ligament is isolated by flexing the knee at 30° and repeating the valgus stress.

Straight Varus Instability

ADDUCTION (VARUS STRESS) TEST. The knee is placed in the same position as for the abduction test, but a medial force (i.e., varus stress) is applied at the knee joint (Fig. 17.26B). Laxity in full extension indicates major instability and damage to the fibular collateral ligament, popliteus, and posterolateral capsule. When testing at 20 to 30° of flexion, which is the true test for one-plane lateral instability, a positive test indicates damage to the fibular collateral ligament.

Anteromedial Rotary Instability

SLOCUM DRAWER TEST. This test is performed in the same position as the anterior drawer test, but with the tibia externally rotated 15° (Fig. 17.27A). In this position, when an anterior drawer force is applied, the majority of anterior translation occurs on the medial side of the knee. If the amount of anterior translation is the same or increases, anteromedial rotary instability is present, indicating injury to the MCL, oblique popliteal ligament, posteromedial capsule, and ACL (posteromedial corner).

Anterolateral Rotary Instability

SLOCUM DRAWER TEST. This test also is performed in the same position as the anterior drawer test, with the tibia internally rotated 25 to 30° (Fig. 17.27B). In this position, the majority of anterior translation occurs on the lateral side of the knee. If the anterior translation increases or does not decrease, ALRI is present.

LATERAL PIVOT SHIFT TEST. This test duplicates the anterior subluxation/reduction phenomenon that occurs during functional activities in ACL-deficient knees. During the test, the tibia moves away from the femur on the lateral side (but rotates medially) and moves anteriorly in relation to the femur. While supine, the hip is flexed at 30° with no abduction. The examiner places one hand behind the head of the fibula, and the other hand holds the foot while internally rotating the lower leg approximately 20°. A valgus force is applied to the knee while maintaining the internal rotation; the knee is moved from extension into flexion (Fig. 17.28).

Pushes forward and applies a valgus stress

Flexion

FIGURE 17.28 Lateral pivot shift test. While the hip is flexed and abducted 30° and is relaxed in slight medial rotation, the examiner places the heel of one hand behind the head of the fibula while the other hand grasps the distal tibia and 20° of internal tibial rotation is maintained. Next, the examiner applies a valgus force while the knee is slowly flexed. When the knee reaches 30 to 40° of flexion, the iliotibial band causes the tibia to reduce or slide backward, giving a noticeable "clunk."

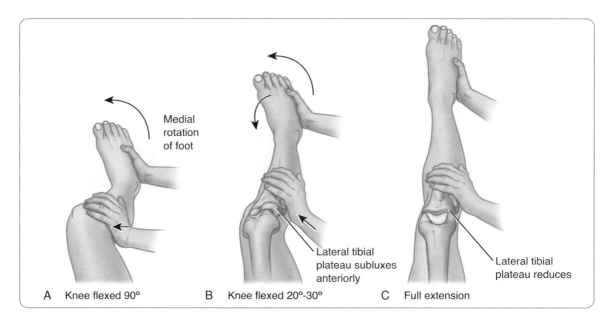

Medial rotation of foot

Lateral tibial plateau subluxes anteriorly

Lateral tibial plateau reduces

A Knee flexed 90°   B Knee flexed 20°-30°   C Full extension

■■■■ FIGURE 17.29 **Jerk test. A,** While the knee is flexed to 90°, the examiner places one hand behind the head of the fibula to produce internal tibial rotation. **B,** When the knee reaches 20 to 30°, the lateral tibial plateau subluxes anteriorly. **C,** When the knee moves into full extension, the lateral tibial plateau reduces.

If the ACL is torn, the femur displaces posteriorly when the knee is placed in 10 to 20° of flexion. As the knee continues to flex, the IT band changes its angle of pull from that of an extensor to that of a flexor. When the knee reaches 30 to 40° of flexion, the IT band causes the tibia to reduce or slide backward, resulting in a noticeable "clunk." This test is highly accurate for detecting acute and chronic ACL injuries.

JERK TEST. Similar to the lateral pivot shift maneuver, the jerk test is performed in the same position, except that the individual's hip is flexed at 45°. Initially, the knee is flexed to 90°. Next, the leg is extended, maintaining medial rotation and a valgus stress (Fig. 17.29). If the test is positive, the tibia jerks (shifts) forward at approximately 20 to 30° of flexion, causing a subluxation of the lateral tibial plateau. If the leg continues into further extension, it spontaneously reduces. Although not as sensitive as the lateral pivot shift test, a positive jerk test indicates injury to the ACL, posterolateral capsule, arcuate–popliteus complex, LCL, and IT band.

SLOCUM ANTEROLATERAL ROTARY INSTABILITY TEST. Although not as sensitive as the pivot shift test, the Slocum ALRI test aids in relaxing the hamstring muscles and is easier to perform on heavy or tense individuals. The individual is placed in a side-lying position (~30° from supine), with the pelvis rotated posteriorly. The bottom leg is the uninvolved leg. Using the involved foot to stabilize the tibia, the examiner applies a valgus force to the knee while the knee is flexed at 25 to 45° (Fig. 17.30). During this range, a subluxation of the tibia is reduced with a noticeable "clunk."

■■■■ FIGURE 17.30 **Slocum anterolateral rotary instability test.** The uninvolved leg is on the bottom. The examiner applies a valgus force to the top, injured knee while the knee is flexed at 25 to 45°. During this range, a subluxation of the tibia is reduced with a "clunk."

CROSS-OVER TEST. The individual is asked to bear weight on the involved limb and step across with the uninvolved leg (Fig. 17.31). Because the foot of the weight-bearing leg remains fixed, the lateral femoral condyle is allowed to displace posteriorly relative to the tibia in the presence of laxity in the lateral capsular restraints. An alternate method involves gently stepping on the involved foot and instructing the individual to rotate the upper torso away from the injured leg to approximately 90° from the fixed foot. Next, the individual is instructed to contract the quadriceps muscles, producing the same symptoms and testing the same structures as in the lateral pivot shift test.

FLEXION-ROTATION DRAWER TEST. This test may be used in an acute injury and tends to be more sensitive than the other ALRI tests. With the individual supine, the examiner holds the individual's ankle between the clinician's trunk and arm, with the hands around the tibia (Fig. 17.32). Next, the knee is flexed to 20 to 30° while maintaining the tibia in neutral rotation. This is followed by pushing the tibia posteriorly, as in a posterior drawer test. This movement reduces the subluxation of the tibia, indicating a positive test for ALRI. If the tibia is alternately pushed posteriorly and released, however, and if the femur is allowed to rotate freely, the reduction and subluxation are seen and felt as the femur rotates medially and laterally.

Posteromedial Rotary Instability

HUGHSTON'S POSTEROMEDIAL DRAWER TEST. The individual is supine with the knee flexed to 80 to 90° and the hip at 45°. The examiner medially rotates the individual's foot and sits on the foot to stabilize it. Next, the examiner pushes the tibia posteriorly. If the tibia displaces or rotates posteriorly on the medial aspect by an excessive amount relative to the normal knee, the test is positive.

POSTEROMEDIAL PIVOT SHIFT TEST. With the individual supine, the examiner passively flexes the knee more than 45° while applying a varus stress, compression, and medial rotation of the tibia. In a positive test, these movements cause subluxation of the medial tibial plateau posteriorly. The examiner then moves the knee into extension. The tibia shifts into the reduced position at approximately 20° to 40° of flexion.

■■ ■ FIGURE 17.31 **Cross-over test.** Stepping across the injured leg determines anterolateral rotary instability. Stepping behind the injured leg can determine anteromedial rotary instability.

■■■ ■ FIGURE 17.32 **Flexion-rotation drawer test.** The knee is flexed to 20 to 30° while maintaining the tibia in neutral rotation. This is followed by pushing the tibia posteriorly, which reduces the subluxation of the tibia, indicating a positive test for anterolateral rotary instability.

Knee flexion
70°
Lateral rotation of foot

=70°

Lateral tibial plateau subluxes posteriorly and drops downward

A

15°

=15°

Lateral tibial plateau shifts anteriorly to reduce subluxation

B

FIGURE 17.33 Reverse pivot shift test. A, A flexed position with lateral rotation causes the lateral tibial tubercle to sublux. **B,** As the knee extends, the lateral tibial tubercle reduces.

Posterolateral Rotary Instability

HUGHSTON'S POSTEROLATERAL DRAWER TEST. The individual is in the same position as the postero-medial drawer test, but with the foot laterally rotated. The tibia is pushed posteriorly. If the tibia displaces or rotates posteriorly on the lateral aspect by an excessive amount relative to the normal knee, this indicates posterolateral rotary instability, but only if the PCL is torn.

REVERSE PIVOT SHIFT TEST. The reverse pivot shift test discerns combination injuries from an isolated PCL injury. The examiner lifts the individual's leg and stabilizes it with one hand on the heel. The other hand is used to support the lateral calf by placing the palm on the proximal fibula. In the first part of the test, the individual's knee is flexed to between 70 and 80°, and the foot is externally rotated, causing the tibia on the injured side to sublux posteriorly (Fig. 17.33A). Next, the leg is extended while applying valgus stress to the knee (Fig. 17.33B). The test is considered to be positive if the subluxation reduces.

EXTERNAL ROTATION RECURVATUM TEST. With the individual supine and the lower limbs relaxed, the examiner gently grasps the big toes of each foot and lifts both feet off the table (Fig. 17.34). The individual is told to keep the quadriceps relaxed. While elevating the legs, the examiner watches the tibial tubercles. If the test is positive, the affected knee goes into relative hyperextension on the lateral aspect, with the tibia and tibial tubercle rotating laterally. The affected knee appears to have genu varum, with damage to the PCL and LCL, arcuate ligament complex, posterolateral joint capsule, and biceps femoris.

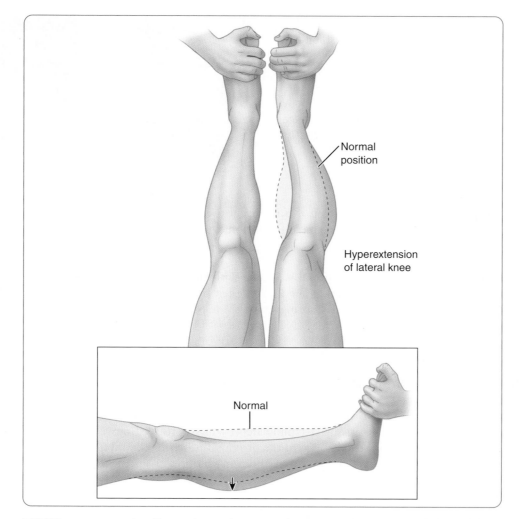

■■■■ FIGURE 17.34 **External rotation recurvatum test.** The examiner grasps the big toes of each foot, then lifts both feet off the table. It is important that the individual keeps the quadriceps relaxed. In a positive test, the affected knee becomes hyperextended on the lateral aspect, with the tibia and tibial tubercle rotating laterally.

Special Tests

A variety of special tests can be used for detecting injury or related pathology involving the knee.

Tests for Meniscal Lesions

MCMURRAY'S TEST. While the individual is supine, the examiner flexes the knee completely against the chest, externally rotates the tibia, and slowly extends the knee and hip (Fig. 17.35). This action attempts to trap the displaced posterior horn of the medial meniscus in the joint and produce an audible and palpable click or thud. Next, the examiner returns the leg to the starting position. During internal rotation and extension of the knee and hip, the posterior horn of the lateral meniscus is trapped. Each test is repeated several times.

APLEY'S COMPRESSION/DISTRACTION TEST. In a prone position with the knee flexed at 90°, the examiner stabilizes the thigh and rotates the leg by applying downward compression in a medial and lateral direction. The test is considered to be positive if pain is produced. This compression test may

■■■ FIGURE 17.35 **McMurray's test.** The hip and knee are flexed, and the examiner stabilizes the lower leg with one hand and laterally rotates the tibia. The other hand is placed over the anterior knee with the fingers on the joint line. The examiner slowly extends the leg. If a loose body is in the medial meniscus, this action causes a snap or click. Internally rotating the leg and repeating the test with the thumb over the lateral joint line tests for lateral meniscus damage.

or may not produce a positive sign even if a meniscal tear is present. Pain should be relieved by repeating the test with the joint distracted. If rotation with distraction produces pain, the lesion probably is ligamentous.

"BOUNCE HOME" TEST. While the individual is supine with the knee fully flexed, the examiner cups the heel of the involved leg in one hand. The knee is then passively allowed to extend. If extension is not complete or a rubbery end feel ("springy block") is present, the individual may have a torn meniscus.

Tests for Tibiofibular Instability

PROXIMAL TIBIOFIBULAR SYNDESMOSIS TEST. While the individual is supine and the knees are flexed at approximately 90°, the examiner stabilizes the tibia with one hand while the other hand grasps the proximal fibular head. In this position, the examiner attempts to displace the fibular head anteriorly and posteriorly. A positive test is indicated by any perceived movement of the fibula on the tibia. An anterior shift indicates damage to the proximal posterior tibiofibular ligament; posterior displacement indicates damage to the proximal anterior tibiofibular ligament.

Plica Tests

MEDIOPATELLAR PLICA TEST. While the individual is supine, the examiner flexes the affected knee to 30°. Next, the examiner moves the patella medially in an effort to cause pain, which would indicate a positive test. The pain is caused by pinching the edge of the plica between the medial femoral condyle and patella.

PLICA "STUTTER" TEST. This is done with the individual seated on the edge of the examination table, with both knees flexed to 90°. The examiner places a finger over the patella and instructs the individual to extend the knee slowly. If the test is positive, the patella stutters or jumps between 45 and 60° of flexion (0° being full extension). The test is only effective if the individual has no joint swelling.

HUGHSTON'S PLICA TEST. While the individual is supine, the examiner flexes the knee and medially rotates the tibia with one arm and hand. The other hand presses the patella medially while palpating the medial femoral condyle with the fingers of the same hand. The individual's knee is passively flexed and extended while the examiner feels for "popping" of the plica band under the fingers, which indicates a positive test.

Tests for Patellofemoral Dysfunction

PATELLA COMPRESSION OR GRIND TEST. To assess articular pain resulting from irritation of subchondral bone, the examiner compresses the patella in the trochlea at various degrees of flexion. Normally, the patella enters the trochlea at 10 to 15° of knee flexion, so pressure applied in full extension does not directly produce articular compression between the patella and trochlea. As such, it is necessary to place a rolled towel under the knee, flexing the knee at approximately 20°. In this position, the

■■ ■■ FIGURE 17.36 **Patellofemoral dysfunction. A,** Patella compression or grind test. Pain on compression of the patella indicates pathology of the patella articular cartilage. **B,** Clarke's sign. Slight compression is applied just proximal to the superior pole of the patella while the individual contracts the quadriceps. The test is positive for chondromalacia patella if the individual has pain or is unable to hold the contraction. **C,** Patellar apprehension test. The examiner gently displaces the patella laterally. The test is positive for a subluxating patella if the individual shows apprehension.

examiner compresses the patella into the patellofemoral groove (Fig. 17.36A). The distal portion of the patella is articulating. Pain with compression in this range suggests a lesion in the distal patellar or proximal trochlear area. Conversely, as knee flexion increases, the patella is drawn distally in the trochlea, causing the area of articulation to be more proximal on the patella. Pain with compression in flexion suggests a more proximal patellar lesion. The test is considered to be positive if pain is felt or a grinding sound is heard, indicating pathology of the patellar articular cartilage.

CLARKE'S SIGN. Using the web of the hand, the examiner places the hand just proximal to the superior pole of the patella (Fig. 17.36B). The individual is instructed to contract the quadriceps while the examiner gently pushes downward. If the individual can hold the contraction without pain, the test is considered to be negative; if the individual has pain and is unable to hold the contraction, the test is considered to be positive for chondromalacia patellae. This test can elicit pain in any individual if the pressure is significant. Therefore, it is imperative to repeat the procedure several times with increasing pressure in full knee extension and at 30, 60, and 90° of knee flexion.

WALDRON TEST. The examiner palpates the patella while the individual does several slow, deep knee bends. Any crepitus, pain, "catching," or improper tracking of the patella should be noted. If any of these signs or symptoms occurs simultaneously, the test is considered to be positive for chondromalacia patellae.

PATELLAR APPREHENSION TEST. While the knee is in a relaxed position, the examiner pushes the patella laterally (Fig. 17.36C). If the individual voluntarily or involuntarily shows apprehension, the test is considered to be positive for a subluxating patella.

Tests for Iliotibial Band Friction Syndrome

NOBLE COMPRESSION TEST. This test is used with Ober's test to determine if IT band friction syndrome is present near the knee (Fig. 17.37A). The individual is supine on a table, with the hip and knee flexed at 90°. The individual slowly lowers the leg and extends the knee, and the examiner applies pressure with the thumb directly over, or 1 to 2 cm proximal to, the lateral epicondyle of the femur. As the knee moves to 30° of knee flexion, a positive response is severe pain similar to that caused during activity.

OBER'S TEST. The individual lies on the side with the lower leg slightly flexed at the hip and knee for stability. The examiner stabilizes the pelvis with one hand to prevent the pelvis from shifting posteriorly during the test. Next, the examiner passively abducts and slightly extends the hip so that the IT band passes over the greater trochanter (Fig. 17.37B). Although the original Ober's test called

■■■■ FIGURE 17.37 **Tests for iliotibial band friction syndrome. A,** Noble compression test. The hip and knee are flexed at 90°. The examiner applies thumb pressure over the lateral epicondyle of the femur as the leg is extended. Pain at or near 30° of flexion indicates iliotibial band (ITB) syndrome. **B,** Ober's test. The examiner passively abducts and slightly extends the hip. Then, the examiner slowly lowers the extended leg. If the ITB is tight, the leg remains in the abducted position.

for the knee to be flexed at 90°, the IT band has a greater stretch if the knee is extended. The examiner slowly lowers the upper leg. If the IT band is tight, the leg will remain in the abducted position.

Neurologic Tests

Neurologic integrity is assessed with isometric muscle testing of the myotomes, reflex testing, and sensation in the segmental dermatomes and peripheral nerve cutaneous patterns.

Myotomes

Isometric muscle testing should be performed in the following motions to test specific segmental myotomes:

- Hip flexion (L_1, L_2)
- Knee extension (L_3)
- Ankle dorsiflexion (L_4)
- Toe extension (L_5)
- Ankle plantar flexion, foot eversion, or hip extension (S_1)
- Knee flexion (S_2)

Reflexes

Reflexes in the lower leg region include the patella (L_3, L_4) and Achilles tendon reflex (S_1) (Fig. 17.38). The patellar reflex is tested with the individual seated on the end of a table so that the knee is flexed at 90°. The examiner strikes the tendon with the flat end of the reflex hammer using a

FIGURE 17.38 Reflex testing. A, The patellar reflex. **B,** The Achilles reflex. **C,** Alternate position for the Achilles reflex.

crisp, wrist-flexion action. A normal reflex exhibits a slight, jerking motion in extension. In testing the Achilles tendon reflex, the examiner slightly dorsiflexes the ankle to place the tendon on stretch and taps the tendon with the flat end of the reflex hammer. An alternate position is to have the individual lie prone on a table or place the knee on a chair, with the foot extended beyond the edge. A normal reflex should elicit a slight plantar flexion jerk.

Cutaneous Patterns

The segmental nerve dermatome patterns for the pelvis, hip, and thigh are demonstrated in Figure 17.39. The peripheral nerve cutaneous patterns are demonstrated in Figure 17.40.

Activity-Specific Functional Tests

Functional tests should be performed before clearing the individual for return to participation. These tests should be performed pain-free, without a limp or antalgic gait. Examples of functional tests include forward running, cross-over stepping, running figure-eights or V-cuts, side-step running, and karioca running. When appropriate, functional braces or protective supportive devices should be used to prevent reinjury.

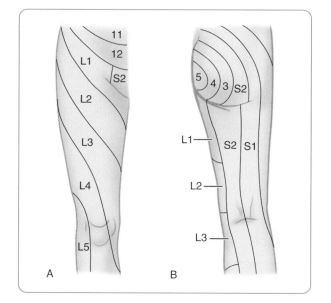

FIGURE 17.39 Segmental nerve dermatome patterns. A, Anterior view. **B,** Posterior view.

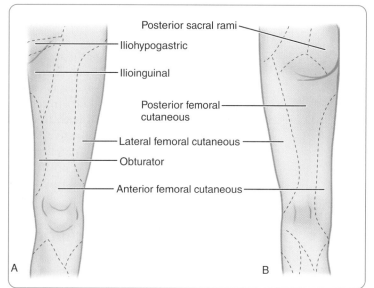

FIGURE 17.40 Peripheral nerve sensory distribution patterns. A, Anterior view. **B,** Posterior view.

The physical examination of the basketball player should include active ROM, passive ROM, and restricted ROM for knee flexion and extension and for internal and external tibial rotation; grind test; Clarke's sign; and Waldron test.

REHABILITATION OF KNEE INJURIES

The basketball player is diagnosed with patellofemoral syndrome. Explain the focus of a rehabilitation program for this condition.

A rehabilitation program attempts to minimize inflammation and the effects of immobilization by initiating early mobilization and controlled movement to allow healing tissues to be stressed gradually and progressively until normal joint function is restored. The rehabilitation program should restore motion and proprioception, maintain cardiovascular fitness, and improve muscular strength, endurance, and power, predominantly through closed-chain exercises. Sample exercise programs for specific injuries are listed in Field Strategies 17.1 to 17.5.

Restoration of Motion

Some loss of motion occurs following most knee injuries. Passive ROM exercises normally can begin on the first day after injury. Because of potential damage to the graft, however, some concern has been raised about the use of continuous passive motion (CPM) machines following autogenous patellar tendon reconstruction of the ACL. The literature does support the early use of the CPM in this population (31). The unit moves the knee through a protected ROM to stimulate the intrinsic healing process. The benefits of CPM following ACL surgery include:

- Maintaining articular cartilage nutrition, and preventing articular cartilage degradation
- Preventing adhesions, joint stiffness, and muscle spasm
- Improving collagen remodeling and joint dynamics
- Reducing pain, thereby reducing amount of pain medication
- Decreasing joint swelling and effusion
- Producing no significant deleterious effects on the stability of the ligament
- Increasing knee ROM sooner

When a CPM machine is not needed, ROM exercises, such as the supine wall slide, heel slide, assisted knee flexion and extension, half squats, or proprioceptive neuromuscular facilitation stretching exercises, can be performed (Fig. 17.41). Extension usually is the most difficult motion to restore, and it is critical in achieving normal gait. The individual is placed prone, with the thigh resting on the table. The lower leg is extended off the end of the table. A weight can be added on the distal tibia so that a gradual stretch is achieved. Following the exercise bout, the knee should be iced in the supine position, with the heel elevated to assist with extension.

In addition to active and passive ROM exercises at the tibiofemoral joint, stretching exercises to improve passive glide of the patellofemoral joint, particularly medial glide, can stretch tight lateral structures to correct patellar positioning and tracking (Fig. 17.42). Normal passive glide of the patellofemoral joint should be restored before full flexion exercises, resisted exercises, or bicycling is initiated.

Restoration of Proprioception and Balance

Proprioception and balance must be regained to return safely to activity. During the early stages following injury, when weight bearing is allowed, closed chain exercises, such as shifting one's weight while on crutches, straight leg raises, bilateral minisquats, or use of a biomechanical ankle platform system (BAPS) board with support, may be helpful. As balance improves, unassisted use

■■■■ FIGURE 17.41 **Range-of-motion exercises. A,** Half-squat. **B,** Assisted heel slide.
C, Assisted knee flexion and hip flexion. **D,** Assisted knee flexion.

of the BAPS board, closed chain exercises, running in place on a minitramp, or use of a slide board may be incorporated along with other closed chain exercises that are used to develop strength.

Muscular Strength, Endurance, and Power

Early emphasis should be placed on strengthening the quadriceps femoris musculature, particularly the vastus medialis and VMO. These muscles aid in the stabilization of the patella both superiorly and medially. Isometric contractions, called quad sets, are performed at or near 0, 45, 60, and 90° of flexion. Isometric hip adduction exercises also are used to recruit the VMO and can be performed by squeezing a rolled towel between the knees in a seated position. Open chain exercises may include straight leg raises in all directions, supplemented by ankle weights or tubing to increase resistance. Knee extension and flexion exercises may be done with free weights or on several commercially available isotonic or isokinetic machines.

Closed chain exercises performed during weight bearing may include terminal knee extension (Fig. 17.43), step-ups, step-downs, lateral step-ups, minisquats from 0 to 40°, leg presses on a machine from 0 to 60°, or use of a stepping machine or stationary bicycle. Several of these exercises are detailed in Field Strategy 17.1. Closed chain exercises can be made progressively more difficult by increasing the resistance or speed of movement or by changing the individual's visual feedback (e.g., looking at the ceiling, looking at the floor, or closing the eyes). Ensuring proper performance of closed chain exercises is critical. For example, when doing a minisquat or leg press, if the hip is not strong enough to control adduction and internal rotation, the knee assumes a valgus alignment,

FIGURE 17.42 Patellar self-mobilization. A, Proximal. **B,** Distal. **C,** Medial. **D,** Lateral.

FIGURE 17.43 Closed chain terminal extension. A, Starting position. **B,** Ending position.

with the foot pronated. This leads to an increased Q-angle, predisposing the individual to patellofemoral pain.

Plyometric jumping during the later stages of rehabilitation can be performed using small boxes and directional changes to improve power and proprioceptive function. Because of the increased eccentric contraction and the associated muscle microtrauma that results from the power maneuvers, these exercises should only be performed two or three times weekly.

Cardiovascular Fitness

Cardiovascular fitness exercises can begin immediately after injury with use of an upper body ergometer or hydrotherapeutic exercise. Running in water and performing sport–specific exercises in deep water can allow the individual to maintain activity-specific functional skills in a non–weight bearing position. When ROM is adequate, a stationary bicycle may be used. The seat should be adjusted so that the knee is flexed by 15 to 30°. The individual should be instructed to pedal with the ball of the foot, using toe clips, and to pull through the bottom of the stroke. A low to moderate workload is recommended to reduce patellofemoral compressive forces. Other exercises, such as walking, light jogging, and functional activities, can progress as tolerated.

Rehabilitation for the basketball player with patellofemoral syndrome should focus on recruiting the VMO, normalizing patella mobility, and increasing flexibility and muscle control of the lower extremity. Resisted terminal knee extension exercises, straight leg raises in hip flexion and adduction, as well as quadriceps isometric, isotonic, and high-speed isokinetic exercises in a 60 to 90° arc may be performed. Closed chain exercises often are preferred because of the decrease in patellofemoral compression forces. Strengthening of the hip muscles to prevent adduction and internal rotation is critical to allow the progression of closed chain exercises. Restoring proprioception also is critical in re-establishing neuromuscular control. Weight training programs that load the patellofemoral joint, such as bent-knee exercises, should be avoided.

SUMMARY

1. The knee (tibiofemoral joint) functions primarily as a modified hinge joint, with some lateral and rotational motions allowed.

2. The cruciate ligaments are intracapsular and extrasynovial. They prevent anterior and posterior translation of the tibia on the femur. The ACL frequently is subject to deceleration injuries, with internal tibial torque being the most dangerous loading mechanism, particularly when combined with an anterior tibial force. The shorter and stronger PCL is considered to be the primary stabilizer of the knee.

3. The collateral ligaments prevent valgus (medial) and varus (lateral) stress at the knee.

4. The menisci aid in lubrication and nutrition of the joint, reduce friction during movement, provide shock absorption by dissipating stress over the articular cartilage, improve weight distribution, and help the capsule and ligaments to prevent hyperextension.

5. Tracking of the patella against the femur is dependent on the direction of the net force that is produced by the attached quadriceps. Factors such as patellar instability, a weak VMO, hypermobility of the patella, anatomical malalignment conditions, plica syndromes, or repetitive minor trauma can lead to chronic patellofemoral pain.

6. Because of its location, the prepatellar bursa is the bursa most commonly injured by compressive forces. The deep infrapatellar bursa often is inflamed by overuse and subsequent friction between the infrapatellar tendon and structures behind it (fat pad and tibia).

7. A straight plane instability implies an instability in one of the cardinal planes. A multidirectional instability involves instability in more than one plane.

8. Isolated anterior instability is rare. Instead, an anteromedial or anterolateral laxity usually occurs. The rate of ACL injuries is higher in women, in part because of an imbalance of muscle strength as well as both intrinsic and extrinsic factors.

9. Menisci become stiffer and less resilient with age. Tears are classified according to age, location, or axis of orientation, and they include longitudinal, bucket-handle, horizontal, and parrot-beak. Because the menisci are not innervated by nociceptors, synovial inflammation and joint effusion may not develop for more than 12 hours after the initial injury.

10. Patellofemoral stress syndrome often occurs when either the VMO is weak or the lateral retinaculum that holds the patella firmly to the femoral condyle is excessively tight. This condition is much more common than chondromalacia patellae, which is a true degeneration in the articular cartilage of the patella.

11. Adolescents are particularly prone to Osgood-Schlatter disease, Sinding-Larsen-Johansson disease, and fractures to the distal femoral epiphysis.

12. Pain in the knee region can be referred from the lumbar spine, hip, or ankle.

13. A rehabilitation program should minimize inflammation and the effects of immobilization by initiating early mobilization and controlled movement to allow healing tissues to be stressed, gradually and progressively, until normal joint function is restored.

14. An individual should be referred to a physician if any of the following conditions are suspected:
   - Obvious deformity suggesting a dislocation or fracture
   - Significant loss of motion or locking of the knee
   - Excessive joint swelling
   - Gross joint instability
   - Reported sounds, such as popping, snapping, or clicking, or giving way of the knee
   - Possible epiphyseal injuries
   - Abnormal or absent reflexes
   - Abnormal sensations in either segmental dermatomes or peripheral cutaneous patterns
   - Absent or weak pulse
   - Weakness in a myotome
   - Any unexplained or chronic pain that disrupts an individual's play or performance

REFERENCES

1. Adirim TA, Cheng TL. Overview of injuries in the young athlete. Sports Med 2003;33(1):75–81.
2. Rath E, Richmond JC. The menisci: basic science and advances in treatment. Br J Sports Med 2000;34:252–257.
3. Mine T, Kimura M, Sakka A, Kawai S. Innervation of nociceptors in the menisci of the knee joint: an immuno-histochemical study. Arch Orthop Trauma Surg 2000;120(3–4):201–204.
4. Shelburne KB, Pandy MG, Anderson FC, Torry MR. Pattern of anterior cruciate ligament force in normal walking. J Biomech 2004:37(6):797–805.
5. Markolf KL, et al. Combined knee loading states that generate high anterior cruciate ligament forces. J Orthop Res 1995;13(6):930–935.
6. Grelsamer RP, Weinstein CH. Applied biomechanics of the patella. Clin Orthop 2001;(389):9–14.
7. Dye SF. Functional morphologic features of the human knee: an evolutionary perspective. Clin Orthop 2003;(410):19–24.
8. Mizuno Y, Kumagai M, Mattessich SM, et al. Q-angle influences tibiofemoral and patellofemoral kinematics. J Orthop Res 2001;19(5):834–840.
9. McClure SK, Adams JE, Dahm DL. Common musculoskeletal disorders in women. Mayo Clin Proc 2005;80(6):796–802.
10. Rubel IF, Schwarzbard I, Leonard A, Cece D. Anatomic location of the peroneal nerve at the level of the proximal aspect of the tibia: Gerdy's safe zone. J Bone Joint Surg Am 2004;86(8):1625–1628.
11. Johal P, Williams A, Wragg P, et al. Tibiofemoral movement in the living knee. A study of weight bearing and non–weight bearing knee kinematics using "interventional" MRI. J Biomech 2005;38(2):269–276.
12. Nakagawa S, Kadoya Y, Kobayashi A, et al. Kinematics of

the patella in deep flexion. Analysis with magnetic resonance imaging. J Bone Joint Surg Am 2003;85(7): 1238–1242.

13. Moro-oka T, Matsuda S, Miura H, et al. Patellar tracking and patellofemoral geometry in deep knee flexion. Clin Orthop 2002;(394):161–168.

14. Escamilla RF. Knee biomechanics of the dynamic squat exercise. Med Sci Sports Exerc 2001;33(1):127–141.

15. Escamilla RF, Fleisig GS, Zheng N, et al. Effects of technique variations on knee biomechanics during the squat and leg press. Med Sci Sports Exerc 2001;33(9): 1552–1566.

16. Costigan PA, Deluzio KJ, Wyss UP. Knee and hip kinetics during normal stair climbing. Gait Posture 2002; 16(1):31–37.

17. Shrive NG, Phil D, O'Connor JJ, Goodfellow JW. Load-bearing in the knee joint. Clin Orthop 1978;131:279–287.

18. Costigan PA, Deluzio KJ, Wyss UP. Knee and hip kinetics during normal stair climbing. Gait Posture 2002; 16(1):31–37.

19. Moul JL. Differences in selected predictors of anterior cruciate ligament tears between male and female NCAA Division I collegiate basketball players. J Ath Train 1998;33(2):118–121.

20. Cardon DA, Tallia AF. Diagnostic and therapeutic injection of the hip and knee. Am Fam Physician 2003; 67(10):2147–2152.

21. Tyler TF, McHugh MP. Neuromuscular rehabilitation of a female Olympic ice hockey player following anterior cruciate ligament reconstruction. J Orthop Sports Phys Ther 2001;31(10):577–587.

22. McDevitt ER, Taylor DC, Miller MD, et al. Functional bracing was no better than nonbracing after anterior cruciate ligament repair. J Bone Joint Surg Am 2005; 87A(8):1890.

23. WalshWM, Vanicek JJ. Knee injuries. In: Mellion MB, Walsh WM, Madden C, Putukian M, Shelton GL, eds. The Team Physician's Handbook. Philadelphia: Hanley & Belfus, 2002.

24. Covey DC. Current concepts review: injuries of the posterolateral corner of the knee. J Bone Joint Surg Am 2001;83(1):106–118.

25. Hale SA. Etiology of patellar tendinopathy in athletes. J Sport Rehab 2005;14(3):258–272.

26. Wall EJ. Osgood-Schlatter disease: practical treatment for a self-limiting condition. Phys Sportsmed 1998;26(3): 29–34.

27. Greis PE, Lahav A, Holmstron MC. Surgical treatment options for patella tendon rupture, Part II: Chronic. Orthopedics 2005;28(8):765–769.

28. Khaund R, Flynn SH. Iliotibial band syndrome: a common source of knee pain. Am Fam Physician 2005;71(8): 1545–1550.

29. Johnson MP. Physical therapy management of an adult with osteochondritis dissecans of the knee. Phys Ther 2005;85(7):665–675.

30. Norkus SA, Swartz EE, Floyd RT. Advantages of the prone Lachman test. Ath Ther Today 2002;7(2):52–56.

31. Weber MD, Woodall WB. Knee rehabilitation. In: Andrews JR, Harrelson GL, Wilk KE, eds. Physical Rehabilitation of the Injured Athlete. Philadelphia: WB Saunders, 2004.

CHAPTER 18

Lower Leg, Ankle, and Foot Conditions

STUDENT OUTCOMES

1. Identify the major bony and soft-tissue structures of the lower leg, ankle, and foot.

2. Identify the various ligamentous structures that support the lower leg, ankle, and foot.

3. Identify the plantar arches and explain their function.

4. Describe the motions of the foot and ankle, and identify the muscles that produce them.

5. Explain the forces that produce the loading patterns responsible for injury to the lower leg, ankle, and foot.

6. Explain the general principles to prevent injuries to the lower leg, ankle, and foot.

7. Describe the common injuries to and conditions of the knee in physically active individuals (including sprains, dislocations, contusions, strains, bursitis, and vascular and neural disorders).

8. Explain the management strategies for common injuries and conditions of the lower leg, ankle, and foot.

9. List the various types of fractures that can occur at the lower leg, ankle, and foot, and explain their management.

10. Describe a thorough assessment of the lower leg, ankle, and foot.

11. Explain the basic principles associated with rehabilitation of injuries to the lower leg, ankle, and foot.

638

ROLE DELINEATION COMPETENCIES

The following Performance Domains and Tasks defined in the National Athletic Trainers' Association Board of Certification *Role Delineation Study*, 5th Edition are addressed in this chapter:

BOC COMPETENCIES

I. Prevention

G. Monitor participants and environmental conditions by following accepted guidelines to promote safe participation.

II. Clinical Evaluation and Diagnosis

A. Obtain a history through observation, interview, and/or review of relevant records to assess current or potential injury, illness, or condition.
B. Inspect the involved area(s) visually to assess the injury, illness, or health-related condition.
C. Palpate the involved area(s) using standard techniques to assess the injury, illness, or health-related condition.
D. Perform specific tests in accordance with accepted procedures to assess the injury, illness, or health-related condition.
E. Formulate a clinical impression by interpreting the signs, symptoms, and predisposing factors of the injury, illness, or condition to determine the appropriate course of action.

III. Immediate Care

A. Employ life-saving techniques through the use of standard emergency procedures in order to reduce morbidity and the incidence of mortality.
B. Prevent exacerbation of non–life threatening condition(s) through the use of standard procedures in order to reduce morbidity.
C. Facilitate the timely transfer of care for conditions beyond the scope of practice of the athletic trainer by implementing appropriate referral strategies to stabilize and/or prevent exacerbation of the condition(s).

IV. Treatment, Rehabilitation, and Reconditioning

E. Reassess the status of injuries, illnesses, and/or conditions using standard techniques and documentation strategies in order to determine appropriate treatment, rehabilitation, and/or reconditioning and to evaluate readiness to return to a desired level of activity.
F. Educate the appropriate individual(s) in the treatment, rehabilitation, and reconditioning of injuries, illnesses, and/or conditions using applicable methods and materials to facilitate recovery, function, and/or performance.

Because of the essential roles played by the lower leg, ankle, and foot during sport and physical activities, injuries to this region are common. Sport participation often places both acute and chronic overloads on the lower extremity, leading to sprains, strains, fractures, and overuse injuries. In particular, basketball, soccer, and football participants sustain a high incidence of injury to this region (1,2). Lateral ankle sprains are the most common of all sports-related injuries, accounting for approximately 25% of injuries to the musculoskeletal system (3). Increasingly, it is being recognized that repeated ankle sprains can result in functional instability of the ankle, which predisposes the individual to further injury (4).

This chapter begins with an anatomical review and biomechanical overview of the lower leg, ankle, and foot. Next, prevention of injury is discussed, followed by details on specific injuries and their management. Finally, a step-by-step injury assessment of the region is presented, and examples of rehabilitative exercises are provided.

ANATOMY OF THE LOWER LEG, ANKLE, AND FOOT

The lower leg, ankle, and foot are comprised of numerous bones and articulations (Fig. 18.1). They provide a foundation of support for the upright body, enabling propulsion through space, adaptation to uneven terrain, and absorption of shock.

Forefoot

The three major regions of the foot are the forefoot, midfoot, and hindfoot. The forefoot is composed of five metatarsals and 14 phalanges, along with numerous joints. In conjunction with the midfoot region, the forefoot forms interdependent longitudinal and transverse arches to support and distribute body weight throughout the foot.

Metatarsophalangeal and Interphalangeal Joints

The metatarsophalangeal (MTP) joint is a condyloid joint with a close-packed position in full extension. The proximal interphalangeal (PIP) and distal interphalangeal (DIP) joints are hinge joints that also have a close-packed position in full extension (see Fig. 18.1). Numerous ligaments reinforce both sets of joints. Each MTP joint is surrounded by an articular and fibrous joint capsule,

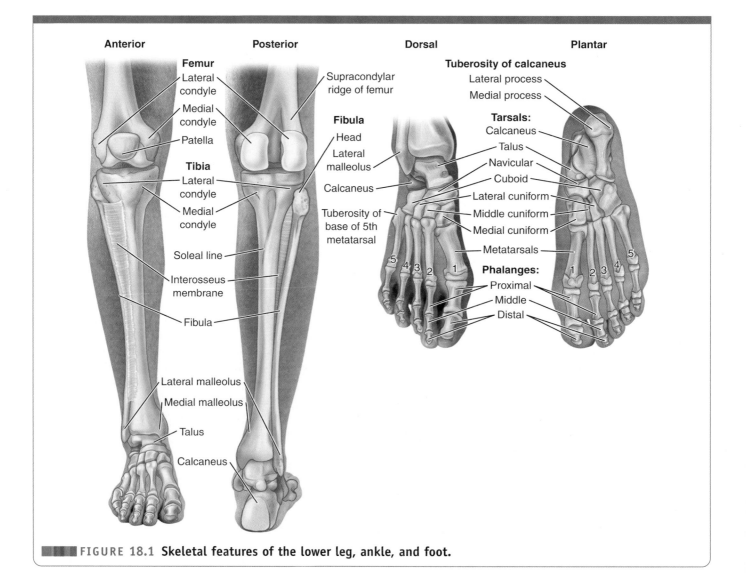

FIGURE 18.1 Skeletal features of the lower leg, ankle, and foot.

the plantar side of which is reinforced by the plantar fascia and thickened portions of the capsule (i.e., plantar ligament). The medial and lateral joint capsules are reinforced by collateral ligaments. The PIP and DIP joints are reinforced by the plantar and dorsal joint capsule and the collateral ligaments. The toes function to smooth the weight shift to the opposite foot during walking and help to maintain stability during weight bearing by pressing against the ground when necessary. The first digit is referred to as the hallux, or "great toe," and is the main body stabilizer during walking or running.

The first MTP joint has two sesamoid bones, which are located on the plantar surface of the joint to share in weight bearing. The sesamoid bones serve as anatomical pulleys for the flexor hallucis brevis muscle and protect the flexor hallucis longus muscle tendon from weight-bearing trauma as it passes between the two bones.

Tarsometatarsal and Intermetatarsal Joints

The deep transverse metatarsal ligament interconnects the five metatarsals. Both the tarsometatarsal and intermetatarsal joints are of the gliding type with the close-packed position in supination. These joints enable the foot to adapt to uneven surfaces during gait.

Midfoot

The midfoot region encompasses the navicular, cuboid, and three cuneiform bones as well as their articulations. The navicular, like its counterpart in the wrist, the scaphoid, helps to bridge movements between the hindfoot and forefoot.

Transverse Tarsal Joint

The transverse tarsal (or midtarsal) joint consists of two side-by-side articulations—namely, the calcaneocuboid joint on the lateral side and the talonavicular on the medial side. Collectively, these two joints are called the transverse tarsal joint, because they are adjacent and function as a unit.

The calcaneocuboid joint is a saddle-shaped joint with a close-packed position in supination. The joint is nonaxial and permits only limited gliding motion. It is supported by the bifurcate ligament, the plantar and dorsal calcaneocuboid ligaments, and the long plantar ligament. The most important of these, the long plantar ligament, extends inferiorly between the calcaneus and the cuboid, then continues distally to the base of the second, third, and fourth metatarsals, contributing significantly to transverse tarsal joint stability.

Because the talus moves simultaneously on the calcaneus and navicular, the term talocalcaneonavicular joint (TCN) often is used to describe the combined action of the talonavicular and subtalar joint. The TCN is a modified ball-and-socket joint with a close-packed position in supination. Movements at the joint include gliding and rotation. Three ligaments support the joint—namely, the plantar calcaneonavicular (spring) ligament inferiorly, the deltoid ligament medially, and the bifurcate ligament laterally (Fig. 18.2).

Because the subtalar joint is mechanically linked to the TCN and transverse tarsal joints, any motion at the subtalar joint produces similar motions at the

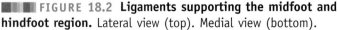 **FIGURE 18.2 Ligaments supporting the midfoot and hindfoot region.** Lateral view (top). Medial view (bottom).

transverse tarsal joints. For example, when the TCN is fully supinated and locked, the midfoot region is supinated and rigid. When the TCN is pronated and loose packed, the midfoot region is mobile and loose.

Other Midtarsal Joints

The remaining joints of the midfoot region include the cuneonavicular, cuboideonavicular, cuneocuboid, and intercuneiform. These joints provide gliding and rotation for the midfoot with a close-packed position in supination. They are bound together by several ligaments. When the midfoot (i.e., TCN) is locked in supination, these joints function in a compensatory manner to pronate the forefoot and increase stability. When the hindfoot is pronated, these joints supinate the forefoot to keep the foot flat on the surface.

Hindfoot

The hindfoot includes the calcaneus and talus. Rising off the anteromedial surface of the calcaneus is the **sustentaculum tali**, which largely supports the talus. Located on the inferior surface of the sustentaculum tali is a groove through which the flexor hallucis longus tendon passes. The peroneal tubercle projects out of the lateral side of the calcaneus and splits the two peroneal tendons as they course inferior to the lateral malleolus. The peroneus brevis tendon runs superior to the tubercle; the peroneus longus tendon runs inferior to the tubercle.

The talus is saddle-shaped and serves as the critical link between the foot and the ankle. It has several functional articulations, the two most important of which being the talocrural joint and the subtalar joint. Both serve a unique role in the integrated function of the lower leg, ankle, and foot.

Talocrural Joint

The talocrural (i.e., ankle) joint is a uniaxial, modified synovial hinge joint formed by the talus, tibia, and lateral malleolus of the fibula. The concave end of the weight-bearing tibia mates with the convex superior surface of the talus to form the roof and medial border of the ankle mortise. The fibula assists with weight bearing, supporting approximately 17% of the load on the leg (5); serves as a site for muscle and ligamentous attachments; and forms the lateral border of the ankle mortise. The lateral malleolus extends farther distally than the medial malleolus; hence, eversion is more seriously limited than inversion. The dome of the talus is wider anteriorly than posteriorly. Therefore, the joint's close-packed position is maximum dorsiflexion.

Although the joint capsule is thin and especially weak anteriorly and posteriorly, a number of strong ligaments cross the ankle and enhance stability (Table 18.1). The four separate bands of the

TABLE 18.1 Ligaments of the Talocrural Joint

	PROXIMAL ATTACHMENT	DISTAL ATTACHMENT
Medial Collateral Ligaments		
Anterior tibiotalar	Anteromedial aspect of medial malleolus	Superior portion of medial talus
Tibiocalcaneal	Apex of medial malleolus	Calcaneus directly below medial malleolus
Posterior tibiotalar	Posterior aspect of medial malleolus	Posterior portion of the talus
Tibionavicular	Distal and slightly posterior to the anterior tibiotalar	Medial aspect of the navicular
Lateral Collateral Ligaments		
Anterior talofibular	Anterolateral surface of lateral malleolus	Talus near the sinus tarsi
Calcaneofibular	Posterior apex of lateral malleolus	Courses 133° inferiorly and posteriorly to attach on calcaneus
Posterior talofibular	Posterolateral border of lateral malleolus	Posterior talus and calcaneus

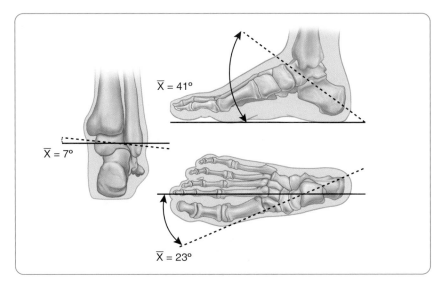

FIGURE 18.3 **Subtalar joint.** The axis of rotation at the subtalar joint lies oblique to the sagittal and frontal planes.

medial collateral ligament (more commonly called the deltoid ligament) cross the ankle medially. The anterior tibiotalar and tibionavicular ligaments are taut when the subtalar joint is plantar flexed, whereas the tibiocalcaneal and posterior tibiotalar ligaments are taut during dorsiflexion. Forces producing stress on the medial aspect of the ankle typically cause an avulsion fracture of the medial malleolus rather than tearing the deltoid ligament.

The lateral side of the ankle is supported by three ligaments. The anterior talofibular ligament (ATFL) is taut and resists inversion during plantar flexion and limits anterior translation of the talus on the tibia. The calcaneofibular ligament (CFL) is taut in the extreme range of dorsiflexion and is the primary restraint of talar inversion within the mid range of motion (ROM). The posterior talofibular ligament is the strongest of the lateral ligaments and limits posterior displacement of the talus on the tibia. The relative weakness of these lateral ligaments as compared with the deltoid ligament, coupled with the fact of less bony stability laterally compared with medially, contributes to a higher frequency of lateral ankle sprains.

Subtalar Joint

As the name suggests, the subtalar joint lies beneath the talus, where facets of the talus articulate with the sustentaculum tali on the superior calcaneus. Obliquely crossing the talus and calcaneus is the tarsal canal, a sulcus that allows attachment of an intra-articular ligament. Because no muscles attach to the talus, the stability of the subtalar joint is derived from several small ligaments. The talocalcaneal interosseous ligament lies in the tarsal canal, and divides the subtalar joint into two articular cavities, serves as an axis for talar tilt, and contributes substantially to joint stability, particularly during supination (Fig. 18.3). Four small talocalcaneal ligaments form interconnections between the talus and calcaneus, and the CFL and tibiocalcaneal fascicle of the deltoid ligament add support. The close-packed position for the joint occurs under vertical loading with internal rotation.

The subtalar joint behaves as a flexible structure, with motion only occurring through stretching of ligaments during weight bearing (6). Motion at the subtalar joint involves "male" ovoid bone surfaces sliding over reciprocally shaped "female" ovoid bone surfaces. Disagreement exists regarding whether the joint functions as a hinge, screw-like, or multiaxial joint (7). The orientation of the subtalar joint axis varies appreciably among individuals.

Tibiofibular Joints

The tibia and fibula articulate at both the proximal and distal ends (see Fig. 18.1). The proximal, or superior, tibiofibular joint is a plantar synovial joint that is tightly reinforced with anterior and

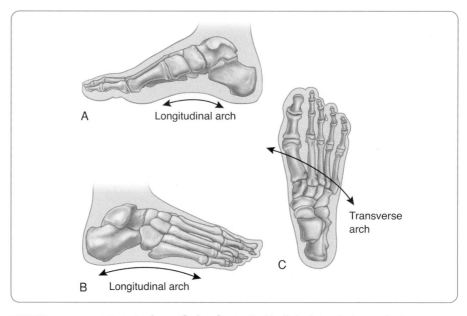

A Longitudinal arch

Transverse arch

B Longitudinal arch

C

FIGURE 18.4 Arches of the foot. A, Medial view. **B,** Lateral view. **C,** Dorsal view.

posterior ligaments. The inferior, or distal, tibiofibular joint is a syndesmosis, where dense fibrous tissue binds the bones together. No joint capsule exists, but the joint is supported by the anterior and posterior tibiofibular ligaments as well as by an extension of the interosseous membrane, the crural interosseous ligament. This structural arrangement allows some rotation and slight abduction (spreading) while still maintaining joint integrity. The strength of the crural interosseous ligament is such that strong lateral stresses often fracture the fibula rather than tear the membrane, although excessive eversion or dorsiflexion can result in sufficient widening of the ankle mortise to injure the ligaments supporting the syndesmosis.

Plantar Arches

The bones and supporting ligamentous structures in the tarsal and metatarsal regions of the foot form interdependent longitudinal and transverse arches (Fig. 18.4). They function to support and distribute body weight from the talus through the foot, through changing weight-bearing conditions, and over varying terrain. The longitudinal arch runs from the anteroinferior calcaneus to the metatarsal heads. Because the arch is higher medially than laterally, the medial side usually is the point of reference, with the navicular bone serving as the point of reference between the anterior and posterior ascending spans.

The transverse arch runs across the anterior tarsals and metatarsals. The foundation of the arch is the medial cuneiform, with the apex of the arch formed by the second metatarsal. The arch is reduced at the level of the metatarsal heads, with all metatarsals aligned parallel to the weight-bearing surface for even distribution of body weight. Structural support is derived from the inter-metatarsal ligaments and the transverse head of the adductor hallucis muscle.

The primary supporting structures of the plantar arches, in order of importance, are the calcaneonavicular (i.e., spring) ligament, long plantar ligament, plantar fascia (i.e., plantar aponeurosis), and short plantar (i.e., plantar calcaneocuboid) ligament (Fig. 18.5). When muscle tension is present, the muscles of the foot, particularly the tibialis posterior, contribute support to the arches and joints as they cross them.

The **plantar fascia**, or plantar aponeurosis, is a specialized, thick, interconnected band of fascia that covers the plantar surface of the foot, providing support for the longitudinal arch (Fig. 18.6). It has three distinct slips. The central slip extends from the posteromedial calcaneal tubercle and inserts into the distal plantar aspects of the proximal phalanges of each toe, where it attaches with

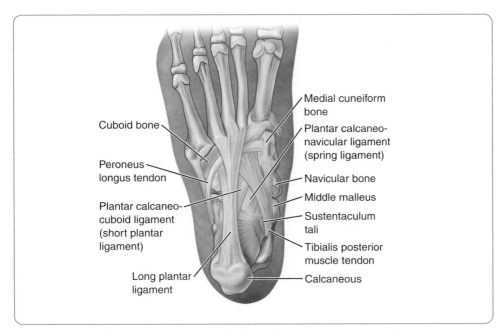

FIGURE 18.5 Medial longitudinal arch. The medial longitudinal arch is supported by the calcaneonavicular (spring) ligament, short plantar ligament, long plantar ligament, plantar aponeurosis, and tibialis posterior muscle tendon.

FIGURE 18.6 Plantar fascia. The plantar fascia stores mechanical energy each time the foot deforms during the weight-bearing phase of the gait cycle.

FIGURE 18.7 Muscles of the lower leg and foot. Lateral and medial view.

deep transverse metatarsal ligaments. As the central slip courses down the length of the foot, it gives off two other slips, one deviating medially and the other laterally. During the weight-bearing phase of the gait cycle, the plantar fascia stretches on the order of 9 to 12% of resting length, functioning like a spring to store mechanical energy that is released to help the foot push off from the surface (8). Stretching the Achilles tendon may elongate the plantar fascia, because both structures attach to the calcaneus.

Muscles of the Lower Leg and Foot

A large number of muscles cross the ankle (Figs. 18.7 and 18.8). Identifying the actions of these muscles is complicated by the fact that several muscles are two-joint muscles (see Table 18.1).

Thick sheaths of fascia divide the muscles of the leg into four compartments—namely, the anterior, deep posterior, superficial posterior, and lateral compartments. The anterior compartment contains the tibialis anterior, extensor digitorum longus, extensor hallucis longus, and peroneus tertius. Muscles in the deep posterior compartment include the tibialis posterior, flexor digitorum longus, tibialis posterior artery, tibial nerve, and flexor hallucis longus The superficial posterior compartment contains the gastrocnemius, soleus, and plantaris, and the lateral compartment contains the peroneus longus and peroneus brevis.

The foot contains both intrinsic and extrinsic muscles. An intrinsic muscle has both attachments contained within the foot (Figs. 18.9 and 18.10), whereas an extrinsic muscle has one attachment outside the foot.

See *Major Muscles of the Foot and Leg*, available on the companion website at thePoint, for a summary of the attachments and primary actions of the major extrinsic muscles of the lower leg, ankle, and foot.

FIGURE 18.8 Muscles of the lower leg and foot. Posterior view.

Nerves of the Lower Leg, Ankle, and Foot

The sciatic nerve and its branches provide primary innervation for the lower leg, ankle, and foot. Traveling down the posterior aspect of the leg from the lumbosacral spine, the sciatic nerve branches into smaller nerves just proximal to the popliteal fossa. The major branches are the tibial nerve, which innervates the posterior aspect of the leg, and the common peroneal nerve, which spawns the deep and superficial peroneal nerves.

The tibial nerve (L_4–S_3) passes through the popliteal fossa and down the leg between the superficial and deep muscles in the posterior compartment of the leg (see Fig. 17.4). It continues medially behind the medial malleolus with the posterior tibial artery to become the medial and lateral plantar nerves. The saphenous nerve (L_2–L_4), which branches from the femoral nerve, supplies cutaneous innervation to the medial aspect of the ankle.

The common peroneal nerve passes laterally around the neck of the fibula to the anterolateral leg, where it splits into the deep and superficial peroneal nerves (see Fig. 17.4). The deep peroneal nerve (L_4–S_1) innervates the anterior compartment, which contains the ankle dorsiflexors and toe extensors, then courses over the dorsum of the foot to innervate the skin between the first and second toes. The superficial peroneal nerve (L_5–S_2) innervates the lateral compartment, which contains the primary everter muscles, and provides cutaneous innervation to the second through fourth toes. The sural nerve (L_4–S_2), a branch from both the common peroneal and tibial nerves, supplies cutaneous innervation to the lateral aspect of the ankle, heel, and foot. Given the extensiveness of the sciatic nerve supply to the lower extremity, it is no surprise that impingement of the sciatic nerve by a herniated disk in the lumbosacral region often results in pain, numbness, and/or impaired function in the foot and ankle region.

Blood Vessels of the Lower Leg, Ankle, and Foot

The blood supply to the lower leg, ankle, and foot enters the lower extremity as the femoral artery (Fig. 18.11). The femoral artery becomes the popliteal artery proximal and posterior to the knee, then branches into the anterior and posterior tibial arteries just distal to the knee. The anterior tibial artery becomes the dorsalis pedis artery to supply the dorsum of the foot. The posterior tibial artery gives off several branches that supply the posterior and lateral compartments and the plantar region of the foot.

FIGURE 18.10 Intrinsic muscles of the foot. Plantar view.

■■ ■ FIGURE 18.11 **Blood supply to the leg, ankle, and foot region. A,** The dorsalis pedis artery is easily palpated in the midfoot region between the second and third tendons of the extensor digitorum longus. **B,** The posterior tibial artery can be palpated just posterior of the medial malleolus.

KINEMATICS OF THE LOWER LEG, ANKLE, AND FOOT

Evaluation of the kinematics of gait during walking and running can provide important clues for the likelihood of injuries. This section describes the kinematics of the lower leg, ankle, and foot, and it identifies the muscles that are responsible for specific movements.

The Gait Cycle

The gait cycle requires a set of coordinated, sequential joint actions of the lower extremity. Despite variation in individual gait patterns, enough commonality exists in human gaits that one can describe the typical gait cycle (Fig. 18.12). The gait cycle begins with a period of single-leg support in which body weight is supported by one leg while the other leg swings forward. The swing phase can be divided into the initial swing, midswing, and terminal swing. The period of double support begins with the contact of the swing leg with the ground or floor. As body weight transfers from the support leg to the swing leg, the swing leg undergoes a loading response and becomes the new support leg. A new period of single support then begins as the swing leg loses ground contact. The time during which body weight is balanced over the support leg is referred to as midstance. As the

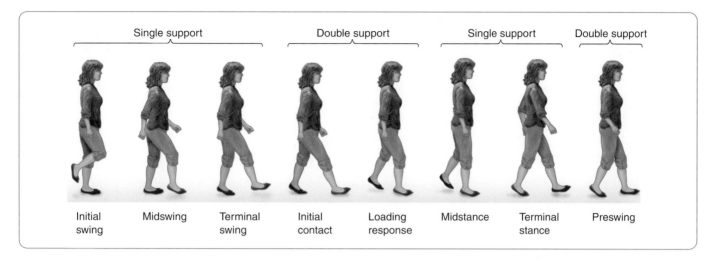

Single support   Double support   Single support   Double support

Initial swing   Midswing   Terminal swing   Initial contact   Loading response   Midstance   Terminal stance   Preswing

FIGURE 18.12 Gait. The gait cycle consists of alternating periods of single-leg support and double-leg support.

body's center of gravity shifts forward, the terminal stance phase of the support leg coincides with the terminal swing phase of the opposite leg.

Differences in running gait have been documented based on both gender and age. Among recreational runners, females appear to have greater hip adduction, hip internal rotation, and knee abduction compared to males (9). A study of elite master sprinters showed an age-related decline in running speed related to reduction in stride length and increase in ground contact time (10).

Toe Flexion and Extension

Several muscles contribute to flexion of the second through fifth toes. These include the flexor digitorum longus, flexor digitorum brevis, quadratus plantae, lumbricals, and interossei. The flexor hallucis longus and brevis produce flexion of the hallux. Conversely, the extensor hallucis longus, extensor digitorum longus, and extensor digitorum brevis are responsible for extension and overextension of the toes.

Dorsiflexion and Plantar Flexion

Motion at the ankle occurs primarily in the sagittal plane, with ankle flexion and extension being termed dorsiflexion and plantar flexion, respectively (Fig. 18.13A). The medial and lateral malleoli serve as pulleys to channel the tendons of the leg muscles either posterior or anterior to the axis of rotation and, in doing so, enable their contributions to either plantar flexion or dorsiflexion. Muscles with tendons passing anterior to the malleoli (i.e., the tibialis anterior, extensor digitorum longus, and peroneus tertius) are dorsiflexors. Those with tendinous attachments running posterior to the malleoli contribute to plantar flexion. The major plantar flexors are the soleus, gastrocnemius, plantaris, and flexor hallucis longus, with assistance being provided by the peroneal longus and brevis and by the tibialis posterior.

Inversion and Eversion

Rotations of the foot in the medial and lateral directions are termed inversion and eversion, respectively (Fig. 18.13B). These movements occur primarily at the subtalar joint, with secondary contributions from gliding movements at the intertarsal and tarsometatarsal joints. The tibialis posterior is the major inverter, with the tibialis anterior providing a minor contribution. The peroneus longus and brevis, with tendons passing behind the lateral malleolus, are primarily responsible for eversion, with assistance being provided by the peroneus tertius.

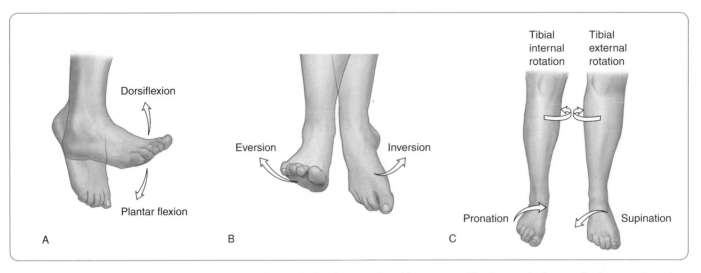

FIGURE 18.13 Motions of the foot and ankle. A, Dorsiflexion and plantar flexion. **B,** Eversion and inversion. **C,** Supination of the subtalar joint results in external rotation of the tibia; pronation is linked with internal rotation of the tibia.

Pronation and Supination

The lower extremity moves through a cyclical sequence of movements during gait. Among these, the action at the subtalar joint during weight bearing has the most significant implications for lower extremity injury potential. During heel contact, the hindfoot typically is somewhat inverted. As the foot rolls forward and the forefoot initially contacts the ground, the foot is plantar flexed. This combination of calcaneal inversion, foot adduction, and plantar flexion is known as **supination**. During weight bearing at midstance, both calcaneal eversion and foot abduction tend to occur as the foot moves into dorsiflexion; these movements are known collectively as **pronation**. Supination of the subtalar joint also results in external rotation of the tibia, with pronation being linked to internal tibial rotation (Fig. 18.13C).

Although a normal amount of pronation is useful in reducing the peak forces sustained during impact, excessive or prolonged pronation can lead to several overuse injuries, including stress fractures of the second metatarsal and irritation of the sesamoid bones, plantar fasciitis, Achilles tendinitis, and medial tibial stress syndrome (11). Normal walking gait typically involves approximately 6 to 8° pronation.

KINETICS OF THE LOWER LEG, ANKLE, AND FOOT

The lower extremity sustains not only the weight of the body but also the weight of any carried loads and the forces of foot impacts during gait as well. Because force is what ultimately causes injury, understanding the kinetic aspects of lower leg, ankle, and foot function is an important foundation for understanding injury mechanisms.

Forces Commonly Sustained by the Lower Leg, Ankle, and Foot

During training, the bones of the lower extremity are subjected to a complex array of loading patterns, including tension, compression, bending, and torsion. During running, the foot sustains impact forces that can reach two- to threefold body weight; the magnitudes of the forces increase with gait speed. Longer stride length promotes shock attenuation, most likely because of the concomitant increased ground contact time (12). Researchers, however, have estimated the strength of lower extremity bones to be two- to fourfold that necessary to withstand the maximum stresses normally sustained during running (13).

Because repeated impact forces that are sustained during overtraining can produce stress fractures in the bones of the lower extremity, researchers have studied the factors associated with stress fracture incidence. Thicker bones generally are more resistant to stress-related injury (14). Women, who tend to have smaller bones than men, also have been found to incur more stress fractures than men, particularly in the tibia and metatarsals. Stress fractures are common in runners, ballet dancers, and gymnasts as well, and they often are secondary to decreased bone mineral density, or **osteopenia**. The **female athlete triad**, involving the simultaneous conditions of osteopenia, disordered eating, and amenorrhea (cessation of menses), is brought on by pressure placed on young women to achieve or maintain an unhealthy, low body weight. The causal linkages among the components of the female athlete triad are not well understood but appear to be related to low levels of circulating estrogen (15,16).

Foot Deformation During Gait

The structures of the foot are anatomically linked, and the load is evenly distributed over the foot during weight bearing. Approximately 50% of body weight is distributed through the subtalar joint to the calcaneus, with the remaining 50% channeled through the transverse tarsal joints to the forefoot (17). The specific anatomical structure of the foot accounts for approximately 35% of the variance in plantar pressure during gait, with the remaining contribution from the dynamics of the gait cycle (18).

If the foot were a more rigid structure, each impact with the support surface would generate extremely large forces of short duration through the skeletal system. Because the foot is composed of numerous bones that are connected by flexible ligaments and are restrained by flexible tendons, it deforms with each ground contact. In doing so, it absorbs much of the shock and transmits a much smaller force of longer duration up through the skeletal system.

The process of foot deformation during weight bearing results in the storage of mechanical energy in the stretched tendons, ligaments, and plantar fasciae. As the tibia rotates forward over the talus during gait, additional energy is stored in the gastrocnemius and soleus as they develop eccentric tension. During the push-off phase, the stored energy in all these elastic structures is released, contributing to the force of push-off and actually reducing the metabolic energy cost of walking or running.

PREVENTION OF LOWER LEG, ANKLE, AND FOOT CONDITIONS

Several steps can reduce the incidence or severity of injury. These include the use of appropriate protective equipment, footwear, and physical conditioning.

Protective Equipment

The use of protective braces and equipment for the lower leg, ankle, and foot is discussed in Chapter 3. Shin pads can protect the anterior tibial area from a direct impact by a ball, bat, stick, or kick from a foot. Commercial ankle braces used to prevent or support a postinjury ankle sprain come in three categories: lace-up brace, semirigid orthosis, or air-bladder brace (see Fig. 3.9). A lace-up brace can limit all ankle motions, whereas semirigid orthoses and air-bladder braces limit only inversion and eversion. In general, ankle braces are more effective than taping the ankle to reduce injuries, are easier for the wearer to apply independently, do not produce some of the skin irritation associated with adhesive tape, provide better comfort and fit, and are more cost-effective and comfortable to wear. Specific foot conditions can be padded and supported with a variety of products, including inner soles, semirigid orthotics, rigid orthotics, antishock heel lifts, heel cups, or commercially available pads and devices. Adhesive felt (e.g., Moleskin), felt, and foam also can be cut to construct similar pads to protect specific areas.

Physical Conditioning

Physical conditioning is one of the strongest defenses against injury. Unfortunately, the foot and lower leg often are neglected. Lack of flexibility can predispose an individual to certain injuries. For example, a tight Achilles tendon has been shown to predispose an individual to plantar fasciitis, Achilles tendinitis, and lateral ankle sprains. Exercises should focus on ensuring normal ROM and may be performed either alone or with a partner using proprioceptive neuromuscular facilitation stretching techniques.

Strengthening exercises for the intrinsic and extrinsic muscles of the region are essential for injury prevention. Foot strength can be improved by picking up marbles or dice with the toes and placing them in a container close to the foot or by placing a tennis ball between the soles of the feet and rolling the ball back and forth from the heel to the forefoot. The lower leg muscles can be strengthened by securing a weight or piece of elastic tubing around the forefoot and by moving through the ROMs for three sets of 10 to 15 repetitions each. Bilateral toe raises and heel raises also may be incorporated. Field Strategy 18.1 demonstrates several exercises that can be used to prevent injuries to the lower leg, ankle, and foot.

Footwear

The demands of a particular activity require adaptations in shoe design and selection. In field sports, shoes may have a flat-sole, long-cleat, short-cleat, or a multicleated design. Cleats should be positioned under the major weight-bearing joints of the foot and should not be felt through the sole of the shoe. Shoe models with flat cleats or screw-in cleats, or pivot-disk models, have been shown to reduce the incidence of anterior cruciate ligament injuries when compared to shoes with the longer, irregular cleats. In individuals with arch problems, the shoe should include adequate forefoot, arch, and heel support. In all cases, individuals should select shoes based on the demands of the activity. Shoe selection and guidelines for fitting shoes are discussed in detail in Chapter 3.

TOE AND FOOT CONDITIONS

A defensive back reports throbbing pain on the plantar side of the great toe of the right foot that has been present for the last 2 days. The athlete does not recall a specific mechanism or time of onset. The pain increases significantly when the athlete pushes off the right foot to block an opponent. For the past 3 days, the team was forced to practice indoors on a composite-type floor. What injury should be suspected, and why?

Many individuals are at risk for toe and foot problems because of a leg-length discrepancy, postural deviation, muscle dysfunction (e.g., muscle imbalance), or malalignment syndrome (e.g., pes cavus, pes planus, pes equinus, and hammer or claw toes) (Fig. 18.14). In particular, pes cavus (e.g., high arch and rigid foot) and pes planus (e.g., flatfoot and mobile foot) are associated with several common injuries (Box 18.1). Typically, when compared to a man's foot, a woman's foot has a narrower hindfoot, a relatively increased forefoot-to-hindfoot width, and increased pronation. Also, because of fashion trends and societal pressures, women tend to wear shoes that are narrower than the women's feet and that have narrow toe boxes. High heels shift the forefoot forward into the toe box, causing crowing of the toes and a tight heel cord. Consequently, women tend to be more prone to hallux valgus deformities, bunionettes, hammer toes, and neuromas (19). Other skin conditions commonly seen at the foot include calluses, corns, athlete's foot, and plantar warts, all of which are discussed in Chapter 28.

Toe Deformities

Most toe deformities are minor and can be treated conservatively. A few deformities require surgical intervention to correct serious structural malalignment.

Hallus Rigidus

Degenerative arthritis in the first MTP joint, associated with pain and limited motion, is known as hallus rigidus. Activities that involve running and jumping may

FIGURE 18.14 Common foot deformities.
A, Pes cavus. **B,** Pes planus.

AU: Is art placed above correct exercise in Field Strategy 18.1?

CHAPTER 18 Lower Leg, Ankle, and Foot Conditions 655

FIELD STRATEGY 18.1

Exercises to Prevent Injury to the Lower Leg

Foot Intrinsic Muscle Exercises

1. **Plantar fascia stretch.** Place a towel around the toes, and slowly overextend the toes. Dorsiflex the ankle to stretch the Achilles tendon.
2. **Towel crunches.** Place a towel between the plantar surfaces of the toes and feet. Push the toes and feet together, crunching the towel between the toes.

3. **Toe curls.** With the foot resting on a towel, slowly curl the toes under, bunching the towel beneath the foot. (Variation: Use two feet or a book or small weight on the towel for added resistance.)
4. **Picking up objects.** Pick up small objects, such as marbles or dice, with the toes, and place them in a nearby container, or use therapeutic putty to work the toe flexors.
5. **Shin curls.** Slide the plantar surface of the foot up the opposite shin, moving distal to proximal.
6. **Unilateral balance activities.** Stand on uneven surfaces with the eyes first open and then closed.

7. **Biomechanical ankle platform system (BAPS) board.** In a seated position, roll the board slowly clockwise and then counterclockwise 20 times.

Ankle/Lower Leg Muscle Exercises

1. **Ankle alphabet.** Using only the ankle and foot, trace the letters of the alphabet from A to Z three times with capital letters and three times with lowercase letters.
2. **Triceps surae stretch.** Keeping the back leg straight and the heel on the floor, lean against a wall until tension is felt in the calf muscles. To isolate the soleus, bend both knees. Point the toes outward, straight ahead, and inward to stretch the various fibers of the Achilles tendon.

3. **Thera-Band or surgical tubing exercises.** Secure the Thera-Band or tubing around a table leg, and do resisted dorsiflexion, plantar flexion, inversion, and eversion.
4. **Unilateral balance exercises.** Balance on the opposite leg while doing Thera-Band exercises.

5. **BAPS board.** In a standing position, balance on the involved foot; repeat several times. Additional challenges, such as using no support or dribbling with a basketball while balancing, can be added.

Box 18.1   Common Injuries Associated with Foot Deformities

Pes Cavus
Plantar fasciitis
Metatarsalgia
Stress fractures of the tarsals and metatarsals
Peroneal tendonitis
Sesamoid disorders
Iliotibial band friction syndrome

Pes Planus
Tibialis posterior tendinitis
Achilles tendinitis
Plantar fasciitis
Sesamoid disorders
Medial tibial stress syndrome
Patellofemoral pain

predispose an individual to this condition as a result of degenerative changes resulting from direct injury, hyperextension injury, or varus/valgus stress (20).

SIGNS AND SYMPTOMS. The individual presents with a tender and enlarged first MTP joint, loss of motion, and difficulty wearing shoes with an elevated heel. A hallmark sign is restricted toe extension (dorsiflexion), usually less than 60°, because of a ridge of osteophytes that can be palpated easily along the dorsal aspect of the metatarsal head.

MANAGEMENT. Conservative management includes ice, wearing low-heeled shoes with adequate width and depth to accommodate the increased bulk of the joint, nonsteroidal anti-inflammatory drugs (NSAIDs), and therapeutic mobilization. Individuals add a Morton's extension to their orthosis or use a rigid insole or shoe to reduce stress across the joint. Steroid injections may help if chronic inflammation is present. If conservative measures fail to resolve the symptoms within 6 months, surgery is indicated. Spurs may be removed through a cheilectomy, which can improve motion and reduce, but not eliminate, pain. An arthrodesis procedure may be suggested to fuse or resect the proximal portion of the proximal phalanx. Both techniques have a good or excellent outcome (21).

FIGURE 18.15 Hallus valgus. Hallux valgus is an abnormality in which the great toe is deviated laterally and may overlap the second toe. An enlarged, painful, inflamed bursa (bunion) may form on the medial side.

Hallus Valgus

Prolonged pressure against the medial aspect of the first MTP joint can lead to thickening of the medial capsule and bursa (i.e., bunion), resulting in a severe valgus deformity of the great toe (Fig. 18.15). The condition may be caused by heredity, metatarsus primus varus, pes planus, rheumatoid arthritis, and neurologic disorders. The most common cause is wearing poorly fitted shoes with a narrow toe box.

SIGNS AND SYMPTOMS. Many individuals with the deformity are asymptomatic. Those with symptoms complain of pain over the MTP joint and have difficulty wearing shoes because of the medial prominence and associated overlapping toe deformity. The condition also may cause the second metatarsal to bear more weight, leading to a callus under the second metatarsal head.

MANAGEMENT. Treatment varies depending on the degree of deformity and the severity of symptoms. Wide, soft shoes with a broad toe box and sufficient insole padding are critical for comfort. Orthoses that support the longitudinal arch and redistribute the pressure areas also may provide some relief. If conservative measures fail, surgery may correct the deformity, but this does not necessarily improve activity performance. Rehabilitation can take from 4 to 6 months (20).

FIGURE 18.16 Toe deformities. A, Hammer toe. **B,** Claw toe. **C,** Mallet toe.

Claw, Hammer, and Mallet Toe

Other lesser toe deformities may be congenital, but more often, they develop because of improperly fitted shoes, neuromuscular disease, arthritis, or trauma. A **hammer toe** is extended at the MTP joint, flexed at the PIP joint, and hyperextended at the DIP joint (Fig. 18.16). **Claw toe** involves hyperextension of the MTP joint and flexion of the DIP and PIP joints. A **mallet toe** is in neutral position at the MTP and PIP joints but flexed at the DIP joint.

SIGNS AND SYMPTOMS. Each condition can lead to painful callus formation on the dorsum of the IP joints. This pressure against the shoe and under the metatarsal head, particularly the second toe, is caused by the retrograde pressure on the long toe.

MANAGEMENT. These conditions are difficult to treat conservatively. A metatarsal pad may help to control symptoms, but surgery may be necessary. Soft-tissue surgery may involve tendon lengthening, capsulotomy, and/or ligament release. For more significant deformities, resection of the head of the proximal phalanx often is necessary to treat the condition.

Turf Toe

Turf toe, or a sprain of the plantar capsular ligament of the first MTP joint, results from forced hyperextension or hyperflexion of the great toe (i.e., jamming the toe into the end of the shoe). Hyperextension causes the sesamoids to be drawn forward to bear weight under the first metatarsal head. Repetitive overload also can lead to injury, particularly when associated with a valgus stress.

Signs and Symptoms

The individual has pain, tenderness, and swelling on the plantar aspect of the MTP joint of the great toe. Extension of the great toe is extremely painful. Because the sesamoid bones are located in the tendons of the flexor hallucis brevis, this condition sometimes is associated with tearing of the flexor tendons, fracture of the sesamoid bones, bone bruises, and osteochondral fractures in the metatarsal head.

Management

Initial treatment for mild sprains involves standard acute care (i.e., ice, compression, elevation, and rest), NSAIDs, and protection from excessive motion. Taping to limit motion at the MTP joint, use of a metatarsal pad to lower stress on the first metatarsal, or use of a rigid shoe or forefoot plate may be helpful. In moderate to severe cases, the individual may need to be restricted from activity until symptoms disappear (i.e., usually 3–6 weeks).

Reverse Turf Toe (Soccer Toe)

Because of forced hyperflexion of the MTP joint while kicking an instep ball strike, soccer players often irritate the dorsal capsular structures of the first MTP joint. The condition can be acute or chronic, and it demonstrates signs and symptoms similar to those of the traditional turf toe, except that pain is noted dorsally over the joint and passive flexion of the toe is painful. Treatment is similar to that of traditional turf toe as well. If taping is applied, however, it should limit flexion, rather than extension, of the MTP joint.

Ingrown Toenail

Although ingrown toenails are common, they are preventable with proper hygiene and nail care. The toenail length should be long enough to extend beyond the underlying skin but short enough so as not to push into the toe box of the shoe. The toenails should be trimmed straight across to prevent the edges from growing under the skin on the side of the nail. In addition, properly fitted shoes and socks should be worn.

Signs and Symptoms

Improper cutting of the nail, improper shoe size, and constant sliding of the foot inside the shoe can traumatize the nail, causing its edge to grow into the lateral nail fold and surrounding skin. The nail margin reddens and becomes painful. If a fungal or bacterial infection is present, the condition is called **paronychia.**

Management

Two methods to treat this condition are discussed in Field Strategy 18.2.

Metatarsalgia

General discomfort around the metatarsal heads is called **metatarsalgia**, or Morton's metatarsalgia. Although often related to participation in sport and physical activity (Box 18.2), other factors, such

---

FIELD STRATEGY 18.2

Management of an Ingrown Toenail

Method 1

- Soak the involved toe in hot water (108–116°F) until the nail bed is soft (usually 10 to 15 minutes).
- Lift the edge of the nail, and place a small piece of cotton or tissue under the nail to elevate the nail out of the skinfold.
- Apply antiseptic to the area, and cover with a sterile dressing.
- Repeat the procedure daily, keeping the area clean and dry.
- *If a purulent infection is present, the individual should be referred to a physician for antibiotics and drainage of the infection.*

Method 2

- Soak the toe as in the preceding, and cut a "V" in the center of the nail.
- As the nail grows, its edges pull toward the center, drawing the nail edges from under the skin.
- Apply an antiseptic, cover with a sterile dressing, and keep the area clean and dry.
- *If a purulent infection is present, the individual should be referred to a physician for antibiotics and drainage of the infection.*

Box 18.2 Factors Leading to Metatarsalgia

Intrinsic Factors
- Excessive body weight
- Limited extensibility of the triceps surae complex
- Fallen metatarsal arch
- Valgus heel
- Hammer toes
- Pes planus or pes cavus

Extrinsic Factors
- Narrow toe box
- Improperly placed shoe cleats
- Improper technique (e.g., in a cyclist, poor foot position or rigid high gears at low cadence)
- Landing incorrectly from a height
- Repetitive jumping or excessive running
- Running style that puts undue pressure on the forefoot

as age, arthritic disease, gout, diabetes, circulatory disease, and some neurologic conditions, can predispose an individual to metatarsal pain.

Signs and Symptoms

Constant overloading of the transverse ligaments leads to flattening of the transverse arch, resulting in callus formation over the middle three metatarsal heads, particularly the second.

Management

Treatment involves reducing the load on the metatarsal heads through activity modification, footwear examination, metatarsal pads or bars, and strengthening the intrinsic muscles of the foot.

Bunions

Bunions generally are found on the medial aspect of the MTP joint of the great toe but also can occur on the lateral aspect of the fifth toe (i.e., a bunionette or tailor's bunion). Pronation of the foot, prolonged pronation during gait, contractures of the Achilles tendon, arthritis, and generalized ligamentous laxity between the first and second metatarsal heads can produce a thickening on the medial side of the first metatarsal head as it is constantly rubbed against the inside of the shoe.

Signs and Symptoms

As the condition worsens, the great toe may shift laterally and overlap the second toe, leading to a rigid, nonfunctional hallux valgus deformity (see Fig. 18.15). This condition is exacerbated by high heels and pointed toe boxes in shoes, which are factors that account for the higher incidence of the condition in women compared to men.

Management

Once the deformity occurs, little can be done to correct the condition. Strapping the great toe as closely to proper anatomical position as possible and wearing wider shoes can provide some relief, but surgical correction is indicated in severe cases.

Retrocalcaneal Bursitis

External pressure from a constrictive heel cup, coupled with excessive pronation or a varus hindfoot, can lead to swelling, erythema, and irritation of the retrocalcaneal bursa located between the Achilles tendon and calcaneus (Fig. 18.17). The posterior calcaneal bursa also can be irritated.

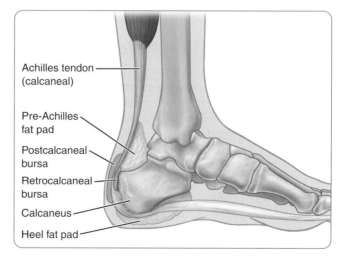

Achilles tendon (calcaneal)

Pre-Achilles fat pad

Postcalcaneal bursa

Retrocalcaneal bursa

Calcaneus

Heel fat pad

■■■ **FIGURE 18.17 Retrocalcaneal bursa.** The retrocalcaneal bursa commonly is inflamed when it is pinched between the Achilles tendon and calcaneus during plantar flexion.

Signs and Symptoms

Pain is elicited on palpation of the soft tissue just anterior to the Achilles tendon, and the skin may be thickened, especially on the lateral side. Active plantar flexion during push-off compresses the bursa between the tendon and bone.

Management

Initial treatment involves standard acute care, NSAIDs, stretching exercises for the Achilles tendon, shoe modification, or a heel lift to relieve external pressure on the bursa. Radiographs may show calcification in the bursa. Excision of the bursa may be indicated if conservative treatment fails. Injection with steroids is not recommended (20).

Occasionally, an inflamed bursa can lead to a dramatic, large mass referred to as a "pump bump," which is common among female figure skaters and runners (i.e., runner's bump). The condition also may be called os calcis exostosis. This bump may be related to an underlying bony spur caused by frequent microtrauma or microavulsions surrounding the distal attachment of the Achilles tendon. An additional Achilles tendinopathy above the insertion often is present when the symptoms have been present for more than 3 months. Conservative treatment is similar to that of retrocalcaneal bursitis. Open (preferably with tendinopathy) or endoscopic excision is recommended. Steroid injections should not be used because of the risk of Achilles tendon rupture (20).

 The defensive back may have a turf toe. The injury could be the result of repeated hyperextension. The change in surface to a more rigid and less giving surface as well as use of inappropriate footwear could have contributed to this injury.

CONTUSIONS

A soccer player was kicked in the anterolateral aspect of the lower leg. The athlete continued to play the remaining 10 minutes of the game. Twenty minutes after the game ended, however, the athlete reported severe pain to the area. Inspection revealed a firm mass and tight skin over the injured site. What condition should be suspected, and what further assessment should be performed?

Contusions of the foot and leg result from direct trauma, such as dropping a weight on the foot or being stepped on, kicked, or hit by a speeding ball or implement. Many of these injuries are minor and easily treated with standard acute care. A few injuries, however, can result in complications, such as excessive hemorrhage, periosteal irritation, nerve damage, or damage to tendon sheaths, leading to tenosynovitis.

Foot Contusions

Compression on the midfoot can be painful and can damage the extensor tendons or lead to a fracture of the metatarsals or phalanges. During weight bearing, contusions of the plantar aspect of the forefoot may result from a loose cleat or spike irritating the ball of the foot. Repairing or replacing the object, along with ice therapy to reduce immediate hemorrhage and discomfort, usually is sufficient to remedy the situation.

A contusion to the hindfoot, called a **heel bruise**, can be more serious. Elastic adipose tissue lies between the thick skin and the plantar aspect of the calcaneus to cushion and protect the inferior portion of the calcaneus from trauma. It is constantly subjected to extreme stress in running, jumping, and changing directions. Excessive body weight, age, poorly cushioned or worn-out running shoes, increases in training, and hard, uneven training surfaces can predispose an individual to this condition. Walking barefoot is particularly painful. Application of cold to minimize pain and inflammation, followed by regular use of a heel cup or doughnut pad, can minimize the condition. Despite excellent care, the condition may persist for months.

Lower Leg Contusions

Contusions to the gastrocnemius result in immediate pain, weakness, and partial loss of motion. Hemorrhage and muscle spasm quickly lead to a tender, firm, easily palpable mass. When applying ice, the muscle should be kept on a stretch to decrease muscle spasm. If the condition does not improve in 2 to 3 days, ultrasound may be used, under the direction of a physician, to assist in breaking up the hematoma.

A contusion to the tibia, commonly called a **shin bruise,** may occur in soccer, field hockey, baseball, softball, football, or activities in which the lower leg is subjected to high-impact forces. The shin is particularly void of natural subcutaneous fat and is vulnerable to direct blows that irritate the periosteal tissue around the tibia. Participants should always wear appropriate shin guards to protect this highly vulnerable area. Although painful, the condition can be managed effectively with ice, compression, elevation, and rest. A doughnut pad over the area and additional shin protection can allow the individual to participate within pain tolerance levels.

Acute Compartment Syndrome

An acute compartment syndrome occurs when a rapid increase in tissue pressure within a nonyielding anatomical space leads to increased local venous pressure and obstructs the neurovascular network. In the lower leg, it tends to be caused by a direct blow to the anterolateral aspect of the tibia or by a tibial fracture. The anterior compartment is particularly at risk, because it is bounded by the tibia medially, the interosseous membrane posteriorly, the fibula laterally, and a tough fascial sheath anteriorly. Although an acute compartment syndrome occurs less frequently than the more common chronic compartment syndrome, the acute syndrome is considered to be a medical and surgical emergency because of the compromised neurovascular functions.

Signs and Symptoms

Signs and symptoms include recent history of trauma, excessive exercise, vascular injury, or prolonged, externally applied pressure. The increasing severe pain and swelling appear to be out of proportion to the clinical situation. A firm mass, tight skin (because it has been stretched to its limits), loss of sensation on the dorsal aspect between the great and second toes, and diminished pulse at the dorsalis pedis are delayed and dangerous signs. A normal pulse, however, does not rule out the syndrome. Acute compartment syndrome can produce functional abnormalities within 30 minutes of the onset of hemorrhage. Immediate action is necessary, because irreversible damage can occur within 12 to 24 hours.

Management

Immediate care involves ice and total rest. Compression is not recommended, because the compartment already is unduly compressed and additional external compression only hastens the deterioration. In addition, the limb must not be elevated, because this decreases arterial pressure and further compromises capillary filling. Referral to a physician for immediate care is absolutely necessary.

If numbness in the foot is present, intercompartmental pressure is measured using either a slit-catheter or a solid-state intracompartment catheter. If the pressure ranges between 30 and 40 mm Hg (normal range, 0–10 mm Hg), the individual is watched carefully, and repeated measurements are taken until symptoms subside. If the pressure ranges from 40 to 60 mm Hg, a surgical release of the fascia (i.e., fasciotomy) is required to prevent permanent tissue damage.

A *The soccer player may have an acute compartment syndrome. In the continued assessment of the athlete, the following should be examined: sensation between the first and second toes on the dorsum of the foot, circulation at the dorsalis pedis pulse, and active ROM, particularly the motions of dorsiflexion and eversion.*

FOOT AND ANKLE SPRAINS

Q *A 30-year-old recreational basketball player has sustained a grade II lateral ankle sprain. What is the immediate management for this condition?*

Sprains to the foot and ankle region are common in sports, particularly among those individuals who play on badly maintained fields. In many sports, cleated shoes become fixed to the ground while the limb continues to rotate around it. In addition, the very nature of changing directions places an inordinate amount of strain on the ankle region. Other methods of injury include stepping in a hole, stepping off a curb, stepping on an opponent's foot, or rolling the foot off the surface.

Toe and Foot Sprains and Dislocations

Sprains and dislocations to the MP and IP joints of the toes may occur by tripping or stubbing the toe. Varus and valgus forces more commonly affect the first and fifth toes rather than the middle three. Pain, dysfunction, immediate swelling, and if dislocated, gross deformity are evident. Radiographs should be taken to rule out possible fracture, but closed reduction and strapping to the next toe for 10 to 14 days usually are sufficient to remedy the problem.

Midfoot sprains often result from severe dorsiflexion, plantar flexion, or pronation. Although the condition is seen in basketball and soccer players, it is more frequent among those who participate in activities where the foot is unsupported, such as in gymnastics or dance (in which slippers are typically worn) or in track athletes who wear running flats. Pain and swelling is deep on the medial aspect of the foot, and weight bearing may be too painful. Depending on the location and severity of pain, adequate strapping, arch supports, and limited weight bearing are warranted during the acute stage. If the condition does not improve, the individual should be referred to a physician to rule out a possible avulsion fracture at the tarsal joints. Reconditioning exercises should include ROM and strengthening for the intrinsic muscles of the foot.

Mechanisms of Injury for Ankle Sprains

Ankle sprains are the most common injury in recreational and competitive sports. They are classified as grade I (first degree), grade II (second degree), and grade III (third degree), based on the progression of the anatomical structures damaged and the subsequent disability (Table 18.2). In basketball, ankle sprains comprise more than 45% of all injuries, and in soccer, up to 31% of all injuries are ankle sprains (22).

Ankle sprains generally are caused by severe medial (i.e., supination or inversion) and lateral (i.e., pronation or eversion) rotation motions. Excessive supination of the foot (i.e., adduction, inversion, and plantar flexion) results when the plantar aspect of the foot is turned inward, toward the midline of the body, which commonly is referred to as an inversion sprain. Excessive pronation (i.e., abduction, eversion, and dorsiflexion) results when the plantar aspect of the foot is turned laterally, which is referred to as an eversion sprain.

Inversion Ankle Sprains

Acute inversion (i.e., lateral) sprains often occur while changing directions rapidly. Interestingly, injury typically involves the unloaded foot and ankle (or, more accurately, just at the moment of loading) with a plantar flexion and inversion force. In plantar flexion, the ATFL is taut and the CFL relatively loose, whereas in dorsiflexion, the opposite is true. The medial and lateral malleoli project

TABLE 18.2 Mechanisms of Common Ankle Sprains and Resulting Ligament Damage			
MECHANISM	**FIRST (MILD)**	**SECOND (MODERATE)**	**THIRD (SEVERE)**
Inversion and plantar flexion	Anterior talofibular stretched	Partial tear of anterior talofibular, with calcaneofibular stretched	Rupture of anterior talofibular and calcaneofibular, with posterior talofibular and tibiofibular torn
Inversion	Calcaneofibular stretched	Calcaneofibular torn, and anterior talofibular stretched	Rupture of calcaneofibular, and anterior talofibular with posterior talofibular stretched
Dorsiflexion eversion	Tibiofibular stretched, deltoid stretched, or an avulsion fracture of medial malleolus	Partial tear of tibiofibular, partial tear of deltoid and tibiofibular	Rupture of tibiofibular, rupture of deltoid, and interosseous membrane with possible fibular fracture above syndesmosis

downward over the talus to form a mortise-tenon joint. The lateral malleolus projects farther downward than the medial, thus limiting lateral talar shifts. As stress is initially applied to the ankle during plantar flexion and inversion, the ATFL first stretches. If the strain continues, the ankle loses ligamentous stability in its neutral position. The medial malleolus acts as a fulcrum to further the inversion and stretches or ruptures the CFL (Fig. 18.18). The overlying inner wall of the peroneal tendon sheath lies adjacent to the CFL and can absorb some strain to prevent injury to this ligament. If the peroneal muscles are weak, however, they are unable to stabilize the joint, leading to tearing of the CFL. In severe injuries, the posterior talofibular ligament also is involved. As the ankle joint becomes unstable, the talus can pinch the deltoid ligament against the medial malleolus, which leads to injury on both sides of the ankle joint.

Signs and Symptoms

The individual usually reports a cracking or tearing sound at the time of injury. In a grade I injury, the individual can bear weight immediately after injury, and pain and swelling are mild. In a grade II injury, swelling and tenderness are localized over the ATFL and may extend over the CFL, and the individual can bear some weight but definitely walks with a limp. If no fracture is involved, bony tenderness is found only at the ligamentous attachments. A complete tear of one or more of the ligaments is considered to be a grade III sprain. Swelling and ecchymosis are rapid and diffuse, and the individual demonstrates functional and clinical instability. Immediate assessment should distinguish the severity of injury, because swelling may soon obscure the level of instability. Table 18.3 summarizes the signs and symptoms of the various grades of lateral ankle sprains.

FIGURE 18.18 **Inversion ankle sprain.** During inversion, the medial malleolus acts as a fulcrum to further invert the talus, leading to stretching or tearing of the calcaneofibular ligament.

Management

Following assessment for possible fracture and ligamentous damage, initial treatment should consist of standard acute care (i.e., cold, compression, elevation, and protected rest) and restricted activity.

TABLE 18.3 Signs and Symptoms of a Lateral Ankle Sprain	
DEGREE	**SIGNS AND SYMPTOMS**
First	Pain and swelling on anterolateral aspect of lateral malleolus
	Point tenderness over anterior talofibular ligament (ATFL)
	No laxity with stress tests
Second	Tearing or popping sensation felt on lateral aspect; pain and swelling on anterolateral and inferior aspect of lateral malleolus
	Painful palpation over ATFL and calcaneofibular ligament; also may be tender over posterior talofibular ligament, deltoid ligament, and anterior capsule area
	Positive anterior drawer and talar tilt test
Third	Tearing or popping sensation felt on lateral aspect, with diffuse swelling over entire lateral aspect, with or without anterior swelling; can be very painful or absent pain
	Positive anterior drawer and talar tilt test

FIELD STRATEGY 18.3

Management Algorithm for a Lateral Ankle Sprain

1. Use a compression wrap to secure crushed ice packs directly to the skin as quickly as possible following the injury; apply the ice for 30 minutes
2. Do not place a towel or elastic wrap (dry or wet) between the crushed ice pack and skin (reduces effectiveness of treatment)
3. Elevate foot and ankle 6 to 10 inches above the level of the heart
4. After initial ice treatment:
   - Remove ice pack.
   - Replace compression wrap.
   - Continue elevation.
5. Apply a horseshoe pad and open basket weave with tape and/or elastic wrap to protect the area
6. Instruct the individual to reapply a crushed ice pack regularly until going to bed:
   - Every 2 hours.
   - Every hour if active between applications (crutch walking, showering).
7. If limping:
   - Fit with crutches.
   - Reassess in the morning.
   - Start rehabilitation.

If fracture is suspected, the individual should be referred to a physician.

Crutches should be used if the individual is unable to bear weight. Individuals with moderate to severe sprains should be referred immediately to a physician. Radiographs can determine damage to the syndesmosis or detect an osteochondral fracture to the dome of the talus. In individuals with a history of ankle sprains, the use of prophylactic taping or bracing in conjunction with a rehabilitation program that includes balance and coordination training for at least 6 weeks after injury can reduce the risk of recurrent sprains (23). The focus of rehabilitation should include strengthening the peroneals, stretching the heel cord, and proprioceptive training. Field Strategy 18.3 summarizes the management of lateral ankle sprains.

Because lateral ankle sprains are common, there may be a tendency to view all injuries around the ankle as being "ankle sprains." Several aspects of the individual's symptoms should lead the examiner to question the possibility of a more serious underlying condition, however, such as a syndesmosis sprain, peroneal tendon injury, loose body, or osteochondral fracture. These aspects include:

- Inability to recall or describe the exact mechanism of injury

- Inability to bear any weight on the foot and ankle

- Any deformity to the foot and ankle

- Severe midfoot swelling or any blistering of skin (i.e., suggesting significant skin stretching caused by associated joint subluxation, dislocation, or fracture)

- In a chronic setting, a primary complaint of pain rather than instability

- Persistent pain exceeding 3 to 4 weeks postinjury

Eversion Ankle Sprains

Eversion (i.e., medial) ankle sprains involve injury to the medial, deltoid-shaped talocrural ligaments (i.e., deltoid ligament). Although an isolated injury to the deltoid ligament may result from forced dorsiflexion and eversion, such as landing from a long jump with the foot abducted or landing on another player's foot. These account for less than 10% of all injuries (22). Most injuries to the deltoid ligament are associated with a fibula fracture, syndesmotic injury, or severe lateral ankle sprain. Individuals with pronated or hypermobile feet tend to be at a greater risk for eversion injuries.

The talar dome is wider anteriorly than posteriorly. During dorsiflexion, the talus fits more firmly in the mortise supported by the distal anterior tibiofibular ligament. During excessive dorsiflexion and eversion, the talus is thrust laterally against the longer fibula, resulting in either a mild sprain to the deltoid ligament or, if the force is great enough, a lateral malleolar fracture. If the force continues after the fracture occurs, the deltoid ligament may be ruptured or may remain intact, avulsing a small bony fragment from the medial malleolus and leading to a bimalleolar fracture. In either case, the distal anterior tibiofibular ligament and interosseous membrane may be torn, producing total instability of the ankle joint and eventual degeneration (Fig. 18.19).

Signs and Symptoms

Signs and symptoms of an isolated eversion sprain depend on the severity of injury. In mild to moderate injuries, the individual often is unable to recall the mechanism of injury. There may be some initial pain at the ankle when it was everted and dorsiflexed. As the ankle returns to its normal anatomical position, however, pain often subsides, and the individual continues to be active. In attempts to run or put pressure on the area, pain intensifies, but the individual may not make the connection between the pain and the earlier injury. Swelling may not be as evident as a lateral sprain, because hemorrhage occurs deep in the leg and is not readily visible. Swelling may occur just posterior to the lateral malleolus, between it and the Achilles tendon. Point tenderness can be elicited over the deltoid ligament and distal anterior tibiofibular ligaments as well as the anterior and posterior joint lines. In severe injuries, passive motion may be pain-free in all motions except dorsiflexion. In a fracture of the malleoli, pain is evident over the fracture site and increases with any movement of the mortise. Percussion and heel strike produce increased pain.

FIGURE 18.19 Eversion ankle sprain. During a severe eversion ankle sprain, the lateral malleolus can fracture, the deltoid ligament can avulse the medial malleolus, and the distal tibiofibular joint can be disrupted.

Management

Initial management is the same as that of a lateral ankle sprain. Appropriate immobilization with a rigid posterior or vacuum splint is necessary. Referral to a physician is warranted. Surgical repair generally is indicated when a fracture or ligamentous disruption of the syndesmosis is involved.

Syndesmosis Sprain

Injury to the distal tibiofibular syndesmosis (i.e., a "high" ankle sprain) often goes undetected, resulting in a longer recovery time and a greater disability than with the more frequent lateral ankle sprain. The incidence of injury is reported as between 1 and 11% of all ankle injuries (24). The mechanism of injury differs from that of an inversion sprain. Often, the foot is dorsiflexed and externally rotated; external rotation injures the structures of the syndesmosis by widening the ankle mortis.

Signs and Symptoms

The area of maximum point tenderness usually is over the anterolateral tibiofibular joint. The degree of pain and swelling can be significant. The individual will have difficulty bearing weight on the injured ankle. The most commonly injured ligament (and a source of anterolateral ankle impingement) is the anterior inferior tibiofibular ligament, and the least injured ligament is the posterior inferior tibiofibular ligament, although the interosseous ligament may also be variably injured (25). Assessment rests on four specific tests:

1. Stabilizing the lower leg with one hand while applying an external rotation force to the ankle (external rotation test)

2. Compressing the proximal tibia and fibula while asking about pain at the ankle (squeeze test)

3. Syndesmosis ligament palpation

4. Passive dorsiflexion test

Management

Initial management is the same as that of a lateral ankle sprain. Referral to a physician is warranted for radiographic confirmation to assess for fractures, bony avulsions (10–50% occur off the tibia), and the mortise alignment of the tibia, talus, and fibula. A grade I high ankle sprain is treated with immobilization in a long, semirigid pneumatic stirrup brace that extends to just below the knee for up to 3 weeks. The individual may return to physical activity with protective taping and a heel lift (25). A grade II injury involves 3 to 6 weeks of non–weight bearing, including stabilization with a fracture brace for 3 to 4 weeks, followed by a pneumatic stirrup brace for an additional 3 weeks. Application of cold should continue until swelling is reduced. Initially, weight bearing should be permitted with crutches, and weaning off of the crutches is done as tolerated. Participation in sports and physical activity may be delayed for up to 3 months after the initial treatment begins. If the injury involves no fracture but widening of the joint mortise is seen on stress radiographs, surgery is recommended.

Subtalar Sprain

The ligaments associated with the lateral subtalar joint are the CFL (spanning both the ankle and subtalar joints), the inferior extensor retinaculum, the lateral talocalcaneal ligament, the cervical ligament (just anterior to the tibiocalcaneal), and the interosseous ligament. The most common mechanism is believed to be dorsiflexion and supination. This position places the CFL in a position of maximal tightness. Further supination can lead to rupture of the CFL, followed by tearing of the cervical ligament and the interosseous tibiocalcaneal ligament (26).

Signs and Symptoms

The individual often complains of a sensation of the ankle "turning inward" or "turning over." Individuals with this problem consistently watch the ground when they walk and are uncomfortable when running on uneven surfaces. Assessment of chronic subtalar instability varies only slightly from that of ankle instability; the conditions may coexist. The anterior drawer test should be negative in isolated subtalar instability but positive with ankle instability. A subtle finding with subtalar instability, however, is increased rotation of the calcaneus under the talus on the anterior drawer test. A definitive diagnosis can be established only with stress radiographs.

Management

Conservative treatment is similar to that of a lateral ankle sprain, including standard acute care, strengthening of the peroneals, stretching the heel cord, proprioceptive training, and use of a brace if needed. High-grade subtalar sprains (as determined by examination and imaging studies) are treated with 2 weeks of non–weight bearing in a below-knee cast, followed by 4 weeks in a commercial walker boot (26). Chronic instability may necessitate surgical repair.

Subtalar Dislocation

Another serious sprain that involves the subtalar joint results from a fall from a height (as in basketball or volleyball). The foot lands in inversion, disrupting the interosseous talocalcaneal and talonavicular ligaments. If the foot lands in dorsiflexion and inversion, the CFL also is ruptured. When the dislocation occurs, the injury is better known as "basketball foot."

Signs and Symptoms

Extreme pain and total loss of function is present. Gross deformity at the subtalar joint may not be clearly visible. The foot may appear to be pale and feel cold to the touch if neurovascular damage is present. The individual may show signs of shock.

Management

Because of the potential for peroneal tendon entrapment and neurovascular damage, leading to reduced blood supply to the foot, this dislocation is considered to be a medical emergency.

> The examiner should activate the emergency action plan, including summoning emergency medical services (EMS). While waiting for EMS to arrive, the examiner should monitor the individual for shock and treat as necessary. Neurovascular function should be monitored as well.

The immediate management of the grade II ankle sprain sustained by the 30-year-old recreational basketball player should include standard acute care (i.e., ice, compression, elevation, and protected rest). Application of a horseshoe pad or open basket weave strapping and an elastic wrap can be used for compression. The individual should be fitted with crutches and referred to a physician.

TENDINOPATHIES OF THE FOOT AND LOWER LEG

A 55-year-old woman preparing to compete in a recreational badminton tournament reports to a sports medicine clinic complaining of pain and swelling behind the medial malleolus and of pain in the arch when arising in the morning. Observation reveals pes planus. During resisted muscle testing, plantar flexion and inversion are weak. What muscle is involved in this injury, and how should this condition be managed?

Tendinopathies of the foot and lower leg are relatively common and encompass a wide spectrum of conditions ranging from tendinitis to tenosynovitis to partial and complete ruptures. The tendons most often involved in the foot and ankle include the Achilles, posterior tibialis, peroneal brevis, and peroneal longus tendons. In contrast to acute traumatic tendinous injury, these injuries most involve repetitive submaximal loading of the tissues, resulting in repetitive microtraumas.

Strains and Tendinitis

Muscle strains seldom occur in the lower extremity, except in the gastrocnemius–soleus complex. Instead, injury occurs to the musculotendinous junction or to the tendon itself. Most of the tendons in the lower leg have a synovial sheath surrounding the tendon; the Achilles tendon, which has a peritendon sheath that is not synovial, is an exception. Several factors can predispose an individual to tendinitis (Box 18.3). Common sites for tendon injuries include:

- The Achilles tendon just proximal to its insertion into the calcaneus
- The tibialis posterior just behind the medial malleolus
- The tibialis anterior on the dorsum of the foot just under the extensor retinaculum
- The peroneal tendons just behind the lateral malleolus and at the distal attachment on the base of the fifth metatarsal

Signs and Symptoms

Common signs and symptoms include a history of stiffness following a period of inactivity (e.g., morning stiffness), localized tenderness over the tendon, possible swelling or thickness in the tendon and peritendon tissues, pain with passive stretching, and pain with active and resisted motion.

Management

In the majority of cases, treatment of muscle strains, tendinitis, or peritendinitis is conservative. If mechanical problems are present, they should be addressed first so that recovery can occur. Early exercises should be within the levels of pain tolerance and should not be too strenuous. Ice massage,

Box 18.3 Predisposing Factors for Tendinitis in the Lower Leg

- Training errors that include:
  - Lack of flexibility in the gastrocnemius–soleus muscles
  - Poor training surface or sudden change from soft to hard surface, or vice versa
  - Sudden changes in training intensity or program (e.g., adding hills, sprints, or distance)
  - Inadequate work-to-rest ratio that may lead to early muscle fatigue
  - Returning to participation too quickly following injury
- Direct trauma
- Infection from a penetrating wound into the tendon
- Abnormal foot mechanics producing friction among the shoe, tendon, and bony structure
- Poor footwear that is not properly fitted to foot

active ROM exercises with elastic tubing for resistance, stretching of the Achilles tendon, and eccentric calf exercises are recommended during the early phase of rehabilitation.

Foot Strains

Foot strains, caused by a direct blow or chronic overuse, often affect the intrinsic and extrinsic muscles of the foot. The tibialis anterior and the toe extensor tendons may be injured as a result of having the feet repeatedly stepped on or by having the shoelaces tied too tightly.

SIGNS AND SYMPTOMS. Pain, localized edema, inflammation, and adhesions may be present. During assessment, the involved tendons have pain on passive stretching and with active and resisted motion. Palpation over the tendon during active motion may reveal a sound similar to that heard when crunching a snowball together; hence, the sound is called **"snowball"** crepitation.

MANAGEMENT. Treatment involves standard acute care, NSAIDs, and strapping to limit active motion of the tendon. Range-of-motion and strengthening exercises should be started after acute pain has subsided.

Peroneal Tendinopathies

Peroneal tendon injuries are less common than injury to the Achilles and posterior tibial tendons. Mechanisms of injury may include forceful passive dorsiflexion, as occurs when a skier catches the tip of the ski and falls forward; exploding off a slightly pronated foot, as when a football player is in a three-point stance and makes a forward surge; or being kicked from behind in the vicinity of the lateral malleolus. Tendonitis of the peroneus longus causes pain as the tendon passes beneath the cuboid toward its insertion on the plantar aspect of the metatarsal. Another problem that may exist involves the retinaculum that holds the tendons in place on the posterior aspect of the lateral malleolus. If this retinaculum gives way, the tendons slip forward over the lateral malleolus but usually return spontaneously. This condition can be overlooked or confused with an ankle sprain, because it gives a feeling of instability and pain over the lateral malleolus. Partial tears of both the peroneus longus and brevis tendons have been linked to persistent lateral ankle pain and chronic lateral ankle instability (27).

SIGNS AND SYMPTOMS. During an acute injury in which the reticulum ruptures, a cracking sensation, followed by intense pain and an inability to walk, is reported. Swelling and tenderness is localized over the posterosuperior aspect of the lateral malleolus rather than the anteroinferior aspect, as in an inversion ankle sprain. A hallmark symptom is extreme discomfort or apprehension during attempted eversion of the foot against resistance. If done immediately after injury, the dislocated tendons may be palpated during resisted dorsiflexion and eversion; however, swelling may soon obscure the dislocation. In a chronic injury, the individual complains primarily of instability, a "giving way," or a slippage around the ankle, with little discomfort.

MANAGEMENT. Treatment is symptomatic with standard acute care. Acute injuries may respond to cast immobilization. External padding and strappings may help to stabilize the tendons, but because of the high rate of recurrence in the active population, surgery often is required.

Posterior Tibialis Tendon Dysfunction

Posterior tibialis tendon dysfunction is a common cause of painful acquired flatfoot deformity and is associated with substantial functional problems leading to significant morbidity. Individuals with a planovalgus foot, or flatfoot with pronation and loss of arch, are predisposed to this common injury. These individuals frequently have a loss of hindfoot inversion and difficulty in negotiating uneven ground and in climbing and descending stairs. Unfortunately, the problem frequently is missed, because progressive pronation is insidious and relatively painless. Overuse occasionally superimposes an acute injury by producing longitudinal tears or tethering, leading to dysfunction.

SIGNS AND SYMPTOMS. Three levels of dysfunction have been identified in the peroneal muscles (28). In stage I, the individual has pain and swelling along the course of the tendon. Pain, tenderness, and swelling also may be present behind the medial malleolus, and there may be an accompanying aching discomfort in the medial longitudinal arch. Because the length of the tendon is normal, a single heel raise can be performed. The flatfoot deformity is minimal, alignment of the hindfoot and forefoot is normal, and the subtalar joint remains flexible.

In stage II, the individual is unable to perform a single heel raise because of attenuation or disruption of the posterior tibial tendon. Weakness is evident in plantar flexion and inversion. The tendon is enlarged, elongated, and functionally incompetent. The foot adopts a pes planovalgus position (flatfoot) with collapse of the medial longitudinal arch, hindfoot valgus and subtalar eversion, and forefoot abduction through the talonavicular joint. The subtalar joint remains flexible, and with the ankle in plantar flexion, the talonavicular joint can be reduced.

Stage III presents with the individual being unable to perform a single heel raise and a more severe flatfoot deformity. The pes planovalgus deformity is fixed, and the laterally subluxed navicular cannot be reduced. If the tendon is ruptured, a painful pop is felt, resulting in an immediate flatfoot deformity (acquired pes planus).

MANAGEMENT. Early treatment of posterior tibialis tendon dysfunction depends on the severity of injury and may include standard acute care, NSAIDs, restricted activity, and a corrective orthoses, such as the University of California Biomechanics Laboratory brace, molded ankle–foot orthoses, articulated molded ankle–foot orthoses, or the Marzano brace (29). The goal of early treatment is to control the progressive valgus of the calcaneus. Modalities (e.g., phonophoresis and iontophoresis, icing, and heat), eccentric strengthening, and hands-on physical therapy also are necessary early in the rehabilitation process. If nonoperative or conservative treatment fails, surgery is indicated, because the progression of dysfunction may be rapid and disabling. In the early states of dysfunction, soft-tissue surgical procedures, such as tendon debridement or tenosynovectomy, may halt the progression of deterioration. Surgical release with tenolysis and/or augmentation by another tendon may be necessary early on to prevent irreversible bony/joint changes (20). Surgical procedures involving osteotomies and arthrodesis are necessary once a flatfoot deformity develops (29).

Gastrocnemius Muscle Strain

Strains to the medial head of the gastrocnemius often are seen in tennis players older than 40 years, hence the nickname "tennis leg." Common mechanisms are forced dorsiflexion while the knee is extended, forced knee extension while the foot is dorsiflexed, and muscular fatigue with fluid-electrolyte depletion and muscle cramping.

If related to muscle cramping, the strain commonly is attributed to dehydration (particularly in the heat), electrolyte imbalance, or prolonged muscle fatigue that stimulates cramping followed by an actual tear in the muscle fibers. Acute spasms may awaken an individual in the night following

FIGURE 18.20

Gastrocnemius muscle strain.
The medial head of the gastrocnemius muscle commonly is strained in individuals older than 40 years. A defect often can be palpated at the musculotendinous junction.

a day of strenuous exercise. Acute cramps are best treated with ice, pressure, and slow stretch of the muscle as it begins to relax. Prevention of this condition involves adequate water intake during strenuous activity and a regular stretching program for the gastrocnemius–soleus complex. When participation extends over 2 hours in hot weather, increased water intake with a weak electrolyte solution should be ensured during and after strenuous activity.

SIGNS AND SYMPTOMS. In an acute strain, the individual experiences a sudden, painful, tearing sensation in the calf muscles, primarily at the musculotendinous junction between the muscles and Achilles tendon or in the medial head of the gastrocnemius muscle (Fig. 18.20). Immediate pain, swelling, loss of function, and stiffness are common. Later, ecchymosis progresses down the leg into the foot and ankle.

MANAGEMENT. Acute management consists of standard acute care to control inflammation, restricted activity, gentle stretching of the gastrocnemius, heel lifts, and a progressive strengthening program. In more severe cases, immobilization and non–weight bearing may be necessary to allow the muscle to heal fully.

Achilles Tendon Disorders

Achilles tendon disorders occur most often in athletes and, of those, most often in individuals who are involved in running sports. Inappropriately generalized as "Achilles tendinitis," posterior heel pain resulting from an overuse injury of the foot and ankle actually encompasses a myriad of distinct and often coexisting pathological disorders with both inflammatory and degenerative etiologies. Common intrinsic risk factors that can predispose an individual to disorders of the Achilles tendon include several foot malalignment and biomechanical faults, such as hyperpronation of the foot, limited mobility of the subtalar joint and limited ROM of the ankle joint, leg-length discrepancy, varus deformity of the forefoot and increased hindfoot inversion, decreased ankle dorsiflexion with the knee in extension, poor vascularity, genetic makeup, and gender, age, endocrine, or metabolic factors. Extrinsic factors that may lead to the disorder include changes in shoes or running surface, a sudden increase in workload (e.g., distance or intensity) or change in exercise environment (e.g., training on hard, slippery, or slanting surfaces), poor technique, and monotonous, asymmetric, and specialized training (30).

When intrinsic and extrinsic factors are involved, microtraumatic changes occur in the Achilles tendon from different force contributions of the gastrocnemius and soleus, producing abnormal loading concentrations within the tendon and frictional forces between the fibrils leading to localized fiber damage. The tendon is relatively avascular at approximately 0.8 inch (2 cm) above its distal insertion into the calcaneus, which is the site of most torque on the tendon. This area is highly vulnerable to partial tears, with secondary nodule formation and degenerative cysts seen in **tendinosis**.

SIGNS AND SYMPTOMS. Acute signs and symptoms include an aching or burning pain in the posterior heel, which increases with passive dorsiflexion and resisted plantar flexion, such as going up onto the toes. Point tenderness and crepitus can be elicited at the bony insertion or 1 to 3 cm above the insertion. There also can be associated retrocalcaneal bursitis. Palpation may reveal local nodules either within the tendon, which moves during dorsiflexion and plantar flexion, or in the periotendon, which does not move during these motions.

Chronic signs and symptoms can include pain that is worse after exercise within days of a change in activity levels or training techniques and that may become constant. The tendon often becomes thickened, and pain is localized on the posterolateral heel. The gastrocnemius–soleus complex is tight, which may result from tendon adhesions, muscle spasm, or inflexibility. Radiographs usually show a prominent posterosuperior calcaneus (Haglund deformity), and calcific spurring often occurs at the bone–tendon interface. Pathologically, the tendon demonstrates chronic degeneration rather than inflammation. Rest may relieve symptoms, but return to activity reactivates the pain, generally within a few training sessions.

A tendinopathy poses the risk of complete rupture of the tendon. Magnetic resonance imaging often is needed for accurate diagnosis.

MANAGEMENT. The goal of treatment is to minimize pain, prevent further degeneration, and allow the individual to return to baseline activity. Initial conservative treatment involves standard acute care, activity modification, and correcting factors that cause load imbalance and repetitive strain on the tendon and surrounding structures. Complete restriction of activity may be necessary for 3 weeks. Active stretching of the Achilles tendon before and after activity, along with a full strengthening program for the gastrocnemius–soleus complex, including eccentric loading, is initiated immediately after acute pain has subsided. Use of oral NSAIDs or steroidal pain relievers to control inflammation remains controversial. Recently, some success has been seen in ultrasound-guided injections of polidocanol, a sclerosing agent, to decrease the neovascularization and symptoms of chronic midportion Achilles tendinosis (31). Operative treatment is recommended for individuals who do not respond to a 3- to 6-month trial of appropriate conservative treatment. Surgery usually involves excision of fibrotic adhesions and degenerated nodules or decompression of the tendon by longitudinal tenotomies.

Achilles Tendon Rupture

Acute rupture of the Achilles tendon probably is the most severe acute muscular problem in the lower leg. It more commonly is seen in individuals from 30 to 50 years of age (32). The usual mechanism is a push-off of the forefoot while the knee is extending, which is a common move in many propulsive activities. Tendinous ruptures usually occur 1 to 2 inches proximal to the distal attachment of the tendon on the calcaneus (Fig. 18.21).

SIGNS AND SYMPTOMS. The individual hears and feels a characteristic "pop" in the posterior ankle and reports a feeling of being shot or kicked in the heel. Clinical signs and symptoms include a visible defect in the tendon, inability to stand on tiptoes or even balance on the affected leg, swelling and bruising around the malleoli, excessive passive dorsiflexion, and positive Thompson's test (see Fig. 18.34). Because the peroneal longus, peroneal brevis, and muscles in the deep posterior compartment are still intact, the individual may limp or walk with the foot and leg externally rotated, because this does not require push-off with the superficial calf muscles.

MANAGEMENT. A compression wrap should be applied from the toes to the knee. The leg and foot can be immobilized in a posterior splint. The individual should be referred immediately to a physician. Nonoperative treatment offers excellent functional results for partial tears in older, noncompetitive individuals. With delayed diagnosis or in highly competitive individuals, surgical repair provides better push-off strength and prevents overelongation of the tendon and, in doing so, lowers the risk for reinjury. The course of action depends on the supervising physician, but in either case, full ROM and strength may not be achieved until 6 months after the injury.

The 55-year-old badminton player has tenosynovitis of the tibialis posterior. Pes planus, along with weakness in plantar flexion and inversion, provide evidence of the muscle involved. Management of the condition includes standard acute care. In addition, the individual should be advised to wear shoes with better arch support. If the condition does not improve, the individual should be referred to a physician.

■■■ ■ FIGURE 18.21 **Achilles tendon rupture.** The Achilles tendon often is ruptured 1 to 2 inches proximal to its distal attachment. This patient's ruptured left Achilles tendon appears to be thickened and less distinct than that on the normal right side, and the patient is unable to plantar flex the left foot.

OVERUSE CONDITIONS

A slightly overweight, novice runner is in the third week of training for a 10K run. He reports the following symptoms: excruciating pain in the anteromedial hindfoot on arising in the morning, which disappears within 5 to 10 minutes; point tenderness just distal to the medial calcaneal tubercle; and pain that increases with weight bearing. What condition may be present, and how should this injury be managed?

Repetitive microscopic injury to tendinous structures can lead to chronic inflammation that overwhelms the tissue's ability to repair itself. Other factors, such as faulty biomechanics, poor cushioning or stiff-soled shoes, or excessive downhill running, also can inflame the tendons. Several overuse conditions are common in specific sports, such as plantar fasciitis in running; medial tibial stress syndrome in football, dance, or running; and exertional compartment syndrome in soccer or distance running. Many individuals complain of vague leg pain but have no history of a specific injury that caused the pain, differentiating these conditions from an acute muscle strain. A common complaint is pain caused by activity.

Plantar Fasciitis

Plantar fasciitis is the most common hindfoot problem in runners, affecting approximately 10% of participants (33). Extrinsic factors that increase the incidence of the condition include training errors, improper footwear, and participating on unyielding surfaces. Intrinsic factors include pes cavus or pes planus, decreased planar flexion strength, reduced flexibility of the plantar flexor muscles (e.g., Achilles tendon), excessive or prolonged pronation, and torsional malalignment. These factors can overload the plantar fascia's origin on the anteromedial aspect of the calcaneus during weight-bearing activities. In a chronic condition, entrapment of the first branch of the lateral plantar nerve can contribute to the pain syndrome. Entrapment of the posterior tibial or medial calcaneal nerve (i.e., tarsal tunnel syndrome) may mimic or complicate the condition.

Signs and Symptoms

The individual reports pain on the plantar, medial heel that is relieved with activity but that recurs after rest. Pain increases with weight bearing. It is particularly severe with the first few steps in the morning, particularly in the proximal, plantar, medial heel, but diminishes within 5 to 10 minutes. Pain and stiffness are related to muscle spasm and splinting of the fascia secondary to inflammation. Pain can radiate up the medial side of the heel and, occasionally, across the lateral side of the foot. Normal muscle length is not easily attained, and reaching normal length can lead to additional pain and irritation. Point tenderness is elicited over or just distal to the medial tubercle of the calcaneus and increases with passive toe extension. Passive extension of the great toe and dorsiflexion of the ankle will increase pain and discomfort. If the lateral plantar nerve is involved, tenderness also is noted at the proximal, superior abductor hallucis muscle. A tight heel cord with decreased dorsiflexion of the ankle is seen in approximately 70% of patients who have unilateral symptoms (33).

Management

Treatment involves standard acute care. Following completion of the inflammatory stage, therapeutic modalities used to alleviate symptoms may include ice, deep friction massage, ultrasound, and electrical muscle stimulation. Achilles tendon stretching exercises, stretching of the toe flexor tendons, strengthening of the peroneal and posterior tibial muscles, NSAIDs, and a soft heel lift may be helpful. A Moleskin® plantar fascia strap or figure-eight arch strapping is an effective means of support. Circular strips of tape around the foot are contraindicated, however, because they may overstretch the fascia and prolong recovery. Use of a viscoelastic heel cushion and/or orthoses along with a corticosteroid injection may be needed. Night splinting to hold the heel cord under mild tension may be used as well. Surgery or noninvasive ultrasonic treatment should be considered after 6 to 12 months (20). Field Strategy 18.4 highlights the management of plantar fasciitis.

FIELD STRATEGY 18.4

Management of Plantar Fasciitis

- Use immediate ice therapy and nonsteroidal anti-inflammatory drugs.
- Use a shock-absorbing soft heel pad or soft plantar arch pad.
- Figure-eight arch strapping or night splints may relieve acute symptoms.
- Use aggressive Achilles tendon stretching for 2 to 4 minutes, three to four times a day, with the toes straight ahead, the toes in, and the toes out.
- Use gentle isometric contractions initially for intrinsic muscles of the foot.
- Progress to active range-of-motion exercise within pain-free ranges: toe curls, marble pick-up, towel crunches, and towel curls.
- Strengthen the intrinsic and extrinsic leg muscles.
- Maintain body fitness and strength, as well as aerobic fitness, with non–weight bearing activities.
- The physician may administer cortisone injections into the plantar fascia aponeurosis.

Medial Tibial Stress Syndrome

Medial tibial stress syndrome is a **periostitis** along the posteromedial tibial border, usually in the distal third, that is not associated with a stress fracture or compartment syndrome. Although originally thought to be related to stress along the posterior tibialis muscle and tendon causing myositis, fasciitis, and periostitis, it is now believed to be related to periostitis of the soleus insertion along the posteromedial tibial border. The soleus makes up the medial third of the heel cord as it inserts into the calcaneus. Excessive or prolonged pronation of the foot causes an eccentric contraction of the soleus, resulting in the periostitis that produces the pain. Other contributing factors include recent changes in running distance, speed, form, stretching, footwear, or running surface.

Signs and Symptoms

Typically seen in runners or jumpers, the pain can occur at any point in the workout and typically is characterized as a dull ache, although it occasionally can be sharp and penetrating. As activity progresses, pain diminishes, only to recur hours after activity has ceased. During later stages, pain is present before, during, and after activity and may restrict performance. Point tenderness is elicited in a 3- to 6-cm area along the distal posteromedial tibial border. Pain is aggravated by resisted plantar flexion or by standing on tiptoe. An associated varus alignment of the lower extremity, including a greater Achilles tendon angle, often is present. In experienced runners, the condition usually is secondary to mechanical abnormalities, such as:

- Increased Achilles tendon angle (during stance phase and while running)
- Greater Achilles tendon angle between heel strike and maximal pronation
- Greater passive subtalar motion in inversion and eversion

Management

Five to 7 days of rest are essential to relieve acute symptoms. Other modalities (e.g., cryotherapy, NSAIDs, cortisone injections, heel pads, casting, crutches, and activity modification) have not been shown to be as effective as rest alone. Pain-free stretching of both the anterior and posterior musculature helps to improve joint mobility, increase muscle and tendon strength as well as coordination, and aid the musculoskeletal system in adapting to the physical demands of a specific sport. If the condition does not improve, possible stress fractures to the tibia should be ruled out through appropriate radiograph or scanning procedures. Analysis of the individual's running motion, foot alignment, running surface, and footwear may prevent recurrence. Field Strategy 18.5 summarizes the management of medial tibial stress syndrome.

FIELD STRATEGY 18.5

Management of Medial Tibial Stress Syndrome

- Five to 7 days of rest is essential.
- Ice, compression, elevation, and nonsteroidal anti-inflammatory drugs may help to relieve acute symptoms.
- Determine if a stress fracture is present.
- Evaluate and correct any foot malalignment or problems in technique.
- Change the running surface and, possibly, shoes.
- Increase muscle flexibility in the anterior and posterior compartments.
- Increase strength in all muscles of the lower leg and foot.

Exertional Compartment Syndrome

Exertional compartment syndrome (ECS) is characterized by exercise-induced pain and swelling that is relieved by rest. The compartments most frequently affected are the anterior (50–60%) and deep posterior (20–30%). The remaining 10 to 20% of cases are divided evenly among the lateral, superficial posterior, and "fifth" compartment around the tibialis posterior muscle (34). Whereas acute ECS generally occurs in relatively sedentary people who undertake strenuous exercise, chronic ECS usually is seen in well-conditioned individuals younger than 40 years (35).

Signs and Symptoms

The typical history of chronic ECS is exercise-induced pain that often is described as a tight, cramp-like, or squeezing ache and a sense of fullness, both of which are felt over the involved compartment. The condition often affects both legs. Symptoms almost always are relieved with rest, usually within 20 minutes of exercise, only to recur if exercise is resumed. Activity-related pain begins at a predictable time after starting exercise or after reaching a certain level of intensity, and the pain increases if the training persists. Many individuals with anterior compartment involvement describe mild foot drop or paresthesia (or both) on the dorsum of the foot and demonstrate fascial defects or hernias, usually in the distal third of the leg over the intramuscular septum.

Evaluation should be performed after the individual has exercised strenuously enough to reproduce the symptoms. The exercise produces swelling and tenderness in the involved compartments and increased leg girth. Tenderness, if present, may be located in the middle third of the tibia, although many individuals have no focal pain. Vibration with a tuning fork produces no pain, as one typically sees in a stress fracture. Likewise, pain is not present in the distal leg, which corresponds with medial tibial stress syndrome. To confirm the diagnosis, intracompartmental pressure must be measured (see Acute Compartment Syndrome).

Management

Treatment involves assessing extrinsic factors (e.g., training patterns, technique, shoe design, and training surface) and intrinsic factors (e.g., foot alignment, especially hindfoot pronation, muscle imbalance, and flexibility). In minor conditions, ice massage, NSAIDs, and occasionally, diuretics may assist, along with stretching and strengthening of the involved compartment muscles, orthotics, and relative rest. If symptoms persist for 6 to 12 weeks of conservative care, or in cases with extreme pressure elevation, fasciotomy is recommended; unlike a fasciotomy for acute ECS, this may be limited to complete release of the involved compartments.

The runner may have plantar fasciitis. As part of the assessment, it is important to check foot alignment, gait, and shoes for problems that may have contributed to the condition. Stretching of the toe flexors and Achilles tendon should be a major part of the treatment plan.

VASCULAR AND NEURAL DISORDERS

A figure skater is complaining of bilateral numbness in the posterolateral aspect of the leg along the Achilles tendon that has been present for the past 2 to 3 weeks. No history of trauma to the ankle is noted. The skater reveals that she routinely spirals her laces tightly around the proximal portion of each boot, then applies several circular bands of white tape to hold them in place. Could this technique impair the vascular or neural function of the lower leg, and how should this situation be managed?

Vascular and neural disorders of the lower leg are rare in sports but can occur. Vascular disorders typically involve occlusion of venous blood in the calf region; neural involvement typically affects the distal ankle and foot region. In either case, any change in circulation, sensation, or function should signal referral to a physician.

Venous Disorders

By way of contraction of smooth and skeletal muscles, blood within the superficial venous system, as well as the deep venous system, is pushed, or "milked," back to the heart and lungs for elimination or metabolism. In some cases, particularly with inactivity following fracture or surgery, prolonged bed rest, and increasing age, this system becomes inefficient, leading to a reduced blood flow. The accumulated blood products may form a clot that can grow in size, depending on the vessel in which it is contained, causing partial or complete blockage. This condition is called a deep venous thrombosis (DVT). The deep calf veins are most frequently involved, but involvement of the popliteal, superficial femoral, and ileofemoral vein segments also is common. An **embolism** occurs when a loosened thrombus circulates from a larger vessel to a smaller one, subsequently obstructing circulation. When the obstruction occurs in the veins of the lungs, it is called a pulmonary embolism. Because the risk factors for DVT include a sedentary lifestyle, smoking, obesity, and prolonged periods of inactivity, DVT rarely is seen in an active population (36).

Signs and Symptoms

Deep venous thrombosis typically is asymptomatic and may not become apparent until a pulmonary embolism occurs. The most reliable signs are paresthesia in the area, chronic swelling and edema in the involved extremity, engorged veins, ecchymosis formation with a blue hue, and a positive Homans' sign (see Fig. 18.35).

Management

Immediate referral to a physician is warranted. Treatment involves anticoagulant therapy, leg elevation, and ambulation in individuals who are clinically stable and for whom it is medically indicated. Functional neuromuscular stimulation of the gastrocnemius and tibialis anterior may help to activate the physiologic muscle pump while moving venous blood back to the central circulation to prevent DVT.

Neurologic Conditions

Impingement of nerves in the lower leg and foot is rare but does happen. Three such conditions involve the compression of the interdigital nerves as they bifurcate at the metatarsal heads (i.e., plantar interdigital neuroma), the posterior tibial nerve beneath the flexor retinaculum and behind the medial malleolus (i.e., tarsal tunnel syndrome), and the sural nerve as it courses behind the lateral malleolus and into the lateral aspect of the foot.

Plantar Interdigital Neuroma

A plantar interdigital neuroma (i.e., Morton's neuroma) is a common source of forefoot pain, especially among middle-aged women. It sometimes is bilateral. Trauma or repetitive stress caused by tight-fitting shoes or a pronated foot can lead to abnormal pressure on the plantar digital nerves as they are compressed between the metatarsal heads and transverse intermetatarsal ligament. It typically occurs at the web space between the third and fourth metatarsals (i.e., second and third intermetatarsal spaces) and, to a lesser extent, between the second and third metatarsals (Fig. 18.22).

SIGNS AND SYMPTOMS. The individual may initially describe a sensation of having a stone in the shoe that worsens when standing. Tingling or burning, radiating to the toes, along with intermittent symptoms of a sharp, shock-like sensation into the involved toes, commonly is reported. Pain subsides when activity is stopped or when the shoe is removed. In fact, the desire to remove the shoe and massage the foot is a classic indicator of a neuroma. The examiner may be able to palpate a painful mass, elicit pain by palpating between the metatarsal heads, or sense a palpable click with lateral compression of the metatarsal heads (see Fig. 18.37).

MANAGEMENT. Conservative management involves placing a metatarsal pad just proximal to the metatarsal heads and wearing a broad, soft-soled shoe with a low heel. The focus is to preserve and maximize flexion at the lesser toe MTP joints to prevent and treat the condition. Local corticosteroid injections or surgical excision of the nerve may be necessary to remedy persistent pain (20).

■■ ■ **FIGURE 18.22 Plantar's neuroma.** Plantar's neuroma (Morton's neuroma) is caused by pinching of the interdigital nerve between the metatarsal heads. While weight bearing in shoes, the individual has an agonizing pain on the lateral side of the foot that is relieved when he or she is barefoot.

Tarsal Tunnel Syndrome

Tarsal tunnel syndrome occurs when the posterior tibial nerve, or one of its branches, becomes constricted beneath the fibrous roof of the flexor retinaculum of the foot (Fig. 18.23). Entrapment most often occurs at the anteroinferior aspect of the canal, where the nerve winds around the medial malleolus. The irritation can be caused by bone, soft tissue, or vascular structures (i.e., varicosity) (20). The lateral plantar nerve branch tends to be affected more frequently than the medial branch. The condition often is linked to excessive pronation or an excessive valgus deformity that leads to stress or traction on the nerve with impingement.

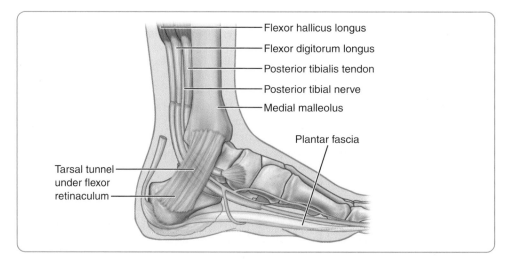

■■ ■ **FIGURE 18.23 Tarsal tunnel syndrome.** The posterior tibial nerve can become constricted beneath the tarsal tunnel roof formed by the flexor retinaculum.

SIGNS AND SYMPTOMS. Clinically, the individual complains of pain at the medial malleolus radiating into the sole and heel (particularly with entrapment of the lateral plantar nerve), paresthesia, dysesthesia, and hyperesthesia in the distribution of the posterior tibial nerve. Hyperdorsiflexion, external rotation, and eversion may reproduce symptoms similar to those during provocative tests for carpal tunnel syndrome. One of the most reliable signs is a positive Tinel's sign—namely, tingling elicited by tapping along the course of the nerve (see Fig. 18.36).

MANAGEMENT. Conservative management involves rest, NSAIDs, orthoses (especially in individuals with hyperpronation), and gradual return to activity. A one-time injection of cortisone and lidocaine without epinephrine may be given into the tarsal tunnel, but if symptoms persist and other causes of heel pain are eliminated, surgical release may be necessary to relieve symptoms. Rehabilitation takes longer than with carpal tunnel syndrome because of the dependent weight-bearing requirements (20).

Sural Nerve Entrapment

The sural nerve, which is formed from branches of the tibial and peroneal nerves, provides cutaneous innervation to the lateral lower leg and foot. It passes distally along the lateral margin of the Achilles tendon to emerge from the fascia of the leg proximal to the lateral malleolus. After providing lateral calcaneal branches to the ankle and heel, the nerve passes behind the lateral malleolus and continues along the lateral border of the foot to extend to the fifth toe as the lateral dorsal cutaneous nerve. In addition to being vulnerable to compression from tight-fitting skates, boots, and shoes, the nerve can be irritated by fibrous adhesions that result from repetitive inversion ankle injuries or by ganglia that may form in the peroneal tendon sheath. Peripheral sural nerve neuropathy related to diabetes also may be a cause of paresthesia in this area.

SIGNS AND SYMPTOMS. Symptoms of sural nerve involvement include numbness in the affected area with decreased temperature sensation along the dorsolateral aspect of the foot, a burning sensation, local tenderness over the sural nerve, and reproduction of the symptoms by compression over the nerve (i.e., positive Tinel's sign).

MANAGEMENT. Conservative treatment may be as simple as changing the lacing of the skates, boots, or shoes; however, surgical intervention may be necessary to correct the problem.

> *The figure skater may have compressed the sural nerve with the tight laces and tape. The individual should be referred to a physician to determine the extent of injury to the nerve. The skater should be advised to change the way that she laces her boots.*

FRACTURES

> *In addition to Sever's disease, what conditions could lead to heel pain in young athletes?*

Fractures in the foot and lower leg region seldom result from a single traumatic episode. Often, repetitive microtraumas lead to apophyseal or stress fractures. Tensile forces associated with severe ankle sprains can lead to avulsion fractures of the fifth metatarsal, or severe twisting can lead to displaced and undisplaced fractures in the foot, ankle, or lower leg. A combination of forces can lead to a traumatic fracture-dislocation.

Freiberg's Disease

Freiberg's disease is a painful avascular necrosis of the second or, rarely, third metatarsal head that often is seen in active adolescents aged 14 to 18 years before closure of the epiphysis. The condition can lead to diffuse pain in the forefoot region. Early detection is best treated by a metatarsal pad or bar to unload the involved metatarsal head and activity modification to eliminate excessive running and jumping. If pain persists and deformity develops with degenerative osteophytes, surgical resection of the distal metatarsal head may be necessary.

Sever's Disease

Sever's disease, or calcaneal apophysitis, frequently is seen in 7- to 10-year-old children. It is associated with growth spurts, decreased heel cord and hamstring flexibility, and other biomechanical abnormalities contributing to poor shock absorption (e.g., forefoot varus, hallux valgus, pes cavus, pes planus, and more commonly, forefoot pronation). Because the apophyseal plate is vertically oriented, it is particularly susceptible to shearing stresses from the gastrocnemius. Hard surfaces, poor-quality or worn-out athletic shoes, being kicked in the region, or landing off-balance also may precipitate the condition.

Signs and Symptoms

The individual complains of unilateral or bilateral, intermittent or continuous, posterior heel pain that occurs shortly after beginning a new sport or season. Pain tends to be worse during and after activity but improves with rest. Although gait may be normal, the child may walk with a limp or exhibit a forceful heel strike. Point tenderness can be elicited at or just anterior to the insertion of the Achilles tendon along the posterior border of the calcaneus. Mediolateral compression (i.e., "squeeze test") of the calcaneus over the lower third of the posterior calcaneus elicits pain, as does standing on the tiptoes (i.e., positive Sever's sign). Heel cord flexibility is tested by passive dorsiflexion of the foot with the knee extended. Other conditions that may lead to heel pain should be ruled out before determining the treatment plan (Box 18.4).

Management

Following standard acute care, the individual should be referred to a physician for further care. The condition usually resolves itself with closure of the apophysis. Until that time, rest, ice, NSAIDs, heel lifts, heel cups, strapping the foot in slight plantar flexion to relieve some strain on the Achilles tendon, and activity modification usually relieve symptoms. Heel cord flexibility and strengthening exercises of the dorsiflexors are recommended. Resistant cases may benefit from a nighttime dorsiflexion splint.

Stress Fractures

Stress fractures often are seen in those who participate in sports that involve running and jumping, particularly after a significant increase in training mileage or a change in surface, intensity, or shoe type. Women with **amenorrhea** of longer than 6 months duration and **oligomenorrhea** have a higher incidence of stress fractures of the foot and leg during sport activity; however, women who use oral contraceptives tend to have significantly fewer stress fractures compared with nonusers (20,37).

Stress fractures can be generally classified as noncritical and critical. Noncritical stress fractures of the lower leg, foot, and ankle include the medial tibia, fibula, and the second, third, and fourth metatarsals. The neck of the second metatarsal is the most common location for a stress fracture, although it also is seen on the fourth and fifth metatarsals. Treatment usually requires relative rest. Physically active individuals may benefit from a short period of immobilization in a walking boot for up to 3 weeks or, in the case of metatarsal stress fractures, from a stiff-sole shoe or steel insert. Return to activity generally is seen in 6 to 8 weeks.

Critical stress fractures require special attention because of a higher rate of nonunion. Common sites include the anterior tibia, medial malleolus, talus, navicular, fifth metatarsal, and sesamoids.

Box 18.4   Differential Diagnosis of Heel Pain in Physically Active, Young Individuals

- Plantar fasciitis
- Heel fat pad syndrome
- Achilles tendinitis/strain
- Retrocalcaneal bursitis
- Calcaneal stress fracture
- Calcaneal exostosis
- Contusion
- Infection
- Tarsal coalition
- Tarsal tunnel syndrome

Stress fractures of the tibia and fibula result from repetitive stress to the leg leading to muscle fatigue. The resulting loss in shock absorption increases stress on the bone and periosteum. In the tibia, most stress fractures occur at the junction of the middle and distal thirds (most common site), the posteromedial tibial plateau, or just distal to the tibial tuberosity. Fibular stress fractures usually occur in the distal metadiaphyseal region. Because the fibula has a minimal role in weight bearing, it is believed that fibular stress fractures result from muscle traction and torsional forces (30).

Stress fractures of the medial malleolus usually present with a history of several weeks of mild discomfort followed by an acute episode that precipitates seeking medical attention. Excessive pronation and accompanying tibial rotation distributes excessive forces to the medial malleolus.

Stress fractures of the talus most commonly involve the lateral body near the junction of the body with the lateral process of the talus. Talar neck stress fractures are considered to be rare. The patient may present with prolonged pain (i.e., several months in duration) following an ankle sprain despite full rehabilitation. Excessive subtalar pronation is felt to predispose an individual to talar stress fractures by allowing impingement of the lateral process of the calcaneus on the concave posterolateral corner of the talus (30).

Stress fractures of the calcaneus produce significant pain on heel strike. The individual often has a history of a substantial increase in the individual's activity level, particularly in distance runners. Palpation reveals maximum pain on the medial and lateral aspects of the plantar-calcaneal tuberosity. The most common site is the upper posterior margin, just anterior to the apophyseal plate and at a right angle to the normal trabecular pattern (30). Squeezing the calcaneus produces pain.

Stress fractures of the navicular are seen in jumpers, ballet dancers, and equestrians because of the nature of foot positions as well as the motions and inevitable stresses that are produced in the midfoot. Often seen in young men, this fracture is difficult to assess. A high degree of suspicion is required when an individual complains of generalized foot pain on the dorsomedial aspect of the midfoot that is brought on by activity and is relieved with rest. During the advanced stages, overlying swelling and pain on walking become evident.

The two sesamoid bones of the great toe can carry threefold the body's weight with leg-based activity. These bones often are fractured as a result of constant weight bearing on a hyperextended great toe or because of prolonged pronation during running. Individuals with pes cavus or tight plantar fascia are predisposed to this injury because of the large tensile forces placed on the bones. Pain and swelling are present on the ball of the foot, and the individual is unable to roll through the foot to stand on the toes. Radiographs may be inconclusive, because it is common for sesamoid bones to be **bipartite**, which are common in the general population.

Signs and Symptoms

Pain from a stress fracture begins insidiously, increasing with activity and decreasing with rest; pain usually is limited to the fracture site. Pain can be elicited with percussion, a tuning fork, or ultrasound. Encircling the forefoot or calcaneus with the hand and squeezing the fingers together produce added discomfort.

Management

Following standard acute care, the individual should be referred to a physician. Frequently, early radiographs are negative, but periosteal reaction or cortical thickening can be seen 2 to 4 weeks later (Fig. 18.24). Bone scans and magnetic resonance images are more sensitive and usually reveal the presence of a fracture long before it becomes evident on radiographs.

Treatment consists of rest until symptoms disappear (i.e., 4–8 weeks or longer), ice therapy, NSAIDs, stretching and

■■■ FIGURE 18.24 **Stress fractures.** Notice the sclerosis and widened cortices associated with bone healing.

■■■■ FIGURE 18.25 Avulsion fractures. A, A type I transverse fracture into the proximal shaft of the fifth metatarsal often is overlooked in cases of an inversion ankle sprain, resulting in a nonunion fracture. **B,** A type II fracture involves the styloid process of the fifth metatarsal.

strengthening exercises, and correcting any mechanical abnormalities that may have contributed to the condition. Protected weight bearing, a stiff shoe, a rigid orthosis, or a walking cast may be indicated in fractures of the metatarsals, calcaneus, or tibia. Wearing stiff-soled shoes or a heel cup may be helpful in cases with stress fractures of the sesamoid bones and calcaneus, respectively. The individual should be completely asymptomatic before returning to participation.

Avulsion Fractures

Avulsion fractures may occur at the site of any ligamentous or tendinous attachment. Severe eversion ankle sprains may cause the deltoid ligament to avulse a portion of the distal medial malleolus rather than tearing of the ligament. Inversion ankle sprains can provide sufficient overload to cause the plantar aponeurosis or peroneus brevis tendon to be pulled from the bone, avulsing the base of the fifth metatarsal (i.e., the so-called dancer's fracture). If the styloid process is avulsed, it is called a type II fracture and has an excellent prognosis, with healing occurring within 4 to 6 weeks.

A much more complicated avulsion fracture that is seen in sprinters and jumpers involves a type I transverse fracture into the proximal shaft of the fifth metatarsal at the junction of the diaphysis and metaphysis, called a **Jones fracture** (Fig. 18.25). It often is overlooked in conjunction with a severe ankle sprain that involves plantar flexion and a strong adduction force to the forefoot. Because of low vascularization and high stresses at this site, Jones fractures are associated with a poor outcome; nonunions and delayed unions are common.

Management

Following standard acute care, the individual should be referred to a physician. Treatment usually involves non–weight bearing immobilization for 6 to 10 weeks, followed by use of a walking cast or orthosis for an additional 4 weeks. Physical activity should be avoided until clinical and radiographic evidence of union appears, typically by 8 to 12 weeks. Displaced fractures may require open reduction and internal fixation. After screw fixation, progressive weight bearing is initiated at 2 weeks, with return to running in 7 weeks. When bone grafting is used, running activities are delayed for 12 weeks to allow bony healing (30).

Osteochondral Fracture of the Talus

Severe ankle sprains can impinge the dome of the talus against the malleoli, leading to a fracture of the cartilaginous cover. Anterolateral fractures comprise 43% of osteochondral lesions, are wafer-shaped, and result from forceful inversion and dorsiflexion. Posteromedial fractures account for 57% of osteochondral fractures and are cup-shaped. They result from forceful inversion and plantar flexion (Fig. 18.26). The fragment may remain nondisplaced or float freely in the joint. Osteochondritis dissecans of the talus can develop if the fragment, particularly one of the corners, floats freely in the ankle joint, thus losing its blood supply.

Signs and Symptoms

Symptoms may be nonspecific, and include a deep, aching pain that is aggravated by activity; recurrent ankle swelling; ankle instability and stiffness; occasional crepitus; clicking; and locking

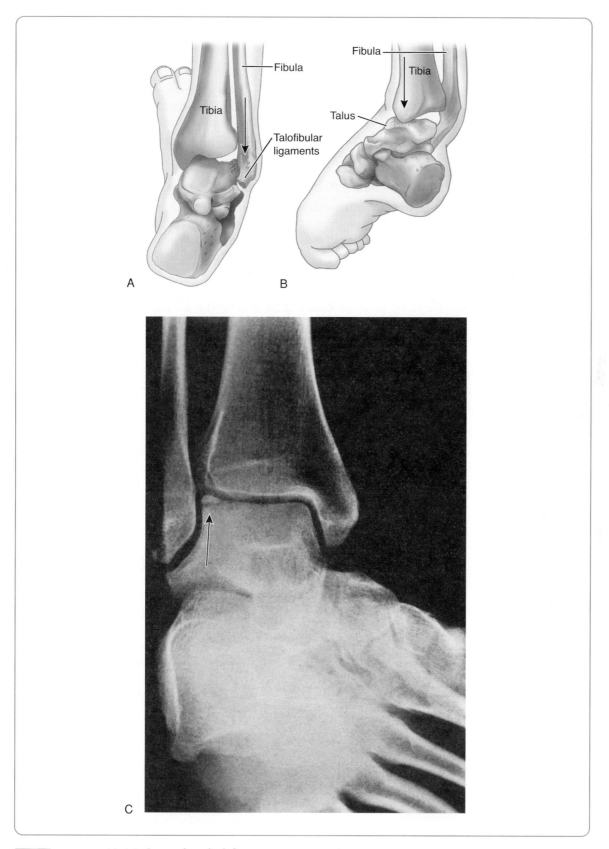

FIGURE 18.26 Osteochondral fractures. A, Forceful inversion of a dorsiflexed ankle can produce damage to the anterolateral talar dome. **B,** Forceful inversion of a plantar flexed ankle can produce damage to the posteromedial aspect of the dome. **C,** Radiograph of an osteochondral lesion on the lateral aspect of the talus.

(if displaced). Passive plantar flexion and palpation of the anterolateral and posteromedial corner of the talus elicits point tenderness. A palpable lesion or crepitus may be felt on the corners.

Management

If pain and joint effusion persist after an inversion ankle sprain or ankle fracture, or if symptoms return after an asymptomatic period, a more serious underlying condition should be suspected, and referral to a physician is warranted. Limited weight bearing (and/or immobilization) and NSAIDs are used to treat undisplaced fractures. Arthroscopic excision or repair usually is necessary in cases with displaced fractures.

Displaced Fractures and Fracture Dislocations

Severe fractures result from direct compression in acute trauma (e.g., falling from a height or being stepped on) or from combined compression and shearing forces (e.g., as occur during a severe twisting action). Because of the proximity of major blood vessels and nerves, many displaced and undisplaced fractures necessitate immediate immobilization and referral to the nearest trauma center.

Forefoot Fractures

Phalangeal fractures are caused by an axial load (e.g., jamming the toe into an immovable object) or direct trauma (e.g., crushing injury). Most are minor injuries, with the exception of a fracture to the great toe. Swelling, ecchymosis, and pain are present; the individual is able to walk but may have problems with footwear. Most tenderness resolves in 3 to 4 weeks. If the bony fragment is nondisplaced, buddy padding, splinting, and wearing a wooden shoe or a shoe with a wide toe box may help.

Metatarsal fractures are classified according to their anatomical location (i.e., neck, shaft, or base). A single fracture tends to be minimally displaced because of the restraining forces of the intermetatarsal ligaments. Swelling and pain are localized over the fracture site, and pain increases with weight bearing.

Tarsal Fractures

A **Lisfranc injury** involves disruption of the tarsometatarsal joint, with or without an associated fracture, and is notorious for delayed diagnosis (Fig. 18.27). The typical mechanism is a severe twisting injury (e.g., a football player falls onto the heel of another player's plantar-flexed foot) that causes an axial load along the metatarsals. The first metatarsal typically is dislocated from the first cuneiform, whereas the other four metatarsals are laterally displaced, usually in combination with a fracture at the base of the second metatarsal (20). Because the supply of blood to the forefoot can be compromised by the dislocation and subsequent swelling, a compartment syndrome may develop and create a serious injury. If assessed soon after the injury, the fracture may appear to be unremarkable until massive swelling sets in. A history of severe midfoot pain, paresthesia, or swelling along the midfoot region with variable flattening of the arch or abduction of the forefoot should signal a serious condition.

The talus often is fractured in a hyperdorsiflexion injury. A fracture of the lateral process of the talus and neck of the talus, which is rare, is caused by acute hyperdorsiflexion with inversion, which leads to severe hindfoot pain and moderate to severe edema, tenderness, and ecchymosis. Because of the

■■■■ FIGURE 18.27 **Lisfranc injury.** Radiograph of a Lisfranc injury: (**a**) first metatarsal, (**b**) second metatarsal, and (**c**) third, fourth, and fifth metatarsals, which have been dislocated laterally.

potential devastating complication of avascular necrosis of the talus, talar neck fractures need immediate immobilization and referral to a physician. Posterior fractures of the talus are seen in individuals aged 15 to 30 years, particularly in those activities requiring forced plantar flexion of the foot, such as ballet or soccer, and may be either acute or stress-related. Posterior pain is present when jumping, running, or kicking with the instep of the foot, and this pain is increased on forced plantar flexion and resisted great toe flexion, stemming from the close proximity of the flexor hallucis longus tendon to the fractured process.

Traumatic fractures of the calcaneus are rare, but when they do occur, such fractures commonly are caused by high-energy axial loads. Occasionally, fractures occur at the anterior process either by forceful plantar flexion and adduction or by compression. Nearly 75% of calcaneus fractures extend into the subtalar joint. Symptoms include severe heel pain, an inability to walk, and palpable, intense pain directly over the process, located just distal to the sinus tarsi. Initial treatment of intra-articular fractures includes immobilization in a bulky dressing and splint, with ice and elevation to control edema.

Tibia–Fibula Fractures

In an inversion sprain, the medial malleolus typically is fractured at the level of the talar dome, or the injury may occur as a spiral fracture at the distal tibial metaphysis. Eversion and dorsiflexion injuries lead to spiral or comminuted fractures of the lateral malleolus. In lateral malleolar fractures, the risks for a bimalleolar fracture are high when the deltoid ligament avulses the medial malleolus (see Fig. 18.19). Often, a crack is heard, and the individual is unable to bear weight on the injured extremity because of intense pain. Deformity may or may not be present.

A **Maisonneuve fracture** is an eversion-type injury of the ankle, with an associated fracture of the proximal third of the fibula, commonly at the junction of the proximal and middle thirds of the shaft (Fig. 18.28). The tibiofibular syndesmosis is disrupted, and either a tear of the tibiofibular ligament or a fracture of the medial malleolus also is present. The more proximal the location of the fibular fracture, the more damage to the interosseous membrane between the tibia and fibula, because the membrane is always disrupted up to the fracture site. The typical mechanism is external rotation of the foot. The individual presents with tenderness over the deltoid ligament and the fracture site on the proximal fibula. Any proximal fibular tenderness after a twisting injury calls for radiographs of the ankle, the tibia, and the fibula. A high fibular fracture often requires open reduction and internal fixation between the distal fibula and tibia to maintain the normal relationship of the bones while ligament healing occurs. The screws generally are removed 8 to 12 weeks after surgery.

Nearly 60% of tibial fractures involve the middle and lower thirds of the tibia. The majority of these fractures are closed (38). Whether open or closed, this fracture is associated with complications such as delayed union, nonunion, or malunion. The most common cause of an isolated tibial fracture is torsional force, resulting in a spiral or oblique fracture of the lower third of the tibia. Gross deformity, gross bone motion at the suspected fracture site, crepitus, immediate swelling, extreme pain, or pain with motion should signal immediate action.

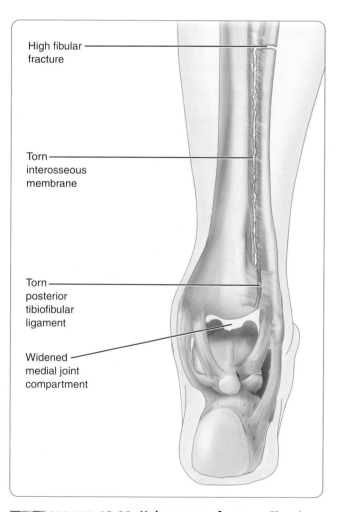

High fibular fracture

Torn interosseous membrane

Torn posterior tibiofibular ligament

Widened medial joint compartment

■■ ■■ FIGURE 18.28 Maisonneuve fracture. The classic fracture occurs at the junction of the proximal and middle thirds of the fibula. The tibiofibular syndesmosis is disrupted, and the interosseous membrane is torn up the level of the fracture. The tibiotalar (medial) joint compartment is widened because of lateral subluxation of the talus.

Ankle Fracture-Dislocations

Fracture-dislocations usually are caused by landing from a height with the foot in excessive eversion or inversion or by being kicked from behind while the foot is firmly planted on the ground. Typically, the foot is displaced laterally at a gross angle to the lower leg, and extreme pain is present. This position can compromise the posterior tibial artery and nerve.

Management of Displaced Fractures and Fracture-Dislocations

Management of lower leg, ankle, and foot fractures involves removing the shoe and sock to expose the injured area. If a fracture is suspected, the examiner should perform percussion, compression, and distraction before any movement of the limb. Depending on the site, the techniques listed in Field Strategy 18.6 may be helpful. The examiner also should assess the neurovascular integrity of the limb before and after immobilization by taking a distal pulse at the posterior tibial artery and/or dorsalis pedis artery or by blanching the toenails to determine capillary refill. The examiner should note the skin color of the foot and toes and should feel the toes for warmth. Sensation can be assessed by using the pulp of the fingers to stroke the top of the distal metatarsal heads and by asking the individual if the stroke was felt. The action is then repeated using the fingernail.

EMS Because shock is possible in serious traumatic fractures, the emergency action plan should be activated. In some settings, this will include summoning EMS to immobilize and transport the individual to the nearest medical facility. Suspected disruption of the tarsometatarsal joint (i.e., Lisfranc fracture) and fractures with suspected neurovascular compromise should be immobilized in a noncircumferential bulky splint to prevent complications from further compression.

If the great toe is fractured, a walking cast with a toe plate, or a wooden shoe and crutches, are helpful; if displaced, surgery may be necessary to prevent osteoarthritis. Metatarsal fractures are treated with a short slipper cast or wooden shoe for 6 weeks, with weight bearing as tolerated. A nondisplaced Lisfranc injury can be treated in a short-leg, nonwalking cast for 6 weeks, followed by 6 weeks in a short-leg, walking cast. Most injuries require open reduction and internal fixation. Nondisplaced extra-articular calcaneal fractures can be treated with a short-leg cast or walking boot for approximately 6 weeks. Most displaced fractures must be repaired surgically, but patients typically experience residual stiffness of their subtalar joint that can adversely affect future athletic performance.

Nondisplaced malleoli fractures are treated conservatively, with cast immobilization for 4 to 6 weeks, followed by a functional brace until the fracture is completely healed. Displaced fractures

FIELD STRATEGY 18.6

Determining a Fracture in the Lower Leg and Foot

- **Percussion.** Tapping on the head of the fibula or tibial shaft can be used to detect a fracture of the malleolus. Tapping on the ends of the toes along the long axis of the bone may detect a phalangeal fracture.
- **Bump test.** Strike the bottom of the heel with the palm to drive the talus into the mortise. Increased pain may indicate an osteochondral fracture, malleolar fracture, or increased mortise spread.
- **Squeeze test.** Compress the tibia and fibula together just distal to the knee. This causes the distal malleoli to distract. Increased pain distally may indicate a fracture.
- **Circumferential squeeze test.** Encircle the midfoot with the hand, and slowly squeeze the metatarsal heads. Increased pain may indicate a tarsal or metatarsal fracture.
- **Vibration.** Place a vibrating tuning fork near the suspected fracture site. Increased localized pain is a positive sign.
- **Compression/distraction.** Compress the ends of the toes and metatarsals along the long axis of the bone. Follow this with distraction along the long axis. If a fracture is present, compression should increase pain, but distraction should decrease pain. If distraction increases pain, the injury may be a joint sprain.

involving joint stability require surgical intervention with open reduction and internal fixation. Healing after surgery usually takes 2 to 3 months or longer, followed by extensive rehabilitation. Internal fixation with plates and screws often is necessary to stabilize tibial fractures; however, these individuals experience a high rate of infection (44%) as a complication of internal fixation (38).

A *In addition to Sever's disease, the following conditions could lead to heel pain in young athletes: plantar fasciitis, heel fat pad syndrome, Achilles tendinitis/strain, retrocalcaneal bursitis, calcaneal stress fracture, calcaneal exostosis, contusion infection, tarsal coalition, and tarsal tunnel syndrome.*

ASSESSMENT OF THE LOWER LEG, ANKLE, AND FOOT CONDITIONS

Q *A cross-country runner reports to the athletic training room complaining of pain along the plantar surface of the left foot. How should the assessment of this injury progress to determine the extent and severity of injury?*

Although pain, discomfort, or weakness may occur at a specific site, the lower extremities work as a unit to provide a foundation of support for the upright body, propulsion through space, absorption of shock, and adaptation to varying terrain. As such, assessment must include the entire lower extremity.

See *Field Strategy: Lower Leg, Ankle, and Foot Evaluation,* available on the companion website at thePoint.

HISTORY

Q *The injury assessment of the cross-country runner should begin with a history. What questions need to be asked to identify the cause and extent of this injury?*

Many conditions in the lower leg, ankle, and foot are related to family history, congenital deformities, poor technique, and recent changes in the training program, surface, or foot attire. The assessment begins by asking questions related to the mechanism of injury, associated symptoms, progression of the symptoms, any disabilities that may have resulted from the injury, and related medical history. For example, an acute onset should lead one to suspect bony trauma or an acute ankle sprain until ruled out. A gradual onset of pain may signal inflammation from overuse of a muscle or the plantar fascia or the development of a stress fracture. Particular attention should be given to recent changes in the distance, duration, or intensity of training; each component can lead to overuse injuries. Medial heel pain may indicate plantar fasciitis or, if in the middle of the plantar heel area, a heel spur. Pain in the medial arch can be a sign of a fallen medial longitudinal arch or tarsal tunnel syndrome. Pain around either malleolus may indicate an ankle sprain. Pain posterior to the lateral malleolus can signify peroneal tendinitis, subluxation, or dislocation or even sural nerve entrapment. Pain posterior to the medial malleolus may reflect tendinitis or rupture of the tibialis posterior.

See *Field Strategy: Developing a History of the Injury,* available on the companion website at thePoint, for specific questions related to the lower leg, ankle, and foot.

A *The cross-country runner should be asked questions that address when, where, and how the injury occurred; intensity, location, and type of pain; when the pain begins (e.g., when you get out of bed, while sitting, while walking, during exercise, or at night); how long the condition been has present; how long the pain lasts; if the pain has changed or stayed the same; if the pain is worse before, during, or after activity; activities that aggravate or alleviate the symptoms; changes in training; changes in footwear; and previous injury, treatment, and medication.*

OBSERVATION AND INSPECTION

Q *The cross-country runner reports pain on the plantar, medial heel that has been present for the past 5 days. The pain is worse after rest but is particularly severe with the first few steps in the morning. The runner indicates that he has increased both the intensity and distance of his daily runs over the past 7 days. Explain the observation component in the ongoing assessment of the cross-country runner.*

Both lower legs should be clearly visible to denote symmetry, any congenital deformity, swelling, discoloration, hypertrophy, muscular atrophy, or previous surgical incisions. The individual should wear running shorts to allow full view of the lower extremity. In addition, the individual should bring the shoes that normally are worn when pain is present so that they can be inspected for unusual wear, which could be indicative of a biomechanical abnormality that may be affecting the knee.

In an ambulatory patient, observation begins with the completion of a postural examination. Any bilateral gross deformity, swelling, or redness in the toes, foot, or ankle should be noted. The foot should be observed for the presence or absence of an arch on weight bearing and non–weight bearing. A supple, or flexible, flatfoot appears to be flattened when weight bearing but produces an obvious arch when non–weight bearing. In contrast, a rigid flatfoot appears to be flattened on weight bearing and non–weight bearing. It is important to note if the foot is in a pronated, neutral, or supinated position (see Box 18.1).

> See *Field Strategy: Postural Assessment of the Lower Leg, Ankle, and Foot*, found on the companion website at thePoint, for specific areas to focus on in the lower extremity.

Next, the examiner should instruct the individual to lie prone on a table with the feet and ankles extended over the end of the table to determine the talar neutral position. In assessing the left foot, the examiner places the right thumb and index finger on the anterior aspect of the foot spanning the talar dome. Using the left hand, the examiner grasps the foot from the lateral side and then inverts and everts the ankle and foot until the neutral position of the foot is determined (Fig. 18.29). The neutral position is identified when the talus is aligned symmetrically between the thumb and index finger. When talar neutral is determined, the relationship of the forefoot and rearfoot alignment should be noted. This may be done in the non–weight bearing position, the weight-bearing position, or both. Conditions that may be present with the calcaneus and talus in neutral position include:

- **Forefoot varus.** The first metatarsal is elevated relative to the fifth metatarsal.

- **Forefoot valgus.** The fifth metatarsal is elevated relative to the first metatarsal.

■■■ **FIGURE 18.29 Assessing the neutral talar position.** The examiner places the thumb and index fingers on the anterior aspect of the foot spanning the talar dome. Using the other hand, the examiner grasps the foot from the lateral side and then inverts and everts the ankle and foot until the neutral position of the foot is determined.

- **Rearfoot varus.** The calcaneus is inverted relative to the long axis of the tibia, which may result from a varus tibial alignment.

- **Rearfoot valgus.** The calcaneus is everted relative to the long axis of the tibia, which may result from a valgus tibial alignment.

The mobility of the first ray (i.e., the first tarsometatarsal joint extending into the first MTP joint) should be assessed. If the first ray is slightly plantar flexed at the tarsometatarsal joint, this causes the ray to be situated inferior to the remaining four rays. This often is associated with a cavus foot, as is a rigid ray. In contrast, hypermobility of the first ray is associated with pes planus.

The examiner should then instruct the individual to walk barefoot and observe the individual from an anterior, posterior, and lateral view. It is important to note any abnormalities in gait, favoring of one limb, heel-toe floor contact, and heel alignment. The gait analysis should be repeated with the individual wearing shoes and any orthoses.

Finally, the injury site should be inspected for obvious deformities, discoloration, edema, scars that might indicate previous surgery, and general condition of the skin. A bilateral comparison should be performed.

Observation of the cross-country runner should include a full postural assessment and gait analysis. The specific injury site should be inspected for obvious deformities, discoloration, edema, scars that might indicate previous surgery, and general condition of the skin.

PALPATION

The observation of the cross-country runner reveals no abnormal findings. Explain palpation specific to the injury sustained by the cross-country runner.

The individual should be seated on an examination table, with the foot and ankle extended beyond the table's edge. Bilateral palpation should be performed to determine temperature, swelling, point tenderness, crepitus, deformity, muscle spasm, and cutaneous sensation. Pulses can be taken at the posterior tibial artery behind the medial malleolus and at the dorsalis pedis artery on the dorsum of the foot.

Palpation should proceed proximal to distal, but the area anticipated to be most painful should be left to last. The following structures should be palpated:

Anterior and Medial Palpation

1. Shaft of the tibia
2. Medial malleolus
3. Posterior tibial artery
4. Tibialis posterior, flexor digitorum longus, and flexor hallucis longus muscles and tendons
5. Deltoid ligament
6. Sustentaculum tali (one finger's width inferior to the medial malleolus)
7. Talar dome and neck (plantar flexion exposes this area)
8. Joint capsule
9. Tibialis anterior, extensor hallucis longus, extensor digitorum longus muscles and tendons, and dorsalis pedis artery
10. Navicular bone and tubercle of the navicular
11. Medial, middle, and lateral cuneiforms
12. Calcaneonavicular ligament (i.e., spring ligament)
13. Medial calcaneus
14. Plantar fascia
15. Head of first metatarsal, sesamoid bones, and great toe
16. Second metatarsal and second toe

Anterior and Lateral Palpation

1. Head of the fibula as well as peroneal longus and brevis
2. Distal tibiofibular joint and ligament
3. Lateral malleolus
4. Anterior and posterior talofibular ligaments, CFL, peroneal tubercle, and peroneal tendons
5. Sinus tarsi (indentation over the talus next to the muscle belly of the extensor digitorum brevis)
6. Joint capsule and dome of the talus (plantar flex the foot)
7. Cuboid bone
8. Styloid process of the fifth metatarsal as well as shafts of the third, fourth, and fifth metatarsals
9. Third through fifth toes

Posterior Palpation

1. Triceps surae and Achilles tendon
2. Calcaneus, calcaneal bursa, and retrocalcaneal bursa
3. Posterior aspect of the heel pad and calcaneus

If a fracture is suspected, percussion, compression, and distraction should be performed before any movement of the limb. Examples of these techniques are provided in Field Strategy 18.6. These tests should be completed before postural or gait analysis.

 In the continued assessment of the cross-country runner, the bony and soft-tissue structures on the plantar aspect of the foot should be palpated for point tenderness, swelling, deformity, sensation, or other signs of trauma.

PHYSICAL EXAMINATION TESTS

The cross-country runner has point tenderness over the medial calcaneal tubercle. Explain the physical examination of the cross-country runner.

Physical examination testing should be performed in a comfortable position, with the individual lying on a table with feet hanging over the end or with the individual sitting. Bilateral comparison is used to assess normal level of function.

Functional Tests

The examiner should determine the available ROM in ankle dorsiflexion-plantar flexion, supination-pronation, toe flexion-extension, and toe abduction-adduction.

Active Movements

Active movements are best performed with the individual sitting on a table, with the leg flexed over the end of the table. The thigh and knee must be stabilized. Actions that may cause pain should be performed last to prevent any painful symptoms from overflowing into the next movement. The motions that should be assessed, and the normal ROM for each, are as follows:

- Dorsiflexion of the ankle (20°)
- Plantar flexion of the ankle (30–50°)
- Pronation (15–30°)
- Supination (45–60°)
- Toe extension
- Toe flexion
- Toe abduction and adduction

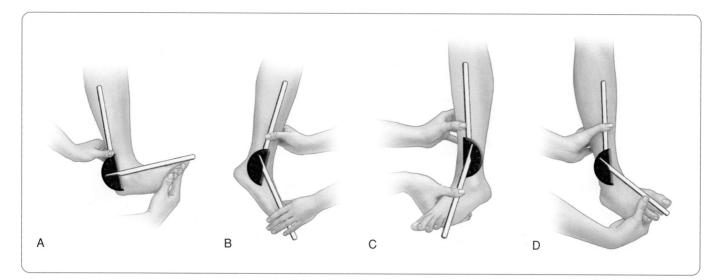

FIGURE 18.30 Goniometry measurement. A and **B,** Ankle dorsiflexion **(A)** and plantar flexion **(B)**. Center the fulcrum over the lateral malleolus. Align the proximal arm along the fibula using the head of the fibula for reference. Align the distal arm parallel to the midline of the fifth metatarsal. **C** and **D,** Pronation **(C)** and supination **(D)**. Center the fulcrum over the anterior ankle midway between the malleoli. Align the proximal arm with the midline of the crest of the tibia. Align the distal arm with the midline of the second metatarsal.

Passive Range of Motion

If the individual is able to perform full ROM during active movements, gentle pressure is applied at the extremes of motion to determine end feel. The end feel for dorsiflexion, plantar flexion, pronation, supination, and toe flexion and extension is tissue stretch. If the individual is unable to perform full active movements, passive movement should be performed to determine available ROM and end feel. Figure 18.30 demonstrates proper positioning for goniometry measurement at the ankle.

Resisted Muscle Testing

The thigh must be stabilized and resisted muscle testing performed throughout the full ROM. The assessment begins with the muscle on stretch, and resistance is applied throughout the full ROM. The examiner should note any muscle weakness when compared with the uninvolved limb. Potentially painful motions should be delayed until last. Figure 18.31 demonstrates the motions that should be tested.

Stress Tests

From information gathered during the history, observation, inspection, and palpation, the examiner determines which tests will assess the condition most effectively. Only those tests that are deemed to be absolutely necessary should be performed.

Anterior Drawer Test

This test assesses collateral ligament integrity of the ankle. While the individual is supine and the foot is extended beyond the table, the examiner stabilizes the tibia and fibula in one hand and cups the individual's heel in the other hand. Testing of both the anterior talofibular and deltoid ligaments involves applying a straight anterior movement with slight dorsiflexion (Fig. 18.32A). If the entire dome of the talus shifts equally forward, it indicates both medial and lateral ligament damage. The ATFL and anterolateral capsule can be isolated by applying a straight anterior movement with slight plantar flexion and inversion. A positive test results in the lateral side of the talus shifting forward, indicating anterolateral rotary instability.

FIGURE 18.31 Resisted manual muscle testing. A, Knee flexion (S_1, S_2). **B,** Dorsiflexion (L_4). **C,** Plantar flexion (S_1). **D,** Pronation. **E,** Supination. **F,** Toe extension (L_5). **G,** Toe flexion.

Talar Tilt

The calcaneofibular and deltoid ligaments are tested in the same position described for the anterior drawer test. Maintaining the calcaneus in normal anatomical position (90° of flexion), the examiner slowly rocks the talus between inversion and eversion (Fig. 18.32B). Inversion tests the CFL, and eversion tests the deltoid ligament.

FIGURE 18.32 Stress tests for the ankle collateral ligaments. A, Anterior drawer test. **B,** Talar tilt test.

External Rotation (Kleiger's) Test

A variation of the talar tilt test for deltoid ligament instability is the external rotation, or Kleiger's, test. Being careful not to compress the joint, the lower leg is stabilized proximal to the distal tibiofibular syndesmosis. While the foot is in a neutral position, the examiner grasps the medial side of the foot and then rotates the foot laterally (i.e., external rotation) (Fig. 18.33). If pain is felt over the medial joint line, it indicates damage to the deltoid ligament, whereas pain in the area of the lateral malleolus indicates injury to the syndesmosis.

Special Tests

A variety of special tests can be used for detecting injury or related pathology involving the lower leg, ankle, and foot.

Thompson's Test for Achilles Tendon Rupture

While the individual is prone on a table, the examiner squeezes the calf muscles. A normal response is slight plantar flexion. A positive test, indicating a rupture of the gastrocnemius–soleus complex or Achilles tendon, is indicated by the absence of plantar flexion (Fig. 18.34). The amount of motion should always be compared with the uninjured side, because some plantar flexion may occur if the plantaris muscle is intact. The magnitude of contraction, however, is significantly reduced compared with that of the uninvolved leg.

■■■■ FIGURE 18.33 **External rotation test.** The examiner passively dorsiflexes the ankle and rotates the foot laterally. Pain in the area of the lateral malleolus indicates injury to the syndesmosis.

Homans' Sign

To test for DVT, the individual must be supine on a table. The examiner dorsiflexes the foot of the involved leg with the knee in extension (Fig. 18.35). Pain in the calf indicates a positive Homans' sign. Tenderness also may be elicited with palpation of the calf. In addition, pallor or swelling in the leg may be accompanied by an absence of the dorsalis pedis pulse.

Tinel's Sign

To determine the presence of tarsal tunnel syndrome, the examiner should tap the posterior tibial nerve as it courses posterior to the medial malleolus (Fig. 18.36). The test is positive if numbness, tingling, and paresthesia occur.

■■■■ FIGURE 18.34 **Thompson's test.** The examiner performs passive compression of the calf muscles. This should produce slight plantar flexion at the ankle. If no plantar flexion occurs, a possible rupture of the gastrocnemius–soleus complex or the Achilles tendon should be suspected.

■■■■ FIGURE 18.35 **Homans' sign.** The examiner passively dorsiflexes the foot with the knee extended. Pain in the calf indicates a possible deep venous thrombosis.

FIGURE 18.36 Tinel's sign. The examiner taps the posterior tibial nerve, which may produce numbing, tingling, and paresthesia, indicating the presence of a possible tarsal tunnel syndrome.

FIGURE 18.37 Morton's test. Sharp pain in the foot caused by transverse compression of the metatarsal heads may indicate the presence of Morton's neuroma or metatarsalgia.

Morton's Test

The patient is in a supine position, with the foot extended over the end of the table. The examiner applies a traverse compression of the heads of the metatarsals (Fig. 18.37). If a sharp pain occurs, the test is positive, indicating metatarsalgia or a Morton's neuroma.

Neurologic Tests

Neurologic integrity is assessed with isometric muscle testing of the myotomes, reflex testing, and sensation in the segmental dermatomes and peripheral nerve cutaneous patterns.

Myotomes

Isometric muscle testing should be performed in the following motions to test specific segmental myotomes:

- Knee extension (L_3)
- Ankle dorsiflexion (L_4)
- Toe extension (L_5)
- Ankle plantar flexion, foot eversion, or hip extension (S_1)

Reflexes

Reflexes in the lower leg region include the patella (L_3, L_4) and Achilles tendon reflex (S_1). These are discussed in Chapter 17 and are demonstrated in Figure 17.38.

Cutaneous Patterns

The segmental nerve dermatome patterns for the pelvis, hip, and thigh are demonstrated in Figure 18.38. The peripheral nerve cutaneous patterns are demonstrated in Figure 18.39.

Activity-Specific Functional Tests

Functional tests should be performed pain-free before clearing any individual for return to activity. These may include any or all of the following:

- Squatting with both heels maintained on the floor
- Going up on the toes at least 20 times without pain
- Walking on the toes for 20 to 30 feet

FIGURE 18.38 Dermatomes for the lower leg, ankle, and foot. A, Anterior. **B,** Posterior.

- Balancing on one foot at a time

- Running straight ahead, stopping, and running backward

- Running figure-eights with large circles that slowly decrease in size

- Running at an angle sideways and making V-cuts

- Jumping rope for at least 1 minute

- Jumping straight up and then going to a 90° squat

 The physical examination of the cross-country runner should include active ROM, passive ROM, and restricted ROM of the foot and ankle; stretching the plantar aspect of the foot by having the athlete extend the toes while passively dorsiflexing the foot; fracture assessment; and performance of functional activities (e.g., walking and running).

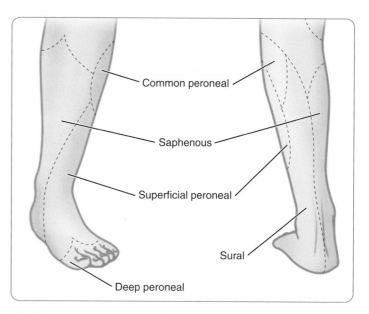

■■ ■■ **FIGURE 18.39 Peripheral nerve distribution in the lower leg, ankle, and foot.**

REHABILITATION

 The cross-country runner has plantar fasciitis. What exercises should now be included in the rehabilitation program?

Rehabilitation exercises for the lower leg, ankle, and foot can be initiated during the acute inflammatory phase so long as the condition is not further irritated. For example, while icing an ankle, the gastrocnemius and soleus can be passively stretched, or strengthening exercises for the foot intrinsic muscles can be started. Pain and swelling dictate the amount of exercise that can be tolerated and may necessitate restricted weight bearing. The rehabilitation program should restore motion and proprioception, maintain cardiovascular fitness, and improve muscular strength, endurance, and power, predominantly through closed chain exercises.

Restoration of Motion

Field Strategy 18.1 provides several ROM exercises that can be performed without weight bearing. For example, towel pulls stretching the Achilles tendon, writing the alphabet in large circles, picking up objects in the toes and combining the action with shin curls, and use of a biomechanical ankle platform system (BAPS) board can each be done in a seated position. As pain subsides and weight bearing is initiated, Achilles tendon stretches, toe raises, balance exercises, and use of a BAPS board can be completed in a standing position.

Restoration of Proprioception and Balance

Proprioception and balance must be regained to allow safe return to sport participation. Early exercises may include shifting one's weight while on crutches, performing bilateral minisquats, or using a BAPS board in a seated position. As balance improves, BAPS board exercises can progress to partial weight bearing while supported by a table, and then to full weight-bearing exercises. Running in place on a minitramp and use of a slide board are closed chain exercises that also improve proprioception and balance.

Muscular Strength, Endurance, and Power

Early emphasis is placed on strengthening the foot's intrinsic muscles. Towel crunches are demonstrated in Field Strategy 18.1. As the condition allows, toe raises and Thera-Band® or surgical tubing exercises are added. Use of a multiaxial ankle machine, toe raises with weights, squats and lunges, and isokinetic exercises continue to strengthen the lower leg musculature. During later stages, jogging, running side to side, and multiangle plyometrics can assist the individual in a gradual return to sport participation.

Cardiovascular Fitness

Maintenance of cardiovascular fitness can begin immediately after injury with use of an upper body ergometer or hydrotherapeutic exercise. Running in deep water and performing sport-specific exercises can provide mild resistance in a non–weight bearing medium. When ROM is adequate, a stationary bicycle may be used. Light jogging, running backward, and running side to side should increase in both intensity and duration to facilitate return to activity. Field Strategy 18.7 lists several rehabilitation exercises that may be incorporated in a complete program for the lower leg.

In addition to exercises, the individual should be assessed for biomechanical anomalies, and appropriate orthotics should be fabricated to correct any malalignment. Following an ankle injury, it may be necessary to provide external support to the ankle region. Following completion of the rehabilitation program and clearance for full participation, a proper maintenance program of stretching and strengthening exercises should be provided.

 The rehabilitation program for the cross-country runner with plantar fasciitis should include aggressive Achilles tendon stretching for 2 to 4 minutes, three to four times a day, with

FIELD STRATEGY 18.7

Rehabilitation Exercises for the Lower Leg

Phase 1. Control inflammation. Minimize inversion and eversion exercises to allow healing. Dorsiflexion and plantar flexion should be performed within the limits of pain. Exercises should be combined with ice therapy or electrical stimulation with elevation. Use those exercises listed in Field Strategy 18.1 as tolerated.

- Plantar fascia stretch
- Towel crunches
- Toe curls
- Picking up objects
- Biomechanical ankle platform system (BAPS) board in seated position
- Triceps surae stretch, non–weight-bearing
- Pool therapy or upper body ergometer (UBE) exercises for cardiovascular fitness

2. **Phase 2.** As pain and tenderness subside, initiate inversion and eversion range of motion. Initiate strengthening exercises as tolerated. Include:

- Shin curls
- Ankle alphabet
- Triceps surae stretch, standing position
- Toe raises
- Elastic tubing exercises in dorsiflexion, plantar flexion, inversion, and eversion
- Unilateral balance BAPS board activities with support
- Pool therapy, upper body ergometer, and stationary bike (if tolerated) for cardiovascular fitness

3. **Phase 3.**

- Toe raises with weights
- Multiaxial ankle machine
- Squats and lunges
- Balance exercises with challenges, such as dribbling while balancing on one leg, performing elastic band exercises while balancing on one leg, or balancing on an uneven surface
- Straight-ahead jogging, if able to walk without a limp

4. **Phase 4.** (Use external support for the ankle as needed.)

- Isokinetic exercises to work functional speeds
- Multiangle plyometrics, including single- and double-limb jumping, front to front, side-to-side, and diagonals
- Side-to-side running
- Running backward
- Jumping for height and distance (long jump)
- Slide board
- Gradual return to activity with protection

toes straight ahead, toes in, and toes out; gentle isometric contractions for intrinsic muscles of the foot, progressing to active ROM exercises within pain-free ranges (e.g., toe curls, marble pick-up, towel crunches, and towel curls) to strengthen the intrinsic and extrinsic muscles of leg; and general fitness (i.e., strength and aerobic conditioning) with non–weight bearing activities.

SUMMARY

1. The true ankle (talocrural) joint is the mortise-tenon joint between the tibia, fibula, and talus. Plantar flexion and dorsiflexion occur at this joint. Motion at the subtalar joint occurs in an oblique direction. The combination of calcaneal inversion, foot adduction, and plantar flexion is known as supination; the combination of calcaneal eversion, foot abduction, and dorsiflexion is known as pronation.

2. The primary supporting structures of the plantar arches are the calcaneonavicular (i.e., spring) ligament, long plantar ligament, plantar fascia (plantar aponeurosis), and short plantar (plantar calcaneocuboid) ligament. In addition, the tibialis posterior provides some support.

3. Congenital abnormalities, leg-length discrepancy, muscle dysfunction (e.g., muscle imbalance), or a malalignment syndrome (e.g., pes cavus, pes planus, pes equinus, and hammer or claw toes) can predispose an individual to several chronic injuries.

4. Generalized forefoot pain may result from intrinsic factors (e.g., excessive body weight, limited flexibility of the Achilles tendon, pronation, valgus heel, hammer toes, fallen metatarsal arch, pes planus, or pes cavus) or from extrinsic factors (e.g., narrow toe box, improperly placed shoe cleats, repetitive jumping or running, or landing poorly from a height).

5. An acute anterior compartment syndrome is a medical emergency. Signs and symptoms include a recent history of trauma; a palpable, firm mass in the anterior compartment; tight skin; and a diminished dorsalis pedis pulse.

6. Ankle sprains are classified as grade I, II, or III based on the progression of the anatomical structures that are damaged and the subsequent disability. In lateral ankle sprains involving plantar flexion and inversion, the ATFL is torn first, followed by the calcaneal fibular ligament. In eversion ankle sprains, the deltoid ligament is injured, and an associated avulsion fracture of one or both malleoli also may be present.

7. Common sites for tendon injuries include the Achilles tendon just proximal to its insertion into the calcaneus, the tibialis posterior just behind the medial malleolus, the tibialis anterior just under the extensor retinaculum, and the peroneal tendons behind the lateral malleolus or at the distal attachment on the styloid process of the fifth metatarsal.

8. Injury to the tibialis posterior results in weakness in plantar flexion and inversion and may lead to acquired pes planus.

9. Risk factors for Achilles tendinitis include a tight heel cord, foot malalignment deformities, recent change in shoes or running surface, sudden increase in workload (e.g., distance or intensity), or changes in the exercise environment (e.g., changing footwear, or excessive hill climbing or impact-loading activities [e.g., jumping]).

10. Medial tibial stress syndrome is a periostitis along the posteromedial tibial border, usually in the distal third, that is not associated with a stress fracture or compartment syndrome. Signs and symptoms include point tenderness in a 3- to 6-cm area along the distal posteromedial tibial border as well as pain and weakness with resisted plantar flexion or standing on tiptoe.

11. Exertional compartment syndrome is characterized by exercise-induced pain and swelling that are relieved by rest. The anterior compartment most frequently is affected, and in such cases, mild foot drop or paresthesia (or both) may be present. Fascial defects or hernias also may be present in the distal third of the leg over the anterior intramuscular septum.

12. Nerve impingement may involve the interdigital nerves as they bifurcate at the metatarsal heads (i.e., plantar interdigital neuroma), posterior tibial nerve beneath the flexor retinaculum and behind the medial malleolus, or sural nerve as it courses behind the lateral malleolus into the lateral foot.

13. Fractures of the lower leg, ankle, and foot may involve:
    - Freiberg's disease (i.e., avascular necrosis of the second metatarsal head)
    - Sever's disease (i.e., calcaneal apophysis)
    - Stress fractures (most commonly the neck of the second metatarsal)
    - Avulsion fractures (e.g., styloid process of the fifth metatarsal and the medial and lateral malleoli)
    - Osteochondral fractures (e.g., talar dome)
    - Displaced fractures or fracture-dislocations

14. Pain may be referred to the lower leg, ankle, and foot from the lumbar spine, hip, or knee.

15. Conditions that warrant special attention include:
    - Obvious deformity suggesting a dislocation, fracture, or ruptured Achilles tendon
    - Significant loss of motion or weakness in a myotome
    - Excessive joint swelling
    - Possible epiphyseal or apophyseal injuries
    - Abnormal reflexes or sensation or an absent or weak pulse
    - Gross joint instability
    - Any unexplained pain

16. Functional tests should be performed pain-free without limp or antalgic gait before clearing any individual for return to activity. In addition, the individual should have bilaterally equal ROM, strength, and proprioception as well as an appropriate cardiovascular fitness level before being allowed to return to activity. When necessary, protective equipment or braces should be used to prevent reinjury.

REFERENCES

1. Puffer JC. The sprained ankle. Clin Cornerstone 2001; 3(5):38–49.
2. McKay GD, Goldie PA, Payne WR, Oakes BW. Ankle injuries in basketball: injury rate and risk factors. Br J Sports Med 2001;35(2):103–108.
3. Cohen RS, Balcom TA. Current treatment options for ankle injuries: lateral ankle sprain, Achilles tendonitis, and Achilles rupture. Curr Sports Med Reports 2003;2(5): 251–261.
4. Caulfield B, Garrett M. Changes in ground reaction force during jump landing in subjects with functional instability of the ankle joint. Clin Biomech 2004;19(6):617–621.
5. Wang Q, et al. Fibula and its ligaments in load transmission and ankle joint stability. Clin Orthop 1997;(330):261–270.
6. Leardini A, Stagni R, O'Connor JJ. Mobility of the subtalar joint in the intact ankle complex. J Biomech 2001; 34(6):805–809.
7. Stagni R, Leardini A, O'Connor JJ, Giannini S. Role of passive structures in the mobility and stability of the human subtalar joint: a literature review. Foot Ankle Int 2003;24(5):402–409.
8. Gefen A. The in vivo elastic properties of the plantar fascia during the contact phase of walking. Foot Ankle Int 2003;24(3):238–244.
9. Ferber R, Davis IM, Williams DS. Gender differences in lower extremity mechanics during running. Clin Biomech 2003;18(4):350–357.
10. Korhonen MT, Mero A, Suominen H. Age-related differences in 100-m sprint performances in male and female master runners. Med Sci Sports Exerc 2003;35(8): 1419–1428.
11. O'Connor KM, Hamill J. The role of selected extrinsic foot muscles during running. Clin Biomech 2004;19(1): 71–77.

12. Mercer JA, Devita P, Derrick TR, Bates BT. Individual effects of stride length and frequency on shock attenuation during running. Med Sci Sports Exerc 2003;35(2):307–313.

13. Klein P, Mattys S, Rooze M. Moment arm length variations of selected muscles acting on talocrural and subtalar joints during movement: an in vitro study. J Biomech 1996;29(1):21–30.

14. Wear KA. Autocorrelation and cepstral methods for measurement of tibial cortical thickness. IEEE Trans Ultrason Ferroelectr Freq Control 2003;50(6):655–660.

15. Kazis K, Iglesias E. The female athlete triad. Adolesc Med 2003;14(1):87–95.

16. Miller KK. Mechanisms by which nutritional disorders cause reduced bone mass in adults. J Women's Health (Larchmt) 2003;12(2):145–150.

17. Norkin CC, Levangie PK. Joint Structure and Function: A Comprehensive Analysis. Philadelphia: FA Davis, 1992.

18. Cavanagh PR, et al. The relationship of static foot structure to dynamic foot function. J Biomech 1997;30(3):243–250.

19. McClure SK, Adams JE, Dahn DL. Common musculoskeletal disorder in women. Mayo Clin Proc 2005;80(6):796–802.

20. McBryde AM, Hoffman JL. Injuries to the foot and ankle in athletes. South Med J 2004;97(8):738–741.

21. Coughlin MJ, Shurnas PS. Hallux rigidus: surgical techniques (cheilectomy and arthrodesis). J Bone Joint Surg Am 2004;86(Suppl 1, Part 2):119–130.

22. Clanton TO, Porter DA. Primary care of foot and ankle injuries in the athlete. Clin Sports Med 1997;16(3):435–466.

23. Olmstead-Kramer LC, Hertel J. Preventing recurrent lateral ankle sprains: an evidence-based approach. Ath Ther Today 2004;9(6):19–22.

24. Norkus SA, Floyd RT. The anatomy and mechanisms of syndesmotic ankle sprains. J Ath Train 2001;36(1):68–73.

25. Smith AH, Bach BR Jr. High ankle sprains. Phys Sportsmed 2004;32(12):39–43.

26. Mullen JE, O'Malley MJ. Sprains—residual instability of subtalar, Lisfranc joints, and turf toe. Clin Sports Med 2004;23(1):97–121.

27. Molloy R, Tisdel C. Failed treatment of peroneal tendon injuries. Foot Ankle Clin 2003;8(1):115–129.

28. Johnson KA, Strom ED. Tibialis posterior tendon dysfunction. Clin Orthop Relat Res 1989;239:196–206.

29. Perry MB, Premkumar A, Venzon DJ, et al. Ultrasound, magnetic resonance imaging, and posterior tibialis dysfunction. Clin Orthop Relat Res 2003;408:225–231.

30. Wilder RP, Sethi S. Overuse injuries: tendinopathies, stress fractures, compartment syndrome, and shin splints. Clin Sports Med 2004;23(1):55–81.

31. Ohbert L, Alfredson H. Ultrasound guided sclerosis of neovessels in painful chronic Achilles tendinosis: pilot study of a new treatment. Br J Sports Med 2002;36(3):173–175.

32. Brown DE. Ankle and leg injuries. In: Mellion MB, Walsh WM, Madden C, Putukian M, Shelton GL, eds. The Team Physician's Handbook. Philadelphia: Hanley & Belfus, 2002.

33. Harmon KG, Rubin A. Plantar fasciitis: prescribing effective treatments. Phys Sportsmed 2002;30(7):21–25.

34. Davey JR, Rorabeck CH, Fowler PJ. The tibialis posterior muscle compartment: an unrecognized cause of exertional compartmental syndrome. Am J Sports Med 1984;12(5):391–397.

35. Edwards P, Myerson MS. Exertional compartment syndrome of the leg: steps for expedient return to activity. Phys Sportsmed 1996;24(4):31–46.

36. Fleming A. Extensive venous thrombosis in a runner. Phys Sportsmed 2005;33(1):34–36.

37. Blue JM, Matthews LS. Leg injuries. Clin Sports Med 1997;16(3):467–478.

38. Garl TC, et al. Tibial fracture in a basketball player: treatment dilemmas and complications. Phys Sportsmed 1997;25(6):41–53.

PART

Systemic Conditions

6

19 Cardiovascular Disorders

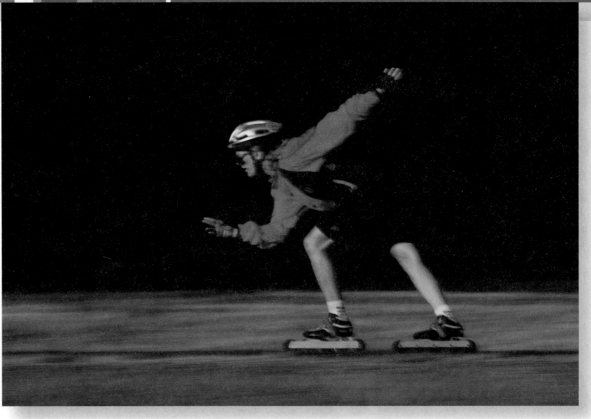

STUDENT OUTCOMES

1. Describe the signs and symptoms of anemia, and explain the potential impact of this blood disorder on sport and physical activity performance.

2. Explain the methods for minimizing the effects of anemia on sport and physical activity performance.

3. Identify the early signs of hemophilia, and describe the treatment of this condition.

4. Describe Reye's syndrome and the strategies for preventing it.

5. Describe the physiologic causes, signs, symptoms, and management of syncope.

6. Describe the basic physiologic principles, signs, symptoms, and management of shock.

7. Identify the four stages of hypertension, and state the predisposing factors or diseases that place an individual at risk for developing hypertension.

8. Identify medications that can adversely elevate blood pressure.

9. Identify the factors and conditions that can lead to hypotension.

10. Describe the management of hypertension and hypotension.

11. Identify the epidemiologic factors and basic physiologic principles associated with sudden death in the physically active population.

12. Identify the cardiac-related causes of sudden death in individuals younger than and older than 30 years.

13. List the risk factors for coronary artery disease and Marfan's syndrome.

14. Identify the noncardiac conditions that can lead to sudden death.

15. Describe the two-tiered approach that is used during a preparticipation physical examination to identify risk factors associated with sudden death.

16. Explain the ethical, legal, and practical considerations that affect the medical decision-making process for determining the eligibility of competitive athletes who have cardiovascular abnormalities.

ROLE DELINEATION COMPETENCIES

The following Performance Domains and Tasks defined in the National Athletic Trainers' Association Board of Certification *Role Delineation Study*, 5th Edition are addressed in this chapter:

BOC COMPETENCIES

II. Clinical Evaluation and Diagnosis

A. Obtain a history through observation, interview, and/or review of relevant records to assess current or potential injury, illness, or condition.
E. Formulate a clinical impression by interpreting the signs, symptoms, and predisposing factors of the injury, illness, or condition to determine the appropriate course of action.
F. Educate the appropriate individual(s) regarding the assessment by communicating information about the current or potential injury, illness, or health-related condition to encourage compliance with recommended care.

III. Immediate Care

A. Employ life-saving techniques through the use of standard emergency procedures in order to reduce morbidity and the incidence of mortality.
B. Prevent exacerbation of non–life threatening condition(s) through the use of standard procedures in order to reduce morbidity.
C. Facilitate the timely transfer of care for conditions beyond the scope of practice of the athletic trainer by implementing appropriate referral strategies to stabilize and/or prevent exacerbation of the condition(s).

IV. Treatment, Rehabilitation, and Reconditioning

D. Administer treatment for general illness and/or conditions using standard techniques and procedures to facilitate recovery, function, and/or performance.
E. Reassess the status of injuries, illnesses, and/or conditions using standard techniques and documentation strategies in order to determine appropriate treatment, rehabilitation, and/or reconditioning and to evaluate readiness to return to a desired level of activity.

Participation in physical activity and sport yields positive effects on an individual's physical, mental, and social health, but participation in any physical activity has inherent risks of injury. Preparticipation physical examinations (PPEs) often can identify conditions that may predispose an individual to injury. Even with a PPE, however, certain conditions may go undetected. As such, the chance exists for severe—and even catastrophic—injury because of preexisting conditions. Blood disorders (e.g., anemia and hemophilia) and cardiovascular disorders (e.g., syncope, hypertension, and hypotension) are conditions that warrant medical attention. If left untreated, these conditions can have serious physical effects on the body and can become even more problematic if they occur during exercise.

This chapter will provide a basic overview of the anatomy of the cardiovascular system, with a focus on the heart. (Discussion on the bronchial trees and lungs are included with Chapter 21.) Next, the causes, identification, and management of various cardiovascular diseases and disorders in the physically active population will be discussed. Recommendations are provided to reduce the risk of these conditions by means of a thorough cardiovascular history as part of preparticipation screening. Finally, issues concerning counseling individuals at risk for sudden death are discussed.

ANATOMY OF THE CIRCULATORY SYSTEM

The circulatory system includes the cardiovascular system and the lymphatic system. The heart and lungs have an intimate relationship both physically and functionally. The heart is positioned obliquely to the left of the midline of the body and is divided into four chambers: the right and left atria superiorly, and the right and left ventricles inferiorly (Fig. 19.1). The heartbeat consists of a simultaneous contraction of the two atria, followed immediately by a simultaneous contraction of the two ventricles. The contraction phase is known as systole; the phase in which the chambers relax and fill with blood is known as diastole. Two pairs of valves within the heart ensure that blood flow is unidirectional. The atrioventricular valves seal off the atria during contraction of the ventricles to prevent the backflow of blood. The aortic and pulmonary semilunar valves prevent the flow of blood from the aorta and pulmonary artery back into the ventricles.

The right side of the heart pumps blood to the lungs, where carbon dioxide and oxygen are exchanged. The left side of the heart receives the freshly oxygenated blood from the lungs and

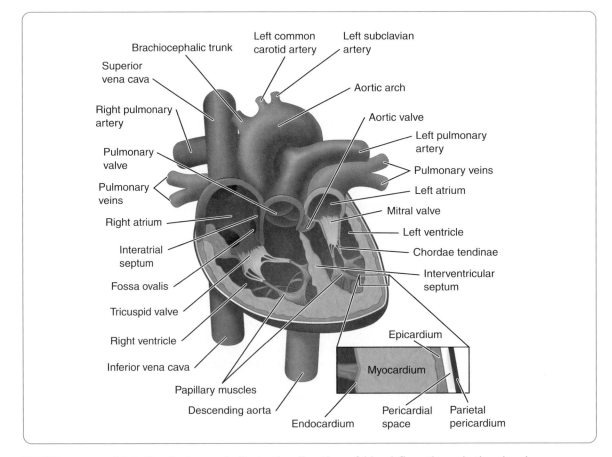

■■■■ FIGURE 19.1 **Heart.** Arrows indicate the direction of blood flow through the chambers.

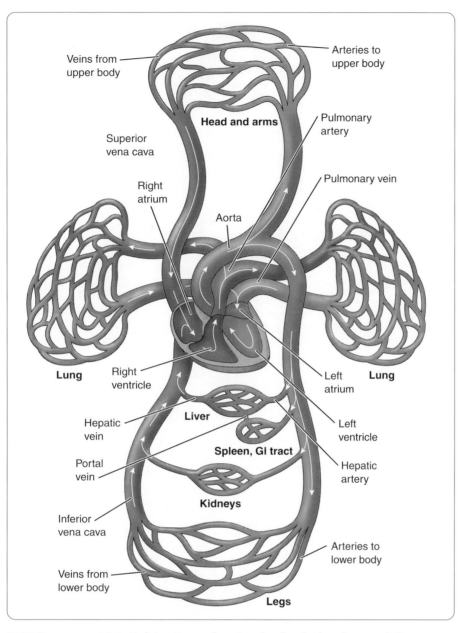

Veins from upper body

Arteries to upper body

Head and arms

Pulmonary artery

Superior vena cava

Right atrium

Pulmonary vein

Aorta

Lung   Right ventricle

Left atrium

Lung

Hepatic vein

Liver

Left ventricle

Portal vein

Spleen, GI tract

Hepatic artery

Kidneys

Inferior vena cava

Veins from lower body

Arteries to lower body

Legs

FIGURE 19.2 Pulmonary and systemic circulation in an adult.

pumps it out to the systemic circulation. The vessels interconnecting the heart and lungs are known as the pulmonary circuit; the vessels that supply the body are known as the systemic circuit (Fig. 19.2). The systemic circulation is composed of numerous and different circuits in parallel, which allows wide variations in regional blood flow without changing the total systemic flow. The heart and blood vessels (e.g., arteries, arterioles, veins, venules, and capillaries) transport oxygen, nutrients, and hormones to cells, remove waste products and carbon dioxide from cells, defend the body against infections, and prevent blood loss through clotting.

Functioning as part of the immune system, the lymphatic system is comprised of lymph capillaries (i.e., lacteals), nodes, vessels, and ducts (Fig. 19.3). This one-way system transports fluids, nutrients (e.g., fats and proteins), and tissue waste back into the bloodstream via connections with major veins, and it flows only toward the heart.

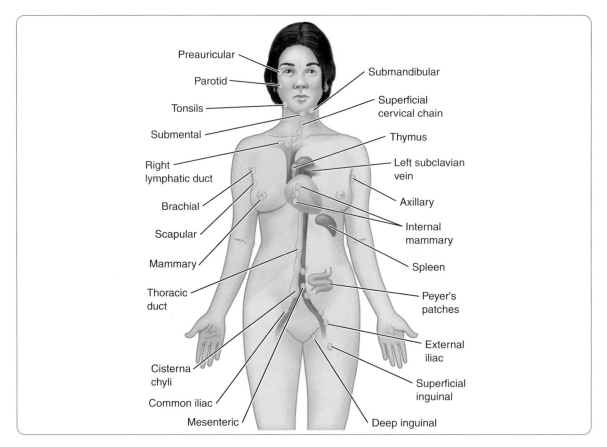

FIGURE 19.3 Lymphatic system with major lymph nodes. The pale green area denotes the body area drained by the right lymphatic duct; the rest of the body is drained by the thoracic duct.

BLOOD AND LYMPH DISORDERS

A 30-year-old female recreational golfer is diagnosed with iron-deficiency anemia attributed to an inadequate diet. What implications will this have on her ability to continue participating in golf on a weekly basis, and what is the management for this condition?

Blood flow is involved in delivering nutrients and wastes to and from cells, gas exchange, absorbing nutrients, and forming urine. Lymphatic vessels return fluids that have leaked from the blood vascular system back to the blood, protect the body by removing foreign material from the lymph stream, and provide a site for immune surveillance. Blood and lymph disorders that are presented in this chapter include anemia, hemophilia, Reye's syndrome, and lymphangitis.

Anemia

Iron, which is present in all human cells, serves several functions, including carrying oxygen from the lungs to the tissues in the form of hemoglobin, facilitating oxygen use and storage in the muscles as myoglobin, serving as a transport medium for electrons within the cells in the form of cytochromes, and playing an integral part of enzyme reactions in various tissues. Insufficient amounts of iron can interfere with these vital functions and lead to serious illness or even death. A reduction in either the red blood cell (RBC) volume (i.e., hematocrit) or the hemoglobin concentration is called **anemia**. Although anemia has five separate classifications, each one is caused by impaired RBC formation, excessive loss, or destruction of RBCs.

The recommended dietary allowance (RDA) for iron is 10 to 15 mg/day, except for pregnant women, in which case the RDA is 30 mg/day. The average diet contains 5 to 7 mg of iron per 1,000 kcal (1).

Therefore, it is necessary to consume 3,000 kcal/day to meet the RDA. A major concern is that many physically active females consume less than 2,000 kcal/day. In addition, individuals consuming a modified vegetarian diet that is low in iron content and low in iron bioavailability may be not be receiving sufficient iron. Good sources of iron include lean animal meat (e.g., liver, beef roasts, tenderloin, lamb, and chicken or turkey legs), tuna, oysters, shrimp, enriched raisin bran or corn flakes, bagels, bran muffins, dried apricots, baked potatoes with the skin, peas, kidney beans, chickpeas, tofu, and molasses.

Anemia reduces maximum aerobic capacity, decreases physical work capability at submaximal levels, increases lactic acidosis, increases fatigue, and decreases exercise time to exhaustion (1,2). Although several predisposing factors can increase the risk of developing anemia (Box 19.1), physically active individuals tend to be more prone to specific anemic conditions.

Stages of Anemia

Iron status is assessed through several laboratory tests. Because each test assesses a different aspect of iron metabolism, the results of one test may not always agree with those of other tests. The hemoglobin concentration and hematocrit commonly are tested, because they measure the amount of functional iron in the body. The concentration of hemoglobin in circulating RBCs is the more direct and sensitive measure. The hematocrit indicates the proportion of whole blood that is occupied by the RBCs, and it decreases only after the hemoglobin concentration falls. Hematologic tests based on the characteristics of RBCs (i.e., hemoglobin, hematocrit, and total iron-binding capacity) are more popular and less expensive than biochemical tests. The biochemical tests (e.g., free erythrocyte protoporphyrin concentration, serum ferritin concentration, and transferrin saturation), however, detect earlier changes in iron status.

Iron deficiency develops gradually, progressing through several stages before anemia is evident. These stages include:

- **Stage I.** Iron depletion is characterized by less than 12 mg/mL of an iron–protein complex known as ferritin, which is an indicator of reduced iron stores in the bone marrow. Other components of iron status—hemoglobin, hematocrit, free erythrocyte protoporphyrin, serum iron, iron-binding capacity, and transferrin saturation—remain normal.

- **Stage II.** Iron-deficiency erythropoiesis follows several months of iron depletion and is characterized by decreased levels of circulating iron, but hemoglobin and hematocrit remain normal.

- **Stage III.** Iron-deficiency anemia follows several weeks of iron-deficient erythropoiesis. Hemoglobin production diminishes, and the individual develops clinically recognized iron-deficiency anemia, which is referred to as frank anemia.

Box 19.1   Predisposing Factors for Development of Anemia

- Personal or family history of anemia, bleeding disorders, or chronic disease
- Intermittent jaundice early in life
- Excessive menstrual flow; increased duration, frequency, or volume
- Chronic blood loss through gastrointestinal bleeding
- Certain drugs and toxins (e.g., chronic use of aspirin or nonsteroidal anti-inflammatory drugs)
- Childbirth
- Disadvantaged socioeconomic background
- Poor diet or dietary restriction (e.g., vegetarian diet, weight loss diets, or fad diets)
- Cancer
- Volunteer blood donor
- Diminished hepatic, renal, or thyroid function

Adapted from Harris SS. Helping active women avoid anemia. Phys Sportsmed 1995;23(5):35–48; with permission.

Iron-Deficiency Anemia

Iron deficiency is characterized by deficient hemoglobin synthesis. It is the most common nutritional deficiency in the United States, affecting 7.8 million adolescent girls and women of childbearing age secondary to menstrual blood loss and increased iron demand during pregnancy (3). Among men 18 years and older and postmenopausal women in the United States, however, iron-deficiency anemia is uncommon. During infancy and early childhood, inadequate diet may be an underlying factor; in older children and adults, blood loss or impaired absorption of iron should be suspected. The condition also is seen in endurance athletes and individuals who maintain a low percentage of body fat.

SIGNS AND SYMPTOMS. Early symptoms include exercise fatigue, tachycardia, blood mixed with feces, pallor, and epithelial abnormalities, such as a sore tongue. Symptoms that can develop at a later time include cardiac murmurs, congestive heart failure, loss of hair, and pearly sclera. Additional signs and symptoms of iron-deficiency anemia include:

- Muscle burning
- Nausea
- Shortness of breath
- Appetite for substances that have little or no nutritional value (e.g., starch, ice, or clay)
- Palpitations
- Spoon-shaped nails (koilonychia)
- Dry scaling and fissures of the lips (angular cheilosis)
- Inflammation of the tongue (glossitis)

MANAGEMENT. Treatment includes dietary iron supplementation (e.g., ferrous sulfate or ferrous gluconate) and ascorbic acid (i.e., vitamin C) to enhance iron absorption. Because caffeine hampers iron absorption, avoid colas, coffee, tea, chocolates, and other caffeine products. If active bleeding is attributed to polyps, ulcers, malignancies, or hemorrhoids, surgery may be necessary.

Exercise-Induced Hemolytic Anemia

Exercise-induced hemolytic anemia, which sometimes is referred to as **runner's anemia,** occurs during exercise when RBCs are destroyed and hemoglobin is liberated into the medium in which the cells are suspended. This process of intravascular hemolysis can occur in both high- and low-impact sports and physical activities. In high-impact activities, such as running, it is posited that the trauma of repetitive, hard foot strikes destroys the RBCs. This condition, which sometimes is referred to as **foot strike hemolysis,** is more commonly observed in marathoners and middle-age distance runners, particularly those who are overweight, run on hard surfaces, wear poorly cushioned shoes, and run with a stomping gait. Intravascular hemolysis, however, also has been reported in competitive swimmers and rowers. As such, damage to the cells could be attributed to other possibilities, including muscle contraction, acidosis, or increased body temperature.

MANAGEMENT. Runner's anemia rarely is severe enough to cause appreciable loss of iron. In general, the condition may be of more concern to highly competitive, world-class athletes, for whom a fractional physiologic difference can result in a competitive disadvantage. Prevention and treatment focuses on encouraging runners to be lean, to run on soft surfaces, to avoid running with a stomping gait, and to wear well-cushioned shoes and insoles.

Sickle Cell Anemia

Sickle cell anemia, most commonly seen in African Americans, results from abnormalities in hemoglobin structure that produce a characteristic sickle- or crescent-shaped RBC that is fragile and unable to transport oxygen. The condition is attributed to inheriting an autosomal recessive gene or to possessing two sickle genes as opposed to having the sickle cell trait, in which only one sickle gene is inherited. Because of their rigidity and irregular shape, sickle cells clump together and block small blood vessels, leading to vascular occlusions, or infarcts, in the central nervous system and organs, such as the heart, lungs, kidneys, and spleen (Fig. 19.4). Although an individual with sickle cell trait may be asymptomatic for his or her entire life, exercising excessively in high heat or humidity or at high altitude may lead to dehydration, increased body temperature, hypoxia, and acidosis, which are predisposing factors for increased protein concentration in the circulating blood cells. This high concentration of protein increases blood viscosity and impairs blood flow, which can lead to a stroke, congestive heart failure, acute renal failure, pulmonary embolism, or sudden death.

SIGNS AND SYMPTOMS. Individuals with sickle cell anemia may be asymptomatic. When manifested, signs and symptoms may include recurrent bouts of swollen, painful, and inflamed hands and feet, irregular heartbeat, severe fatigue, headache, pallor, muscle weakness, and severe pain because of oxygen deprivation. The sclera of the eye also may appear to be jaundiced.

MANAGEMENT. Currently, no treatment is known to reverse the condition. Because dehydration can complicate the condition, individuals should hydrate maximally before, during, and after exercise or physical exertion. Liquids with caffeine should be avoided because of their diuretic effect. Individuals with sickle cell trait should limit running to no more than 1 mile without rest and avoid activity in extremely hot, humid weather and at altitudes of greater than 2,500 feet (2).

Normal red blood cells

Lumen blocked by sickle cells

▬▬ ▬ FIGURE 19.4 Sickle cell. Sickle cells are abnormal red blood cells that are fragile and unable to transport oxygen. Because of their rigidity and irregular shape, they often clump together and block small blood vessels, leading to vascular occlusions in the vital organs.

Hemophilia

Hemophilia is a bleeding disorder that is characterized by a deficiency of selected proteins in the body's blood-clotting system. Three categories of blood proteins play a role in blood clotting:

1. Procoagulant proteins help to form clots.

2. Anticoagulant proteins prevent the formation of clots.

3. Fibrinolytic proteins help to dissolve clots that have formed.

The clotting process involves blood particles, called platelets, and procoagulant plasma proteins, called clotting factors. The process begins with the platelet phase, during which the platelets stick to a blood vessel at the site of an injury. An intricate cascade of enzyme reactions occurs, producing a web-like protein network that encircles the platelets and holds them in place. This is followed by the coagulation phase in which clot formation begins. In this cascade, each clotting factor is transformed from an inactive to an active form.

Hemophilia occurs in three types, which are differentiated by the deficient clotting factor. Hemophilias A, B, and C are inherited diseases. Because of the pattern of inheritance, hemophilias A and B occur almost always in males; hemophilia C can occur in both males and females. All three types, however, can cause prolonged bleeding. Complications may occur from the disease or from treatment of the disease (Box 19.2) (4).

Signs and Symptoms

Signs and symptoms may include many large or deep bruises, joint pain and swelling caused by internal bleeding, intramuscular bleeding, blood in the urine or stool, and prolonged bleeding from cuts or injuries, surgical procedures, or tooth extraction. During infancy, hemophilia appears to be asymptomatic because of limited mobility. As the child begins to fall and bump into things, superficial bruises may occur. Soft-tissue bleeding becomes more frequent as the child becomes more

Box 19.2   Complications of Hemophilia

- **Deep internal bleeding.** Hemophilia may cause deep-muscle bleeding. Swelling of a limb may press on nerves and lead to numbness or pain, which may result in reluctance to use the limb.
- **Damage to joints.** Internal bleeding may put pressure on and damage joints. Pain may be severe, resulting in reluctance to use a limb or joint. If bleeding occurs frequently and goes untreated, the irritation to a joint may lead to destruction of that joint or to the development of arthritis.
- **Infection.** People with hemophilia are more likely to receive blood transfusions and, as such, are at a greater risk of receiving contaminated blood products. Although risk of infection through blood products has decreased substantially since the introduction of genetically engineered clotting products, called recombinant factors, that are free of infection, it is still possible for people who rely on blood products to contract other diseases, such as infection with the human immunodeficiency virus and hepatitis.
- **Adverse reaction to clotting factor treatment.** Some people with hemophilia develop proteins in their blood that inactivate the clotting factors used to treat bleeding.

active. In most cases, the bumps and bruises do not require medical treatment. Signs and symptoms that would indicate an emergency situation include:

- Suspected bleeding into the head, neck, or digestive tract
- Sudden pain, swelling, and warmth of extremity muscles and large joints, such as the knees, elbows, hips, and shoulders
- Persistent bleeding from an injury, especially if the individual has a severe form of hemophilia

Management

Treatment of hemophilia varies with its severity. Mild hemophilia A is treated with prescribed injections of desmopressin to stimulate a release of the body's natural clotting factors to stop the bleeding (4). Occasionally, desmopressin is given as a nasal medication. Management of bleeding from severe hemophilia A or hemophilia B typically requires an infusion of clotting factors derived from donated human blood or genetically engineered products called recombinant clotting factors. If the internal bleeding is serious, repeated infusions could be necessary. Plasma infusions are needed to stop bleeding episodes in individuals with hemophilia C. Infusion of a clotting factor two or three times per week may help to prevent bleeding episodes.

Reye's Syndrome

Reye's syndrome is a rare but serious, acute illness that disrupts the body's urea cycle. The result is an accumulation of ammonia in the blood, hypoglycemia, severe brain edema, and critically high intracranial pressure. The disease almost exclusively affects individuals between 2 and 16 years of age (5).

Reye's syndrome tends to occur in previously healthy children and almost always follows an upper respiratory viral infection. In particular, the condition is associated with type B influenza and varicella (chickenpox), but it may develop after a common cold. Reye's syndrome can be an asymptomatic metabolic condition that is unmasked by the viral illness. The precise cause of the condition is unknown, but using aspirin to treat the viral illness or infection may trigger the condition in children. In Reye's syndrome, the level of ammonia and acidity in the blood typically rises while the level of sugar drops. At the same time, the liver may swell and develop fat deposits. Swelling also may occur in the brain and cause seizures or convulsions and, eventually, lead to a coma and brain death.

Signs and Symptoms

Reye's syndrome progresses quickly and can result in permanent liver damage, irreversible neurologic damage, coma, and even death. The signs and symptoms typically begin approximately 1 week after a viral infection (e.g., influenza, chickenpox, or a cold). Following appearance of recovery from an illness, a child may become much more seriously ill. The condition typically progresses through five stages (5):

- **Stage I.** Lethargy, vomiting, and hepatic dysfunction, followed by a few days of recovery

- **Stage II.** Hyperventilation, delirium, and hyperactive reflexes

- **Stage III.** Coma and rigidity of organ cortices

- **Stage IV.** Deepening coma, large and fixed pupils, and loss of cerebral functions

- **Stage V.** Seizures, loss of deep tendon reflexes, flaccidity, and respiratory arrest

Management

Children with Reye's syndrome require hospitalization and intensive treatment to restore blood sugar levels, control cerebral edema, and correct acid-base imbalances. Drug treatments may include (5):

- Intravenous medications, such as glucose to increase low blood sugar; electrolyte solutions containing sodium, potassium, and chloride to correct blood chemistry values; and basic solutions to treat acidity

- Small amounts of insulin to increase glucose metabolism

- A corticosteroid (e.g., dexamethasone) to reduce brain swelling and inflammation

- A diuretic (e.g., mannitol) to increase fluid loss through urination and help reduce brain swelling

If Reye's syndrome reaches an advanced stage, treatment may include endotracheal intubation and mechanical ventilation to assist with breathing. In some cases, surgery may be indicated to decrease intracranial pressure.

Lymphangitis

Lymph nodes or glands filter the lymph fluid. **Lymphangitis** is an inflammation of the lymphatic channels that occurs as a result of infection at a site distal to the channel. Pathogenic organisms invade the lymphatic vessels, either directly, through an abrasion or wound, or as a complication of an infection, and then spread along these channels toward regional lymph nodes.

Signs and Symptoms

Once the organisms enter the channels, local inflammation and subsequent infection ensue, manifesting as red streaks that are visible along the course of the vessels. The inflammation or infection then extends proximally, toward regional lymph nodes. Individuals often complain of headache, loss of appetite, fever, chills, malaise, and muscle aches. The condition can progress rapidly, particularly when caused by group A streptococci, to bacteremia and disseminated infection and sepsis.

Management

Immediate referral to a physician is required, and hospitalization usually is necessary. If possible, the affected area should be elevated and immobilized to reduce swelling, pain, and spread of infection. Hot, moist compresses may help to reduce inflammation and pain. Prescribed antimicrobial and antibiotic agents should be administered, and analgesics or anti-inflammatory medications can be used to reduce pain, inflammation, and swelling. An abscess may require surgical drainage.

A *Anemia can reduce maximum aerobic capacity, decrease physical work capability at submaximal levels, increase lactic acidosis, increase fatigue, and decrease exercise time to exhaustion. Because the golfer's anemia was attributed to her eating habits, management of the condition should include a diet rich in iron content as well as dietary iron supplementation and ascorbic acid to enhance iron absorption.*

SYNCOPE

Q *Following 60 minutes of an intense, running workout on a treadmill, a healthy, 25-year-old man steps off the treadmill, suddenly collapses, and becomes unconscious. What might explain this sudden unconsciousness, and how should this condition be managed?*

Syncope is a sudden, transient loss of consciousness (LOC), described as "fainting," that often occurs in healthy individuals and is not associated with seizures, coma, shock, or other states of altered consciousness. **Near syncope** is a sense of impending LOC or weakness. It appears more frequently than syncope and provides a better source of injury/illness history, because the patient usually has better recollection of the event (6). Questions concerning syncope should be part of the medical history during the PPE. If a history of syncope is noted, the individual should be referred to a physician for further evaluation.

Syncope and near syncope have five primary causes:

1. Cardiac and circulatory

2. Metabolic

3. Neurologic

4. Reflex syncope resulting from impaired right-sided heart filling and global cerebral hypoperfusion.

5. Miscellaneous causes (e.g., cough syncope, psychogenic, severe visceral or ligamentous pain, or vertigo)

See Causes of Syncope and Near Syncope, available on the companion website at thePoint.

The most frequent cause of syncope is neural-mediated syncope, which also is called neurocardiogenic, vasovagal, vasodepressor, or reflex-mediated syncope. This condition is more common in children and young adults, although it can occur at any age. A sudden drop in blood pressure reduces blood circulation to the brain and leads to LOC. Other causes may be related to heat illness (e.g., **heat syncope**), dehydration, emotional stress, irregular cardiac rhythm, and changes in blood volume or blood distribution. Syncope also may result from cardiac, neurological, psychiatric, metabolic, and various lung disorders (7).

Signs and Symptoms

Typical neural-mediated syncope occurs while standing and often is preceded by prodromal symptoms, including restlessness, pallor, weakness, sighing, yawning, diaphoresis, and nausea. These symptoms may be followed by light-headedness, blurred vision, collapse, and LOC. Occasionally, mild clonic seizures occur, but unless other signs indicate, a detailed seizure evaluation is not indicated. Other signs and symptoms may include dizziness, profuse sweating, paresthesia of the hands or feet, and unilateral or bilateral chest pain (8). Some forms of syncope suggest a serious disorder, including those occurring with exercise, those associated with palpitations or irregularities of the heart, and those associated with a family history of recurrent syncope or sudden death.

Management

Neural-mediated syncope usually responds well to avoidance of stimuli that trigger the event. If syncope does occur, initial management includes assessment of the individual's vital signs. The individual should be placed in a safe, lying-down position. Recovery usually occurs within minutes. If the individual does not regain consciousness within a few minutes or demonstrates signs of breathing or cardiac impairment, the emergency action plan, including summoning emergency medical services (EMS), should be activated.

A thorough medical evaluation should be conducted in the following cases:

- Syncope reoccurs

- Syncope occurs with exercise

- Syncope is associated with palpitations or irregularities of the heart

- Family history of syncope

In cases of severe syncope, β-blockers, cardiac pacing, and antidepressants may be recommended; however, the success rate is poor.

The exerciser may have experienced syncope as a result of dehydration or heat illness. The individual's vital signs should be measured and monitored. If he does not regain consciousness within a few minutes, the emergency action plan, including summoning EMS, should be activated.

SHOCK

Following a slide into home plate that resulted in a collision with the catcher, a baseball player sustains a compound fracture to the tibia. The athletic trainer activated the emergency action plan, including summoning EMS. The athletic trainer also immobilized the leg. What possible complications might occur as a result of this traumatic injury? What other treatment should the athletic trainer provide while waiting for EMS to arrive?

Shock occurs if the heart is unable to exert adequate pressure to circulate enough oxygenated blood to the vital organs. This condition may result from a damaged heart that fails to pump properly, low blood volume from blood loss or dehydration, or dilation of blood vessels that leads to blood pooling in larger vessels away from vital areas (Fig. 19.5). The result is a lack of oxygen and nutrition at the cellular level. The heart pumps faster, but because of reduced volume, the pulse rate is weakened and the blood pressure drops (i.e., **hypotension**). A rapid, weak pulse is the most prominent sign of shock. As an individual's condition deteriorates, breathing becomes rapid and shallow, and sweating is profuse. Vital body fluids pass through weakened capillaries, thereby causing further circulatory distress. If not corrected, circulatory collapse can lead to unconsciousness and even death.

Shock occurs with injuries involving severe pain, bleeding, the spinal cord, fractures, or intra-abdominal or intrathoracic regions, but shock also may occur, to some degree, with minor injuries. The severity of shock depends on age, physical condition, pain tolerance, fatigue, dehydration, presence of any disease, extreme cold or heat exposure, or handling of an injured area. Types of shock include anaphylactic, cardiogenic, hypovolemic, metabolic, neurogenic, respiratory, psychogenic, and septic (Box 19.3).

FIGURE 19.5 Shock. The diameter of an arteriole blood vessel is controlled by circular layers of smooth muscles that either constrict or relax to regulate peripheral blood flow (**A**). Blood vessels dilate during shock. This action increases the size of the vascular bed and decreases the resistance to blood flow, resulting in blood pooling in larger vessels, depriving the brain and vital organs of needed oxygen. As a result, heart rate increases, giving the characteristic rapid, weak pulse that often is the first sign of shock (**B**).

Signs and Symptoms

Signs and symptoms of shock can develop over time (Box 19.4). Initially, the individual may have a feeling of uneasiness or restlessness, increased respirations, and increased weakened heart rate. The skin turns pale and clammy, which usually is accompanied by profuse sweating. The lips, nail beds, and membranes of the mouth appear to be cyanotic. Thirst, weakness, nausea, and vomiting may then become apparent. During later stages, a rapid, weak pulse and labored, weakened respirations may lead to decreased blood pressure and possible unconsciousness.

Box 19.3 Types and Causes of Shock

- **Hypovolemic.** From excessive blood or fluid loss leading to inadequate circulation and oxygen supply to all body organs. Possible causes include hemorrhage, dehydration, multiple trauma, and severe burns.
- **Respiratory.** From insufficient oxygen in the blood as a result of inadequate breathing. Possible causes are spinal injury to the respiratory nerves, airway obstruction, or chest trauma, such as from a pneumothorax, hemothorax, or punctured lung.
- **Neurogenic.** Occurs when peripheral blood vessels dilate and an insufficient blood volume cannot supply oxygen to the vital organs. This may occur in a spinal or head injury when nerves that control the vascular system are impaired, thereby altering the integrity of blood vessels.
- **Psychogenic.** Refers to a temporary dilation of blood vessels, resulting in the draining of blood from the head with pooling of blood in the abdomen. A common example is an individual fainting from the sight of blood.
- **Cardiogenic.** Occurs when the heart muscle is no longer able to sustain enough pressure to pump blood through the system. Possible causes are injury to the heart or previous heart attack.
- **Metabolic.** Results from a severe loss of body fluids because of an untreated illness that alters the biochemical equilibrium. Possible causes are insulin shock, diabetic coma, vomiting, or diarrhea.
- **Septic.** Derives from severe, usually bacterial, infection whereby toxins attack the walls of small blood vessels, causing them to dilate and, therefore, decreasing blood pressure.
- **Anaphylactic.** Refers to a severe allergic reaction of the body to a foreign protein that is ingested, inhaled, or injected (e.g., foods, drugs, or insect stings).

Management

EMS The emergency action plan, including summoning EMS, should be activated. While waiting for EMS to arrive, the examiner should maintain the airway, control any bleeding, splint any fractures, and maintain normal body temperature. If a head or neck injury is not suspected, the feet and legs should be elevated 8 to 12 inches. Vital signs should be taken and recorded every 5 minutes. Field Strategy 19.1 summarizes the immediate care of shock.

A *The compound fracture sustained by the baseball player can lead to shock. Shock is considered to be a medical emergency. As such, the emergency action plan, including summoning EMS, should be activated. While waiting for EMS to arrive, the examiner should maintain the airway, maintain normal body temperature, and position the athlete lying down with the leg raised after—and only if—it has been properly immobilized.*

Box 19.4 Signs and Symptoms of Shock

- Restlessness, anxiety, fear, or disorientation
- Cold, clammy, moist skin
- Profuse sweating
- Extreme thirst
- Eyes are dull, sunken, and with the pupils dilated
- Skin that is chalk-like but that later may appear to be cyanotic

- Nausea and/or vomiting
- Shallow, irregular breathing; breathing also may be labored, rapid, or gasping
- Dizziness
- Rapid and weak pulse

FIELD STRATEGY 19.1

Management of Shock   [AU: Add EMS icon?]

- Activate emergency action plan, including summoning emergency medical services (EMS). Secure and maintain an open airway. Control any major bleeding. Monitor vital signs.
- If a head or neck injury or a leg fracture is not suspected, elevate the feet and legs 8 to 12 inches. With breathing difficulties, the individual might be more comfortable with the head and shoulders raised in a semireclining position. If a head injury is suspected, elevate the head and shoulders to reduce pressure on the brain. The feet also may be slightly elevated. In a suspected neck injury, keep the individual lying flat.
- An individual who vomits or is unconscious should be placed on their side to avoid blocking the airway with any fluids. This allows the fluids to drain from the mouth.
- Splint any fractures. This reduces shock by slowing bleeding and helps to ease pain. If the individual has a leg fracture, keep the leg level while splinting the fracture. Raise the leg only after it has been properly immobilized.
- Maintain normal body temperature. This action may require removing any wet clothing, if possible, and covering the individual with a blanket. Keep the individual quiet and still. Avoid rough or excessive handling of the individual.
- Do not give the individual anything by mouth.
- Monitor vital signs every 2 to 5 minutes until EMS arrives.

BLOOD PRESSURE DISORDERS

Q *A senior athlete reports feeling dizzy when getting up from a lying position and when suddenly changing body positions while playing tennis. What might this person be experiencing, and what is the management for this condition?*

Blood pressure (BP) is the force per unit area exerted on the walls of an artery, generally considered to be the aorta. It is the result of two factors—namely, cardiac output and total peripheral resistance. Cardiac output is determined by heart rate, myocardial contractility (i.e., force of contraction), blood volume, and venous return. Peripheral resistance is determined by arteriolar constriction. As one of the most important vital signs, blood pressure reflects the effectiveness of the circulatory system.

Although blood pressure varies among individuals, normal blood pressure is considered to be 120 mm Hg systolic blood pressure (SBP) and 80 mm Hg diastolic blood pressure (DBP). **Systolic blood pressure** is measured when the left ventricle contracts and expels blood into the aorta. **Diastolic blood pressure** is the residual pressure in the aorta between heartbeats. It is not unusual for a relatively physically fit person to have a blood pressure of 90/70 mm Hg. Blood pressure may be affected by gender, weight, race, lifestyle, and diet, and it can vary throughout the day, depending on the time of day and the individual's fitness level. Blood pressure is measured in the brachial artery with a sphygmomanometer and stethoscope (refer to Field Strategy 2.1).

Any change in either cardiac output or peripheral resistance results in an increase or decrease in blood pressure. **Hypertension** is defined as a sustained, elevated blood pressure greater than 140 mm Hg SBP or greater than 90 mm Hg DBP. A fall of 20 mm Hg or more from a person's normal baseline SBP characterizes **hypotension**.

Hypertension

Hypertension affects approximately 50 million individuals in the United States and approximately 1 billion individuals worldwide (9). The higher the blood pressure, the greater the chance of myocardial infarction, heart failure, stroke, and kidney disease. For individuals 40 to 70 years of age, each increment of 20 mm Hg in SBP or of 10 mm Hg in DBP doubles the risk of cardiovascular disease across the entire blood pressure range of 115/75 to 185/115 mm Hg (9).

Several factors increase the risk of developing hypertension (Table 19.1). Onset generally is between the ages of 20 and 50 years, with the frequency being greatest in African Americans. Hypertension can be caused by a variety of substances, including:

- Certain prescribed medications
- Oral contraceptives
- Anabolic steroids
- Amphetamines
- Chronic alcohol use
- Nasal decongestants containing sympathomimetic amines
- Some nonsteroidal anti-inflammatory drugs
- Sleep apnea
- Chronic kidney disease
- Renovascular disease
- Coarctation of the aorta
- Thyroid or parathyroid disease

Hypertension is classified into prehypertension, stage 1 hypertension, and stage 2 hypertension (Table 19.2). This categorization applies to adults 18 years of age and older who are not taking antihypertensive medication and are not acutely ill. When SBP and DBP fall into different categories, the higher category is used to classify the individual's blood pressure status. For more detailed standards in children and adolescents, refer to Chapter 2.

Categories of Hypertension

Classifications of hypertension are based on the mean of two or more properly measured, seated blood pressure readings on each of two or more occasions. In contrast to past standards, new standards classify a designated prehypertension category to identify patients who are at increased risk for progression to hypertension. Individuals in the 130/80 to 139/89 mm Hg range are at twice the risk of developing hypertension compared with those who have lower values (9).

TABLE 19.1 Risk Factors for Developing Hypertension

RISK FACTOR	REASON
Age	Arteries lose their elasticity, and blood pressure increases with age. High incidence of hypertension after age 60.
Diabetes	High incidence in those with diabetes is attributed to insulin resistance promoted by abdominal obesity.
Heredity	Higher incidence with a family history of hypertension and heart disease in women (<65 years) and men (<55 years).
High blood lipids	High blood lipids contribute to atherosclerosis and hypertension. A high-fat diet also contributes to hypertension.
Obesity	Excess body fat, especially abdominal fat, is closely associated with hypertension.
Race	Prevalence differs among racial and ethnic groups, but incidence in African Americans is among the highest in the world.
Sex	Higher incidence in men and postmenopausal women.
Smoking	Smoking increases the workload of the heart and, as such, increases blood pressure.

TABLE 19.2 Classification of Blood Pressure for Adults 18 Years or Older

CLASSIFICATION	SYSTOLIC (MM HG)[a]		DIASTOLIC (mm HG)[a]	Lifestyle Modification
Normal	<120	and	<80	Encourage
Prehypertension	120–139	or	80–89	Yes
Stage 1 hypertension	140–159	or	90–99	Yes
State 2 hypertension	≥160	or	≥100	Yes

[a]Treatment determined by highest category.

Standards from The Seventh Report of the Joint National Committee on Prevention, Detection, Evaluation, and Treatment of High Blood Pressure. JAMA 2003;289(19):2560–2572.

Hypertension is divided into two categories. Primary, or essential, hypertension is a chronic, progressive disorder with no identifiable cause that often attacks the heart, brain, kidneys, and eyes and that is associated with increased morbidity and mortality. The condition can be treated successfully with medication, diet modification, and exercise. Secondary hypertension has an identified cause, which often is associated with chronic renal disease, renovascular disease, **coarctation**, and other conditions. If the cause is identified, secondary hypertension can be controlled.

Clearance for Sport and Physical Activity Participation

An individual who has mild or moderate hypertension should not participate in competitive sports and physical activity until he or she is cleared by a physician. These individuals often are given physician clearance to participate in activity if their blood pressure is well controlled and no target organ damage or heart disease is present. These individuals should have their blood pressure rechecked by the athletic trainer on a weekly basis and by the physician every 2 to 4 months. For individuals with stage 2 hypertension, physical activity is restricted, especially in sports or activities with a high static component (e.g., wrestling, gymnastics, weight lifting, rock climbing, and rowing) until the hypertension is well controlled.

Management of Hypertension

Treatment of hypertension focuses on reducing SBP and DBP as well as on preventing long-term complications. Target blood pressure readings of less than 140/90 mm Hg are associated with a decrease in cardiovascular complications. The target for a patient with hypertension along with diabetes or renal disease is less than 130/80 mm Hg (9). Nonpharmaceutical treatment includes lifestyle modifications and aerobic exercise. Pharmaceutical treatment may involve antihypertensive medications.

LIFESTYLE MODIFICATIONS. Because hypertension has a significant impact on risk for cardiovascular disease, individuals with hypertension should be encouraged to establish lifestyle modifications in collaboration with an exercise program. These steps may include measures such as the following (9,10):

- Lose weight if overweight or obese.

- Engage in regular aerobic physical activity, such as brisk walking

- Limit alcohol intake. For most males, alcohol intake should be no more than two drinks per day (<1 oz/day of ethanol [e.g., 24 oz of beer, 10 oz of wine, or 3 oz of 80-proof whiskey]); females and lighter-weight males should not have more than 1 drink per day.

- Reduce sodium intake to less than 100 mmol/day (<2.4 g of sodium or <6 g of sodium chloride).

- Consume a diet rich in fruits, vegetables, and low-fat dairy products, with a reduced content of saturated and total fats.

- Maintain adequate dietary potassium, calcium, and magnesium intake.

- Do not smoke cigarettes.

Diet modifications should include a diet low in saturated fats, with total dietary fat not exceeding 30% of total caloric intake, and increased potassium, calcium, and magnesium intake. In severe cases of hypertension, more significant sodium and alcohol restrictions, weight loss, and reduction of other cardiovascular risk factors must be incorporated into the program.

EXERCISE PROGRAM. Aerobic exercise has a positive effect on the blood pressure of individuals with hypertension by lowering resting SBP an average of 4 to 9 mm Hg and DBP an average of 6 mm Hg. Specific mechanisms for this response are still unknown (9,11), but significant contributing factors may include:

- Reduced activity of the sympathetic nervous system, which decreases peripheral resistance and blood flow

- Altered renal function, which facilitates the elimination of sodium by the kidneys, subsequently reducing fluid volume and blood pressure

- Decreased body fat

- Decreased smoking and alcohol consumption that often accompany exercise conditioning

- Increased relaxation during exercise

Thirty minutes of aerobic exercise at 55 to 70% of maximum heart rate (MHR), five to six sessions per week, is recommended. In older or less fit individuals, initial exercise targets should be 55 to 60% of MHR; it may be appropriate for some individuals who have a good fitness level to have a target of 65 to 70% of MHR (12). (Chapter 2 provides information on measuring MHR.) Individuals with hypertension should avoid isometric exercises and heavy resistance training. Field Strategy 19.2 provides an exercise program for individuals with hypertension.

PHARMACEUTICAL MEDICATIONS. When lifestyle modifications, diet, and physical activity fail to control hypertension, diuretics and antihypertensive agents often are prescribed. Most patients require two or more antihypertensive medications to achieve a desirable blood pressure. Thiazide diuretics, which are used in the initial therapy for most patients, enhance the antihypertensive efficacy of multidrug regimens, can be useful in achieving blood pressure control, and are more affordable than

FIELD STRATEGY 19.2

Hypertension Exercise Program

- Have a physical examination before beginning an exercise program.
- If taking medication, make sure the medication does not negatively interact with the exercise program.
- Initially, perform aerobic exercise (e.g., walking, jogging, cycling, or swimming) three or more times per week, progressing to five to six times per week, at a rate of 55 to 70% of maximum heart rate.
- Begin the exercise bout with a 5-minute warmup, followed by 25 to 30 minutes of exercise and ending with a 5-minute cool-down period.
- Progressively increase the intensity of the program as tolerated.
- Do not perform isometric or heavy resistance exercises.
- Stop exercise immediately on experiencing any of the following: pain in the chest, jaw, or arm; dizziness; or unusual shortness of breath.

other antihypertensive agents. Diuretics lower blood pressure by increasing fluid loss; however, some diuretics can lead to a potassium deficiency. As such, individuals should be aware of the signs of potassium imbalance, including weakness (particularly of the legs), unexplained numbness or tingling sensations, cramps, irregular heartbeats, and excessive thirst and urination. Other antihypertensive agents, such as calcium channel blockers and angiotensin-converting enzyme inhibitors, are used to manage hypertension (9,13). Angiotensin-converting enzyme inhibitors are the pharmaceutical interventions that are least likely to interact negatively with exercise, but they are not recommended for individuals with exercise-induced bronchospasm or pregnant women. Taking calcium channel blockers while exercising may cause orthostatic problems, but a thorough cool-down following all exercise activities can prevent such problems from occurring.

Hypotension

When arterial blood pressure is lower than normal, inadequate blood is circulated to the heart, brain, and other vital organs. The result often is a collapse of bodily functions. Hypotension, or low blood pressure, is defined as a decrease of 20 mm Hg or more in an individual's normal SBP. It can be caused by a variety of factors, including shock, acute hemorrhage, dehydration, **orthostatic hypotension, postural hypotension,** or overtreatment of hypertension (Box 19.5).

Orthostatic hypotension is not unusual. Estimated to occur in approximately half of all elderly people, it can lead to fainting and falls (14). In the absence of symptoms, however, treatment is not required. Symptoms that indicate a medical referral include dimming or loss of vision, light-headedness, dizziness, excessive perspiration, diminished hearing, pallor, nausea, and weakness (15). It should be noted that certain medications (e.g., vasodilators and antidepressants) may cause orthostatic hypotension. This complication can be addressed by having a physician change the medication or dosage.

Physically active people do not usually need to be concerned about hypotension. In general, the lower the blood pressure, the better—as long as the person feels well. Older individuals, however, should always check with their physician before performing heavy resistance exercises. Nonpharmaceutical steps that can be taken to reduce the effects of orthostatic hypotension include:

- Avoid:
  - Prolonged standing.
  - Vigorous exercise.
  - Alcohol.
  - Hot environments; hot showers or baths.
- Execute slow, careful changes in position, especially when arising in the morning.
- Eat multiple, small meals.
- Schedule physical activities in the afternoon.
- Increase salt and fluid intake.

Box 19.5   Nonneurogenic Causes of Hypotension

- Shock as a response to stress or trauma
- Hemorrhage
- Diabetes mellitus
- Allergic drug reaction
- Dehydration
- Low-salt diets
- Diarrhea
- Heat (e.g., hot environments, hot showers and baths, or fever)
- Drug toxicity (e.g., alcohol, anesthesia, diuretics, analgesics, or vasodilators)
- Overtreatment of hypertension (e.g., diuretics, antihypertensives, or vasodilators)
- Orthostatic or postural hypotension
- Straining on heavy lifting, urination, or defecation
- Vasovagal syncope (fainting)

The senior athlete most likely has experienced orthostatic hypotension. Management for this condition can include avoiding prolonged standing, vigorous exercise, alcohol, and hot environments; slowly and carefully changing body positions; eating multiple, small meals; scheduling physical activities in the afternoon; and increasing salt and fluid intake.

SUDDEN CARDIAC DEATH

A little league baseball pitcher receives a line drive to his chest. He immediately collapses. What condition should be suspected, and how should this condition be managed?

Sudden cardiac death (SCD) has been termed the "silent killer." It is defined as an unexpected death resulting from sudden cardiac arrest within 6 hours of an otherwise normal, healthy clinical state (16).

Epidemiology

The prevalence of SCD during physical activity is uncertain. It is estimated that 1 in 180,000 high school–aged athletes experience sudden death. Males have an estimated death rate fivefold that of females, with the highest rates being seen in basketball and football players (16). Explanation for the low occurrence in female athletes is inconclusive; however, some researchers postulate that the decreased incidence can be attributed to the following (17–19):

- Fewer females participate in sports.

- Fewer females participate in highly intense sports that require full-body protective equipment (e.g., football or ice hockey).

- Gender differences exist regarding cardiac adaptation to training demands.

- Females have smaller hearts.

Sudden cardiac death often is precipitated by physical activity and may be caused by an array of cardiovascular conditions, the most common of which is hypertrophic cardiomyopathy. Noncardiac causes include commotio cordis, heat stroke, pulmonary complications, and drug abuse (17). The age of the individual appears to dictate the underlying physiologic pathology for the occurrence of SCD. Congenital cardiac abnormalities are responsible for the vast majority of SCDs in individuals under the age of 30 years, whereas atherosclerotic coronary artery disease is the leading cause for individuals older than 35 years, accounting for up to 80% of such events (20).

Cardiac Causes of Sudden Cardiac Death

Cardiac anomalies are the most direct cause of SCD in individuals younger than 30 years, with hypertrophic cardiomyopathy being the most common. Other reported cardiac-related causes include cardiac mass, mitral valve prolapse, myocarditis, acquired valvular heart disease, coronary artery anomalies, ruptured aortic aneurysm (often from intrinsic aortic weakness with Marfan's syndrome), Wolff-Parkinson-White syndrome, and arrhythmogenic right ventricular dysplasia. Other rare cardiac conditions that can contribute to sudden death involve abnormalities of the cardiac conduction system (i.e., long QT syndrome), which can result in lethal cardiac rhythm problems.

Hypertrophic Cardiomyopathy

Hypertrophic cardiomyopathy (HCM), which is characterized by an abnormal thickening of the left ventricle wall, develops before 20 years of age. It is the leading cause of sudden death in young, physically active individuals. Hypertrophic cardiomyopathy typically goes undetected during routine physical examination. By definition, HCM is a hypertrophied, nondilated left ventricle in the absence of another cardiac or systemic disease capable of producing the degree of hypertrophy that is present. A normal left ventricle is approximately 1 cm thick. In HCM, the wall thickness typically ranges from 2 to 4 cm—and can be greater than 15 cm (21). This abnormal thickness can lead to electrical problems and abnormal rhythms, including ventricular fibrillation and lethal rhythm.

Hypertrophic cardiomyopathy occurs in approximately 0.2% of the young adult population and usually is transmitted genetically (22). The condition appears during childhood and adolescence, reaching full development by the time of physical maturity. Symptoms of cardiac dysfunction, which do not appear until early adulthood (if at all), result in impaired ventricle filling. As a result, periods of **arrhythmia** or blood flow obstruction may produce syncope during physical exertion.

Physical examinations should include a thorough cardiac history and cardiac examination (see *Cardiovascular Preparticipation Screening*). Unfortunately, HCM often goes undetected during routine physical examinations. Individuals may engage in physical activity and sports for years without demonstrating signs or symptoms of HCM. Any individual who complains of prodromal symptoms, such as syncope, dizziness, or undue fatigue during or after exercise, should be seen by a physician or a cardiologist.

Mitral Valve Prolapse

Mitral valve prolapse is not a frequent cause of sudden death but can affect 2 to 5% of the population, spanning all ages (23). Mitral valve prolapse is a condition in which redundant tissue is found on one or both leaflets of the mitral valve. During a ventricular contraction, a portion of the redundant tissue on the mitral valve pushes back beyond the normal limit and, as a result, produces an abnormal sound. This sound is followed by a systolic murmur as blood is regurgitated back through the mitral valve into the left atrium. Because of the characteristic sound, this condition often is referred to as a "click-murmur syndrome." Individuals with mitral valve prolapse usually experience some degree of chest pain, dyspnea, palpitations, and fatigue with exertion (24).

Myocarditis

Myocarditis is an inflammatory condition of the muscular walls of the heart that can result from a bacterial or viral infection. The condition is characterized by the infiltration of inflammatory cells into the myocardium, leading to an abnormally enlarged left ventricle. Sudden cardiac death occurs when the inflammatory changes in the myocardium lead to degeneration or death of adjacent muscle cells, resulting in electrical instability and life-threatening arrhythmias. Although some individuals may be asymptomatic, others exhibit symptoms commonly associated with viral infections, including fever, body aches, fatigue, cough, or vomiting; this similarity often impedes establishing the diagnosis. Exercise intolerance, shortness of breath, and more serious cardiac symptoms, including **palpitations** or syncope, may occur without warning.

Acquired Valvular Heart Disease

Acquired valvular heart disease stems from a defect or insufficiency in a heart valve that can lead to improper blood flow through the heart. The condition is manifested as either **valvular stenosis**, which is a narrowing of the orifice around the cardiac valves, or **regurgitation**, which involves a backward flow of blood. The condition is named according to the affected valve (e.g., mitral valve, aortic valve, and tricuspid valve). If more than one valve is affected, the condition is called **multivalvular disease**, which occurs in the context of rheumatic heart disease. The characteristic murmurs associated with this condition are detected during a physical examination.

Individuals with mild to moderate mitral and tricuspid valve stenosis or regurgitation typically can participate in sports and physical activity. Each case, however, must be evaluated on an individual basis.

Initially, experts posited that aortic stenosis was a common cause of sudden death; however, new research has not supported their theory. Aortic stenosis, like other valve conditions, often can be detected early through physical examination. Individuals with mild aortic stenosis may participate in physical activity and competitive sports. Individuals with mild or moderate asymptomatic aortic stenosis and a history of **supraventricular tachycardia** (i.e., rapid heartbeats proximal to the ventricles in the atrium or atrioventricular node) or ventricular arrhythmias at rest should participate only in low-intensity physical activity and sports. Individuals with severe aortic stenosis or symptomatic, moderate stenosis should not engage in any competitive sport (25).

Coronary Artery Disease

The most common cause of sudden death in individuals older than 30 years is coronary artery disease, also referred to as **atherosclerosis**. An excessive buildup of cholesterol within the coronary arteries narrows the diameter of the arteries and impedes the flow of blood, which in turn reduces the amount of oxygen supplied to the heart. Subsequent to the diminished oxygen, **angina** is a common symptom. If excessive cholesterol buildup blocks a coronary artery, the person is at risk for a **myocardial infarction**. If the blockage is in a major coronary artery, death often occurs.

Unlike young individuals, who rarely know if they have a cardiac anomaly that may put them at risk for sudden death, physically active individuals older than 30 years usually have experienced prodromal cardiovascular symptoms or have a known medical history of coronary artery disease. Therefore, individuals older than 30 years can choose:

- To ignore the symptoms and continue participating at the same level, placing them at risk for sudden death.

- To change their lifestyle according to coronary artery disease recommendations and continue to participate in limited activity.

- To no longer participate in physical activity.

The American College of Sports Medicine (ACSM) has developed a list of risk factors for coronary artery disease (26) (Table 19.3). The criteria should be used to identify individuals who are at risk for a heart attack. These individuals should have an exercise **electrocardiogram** or a treadmill stress test before beginning an exercise program. The ACSM recommends an exercise electrocardiogram before beginning a moderate or vigorous exercise program for anyone who has had a history of angina, palpitations, syncope, or dyspnea during physical activity.

Marfan's Syndrome

Marfan's syndrome does not necessarily lead to SCD. When SCD does occur, it usually is caused by the condition's hallmark characteristic—namely, a weakened aorta. Marfan's syndrome is a genetic

TABLE 19.3 American College of Sports Medicine (ACSM) Coronary Artery Disease Risk Factors

POSITIVE RISK FACTORS	DEFINING CRITERIA
Family history	Myocardial infarction, coronary revascularization, or sudden death before 55 years of age in father or other male first-degree relative (i.e., brother or son) or before age 65 years of age in mother or other first-degree female relative (i.e., sister of daughter)
Cigarette smoking	Current cigarette smoker or someone who quit within the previous 6 months
Hypertension	Systolic blood pressure ≥ 140 mm Hg or diastolic blood pressure ≥ 90 mm Hg confirmed by measurements on at least two separate occasions, or using antihypertensive medication
Hypercholesterolemia	Total serum cholesterol > 200 mg/dL (5.2 mmol/L) or high-density lipoprotein cholesterol < 35 mg/dL (0.9 mmol/L), or on lipid-lowering medication. If low-density lipoprotein cholesterol is available, use > 130 mg/dL (3.4 mmol/L) rather than total cholesterol > 200 mg/dL
Impaired fasting glucose	Fasting blood glucose of ≥ 110 mg/dL (6.1 mmol/L) confirmed by measurements on at least two separate occasions
Obesity	Body mass index ≥ 30 kg/m2, or waist girth > 100 cm
Sedentary lifestyle	Persons comprising the least active 25% of the population, as defined by the combination of a sedentary job involving sitting for a large part of the day and no regular exercise or active recreational pursuits
NEGATIVE RISK FACTOR	**DEFINING CRITERIA**
High serum high-density lipoprotein cholesterol	>60 mg/dL (1.6 mmol/L)

From American College of Sports Medicine. ACSM's Guidelines for Exercise Testing and Prescription. 6th Ed. Baltimore: Lippincott Williams & Wilkins, 2000; with permission.

disorder of the connective tissue that can affect the skeleton, lungs, eyes, heart, and blood vessels. A single mutant gene is linked to the condition. Although usually inherited, one-third of all cases have no family history (27).

Individuals with Marfan's syndrome are tall in stature, with overly long extremities; the arm span exceeds the person's height. Joints usually are hypermobile, and the person may have a pigeon (sunken) chest, stretch marks, scoliosis, and increased incidence of hernias. A positive thumb test and wrist test are classic signs of Marfan's syndrome. The thumb test involves adduction of the thumb across the palm of the hand and flexion of the fingers around the thumb; the test is positive if the thumb extends past the fifth finger. The wrist test involves the person encircling a wrist with the thumb and fifth finger of the opposite hand; the test is positive if the thumb and fifth finger overlap. In addition to orthopaedic anomalies, it is not unusual to find an excessively high palate, eye defects (i.e., myopia or nearsightedness), mitral valve prolapse, and defects in the connective tissue layers of the aorta. As a result of the defect in the aorta tissues, death from Marfan's syndrome usually is associated with an aortic dissection or rupture.

Screening for Marfan's syndrome includes a musculoskeletal and eye examination as well as an echocardiogram to determine abnormalities of the aorta. Marfan's syndrome has no cure, but with careful medical management, most people can live a normal life. An individual with Marfan's syndrome should avoid contact activities because of the risk of injury to the eyes and aorta. Individuals with a family history of premature SCD and without evidence of aortic root dilation may participate in moderate, low-static, and low-dynamic activities, such as brisk walking, leisure bicycling, golf, slow jogging, and slow-paced tennis.

Individuals with aortic root dilatation may participate only in low-intensity physical activities—specifically, noncompetitive, nonstrenuous aerobic activities that do not exceed 50% of aerobic capacity. In addition, isometric exercise is contraindicated for these individuals (28,29).

> See Screening for Marfan's Syndrome, *available on the companion website at thePoint.*

Rare Cardiac Conditions

Other rare cardiac conditions, such as a long QT syndrome and right ventricular dysplasia, may contribute to SCD. Both conditions produce serious arrhythmias. Long QT syndrome, which usually affects children and young adults, is a hereditary disorder of the heart's electrical system. The individual is susceptible to arrhythmia, which produces inefficient contraction of the heart. The result is the reduction of normal blood volume in the body and the brain. Inability of the heart to regain its normal rhythm can lead to ventricular fibrillation, which is a fatal arrhythmia.

Right ventricular dysplasia, a disorder of the right ventricle, is characterized by the formation of adipose or fibrous tissue extending from the epicardium to the endocardium. This abnormal growth of tissue increases the risk of ventricular fibrillation. Any unstable ventricular heart rhythm, such as ventricular tachycardia or ventricular fibrillation, can lead to death. In fact, most cardiac conditions that produce SCD are the result of an abnormal ventricular rhythm (17,23,30).

Wolff-Parkinson-White syndrome is an abnormality of cardiac rhythm that manifests as a supraventricular tachycardia. The condition is associated with an accessory electrical pathway in the heart proximal to the ventricles that can spontaneously produce episodes of rapid twitching of the atrium muscle fibers within a range of 200 to 300 heartbeats per minute. The condition often is seen in asymptomatic, healthy individuals during electrocardiographic examination. Although rarely associated with sudden death, the condition may complicate other heart conditions, such as myocarditis or ischemic heart disease.

Congenital coronary artery anomalies are another cause of sudden death in young athletes. The most common anomaly is an abnormal origin of the left coronary artery. The anomaly necessitates an acute take-off angle, forcing the artery to pass between the aorta and the pulmonary artery, both of which can decrease blood flow to the heart. Other anomalies may involve an abnormal origin of the right coronary artery, presence of a right coronary artery without a left coronary artery, and abnormal coronary artery spasm. Congenital coronary artery anomalies may not be detected during exercise because symptoms, such as syncope, near syncope, and chest pain, are intermittent and unpredictable.

Noncardiac Causes of Sudden Death

Sudden cardiac death usually is directly related to cardiac conditions. Noncardiac conditions, however, also can lead to SCD; these include commotio cordis, substance abuse, head injuries, heat illness, exertional hyperthermia, exercise-induced anaphylaxis, exertional rhabdomyolysis, and sickle cell trait. Often, noncardiac conditions are more easily identifiable through physical examination and field evaluation. As such, if a condition can be identified, it usually can be treated.

. In   Van Camp and colleagues (16) conducted a study to determine the frequency and causes of nontraumatic, sport-related deaths in high school and college athletes. Between the years 1983 and 1993, 160 nontraumatic deaths were reported, of which 124 were high school athletes and 36 were collegiate athletes. Adequate information regarding cause of death was available for 136 of the 160 athletes. Fivefold more deaths occurred in male than in female athletes at both levels of competition. Cardiovascular conditions were the most common cause of sudden death (74%), but other causes (22%) included exertional hyperthermia; **exertional rhabdomyolysis,** in which cellular contents of damaged skeletal muscle enter the circulation; status asthmaticus, which is a state of prolonged asthma; and electrocution from lightning (16).

Commotio Cordis

Cardiac arrest from a low-impact, blunt blow to the chest in the absence of a structural cardiovascular disease is rare in sports. The U.S. Commotio Cordis Registry has catalogued 128 cases as of September 2001 (31). The majority of cases occurred in young individuals (average age, 13.6 years) who were engaged in competitive sports (62%). Ninety-five percent of the affected individuals were male. The leading mechanism of injury was from a projectile striking the chest, including baseballs (41% of all cases), softballs (11%), hockey pucks (7.8%), and lacrosse balls (3.9%). Other less frequent projectiles were a soccer ball and a cricket ball (31).

Postmortem analyses of individuals dying from commotio cordis revealed no structural damage to the heart or overlying protective structures (e.g., sternum or ribs), but soft-tissue contusions of the left chest wall commonly were visualized (32). This suggests that sudden death in these cases resulted from blunt force–induced conduction abnormalities. Because commotio cordis usually is a fatal event, focus has been aimed at prevention. Possible prevention strategies include the use of protective padded equipment that covers the area of the chest over the heart and switching to balls or pucks made of softer materials.

Substance Abuse

Certain types of drug abuse can lead to cardiac changes that predispose an individual to SCD. Amphetamines are central nervous system stimulants that increase heart rate, respiration rate, and blood pressure. Cocaine, which is an anesthetic, constricts coronary arteries and has been known to lead to myocardial infarction in those with and in those without coronary artery disease. In addition, myocarditis has been found in autopsy reports of cocaine-related SCD cases. It must be noted that a massive dose of cocaine is not required to produce cardiac or respiratory consequences. Several reported cases of SCD have involved anabolic steroid users, although a direct relationship between steroid use and sudden death has not yet been established.

Produced in the kidneys, **erythropoietin** is a hormone that stimulates bone marrow to increase production of RBCs. Erythropoietin (EPO/EPOGEN) became synthetically available in the late 1980s when its use as an ergogenic aid for endurance athletes was first documented. The use of EPO is equal to blood doping and, like blood doping, can increase blood volume and viscosity of the blood, leading to decreased circulation, thrombosis, and myocardial infarction. These adverse cardiovascular effects have led to SCD; EPO may be one of the most deadly ergogenic aids available (33).

Head Injuries

Catastrophic brain injuries that can lead to SCD include skull fracture, epidural hematoma, acute and subacute subdural hematoma, second-impact syndrome, or various other brain hemorrhage conditions (34). Individuals should be observed closely after sustaining any type of head injury, regardless of the level of consciousness. Signs of rapidly increasing intracranial pressure include a dilated or irregular pupil or pupils, reduced pulse, nausea or vomiting, dyspnea, **photophobia,** mood swings, muscle weakness, and decreased level of consciousness. **Decortication**, a condition that presents as extension of the legs with flexion of the elbows, wrists, and fingers, or **decerebration**, a condition that presents as extension of all four extremities, often is present in severe injuries (see Chapter 5). An individual who is unable to remember events leading up to (i.e., **retrograde amnesia**) or following the injury (i.e., **anterograde amnesia**) should not be permitted to continue activity and should be referred immediately to a physician. Additional information concerning head injuries can be found in Chapter 9.

Heat Illness

Heat illness is one of the most preventable causes of SCD, yet individuals die from exertional hyperthermia each year. In football, heat stroke is second only to head injuries as the most frequent cause of death. The condition also is seen in distance runners and wrestlers who are dehydrated through weight loss. Heat stroke almost always is preceded by prolonged, strenuous physical exercise in individuals who are poorly acclimatized or in situations during which evaporation of sweat is inhibited.

The individual often complains of a feeling of "burning up." Deep breaths, irritability, hysterical behavior, and an unsteady gait may be present. As the condition deteriorates, the skin is hot and dry and appears to be red or flushed, and the pulse becomes rapid and strong (as high as 150–170 heartbeats per minute). Brain tissue damage by excessive body heat leads to vasomotor collapse, shallow breathing, decreased blood pressure, and a rapid and weak pulse. Muscle twitching or seizures may occur just before the individual lapses into coma. This condition is a medical emergency and, as such, warrants activation of the emergency action plan, including summoning EMS. Further information concerning heat illness is presented in Chapter 24.

Sickle Cell Trait

Sickle cell trait is an inherited disorder in which RBCs tend to form into a sickle-shaped structure (see Fig. 19.4). This sickling formation of RBCs prevents efficient transportation of oxygen to the tissues and can lead to vascular occlusion, coagulation, and even death. Eight percent of all African Americans have sickle cell trait, and individuals in the 23- to 30-year-old age range have a 1.3 in 1,000 chance of dying from sudden death during exertional activities, particularly during extreme conditions of heat, humidity, and increased altitude (35). Unexpected death is almost always associated with severe exertional **rhabdomyolysis**, a fatal disease stemming from renal failure caused when cellular contents of damaged skeletal muscle (myoglobin) enter the circulation. Sickle cell anemia is easily screened through laboratory testing. As such, recommendations can be made to ensure that individuals with sickle cell anemia can safely participate in sport and physical activity.

A *Following the collapse of the little league baseball player, an immediate assessment of ABCs is essential. If the athlete is not breathing or does not have a pulse, the emergency action plan, including summoning EMS, should be activated and cardiopulmonary resuscitation administered. The player may have experienced cardiac arrest from the blow to the chest. The condition, known as commotio cordis, results in conduction abnormalities. Because it usually is fatal, focus has been on prevention rather than treatment.*

CARDIOVASCULAR PREPARTICIPATION SCREENING

Q *In preparation for PPEs of high school and college athletes, several areas must be addressed, including obtaining a cardiovascular history. What questions should be asked as part of the medical history to assist in screening for those at risk of sudden death?*

Identification of the risks associated with SCD requires the implementation of a two-tiered approach. First, a standard screening examination should be done 6 to 8 weeks before engaging in physical activity or sport and then every 2 years thereafter (36,37). Screening should be performed by a health care provider with the medical skills, requisite training, and clinical experience to obtain a detailed cardiovascular history, to perform an extensive physical examination, and to recognize potential heart disease or cardiac anomalies.

Box 19.6 Recommendations for Sudden Cardiac Death Screening

1. Medical history questions
   - Previous chest pain during physical exertion
   - Exercise-induced syncope or near syncope
   - Excessive unexplained shortness of breath, fatigue, or dizziness with exercise
   - History of heart murmur or increased blood pressure
   - Family history of death from cardiovascular disease in a relative younger than 50 years
   - Family history of hypertrophic cardiomyopathy, dilated cardiomyopathy, long QT syndrome, or Marfan's syndrome

2. Physical examination
   - Screening for Marfan's syndrome
   - Cardiovascular examination emphasizing:
     - Brachial artery blood pressure measurement
     - Precordial auscultation in both the supine and standing positions
     - Assessment of the femoral artery pulse

According to recommendations from a joint summit on sudden death sponsored by the National Athletic Trainer's Association Research and Education Foundation (36) and the ACSM 26th Bethesda Conference (38), a cardiac history should include extensive questions regarding previous symptomatic episodes and family history. In addition to the medical history, the physical examination should include, but need not be limited to, precordial auscultation to identify heart murmurs, assessment of the femoral artery pulses, checking for signs of Marfan's syndrome (Box 19.6), and measuring brachial blood pressure. Unfortunately, many experts believe that a personal cardiac history does little to detect abnormalities in young athletes; however, an extensive medical history has been found to be advantageous in older athletes (38,39).

Identification of a possible cardiovascular abnormality during the cardiac history or standard physical examination is the first tier of recognition. Many of these conditions were listed in Box 2.3. The second tier involves referral to a cardiologist for more extensive screening, including an echocardiogram, particularly when seeking detection of HCM.

The decision regarding whether to permit an individual to participate after identifying a cardiovascular abnormality must be resolved on an individual basis under the Americans with Disabilities Act of 1990, the Rehabilitation Act of 1973, and similar state statutes prohibiting unjustified discrimination against the physically impaired. These laws permit an individual with the physical capabilities and skills to participate in a sport despite the fact that a cardiovascular abnormality is present. Exclusion from participation must be based on reasonable medical judgments, given the state of scientific research on the specific condition. These laws require careful balancing of the individual's right to participate, the physician's evaluation of the medical risks of participation, and an organization's interest in conducting a safe athletic program.

The ACSM, at its 26th Bethesda Conference, established eligibility guidelines for the determination of athletic participation (38). These guidelines, regarding the acceptable medical risks of athletic participation with known cardiovascular abnormalities, are directed toward team physicians, athletes, team officials, athletic governing bodies, and the courts. In addition, the National Collegiate Athletic Association Committee on Competitive Safeguards and Medical Aspects of Sports has firmly stated that the team physician should be the final authority in determining whether a collegiate athlete is eligible for competition. It is essential that the team physician use all available resources to reach an appropriate decision. These resources may include consultation with recognized cardiologists, either locally or nationally; discussion with ancillary administrative, medical, and coaching staffs; and input from the athlete and family. Certainly, the more elite the athlete, the more complex

See *Diagnostic Testing for Various Causes of Sudden Cardiac Death,* available on the companion website at thePoint.

and difficult the decisions regarding eligibility. The key players in this relationship, however, remain the team physician and the athlete. Clearly, it is in the best interest of the physician charged with the responsibility of determining medical clearance for an athlete with known cardiovascular abnormalities to know and to follow the ACSM Bethesda Conference guidelines (40).

As part of a well-defined emergency action plan, every facility should establish catastrophic incident guidelines that address the immediate action plan, chain of command responsibilities, standards for documentation of the event, and long-term support for individuals who may be affected by SCD (41). It is critical to have an emergency action plan in place to help any facility or sport program work through an emotional and highly visible situation.

(A) *The medical history for cardiovascular conditions should include questions regarding previous chest pain during physical exertion; exercise-induced syncope or near syncope; excessive, unexplained shortness of breath, fatigue, and dizziness with exercise; history of heart murmur; history of hypertension; family history of death of cardiovascular disease in a relative younger than 50 years; and family history of HCM, dilated cardiomyopathy, long QT syndrome, or Marfan's syndrome.*

SUMMARY

1. Anemia is a reduction in either the RBC volume (hematocrit) or hemoglobin concentration. Anemia reduces maximum aerobic capacity, decreases physical work capability at submaximal levels, increases lactic acidosis, increases fatigue, and decreases exercise time to exhaustion.

2. Hemophilia occurs in three types—namely, A, B, and C. These types are distinguished by the clotting factor that is deficient. All three types can cause prolonged bleeding.

3. Reye's syndrome is a rare but serious, acute illness that disrupts the body's urea cycle, resulting in the accumulation of ammonia in the blood, hypoglycemia, severe brain edema, and critically high intracranial pressure. The disease almost exclusively affects individuals from 2 to 16 years of age. It is linked to the use of aspirin to treat a viral infection.

4. Syncope is a transient LOC, described as "fainting," that often occurs in healthy individuals.

5. Shock occurs when the heart is unable to exert adequate pressure to circulate enough oxygenated blood to vital organs.

6. A rapid and weak pulse is the most prominent sign of shock, but other signs include rapid and shallow breathing, profuse sweating, and cold, clammy skin.

7. Neural-mediated syncope is the most common type of syncope that produces fainting and results from a sudden drop in blood pressure, which reduces blood circulation to the brain, leading to a LOC.

8. Blood pressure is the force per unit area exerted on the walls of an artery, generally considered to be the aorta. It is the result of two factors—namely, cardiac output and total peripheral resistance.

9. Blood pressure varies among individuals, but normal is considered to be 120 mm Hg SBP over 80 mm Hg DBP. Hypertension is defined as a sustained, elevated blood pressure of greater than 140 mm Hg SBP or greater than 90 mm Hg DBP. Hypotension is characterized by a fall of 20 mm Hg or more from a person's normal baseline SBP.

10. An individual in stage 1 or 2 hypertension should not participate in sport and physical activity until he or she is cleared by a physician. Individuals with stage 1 hypertension usually can participate if the blood pressure is well controlled and no target organ damage or heart disease is present. The blood pressure should be rechecked every week by a qualified specialist (e.g., athletic trainer) and every 2 to 4 months by the physician.

11. For individuals in stage 2 hypertension, restrictions are placed on physical activity, especially in sports or activities with a high static component.

12. Diet modifications for hypertension include limiting sodium and saturated fats, with the total dietary fat not to exceed 30% of the total caloric intake, and increasing potassium, calcium, and magnesium intake.

13. Aerobic exercise has been shown to reduce blood pressure among individuals in the prehypertension stage and in stage 1 hypertension.

14. Orthostatic hypotension is not unusual; however, a physician should be consulted if dizziness or light-headedness becomes more frequent with a sudden change in body position.

15. Physically active people do not usually need to be concerned with hypotension. In general, a lower blood pressure is desirable as long as the person feels well.

16. Sudden cardiac death is rare. When it does occur, however, the on-site personnel should immediately activate the emergency action plan and begin cardiopulmonary resuscitation.

17. Hypertrophic cardiomyopathy is the most common cardiac-related cause of sudden death.

18. Other cardiac-related causes of SCD include mitral valve prolapse, myocarditis, acquired valvular heart disease, coronary artery disease, Marfan's syndrome, long QT syndrome, Wolff-Parkinson-White syndrome, and arrhythmogenic right ventricular dysplasia.

19. Noncardiac causes of SCD include commotio cordis, heat illness, head injuries, substance abuse, exertional hyperthermia, exercise-induced anaphylaxis, exertional rhabdomyolysis, and sickle cell anemia.

20. The risk of SCD in physically active individuals can be reduced by using a two-tiered system. First, a PPE should include an extensive cardiac medical history and physical examination. If a cardiac abnormality is identified, the individual should then be referred to a specialist for further evaluation.

21. Determination of continued participation in sports should rest with the individual and the team physician after consultation with expert cardiologists, family, and team officials.

22. Clearance for participation should follow the ACSM 26th Bethesda Conference recommendations for determining the eligibility of athletes with cardiovascular abnormalities.

REFERENCES

1. Harris SS. Helping active women avoid anemia. Phys Sportsmed 1995;23(5):35–48.
2. Fields KB. Anemia in athletes. In: Mellion MB, Walsh WM, Madden C, Putukian M, Shelton GL, eds. The Team Physician's Handbook. Philadelphia: Hanley & Belfus, 2002.
3. Recommendations to prevent and control iron deficiency in the United States. MMWR 1998;47(RR-3):1–29.
4. Bolton-Maggs PHB, Pasi KJ. Hemophilias A and B. Lancet 2003;361(9371):1801–1810.
5. Tamparo CD, Lewis MA. Diseases of the Human Body. Philadelphia: FA Davis, 2000.
6. Henderson MC, Prabhu SD. Syncope: current diagnosis and treatment. Curr Probl Cardiol 1997;22(5):242–296.
7. Kapoor WN. Evaluation and management of the patient with syncope. JAMA 1992;268(18):2553–2560.
8. Meyer MD, Handler J. Evaluation of the patient with syncope: an evidence-based approach. Emerg Med Clin North Am 1999:17(1):189–201.
9. Chobanian AV, Bakris GL, Black HR, et al. The Seventh Report on the Joint National Committee on Prevention, Detection, Evaluation, and Treatment of High Blood Pressure. JAMA 2003;289(19):2560–2572.
10. Hollenberg NK, Braunwald E, eds. Atlas of Heart Diseases. Hypertension: Mechanisms and Therapy. Philadelphia: Current Medicine, 1998.
11. Bove AA, Sherman C. Active control of hypertension. Phys Sport Med 1998;26(4):45–53.
12. Massie BM. To combat hypertension, increase activity. Phys Sportsmed 1992;20(5):89–111.
13. Martin M, Yates WN. Therapeutic Medications in Sports Medicine. Baltimore: Williams & Wilkins, 1998.
14. Parson Y. Feeling faint: sudden changes in blood pressure can lead to falls. Contemp Long-Term Care 1997;220(6):13.
15. Engstrom JW. Evaluation and treatment of orthostatic hypotension. Am Fam Physician 1997;56(5):1378–1385.
16. Van Camp SP, Bloor CM, Mueller FO, et al. Nontraumatic sports death in high school and college athletes. Med Sci Sports Exerc 1995;27(5):641–647.
17. Maron BJ, Shirani J, Poliac LC, et al. Sudden death in young competitive athletes: clinical, demographic, and pathological profiles. JAMA 1996;276(3):199–204.
18. Kronisch RL. Sudden cardiac death in sports. Ath Ther Today 1996;1(4):39–41.

19. Thompson PD. The cardiovascular complications of vigorous physical activity. Arch Intern Med 1996;156(20):2297–2302.

20. Hosey RG, Armsey TD. Sudden cardiac death. Clin Sports Med 2003;22(1):51–66.

21. Pelliccia A, Maron BJ, Culasso F, et al. Athlete's heart in women. JAMA 1996;276(3):211–215.

22. Elliott P, McKenna WJ. Hypertrophic cardiomyopathy. Lancet 2004;363(9424):1881–1891.

23. Hayek E, Gring CH, Griffin BP. Mitral valve prolapse. Lancet 2005;365(9458):507–518.

24. Kenny A, Shapiro LM. Sudden cardiac death in athletes. Br Med Bull 1992;48(3):534–545.

25. Cheitlin MD, Douglas PS, Parmley WW. Acquired valvular heart disease. Med Sci Sports Exerc 1994;26(10):S254–S260.

26. American College of Sports Medicine. ACSM's Guidelines for Exercise Testing and Prescription. Baltimore: Lippincott Williams & Wilkins, 2000.

27. Lopez R. Sudden cardiac death: what athletic directors, coaches and trainers should know. Int Sports J 2003; 7(2):1–17.

28. The Marfan Syndrome Fact Sheet. Washington, DC: National Marfan Foundation, 1997.

29. Mitchell JF, Haskell W, Raven PB. Classification of sports. Med Sci Sports Exerc 1994;26(10):S242–S245.

30. Sudden Death in Sports. Champaign, IL: Human Kinetic and National Athletic Trainer's Association Research and Education Foundation, 1997.

31. Maron BJ, Gohman TE, Kyle SB, et al. Clinical profile and spectrum of commotio cordis. JAMA 2002:287(9): 1142–1146.

32. Maron BJ, Poliac LC, Kaplan JA, et al. Blunt impact to the chest leading to sudden death from cardiac arrest during sports activities. N Engl J Med 1995; 333(6):337–342.

33. Cowart VS. Erythropoietin: a dangerous new form of blood doping. Phys Sportsmed 1989;17(8):115–118.

34. Cantu RC. Cerebral concussion in sport management and prevention. Sports Med 1992;14(1):67–74.

35. Kerle KK, Nishimura KD. Exertional collapse and sudden death associated with sickle cell trait. Am Fam Physician 1996;54(1):237–240.

36. Van Camp SP, Luckstead EF, Palacios L, et al. Sudden Death in Athletes: Summit Statement. Dallas: National Athletic Trainer's Association Research and Education Foundation, 1997.

37. Maron BJ, Thompson PD, Puffer JC, et al. Cardiovascular preparticipation screening of competitive athletes. Washington, DC: American Heart Association, 1996.

38. Mitchell JG, Maron BJ, Raven PB, eds. American College of Sports Medicine, American College of Cardiology 26th Bethesda Conference. Recommendations for determining eligibility for competition in athletes with cardiovascular abnormalities. Med Sci Sports Exerc 1994;26(10): S223–S283.

39. Maron BJ, Pelliccia A, Spirito P. Cardiac disease in young trained athletes: insights into methods for distinguishing athlete's heart from structural heart disease, with particular emphasis on hypertrophic cardiomyopathy. Circulation 1995;91(5):1596–1601.

40. Mitten MJ, Maron BJ. Legal considerations that affect medical eligibility for competitive athletes with cardiovascular abnormalities and acceptance of Bethesda conference recommendations. Med Sci Sports Exerc 1994;26(10):S238–S241.

41. Hunt V. Can guidelines ease the aftermath of tragedy? NATA News 2003;May:10–14.

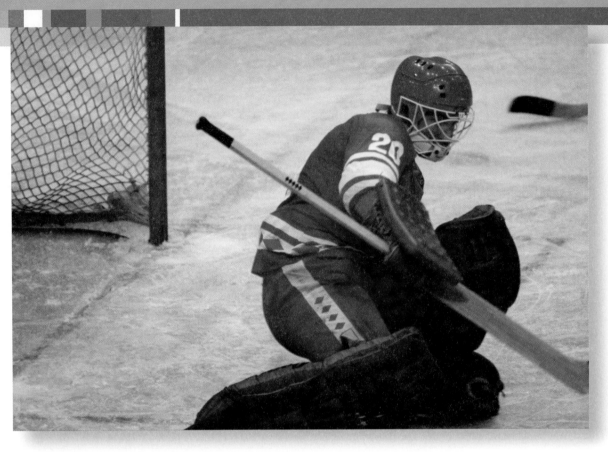

STUDENT OUTCOMES

1. Describe the pathophysiology of migraine headaches.

2. List the signs and symptoms of various types of migraine headaches.

3. Describe the prevention and management of migraine headaches.

4. Differentiate between a seizure disorder and epilepsy.

5. Identify the causes of epilepsy.

6. List the types of generalized and partial seizures.

7. Describe the characteristics and management of common seizures.

8. Describe the seizure situations that constitute a medical emergency.

9. Explain the exercise guidelines for individuals with controlled seizures.

ROLE DELINEATION COMPETENCIES

The following Performance Domains and Tasks defined in the National Athletic Trainers' Association Board of Certification *Role Delineation Study*, 5th Edition are addressed in this chapter:

BOC COMPETENCIES

II.   Clinical Evaluation and Diagnosis

E. Formulate a clinical impression by interpreting the signs, symptoms, and predisposing factors of the injury, illness, or condition to determine the appropriate course of action.

F. Educate the appropriate individual(s) regarding the assessment by communicating information about the current or potential injury, illness, or health-related condition to encourage compliance with recommended care.

III.   Immediate Care

A. Employ life-saving techniques through the use of standard emergency procedures in order to reduce morbidity and the incidence of mortality.

B. Prevent exacerbation of non–life threatening condition(s) through the use of standard procedures in order to reduce morbidity.

C. Facilitate the timely transfer of care for conditions beyond the scope of practice of the athletic trainer by implementing appropriate referral strategies to stabilize and/or prevent exacerbation of the condition(s).

IV.   Treatment, Rehabilitation, and Reconditioning

D. Administer treatment for general illness and/or conditions using standard techniques and procedures to facilitate recovery, function, and/or performance.

E. Reassess the status of injuries, illnesses, and/or conditions using standard techniques and documentation strategies in order to determine appropriate treatment, rehabilitation, and/or reconditioning and to evaluate readiness to return to a desired level of activity.

The body's nervous system includes the brain, spinal cord, and nerves. It regulates and coordinates body activities, and it brings about responses by which the body adjusts to changes in its internal and external environment. Initially, this chapter explores migraine headaches—namely, their types, signs, symptoms, and management. Next, the various types of seizure disorders are presented followed by signs, symptoms, management, and physical activity guidelines for those who suffer from a seizure disorder. Finally, information is presented regarding infections of the central nervous system and reflex sympathetic dystrophy.

HEADACHES

A female collegiate basketball player complains of a pounding headache with nausea. Two weeks earlier, she reported a similar headache that was accompanied by light sensitivity. Should this individual be referred to a physician for further assessment and care?

It is estimated that 93% of men and 99% of women have experienced one or more severe headaches. Migraine headaches in particular afflict approximately 6% of men and 18% of women in the United States (1). In addition, 20 to 54% of preadolescent children have had at least one headache, and 4% have had migraine headaches (2). Headaches may be chronic or acute, and they often signal nothing more than fatigue, stress, or tension. In some cases, however, headaches can indicate a serious disease (Box 20.1).

Box 20.1   Red Flags That Require Further Examination

- Serious headaches after 50 years of age
- Sudden onset of a headache
- Change in pattern in a headache (e.g., increased severity and frequency)
- New-onset headache in immunocompromised patients
- Headache associated with systemic illness, fever, or neck stiffness

- Headache associated with focal neurologic deficits
- Papilledema (i.e., edema of the optic disk)
- Headache associated with trauma
- Headache associated with antalgic gait, amnesia, or altered consciousness
- Early morning nausea and vomiting without headache

Headaches are caused by irritation of one or more of the pain-sensitive structures or tissues in the head and neck. These structures include the cranial arteries and veins, the cranial and spinal nerves, the cranial and cervical muscles, and the meninges. The condition may stem from organic disorders (e.g., toxins, systemic diseases, or diseases in specific systems of the body), psychoneurologic problems (e.g., nervous tension, fatigue, worry, excitement, or psychoneuroses), and environmental insults (e.g., head trauma, bright lights, noise, rapid altitude change, sunstroke, motion sickness, or irritants such as smoke, dust, or pollen) (3). The most common types of headaches are migraine, cluster, tension-type, analgesic rebound, and drug-induced.

Migraine Headache

A migraine headache is defined by the International Headache Society as an idiopathic, episodic headache disorder with attacks lasting from 4 to 72 hours. The exact cause is unknown, but many medical professionals believe the primary cause to be a central nervous system event and not a vascular event (4). Women are threefold more likely than men to suffer from migraine headaches. Approximately 70% of females show a relationship between migraine headaches and their menstrual cycle. Menstrual migraines are thought to be triggered by a change in estrogen levels that accompanies the menstrual cycle (5). This fluctuation in hormone level is considered one of many **triggers** or conditions that hasten, worsen, or lengthen the duration of a migraine. Other common triggers include aspartame, caffeine (i.e., use or withdrawal), monosodium glutamate, nicotine, nitrates, alcohol, cheese, chocolate, missed meals, perfume, red grapes, too much or too little sleep, stress, bright lights, strong odors, or a change in altitude (2,6).

Classifications of Migraine Headaches

Migraines are classified into three main subgroups:

1. Migraine with aura

2. Migraine without aura

3. Complicated migraine

Migraine with aura, commonly referred to as a classic migraine, is characterized by a forewarning, also known as an **aura,** that usually precedes the onset of a migraine by less than an hour. Some of the most common auras include seeing flashes, losing part of the visual field, smelling a specific odor, tasting a specific taste, or feeling dizzy. These symptoms usually disappear once the migraine headache begins. Other classifications are described in Box 20.2.

Signs and Symptoms

If an aura does occur, it often is visual, lasting from 20 to 60 minutes before the headache. Migraine headaches typically are unilateral (but also can be bilateral), pulsating, of moderate to severe intensity, exacerbated by activity, and associated with nausea, vomiting, photophobia, phonophobia, and the desire to lie down in a dark, quiet room. Migraine headaches can last from 4 hours to 3 days.

Box 20.2   Classifications of Migraine Headaches

- **Migraine with Aura.** Characterized by a forewarning, or aura, that usually precedes the onset of a migraine by less than an hour.
- **Migraine without Aura.** Accounting for more than 80% of all migraine headaches, this type of migraine occurs without forewarning symptoms.
- **Complicated Migraine.** Neurologic symptoms occur throughout the entire headache, which can last for several days or weeks.
- **Hemiplegic Migraine.** Characterized by difficulty speaking, drowsiness, vomiting, weakness, and numbness on one side of the body with headache pain, which can last for several days to weeks.
- **Ophthalmoplegic Migraine.** Characterized by headache pain, double vision, drooping eyelids, dilated pupils, and turning of eyes in one direction lasting for several minutes to several days.
- **Basilar Artery Migraine.** Characterized by headache pain in the occipital area associated with blurred or tunnel vision, weakness, numbness, bilateral paresthesia or paresis, nausea or vomiting, vertigo, and slurred speech.

Approximately 25% of individuals who experience migraines have fewer than five headaches each month, and approximately 25% experience more than 24 headaches each year (7).

Cluster Headache

Cluster headaches are defined as severe unilateral pain, either orbitally, supraorbitally, or temporally, that last from 15 to 180 minutes. They occur from every other day to eight times per day and often wake the individual from sleep (2). Although less common than migraines, cluster headaches tend to occur more often in males between the ages of 30 and 50 years.

Signs and Symptoms

The pain is often described as unilateral "stabbing," "boring," or "burning." Pain is clustered, or grouped, and can last from 3 weeks to 3 months, followed by headache-free periods that last from months to years. The episodes often are associated with at least two of the following:

- Ipsilateral conjunctival injection
- Lacrimation
- Nasal congestion
- Rhinorrhea
- Forehead and facial sweating
- Pupillary contraction
- Lid drooping
- Eyelid edema.

Alcohol may trigger the headache.

Tension-Type Headache

This type of headache is characterized by bilateral, mild to moderate pain that is of a "pressing" or "tightening" quality in the bitemporal or occipital region.

Signs and Symptoms

Pain lasts from 30 minutes to 7 days and may be associated with mild nausea, phonophobia, and photophobia. Chronic tension-type headaches are present at least 15 days per month for at least 6 months (2).

Analgesic Rebound Headache

Daily analgesic rebound headaches often are caused by over-the-counter medications (e.g., aspirin or acetaminophen) or prescription drugs (e.g., butalbital-containing compounds or opiates).

Signs and Symptoms

The pain often begins early in the morning. The location and severity may change from day to day, and the pain is characterized by a mild, dull headache that may last from 6 to 24 hours. Other associated symptoms include nausea, anxiety, irritability, depression, or problems sleeping. Discontinuance of the analgesic medication is paramount in treating the condition (8).

Drug-Induced Headache

Drug-induced headaches may result from substances such as monosodium glutamate, nitrates, carbon monoxide, alcohol, cocaine, and chronic substance use. Acute headaches may stem from vasodilators, nonsteroidal anti-inflammatory drugs (NSAIDs), serotonin antagonists, amino acids, sex hormones, ethanol, chemotherapeutic drugs, immunomodulating drugs, and antimicrobial as well as antimalarial drugs.

Exertional Headache

Intense physical activity can lead to an exertional headache. It is defined as a vascular or tension-type headache, but the pain is brought on by exercise.

Signs and Symptoms

Individuals who are susceptible to migraines may develop a bilateral, throbbing pain that lasts from 5 minutes to 24 hours and may develop migraine-like symptoms. This type of headache can be prevented by avoiding excessive exercise, particularly in hot weather or at high altitudes.

Posttraumatic Headache

Posttraumatic headache is the most common neurologic symptom following head trauma. It can be any form of headache (e.g., migraine, cluster, or tension) that occurs after head trauma. It has been reported in up to 50% of patients after mild head injury (2).

Signs and Symptoms

Acute posttraumatic headache occurs within 14 days of trauma and disappears within 8 weeks. Chronic posttraumatic headache can last for more than 8 weeks. The condition is suspected in those with a loss of consciousness, posttraumatic amnesia that lasts more than 10 minutes, or two abnormalities found on the following: neurologic examination, skull radiograph, evoke potentials, vestibular function test, or neuropsychological testing (2). Ruling out the organic bases of the symptoms is an essential part of assessment. An individual should never be returned to activity if symptoms are present. Concerns include second-impact syndrome, vascular abnormalities, tumors, and other neurologic disorders.

Treatment of Headaches

Treatment begins with a history and description of the headache while ruling out metabolic and structural etiologies. Most headaches are treated with drug therapy; however, the longer that symptoms go untreated, the less likely that medication will relieve the pain. Over-the-counter pain relievers, such as ibuprofen, naproxen, and caffeine, or NSAIDs may be sufficient. Prescription medications used for intense headaches include drugs intended to prevent the migraine from occurring and abortive drugs to stop the headache after it begins.

Preventive treatment may be warranted if headaches interfere with daily activities or occur more than four times per month. A number of drugs and alternative therapeutic techniques can be used, including β-blockers, calcium channel blockers, antidepressants, selective serotonin-reuptake inhibitors, monoamine oxidase inhibitors, NSAIDs, and corticosteroids. Stress reduction and biofeedback techniques also have been successful for some patients. If medications and stress reduction techniques are not helpful, a computed tomographic scan or magnetic resonance image may be necessary to determine if a structural disorder of the central nervous system is causing the pain (5).

The female basketball player most likely has a migraine headache. Her history is consistent with a migraine headache, including throbbing or pounding headache pain associated with light sensitivity, loss of appetite, and/or nausea four or more times per month. If the headache does not respond to an over-the-counter anti-inflammatory or analgesic medication, referral to a physician is warranted.

SEIZURE DISORDERS AND EPILEPSY

What issues should be addressed in determining the sport participation level of an individual with a seizure disorder?

A **seizure** is an abnormal electrical discharge in the brain. A **seizure disorder** entails recurrent episodes of sudden, excessive charges of electrical activity in the brain, whether from known or idiopathic causes. **Epilepsy** is a general term used to describe only recurrent (at least two) idiopathic episodes of sudden, excessive discharges of electrical activity in the brain (9,10). The discharge may trigger altered sensation, perception, behavior, mood, level of consciousness, or convulsive movements. Seizures and epilepsy often are used interchangeably; however, it is important to understand their definitions.

Causes of Epilepsy

Epilepsy appears to be directly related to age of onset and generally is categorized as provoked or unprovoked (Box 20.3). Seizures that begin before 5 years of age usually are associated with mental or neurologic impairment. Seizures that begin between 5 and 15 years of age are not usually associated with a known metabolic or structural cause and are called idiopathic or unprovoked seizures. These seizures respond very well to treatment, and individuals usually can participate in physical activity with little to no restrictions. Trauma and tumors are responsible for most seizures in young adults; strokes are the most frequent cause in those 40 years and older (9,11).

Box 20.3   Causes of Epilepsy

1. Unprovoked or idiopathic (no cause of the seizure is identified)
2. Provoked:
   - Posttraumatic (e.g., skull fracture, intracranial hematoma)
   - Metabolic (e.g., hyponatremia, hypocalcemia, hypoglycemia, hypomagnesemia, dehydration)
   - Drug and drug withdrawal (e.g., alcohol, cocaine)
   - Infections (e.g., meningitis, encephalitis, brain abscess)
   - Anoxia and hypoxia
   - Cerebrovascular (e.g., stroke, intracerebral or subarachnoid hemorrhage, sinus thrombosis)
   - Hyperthermia
   - Sleep deprivation
   - Febrile seizures
   - Neoplasms (e.g., primary intracranial, carcinomatous meningitis, metastatic, lymphoma, leukemia)
   - Perinatal or hereditary (e.g., congenital anomalies, genetic and hereditary disorders, perinatal trauma)

Types of Seizures

Seizures can be divided into three basic types:

1. Partial or focal

2. Generalized

3. Special epileptic syndromes

Box 20.4 summarizes the classifications of seizures.

Partial or Focal Seizures

Partial or focal seizures have a localized onset, are focused in one particular area of the brain, and are restricted to specific areas of the body (10). Partial seizures may be subdivided into simple, in which consciousness is retained, and complex, in which consciousness is impaired.

SIGNS AND SYMPTOMS. A simple partial seizure is relatively common. It is classified according to the main clinical manifestations. The sensory manifestation includes bodily sensations and discomforts, such as tingling, numbness, "pins and needles," or loss of feeling. A motor manifestation is characterized by involuntary movements of the face, limbs, or head and may involve an inability to speak. The seizures, which can last for minutes or hours, may be followed by localized weakness or paralysis of the body part in which the seizure occurs; this condition is termed **Todd's paralysis.** The individual may experience powerful emotions, such as fear, anxiety, depression, or embarrassment, for no apparent reason. In some cases, a feeling of the mind and body separating may be reported. The person also may experience visual, olfactory, and auditory hallucinations. Psychic symptoms may include disturbing memory flashbacks or frequent, disconcerting feelings of déjà vu, in which something or someone unfamiliar seems to be familiar, or jamais vu, in which something or someone familiar seems to be unfamiliar. Time distortions, out-of-body experiences, sudden nausea, or stomach pain may occur. Consciousness is not impaired; however, a partial or focal seizure may precede a generalized seizure and serve as an aura that consciousness is about to be altered (12).

Complex partial seizures affect a larger area of the brain and, therefore, impair consciousness. They also are referred to as temporal lobe epilepsy or psychomotor seizures and are characterized by attacks of purposeful movements or experiences followed by impairment of consciousness. In other words, although appearing to be conscious, the individual is in an altered state of consciousness, an almost trance-like state. These purposeful activities and experiences may include (11):

- Emotions (e.g., depression, fear, paranoia, or crying out)

- Simple automatism (e.g., chewing, swallowing, lip smacking, chewing, or saying the same words over and over)

- Complex automatism (e.g., walking into a room, undressing, or arranging objects)

- Hallucinations (e.g., auditory, visual, gustatory, or olfactory)

Box 20.4 Classification of Seizures

1. Partial or focal seizures:
   - Simple (i.e., consciousness not impaired)
   - Complex (i.e., impairment of consciousness)
   - Partial with secondary generalization

2. Generalized seizures:
   - Tonic-clonic (i.e., grand mal)
   - Intermittent seizure
   - Continuous seizure (i.e., status epilepticus)
   - Absence (i.e., petit mal)
   - Myoclonic epilepsy
   - Posttraumatic

3. Special epileptic syndromes:
   - Febrile seizures
   - Hysterical seizures
   - Reflex epilepsy

If engaged in activity, an individual's movements usually are disorganized, confused, and unfocused, but observers may find it hard to believe that the individual does not know of his or her actions. The average seizure lasts from 1 to 5 minutes. The individual is unresponsive to verbal stimuli and may exhibit disorientation or confusion. Afterward, the individual is unable to recall the actions that took place. These types of seizures usually start between 10 and 30 years of age.

Generalized Seizures

Generalized seizures can affect the entire brain. These seizures may be further subdivided into convulsive and nonconvulsive types.

The tonic-clonic, or grand mal, seizure, is the most common and severe seizure of the convulsive type. It may occur in an intermittent or a continuous form. **Tonic** refers to prolonged contractions of skeletal muscles, whereas **clonic** refers to rhythmic contractions and relaxation of muscles in rapid succession.

An intermittent seizure may be tonic, clonic, or both, and it often is associated with loss of consciousness. Many individuals experience a sensory phenomenon (aura), such as a particular taste or smell, before the seizure. The average seizure lasts from 50 to 90 seconds but may extend up to 5 minutes. Because the unconscious, seizing individual is overtaken by the excessive electrical discharge during the seizure, control of bladder and bowel functions may be lost, resulting in urination or defecation. This action typically is embarrassing and unpleasant but not unexpected. When the seizure ends, the brain may shift into a sleep pattern. As such, the individual may be unarousable for a brief period of time (i.e., seconds to a few minutes). The muscles relax during this period, and the person awakens. Following the seizure, the person often is disoriented, confused, and lethargic and may not remember what happened.

A continuous tonic-clonic seizure (status epilepticus) is a medical emergency. Continuous convulsions can last 30 minutes or longer, or recurrent generalized convulsions can occur without the person regaining full consciousness between attacks. If the convulsions exceed 60 minutes, irreversible neuronal damage may occur. Any seizure that lasts longer than 5 minutes should be seen as indicating a serious problem. Accordingly, the emergency action plan, including summoning of emergency medical services (EMS), should be activated.

Myoclonic seizures are characterized by sporadic or continuous clonus of muscle groups. They are associated with progressive mental deterioration. These types of seizures are seldom seen in the physically active population.

Posttraumatic seizures are provoked by head trauma and are classified as impact, immediate, early, and late. Impact seizures occur at the time of trauma and are considered to result from electrochemical changes induced by the trauma. Immediate seizures occur within the first 24 hours of trauma. Early seizures occur within the first week after head trauma and often are associated with prolonged posttraumatic amnesia lasting more than 24 hours. A late seizure occurs after the first week of head trauma but primarily within 1 year, and it may be associated with a history of childhood epilepsy (5).

The typical absence, or petit mal, attack is characterized by a slight loss of consciousness, or blank staring into space, for 3 to 15 seconds without loss of body tone or falling. Slight twitching of the facial muscles, lip smacking, or fluttering of the eyelids may occur. Onset of the condition usually is between 4 and 8 years of age; it tends to resolve by age 30.

Special Epileptic Syndromes

A third category of seizures includes febrile seizures during infancy and childhood. Febrile seizures have their onset during the course of a fever usually greater than 38.9°C (102°F) and are most likely to happen while the temperature is rising rapidly. Other seizures in this category include hysterical seizures and reflex epilepsy. These conditions represent a small subgroup of seizures that occur only in response to specific stimuli, such as flickering lights, specific sounds, sudden movements, eating, or reading of words or numbers (10).

Immediate Management of Seizures

It is important that the examiner note the time at the onset and the end of a seizure. Seconds may seem like minutes; unless accurately timed, the actual length of the seizure may be exaggerated. Management of any seizure is directed toward protecting the individual from injury. Nearby objects

EMS It is essential to document the length of time of the seizure and the amount of time the individual sleeps. If a single, continuous seizure or a series of intermittent seizures exceeds 5 minutes, the emergency action plan, including summoning EMS, should be activated. If the individual has a known seizure disorder, the athletic trainer should attempt to discern the reason for the seizure. If possible, the individual should be questioned about his or her use of prescribed medication; this information should be provided to EMS on their arrival. Field Strategy 20.1 summarizes the management of a seizure.

should be removed or padded so that the individual does not strike them during uncontrollable muscle contractions. The individual should not be restrained, but the head should be protected at all times. Although the individual may bite the tongue during the seizure, nothing (e.g., fingers or any object) should be placed into the mouth. In an effort to avoid embarrassment to the individual, any observers or spectators should be removed from the area, if possible, to allow privacy. When the seizure ends, it is not unusual for the individual to fall into a sleep pattern. The examiner should ensure an adequate airway and wait until the individual awakens.

Medications and Epilepsy

Antiepileptic and anticonvulsive medications are the agents of choice for those with seizure disorders and epilepsy. These medications should be taken at least 1 to 2 hours before physical activity. The long-term goal is to control or eliminate seizure activity with the lowest doses of the fewest medications. Because anticonvulsive agents have long half-lives, they clear the body slowly and take time to build up to the therapeutic range. As such, regular, long-term administration (i.e., months to years to a lifetime) of medication is needed to keep the body level of the medication in the therapeutic range. Failure to take medication over several days can result in

FIELD STRATEGY 20.1

Management of Seizures

During the Seizure

1. Note the time that the seizure began.
2. Help the individual to a supine position; protect the head.
3. Remove glasses and loosen clothing.
4. Do not:

   ▪ Stop or restrain the person.
   ▪ Place fingers or any object in the mouth.

After the Seizure

1. Ensure an adequate airway.
2. Turn the individual to one side to allow saliva to drain from mouth.
3. Protect the person from curious bystanders.
4. Do not leave until the individual is fully awake.
5. If this is:

   A first-time seizure
   The individual should be seen
   by a physician

   A continuous seizure, or if another seizure occurs in rapid succession
   Activate the emergency action plan, including summoning emergency medical services

6. Send documentation, including a written description of:

   ▪ Type of seizure; localized or generalized.
   ▪ How it started.
   ▪ Length of time from onset until return of consciousness.
   ▪ Number of seizures.

falling out of the effective therapeutic range. Serum levels should be checked frequently for two reasons:

1. To ensure that the medication is within the therapeutic range

2. If the individual is physically active, to ensure that increased fitness levels have not altered the drug metabolism

If serum levels are too low, the risk of seizures is increased. If levels are too high, the toxic effects of the medication may depress brain activity, and as such, vital functions may not be supported. Some anticonvulsant agents may cause fatigue, headache, or nausea, whereas others may cause ataxia (13). These agents should be avoided in competitive athletes, although many anticonvulsive agents are approved by the National Collegiate Athletic Association (NCAA) and the U.S. Olympic Committee (USOC).

Physical Activity Guidelines

In nearly all instances, seizure disorders can be controlled with proper medication. Traditionally, good seizure control has been identified as being seizure-free for 6 months or a year. Participation in physical activity and sports, particularly those sports with a danger of falling, contact sports, and water sports, should be carefully evaluated by a neurologist before such participation is allowed. Several issues must be addressed in determining participation levels:

- What type of physical or sport activity is being performed?

- Is there a risk of death or severe injury if the individual has a seizure during activity?

- Is there a preexisting brain injury or any neurologic dysfunction?

- Is there a risk of potential brain injury from participation in the activity (e.g., concussion or intracranial hematoma)?

- Will exercise adversely affect seizure control?

- What are the potential effects of anticonvulsive medications on performance (e.g., impaired judgment or delayed reaction time)?

Head injury during activity participation can certainly precipitate seizures. Individuals with epilepsy, however, are no more prone to seizures after a head injury than are individuals without epilepsy. In addition, epilepsy does not increase the risk of injury while participating in sports (14), although certain activities (e.g., football, scuba diving, mountain climbing, and automobile racing) should be discouraged if they put the individual or others at risk should a seizure occur. Any individual with a history of seizures should be prohibited from boxing, regardless of seizure control. Individuals who experience frequent seizures should choose physical activities accordingly. It is highly recommended that children with seizure disorders be allowed to participate in physical activity and sports provided that good seizure control and proper supervision are available at all times.

A *In determining the sport participation level of an individual with a seizure disorder, the following areas should be addressed: the type of sport being played (i.e., contact or collision versus noncontact), the risk of death or severe injury if the individual has a seizure during activity, the presence of a preexisting brain injury or any neurologic dysfunction, the risk of potential brain injury from participation in the sport (e.g., concussion, intracranial hematoma), any adverse affect of exercise on seizure control, and the potential effects of anticonvulsive medications on sport performance (e.g., impaired judgment or delayed reaction time).*

OTHER CENTRAL NERVOUS SYSTEM DISORDERS

Q *A 35-year-old male recreational soccer player sustained an ankle injury. He reported to a sports medicine clinic for evaluation and treatment. Assessment indicated a mild inversion ankle sprain, and standard acute management was initiated. During the 2 weeks postinjury,* *the pain intensified (related as a 10+ on a scale of 1 to 10); he was unable to walk, to put any pressure on the left leg, to ascend or descend stairs, or to put any type of material (e.g., sheets, blankets, or clothes) on the ankle. He reports getting only 2 to 4 hours of sleep each night. He has been taking naproxen for the pain, but the naproxen appears to be causing nausea, vomiting, and dizziness. After completing a thorough reassessment of the ankle, the presence of an injury that supports the level of pain and dysfunction cannot be confirmed. How should this condition be managed?*

Three rare but serious central nervous system disorders can impact the physically active participant. Meningitis, an infection and inflammation of the membranes (i.e., meninges) and fluid (i.e., cerebrospinal fluid) surrounding the brain and spinal cord, most often is caused by bacteria or viruses. Encephalitis is an inflammation of the brain caused by a viral infection; the disease often is spread by insects, particularly mosquitoes that feed on infected birds and animals. Complex regional pain syndrome (CRPS), sometimes referred to as reflex sympathetic dystrophy, is an uncommon disturbance of the sympathetic nervous system (i.e., the part of the nervous system that controls blood flow and sweat glands). If not recognized early and treated immediately, each condition can have devastating effects on an individual.

Meningitis

Most cases of meningitis are caused by bacteria or a virus, but meningitis also can result from a fungal infection; parasites; a blow to the head; some types of cancer; inflammatory diseases, such as lupus; a sensitivity reaction to certain medications, especially ibuprofen (e.g., Advil or Motrin); and an infusion of gamma globulins used to treat other conditions.

Acute bacterial meningitis, which is caused primarily by the bacterium *Streptococcus pneumoniae* (pneumococcus), is considered to be a medical emergency. Acute bacterial meningitis usually is much more serious than viral meningitis and can be caused by various bacteria. Most cases occur when bacteria from an infection in another part of the body (e.g., osteomyelitis, pneumonia, or endocarditis) travels through the bloodstream to the brain and spinal cord. Bacteria also can spread directly to the brain or spine from a severe head injury (e.g., skull fracture); from an infection in the paranasal sinus, middle ear, nose, or teeth; neurosurgical procedures (e.g., cerebrospinal fluid diversion shunts); or penetrating wounds (15). The condition is contagious through exposure to the bacteria when someone with meningitis coughs or sneezes. The bacteria also can be spread through kissing or sharing eating utensils, a toothbrush, or a cigarette.

See Causes of Acute Bacterial Meningitis, available on the companion website at thePoint.

Viral meningitis, also called aseptic meningitis, usually is mild and often clears on its own in 1 to 2 weeks. Common intestinal viruses cause approximately half the cases in the United States. Viruses associated with mumps, herpes infection, or other diseases as well as polluted water also can cause viral meningitis.

Cryptococcal meningitis is a fungal form of the disease that affects approximately 10% of people with acquired immunodeficiency syndrome. Although cryptococcal meningitis can be treated effectively with antifungal medications, it tends to recur in nearly half of those affected. In these cases, a physician may recommend long-term antifungal therapy with drugs such as fluconazole (e.g., Diflucan).

Signs and Symptoms

Early symptoms of bacterial and viral meningitis are similar to those of the flu but tend to have a sudden onset (Box 20.5). Symptoms can include a high fever, severe headache, vomiting, stiffness of the neck and back, sensory disturbances, and mental confusion (6,16). During assessment, a positive Kernig's or Brudzinski's sign may be present (see Chapter 11). In older patients, **nuchal rigidity** is a classic sign.

As the disease progresses, the brain swells and may begin to bleed. Initial drowsiness may progress to stupor or coma. Meningitis is fatal in approximately 10% of cases. Unfortunately, those who survive may have serious long-term neurologic complications (e.g., deafness, blindness, loss of speech, learning disabilities, and behavior problems) or nonneurologic complications (e.g., kidney and adrenal gland failure) (15).

Box 20.5   Signs and Symptoms of Acute Bacterial Meningitis

- High fever that prevents one from eating or drinking
- Severe headache
- Chills
- Photophobia
- Vomiting
- Confusion
- Convulsion or seizure

- Irritability
- Delirium
- Progressive lethargy
- Drowsiness
- Nuchal rigidity associated with positive Kernig's and Brudzinski's signs
- An accompanying skin rash, especially near the axilla or on the hands or feet
- Rapid progression of small hemorrhages under the skin

Chronic (ongoing) forms of meningitis occur when slow-growing organisms, such as the microorganisms that cause tuberculosis, invade the membranes and fluid surrounding the brain. Although acute meningitis strikes suddenly, chronic meningitis develops over weeks or months. Nevertheless, the symptoms of chronic meningitis (i.e., headaches, fever, vomiting, and mental cloudiness) are similar to those of acute meningitis.

Management

Acute bacterial meningitis requires prompt treatment with intravenous antibiotics to ensure recovery and reduce the risk of complications. The choice of antibiotics depends on the degree of penetration of the agent through the blood-brain barrier and the bactericidal effect of the agent. Often, analyzing a sample of cerebrospinal fluid can help to identify the causative agent. In general, intravenous treatment against

Meningitis is a medical emergency. The recovery rate depends on the length of time that elapses before the patient receives treatment. If meningitis is suspected, the emergency action plan should be activated.

S. pneumoniae should extend for 10 to 14 days, followed by a course of oral antibiotics (16). Also, corticosteroids can be administered to help prevent hearing loss, which is the most common complications of the disease.

Mild cases of viral meningitis usually are treated with bed rest, plenty of fluids, and analgesics to reduce fever and relieve body aches. If meningitis is caused by the herpes virus, treatment may include a herpes group antiviral medication. Not all viruses that cause meningitis, however, have antiviral agents available for use.

Encephalitis

Encephalitis is an inflammation of the brain, especially the cerebral hemisphere, cerebellum, or brainstem, caused by a viral infection. It may occur in epidemic outbreaks. The disease often is spread by insects, particularly mosquitoes that feed on infected birds and animals. Encephalitis takes two forms:

- **Primary.** Caused by a direct viral invasion of the brain and spinal cord, the condition can be sporadic or epidemic. The most common sporadic form, herpes simplex encephalitis, may start as a minor illness with headache and fever, followed by more serious symptoms. Epidemic varieties commonly are caused by mosquito-borne viruses. The major types of mosquito-borne encephalitis that infect people in the United States are eastern equine encephalitis, western equine encephalitis, St. Louis encephalitis, La Crosse encephalitis, and more recently, West Nile encephalitis.

- **Secondary (postinfectious).** This form follows or occurs with a viral infection in another part of your body, such as chickenpox, measles (rubeola), mumps, rubella, or polio. The cause of encephalitis in some secondary cases may be a hypersensitivity reaction manifested as an overreaction of your immune system to a foreign substance.

Primary encephalitis is the most serious kind of encephalitis, but the secondary form is more common. A few thousand cases of encephalitis are reported annually in the United States. In addition, many cases likely go unreported, because people experience only mild or nonspecific symptoms. Even though mosquito-borne encephalitis is rare, encephalitis is the most common mosquito-borne disease in the United States.

Signs and Symptoms

Signs and symptoms vary with the age of the patient. In infants, there may be a sudden onset of fever, convulsions, and bulging in the soft spots (i.e., fontanelles) of the skull. Children may experience headache, fever, and drowsiness, followed by nausea, vomiting, photophobia, muscular pain, and nuchal rigidity. Adults often experience a sudden onset of fever, nausea, and vomiting accompanied by severe headache, muscle aching that may progress to tremors, and photophobia. Mental confusion and disorientation are hallmark symptoms in adults.

Management

In treating herpes simplex encephalitis, an antiviral agent, such as acyclovir, may be prescribed initially. In some cases, an anticonvulsant medication is prescribed. Anti-inflammatory drugs or medications that reduce pressure within the skull may be used as well. Because viruses that cause encephalitis do not respond to antibiotics, supportive treatment may consist of rest and a healthy diet, including plenty of liquids to help the immune system fight the virus. In some cases, physical and speech therapy may be a part of the treatment plan.

Complex Regional Pain Syndrome

Complex regional pain syndrome is the new term for pain disorders formerly called **reflex sympathetic dystrophy**. Complex regional pain syndrome requires the presence of regional pain and sensory changes following a noxious event. The pain is associated with findings such as abnormal skin color, temperature changes, abnormal sweating, hypersensitivity in the affected area, abnormal edema, and significant impairment of motor function (e.g., muscle weakness in the affected limb). The combination of these findings exceeds their expected magnitude in response to known physical damage (17). Complex regional pain syndrome is more likely to affect women (60–81% of cases) than men, and although the condition can occur at any age, it is most common in people between 40 and 60 years (18,19).

Complex regional pain syndrome occurs in two types, with similar signs and symptoms but different causes. Type I, previously known as reflex sympathetic dystrophy, occurs following an illness or injury that has not directly damaged the nerves in the affected limb. This injury could be as simple as a splinter, ankle sprain, intravenous catheter insertion, or back strain or as complex as a myocardial infarction, surgery, or infection. Type II, once referred to as **causalgia**, follows a distinct nerve injury (18). The diagnosis of CRPS is excluded by the existence of painful conditions with known pathology that could account for the degree of pain and dysfunction at the injured site.

The nature of CRPS is puzzling, and the cause is not clearly understood. It is thought that the initiating event, often minor trauma, sensitizes C-nociceptive fibers. These small-diameter axons with slow conduction velocities are polymodal, responding to mechanical, thermal, and chemical stimuli. The activation of the sympathetic nervous system permits the body to respond appropriately to injury by activating the inflammatory response. Normally, this activity decreases within minutes to hours after the injury. In CRPS, however, the sympathetic impulses do not shut off. This triggers a constant inflammatory response, causing vessels to spasm and leading to continual release of neurotransmitters, increased pain, and tissue destruction.

Signs and Symptoms

Signs and symptoms of both types of CRPS develop in three stages (Box 20.6). Some people never progress past stage 1, and only a small percentage of those affected advance to stage 3. Signs and symptoms initially appear only near the site of the injury. Pain, usually located in the distal part of an extremity, is described as burning or aching and is aggravated by movement or lowering the affected limb. Tapping on the skin (i.e., Tinel's sign) may increase pain, or sudden jolts of sharp pain may occur, especially at trigger points (18).

Box 20.6 Signs and Symptoms of Complex Regional Pain Syndrome

Stage 1: Generally lasts from 1 to 3 months and is characterized by:
- Severe burning or aching pain, tenderness, and swelling limited to the site of injury
- Changes in skin temperature, color, and texture. The skin may be sweaty or cold. Skin color can range from white and mottled to red or blue. The skin may become tender, thin, or shiny in the affected area
- Increased hair and nail growth
- Muscle cramps or spasms
- Edema and joint stiffness restrict mobility

Stage 2: Generally lasts from 3 to 6 months and is marked by:
- Pain intensifies and spreads; pain is disproportionate to the injury
- Edema increases
- More pronounced changes in skin color and texture
- Hair becomes coarse, then scant; nails become brittle, cracked, and grooved
- Muscle and joint stiffness increases; atrophy occurs

Stage 3: Permanent damage occurs. Signs and symptoms may include:
- Debilitating pain that may now affect an entire limb
- Muscle atrophy and advanced joint damage, causing reduced mobility in the affected part of your body
- Flexion tendon contractures
- Irreversible skin damage
- Osteoporosis

Initially, the affected limb usually is warmer, shows a red and sometimes mottled discoloration, and has pronounced distal edema. Skin temperature can shift from hyperthermic to hypothermic during the later course of the disease. Substantial muscle weakness in the affected limb that is disproportionate to the injury also can be reported. Nails become brittle and grooved, and regional hair growth increases. The skin appears to be thin and glossy; eventually, hyperkeratosis and palmar or plantar fibrosis may be present (17).

The illness can spread from its source to elsewhere in the body in the following patterns:

- **Continuity type.** Symptoms may migrate from the initial site of the pain; for example, from the hand to the shoulder, trunk, and face, affecting a quadrant of the body.

- **Mirror-image type.** Symptoms may spread from one limb to the opposite limb.

- **Independent type.** Symptoms may leap to a distant part of the body.

Management

Dramatic improvement and even remission of CRPS are possible if treatment begins within a few months of the initial symptoms. The main goal of the treatment plan is pain relief, functional recovery, and psychological improvement. Over-the-counter NSAIDs, such as aspirin, ibuprofen (e.g., Advil or Motrin), and naproxen sodium (e.g., Aleve), may ease pain and inflammation. Prescription pain relievers may be recommended in some cases. Because hypersensitivity to heat is one of the most consistent symptoms in patients with acute CRPS, cryotherapy may provide substantial relief of pain, swelling, and sweating. If the affected area is cool, applying heat may offer relief. Gentle, guided exercising of the affected limbs may improve range of motion and strength.

If the preceding treatments are not effective, the supervising physician may recommend use of the corticosteroid prednisone to reduce inflammation or may inject an anesthetic to block pain fibers in the affected nerves. Vasodilators, which traditionally are used to treat high blood pressure, may help to relieve pain in affected areas by easing blood vessel constriction. Transcutaneous electrical nerve stimulation (TENS) may be used to ease chronic pain, or biofeedback techniques may help the patient to relax the body and relieve pain symptoms. In rare cases, surgically cutting the nerves in the affected area may be recommended. This procedure is controversial, however, because it also may destroy other sensations (17).

The 35-year-old male recreational soccer player sustained an ankle inversion sprain that did not correspond to the level of the reported symptoms. The individual may be experiencing CRPS. As such, the individual should be referred to a physician for further evaluation.

SUMMARY

1. Migraine headaches are characterized by moderate to severe throbbing or pounding pain often accompanied by light sensitivity, nausea or vomiting, loss of appetite, and abdominal pain.

2. Treatment for migraine headaches is based on the type, frequency, and cause of the migraine. Most often, migraines are treated with various drug therapies.

3. A seizure disorder entails recurrent episodes of sudden, excessive charges of electrical activity in the brain, whether from known or unknown (idiopathic) causes. Epilepsy is a general term used to describe only recurrent idiopathic episodes (at least two) of sudden, excessive discharges of electrical activity in the brain. The discharge may trigger altered sensation, perception, behavior, mood, or level of consciousness or may lead to convulsive movements.

4. Seizures are classified as partial, generalized, or special epileptic syndromes.

5. The most serious seizure is the tonic-clonic seizure, which may occur in an intermittent or a continuous form. An intermittent seizure, which usually only lasts from 50 to 90 seconds but may extend to 5 minutes, often is preceded by a particular taste or smell (aura).

6. The typical absence (petit mal) attack is characterized by a slight loss of consciousness or blank staring into space for 3 to 15 seconds without loss of body tone or falling.

7. The simple partial seizure is characterized by involuntary movements of the face, limbs, or head, and the individual may experience tingling or numbness. The localized motor seizures may be followed by localized weakness or paralysis of the body part in which the seizure occurs.

8. Complex partial (psychomotor) seizures are characterized by purposeful movements or experiences followed by impairment in consciousness.

9. Management of any seizure is directed toward protecting the individual from injury. The area surrounding the individual should be clear of objects; immovable objects should be padded. The individual should not be restrained, but the head should be protected at all times. Nothing should be placed in the mouth of an individual having a seizure. When the seizure ends, an adequate airway should be ensured. If the time of the seizure exceeds 5 minutes, activation of the emergency action plan is warranted.

10. In the majority of cases, individuals with a seizure disorder can be allowed to participate in certain physical activities and sports provided that good seizure control and proper supervision are available at all times.

11. Certain activities (e.g., football, scuba diving, mountain climbing, and automobile racing) may put the individual or others at risk if a seizure occurs. Participation in these activities should be discouraged.

12. Meningitis, an infection and inflammation of the membranes (meninges) and fluid (cerebrospinal fluid) surrounding the brain and spinal cord, most often is caused by bacteria or viruses.

13. Encephalitis is an inflammation of the brain caused by a viral infection. The disease often is spread by insects, particularly mosquitoes that feed on infected birds and animals.

14. Complex regional pain syndrome, sometimes referred to as reflex sympathetic dystrophy, is an uncommon disturbance of the sympathetic nervous system. The condition often is associated with intense pain, abnormal skin color, temperature changes, hypersensitivity to touch, edema, and motor dysfunction not proportionate to the injury.

REFERENCES

1. Lipton RB, Scher AI, Kolodner K, et al. Migraine in the United States epidemiology and patterns of health care. Neurology 2002;58(6):885–894.
2. Putukian M. Headaches in the athlete. In: Mellion MB, Walsh WM, Madden C, Putukian M, Shelton GL, eds. The Team Physician's Handbook. Philadelphia: Hanley & Belfus, 2002.
3. Tamparo CD, Lewis MA. Diseases of the Human Body. Philadelphia: FA Davis, 2000.
4. Goadsby PJ. Migraine: current understanding and therapy. N Engl J Med 2002;346(4):257–270.
5. Robbins L, Lang SS. Headache Help: A Complete Guide to Understanding Headaches and the Medicines that Relieve Them. MA: Houghton Mifflin. National Headache Foundation, 1998.
6. Diamond S, Still B, Still C. Migraines and Other Headaches. MA: Houghton Mifflin. National Headache Foundation, 1995.
7. Lawrence EC. Diagnosis and management of migraine headaches. South Med J 2004;97(11):1069–1077.
8. American Academy of Family Physicians. Rebound headaches. Today's Fam Physician 2004;70(12): 2313–2314.
9. Lang D. Seizure disorders and physical activity. Your Patient and Fitness 1996;10(5):24e–24k.
10. Agnew CM, Nystul MS, Conner MC. Seizure disorders: an alternative explanation for students' inattention. Prof Sch Coun 1998;2(1):54–60.
11. Jordan BD, Sundell R. Epilepsy and the athlete. In: Mellion MB, Walsh WM, Madden C, Putukian M, Shelton GL, eds. The Team Physicians' Handbook. Philadelphia: Hanley & Belfus, 2002.
12. Kistner D, DeWeaver KL. Nonconvulsive seizure disorders: importance and implications for school social workers. Soc Work Ed 1997;19(2):73–86.
13. Martin M, Yates WN. Therapeutic Medications in Sports. Baltimore: Williams & Wilkins, 1998.
14. Nakkan KO, et al. Effect of physical training on aerobic capacity, seizure occurrence, and serum level of antiepileptic drugs in adults with epilepsy. Epilepsia 1990;31(1):88–94.
15. Saez-Lioren X, McCracken GH Jr. Bacterial meningitis in children. Lancet 2003;361(9375):2139–2148.
16. Choi C. Bacterial meningitis in aging adults. Aging Infect Dis 2002;33(8):1380–1385.
17. Vacariu G. Complex regional pain syndrome. Disabil Rehab 2002;24(8):435–442.
18. Miller RLS. Reflex sympathetic dystrophy. Orthop Nursing 2003;22(2):91–99.
19. Ghai B, Dureja GP. Complex regional pain syndrome: a review. J Postgrad Med 2004;50(4):300–307.

Respiratory Tract Conditions

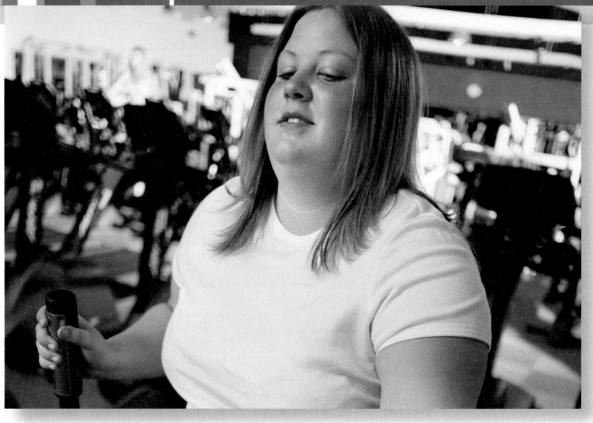

STUDENT OUTCOMES

1. Explain the physiologic factors associated with common respiratory tract conditions.

2. Identify the signs and symptoms of common upper respiratory tract conditions, including the common cold, sinusitis, pharyngitis, laryngitis, tonsillitis, and allergic rhinitis.

3. Describe the strategies that can be used to prevent the common cold.

4. Identify the signs and symptoms of general respiratory conditions, including bronchitis, bronchial asthma, exercise-induced bronchospasm, influenza, and pneumonia.

5. Describe the management of common respiratory tract conditions.

6. Explain the use of metered-dose inhalers and peak flowmeter in the management of asthma.

ROLE DELINEATION COMPETENCIES

The following Performance Domains and Tasks defined in the National Athletic Trainers' Association Board of Certification *Role Delineation Study*, 5th Edition are addressed in this chapter:

BOC COMPETENCIES

II.   Clinical Evaluation and Diagnosis

E. Formulate a clinical impression by interpreting the signs, symptoms, and predisposing factors of the injury, illness, or condition to determine the appropriate course of action.

F. Educate the appropriate individual(s) regarding the assessment by communicating information about the current or potential injury, illness, or health-related condition to encourage compliance with recommended care.

III.   Immediate Care

A. Employ life-saving techniques through the use of standard emergency procedures in order to reduce morbidity and the incidence of mortality.

B. Prevent exacerbation of non–life threatening condition(s) through the use of standard procedures in order to reduce morbidity.

C. Facilitate the timely transfer of care for conditions beyond the scope of practice of the athletic trainer by implementing appropriate referral strategies to stabilize and/or prevent exacerbation of the condition(s).

IV.   Treatment, Rehabilitation, and Reconditioning

D. Administer treatment for general illness and/or conditions using standard techniques and procedures to facilitate recovery, function, and/or performance.

E. Reassess the status of injuries, illnesses, and/or conditions using standard techniques and documentation strategies in order to determine appropriate treatment, rehabilitation, and/or reconditioning and to evaluate readiness to return to a desired level of activity.

Healthy lungs consist of an elastic network of air passageways and spaces that are bound together by connective tissue. Although the lungs occupy the majority of the thoracic cavity, each lung only weighs approximately 0.6 kg (1.25 lb). The left lung is smaller than the right lung, because it contains a concavity known as the cardiac notch, in which the heart is nestled. The lungs extend distally to the level of, or slightly below, the 12th rib in 80% of people and to the L_1 spinal level in approximately 18% of individuals. The primary bronchial tubes branch obliquely downward from the trachea, then branch into approximately 23 levels until the terminal bronchioles are reached (Fig. 21.1). These tiny air sacs, called alveoli, serve as diffusion chambers where oxygen from the lungs enters adjacent capillaries and carbon dioxide from the blood is returned to the lungs.

Conditions of the respiratory tract are common. Resistance to these conditions can be suppressed by a variety of factors, including fatigue, chronic inflammation from a localized infection, environment (e.g., allergens, dust, and smog), and psychological stress. In this chapter, common upper respiratory tract infections and general respiratory conditions are discussed.

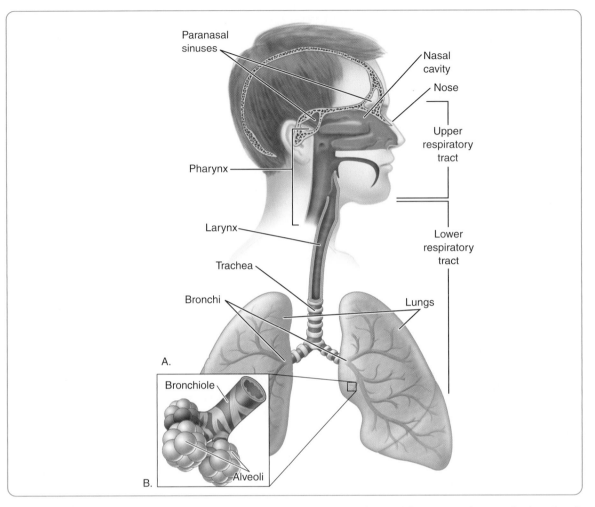

Upper
respiratory
tract

Lower
respiratory
tract

A.

B.

▬▬ ▮▮ FIGURE 21.1 **Respiratory system. A,** The trachea, bronchi, and lungs. **B,** The terminal ends of the bronchial tree are alveolar sacs, where oxygen and carbon dioxide are exchanged.

UPPER RESPIRATORY TRACT INFECTIONS

A swimmer appears to have a common cold. What additional signs and symptoms would suggest that the swimmer has sinusitis?

Viral conditions often are referred to as upper respiratory infections (URIs). These conditions, although minor, can clearly impact one's performance, especially if a fever is present. In general, individuals should not participate in physical activity if they have a fever (≥100.5°F), severe **malaise, myalgias,** weakness, shortness of breath, and/or severe cough or if they are dehydrated (1). Fever decreases strength, aerobic power, endurance, coordination, and concentration, and it can lead to injury or heat illness. Dehydration magnifies the effects of fever and also can lead to heat illness. In this section, the common cold, sinusitis, pharyngitis, laryngitis, tonsillitis, and allergic rhinitis (i.e., hay fever) are discussed.

Common Cold

The average adult has from one to six colds each year, with human rhinoviruses accounting for 40 to 50% of these infections. The majority of colds occur during the fall and spring months (2). The condition may be triggered by aspirin sensitivity, use of oral contraceptives, topical decongestant abuse, cocaine abuse, presence of nasal polyps or a deviated septum, or allergic conditions. A

Box 21.1 Strategies to Reduce the Risk of Getting a Cold

- Avoid contact with individuals who have upper respiratory infections (URIs), particularly children, who tend to have more frequent URIs.
- In the presence of individuals who have URIs, avoid touching objects or sharing objects that they have touched.
- Wash the hands frequently during cold season, and avoid touching the eyes and nose with the fingers. This will prevent many viruses from reaching the mucus membranes.
- Drink plenty of clear, nonalcoholic fluids.
- Although vitamin C supplements will not decrease the incidence of colds, they will decrease the duration and severity of symptoms.
- Reduce environmental factors (e.g., dust, smog, allergens) that may be a predisposing factor for rhinitis.
- Reduce stress.
- If using a topical decongestant, follow the instructions carefully. Do not prolong its use, because rebound rhinitis may occur. Use decongestants during the day and, because of their sedative effect, antihistamines at night.
- If cold symptoms are mild, exercise is safe. If, however, symptoms include headache, fever, muscule aches, hacking productive cough, or loss of appetite, then exercise should cease. Rest is best.

cold can be quite contagious and can be transmitted either by person-to-person contact or by airborne droplets; however, several strategies can be implemented to reduce the risk of getting a cold (Box 21.1).

Upper respiratory symptoms usually begin 1 to 2 days after exposure and generally last for 1 to 2 weeks. Viral shedding and contagion, however, can continue for another 2 or 3 weeks (3). Although many individuals feel that performance in sport and physical activity is hindered by a cold, a recent study of male and female athletes who underwent a resting pulmonary function test and submaximal exercise test during a healthy state and a state of peak illness found no significant impairment of pulmonary function, maximum oxygen consumption, maximum heart rate, or rate of perceived exertion (4).

Signs and Symptoms

Symptoms include a rapid onset of **rhinorrhea**, nasal itching, sneezing, nonproductive cough, and associated itching and puffiness of the eyes. **Malaise**, a mild sore throat, chills, and, in some cases, low-grade fever also may be present. Although most cold symptoms are benign and confined to the upper respiratory tract, colds can lead to middle ear infections and bacterial sinusitis when airflow is obstructed by swollen nasal membranes.

Management

Although no cure for the viral common cold is known, over-the-counter (OTC) medications can alleviate or lessen the symptoms. Vitamin C supplements can decrease the duration of cold episodes and the severity of symptoms. Likewise, zinc gluconate in the form of throat lozenges also has been shown to decrease the duration of cold episodes and the severity of symptoms if started within 24 to 48 hours of onset (5). If environmental factors, allergens, bacterial infections, or stressful life events are the cause, treatment involves rest, reducing contributing factors, and using topical therapy delivered through pump sprays rather than systemic therapy. When compared to OTC squeeze containers, pump sprays offer better dosage control and provide less irritation to the interior nose, particularly the septum. Topical medications may include antiasthmatic agents (e.g., cromolyn sodium [NasalCrom]), corticosteroids (e.g., beclomethasone or flunisolide), and anticholinergics (e.g., nasal ipratropium or atropine in saline). Caution should be observed when any of the preceding medications are used by competitive athletes, however, because an agent may be on the list of banned substances, particularly at high competitive levels.

FIGURE 21.2 Facial sinuses. The frontal and ethmoid sinuses are more commonly involved in sinusitis.

Sinusitis

Sinusitis is an inflammation of the paranasal sinus caused by a bacterial or viral infection, allergy, or environmental factors (Fig. 21.2). Sinusitis can be acute, lasting for less than 30 days; subacute, lasting for 3 weeks to 2 months; or chronic, lasting for longer than 2 months. The condition often is triggered by an obstruction of the passageway between the sinuses (i.e., ostium) because of local mucosal swelling and insult or by mechanical obstruction. Local mucosal swelling may be secondary to an upper respiratory tract infection, allergy, or direct trauma. Mechanical obstruction may be caused by a deviated septum; concha bullosa, which is the vesicle of serum or blood located on the concha inside the nose; or nasal masses from polyps or tumors.

Signs and Symptoms

A sinus infection should be suspected when cold symptoms last for longer than 7 to 10 day or if cold symptoms start to improve but then become worse once again. Nasal congestion, facial pain or pressure over the involved sinus, pain in the upper teeth, or pain and pressure behind the eyes (i.e., retro-orbital) are present. Other symptoms may include purulent nasal discharge, palpable pain over the involved sinus, nighttime and daytime coughing, and in severe cases, perinasal and eyelid swelling, fever, and chills. Drainage with bacterial infections most likely is dark in color, whereas drainage from other causes usually is clear. Chronic sinusitis is characterized by chronic nasal congestion, rhinorrhea or postnasal discharge accompanied by perinasal pressure, and headache not associated with migraine or muscle tension. The individual often pinches the bridge of the nose to demonstrate the area of discomfort or reports discomfort that is aggravated by eyeglasses.

Management

Treatment involves controlling the infection, reducing mucosal edema, and allowing nasal discharge. Oral antibiotics, such as amoxicillin, penicillin, or erythromycin, may be prescribed; however, some patients may not see significant benefits with antibiotics (6). Topical agents, such as phenylephrine hydrochloride (e.g., Neo-Synephrine) or oxymetazoline hydrochloride (e.g., Afrin), can be used during the first 3 to 4 days of treatment to facilitate drainage. Longer use of decongestants, however, can lead to a rebound effect, whereby excessive production of mucus and edema are increased. In severe cases, surgical intervention may be necessary to drain the sinuses.

Pharyngitis (Sore Throat)

Pharyngitis may be caused by a viral, bacterial, or fungal infection of the pharynx, leading to a sore throat. The condition may result from a common cold, influenza, streptococcal infection, diphtheria, herpes simplex virus types 1 and 2, Epstein-Barr virus, gonococcal bacteria, chlamydia, or candidiasis. If caused by the bacteria *Streptococcus pyogenes* (i.e., strep throat) and inadequately treated, peritonsillar abscess, scarlet fever, rheumatic fever, or rheumatic heart disease may result. Peak seasons for pharyngitis include the late winter and early spring (7).

Signs and Symptoms

The throat typically appears to be dark red and the tonsils red and swollen, and a pus discharge may be present. Throat pain is aggravated by swallowing and may radiate along the distribution of the glossopharyngeal nerve (i.e., cranial nerve IX) to the ears. Other symptoms include rhinorrhea, swollen lymph glands, hoarseness, headache, cough, conjunctivitis, low-grade fever, and malaise. Individuals with bacterial pharyngitis generally do not have rhinorrhea, cough, or conjunctivitis (7).

Management

Treatment for streptococcal pharyngitis includes antibiotics, such as penicillin or erythromycin. Other antibiotics that may be used are amoxicillin, cephalosporins, macrolides, or clindamycin (1). In cases that do not involve streptococcal pharyngitis, treatment involves bed rest, drinking fluids, warm saline gargles, throat lozenges, and mild analgesics (e.g., aspirin or ibuprofen).

Laryngitis

In **laryngitis**, the tissues below the level of the epiglottis are swollen and inflamed. This causes swelling around the area of the vocal cords so that they cannot vibrate normally, resulting in a characteristic hoarseness of the voice. Laryngitis is a common problem, and it often occurs during the course of an upper respiratory tract infection (e.g., cold). The condition also may stem from general irritation of straining the vocal cords, as may occur in singers, politicians, cheerleaders, or other individuals who shout excessively while playing or working. Environmental causes, such as smoking, being in an environment with second-hand tobacco smoke, or being exposed to irritating chemicals, can lead to similar symptoms.

Signs and Symptoms

Laryngitis is characterized by a weak, hoarse, gravely voice as well as by sore throat, fever, cough (usually dry and nonproductive), a tickling in the back of the throat, and difficulty swallowing. Children's croup, or **acute epiglottis**, can, however, present like laryngitis. Similar to a cough, laryngitis may persist after the acute infection is over. This can be recognized by noting that the fever and ill feeling subside but the hoarseness continues for another several days to a week or longer.

Management

Laryngitis is self-limiting under most conditions. The individual should attempt to speak softly, so as not to further strain the vocal cords. Drinking warm liquids; sucking on a cough drop, throat lozenge, or hard candy; or gargling with a warm salt solution (half a teaspoon of salt in 1 cup of water) may relieve some of the symptoms. One should avoid smoking or places where cigarettes are smoked. Use of a humidifier, preferably a cool mist ultrasonic humidifier, may ease symptoms. This type of humidifier is more expensive than the usual vaporizer, but it also is safer and more effective. Standing for extended periods in a hot, steamy shower also may be helpful. Aspirin, ibuprofen, or acetaminophen may be used to reduce the fever, muscle discomfort, and pain. Aspirin, however, should not be used in someone younger than 19 years, because it can trigger an attack of **Reye's syndrome**.

The individual should be seen by a physician if any of the following conditions are present, because these symptoms may indicate a more serious underlying problem:

- Difficult breathing or swallowing
- Fever of more than 101°F
- In a young child, a deep cough like the bark of a seal
- Presence of brown, green, or yellow sputum
- Hoarseness that lasts for 1 month without any identifiable cause

Tonsillitis

The tonsils are lymph glands or nodes located at the back of the throat that help to protect the pharynx by filtering disease-producing bacteria before they enter the breathing passage. During the filtering process, the tonsils themselves may become inflamed and acutely or chronically infected. This condition, called **tonsillitis**, most often is caused by a bacterial streptococcal infection, but it also may result from viral infections, such as the flu, common cold, mononucleosis, or herpes simplex. All forms of tonsillitis are contagious and generally spread from person to person in coughs, sneezes, and nasal fluids.

Signs and Symptoms

Tonsillitis is an infectious condition that is characterized by inflamed and enlarged tonsils, fever, painful swallowing, sore throat, and a slight change in voice. Tissues surrounding the tonsils frequently form pus during acute attacks of tonsillitis, particularly streptococcal tonsillitis, causing the tonsils to show white specks or become coated with whitish exudate. Other symptoms include swollen lymph nodes, headache, and bad breath. Nausea, vomiting, and abdominal pain may occur in younger children. Pharyngitis often occurs along with tonsillitis.

Management

Acute cases of bacterial tonsillitis can be treated with antibiotics, such as penicillin, but viral tonsillitis cannot. Chronic recurrent tonsillitis may be treated by surgical removal of the tonsils, a procedure known as a tonsillectomy.

Allergic Rhinitis (Hay Fever)

Allergic rhinitis is an inflammation of the nasal mucous membranes that affects nearly 20% of children and adults in the United States (8). The risk of rhinitis increases throughout childhood and adolescence, then peaks during the late twenties and early thirties. It often is divided into seasonal allergic rhinitis, or "hay fever," and perennial allergic rhinitis. Hay fever usually involves a specific period of symptoms during successive years caused by airborne pollens or fungal spores associated with that season. In contrast, perennial allergic rhinitis occurs year-round if the individual is continually exposed to allergens such as food (e.g., shellfish or bread mold), dust, and animal emanations (e.g., hair or feathers).

Signs and Symptoms

Postnasal drainage leads to a chronic sore throat and bronchial infection. In addition, the phalangeal openings of the eustachian tubes can become blocked by swollen mucosa, enlarged lymphoid tissue, or exudate. Without normal airflow, increasing negative pressure in the middle ear results in fluid accumulation, leading to partial hearing loss and recurrent middle ear infections.

Taking a complete history is the key to differentiating allergic rhinitis from other respiratory conditions. Questions should focus on the relationship of symptoms to seasons or exposures that trigger symptoms. For example, if symptoms increase while the individual is outdoors, pollen may be the triggering agent; if symptoms increase while the individual is indoors, mold could be the culprit. In addition, certain geographic areas may have more environmental allergens than others. Individuals should try to limit their exposure to allergens when participating in different environments. Allergy tests (i.e., skin or intradermal testing) may not be necessary if a history uncovers allergens to specific environmental factors.

Management

Management involves limiting exposure to the allergen or irritant, suppressive medication to alleviate symptom severity, and specific hypersensitization to reduce responsiveness to unavoidable allergens. For example, if dust is an allergen, then having bare floors, pillows, and mattresses encased in plastic covers, minimizing cloth curtains, and avoiding cluttered tabletops can reduce the amount of dust in a home. Antihistamine drugs (e.g., Benadryl, Tavist-1, or Chlor-Trimeton) are effective agents in reducing symptoms of allergic rhinitis; however, drowsiness, lethargy, mucous membrane dryness, and occasional nausea and light-headedness may be unwanted side effects in physically active individuals. Medications, including ephedrine (e.g., Fedrine, Ephedd II, or Efedron nasal jelly), isoephedrine, and phenylpropanolamine, acting as mucosal decongestants can offset sedative effects of antihistamine agents. Cromolyn sodium can reduce the symptoms of allergic rhinitis and conjunctivitis. Caution should be observed when any of the preceding medications are used by competitive athletes, however, because an agent may be on the list of banned substances, particularly at high competitive levels.

In addition to the signs and symptoms associated with the common cold, sinusitis would be suggested if the swimmer exhibits nasal congestion, facial pain over the sinus region, pain behind the eyes, and coughing.

GENERAL RESPIRATORY CONDITIONS

 A softball player has exercise-induced bronchospasm. What conditions might contribute to the severity of this respiratory problem?

General respiratory conditions may result from infection or irritation from inhaled particles and substances. Bronchitis, bronchial asthma, and exercise-induced bronchospasm (EIB; formerly called exercise-induced asthma), influenza, and pneumonia are discussed.

Bronchitis

Bronchitis is inflammation of the mucosal lining of the tracheobronchial tree. The condition results from infection or inhaled particles and substances. It may be acute or chronic. The most common causes stem from viruses (e.g., parainfluenza, respiratory syncytial, adenoviruses, rhinoviruses, influenza viruses, or enteroviruses) and bacteria (e.g., *Mycoplasma pneumoniae*, *Chlamydia pneumoniae*, or *Bordatella pertussis*) (1).

Signs and Symptoms

Acute bronchitis, which commonly is seen in physically active individuals, involves bronchial swelling, mucus secretion, and increased resistance to expiration. Coughing, wheezing, and large amounts of purulent mucus are present. Once the stimulus is removed, however, the swelling decreases and the airways return to normal.

Chronic bronchitis is characterized by a productive daily cough for at least three consecutive months in two successive years. Irritation may result from cigarette smoke, air pollution, or infections. This condition can progress to increased airway obstruction, heart failure, and cellular changes in respiratory epithelial cells that may become malignant. Signs and symptoms include marked cyanosis, edema, large production of sputum, and abnormally high levels of carbon dioxide as well as low levels of oxygen in the blood. This condition often is seen simultaneously with emphysema.

Management

No specific therapy is available for most types of viral bronchitis. Most cases, however, subside after a few days or a week. Limited prescribed medication is available if the cause stems from influenza viruses. Bacteria-related bronchitis is treated more effectively with macrolides. Fever associated with the conditions may be managed with acetaminophen or ibuprofen. Aspirin, however, should not be used for individuals younger than 19 years, because it increases the incidence of Reye's syndrome (1).

Bronchial Asthma

Asthma is caused by a constriction of bronchial smooth muscles (bronchospasm), increased bronchial secretions, and mucosal swelling, all leading to an inadequate air-flow during respiration (especially expiration) (Fig. 21.3). The condition is classified as intermittent, seasonal, or chronic. Intermittent asthma usually is of relatively short duration, occurring less than 5 days per month with extended, symptom-free periods. Symptoms of seasonal asthma occur for prolonged periods as a result of exposure to seasonal inhalant allergens. Chronic asthma occurs daily or near daily, with an absence of extended, symptom-free periods.

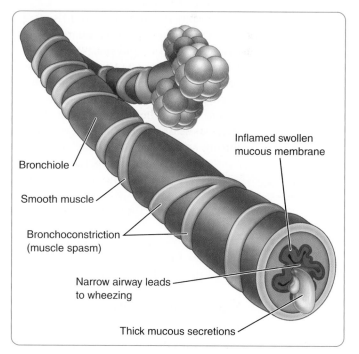

FIGURE 21.3 Bronchospasm. An asthma attack is caused by bronchospasm that constricts the bronchiolar tubes. This spasm, combined with increased bronchial secretions and mucosal swelling, results in a characteristic, loud wheezing sound that is heard during expiration.

Signs and Symptoms

Wheezing is a common sign that results from air squeezing past the narrowed airways. Because the airways cannot fill or empty adequately, the diaphragm tends to flatten, and the accessory muscles must work harder to enlarge the chest during inspiration. This increased workload leads to a rapid onset of fatigue when the individual can no longer hyperventilate enough to meet the increased oxygen need. Acute attacks may occur spontaneously, but they often are provoked by a viral infection.

A large amount of thick, yellow or green sputum is produced by the bronchial mucosa. As dyspnea continues, anxiety, loud wheezing, sweating, rapid heart rate, and labored breathing develop. In severe cases, respiratory failure may be indicated by cyanosis, decreased wheezing, and decreased levels of consciousness.

Management

Individuals who are diagnosed with asthma typically carry medication that is delivered by a compressor-driven nebulizer or inhaler to alleviate the attack. The value of bronchodilators in children and young adults, however, continues to be debated. Medications involve selective bronchodilators, aerosol corticosteroids, and cromolyn sodium, which is an antihistamine drug that prevents the release of chemical mediators that cause bronchospasms and inflammatory changes of the mucous membrane. Once the attack has subsided, the lungs usually return to normal.

Exercise-Induced Bronchospasm

Exercise-induced bronchospasm affects up to 90% of those with asthma and up to 35% of those without known asthma. Factors contributing to the severity of EIB include ambient air conditions (e.g., cold air, low humidity, and pollutants); duration, type, and intensity of exercise; exposure to allergens in sensitized individuals; overall control of asthma; poor physical conditioning; respiratory infections; time since the last episode of EIB; and any underlying bronchial hyperreactivity (9). Individuals suffering from allergies, sinus disease, or hyperventilation may be at increased risk for EIB, and symptoms can be exacerbated for those with bronchitis, emphysema, and other diseases affecting the bronchial tubes.

Despite the prevalence of EIB, the precise mechanisms that are responsible for it remain unknown. Theories include hyperventilation resulting in airway heat and water loss, carbon dioxide loss with hyperventilation, and release of chemical mediators causing bronchospasm; however, these theories have not been substantiated. It is thought that breathing dry, cold air through the mouth stimulates bronchospasm. As such, breathing through the nose or covering the nose and mouth when exercising in cold weather can warm and humidify the air and lessen the onset of symptoms. Swimming in an indoor pool, where the air typically is warm and humid, also may prevent the onset of symptoms. Regardless of the mechanism, the amount of ventilation and the temperature of the inspired air both during and after exercise are important factors in determining the severity of EIB. The greater the ventilations (i.e., volume of air inspired) in cold, dry, air, the greater the risk of EIB, and the more strenuous the exercise, the greater the ventilations.

See *Field Strategy: Use of a Peak Flowmeter,* available on the companion website at thePoint.

Recently, EIB has been diagnosed according to forced expiratory volume at 1 second (FEV_1) using a peak flowmeter. Normally, individuals can have up to a 10% decrease in FEV_1 postexercise. When FEV_1 drops by 10 to 20%, however, the individual is considered to have mild EIB. A drop of 20 to 40% indicates moderate to severe EIB, and a drop of more than 40% indicates severe EIB (10). Several questions can be asked during the history to help screen for EIB (Box 21.2).

Signs and Symptoms

EIB occurs in three distinct phases. In the first phase, symptoms peak 5 to 10 minutes after exercise begins, and they last for 30 to 60 minutes. Common signs and symptoms of EIB include chest pain, chest tightness, or a burning sensation with or without wheezing; a regular, dry cough; shortness of breath shortly after or during exercise; and stomach cramps after exercise. Exercise-induced bronchospasm symptoms typically appear after 8 to 10 minutes of vigorous exercise and may worsen after activity is terminated. Episodes usually remit completely within 30 to 60 minutes and

Box 21.2 History Questions to Screen for EIB

- Have you ever been told that you have asthma or exercise-induced bronchospasm?
- Do you ever have chest pain or tightness during or following exercise?
- Do you ever wheeze during or after moderate exercise?
- Do you ever have shortness of breath during or after exercise?
- Do you ever have itching of the nose or throat, or sneezing episodes during or after exercise?
- Have you ever experienced stomach cramps after exercise?
- Have you ever missed work or school because of chest pain, chest tightness, coughing, wheezing, or prolonged shortness of breath?

do not increase airway reactivity or induce long-term deterioration in lung function. Approximately 50% of individuals with EIB experience the second phase, a "refractory" period. This phase starts 30 minutes to 4 hours after exercise begins and is associated with limited to no bronchospasm. During this period, it may be possible to exercise longer and more strenuously without difficulty. The final phase involves symptoms similar to those experienced during the first phase, but these symptoms are less severe. Symptoms recur 12 to 16 hours after exercise is completed and usually remit within 24 hours (11–13).

Management

Management includes medications used in regular asthma treatment, such as short-acting bronchodilators, cromolyn sodium, nedocromil sodium, oral theophylline, and the leukotriene modifiers zafirlukast and zileuton (9,12). Competitive athletes, however, should consult with the appropriate governing sport body to ensure the medication is legal for competition.

See *Field Strategy: Use of a Metered-Dose Inhaler*, available on the companion website at thePoint.

Children and young adults who have asthma, are physically fit, and are free of significant airway obstruction respond to exercise similar to individuals without asthma. Many strenuous physical activities are well tolerated when preceded by a 10- to 15-minute warm-up period at 60% of maximum heart rate performed a half-hour before the more intense activity. Following the warm-up period, a short-acting inhaler should be used to protect against an attack for 2 to 6 hours. Using an inhaler by itself does not always allow a full dose of medication to be delivered to the lungs; as such, adjunct medications can be used with metered-dose inhalers to enhance the delivery and more evenly distribute the medication to the bronchial tubes and lungs. Following activity, a cool-down period allows a gradual rewarming of the airways and makes postactivity symptoms less likely (12). *Field Strategy 21.1* presents a management algorithm for individuals with EIB.

Influenza

Influenza, or "the flu," is a specific viral bronchitis caused by *Haemophilus influenza* type A, B, or C. It often occurs in epidemic proportions, particularly among school-aged children. Immunization for the type A and B viruses is available for individuals who are at high risk, including pregnant women; individuals with chronic illness, such as diabetes mellitus and disorders of the pulmonary or cardiovascular system; children; and those with immunocompromised systems. Individuals with a fever should not be immunized until the fever has passed.

Signs and Symptoms

A fever of 39 to 39.5°C (102–103°F), chills, malaise, headache, general muscle aches, hacking cough, and inflamed mucous membranes may be present. Rapid onset of symptoms can occur within 24 to 48 hours after exposure to the virus. Sore throat, watery eyes, photophobia, and a nonproductive cough may linger for up to 5 days. In some cases, the cough may progress to bronchitis.

FIELD STRATEGY 21.1

Management Algorithm for Exercise-Induced Bronchospasm

General Recommendations

- Consult a physician before beginning an exercise program
- Take medication for asthma as prescribed to achieve overall control of asthmatic symptoms, including those caused by exercise and airborne allergens
- Use a peak flowmeter as directed by a physician
- Avoid exposure to air pollutants and allergens whenever possible
- Avoid exercise during the early morning hours, when the concentration of ragweed is highest

Exercise Routine

- Use a bronchodilator before exercise
- Perform a 5- to 10-minute warm-up period of moderate stretching, and work out slowly for another 10 to 15 minutes, keeping the pulse rate below 60% of maximum heart rate
- Increase the time and intensity of the workout as tolerated, especially if the activity is new
- Breathing:
  - Breathe slowly through the nose to warm and humidify the air. Exercise in a warm, humid environment, such as a heated swimming pool.
  - In cold, dry environments, breathe through a mask or a scarf. Alternatively, consider different locations and types of exercise during winter months, such as swimming, running, or cycling indoors.
- Perform a gradual 10- to 30-minute cool-down period after a vigorous workout:
  - This avoids rapid thermal changes in the airways.
  - This can be achieved by slowing to a less intense pace while jogging, cycling, swimming, and stretching.

Management

Initial treatment consists of rest, plenty of fluids, saltwater gargles, cough medication, and analgesics to control fever, aches, and pains. If the temperature does not return to near normal within 24 hours, the individual should be seen immediately by a physician to rule out other infectious conditions.

Pneumonia

Pneumonia is an inflammation and infection of the lungs that may be caused by bacteria, viruses, mycoplasmas, or other infectious agents, such as fungi, including *Pneumocystis* sp., and by various chemicals. Individuals at an increased risk of pneumonia include those age 65 or older; very young children, whose immune systems are not fully developed; those with an immunodeficiency disease (e.g., acquired immunodeficiency syndrome [AIDS]) or a chronic illness (e.g., cardiovascular disease, emphysema, or diabetes); individuals who have had their spleen removed; and individuals whose immune system has been impaired by chemotherapy or long-term use of immunosuppressant drugs. Smoking and abusing alcohol or drugs also can place one at higher risk. Smoking damages the airways, and alcohol interferes with the action of the white blood cells that fight infection. Use of intravenous drugs can lead to injection-site infections that can travel through the bloodstream to the lungs. In addition, exposure to air pollutants or toxic fumes from certain agricultural, construction, and industrial chemicals may contribute to some types of pneumonia.

Pneumonia bacteria are present in some healthy throats. When body defenses are weakened in some way, such as by illness, old age, malnutrition, general debility, or impaired immunity, the bacteria can multiply and cause serious damage. Usually, when a person's resistance is lowered, bacteria work their way into the lungs and inflame the alveoli. The alveoli then fill with pus and other liquids, preventing oxygen from transferring into the bloodstream. The tissue from either part of a lobe of the lung, an entire lobe, or most of the lung's five lobes becomes completely filled with liquid. The infection quickly spreads through the bloodstream, and the whole body is invaded. In some cases, this may lead to death. *Streptococcus pneumoniae* is the most common cause of bacterial pneumonia, and it is one form of pneumonia for which a vaccine is available. Pneumonia can affect one or both lungs. Infection of both lungs is popularly referred to as double pneumonia.

Signs and Symptoms

The signs and symptoms of pneumonia vary greatly, depending on the type of organism causing the infection and any underlying conditions that may be present. Bacterial pneumonia often follows a URI, such as a cold or flu. Signs and symptoms are likely to present suddenly and include shaking, chills, high fever, sweating, chest pain (pleurisy), and a cough that produces thick phlegm that is rust, green, or yellow in color. Symptoms may be fewer or milder in older adults or in those with a chronic illness (1).

Viral pneumonia, which is caused by some of the same viruses that cause influenza, strikes primarily during the fall and winter and tends to be more serious in people with cardiovascular or lung disease. It usually starts with a dry and nonproductive cough, headache, fever, muscle pain, and fatigue. As the condition progresses, the individual may become breathless, develop a cough that produces phlegm, and run the risk of developing a secondary bacterial pneumonia as well.

Mycoplasmas are tiny organisms that cause symptoms similar to those of both bacterial and viral pneumonia, although these symptoms appear more gradually and often are milder. Mycoplasmas often cause the type of pneumonia seen in individuals with walking pneumonia. The individual is not sick enough to stay in bed and, therefore, may not seek medical care. This type of pneumonia spreads easily in situations where people congregate and is common in child-care centers and among school children and young adults.

Certain types of fungus also can cause pneumonia, especially *Histoplasma capsulatum*, which is common in the Mississippi and Ohio River valleys. Some people experience no symptoms after inhaling this fungus. Others develop symptoms of acute pneumonia, and still others may develop a chronic pneumonia that persists for months.

Pneumonia caused by a parasite, *Pneumocystis carinii*, commonly affects Americans with AIDS. The signs and symptoms of *Pneumocystis carinii* pneumonia include an ongoing cough, fever, and trouble breathing.

Management

Treatment for pneumonia varies, depending on the type of pneumonia and on the severity of symptoms. Bacterial pneumonia usually is treated with antibiotics; however, antibiotics are not effective against viral forms of pneumonia. Although viral pneumonia may be treated with antiviral medications, the recommended treatment is the same as that for the flu (i.e., rest and plenty of fluids). Mycoplasmal pneumonias are treated with antibiotics. Regardless, it may take 4 to 6 weeks to recover completely if the pneumonia is serious. In some cases, fatigue may continue long after the infection itself has cleared. In addition to these treatments, the physician may recommend OTC medications to reduce fever, treat aches and pains, and soothe the cough associated with pneumonia. The aim is not to suppress the cough completely, however, because coughing helps to clear the lungs.

Conditions that could contribute to the severity of exercise-induced bronchospasm (EIB) include ambient air conditions, exposure to allergens, poor physical conditioning, respiratory infections, and amount of time since the last episode of exercise-induced bronchospasm.

SUMMARY

1. Viral conditions often are referred to as upper respiratory infections (URIs).

2. The common cold is an acute viral infection that may be triggered by aspirin sensitivity, use of oral contraceptives, abuse of topical decongestants, abuse of cocaine, presence of nasal polyps or a deviated septum, and allergic conditions.

3. Sinusitis is an inflammation of the paranasal sinus caused by a bacterial or viral infection, an allergy, or environmental factors.

4. If pharyngitis is caused by the bacteria *Streptococcus pyogenes* and is inadequately treated, peritonsillar abscess, scarlet fever, rheumatic fever, or rheumatic heart disease may result.

5. In laryngitis, the tissues below the level of the epiglottis are swollen and inflamed, preventing the vocal cords from vibrating normally, which results in hoarseness of the voice.

6. Tonsillitis is an infectious condition characterized by inflamed and enlarged tonsils, fever, painful swallowing, sore throat, and a slight change in voice.

7. Hay fever may be seasonal (i.e., caused by airborne pollens and fungal spores associated with that season) or perennial (i.e., occurs year-round if the individual is continually exposed to allergens).

8. Bronchitis may be acute or chronic, and it is characterized by bronchial swelling, mucus secretion, and increased resistance to expiration.

9. Asthma is caused by a constriction of bronchial smooth muscles (bronchospasm), increased bronchial secretions, and mucosal swelling, each leading to inadequate airflow during respiration (especially during expiration). Wheezing, a common sign of asthma, results from air squeezing past the narrowed airways. The condition is classified as intermittent, seasonal, or chronic, and it is managed with bronchodilators, aerosol corticosteroids, and cromolyn sodium.

10. Exercise-induced bronchospasm (EIB) affects up to 90% of those with asthma and up to 35% of those without known asthma. Key signs are a dry, regular cough within 8 to 10 minutes of the start of moderate exercise as well as stomach cramps after exercise.

11. Rapid onset of fever, chills, malaise, headache, general muscle aches, hacking cough, and inflamed mucous membranes indicates the onset of influenza, or "the flu." Initial treatment consists of rest, plenty of clear fluids, saltwater gargles, cough medication, and analgesics to control fever, aches, and pains.

12. Viral pneumonia, which strikes primarily during the fall and winter, tends to start with a dry and nonproductive cough, headache, fever, muscle pain, and fatigue. As the condition progresses, the individual becomes short of breath, develops a cough that produces phlegm, and runs the risk of developing a secondary bacterial pneumonia.

REFERENCES

1. Martin TJ. Infections in athletes. In: Mellion MB, Walsh WM, Madden C, Putukian M, Shelton GL, eds. The Team Physician's Handbook. Philadelphia: Hanley & Belfus, 2002.
2. Weidner TG, Gehlsen G, Schurr T, Dwyer GB. Effects of viral upper respiratory illness on running gait. J Ath Train 1997;32(4):309–314.
3. Swain RA, Kaplan B. Upper respiratory infections: treatment selection for active patients. Phys Sportsmed 1998;26(2):85–96.
4. Weidner TG, Anderson BN, Kaminsky LA, et al. Effect of a rhinovirus caused upper respiratory illness on pulmonary function test and exercise response. Med Sci Sports Exerc 1997;29(5):604–609.
5. Mossad SB, Macknin ML, Medendorf SV, et al. Zinc gluconate lozenges for treating the common cold. A randomized, double-blind, placebo-controlled study. Ann Intern Med 1996;125(2):81–88.
6. Merenstein D, Wittaker C, Chadwell T, et al. Are antibiotics beneficial for patients with sinusitis complaints: a randomized double-blind clinical trial. J Fam Pract 2005;54(2):144–150.
7. Vincent MT, Celestin N, Hussain AN. Pharyngitis. Am Fam Physician 2004;69(6);1465–1470.
8. Ferguson BJ. Allergic rhinitis: recognizing signs, symptoms, and triggering allergens. Postgrad Med 1997;101(5):110–116.
9. Rupp NT. Diagnosis and management of exercise-induced asthma. Phys Sportsmed 1996;24(1):77–87.
10. Randolph C. Exercise-induced asthma: update on pathophysiology, clinical diagnosis, and treatment. Curr Prob Pediatr 1997;27(2):53–77.
11. Tan RA, Sheldon SL. Exercise-induced asthma. Sport Med 1998;25(2):1–6.
12. Disabella V, Sherman C. Exercise for asthma patients: little risk, big rewards. Phys Sportsmed 1998;26(6):75–84.
13. Hermansen CL, Kirchner JT. Identifying exercise-induced bronchospasm. Postgrad Med 2004;115(6):15–20.

Gastrointestinal Conditions

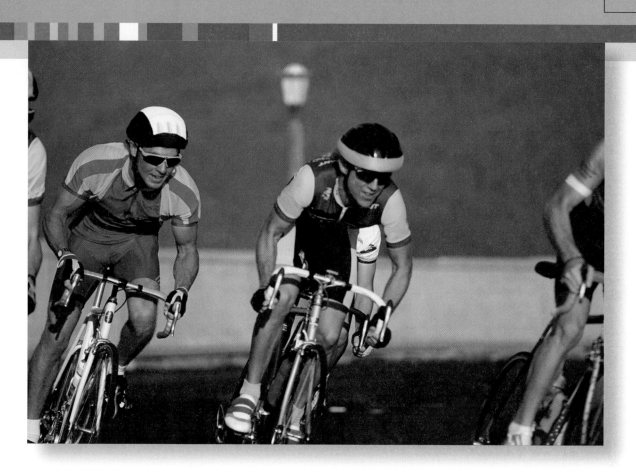

STUDENT OUTCOMES

1. Explain the physiologic factors associated with common gastrointestinal (GI) conditions.

2. Identify the common signs and symptoms associated with upper GI conditions, including dysphagia, gastroesophageal reflux, dyspepsia (indigestion), gastric (peptic) ulcers, gastritis, and gastroenteritis.

3. Identify the common signs and symptoms associated with lower GI conditions, including irritable bowel syndrome, Crohn's disease, ulcerative colitis, diarrhea, constipation, and hemorrhoids.

4. Describe the general management of upper and lower GI conditions.

5. Explain the factors that may not be related to an injury or condition specific to the upper or lower GI tract but that can adversely affect the entire GI tract.

ROLE DELINEATION COMPETENCIES

The following Performance Domains and Tasks defined in the National Athletic Trainers' Association Board of Certification *Role Delineation Study*, 5th Edition are addressed in this chapter:

BOC COMPETENCIES

II. Clinical Evaluation and Diagnosis

E. Formulate a clinical impression by interpreting the signs, symptoms, and predisposing factors of the injury, illness, or condition to determine the appropriate course of action.

F. Educate the appropriate individual(s) regarding the assessment by communicating information about the current or potential injury, illness, or health-related condition to encourage compliance with recommended care.

III. Immediate Care

A. Employ life-saving techniques through the use of standard emergency procedures in order to reduce morbidity and the incidence of mortality.

B. Prevent exacerbation of non–life threatening condition(s) through the use of standard procedures in order to reduce morbidity.

C. Facilitate the timely transfer of care for conditions beyond the scope of practice of the athletic trainer by implementing appropriate referral strategies to stabilize and/or prevent exacerbation of the condition(s).

IV. Treatment, Rehabilitation, and Reconditioning

D. Administer treatment for general illness and/or conditions using standard techniques and procedures to facilitate recovery, function, and/or performance.

E. Reassess the status of injuries, illnesses, and/or conditions using standard techniques and documentation strategies in order to determine appropriate treatment, rehabilitation, and/or reconditioning and to evaluate readiness to return to a desired level of activity.

The gastrointestinal (GI) tract extends from the mouth to the anus. It functions to absorb nutritional substances from ingested food and to expel waste (Fig. 22.1). In an active population, exercise alone can induce both upper and lower GI symptoms and problems. During the first few minutes of exercise, up to 15% of the central blood volume is shunted away from the visceral organs to the working muscles. As core temperature rises, 20% of central blood volume is shunted to the skin for cooling. This can result in the reduction of normal intestinal blood flow by as much as 80% for the purpose of maintaining an adequate central blood volume (1). Exercise-induced shunting, as it often is called, can lead to decreased esophageal motility, erosive hemorrhagic gastritis, delayed gastric emptying, diarrhea, or intestinal bleeding. Dehydration, high ambient temperature, and lack of acclimatization to exercise in the heat can exacerbate this hypoperfusion of the GI tract. Nervous tension also can lead to indigestion, diarrhea, or constipation and can adversely affect sport and physical activity. Many disorders may appear to be minor, but they can be the first sign of more serious underlying conditions.

In this chapter, disorders affecting the upper and lower GI region are discussed. Factors not specific to the upper or lower GI tract but affecting the entire GI tract also are presented.

UPPER GASTROINTESTINAL DISORDERS

Before the start of a rehabilitation session at a sports medicine clinic, a middle-aged man indicates that he has a mild fever, upset stomach, and abdominal cramps. He also states that during the previous night, he had diarrhea and experienced nausea but did not vomit. What condition might be present, and how should this situation be managed?

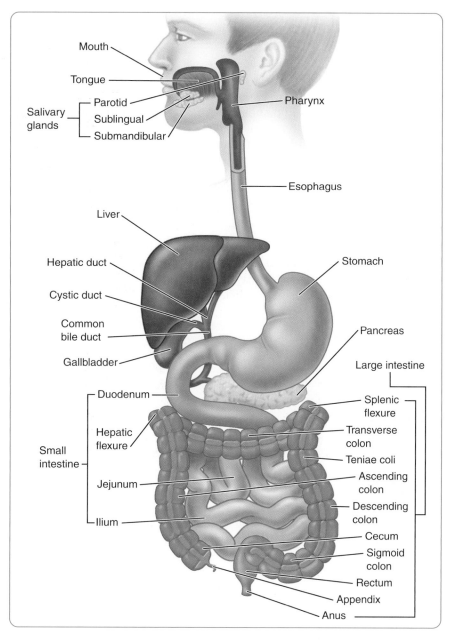

FIGURE 22.1 **The digestive system.**

Upper GI disorders (i.e., stomach and above) are caused by local irritation resulting from a variety of factors, including stress and the ingestion of caffeine, alcohol, and tomato and citric acid products. This irritation can lead to nausea, **emesis** (i.e., vomiting), bloating, abdominal cramps, and heartburn. General management includes agents containing **antacids** and diet modification.

Dysphagia

Dysphagia is associated with labored swallowing actions. Predisposing factors include a narrowing of the esophagus as well as paralysis or muscle spasms of the esophageal or pharyngeal muscles.

Signs and Symptoms

The individual will have difficulty swallowing or be unable to swallow.

Management

Any individual who exhibits dysphagia should discontinue activity and be referred immediately to a physician for further evaluation.

Gastroesophageal Reflux

When gastric juice, an extremely acidic substance, regurgitates into the esophagus, it is called **gastroesophageal reflux**. The condition is most likely to occur when an individual has eaten or drunk to excess, but it also is caused by conditions that force abdominal contents superiorly, such as obesity, pregnancy, and running. In the condition referred to as runner's reflux, the stomach contents splash upward with each step. Increasing the intensity of exercise can result in a decrease in the frequency, amplitude, and duration of esophageal contractions.

Signs and Symptoms

Gastroesophageal reflux is associated with mild heartburn, which is a burning, radiating, substernal pain. When gastroesophageal reflux is caused by a chronic exposure to gastric juices, reflux leads to physical complications, such as severe heartburn and upper chest pain. Symptoms are so similar to those of a heart attack that many first-time sufferers are rushed to the nearest medical facility.

Management

Initial management involves use of antacids 4 hours before exercise as well as changes in diet, timing of meals before exercise, and type of activity.

Dyspepsia (Indigestion)

Dyspepsia, or indigestion, is associated with upper GI pain that has no identified etiology but has been attributed to excessive acid accumulation in the stomach and overconsumption of alcohol.

Signs and Symptoms

Irregularly occurring symptoms can range from a sense of fullness after eating to feeling as though something is lodged in the esophagus to heartburn, nausea, vomiting, and loss of appetite. Pain and discomfort at the xiphoid region during digestion are the most common symptoms.

Management

Use of antacids 4 hours before exercise and activity modification may help with the discomfort. If symptoms persist, immediate referral to a physician is warranted to rule out more serious abdominal conditions or diseases.

Gastric (Peptic) Ulcer

Gastric ulcers occur at the lower end of the esophagus, in the stomach, or in the duodenum. Excessive production of gastric acid usually is a precursor, along with consumption of excessive alcohol, spicy or salty foods, pepper or caffeinated drinks, salicylates, and use of tobacco products, particularly cigarettes and cigars (2). The resulting open lesion is further exposed to the effects of gastric acids and pepsins released within the stomach. In essence, the stomach begins digesting itself.

Signs and Symptoms

The most common symptom is a gnawing epigastric pain that typically occurs within 1 to 3 hours of eating and after the consumption of orange juice, coffee, aspirin, or alcohol. The pain often is relieved by eating again. Dyspepsia, nausea, vomiting, heartburn, and diarrhea also may be present. The danger with a peptic ulcer is perforation of the stomach wall, followed by peritonitis and, potentially, massive hemorrhage.

Management

Treatment is aimed at reducing acid secretions, healing the mucosal lining, and relieving symptoms. When taken on an empty stomach or 1 hour after a meal, antacids reduce acidity within 30 minutes and continue to reduce it for up to 3 hours. Bland diets may have some limited benefit. In addition, individuals should be advised to avoid alcohol, caffeine, and smoking. If over-the-counter (OTC) antacids fail to reduce the pain and discomfort, the individual should be referred to a physician. Hemorrhaging and perforations, which may be present, can result in an emergency situation; these individuals should be under a physician's supervision.

Gastritis

Gastritis, the most common stomach ailment, occurs when the stomach lining becomes inflamed, leading to erosion of the gastric mucosa. It may be induced by anxiety, exercise-related hypoperfusion, use of nonsteroidal anti-inflammatory drugs, or excessive consumption of caffeine or alcohol.

Signs and Symptoms

After consumption of an offending substance, acute gastritis may present with GI bleeding, belching, epigastric pain, and vomiting, including **hematemesis.** Chronic gastritis may exhibit similar symptoms, mild discomfort, or no symptoms. When present, symptoms range from a loss of appetite to a "full" feeling in the stomach or vague epigastric pain.

Management

Symptoms are relieved by eliminating the irritant or cause. Anticholinergics and antacids may relieve distress, but with severe bleeding, blood replacement may be necessary. Antacids may be contraindicated if gastric bleeding is present. If gastric bleeding does occur, exercise is contraindicated, and the individual should be referred to a physician.

Gastroenteritis

The incidence of gastroenteritis, an acute inflammation of the mucous membrane of the stomach or small intestine, is second only to that of upper respiratory tract infections in adolescents and young adults (1). The condition also may be called intestinal flu, traveler's diarrhea, or food poisoning. The condition may be caused by a viral or bacterial infection, allergic reaction, medication, parasites, contaminated food (food poisoning), or emotional stress.

Signs and Symptoms

In mild cases, increased secretion of hydrochloric acid in the stomach may lead to indigestion, nausea, flatulence (gas), and a sour stomach. In moderate to severe cases, abdominal cramping, diarrhea, fever, and vomiting can lead to fluid and electrolyte imbalance.

Management

The condition often is self-limiting and usually clears in 2 to 3 days. Treatment includes eliminating irritating foods from the diet, avoiding factors that bring on anxiety and stress, and avoiding dehydration by drinking clear fluids or electrolyte-containing fluids. Antimotility drugs (e.g., Imodium, Lomotil, and Diasorb) reduce movement in the small intestines and may be effective for abdominal cramps and diarrhea, but these drugs also may prolong some infections. The individual's return to activity is limited by his or her hydration status, the nature of the infection, the complexity of the symptoms (e.g., frequent diarrhea), and reconditioning. Children and senior athletes should be carefully monitored for fluid and electrolyte imbalance during exercise.

 The male patient had a mild fever, upset stomach, abdominal cramps, diarrhea, and nausea. He may have gastroenteritis. He should be encouraged to rest and increase his intake of clear or electrolyte-containing fluids. He also should be advised to see a physician if the condition does not improve in 2 to 3 days.

LOWER GASTROINTESTINAL DISORDERS

 What treatment should be suggested to a triathlete who is experiencing chronic diarrhea while running?

Lower GI disorders occur distal to the stomach. Common conditions associated with lower GI problems include irritable bowel syndrome, Crohn's disease, ulcerative colitis, diarrhea, constipation, and hemorrhoids. Many lower GI disorders are managed by increasing dietary fiber and avoiding irritating foods.

Irritable Bowel Syndrome

Irritable bowel syndrome (IBS) is marked by abdominal pain and altered bowel function (i.e., constipation, diarrhea, or alternating constipation and diarrhea) for which no organic cause can be determined. It affects up to 20% of the North American population, with women twice as likely as men to be affected (3). This chronic condition, which sometimes is referred to incorrectly as "spastic colon," usually begins during early adulthood, lasting intermittently for years. It commonly presents with symptoms between ages 30 and 50 (4).

Signs and Symptoms

The most prominent symptom with IBS is abdominal pain or discomfort that lasts for at least 12 weeks (which need not be consecutive) of the preceding 12 months and includes at least two of the three following features: relief is achieved with defecation, onset is associated with a change in frequency of stool, and/or onset is associated with a change in the form and appearance of the stool (3). The stool may be covered with mucus. Heartburn, abdominal distension, back pain, weakness, and faintness also may occur. Acute attacks may subside within 1 day, but recurrent exacerbation is likely.

Management

This individual should be referred to a physician to rule out more serious conditions. A complete blood count and stool examination should be administered to identify occult blood, ova, parasites, and pathogenic bacteria that may be linked to related conditions. No single successful treatment is available for IBS. Dietary modification may involve eliminating irritating foods (i.e., dairy products, gas-forming foods, caffeine, and artificial sweeteners) or, if constipation is a symptom, adding fiber. Adequate rest and exercise is encouraged, along with reduction of stress. A sedative or antispasmodic medication may be used (5).

Crohn's Disease

Crohn's disease (i.e., regional enteritis) is a serious, chronic inflammation, usually of the ileum, although it may affect any portion of the intestinal tract. Its cause is unknown. The condition is distinguished from IBS by its inflammatory pattern. The inflammation extends through all layers of the intestinal wall, resulting in a characteristic thickening or toughening of the wall and a narrowing of the intestinal lumen. The inflammation tends to be patchy or segmented. The disease may be mild, moderate, severe, or in remission.

Signs and Symptoms

The individual often experiences colicky or steady abdominal pain in the right lower quadrant, diarrhea 10 to 20 times per day, loss of appetite, and weight loss. A variety of sores, fissures, or **fistulas** may appear in the anal region. The disease can lead to complications outside the digestive tract, such as joint pain, eye problems, skin rash, or liver disease, suggesting a possible immune system response.

Management

This individual should be referred to a physician. A barium enema, sigmoidoscopy, and colonoscopy may be necessary to rule out other conditions. Only a biopsy, however, can provide a definitive diagnosis. Treatment is symptomatic and supportive. It involves medications to prevent flare-ups or maintain remission of the disease. Mild symptoms may respond to an antidiarrheal medication, such as loperamide (e.g., Imodium), which slows or stops the painful spasm. For mild to moderate symptoms, aminosalicylates (e.g., sulfasalazine or mesalamine) also may be used to manage the condition or to prevent relapses. Corticosteroids, which can be administered orally, rectally, or by injection, are given when symptoms are more severe (2). Fistulas are treated with antibiotics. If the immune system is impacted, immunomodulator medications may be prescribed.

Ulcerative Colitis

Colitis is another chronic, inflammatory ulceration of the colon, often beginning in the rectum or sigmoid colon and extending upward into the entire colon. Unlike Crohn's disease, in which the inflammatory pattern extends into all layers of the intestinal wall and is patchy or segmented, the inflammation in ulcerative colitis tends to involve only the mucosal lining of the colon. The affected part of the colon is uniformly involved and exhibits erythema and numerous hemorrhagic ulcerations, with no patches of healthy mucosal tissue being evident (2).

Signs and Symptoms

Recurrent bloody diarrhea is a classic symptom. The stool often contains pus and mucus. Abdominal pain and severe urgency to move the bowels also are characteristic. Other symptoms include fever, weight loss, and signs of dehydration. Periodic exacerbation of the disease followed by remission of symptoms is common.

Management

Management of colitis focuses on suppressing the inflammatory response to relieve symptoms and permit healing. Mild symptoms may respond to an antidiarrheal medication, such as loperamide (e.g., Imodium A-D), and to changes in the diet. Usually, corticosteroids (e.g., hydrocortisone or prednisone) are given for a few weeks to control the active disease. When symptoms are under control, aminosalicylates (e.g., sulfasalazine or mesalamine) may be used to keep the disease in remission. Moderate to severe symptoms usually require corticosteroids to control inflammation. Anti-inflammatories and corticosteroid treatment also can be effective (2). If the immune system is impacted, immunomodulator medications may be prescribed.

Diarrhea

Anxiety and precompetition jitters commonly result in "nervous diarrhea." A common and troublesome disorder, **diarrhea** is characterized by abnormally loose, watery stools. This is caused by food residue running through the large intestine before the organ has had sufficient time to absorb the remaining water. Diarrhea in adults may result from malabsorption syndrome, gastritis, lactose intolerance, IBS, Crohn's disease, ulcerative colitis, GI tumors, diverticular disease, viral and bacterial infections of the intestine, parasitic infections, psychogenic disorders, food allergies, and a variety of medications (2). Prolonged diarrhea can lead to dehydration and depletion of electrolytes, particularly sodium, bicarbonate, and potassium. Common among runners, runner's diarrhea, or runner's trots, is caused by increased intestinal motility that can lead to several patterns of bowel dysfunction (Box 22.1). If this is a known problem, the individual should perform light exercise before activity to help empty the bowels and drink extra water to maintain hydration.

Signs and Symptoms

Abnormally loose and watery stools may be accompanied by flatulence, abdominal distension, fever, headache, vomiting, malaise, and **myalgia**.

Management

Diarrhea may respond to certain antidiarrheal medications, which reduce intestinal movement, increase fluid absorption, modify intestinal bacteria, or reduce inflammation associated with diarrhea. Pepto-Bismol, loperamide (e.g., Imodium), or diphenoxylate with atropine (e.g., Lomotil) may help; however, these products should not be used on a regular basis. An attempt should be made

Box 22.1 Patterns of Bowel Dysfunction Found in Runners

1. Nervous diarrhea before competition
   - More common in women
   - Occurs in runners with:
     - Irregular bowel function when not running
     - History of lactose intolerance
2. The need to stop and have a bowel movement while training
   - More common in men during the first few miles of a run
   - Occurs in runners:
     - With irregular bowel function
     - Who eat before running
     - Who take a morning run before breakfast
3. Cramps and diarrhea without blood in the stool after hard run
   - Common in runners; associated with severe lower abdominal cramps, nausea, and vomiting
4. Cramps and diarrhea with blood in the stool after hard run
   - Associated with diarrhea, severe lower abdominal cramps, and rectal bleeding

to defecate at a regular daily time, taking advantage of the morning **gastrocolic reflex**, a propulsive reflex in the colon that stimulates defecation. Peristalsis and defecation can be stimulated by drinking coffee or tea, having a light meal before competition, and jogging to stimulate the gastrocolic reflex. Exercise—specifically, more than what the body is accustomed to—increases intestinal activity; therefore, individuals may want to:

- Immediately decrease the level of training and competition by 20 to 40% in both mileage and intensity until the episode passes, and then build back up slowly.

- Eliminate foods that trigger bowel irritation, including dairy products if lactose intolerance is involved, excessive juices, fresh fruits, raisins and other dried fruits, beans, and lentils.

- Limit the amount of sugar-free gum and hard candies that contain sorbitol, which can cause diarrhea.

- Improve hydration before and during exercise to increase plasma volume and decrease intestinal mucosal ischemia.

Individuals on a low-fiber diet may benefit from adding fiber to absorb excess fluids. In contrast, individuals on a high-fiber diet may benefit by reducing fiber to decrease stimulation of intestinal motility. Food triggers can be identified by keeping a food/diarrhea chart. This can be done by taking away any suspected food for a few days, followed by eating a large portion of the food and observing any changes in bowel movements. Food usually moves through the intestines in 2 to 4 days. A simple way to identify the body's "transit time" is to eat foods that can be seen in the feces, such as corn, sesame seeds, or beets. An increase in clear liquids for 24 to 48 hours should be followed by readjustment to a regular diet (1,6).

Constipation

Constipation occurs when stools are difficult to pass. Some people are overly concerned with the frequency of their bowel movements, because they have been taught that a healthy person has a bowel movement every day. This is not true. Most people pass stools anywhere from 3 times a day to 3 times a week. If the stools are soft and pass easily, an individual is not constipated.

Signs and Symptoms

Constipation is present if an individual has two or fewer bowel movements each week. Infrequent or incomplete bowel movements are not a disease but, rather, are a description of symptoms that may indicate a more serious underlying condition. Potential causes include lack of fiber in the diet, improper bowel habits, lack of exercise, emotional distress, diabetes mellitus, pregnancy, laxative abuse, and drug effects (e.g., diuretics, bile acid binders, calcium supplements, aluminum antacids, antidepressants, antihistamines, antihypertensives, antispasmodics, and narcotic pain relievers) (7,8).

Management

Management depends on the origin of the condition. Individuals who have a low-fiber diet should gradually increase their intake of high-fiber foods. Fiber absorbs water and makes feces softer and easier to eliminate. Bran cereals are the foods that are richest in fiber, even superior to salads, vegetables, and fruits. Increasing daily exercise, particularly aerobic exercise, and ensuring adequate fluid intake can help to alleviate symptoms. Laxatives or suppositories are useful but should be used sparingly and only for short-term treatment. Laxatives stimulate and promote bowel emptying. They work by holding water and swelling in the intestines, whereas stool softeners work by mixing fat and water into fecal matter. Some common OTC stool softeners include Dulcolax, Senokot, Metamucil, and Citrucel.

In addition to medications, drinking warm, clear fluids (e.g., juice, soda, or broth), particularly in the morning, can stimulate bowel activity. The body naturally wants to defecate approximately half an hour after consuming a warm beverage in the morning. Time should be allotted to relax and honor this urge. It is advisable to drink plenty of fluids throughout the day, but no more than half a cup of prune juice. Signs suggesting that sufficient fluid is being consumed include urination every 2 to 4 hours and urine that is light in color, like lemonade, and not dark, like apple cider. Surgical intervention may be necessary in cases of chronic constipation.

Hemorrhoids (Piles)

Hemorrhoids are dilations of the venous plexus surrounding the rectal and anal area. They are most common during pregnancy and in those who are older than 30 years. The dilated sacs become exposed if they protrude internally into the rectal and anal canals (i.e., polyps) or externally around the anal opening. Several factors increase the incidence of hemorrhoids, including constipation, diarrhea, straining during physical exertion, pelvic congestion, enlargement of the prostate, uterine fibroids, rectal tumors, varicose veins, and pregnancy.

Signs and Symptoms

Pain, itching, and passing small amounts of bright red blood on defecation, separate from the feces, are the most common signs and symptoms.

Management

The condition normally heals within 2 to 3 weeks. Medicated rectal anesthetic preparations can be used to relieve pain, itching, and irritation. Forms of medication include suppository, cream, ointment, and aerosol foam. Preparation-H, Proctofoam, Tucks Pads, and Tronolane are OTC rectal preparations. Pain or swelling also can be relieved by following the suggestions listed in Box 22.2.

If these suggestions are not successful, physician referral is indicated. Prescribed nitroglycerin ointment applied over the inflamed area has been found to relieve hemorrhoid pain in approximately 5 minutes (9). In severe cases, however, surgery may be necessary.

Athletes who participate in contact or collision sports (e.g., boxing, football, and ice hockey) normally may experience small amounts of blood on defecation. In many endurance runners, blood in fecal material is caused by GI bleeding and is quite common and normal. This bleeding can lead to iron-deficiency anemia. If moderate amounts of blood are mixed with feces, however, a full evaluation by a physician should be conducted.

(A) Treatment for the triathlete experiencing chronic diarrhea while running should include taking antidiarrheal medications (e.g., Pepto-Bismol, Imodium, or Lomotil), eliminating foods that trigger bowel irritation, improving hydration before and after exercise, eating a low-fiber diet 24 to 36 hours before exercise, decreasing the intake of coffee or tea before exercise. If the condition continues, refer the individual to a physician for further evaluation.

Box 22.2 Reducing the Inflammation of Hemorrhoids

- Take warm sitz baths for 15 minutes several times a day, especially after bowel movements.
- Use stool softeners to prevent constipation and products to ease friction (i.e., petroleum jelly applied around the anus).
- Increase fiber in the diet by adding unprocessed bran to breakfast cereals and eating other high-roughage food.
- Drink plenty of water and other clear fluids.
- Do not ignore the urge for bowel movements, because a delay allows pressure to build up in the rectum and increases the chance of constipation and development of hemorrhoids.
- Exercise to promote good abdominal muscle tone.
- Avoid pushing too hard or long during bowel movements.

OTHER GASTROINTESTINAL PROBLEMS

Two hours after eating at a fast-food restaurant, while on the bus trip home from a game, several baseball players report varying levels of abdominal gas and pain, nausea, vomiting, low-grade fever, and diarrhea. What condition should be suspected, and what is the management for this condition?

Certain factors, although they may not be related to an injury or condition specific to the upper or lower GI tract, may affect the entire GI tract. Anxiety and stress, vomiting, and food poisoning are such conditions.

Anxiety and Stress Reaction

Performance anxiety and pregame stress are common in competing athletes. Upper GI tract function can be affected through decreased acid secretion in the stomach, slowed intestinal motility, or decreased blood flow. Continued anxiety can lead to hypersecretion of stomach acids, increased motility, or decreased transit time.

Signs and Symptoms

Common symptoms include dry mouth, dyspepsia, gastroesophageal reflux, heartburn, abdominal cramping, or diarrhea.

Management

Treatment involves reassurance and education about the body's processes; relaxation techniques, such as deep breathing, passive and active relaxation, soothing music, and therapeutic massage; and behavior modification using cognitive restructuring, concentration skills, confidence training, coping rehearsal, imagery, and positive self-talk. Many of these intervention strategies are discussed in Chapter 8.

Vomiting

Nausea is an unpleasant, wave-like feeling in the back of the throat and/or stomach that may or may not result in vomiting. Vomiting is the forceful elimination of the contents of the stomach through the mouth. Retching is the movement of the stomach and esophagus without vomiting and is also called "dry heaves."

Signs and Symptoms

Vomiting involves the oral ejection of stomach contents from reverse peristaltic contractions of voluntary and involuntary muscles. It often is preceded by a watering mouth and nausea. It often results from the intake of irritating foods and other intestinal irritants, stress, excessive consumption of alcohol or other drugs, or food poisoning.

Management

Vomiting is best managed by comforting the individual and maintaining a clear airway. The mouth should be rinsed and monitored for repeated vomiting, followed by administration of antinausea medication and clear fluids to prevent dehydration. If food poisoning is expected or blood is found in the vomit, immediate referral to a physician is necessary. Vomiting also can be an early sign of pregnancy, particularly if it occurs in the morning hours.

Food Poisoning

The most common cause of food poisoning is contaminated food. Food poisoning, however, also can stem from insecticides or infectious organisms (e.g., bacteria from the salmonella group, certain staphylococci, streptococci, or dysentery bacilli) from food that is undercooked or decomposed.

Signs and Symptoms

Food poisoning includes varying levels of abdominal gas and pain, nausea, vomiting, low-grade fever, and diarrhea. These signs and symptoms can begin from 1 to 6 hours after ingestion of contaminated foods and may last for 1 to 3 days. Dehydration from the vomiting and diarrhea can lead to weakness, fatigue, and increased risk of heat illness.

Management

Mild symptoms are treated conservatively, with rapid replacement of fluids and electrolytes and administration of an antidiarrheal agent. If tolerated, light fluids, broth, or bouillon with a small amount of salt as well as poached eggs or bland cereals may be given.

> Severe cases of food poisoning require activation of the emergency action plan, including summoning emergency medical services. Fluids must be replaced intravenously, and pumping of the stomach contents may be necessary. If possible, samples of the vomitus should be provided to the physician; the sample can aid in identifying the food that is responsible for the poisoning.

The symptoms reported by the baseball players suggest food poisoning. The athletes should continue to be monitored to determine the severity of the condition. Mild symptoms are treated conservatively, with rapid replacement of fluids and electrolytes and administration of an antidiarrheal agent. Severe cases require intravenous fluid replacement, and pumping of the stomach contents may be necessary. As such, activation of the emergency action plan, including summoning emergency medical services, is warranted.

SUMMARY

1. Exercise-induced shunting can lead to decreased esophageal motility, erosive hemorrhagic gastritis, delayed gastric emptying, diarrhea, or intestinal bleeding. Dehydration, high ambient temperatures, and lack of acclimatization can exacerbate hypoperfusion of the GI tract.

2. Many upper GI tract disorders are caused by irritation attributed to stress or to the ingestion of caffeine, alcohol, or tomato and citric acid products, leading to nausea, vomiting, bloating, abdominal cramps, and heartburn.

3. Gastroesophageal reflux is associated with regurgitation of gastric juices into the esophagus. Dyspepsia, or indigestion, is associated with upper GI pain that has no identified etiology. Both are treated with antacids taken 4 hours before physical activity.

4. Peptic ulcers generally occur at the lower end of the esophagus, in the stomach, or in the duodenum. Antacids may reduce or neutralize stomach acids and prevent them from moving into the esophagus, reducing heartburn and discomfort.

5. Gastroenteritis is second in incidence only to upper respiratory tract infections in adolescents and adults. It is caused by viral or bacterial infection, allergic reaction, medication, contaminated

food, or emotional stress. The condition is self-limiting and usually clears in 2 to 3 days. Treatment includes eliminating irritating foods from the diet, avoiding factors that bring on anxiety and stress, and avoiding dehydration.

6. Diarrhea, which is common among runners, is caused by increased intestinal motility. Antidiarrheal medications reduce intestinal movement, increase fluid absorption, modify intestinal bacteria, or reduce inflammation associated with diarrhea. If this is a known problem, the individual should try to defecate before exercise and should not eat before running.

7. Hemorrhoids are dilations of the venous plexus surrounding the rectal and anal area. Pain, itching, and passing small amounts of bright red blood on defecation, separate from the feces, are the most common signs and symptoms. Medicated rectal anesthetic preparations can be used to relieve pain, itching, and irritation. The condition normally heals within 2 to 3 weeks.

8. Anxiety and stress can lead to decreased acid secretion in the stomach, slower intestinal motility, or decreased blood flow. Continued anxiety can lead to hypersecretion of stomach acids, increased motility, or decreased transit time. Treatment involves reassurance and education about the body's processes, relaxation techniques, and behavior modification.

9. Vomiting may be caused by irritating foods and other intestinal irritants, stress, excessive alcohol or drug consumption, or food poisoning. Although it often can be treated conservatively with antinausea medication and clear fluids to prevent dehydration, vomiting may be an early sign of pregnancy, particularly if it occurs in the morning hours. Persistent vomiting signals a more serious condition, in which case immediate referral to a physician is warranted.

REFERENCES

1. Balakrishnan N, Torres JL, Mellion MB. Gastrointestinal problems. In: Mellion MB, Walsh WM, Madden C, Putakian M, Shelton GL, eds. The Team Physician's Handbook. Philadelphia: Hanley & Belfus, 2002.
2. Tamparo CD, Lewis MA. Diseases of the Human Body. Philadelphia: FA Davis, 2000.
3. Brandt LJ, Bjorkman D, Fennerty MB, et al. Systematic review on the management of irritable bowel syndrome in North America. Am J Gastroenterol 2002;97(11 Suppl): S7–S26.
4. Bennett G, Talley NJ. Irritable bowel syndrome in the elderly. Best Pract Res Clin Gastroenterol 2002;16(1):63–76.
5. Ehrenpreis ED. Irritable bowel syndrome in older adults. Geriatric 2005;60(1):25–28.
6. Clark N. Process of elimination. Am Fitness 1998;16(3): 58–59.
7. Martin M, Yates WN. Therapeutic Medications in Sports Medicine. Baltimore: Williams & Wilkins, 1998.
8. Consumers Union. Pillbox: laxatives and alternatives. Consumer Reports Health 1998;10(4):8–9.
9. Fast relief from a pain in the butt. Men's Health 1997; 12(9):144.

Endocrine Conditions

STUDENT OUTCOMES

1. Describe the signs and symptoms of hyperthyroidism and hypothyroidism, and explain the management of thyroid disorders.

2. Describe the signs and symptoms of acute and chronic pancreatitis, and explain the management of both conditions.

3. Explain the insulin regulation of blood glucose levels.

4. Explain the physiologic basis of diabetes.

5. Describe the four types of diabetes mellitus.

6. Describe the circulatory and neural complications that can result from diabetes mellitus.

7. Describe the signs and symptoms of insulin shock and diabetic coma, and explain the management of insulin shock and diabetic coma.

8. Explain the nutritional recommendations for physically active individuals with type 1 and type 2 diabetes.

9. Identify physical activities that are indicated and contraindicated for a physically active individual with diabetes.

ROLE DELINEATION COMPETENCIES

The following Performance Domains and Tasks defined in the National Athletic Trainers' Association Board of Certification *Role Delineation Study*, 5th Edition are addressed in this chapter:

BOC COMPETENCIES

I. Prevention

A. Educate the appropriate individual(s) about risks associated with participation and specific activities using effective communication techniques to minimize the risk of injury and illness.

B. Interpret preparticipation and other relevant screening information in accordance with accepted guidelines to minimize the risk of injury and illness.

G. Monitor participants and environmental conditions by following accepted guidelines to promote safe participation.

II. Clinical Evaluation and Diagnosis

E. Formulate a clinical impression by interpreting the signs, symptoms, and predisposing factors of the injury, illness, or condition to determine the appropriate course of action.

F. Educate the appropriate individual(s) regarding the assessment by communicating information about the current or potential injury, illness, or health-related condition to encourage compliance with recommended care.

G. Share assessment findings with other health care professionals using effective means of communication to coordinate appropriate care.

III. Immediate Care

A. Employ life-saving techniques through the use of standard emergency procedures in order to reduce morbidity and the incidence of mortality.

B. Prevent exacerbation of non–life threatening condition(s) through the use of standard procedures in order to reduce morbidity.

C. Facilitate the timely transfer of care for conditions beyond the scope of practice of the athletic trainer by implementing appropriate referral strategies to stabilize and/or prevent exacerbation of the condition(s).

IV. Treatment, Rehabilitation, and Reconditioning

D. Administer treatment for general illness and/or conditions using standard techniques and procedures to facilitate recovery, function, and/or performance.

E. Reassess the status of injuries, illnesses, and/or conditions using standard techniques and documentation strategies in order to determine appropriate treatment, rehabilitation, and/or reconditioning and to evaluate readiness to return to a desired level of activity.

F. Educate the appropriate individual(s) in the treatment, rehabilitation, and reconditioning of injuries, illnesses, and/or conditions using applicable methods and materials to facilitate recovery, function, and/or performance.

G. Provide guidance and/or counseling for the appropriate individual(s) in the treatment, rehabilitation, and reconditioning of injuries, illnesses, and/or conditions through communication to facilitate recovery, function, and/or performance.

The endocrine system is one of the most critical systems for maintaining a healthy body. The endocrine system is a series of ductless organs that secrete hormones into the blood to be transported throughout the body (Fig. 23.1). The endocrine glands include the pituitary, thyroid, parathyroid, adrenal, pineal, and thymus glands. In addition, several organs of the body contain discrete areas of endocrine tissue and produce hormones. Such organs include the pancreas, gonads (i.e., ovaries and testes), and hypothalamus. When hormones are not produced in the proper level, serious conditions may occur. In this chapter, thyroid disorders, such as hyperthyroidism and hypothyroidism, are discussed, as are pancreatitis and diabetes mellitus.

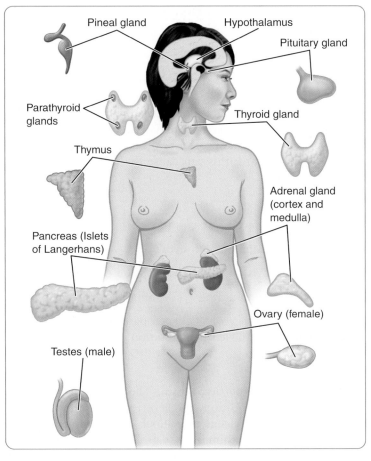

FIGURE 23.1 Location of the major endocrine glands.

THYROID DISORDERS

The thyroid is a butterfly-shaped gland located at the base of the neck, just below the Adam's apple. The thyroid gland produces two main hormones, thyroxine and triiodothyronine. These hormones maintain the rate at which the body uses fats and carbohydrates, regulate the body temperature, influence the heart rate, and help to regulate the production of protein. The thyroid gland also produces calcitonin, a hormone that regulates the amount of calcium in the blood. The rate at which hormones are released is controlled by the pituitary gland and the hypothalamus, an area at the base of the brain that acts as a thermostat for the body.

As long as the thyroid produces the necessary amount of hormones, metabolism functions normally. Occasionally, the thyroid gland produces too much of the hormone thyroxine, a condition known as hyperthyroidism (i.e., overactive thyroid disease). This condition can accelerate the body's metabolism by as much as 60 to 100%, causing sudden weight loss, rapid or irregular heartbeat, nervousness, or irritability. In contrast, if too little thyroxine is produced, hypothyroidism occurs.

Hyperthyroidism

Hyperthyroidism is caused by the overproduction of thyroxine. This condition frequently produces a cluster of symptoms called thyrotoxicosis. Hyperthyroidism can result from a number of conditions and diseases, most commonly **Graves' disease**. In turn, Graves' disease may result from genetic and immunologic factors and is marked by an enlarged thyroid gland (i.e., goiter), characteristic changes in the structure of the eyes (i.e., ophthalmopathy), and rarely, characteristic skin lesions (i.e., dermopathy) (1). Graves' disease affects more women than men, and it typically appears between 30 and 50 years of age (2).

Signs and Symptoms

The classic manifestations of hyperthyroidism are goiter, symptoms of thyrotoxicosis, ophthalmopathy, and dermopathy (Table 23.1). The symptoms of thyrotoxicosis include nervousness, increased heart rate, loss of sleep, fatigue during ordinary activities, excessive perspiration, and heat intolerance. As a result, sport and physical activity may be contraindicated. Ophthalmopathy results in the eyeball protruding beyond its normal protective orbit when the tissues and muscles behind the eyes swell and push the eyeball forward; this can cause the front surface of the eyeball to become very dry. Other symptoms include:

- Red or swollen eyes
- Widening of the space between the eyelids
- Excessive tearing or discomfort in one or both eyes
- Light sensitivity, blurry or double vision, and inflammation or reduced eye movement
- Inflammation of the muscles surrounding the eye leading to persistent blinking

Dermopathy is marked by the appearance of thickened patches of skin, usually on the feet or legs, having an "orange skin" texture and uneven pigmentation (2).

Management

Several treatments are available for hyperthyroidism. The choice of a specific approach depends on the individual's age, sex, physical condition, and severity of the disorder. One approach involves the use of antithyroid medication (i.e., drugs that block hormone production within the thyroid gland), such as propylthiouracil and methimazole (e.g., Tapazole). Symptoms usually improve in 6 to 8 weeks, but it may be necessary to continue the use of antithyroid medications for a year or more (1).

TABLE 23.1 Signs and Symptoms of Thyroid Disorders

HYPERTHYROIDISM	HYPOTHYROIDISM
Sudden weight loss, even when appetite and food intake remain normal or increase	Unexplained weight gain
Rapid or irregular heartbeat (arrhythmia) or pounding of the heart	Elevated blood cholesterol levels
Nervousness, irritability, tremor	Depression
Sweating	Pale, dry skin; puffy face
Changes in menstrual patterns	Heavier-than-normal menstrual periods
Increased sensitivity to heat	Increased sensitivity to cold
Changes in bowel patterns, especially more frequent bowel movements	Constipation
An enlarged thyroid (goiter), which may appear as a swelling at the base of the neck	Goiter
Fatigue, muscle weakness	Headache
Difficulty sleeping	Sleep apnea
	Brittle nails; coarse hair
	Hypertension
	Paresthesia

Another approach is to alter the structure of the thyroid gland, either through surgery or with **radioactive iodine**. Radioactive iodine, which is the most common treatment method in the United States, is taken orally. It is absorbed by the thyroid gland, causing the gland to shrink and the symptoms to subside. The process usually occurs within 2 to 3 months. Because this treatment causes thyroid activity to slow considerably, however, the individual eventually may need to take a medication every day to replace thyroxine (1).

Hypothyroidism

Hypothyroidism may be caused by an insufficient quantity of thyroid tissue or by the loss of functional thyroid tissue. An insufficient quantity of thyroid tissue may result from thyroid surgery, in which a portion of the gland is removed; radioactive iodine therapy for another thyroid disease, such as hyperthyroidism or Graves' disease; or a congenital thyroid abnormality. The progressive loss of functional thyroid tissue generally is idiopathic, but it is thought to have strong ties to an autoimmune disorder, such as Hashimoto's thyroiditis, which is the leading cause of hypothyroidism (3). The principal symptom of Hashimoto's thyroiditis is goiter. Other causes may include iodine deficiency, radiation therapy for cancers of the head and neck, a pituitary disorder whereby the pituitary gland fails to produce enough thyroid-stimulating hormone, or pregnancy. Some women develop hypothyroidism during or after pregnancy, often because they produce antibodies to their own thyroid gland. Left untreated, hypothyroidism increases the risk of miscarriage, premature delivery, and preeclampsia. It also can seriously affect the developing fetus (2).

Hypothyroidism occurs mainly in women older than 40 years, and the risk of developing the disorder increases with age (4). Others at risk for the condition include those with a close relative, such as a parent or grandparent, who has an autoimmune thyroid disorder; those with previous head and neck or thyroid irradiation or surgery; those with other autoimmune endocrine conditions, such as type 1 diabetes mellitus, adrenal insufficiency, and ovarian failure; and those with some other nonendocrine autoimmune disorders (e.g. celiac disease, vitiligo, pernicious anemia, and multiple sclerosis), primary pulmonary hypertension, and Down's and Turner's syndromes (4).

Signs and Symptoms

The signs and symptoms of hypothyroidism vary widely, depending on the severity of the hormone deficiency and on the age of the patient (see Table 23.1). In children, retarded growth, delayed emergence of secondary sexual characteristics, impaired intelligence, and one or more of the adult symptoms of hypothyroidism may be present. In adults, the initial onset of symptoms such as fatigue, constipation, intolerance to cold, muscle cramps, **menorrhagia** (prolonged or profuse menses), and sluggishness are barely noticeable and may be attributed simply to the individual getting older. Additional symptoms, however, develop as the metabolism continues to slow; these additional symptoms include mental clouding, diminished appetite, and weight gain. The skin may become dry, and the hair and nails may become brittle. During the advanced stages of the disease, the affected individual may have an expressionless face, sparse hair, and an enlarged thyroid (goiter) (3). Hypothyroidism also may be associated with increased risk of heart disease, primarily because high levels of low-density lipoprotein (LDL) cholesterol (considered to be the "bad" cholesterol) can occur in people with an underactive thyroid. Hypothyroidism also can lead to an enlarged heart, bouts of depression, dementia, and decreased sexual desire (libido).

Management

The treatment of choice for hypothyroidism involves hormone replacement therapy with the synthetic thyroid hormone levothyroxine sodium (LT_4) or animal-derived thyroid hormones. The oral medication restores adequate hormone levels, reduces fatigue, gradually lowers cholesterol levels elevated by the disease, and may reverse any weight gain. Overtreatment of LT_4 may cause subclinical hyperthyroidism, which increases the risk of osteoporosis and atrial fibrillation. Undertreatment with LT_4 causes subclinical hypothroidism, which may increase cardiovascular risk (5). Treatment with LT_4 usually is lifelong.

PANCREATITIS

The pancreas is a long, flat gland that lies horizontally behind the stomach. The head of the pancreas rests against the upper part of the small intestine (duodenum), and its tail reaches toward the spleen. The pancreas has two main functions:

1. The pancreas produces digestive juices and enzymes to help break down fats, carbohydrates, and proteins (pancreatic exocrine function). Once produced, these juices and enzymes are then transported through a small duct that opens into the duodenum.

2. The pancreas secretes the hormones insulin and glucagon into the bloodstream, along with somatostatin, another hormone that helps to regulate their function. The primary role of insulin and glucagon is to regulate the metabolism of carbohydrates and to control the level of blood sugar.

When inflammation develops in the pancreas, these functions are disrupted. The inflammation can be acute or chronic. Symptoms in most cases are mild to moderate, but in approximately 20% of cases, symptoms can be severe.

Acute Pancreatitis

Gallstones are the leading cause of acute pancreatitis in developed countries and account for more than 90% of cases worldwide (6). These stones migrate out of the gallbladder through the common bile duct, which merges with the pancreatic duct near the entrance to the duodenum. At this junction, gallstones can lodge in or near the pancreatic duct and block the flow of pancreatic juices into the duodenum. Digestive enzymes then become active in the pancreas instead of in the digestive tract, causing acute pancreatitis.

Alcohol abuse typically is cited as the second major cause of acute pancreatitis. Other causes of the disorder include drug reactions, viral infections, systemic immunologic disorders, pancreatic cancer, or complications from a duodenal ulcer. In some cases, the cause is unknown.

Signs and Symptoms

The main symptom of acute pancreatitis is the sudden onset of persistent, mild to severe abdominal pain centered over the epigastric region that may radiate to the back and, occasionally, the chest. It can persist for hours or days without relief. Drinking alcohol or eating worsens the pain. Many people with acute pancreatitis sit up and bend forward or curl up in a fetal position, because these positions seem to relieve the pain. Severe attacks also may cause abdominal distention or bruises from internal bleeding, persistent vomiting, fever, and tachycardia. Vital signs show rapid and shallow respirations, drop in blood pressure, and elevated temperature.

Management

Acute pancreatitis requires immediate medical care to avoid possibly fatal complications. Treatment largely is symptomatic. The aim is to maintain circulation and fluid volume, decrease pain and pancreatic secretions, and control any complications. Analgesic drugs, intravenous administration of fluids, and fasting may be necessary. Acute pancreatitis usually is self-limiting, and pancreatic function eventually is restored.

Chronic Pancreatitis

Unlike acute pancreatitis, which may improve spontaneously and without long-term complications, chronic pancreatitis is characterized by permanent damage in terms of structure, function, or both because of progressive inflammation. Alcohol abuse is thought to be the leading cause. Less common causes include autoimmune disease, systemic immunologic disorders, obstruction of the pancreatic duct by tumor, and genetic abnormalities. The disease usually presents itself in adults from 50 to 70 years of age, but some patients present before the age of 30 years (6).

As the inflammation persists, it slowly destroys the pancreas, and the organ becomes less able to secrete the enzymes and hormones that are needed for proper digestion. This leads to poor absorption (malabsorption) of nutrients, particularly fat, causing weight loss and passage of fat-containing stools that are loose, malodorous, and oily in appearance. Eventually, the cells that produce insulin are impaired, causing diabetes. Chronic pancreatitis, especially the hereditary form, also is linked to increased risk for pancreatic cancer (6).

Signs and Symptoms

Chronic pancreatitis differs acute pancreatitis in that the inflammation is a slow, progressive destruction of the tissues, often over many years. This disease usually is less obvious, and during its early stages, the signs and symptoms can be difficult to recognize. Some people with chronic pancreatitis have no pain. Others have intermittent periods of mild to moderate abdominal pain linked to recurrent bouts of acute pancreatitis, often worsening after drinking alcohol or eating a meal. Other symptoms may include nausea, vomiting, fever, bloating, gas, weight loss, malabsorption, and hyperglycemia.

Management

Treatment of chronic pancreatitis is aimed at managing pain and correcting any nutritional disorders that result from malabsorption. A low-fat diet is recommended. Pain may be relieved through medication or various surgical procedures. Pancreatic enzyme replacement therapy may help to correct malabsorption problems and provide additional pain relief. If the condition is caused by alcoholism, the mortality rate is high (1).

DIABETES MELLITUS

Q *During a rehabilitation session, a patient becomes very dizzy, complains of a headache, and reports being very hungry. The individual is sweating profusely, the skin appears to be pale and clammy, and movement is somewhat clumsy. In addition, the person appears to be swallowing an excessive number of times. What condition should be suspected, and how should the conditioned be managed?*

Diabetes mellitus (DM) is a chronic metabolic disorder characterized by a near or absolute lack of the hormone insulin, insulin resistance, or both. The disease affects approximately 15 million Americans and ranks fifth among the leading causes of death in the United States. It is estimated that approximately 2.7 million or 11.4% of African Americans aged 20 years or older have diabetes. The most life-threatening consequences of diabetes are heart disease and stroke, which strike people with diabetes more than twice as often as they do those without the disorder (7). Several factors increase the risk and severity of diabetes, including heredity, increasing age, minority ethnicity, obesity, female gender, stress, infection, a sedentary lifestyle, and a diet high in carbohydrates and fat.

Physiologic Basis of Diabetes

Carbohydrates in human nutrition supply the body's cells with glucose to deliver energy to the body's systems. Eating causes the blood glucose (BG) to rise, stimulating the pancreas to release insulin. Under normal conditions, BG ranges between 80 and 120 mg/dL. The main effect of insulin is lowered blood sugar levels, but it also stimulates amino acid uptake, fat metabolism, and protein synthesis in muscle tissue. Insulin lowers blood sugar by enhancing membrane transport of glucose and other simple sugars from the blood into body cells, especially the skeletal and cardiac muscles (Fig. 23.2). It does not accelerate the entry of glucose into liver, kidney, and brain tissue, all of which have easy access to BG regardless of insulin levels. After glucose enters the target cells, insulin:

- Promotes the oxidation of glucose for adenosine triphosphate production.

- Joins glucose together to form glycogen.

- Converts glucose to fat for storage, particularly in adipose tissue.

As a general rule, energy needs are met first, and then liver and muscle cells can assemble the excess single glucose cells into long, branching chains of glycogen for storage. The liver cells also

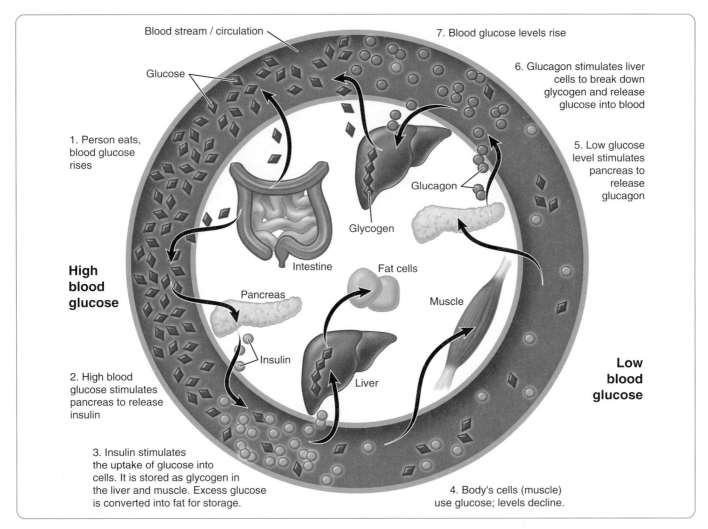

Blood stream / circulation

7. Blood glucose levels rise

Glucose

6. Glucagon stimulates liver
cells to break down
glycogen and release
glucose into blood

1. Person eats,
blood glucose
rises

5. Low glucose
level stimulates
pancreas to
release
glucagon

Glucagon

Glycogen

**High
blood
glucose**

Intestine

Fat cells

Muscle

Pancreas

**Low
blood
glucose**

Insulin

2. High blood
glucose stimulates
pancreas to release
insulin

Liver

3. Insulin stimulates
the uptake of glucose into
cells. It is stored as glycogen in
the liver and muscle. Excess glucose
is converted into fat for storage.

4. Body's cells (muscle)
use glucose; levels decline.

FIGURE 23.2 Maintaining a balance of blood glucose. Insulin must be available to stimulate uptake of blood glucose (BG) into the body's cells. As the cells use glucose, blood levels decline, and the liver responds by releasing glucagon into the bloodstream. Glucagon stimulates liver cells to break down stored glycogen and releases glucose into the blood and, in doing so, raises BG to normal levels.

are able to convert excess glucose to fat for export to other cells. High BG levels return to normal as excess glucose is stored as glycogen, which can be converted back to glucose, and as fat, which cannot be converted back to glucose.

When BG falls, as occurs between meals, other special cells of the pancreas respond by secreting **glucagon** into the blood. Glucagon raises BG by stimulating the liver to dismantle its glycogen stores and release glucose into the blood for use by the body's cells. Epinephrine, another hormone, also can stimulate the liver cells to return glucose to the blood from liver glycogen. This "fight-or-flight" response often is triggered when a person experiences stress.

When insulin activity is absent or deficient, as in those with diabetes, the level of blood sugar remains high after a meal, because glucose is unable to move into most tissue cells, causing BG levels to increase to abnormally high levels. Increased osmotic blood pressure drives fluid from the cells into the vascular system, leading to cell dehydration. The excess glucose is passed into the kidneys, resulting in **polyuria**, a huge urine output of water and electrolytes that leads to decreased blood volume and further dehydration. Serious electrolyte losses also occur as the body rids itself of excess ketones. Because ketones are negatively charged ions, they carry positive ions out with them; as a result, sodium and potassium ions are lost. An electrolyte imbalance leads to abdominal pains, possible vomiting, and the stress reaction spirals. Dehydration stimulates the hypothalamic thirst centers, causing **polydipsia,** or excessive thirst. In response, the body shifts from carbohydrate metabolism to fat metabolism for energy. The final cardinal sign, **polyphagia,** refers to excessive hunger and food consumption—a sign that the person is "starving." As such, although plenty of glucose is available, it cannot be used. In severe cases, blood levels of fatty acids and their metabolites rise dramatically, producing an excess of ketoacids that, in turn, results in acidosis. Acetone, formed as a by-product of fat metabolism, is volatile and blown off during expiration, which gives the breath a sweet or fruity odor. If the condition is not rectified with insulin injection, further dehydration and **ketoacidosis** result as the ketones begin to spill into the urine (i.e., **ketonuria**). If untreated, ketoacidosis disrupts virtually all physiologic processes, including heart activity and oxygen transport. Severe depression of the nervous system leads to confusion, drowsiness, coma, and finally, death.

Types of Diabetes

The National Diabetes Data Group and the World Health Organization recognize four types of DM:

1. Type 1

2. Type 2

3. Gestational DM

4. Diabetes secondary to other conditions

Each group is characterized by high BG levels, or **hyperglycemia.** For individuals with symptoms of DM, such as excessive thirst and urination or unexplained weight loss, only an elevated fasting plasma glucose of greater than 126 mg/dL, or a random venous plasma glucose of greater than 200 mg/dL, is required to confirm the diagnosis (8). High blood pressure, LDL cholesterol, and glucose levels are linked to serious complications in the diabetic. Recently, the American College of Physicians, National Institutes of Health, and American Diabetes Association established new guidelines for monitoring those with diabetes. In addition to traditional glucose testing that measures blood sugar levels, a new gold standard is the A1C test, which measures levels of a substance in the blood called hemoglobin A1C. The A1C test reports control of glucose levels for the past 3 months. The U.S. Federal Drug Administration has approved several A1C monitors for home use, and the ideal parameters for diabetics are as follows (9):

- A1C < 7%

- Blood pressure < 135/80 mm Hg

- LDL cholesterol < 100 mg/dl

Because athletic trainers most likely encounter physically active individuals with type 1 or type 2 DM, these conditions receive more focus and are compared in Table 23.2.

Type 1 Diabetes Mellitus

In type 1 DM, the pancreas cannot synthesize insulin. As such, the individual must obtain insulin to assist the cells in taking up the needed fuels from the blood. This insulin must be injected. It cannot be taken orally, because insulin is a protein and the gastrointestinal enzymes would digest it. Type 1 DM (formerly called insulin-dependent diabetes or juvenile diabetes) is considered to be an autoimmune disorder and is one of the most frequent chronic childhood diseases. The onset usually is acute, developing over a period of a few days to weeks. More than 95% of individuals who develop type 1 DM are younger than 25 years, with an equal incidence in both sexes and an increased prevalence in the white population (10). A family history of type 1 DM or other endocrine disease is found in a small number of cases. The disease typically has an onset before 30 years of age in people who typically are not obese; however, it can begin at any age. Obese individuals generally have a more severe time balancing glucose levels. In addition, the effects of exercise on the metabolic state are more pronounced in these individuals, and the management of exercise-related problems is more difficult.

TABLE 23.2 Comparison of Type 1 and Type 2 Diabetes Mellitus

	TYPE 1	TYPE 2
Former names	Juvenile-onset diabetes	Adult-onset diabetes
	Insulin-dependent diabetes mellitus	Non–insulin dependent diabetes mellitus
Age of onset	Usually before 30 years	Usually after 30 years
Type of onset	Abrupt (i.e., days to weeks)	Usually gradual (i.e., weeks to months)
Nutritional status	Almost always lean	Usually obese
Insulin production	Negligible to absent	Present, but may be in excess and ineffective because of obesity
Insulin	Needed for all patients	Necessary in only 20–30% of patients
Diet	Mandatory, along with insulin for control of blood glucose	Diet alone frequently is sufficient to control blood glucose
High incidence	White population	Women with a history of gestational diabetes, Blacks, Native Americans, Hispanics
Family history	Minor	Common link

Type 2 Diabetes Mellitus

Formerly called non–insulin dependent diabetes or adult-onset diabetes, type 2 DM is the most common form of diabetes (90–95% of all cases) (11,12). It is associated with a family history of diabetes, older age, obesity, and lack of exercise. It also is more common in women with a history of gestational diabetes and in African Americans, Hispanics, and Native Americans (10). Although the exact cause of type 2 DM is unknown, high BG and insulin resistance are major contributing factors. The insulin resistance is related to an insulin secretory defect of the beta cells, which prohibit or limit the transfer of insulin across the cellular membrane. As such, the individual actually may have higher-than-average insulin levels, but the cells respond less sensitively to it—in essence, they become insulin resistant. As in type 1 DM, BG rises to an inappropriate level (i.e., hyperglycemia). The high BG stimulates the pancreas to make insulin, exhausting these cells and reducing their ability to continue making insulin. Therefore, type 2 DM appears to be a self-aggravating condition.

Onset is typically after 40 years of age, but type 2 DM also is seen in obese children. Obesity, a major factor in adults, affects nearly 90% of adults with type 2 DM. Compared to normal-weight individuals, obese people require much more insulin to maintain a normal BG level. More insulin is produced, but as body fat increases, insulin receptors are reduced in number and ability to function. Consequently, insulin resistance increases, and adipose and muscle tissues become less able to take up glucose. At some point, the body cannot supply enough insulin to keep up, and type 2 DM develops.

Gestational Diabetes Mellitus

Gestational DM is an operational classification (rather than a pathophysiologic condition) that identifies women who develop DM during **gestation**. The condition is associated with older age, obesity, and a family history of diabetes. Women who are diagnosed with DM before pregnancy are not included in this group. Women who develop type 1 DM during pregnancy and women with undiagnosed, asymptomatic, type 2 DM that is discovered during pregnancy are classified as having gestational DM. Most women who are classified as having gestational DM have normal glucose homeostasis during the first half of the pregnancy, but the mother's BG rises because of hormones secreted during the latter half of the pregnancy. As a result, the mother cannot produce enough insulin to handle the higher BG, leading to hyperglycemia. The hyperglycemia usually resolves after delivery, but it places the woman at risk for developing type 2 DM later in life.

Diabetes Secondary to Other Conditions

Types of DM from various known causes are grouped together to form the classification called "other specific types." This group includes those with genetic defects of beta-cell function (formerly called maturity-onset diabetes in youth) or with defects of insulin action and persons with pancreatic disease, hormonal disease, and drug or chemical exposure (11).

Complications of Diabetes Mellitus

In both type 1 and type 2 DM, glucose fails to enter into the cells and accumulates in the blood, which can lead to both acute and chronic complications. Figure 23.3 illustrates some of the metabolic consequences of untreated diabetes. Over the long term, these metabolic changes can lead to serious chronic complications. Chronically elevated BG levels can damage the blood vessels and nerves, leading to circulatory and neural damage. Failure to adequately balance nutrition, exercise, insulin injections, and BG levels also can cause a physically active individual to experience insulin shock or diabetic coma.

Circulatory Complications

Coronary heart disease, the most common form of cardiovascular disease, usually involves atherosclerosis and hypertension. Atherosclerosis is the accumulation of lipids and other materials in the arteries. The condition begins with the accumulation of soft, fatty deposits along the inner arterial wall, especially at branch points. These deposits eventually enlarge and become hardened with minerals, forming plaque, which in turn hardens and narrows the arteries. Blood platelets cause clots to form whenever an injury occurs. Under normal conditions, these clots form and dissolve in blood all the time, but with atherosclerosis, clots form faster than they are dissolved. In those with diabetes, atherosclerosis tends to develop early, progress rapidly, and be more severe. More than 80% of people with diabetes die as a result of cardiovascular diseases, especially heart attacks (12). Complications in the capillaries also may lead to impaired kidney function and retinal degeneration with accompanying loss of vision. Approximately 85% of people with diabetes have impaired kidney function, loss of vision, or both (12). Consequently, diabetes is the leading cause of kidney failure and blindness.

Nerve Complications

Diabetes causes nerves to deteriorate. The initial symptom often is a painful, prickling sensation in the arms and legs. Later, loss of sensation may occur in the hands and feet. Injuries to these areas may go unnoticed, and infections can progress rapidly. Undetected injuries and infection may lead to aseptic necrosis of tissue (i.e., **gangrene**), necessitating amputation of the involved limbs (most often the feet or legs). For this reason, it is critical that those with diabetes take very good care of their feet and visit a podiatrist regularly. As a preventive measure, silica gel shoe inserts should be used and cotton-polyester socks worn to prevent blisters and keep the feet dry. All open wounds should be treated promptly, cleaned daily, and carefully checked for infection.

Nerve damage also can retard gastric emptying. When the stomach empties slowly after a meal, the person may experience a premature feeling of fullness. This can lead to bloating, nausea, vomiting, weight loss, and poor control of BG resulting from irregular nutrient absorption.

Hypoglycemia

Hypoglycemia, which is common in those with type 1 insulin-treated diabetes, can range from very mild, lower levels of glucose

■■■ FIGURE 23.3 **Metabolic consequences of untreated diabetes.** The metabolic consequences of type 1 diabetes mellitus are more rapid and severe than those of type 2 diabetes mellitus. In type 1, no insulin is available to allow glucose to enter the cells, resulting in a cascade of metabolic changes. In type 2, some glucose enters the cells. Because the cells are not "starved" for glucose, the body does not shift into the metabolism of fasting (i.e., losing weight and producing ketones).

(60–70 mg/dL) with minimal or no symptoms to severe hypoglycemia with very low levels of glucose (<40 mg/dL) and neurologic impairment. Although hypoglycemia can occur with any individual, it is critical in a person with type 1 DM, because the ability to recover from it is limited. Recovery is mediated by the release of epinephrine, norepinephrine, and glucagon (13). In a person with diabetes, hypoglycemia associated with insulin therapy may be related to errors in dosage, delayed or skipped meals, exercise, intensity of BG control, variation in absorption of insulin from subcutaneous injection sites, variability of insulin binding, impairment of counter-regulation, and possibly, use of human insulin (11). When left untreated, this condition can lead to insulin shock.

Insulin Shock

Exercise lowers blood sugar; as such, any exercise must be counterbalanced with increased food intake or decreased amounts of insulin. Hypoglycemia results if BG falls below normal levels. Although any individual can experience hypoglycemia, it is particularly critical for the physically active person with diabetes to address the situation immediately.

SIGNS AND SYMPTOMS. Contrary to the slow onset of a diabetic coma, hypoglycemia has a rapid onset. Signs and symptoms include dizziness; headache; intense hunger; aggressive behavior; pale, cold, and clammy skin; profuse perspiration; salivation; drooling; and tingling in the face, tongue, and lips. Other observable signs may include a staggering gait, clumsy movements, confusion, and a general decrease in performance.

MANAGEMENT. Because glucose levels in the blood are low compared to high levels of insulin, treatment focuses on getting 10 to 15 g of a fast-acting carbohydrate into the system quickly. This can be found in 4 ounces of regular cola or 6 ounces of ginger ale, 4 ounces of apple or orange juice, four packets of table sugar, or two tablespoons of raisins (13,14). Chocolates, which contain a high level of fat, should not be used for treating a hypoglycemic reaction, because the fat interferes with the absorption of sugar. If the person is unconscious or unable to swallow, the individual should be rolled on his or her side, and close attention should be given to the airway so that saliva drains out of the mouth, not into the throat. Sugar or honey should be placed under the tongue, because it is absorbed through the mucous membrane. Recovery usually is rapid.

After initial recovery, the individual should wait 15 minutes and check the blood sugar level. If the level is still less than 70 mg/dL or no meter is available and the individual still has symptoms, another 10 to 15 g of carbohydrates should be administered. Blood testing and treatment should be repeated until the BG level has normalized (13). Even when the BG level has returned to normal, however, physical performance and judgment may still be impaired, or the individual may relapse if the quick sugar influx is rapidly depleted. After the symptoms resolve, the individual should be instructed to have a good meal as soon as possible to increase carbohydrates in the body.

Many individuals with diabetes who experience repeated bouts of hypoglycemia have glucagon injection kits that contain a syringe prefilled with a diluting solution and a vial of glucagon powder. Once the solution and powder are mixed, they are injected into the upper arm, thigh, or buttock. Although the individual may instruct friends and family members on how to mix, draw up, and inject the glucagon, athletic trainers may not automatically be included in the process. It is critical, however, that athletic trainers know whether and under what circumstances a glucagon injection should be administered as well as when to activate the emergency plan. The athletic trainer should be properly trained by the individual's physician or designee, and permission to administer the solution should be documented.

Diabetic Coma

Without insulin, the body is unable to metabolize glucose, leading to hyperglycemia. As the body shifts from carbohydrate metabolism to fat metabolism, an excess of ketoacids in the blood can lower the blood pH to 7.0 (i.e., normal pH is 7.35–7.45), leading to a condition called diabetic ketoacidosis. This is manifested by ketones in the breath, **ketonemia**, and **ketonuria**.

SIGNS AND SYMPTOMS. Symptoms appear gradually and often occur over several days. The individual becomes increasingly restless and confused and complains of a dry mouth and intense thirst. Abdominal cramping and vomiting are common. As the individual slips into a coma, signs include dry, red, warm skin; eyes that appear deep and sunken; deep, exaggerated respirations; a rapid, weak pulse; and a sweet, fruity acetone breath similar to nail polish remover.

MANAGEMENT. It is not usually possible to diagnose with certainty whether an individual is in a diabetic coma or insulin shock. As such, a conscious individual should be given glucose or orange juice. If recovery is not rapid, a medical emergency exists, and the emergency plan should be activated. The additional glucose will not worsen the condition provided that the individual is transported immediately. If the person is unconscious or semiconscious, nothing should be given orally. Instead, an open airway should be maintained, the person treated for shock, and the emergency plan activated. Field Strategy 23.1 summarizes the management of insulin shock and diabetic coma.

> As the name implies, diabetic coma is a serious condition and is considered to be a medical emergency. The emergency plan, including summoning emergency medical services, should be activated.

FIELD STRATEGY 23.1

Management Algorithm for Diabetic Emergencies

Look for a medic alert tag

Is the person conscious?

Yes	**No**
Administer 10–15 g of fast-acting carbohydrate:	*Activate the emergency plan, including summoning emergency medical services.*
▪ 4 oz of regular cola	
▪ 6 oz of ginger ale	Roll the individual on his or her side so that saliva will drain out of the mouth.
▪ 4 oz of apple or orange juice	
▪ 4 packets of table sugar	
▪ 2 tablespoons of raisins	Maintain an open airway.

Does the individual show signs of improvement after the initial carbohydrates?

Yes	**No**
Wait 15 minutes, and check the blood sugar level.	*Activate the emergency plan, including summoning emergency medical services.*

Place sugar or fast-acting carbohydrates under the tongue.

Do not give liquids.

If the blood glucose level is still below 70 mg/dL or if symptoms persist:
▪ Give another 10–15 g carbohydrates.
▪ Repeat blood testing and treatment until blood glucose is normalized.

After the symptoms resolve:
The individual should eat a good meal as soon as possible

Nutrition and Exercise Recommendations

Control of diabetes depends on a balance of glucose levels, insulin production, nutrition, and exercise. Before initiating an exercise program, a physician should be consulted about diet and normal BG levels documented, because strenuous exercise is contraindicated for some individuals with diabetes. With the advent of BG self-monitoring, exercise is encouraged if certain precautions are followed. BG levels should be taken 30 minutes before and 1 hour after exercise to determine the effects of exercise on BG; this allows better regulation of food intake and insulin dosage.

Nutritional Recommendations for Type 1 Diabetes

Normally, the body secretes a constant, baseline amount of insulin at all times, and it secretes more insulin as the BG level rises following meals. Individuals with type 1 DM must learn to adjust their insulin doses and administration schedule to accommodate meals, physical activity, and health status. Recommendations for maintaining optimal nutritional status focus on controlling BG levels, achieving a desirable blood lipid profile, controlling blood pressure, and preventing and managing complications from diabetes. The diet should provide a consistent daily intake of carbohydrates at each meal and each snack to minimize fluctuations in the BG level. A meal should be ingested 1 to 3 hours before physical activity, and the individual should have approximately 10 to 15 g of additional carbohydrates 30 minutes before moderate activity or approximately 20 to 30 g of carbohydrates before vigorous activity (12). During intense exercise, 15 to 30 g of carbohydrates should be ingested every 30 minutes. A snack of carbohydrates should follow the exercise period; carbohydrates are readily available from fruits, fruit juices, yogurt, crackers, and other starches.

When exercise lasts for several hours, insulin requirements decrease; as such, total insulin dosage should be decreased 20 to 50%. Injection administration should be timed so that peak activity does not take place when high insulin levels are present (i.e., 2–4 hours after injection). If this is not possible, the individual should eat a high-carbohydrate snack, like juice and crackers or milk and cookies, approximately 30 minutes before the resumption of activity (15). In addition, food should always be available for supplemental feeding (e.g., in the locker room, on the bus, and in the athletic training kit).

Nutritional Recommendations for Type 2 Diabetes

As with type 1 DM, an individual with type 2 DM must maintain a near-normal BG level by delivering the same amount of carbohydrates each day, spaced evenly throughout the day. Eating too much carbohydrate at one time can raise BG too high, stressing the already-compromised insulin-producing cells. Eating too little carbohydrate can lead to hypoglycemia. In addition, those who have elevated blood lipids may need to watch not only their carbohydrates but also their fat intake. When an individual lowers his or her fat intake, the percentage of calories from carbohydrates increases. A high-carbohydrate diet raises triglycerides and lowers high-density lipoprotein. For those individuals accustomed to a high-fat diet, complying with a low-fat diet may be difficult. When combined with regular exercise, even moderate weight loss (i.e., 10–20 pounds) can improve BG control and blood lipid profiles, help to reverse insulin resistance, and reduce blood pressure (12).

Exercise Recommendations

Exercise is a critical component in managing diabetes. Aerobic exercise can decrease the requirements of insulin and increase the body's sensitivity to it. Exercise also can help an individual to attain and maintain ideal body weight; decrease the risk for hypertensive diseases, including cardiovascular and peripheral vascular disease; and slow the progression of **diabetic nephropathy**. It is recommended that physically active individuals with diabetes follow the guidelines listed in Box 23.1.

Despite the benefits of exercise, individuals with type 2 DM who have lost protective neural sensation should not participate in treadmill walking, prolonged walking, jogging, or step exercises. Recommended exercises include low-resistance walking, swimming, bicycling, rowing, chair exercises, arm exercises, and other non–weight bearing exercises. Activities that require resistance strength training are permissible as long as no indications of retinopathy or nephropathy are present. Scuba diving, rock climbing, and parachuting are strongly discouraged.

Box 23.1   Guidelines for Safe Exercise by Physically Active Individuals with Diabetes

- Have a routine medical examination, and be cleared for activity.
- Develop a balanced program of diet and exercise under a physician's supervision.
- Wear identification (e.g., bracelet or necklace) indicating that the individual has diabetes.
- Eat at regular times throughout the day.
- Avoid exercising at the peak of insulin action and in the evening, when hypoglycemia is more apt to occur.
- Adjust carbohydrate intake and insulin dosage before physical activity.
- Check blood glucose levels before, during (if possible), and after physical activity.
- Prevent dehydration by consuming adequate fluids before, during, and after physical activity.
- Have access to fast-acting carbohydrates during exercise to prevent hypoglycemia.
- Avoid alcoholic beverages, or drink them in moderation.
- Avoid cigarette smoking.

A *Hypoglycemia, or low blood sugar, should be suspected. It is necessary to get sugar into the system quickly. This can be accomplished by giving the individual table sugar, honey, sugared candy, orange juice, or a regular soda. Recovery should be rapid. The individual should be instructed to have a good meal as soon as possible. Finally, the individual should be closely monitored for any relapse.*

SUMMARY

1. Hyperthyroidism is caused by overproduction of thyroxine, leading to a cluster of symptoms called thyrotoxicosis. The symptoms of thyrotoxicosis include nervousness, increased heart rate, loss of sleep, fatigue during ordinary activities, excessive perspiration, and heat intolerance.

2. Hypothyroidism may be caused by an insufficient quantity of thyroid tissue or by the loss of functional thyroid tissue. In adults, the initial onset of symptoms such as fatigue, constipation, intolerance to cold, muscle cramps and menorrhagia, and sluggishness are barely noticeable. As the metabolism continues to slow, however, symptoms include mental clouding, diminished appetite, and weight gain.

3. Gallstones are the leading cause of acute pancreatitis. Alcohol abuse also is a leading cause of the disease.

4. The main symptom of acute pancreatitis is the sudden onset of persistent, mild to severe abdominal pain centered over the epigastric region that may radiate to the back and, occasionally, the chest.

5. Alcohol abuse is thought to be the leading cause of chronic pancreatitis.

6. Insulin is needed after carbohydrate ingestion to transfer glucose from the blood into the skeletal and cardiac muscles. It also promotes glucose storage in the muscles and liver in the form of glycogen. If little or no insulin is secreted by the pancreas, glucose bypasses the body cells and rises to abnormally high levels in the blood. The excess glucose is excreted in the urine, drawing with it large amounts of water and electrolytes and leading to weakness, fatigue, malaise, and increased thirst.

7. When glucose cannot enter the cells, the cells shift from carbohydrate metabolism to fat metabolism for energy, resulting in dehydration and ketoacidosis, which can depress cerebral function. Acetone, formed as a by-product of fat metabolism, is volatile and blown off during expiration, giving the breath a sweet or fruity odor.

8. There are four types of DM:

  - Type 1 (insulin-dependent) DM has an onset before age 30 in people who are not obese.

  - Type 2 (non–insulin dependent) DM has an onset after age 40 and is the most common form. It is highly associated with a family history of diabetes, older age, obesity, and lack of exercise.

  - Gestational DM occurs when a pregnant woman cannot produce enough insulin to handle the higher BG level because of hormones secreted during the latter half of pregnancy. The condition usually resolves after delivery, but it places the woman at risk for developing type 2 DM later in life.

  - Diabetes secondary to other conditions includes individuals with genetic defects of beta-cell function or with defects of insulin action and persons with pancreatic disease, hormonal disease, and drug or chemical exposure.

9. Chronic diabetes can lead to atherosclerosis and coronary heart disease, kidney failure, blindness, and impaired neural function, whereby the individual may become unaware of injuries or infections of the hands and feet.

10. Severe hypoglycemia can lead to insulin shock. The signs and symptoms include a rapid onset with dizziness; headache; intense hunger; aggressive behavior; pale, cold, and clammy skin; profuse perspiration; salivation; drooling; and tingling in the face, tongue, and lips.

11. An individual progresses into a diabetic coma (i.e., hyperglycemia) over a long period of time. Common symptoms include dry mouth, intense thirst, abdominal pain, confusion, and fever. Severe signs include deep respirations; rapid, weak pulse; dry, red, warm skin; and a sweet, fruity acetone breath.

12. Because it may be difficult to determine which condition is present, a fast-acting carbohydrate should be given to the individual. If the individual is in insulin shock, recovery usually is rapid. If recovery does not occur, the emergency plan should be activated.

13. An individual with diabetes should have a consistent daily intake of carbohydrates at each meal and snack to minimize BG fluctuations. A preactivity meal should be eaten 1 to 3 hours before activity, and 10 to 15 g of carbohydrates should be ingested 30 minutes before moderate activity or 20 to 30 g before vigorous activity. In addition, 15 to 30 g of carbohydrates should be ingested every 30 minutes during activity.

14. Aerobic, low-resistance exercise is recommended for the individual with diabetes. The program should be established under the guidance of a supervising physician.

REFERENCES

1. Ginsberg J. Diagnosis and management of Graves' disease. Can Med Assoc J 2003;168(5):575–586.
2. Tamparo CD, Lewis MA. Disease of the Human Body. Philadelphia: FA Davis, 2000.
3. Guha B, Krishnaswamy G, Peiris A. The diagnosis and management of hypothyroidism. South Med J 2002;95(5):475–481.
4. Roberts CGP, Ladenson PW. Hypothyroidism. Lancet 2004;363(9411):793–803.
5. Godfrey J. Toward optimal health: the experts discuss thyroid dysfunction. J Women's Health 2004;13(2):141–146.
6. Mitchell RMS, Byrne MF, Baillie J. Pancreatitis. Lancet 2003;361(9367):1447–1456.
7. Diabetes: New ways to deal with an old problem. Ebony 2003;58(5):64–68.
8. Birrer RB, Sedaghat VD. Exercise and diabetes mellitus. Phys Sportsmed 2003;31(5):10–14.
9. Gorman C. The ABCs of diabetes. Time 2003;161(15):104.
10. Mayfield M. Diagnosis and classification of diabetes mellitus: new criteria. Am Fam Physician 1998;58(6):1355–1363.
11. National Institutes of Health. Diabetes in America. Washington, DC: National Institute of Diabetes and Digestive and Kidney Diseases, 1995.
12. Whitney EN, Rolfes SR. Understanding Nutrition. Belmont, CA: Wadsworth, 1999.
13. Jimenez CC. Diabetes and exercise: the role of the athletic trainer. J Ath Train 1997;32(4):339–343.
14. Seitzman A, Anderson C. Lower your risk for lows. Diabetes Forecast 1998;51(6):60–65.
15. Small E, Bar-Or O. The young athlete with chronic disease. Clin Sports Med 1995;14(3):709–726.

Special Considerations

7

STUDENT OUTCOMES

1. Describe the activation of heat-regulating mechanisms in the body, including the methods used to generate heat via internal and external sources.

2. Demonstrate measurement of the heat stress index using a sling psychrometer.

3. Explain the methods used to prevent heat illness.

4. Identify the signs and symptoms of heat-related conditions.

5. Describe the appropriate management of heat-related conditions.

6. Describe the body's production of internal heat during cold ambient temperatures.

7. Differentiate between frostbite and systemic cooling, and describe the appropriate management of each condition.

8. Explain the impact of high altitude and poor air quality on exercise and sport performance.

9. Explain the dangers of lightning, and list the lightning safety guidelines for sport and exercise participation.

ROLE DELINEATION COMPETENCIES

The following Performance Domains and Tasks defined in the National Athletic Trainers' Association Board of Certification *Role Delineation Study*, 5th Edition are addressed in this chapter:

BOC COMPETENCIES

I. Prevention

A. Educate the appropriate individual(s) about risks associated with participation and specific activities using effective communication techniques to minimize the risk of injury and illness.

B. Interpret preparticipation and other relevant screening information in accordance with accepted guidelines to minimize the risk of injury and illness.

G. Monitor participants and environmental conditions by following accepted guidelines to promote safe participation.

II. Clinical Evaluation and Diagnosis

E. Formulate a clinical impression by interpreting the signs, symptoms, and predisposing factors of the injury, illness, or condition to determine the appropriate course of action.

F. Educate the appropriate individual(s) regarding the assessment by communicating information about the current or potential injury, illness, or health-related condition to encourage compliance with recommended care.

G. Share assessment findings with other health care professionals using effective means of communication to coordinate appropriate care.

III. Immediate Care

A. Employ life-saving techniques through the use of standard emergency procedures in order to reduce morbidity and the incidence of mortality.

B. Prevent exacerbation of non–life threatening condition(s) through the use of standard procedures in order to reduce morbidity.

C. Facilitate the timely transfer of care for conditions beyond the scope of practice of the athletic trainer by implementing appropriate referral strategies to stabilize and/or prevent exacerbation of the condition(s).

IV. Treatment, Rehabilitation, and Reconditioning

D. Administer treatment for general illness and/or conditions using standard techniques and procedures to facilitate recovery, function, and/or performance.

E. Reassess the status of injuries, illnesses, and/or conditions using standard techniques and documentation strategies in order to determine appropriate treatment, rehabilitation, and/or reconditioning and to evaluate readiness to return to a desired level of activity.

F. Educate the appropriate individual(s) in the treatment, rehabilitation, and reconditioning of injuries, illnesses, and/or conditions using applicable methods and materials to facilitate recovery, function, and/or performance.

G. Provide guidance and/or counseling for the appropriate individual(s) in the treatment, rehabilitation, and reconditioning of injuries, illnesses, and/or conditions through communication to facilitate recovery, function, and/or performance.

Environmental conditions affect even the best-conditioned individuals. Athletic practices and contests can be held on hot, humid days or on cold, windy days, which predisposes individuals to hyperthermia and hypothermia, respectively. In addition, exercising during thunderstorms that produce lightning can be extremely dangerous. These environmental conditions as well as altitude and air quality are discussed in this chapter.

HEAT-RELATED CONDITIONS

Q *Field-hockey practice is scheduled for this afternoon. The U.S. Weather Bureau is forecasting 90°F (air temperature), with a relative humidity of 80% during the practice time. Based on this information, what measures should be taken to reduce the risk of heat-related illness?*

The process by which the body maintains body temperature is called **thermoregulation.** It is controlled primarily by the **hypothalamus,** which is a region of the diencephalon forming the floor of the third ventricle of the brain. **Hyperthermia,** or elevated body temperature, occurs when internal heat production exceeds external heat loss (Fig. 24.1). The hypothalamus is a gland that maintains **homeostasis,** or a state of equilibrium within the body, by initiating cooling or heat-retention mechanisms to achieve a relatively constant body core temperature between 36.1 and 37.8°C (97–100°F). The body core encompasses the skull, thoracic, and abdominal area. Heat-regulating mechanisms, such as perspiring or shivering, are activated by two means:

1. Stimulation of peripheral thermal receptors in the skin

2. Changes in blood temperature as it flows through the hypothalamus.

Internal Heat Regulation

During exercise, the body gains heat either from external sources (i.e., environmental temperatures) or from internal processes (Fig. 24.2). Much of the internal heat is generated during muscular activity through energy metabolism. The act of shivering can increase the total metabolic rate by three- to fivefold. During sustained, vigorous exercise, the metabolic rate can increase by 20- to 25-fold above the resting level. Theoretically, such a rate can increase core temperature by approximately 1°C (1.8°F) every 5 to 7 minutes.

During exercise, the circulatory system must deliver oxygen to the working muscles and heated blood from deep tissues (i.e., core) to the periphery (i.e., shell) for dissipation. The increased blood

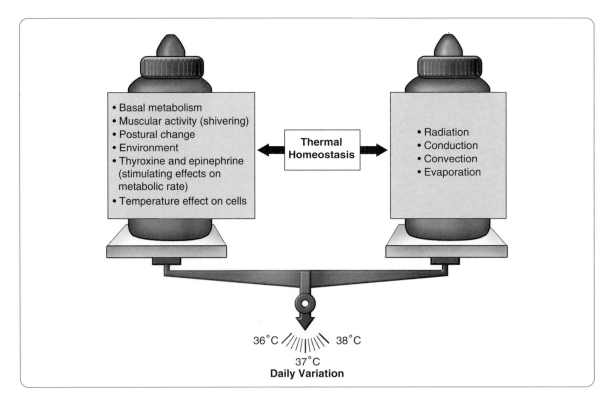

FIGURE 24.1 Thermal homeostasis. Homeostasis is achieved when internal heat production and heat loss are properly balanced to maintain a relatively constant body core temperature.

flow to the muscles and skin is made possible by increasing cardiac output and redistributing regional blood flow (i.e., blood flow to the visceral organs is reduced). As exercise begins, heart rate and cardiac output increase while superficial venous and arterial blood vessels dilate to divert warm blood to the skin surface. Heat is dissipated when the warm blood flushes into skin capillaries. This is evident when the face becomes flushed and reddened on a hot day or after exercise. When the individual is in a resting state and the air temperature is less than 30.6°C (87°F), approximately two-thirds of the body's normal heat loss results from conduction, convection, and radiation. As air temperature approaches skin temperature and exceeds 30.6°C, evaporation becomes the predominant means of heat dissipation.

Radiation

Radiation is the loss of heat from a warmer object to a cooler object in the form of infrared waves (i.e., thermal energy) without physical contact. Usually, body temperature is warmer than the environment, and radiant heat is dissipated through the air to surrounding solid, cooler objects. When the temperatures of surrounding objects, such as hot artificial turf, exceed skin temperature, radiant heat is absorbed. Participating in a shaded area is one means of reducing the effects of radiant heat during activity.

Conduction

Conduction is the direct transfer of heat through a liquid, solid, or gas from a warm to a cooler object. For example, a football player can absorb heat through the feet simply by standing on hot artificial turf. The rate of conductive heat loss depends on the temperature gradient (i.e., difference) between the skin and surrounding surfaces and on the thermal qualities of both surfaces. For example, heat loss in water can be considerable.

FIGURE 24.2 Heat gain and loss. Heat produced within working muscles is transferred to the body's core and skin. During exercise, body heat is dissipated into the surrounding environment by radiation, conduction, convection, and evaporation. Straight lines represent heat gain, and wavy lines indicate heat loss.

Convection

Convection depends on conduction from the skin to the water or the air next to it. The effectiveness of heat loss by convection is dependent on the speed at which the air (or water) next to the body is exchanged. If air movement is slow, air molecules next to the skin are warmed and act as insulation. In contrast, if warmer air molecules are continually replaced by cooler air molecules, as occurs on a breezy day or in a room with a fan, heat loss increases as the air currents carry heat away. Convection cools the body as air currents pass by while the individual is running or cycling. For example, air currents at 4 miles per hour are approximately twice as effective for cooling as air currents moving at 1 mile per hour. This is the basis of the wind-chill index (see Fig. 24.4), which shows the equivalent still-air temperature for a particular ambient temperature at different wind velocities. In water, the body loses heat more rapidly by convection while swimming than lying motionless in the water.

Evaporation

Evaporation is the most effective heat loss mechanism for cooling the body. During rest, sweat glands assist thermoregulation by secreting unnoticeable amounts of sweat (i.e., ~500 mL/day). Sweat is a weak saline solution, largely composed of water (99%), which evaporates when molecules in the water absorb heat from the environment and become energetic enough to escape as a gas. As core temperature rises during exercise or illness, peripheral blood vessels dilate, and sweat glands are stimulated to produce noticeable amounts of sweat, which can be responsible for a loss of 1.5 to 2.5 liters of body water in 1 hour (1). On a hot, dry day, sweating is responsible for more than 80% of heat loss. Sweating, however, does not cool the body; the evaporation of the sweat is what cools the body. The total sweat that is vaporized from the skin depends on three factors:

1. The skin surface exposed to the environment

2. The temperature and relative humidity of the ambient air

3. The convective air currents around the body

Relative humidity is the most important factor in determining the effectiveness of evaporative heat loss. Relative humidity is the ratio of water in the ambient air to the total quantity of moisture that can be carried in air at a particular ambient temperature. It is expressed as a percentage. For example, 65% relative humidity means that ambient air contains 65% of the air's moisture-carrying capability at the specific temperature. When humidity is high, the ambient vapor pressure approaches that of the moist skin, and evaporation is greatly reduced. Therefore, this avenue for heat loss is closed, even though large quantities of sweat bead on the skin and, eventually, roll off. In this form, sweating represents a useless water loss that can lead to a dangerous state of dehydration and overheating.

In addition to heat loss through sweating, a basal level of body heat loss exists because of the continuous evaporation of water from the lungs, from the mucosa of the mouth, and through the skin. This averages approximately 350 mL of water as it seeps through the skin every day, as well as another 300 mL of water vaporized from mucous membranes in the respiratory passages and mouth. The latter is illustrated when you "see your breath" in very cold weather. In total, it is not uncommon for an individual to lose 1.5 to 2.5 L/hour of water during exercise. This translates into a loss of 3 to 6 pounds of body weight per hour. During a 2- to 3-hour workout, an individual could lose from 6 to 12 pounds of body weight. Although an individual may continually drink water throughout an exercise bout, less than 50% of the fluid lost is replenished. This "voluntary dehydration" was recognized long ago and continues to be characterized by researchers (1). Accordingly, a physically active individual should drink as much fluid as possible before exercise and before thirst is perceived during exercise. It is critical to drink beyond the perception of satisfying one's thirst to **hyperhydrate** the body to prevent voluntary dehydration.

Measuring the Heat-Stress Index

The heat-stress index is a measure of ambient air temperature, humidity, and solar radiant energy. The most commonly used heat-stress index, the Wet-Bulb-Globe Temperature Index (WBGT), consists of the measurement of ambient temperature (T_a), wet-bulb temperature (T_w) and black globe temperature (T_g) as follows:

1. For outdoor use:

$$\text{WBGT} = (0.1 \times T_a) + (0.7 \times T_w) + (0.2 \times T_g)$$

2. For indoor use:

$$\text{WBGT} = (0.3 \times T_a) + (0.7 \times T_w)$$

Currently, the WBGT is the most widely used index of determining heat stress for indoor and outdoor use. It is used in military and industrial settings to determine safe limits for physical activity. The index is limited, however, in that it fails to take into account the impact of wearing clothing. Clothing that is impermeable or semipermeable can impede or prevent sweat evaporation, and as such, a higher heat stress level is generated. In addition, many individuals find it inconvenient and impractical to measure black globe temperature (2).

Wet-bulb temperature (T_w) is the temperature recorded by a thermometer with the mercury bulb surrounded by a wet wick. Globe temperature (T_g) is the temperature recorded by a thermometer with a mercury bulb encased in a sphere that is painted black. The black globe absorbs radiant

TABLE 24.1 Wet-Bulb-Globe Temperature Risk Chart

WET-BULB-GLOBE TEMPERATURE	FLAG COLOR	LEVEL OF RISK	COMMENTS
<65°F (<18°C)	Green	Low	Risk low but still exists on the basis of risk factors
65–73°F (18–23°C)	Yellow	Moderate	Risk increases as the event progresses through the day
73–82°F (23–28°C)	Red	High	Everyone should be aware of injury potential; individuals at risk should not participate in physical activity
>82°F (28°C)	Black	Extreme or hazardous	Consider rescheduling or delaying the event until safer conditions prevail; if the event must take place, a high alert condition exists

energy from the environment to obtain a measure that is not available using dry- and wet-bulb thermometers.

A sling psychrometer measures heat stress by exposing dry- and wet-bulb thermometers to rapid airflow. One thermometer is ordinary (i.e., a dry-bulb thermometer); the other thermometer has a cloth wick over its bulb (i.e., a wet-bulb thermometer). After whirling the instrument in the air for several minutes, the temperatures of both thermometers are read. If the surrounding air is holding as much moisture as possible (i.e., relative humidity of 100%), no difference exists between the two temperatures. In contrast, greater differences in the recorded temperatures indicate a high rate of evaporation and low humidity.

See *Field Strategy: Using a Sling Psychrometer to Determine Relative Humidity*, available on the companion website at thePoint, for further information on use of a sling psychrometer.

In 2002, the National Athletic Trainers' Association (NATA) published a position statement on exertional heat illnesses (3). This statement served as a basis for an additional document in 2003 released by the Inter-Association Task Force on Exertional Heat Illness (4), a group that convened at the request of the NATA to develop universal guidelines for reducing the risk of heat illness. The document from the Inter-Association Task Force received the support of the American Academy of Pediatrics, American College of Emergency Physicians, American Orthopaedic Society for Sports Medicine, and American College of Sports Medicine, among other prestigious organizations. Both documents should be used to develop policies for ensuring a safe exercise environment for sport participants based on their geographic location. For example, in certain geographic locations, such as the southeastern United States, the WBGT is routinely high, extreme, or hazardous throughout a large portion of the year; as such, appropriate steps should be taken to reduce increased risk of heat illness. Table 24.1 lists recommendations for activities when temperature, humidity, and radiation are measured using the WBGT index.

Factors That Modify Heat Tolerance

Several factors can affect an individual's tolerance to heat. Acclimatization and proper hydration are among the most critical in preventing heat illness.

Acclimatization

Exercising moderately during repeated heat exposures can result in physiologic adaptation to a hot environment, which can improve performance and heat tolerance (Box 24.1). In general, the major acclimatization occurs during the first week of heat exposure and is complete after 10 to 14 days. Only 2 to 4 hours of daily heat exposure is required. The first several exercise sessions should be light and last approximately 15 to 20 minutes. Thereafter, exercise sessions can progressively increase in duration and intensity. Well-acclimatized individuals should train for 1 to 2 hours under the same heat conditions that will be present during their competitive event (3). Proper hydration is essential for the acclimatization process to be effective.

Heat acclimatization is lost rapidly, however. As a general rule, 1 day of heat acclimatization is lost over 2 to 3 days without heat exposure, with the major benefits being lost within 2 to 3 weeks after returning to a more temperate environment.

Box 24.1 Physiologic Changes Seen After 10 Days of Heat Exposure

- Heart rate and body temperature decrease.
- Peripheral blood flow and plasma volume increase.
- Sweating capacity nearly doubles.

- Sweat becomes more diluted (i.e., less salt is lost).
- Sweat is distributed more evenly over the skin surface.
- The increased perspiration rate is sustained over a longer period of time.

Fluid Rehydration

The primary objective of fluid replacement is to maintain plasma volume so that circulation and sweating occur at optimal levels. Dehydration progressively decreases plasma volume, peripheral blood flow, sweating, and stroke volume (i.e., the quantity of blood ejected with each heartbeat), and it leads to a compensatory increase in heart rate. The general deterioration in circulatory and thermoregulatory efficiency increases the risk of heat illness, impairs physiologic functions, and decreases physical performance.

Thirst is not an adequate indicator of water needs during exercise. Physically active individuals may not become thirsty until systemic water loss equals 2% of body weight (5). Rather, thirst develops in response to increases in osmolality and blood sodium concentrations and decreases in plasma volume caused by dehydration.

It is essential that physically active individuals begin an exercise session when they are well hydrated and have ready access to adequate water replacement throughout the exercise session to prevent dehydration. Pre-exercise hydration should involve 17 to 20 ounces of water or a sports drink 2 to 3 hours before exercise and 7 to 10 ounces of water or a sports drink 10 to 20 minutes after exercise (6). Cold liquids, especially water, empty from the stomach and small intestines significantly faster than warm fluids do. Fluid replacement during exercise should approximate the losses of sweat and urine, resulting in a loss of body weight no greater than 2% weight. This generally requires 7 to 10 ounces of fluid every 10 to 20 minutes (6). Postexercise hydration should be completed within 2 hours of the exercise bout. This should include water, carbohydrates to replenish glycogen stores, and electrolytes to speed rehydration. Several steps can be taken to ensure adequate hydration before, during, and after exercise (Box 24.2).

See Recommended Fluid Intake for a Strenuous 90-Minute Exercise Bout, found on the companion website at thePoint.

Box 24.2 Strategies To Reduce the Risk of Dehydration

Healthy Population
- Drink 8 to 12 cups (8 oz/cup) of fluid at least 24 hours before an event.
- Drink at least 16 oz of fluid 2 hours before exercise and again approximately 20 minutes before exercise.
- Have unlimited fluid available during exercise.
- When exercising for 1 hour or more, drink at least 5 to 10 oz of fluid every 15 to 20 minutes. Drink beyond thirst.
- Drink cool fluids containing less than 8% carbohydrates.
- Use individual water bottles to accurately measure fluid consumption.
- Freeze fluid in plastic bottles before exercise; the bottles will thaw and stay cool during exercise sessions.
- Record pre- and postexercise weight to determine if excessive and unsafe weight loss has occurred.
- Replenish lost fluid with at least 24 oz of fluid for every pound of body weight lost.
- Avoid caffeine, alcohol, and carbonated beverages.

Children (in Addition to Above)
- Allow 10 to 14 days of acclimatization.
- Reduce intensity of prolonged exercise.

To prevent dehydration, fluids must be ingested and absorbed by the body. Running through sprinklers or pouring water over the head may feel cool and satisfying, but it does not prevent dehydration. A standard rule is to drink until thirst is quenched—and then drink a few more ounces.

An easy method to determine if enough fluids are being consumed is to monitor the color and volume of the urine. An average adult's urine amounts to 1.2 quarts in a 24-hour period. Urination of a full bladder usually occurs four times each day. Within 60 minutes of exercise, passing light-colored urine of normal to above-normal volume is a good indicator of adequate hydration. If the urine is dark yellow in color, of a small volume, and of strong odor, the individual needs to continue drinking. Ingesting vitamin supplements often can result in a dark-yellow urine; as such, urine color, volume, and odor must all be considered when determining hydration status (1,5).

Electrolyte Replacement

The minerals sodium, chloride, magnesium, and potassium are called electrolytes, because they are dissolved in the body as electrically charged particles called ions. Electrolytes regulate fluid balance, nerve conduction, and muscle contractions. Sweat contains high levels of sodium and chloride but little potassium, calcium, or magnesium. Ionic concentrations in sweat are greatly influenced by the rate of perspiration and acclimatization. Four liters of perspiration equal an approximately 5.8% loss of body weight. Such a loss can lower the body's content of sodium and chloride by 5 to 7% and of potassium by less than 1.2% (7). Because the body loses more water than electrolytes, the ionic concentration of these minerals in the body fluids rises. Accordingly, during periods of heavy perspiration, the need to replace body water is greater than the need to replace electrolytes. Lost electrolytes are readily replenished by adding a slight amount of salt to food or by eating potassium-rich foods, such as citrus fruits and bananas. A glass of orange or tomato juice replaces almost all the potassium, calcium, and magnesium excreted in approximately 3 L of sweat.

Electrolyte solutions are unnecessary for individuals with normal diets. Individuals demanding peak performance in competitions of greater than 1 hour or during intense intermittent exercise, however, may benefit from carbohydrate drinks (6,8). Commercial drinks may be used but should be cooler than ambient temperature (10–15°C [50–59°F]), flavored to enhance palatability, range between 4 and 8% of multiple transportable carbohydrate, and contain a small amount of sodium chloride (6,8,9). Electrolyte drinks should be consumed during the pre-exercise hydration session (2–3 hours pre-exercise) and 30 minutes before exercise. During exercise, 1 L of a 6% carbohydrate drink is recommended every hour. Fruit juices, carbohydrate gels, sodas, and some sports drinks have carbohydrate concentrations of greater than 8% and are not recommended during an exercise session as the sole beverage (6). While maintaining hydration, the participant should avoid **diuretics**, such as excessive amounts of protein, caffeinated drinks (e.g., soda, tea, and coffee), chocolate, and alcoholic beverages.

Clothing

Light-colored, lightweight, porous clothing is preferred to dark, heavyweight, nonporous material. Clothing made of 100% cotton is not recommended, especially in hot climates, because moisture in sweat-soaked cotton does not evaporate easily. Evaporative heat loss occurs only when clothing is thoroughly wet and perspiration can evaporate. Changing into a dry shirt simply prolongs the time between sweating and cooling. Heavy sweat suits or rubberized plastic suits produce high relative humidity close to the skin and retard evaporation, severely increasing the risk of heat illness. Even when wearing only football helmets and loose-fitting, porous jerseys and shorts, 50% of the body surface of football players can be sealed and evaporative cooling limited. The increased metabolic rate that is needed to carry the weight of the equipment and the increased temperature on artificial surfaces also can increase the risk of heat illness. As such, football players should initially practice in t-shirts, shorts, and low-cut socks. On hot, humid days, uniforms should not be worn, and if possible, shoulder pads and helmets should be removed often to allow radiation and evaporative cooling. Because much of the body's heat escapes through the head, helmets used in noncontact sports (e.g., cycling) should allow adequate airflow and evaporation.

Age

Children have a lower sweating capacity and a higher core temperature during exposure to heat as compared to adolescents and adults. This occurs even though children have a higher number of heat-activated sweat glands per unit of skin. Sweat composition in children also differs. Children excrete higher concentrations of sodium and chlorine and lower concentrations of lactate and potassium. Therefore, children do not benefit from electrolyte beverages and should use only cool water for fluid replacement (10). In addition, children require a longer time to acclimatize to heat as compared to adolescents and young adults.

In general, middle-aged and older men and women are less tolerant to exercising in heat. When compared to younger men and women, older men and women develop higher heart rates, higher skin and core temperatures, and lower sweat rates during exercise in heat. Aging can lead to a limited peripheral vascular response that can impair local vasodilation. Onset of sweating also appears to be delayed with advancing age, and the sweating response appears to be blunted. This may result from either a limitation in sweat gland output or a dehydration-limited sweat output if fluid replacement is insufficient. In addition, older individuals do not recover from dehydration as effectively as younger individuals do, which may be related to a blunted thirst drive. This may make older individuals more prone to dehydration that could adversely affect the thermoregulatory capacity (2).

Sex

The general consensus is that women can tolerate the physiologic and thermal stress of exercise at least as well as men of comparable fitness and level of acclimatization. Both sexes can acclimatize to a similar degree; however, sweating does differ. Although women possess more heat-activated sweat glands per unit of skin area as compared to men, women sweat less than men do. Compared with men, women begin to sweat at higher skin and core temperatures, produce less sweat for a comparable heat-exercise load, yet show an equivalent heat tolerance. Women probably rely more on circulatory mechanisms for heat dissipation, whereas men rely on evaporative cooling. The production of less sweat to maintain thermal balance can provide women with significant protection from dehydration during exercise at a high ambient temperature.

Diuretics, Supplements, and Medications

Individuals taking diuretics or laxatives should be carefully observed for dehydration. These agents increase fluid loss, reduce plasma volume, and may adversely affect thermoregulation and cardiovascular function. Substances used to induce vomiting and diarrhea also leads to dehydration and may cause excessive electrolyte loss with accompanying muscle weakness. Some nutritional supplements, such as creatine phosphate, require additional fluids to decrease the risk of heat cramps and other associated heat illnesses. Medications, such as β-adrenergics, anticholinergics, antihistamines, β-blockers, calcium channel blockers, and tricyclic antidepressants can impair the body's normal mechanisms of dissipating heat, which may result in a dangerously high core temperature (11). Before taking supplements or medications, an individual should be fully informed regarding the proper use and possible side effects of the substances.

Practice Schedules

On hot, humid days, workouts, practices, and competitions should be scheduled during early morning or evening hours to avoid the worst heat of the day (i.e., 11:00 AM to 3:00 PM). It also may be necessary to allow frequent water breaks (i.e., 10 minutes every half an hour), shorten practices, and lessen the exercise intensity. Whenever possible, participants should be moved out of direct sunlight (e.g., shade trees and tents), and restrictive equipment (e.g., pads and helmets) should be removed frequently.

Weight Charts

Measuring pre- and postexercise weight can decrease the risk of heat illness. A fluid loss equivalent to as little as 1% of body mass is associated with a significant increase in rectal temperature. For each liter of sweat-loss dehydration, the heart rate can increase by approximately eight beats per minute, with a corresponding decrease in cardiac output. When water loss reaches 4 to 5% of body mass, a definite impairment is noted in physical work capacity, physiologic function, and thermoregulation. A rule of thumb is that for every pound of water lost, 24 oz (i.e., three cups) of fluid should be ingested, meaning that 150% of the fluid loss during exercise is replenished (7).

In addition to fluids, carbohydrates also should be ingested within 30 minutes postexercise, especially those with high water content (e.g., melons or tomatoes). Even under the best circumstances, 24 hours are needed to fully restore the fluids and muscle glycogen that are used during just 2 hours of strenuous exercise. Before the next exercise period, the individual should ingest 3.5 to 4.5 g of carbohydrates per pound of body weight. Alcohol should be avoided. Lost fluid should be replaced and weight normalized before the next episode of exercise.

Identifying Individuals at Risk

Healthy individuals at risk for heat illness include those who are poorly acclimated or conditioned, those who are inexperienced with heat illness, those with large muscle mass, children, wheelchair athletes, Special Olympians, and elderly people. Others who are at risk are listed in Box 24.3.

Heat Illnesses

If the signs and symptoms of heat stress (e.g., thirst, fatigue, lethargy, flushed skin, headache, and visual disturbances) are not treated, cardiovascular compensation begins to fail, and a series of progressive complications, termed heat illness, can result. The various forms of heat illness, in order of severity, include exercise-associated muscle (heat) cramps, exercise (heat) exhaustion, and exertional heat stroke. Although symptoms often overlap between the conditions, failure to take immediate action can result in severe dehydration and possible death.

Box 24.3 Individuals at Risk for Heat Illness

Healthy individuals:
- Age extremes (children, elderly persons)
- Excessive muscle mass, large, or obese
- Poorly acclimatized or conditioned
- Previous history of heat illness
- Salt or water depletion
- Sleep deprived

Those with acute illnesses:
- Illnesses that involve fever
- Gastrointestinal illnesses

Those with chronic illnesses:
- Alcoholism and substance abuse (e.g., amphetamines, cocaine, hallucinogens, laxatives, diuretics, narcotics)
- Cardiac disease
- Certain nutritional supplements (e.g., creatine phosphate)
- Cystic fibrosis
- Eating disorders
- Medications (e.g., anticholinergics, antidepressants, antihistamines, diuretics, neuroleptics, β-blockers)
- Skin problems with impaired sweating (e.g., miliaria rubra or miliaria profunda)
- Uncontrolled diabetes mellitus or hypertension
- Using oil- or gel-based sunscreens that block evaporative cooling

Wheelchair athletes who:
- Have a spinal cord injury (alters thermoregulation)
- Limit water intake to avoid going to the bathroom

Exercise-Associated Muscle (Heat) Cramps

Heat cramps are painful, involuntary muscle spasms caused by excessive water and electrolyte loss during and after intense exercise in the heat. Paradoxically, the condition most frequently occurs in well-conditioned, acclimatized, physically active individuals who have overexerted themselves in hot weather and rehydrated only with water. Predisposing factors include lack of acclimatization, use of diuretics or laxatives, and sodium depletion in the normal diet. The condition can be prevented by ingesting copious amounts of water and increasing the daily intake of salt through a normal diet several days before the period of heat stress.

SIGNS AND SYMPTOMS. Exercise-associated muscle cramps commonly occur in the calf and abdominal muscles, but they also may involve the muscles of the upper extremity. Signs and symptoms mimic dehydration and include thirst, sweating, transient muscle cramps, and fatigue. Body temperature is not usually elevated, and the skin remains moist and cool. Pulse and respiration may be normal or slightly elevated. Dizziness may be present.

MANAGEMENT. The individual should stop activity, replace lost fluids with sodium-containing fluids, and begin mild, passive stretching of the involved muscle(s) and ice massage over the affected area. The individual should ingest enough cool carbohydrate fluids to drink beyond the point of satisfying thirst. A recumbent position may allow more rapid redistribution of blood flow to cramping leg muscles (3). The individual should be watched carefully, because this condition may precipitate heat exhaustion or heat stroke.

Exercise (Heat) Exhaustion

Exercise (heat) exhaustion usually occurs in unacclimatized individuals during the first few intense exercise sessions on a hot day. Those who wear protective equipment or heavy uniforms also are at greater risk, because evaporation through the material may be retarded. It is a "functional" illness and is not associated with organ damage. Heat exhaustion is caused by ineffective circulatory adjustments compounded by a depletion of extracellular fluid, especially plasma volume, as a result of excessive sweating. Blood pools in the dilated peripheral vessels, which dramatically reduces the central blood volume necessary to maintain cardiac output.

SIGNS AND SYMPTOMS. Thirst, headache, dizziness, light-headedness, mild anxiety, fatigue, profuse sweating, weak and rapid pulse, and low blood pressure in the upright position are common signs and symptoms. The individual may appear to be ashen and gray, with cool, clammy skin. An uncoordinated gait often is present. Urine output may be small (Fig. 24.3A). Sweating may be reduced if the person is dehydrated, but body temperature generally does not exceed 39.5°C (103°F). The individual may have an urge to defecate or may experience diarrhea. Significant neurological impairment is absent.

MANAGEMENT. The individual should be moved immediately to a cool place. All equipment and unnecessary clothing should be removed. Rapid cooling of the body should be initiated. Two effective cooling methods are evaporative cooling and ice immersion. Evaporative cooling involves spraying copious amounts of tap water over the patient's skin with air fanning. The average cooling rate through this technique is 0.14°C/min. (12). Ice immersion involves placing the patient into a pool or tub of cold water (~1–15°C [35–59°F]) (3,14). Circulation of the water may enhance cooling. If immersion in ice water is not available, other cooling methods should be used. These may include wrapping in cool, wet, iced towels; using fans; and applying crushed-ice packs to the neck, axilla, and groin. Fans and cool-mist machines, however, have limited use during humid conditions. It is essential to administer copious amounts of cool fluids with a diluted electrolyte solution as quickly as possible. Elevating the legs to reduce postural hypotension also can be effective. If recovery is not rapid and uneventful, the individual should be transported to the closest medical facility; intravenous fluids may need to be administered. Some patients, particularly endurance athletes exercising in the heat, may require as much as 4 L of fluid replacement (13). Physical activity should not be resumed until the individual has returned to the pre-dehydrated state and been cleared by a physician.

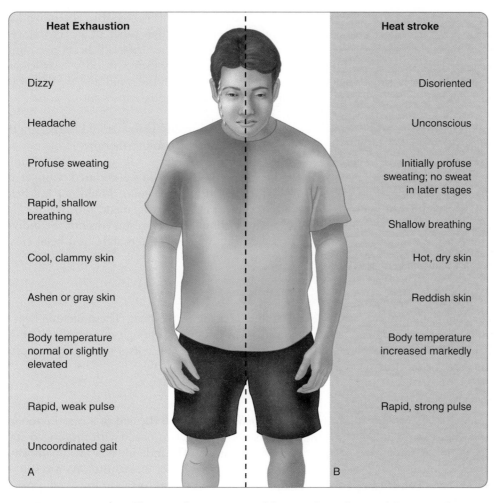

Heat Exhaustion

Dizzy

Headache

Profuse sweating

Rapid, shallow breathing

Cool, clammy skin

Ashen or gray skin

Body temperature normal or slightly elevated

Rapid, weak pulse

Uncoordinated gait

A

Heat stroke

Disoriented

Unconscious

Initially profuse sweating; no sweat in later stages

Shallow breathing

Hot, dry skin

Reddish skin

Body temperature increased markedly

Rapid, strong pulse

B

▪▪▪▪ FIGURE 24.3 **Signs and symptoms of heat exhaustion and heat stroke.**
A, Heat exhaustion. **B,** Heat stroke.

Exertional Heat Stroke

Exertional heat stroke is the least common, but most serious, heat-related illness. In football, heat stroke is second only to head injuries as the most frequent cause of death. The condition also is seen in dehydrated distance runners and wrestlers. Heat stroke almost always is preceded by prolonged, strenuous physical exercise in individuals who are poorly acclimatized or seen in situations during which evaporation of perspiration is blocked.

During exercise, metabolic heat continues to rise. Decreased blood plasma volume causes the heart to beat faster and work harder to pump blood through the circulatory system. The thermoregulatory system is overloaded, and the body's cooling mechanisms fail to dissipate the rising core temperature. The hypothalamus shuts down all heat-control mechanisms, including the sweat glands in an effort to conserve water loss. A vicious circle is created in which, as temperature increases, the metabolic rate increases, which in turn increases heat production. The skin becomes hot and dry. As the temperature continues to rise, permanent brain damage may occur. Core temperature can rise to 40.6°C (105°F), and it has been known to reach 41.7 to 42.2°C (107–108°F). If untreated, death is imminent. Mortality is directly related to the magnitude and duration of the hyperthermia.

SIGNS AND SYMPTOMS. By definition, the condition occurs when body temperature is elevated to a level that causes characteristic clinical and pathological damage to body tissues and affects multiple organs. Initial symptoms include a feeling of burning up, confusion, disorientation, irrational behavior, agitation, profuse sweating, and an unsteady gait. As the condition deteriorates, sweating ceases.

The skin is hot and dry and appears to be reddened or flushed (Fig. 24.3B). The individual hyperventilates or breathes deeply and has dilated pupils, giving the appearance of a glassy stare. As core temperature rises, the pulse becomes rapid and strong (as high as 150–170 beats per minute). The individual may become hysterical or delirious. Tissue damage by excessive body heat leads to vasomotor collapse, shallow breathing, decreased blood pressure, and a rapid and weak pulse. Muscle twitching, vomiting, or seizures may occur just before the individual lapses into a coma.

MANAGEMENT. Mortality and organ damage appear to be directly proportional to the length of time between elevation of core body temperature and initiation of cooling therapy.

The individual should be moved immediately to a cool place. All equipment and unnecessary clothing should be removed, and rapid cooling of the body should be initiated. Core temperature should be measured every 5 to 10 minutes and, to avoid hypothermia, should not fall below 38°C (101°F) (3,15). Victims of heat stroke usually require airway management, intravenous fluids, and in severe cases, circulatory support. Physical activity should not be resumed until the individual has returned to the pre-dehydrated state and been cleared by a physician.

 The emergency plan, including summoning emergency medical services (EMS), should be activated.

Other Heat Conditions

Four other common conditions may result from exercising in the heat. These include heat syncope, exertional hyponatremia, miliaria rubra, and miliaria profunda. Although not usually life-threatening, they can be bothersome to a competitive individual. Table 24.2 lists the signs, symptoms, and immediate care for all heat-related conditions.

Heat Syncope

Heat syncope (i.e., fainting) or light-headedness usually is seen at the end of a race in nonacclimated individuals who may or may not be under heat stress. It also can occur with prolonged standing or with standing up suddenly from a sitting or a lying position. The individual is maximally vasodilated; when activity stops, much of the blood volume pools in the lower extremities. As a result, the heart has too little venous return to pump an adequate supply of blood to the brain. Predisposing factors

TABLE 24.2 Management of Heat-Related Conditions

CONDITION	SIGNS/SYMPTOMS	TREATMENT
Heat cramps	Involuntary muscle spasms or cramps; normal pulse and respirations; profuse sweating and dizziness	Rest in cool place; massage the cramp with ice and passive stretching; drink cool water with diluted electrolyte solution
Heat syncope	Weakness; fatigue; hypotension; blurred vision; fainting; elevated skin and core temperature	Place supine in cool place; elevate legs; give oral saline if conscious; record blood pressure and body temperature
Miliaria rubra and miliaria profunda	Pruritic, inflamed skin eruptions	Cool and dry the affected skin; control infection; avoid reexposure until lesions have healed
Heat exhaustion	Thirst; headache; weakness; confusion; profuse sweating; skin is wet, cool, and clammy and may appear ashen; breathing is rapid and shallow; pulse is weak	Rest in cool place; remove equipment and clothing; execute rapid cooling of body; sponge or towel with cool water, or use a fan; intravenous fluids; discontinue activity until thoroughly recovered and cleared by a physician
Heat stroke	Sweating ceases; irritability progresses to confusion and hysteria; unsteady gait; pulse is rapid and strong; skin is hot, dry, red, or flushed; blood pressure falls; convulsions; seizures; coma	Activate the emergency plan, including summoning emergency medical services; rapidly cool body with immersion in ice water, or place crushed-ice packs on the neck, axilla, and groin

include dehydration, lack of acclimatization, ending the exercise bout without a cool-down, or moving quickly from the cold (e.g., a cold bath) into a hot sauna or whirlpool.

SIGNS AND SYMPTOMS. Signs and symptoms include dizziness, low blood pressure (hypotension), blurred or tunnel vision, pale or sweaty skin, weakness or fatigue, reduced pulse rate, and elevated skin temperature. Core temperature may not be elevated (3).

MANAGEMENT. Treatment involves placing the individual in a supine position in a shaded or cool area, elevating the legs above the level of the head, monitoring vital signs, and replacing any water deficit.

Exertional Hyponatremia

Exercising for long periods may cause low blood sodium (i.e., **hyponatremia**), which is a potentially fatal condition. Low blood sodium occurs when an individual drinks excessive amounts of water, thus diluting the sodium content of blood. Inadequate sodium intake also may play a role; however, low blood sodium is most likely to occur during prolonged exercise in dehydrated individuals who lose large amounts of sodium through sweating.

SIGNS AND SYMPTOMS. Hyponatremia is characterized by headache, confusion, nausea, cramping, bloated stomach, altered consciousness, significant mental compromise, swelling in the extremities (e.g., fingers and ankles), and seizures. In severe cases, the individual may experience respiratory changes as a result of cerebral and/or pulmonary edema (4).

MANAGEMENT. The individual should not resume activity until cleared by a physician and instructed in an individual-specific hydration protocol to ensure that the proper level and type of beverages and meals are consumed before, during, and after exercise (4).

> The emergency plan, including summoning EMS, should be activated. Blood sodium levels need to be monitored. Use of certain diuretics or intravenous solutions may be necessary.

Miliaria Rubra and Miliaria Profunda

Miliaria rubra (i.e., heat rash or prickly heat) is an inflamed, itchy (i.e., **pruritic**) skin eruption that arises when active sweat glands become blocked by organic debris. It often is seen in humid climates or with skin that is totally covered by clothing, resulting in a highly humid environment. Treatment involves cooling and drying the skin and relieving the itching. Cool baths and topical antipruritics, such as pramoxine and calamine lotion, can provide relief. The rash usually subsides if a person avoids sweating for 1 or 2 days (16).

If miliaria rubra becomes generalized and prolonged, it is called miliaria profunda. The condition can lead to heat exhaustion, because the sweat glands are occluded and can no longer produce sweat for evaporation. The lesions are truncal, noninflamed, and **papular**. Individuals with profunda are less heat tolerant than the general population; therefore, they are at a higher risk for heat illnesses (17). The condition is managed in a similar manner as miliaria rubra.

> *Because the U.S. Weather Bureau is forecasting 90°F (air temperature) with a relative humidity of 80% during the scheduled time for field-hockey practice, the following measures should be taken to reduce the risk of heat-related illness: Practice should be shortened and the intensity of some activities reduced; water should be available at any time throughout practice; and scheduled water breaks should take place every 20 minutes.*

COLD-RELATED CONDITIONS

> *The weather for a scheduled soccer game is forecast to be in the low 40s, with winds gusting up to 25 miles per hour. What measures can be taken to prevent cold-related conditions?*

Hypothermia, or reduced body temperature, occurs when the body is unable to maintain a constant core temperature. In cold weather, three primary heat-promoting mechanisms attempt to maintain or increase core temperature. The initial response is cutaneous vasoconstriction to prevent blood from shunting to the skin. Because the skin is insulated with a layer of subcutaneous fat, heat loss is reduced. The second response is to increase metabolic heat production by shivering, which is an involuntary contraction of skeletal muscle, or to increase physical activity. During vigorous exercise, skeletal muscles can produce 30- to 40-fold the amount of heat produced at rest. During gradual, seasonal changes, an increased amount of the hormone thyroxine is released by the thyroid gland, which serves as the third avenue to increase metabolic rate.

Because of their larger ratio of surface area to body mass and smaller amount of subcutaneous fat, children are more prone to heat loss during cold exposure than adults are. Cold exposure also increases the risk for exercise-induced bronchospasm, which being seen increasingly in children. Women are less able to produce heat through exercise or shivering because of their lower percentage of lean body mass, although the additional subcutaneous fat does provide more tissue insulation. Men tend to maintain lower heart rate, higher stroke volume, and higher mean arterial blood pressure than women do, but no distinct differences are seen in cold tolerance when genders are matched for aerobic fitness at the same relative workload. Elderly people, however, have a decreased capacity for metabolic heat production and vasoconstriction. Alcohol dulls mental awareness of cold and inhibits shivering, perhaps by causing hypoglycemia (2).

Preventing Cold-Related Injuries

During cold weather, body heat is lost through respiration, radiation, conduction, convection, and evaporation. Although the body attempts to generate heat through heat-producing mechanisms, this may be inadequate to maintain a constant core temperature. Box 24.4 lists predisposing factors that contribute to cold-related injuries.

Several steps that can be taken to prevent heat loss are summarized in Box 24.5. The "layered principle" of clothing allows several (i.e., three or more) thin layers of insulation rather than one or two thick ones. Fabrics should be light yet porous enough to allow free exchange of perspiration, and they should not restrict movement. Fabrics may include wool, wool/synthetic blends, polypropylene, treated polyesters (e.g., Capilene), and hollow polyesters (e.g., Thermastat) (18). Cotton has poor insulating ability that is markedly decreased when saturated with perspiration. Pile garments that contain down (e.g., Dacron, Hollofil, Thinsulate, or Quallofil) are more useful when worn during warm-up, time-outs, or cool-down periods following exercise. Jackets with a hood and drawstring as well as pants made of wind-resistant material (e.g., Gore-Tex, nylon, or 60/40 cloth) can protect against the wind.

A ski cap, face mask, and neck warmer can protect the face and ears from frostbite. Ski goggles can protect the eyes; goggles must be well ventilated to prevent fogging and be treated with antifog preparations. Polypropylene gloves or, in extreme temperatures, woolen mittens can be worn with windproof outer mittens of Gore-Tex or nylon. Athletic shoes should be large enough to accommodate

Box 24.4 Predisposing Factors for Cold-Related Injuries

- Inadequate insulation from cold and/or wind
- Restrictive clothing or arterial disease that prevents peripheral circulation, especially in the feet
- Diet lacking adequate carbohydrates or fat
- Presence of chronic metabolic disorders
- Spinal cord injury (cannot vasoconstrict peripheral arterioles in the skin and has a blunted shivering response to cold)
- Pre-existing fatigue or general weakness
- Use of alcohol, tobacco products (especially smoking tobacco), and other medications, such as barbiturates, phenothiazines, reserpine, and narcotics
- Age (very young or old)
- Decreased circulation

Box 24.5   Reducing the Risk of Cold-Related Injuries

- Check weather conditions, and consider possible deterioration.
- Identify individuals who may be susceptible to cold, and observe closely.
- Dress in several light layers.
- Wear windproof, dry, well-insulated clothing that allows water evaporation; wool, polypropylene, or polyesters (e.g., Capilene, Thermastat) are recommended.
- Carry windproof pants and jacket if conditions warrant; keep your back to the wind.
- Wear well-insulated, windproof mittens, gloves, hats, and scarves.
- Wear well-insulated footwear that keeps the feet dry.
- Avoid dehydration. Do not drink alcoholic beverages or eat snow, because these worsen hypothermia.
- Carry nutritious snacks that contain predominantly carbohydrates.
- Eat small amounts of food frequently.
- Do not stand in one position for extended periods of time. Wiggle your toes, and keep moving to bring warm blood to various areas of the body.
- Stay dry by wearing appropriate rain gear or protective clothing. If you get wet, change into dry clothing as soon as possible.
- Breathe through your nose, rather than your mouth, to minimize heat and fluid loss.
- Watch your face, ears, and fingers for signs of frostbite.

an outer pair of heavy wool socks. It is important to avoid getting wet, because heat loss can be increased by evaporation. The insulating ability of clothing can be decreased by as much as 90% when saturated either with external moisture or condensation from perspiration. If weather conditions are bad enough, it is better to cancel the practice or event for the day.

Cold Conditions

People tend to adapt less readily to cold than to heat. Even inhabitants of cold regions show only limited evidence of adaptation, such as a higher metabolic rate. Like heat illness, cold-related injuries range from minor problems, such as Raynaud's syndrome, cold-induced bronchospasm, or frostbite, to the more severe, general systemic cooling, or hypothermia, which can be life threatening. Cold emergencies occur in two ways. In one, the core temperature remains relatively constant, but the shell temperature decreases. This results in localized injuries from frostbite. In the other, both core temperature and shell temperature decrease, leading to general body cooling. All body processes slow down, and systemic hypothermia results. If left unabated, death is imminent.

Raynaud's Syndrome

Raynaud's syndrome is seen in young individuals, especially females, and is characterized by bilateral episodes of spasms of the digital blood vessels in response to emotion or cold exposure. It can be caused by an underlying disease or anatomical abnormality, and it can be a long-term complication of frostbite. Usually, however, its source is unknown. Initially, during the ischemic phase, the affected digits (usually the fingers) become cold, pale, and numb. This is followed by **hyperemia** with redness, throbbing pain, and swelling. The condition is treated by warming the affected extremity. A physician should evaluate the individual to rule out an underlying condition. Cigarette smoking should be avoided, because it compromises circulation.

Cold-Induced Bronchospasm

Cold-induced bronchospasm is a condition seen frequently in young people. It is brought on by exposure to cold, dry air during cold-weather sports. Linked to exercise-induced bronchospasm, the individual experiences difficulty breathing, as manifested by shortness of breath, coughing, chest tightness, and wheezing. Attacks can be prevented by the use of bronchodilators or cromolyn sodium. Salmeterol, a more recent, long-acting bronchodilator, administered 30 to 60 minutes before exercise appears to protect many individuals for up to 12 hours (18). Chapter 21 provides information on exercise-induced bronchospasm.

Frostbite Injuries

Frostbite is caused by the freezing of soft tissue. Individuals who have cold urticaria (cold allergy) or Raynaud's syndrome are at higher risk for frostbite. Frostbite is classified on a continuum of three degrees (Table 24.3). First-degree, or superficial, frostbite involves the skin and underlying tissues, but the deeper tissues are soft and pliable. If damage extends into the subcutaneous tissues, it is classified as second-degree frostbite. Third-degree, or deep, frostbite involves the tissues deep to the subcutaneous layers and may result in complete destruction of the injured tissue, including damage to bones, joints, and tendons (19). Damage depends on the depth of cold penetration that results from the duration of exposure, temperature, and wind velocity. Areas commonly affected are the fingertips, toes (especially when wearing constricting footwear), earlobes, and tip of the nose.

SIGNS AND SYMPTOMS. In superficial frostbite, the area may feel firm to the touch, but the tissue beneath is soft and resilient. The skin initially appears red and swollen, and the individual complains of diffuse numbness that may or may not be preceded by an itchy or prickly sensation. If the frostbite extends into the subcutaneous or deep layers, the skin feels hard, because it actually is frozen tissue. The area then turns white, with a yellow or blue tint that looks waxy.

MANAGEMENT. A person with superficial frostbite should be removed from the cold and taken indoors immediately, then treated with careful, rapid warming of the area. Clothing, jewelry, or rings should be removed and the injured area immersed in water heated to between 39 and 45°C (102–113°F) for 30 to 45 minutes (20). A whirlpool is ideal, but if one is unavailable, a basin large enough to prevent the skin from touching the sides of the container should be used. Hot water should be avoided, because it may cause burns. If frostbite is superficial, rewarmed skin may have clear blisters, whereas with deep frostbite, the rewarmed skin has hemorrhagic blisters (19). The involved area should be dried and a sterile dressing applied. If fingers or toes are involved, sterile dressings should be placed between the digits before covering. The entire area can be covered with towels or a blanket to keep it warm, and the individual should be transported to the nearest medical center, with the affected limb slightly elevated.

 EMS Deep frostbite is best rewarmed under controlled conditions in a hospital. The emergency plan, including summoning EMS, should be activated. During transport, the individual should be kept warm, but active rewarming of the frozen part should not occur.

If the frostbite is severe, hemorrhagic blisters may form over the area, and gangrene may develop within 2 to 3 weeks. Throbbing, aching pain as well as burning sensations may last for weeks. The skin may remain permanently red, tender, and sensitive to reexposure to cold.

Systemic Body Cooling (Hypothermia)

Hypothermia is more of a danger to individuals who are exposed to cold for long periods of time, such as long distance runners and Nordic ski racers, especially those who are slowing down late in a race because of fatigue or injury. Any injured or ill individual who has been exposed to cold weather or cold water should be suspected of having hypothermia until proved otherwise.

TABLE 24.3	Signs and Symptoms of Frostbite
First degree	Skin is soft to the touch and appears initially red, then white, and usually is painless. The condition typically is noticed by others first.
Second degree	Skin is firm to the touch, but tissue beneath is soft and initially appears red and swollen. Diffuse numbness may be preceded by an itchy or prickly sensation. White or waxy skin color may appear later.
Third degree	Skin is hard to the touch, totally numb, and appears blotchy white to yellow-gray or blue-gray.

Temperature (°F)																	
Calm	40	35	30	25	20	15	10	5	0	-5	-10	-15	-20	-25	-30	-35	-40	-45
5	36	31	25	19	13	7	1	-5	-11	-16	-22	-28	-34	-40	-46	-52	-57	-63
10	34	27	21	15	9	3	-4	-10	-16	-22	-28	-35	-41	-47	-53	-59	-66	-72
15	32	25	19	13	6	0	-7	-13	-19	-26	-32	-39	-45	-51	-58	-64	-71	-77
20	30	24	17	11	4	-2	-9	-15	-22	-29	-35	-42	-48	-55	-61	-68	-74	-81
25	29	23	16	9	3	-4	-11	-17	-24	-31	-37	-44	-51	-58	-64	-71	-78	-84
30	28	22	15	8	1	-5	-12	-19	-26	-33	-39	-46	-53	-60	-67	-73	-80	-87
35	28	21	14	7	0	-7	-14	-21	-27	-34	-41	-48	-55	-62	-69	-76	-82	-89
40	27	20	13	6	-1	-8	-15	-22	-29	-36	-43	-50	-57	-64	-71	-78	-84	-91
45	26	19	12	5	-2	-9	-16	-23	-30	-37	-44	-51	-58	-65	-72	-79	-86	-93
50	26	19	12	4	-3	-10	-17	-24	-31	-38	-45	-52	-60	-67	-74	-81	-88	-95
55	25	18	11	4	-3	-11	-18	-25	-32	39	-46	-54	-61	-68	-75	-82	-89	-97
60	25	17	10	3	-4	-11	-19	26	-33	-40	-48	-55	-62	-69	-76	-84	-91	-98

Wind (mph)

Wind Chill (°F) = 35.74 + 0.6215 T - 35.75 (V$^{0.16}$) + 0.4275 T (V$^{0.16}$)
Where, T = Air Temperature (°F); V = Wind Speed (mph)

Little Danger   Frostbite Times: ■ 30 minutes ■ 10 minutes ■ 5 minutes

FIGURE 24.4 Wind-chill index.

Most of the body heat is lost through radiation involving the exposed surfaces on the hands, face, head, and neck. When the temperature is 4.4°C (40°F), more than half the body's generated heat can be lost from an uncovered head. If the temperature is –15°C (5°F), up to 75% of the body's heat is lost through the head. Air movement coupled with cold produces a wind-chill factor that causes heat loss from the body much faster than occurs in still air. The faster the wind, the higher the wind-chill factor (Fig. 24.4).

When core temperature falls below 34.4°C (94°F), essential biochemical processes begin to slow. Heart and respiration rates slow, cardiac output and blood pressure fall, and as the skin and muscles cool, shivering increases violently. Numbness sets in, and even the simplest task becomes difficult to perform. If core temperature continues to drop below 32°C (90°F), shivering ceases, and muscles become cold and stiff. Cold diuresis (i.e., polyuria) occurs as blood is shunted away from the shell to the core in an effort to maintain vascular volume. This leads to excessive excretion of urine by the kidneys. If intervention is not initiated, death is imminent.

See *Signs and Symptoms of Hypothermia*, available on the companion website at thePoint, for highlights of the stages of systemic hypothermia.

SIGNS AND SYMPTOMS. Individuals with hypothermia are divided into those with mild hypothermia (rectal temperature < 32°C [90°F]) and those with moderate to severe hypothermia (rectal temperature = 32°C [90°F]).[AU: Please clarify/confirm. Symbol (i.e., =) OK as added for clarity in the second rectal temperature listing?] In mild hypothermia, the individual is still shivering. The individual may appear to be clumsy, apathetic, or confused and have slurred speech, stumble, and drop things. An individual with moderate to severe hypothermia does not feel any sensation or pain, is not shivering, and likely is colder than 32°C (90°F). The individual's movements will become jerky, and the individual becomes unaware of their surroundings.

MANAGEMENT

In cases of mild hypothermia, the individual should be moved carefully into a warm shelter. Re-warming can be accomplished by allowing the individual to shiver inside a sleeping bag or by using external rewarming devices, such as hot-water bottles or heating pads. Hot tubs can be used if available. The water should be approximately 43°C (110°F) (18). Hot drinks (preferably noncaffeinated) may be useful after the individual is partly rewarmed and able to swallow. The individual should continue to be rewarmed en route to the nearest medical facility.

The emergency medical plan, including summoning EMS, should be activated.

If hypothermia is moderate to severe, on-site rewarming should not be attempted. Once rewarming begins, serious electrolyte, metabolic, and cardiovascular changes occur that cannot be treated in the field. As such, while waiting for EMS to arrive, treatment involves preventing any further cooling and monitoring and treating for shock as necessary.

The effects of cold can be minimized by dressing in several layers of insulating clothing under the uniforms. Jackets with a hood and drawstring as well as pants made of wind-resistant material can protect against the wind. Wool socks and gloves also may keep the player warm.

OTHER ENVIRONMENTAL CONDITIONS

The threat exists for thunderstorms to pass through the area during a scheduled afternoon lacrosse game. Based on this information, what actions should be taken before the game, and how should a decision to suspend the game be determined?

The ever-changing environment presents a unique challenge for individuals participating in sport and physical activity. Individuals must cope with heat, humidity, cold, rain, lightning, altitude, and air pollution. A basic understanding of these situations can help to facilitate the performance of participants.

Altitude Disorders

The percentage of oxygen in the atmosphere at an altitude of 10,000 feet is exactly the same as that at sea level. The density of air, however, decreases progressively with ascension above sea level. The decreased partial pressure of ambient oxygen, or density of oxygen molecules, makes it more difficult to deliver oxygen to working muscles of the body. This leads to a reduction in work capacity that is directly proportional to altitude. This factor has little, if any, effect on short bursts of energy, but it can have significant impact on sustained aerobic activities. In some cases, individuals are unaware of the impact that altitude exposure can have on their performance and, in compensating for the decrease in maximum oxygen uptake, experience hyperventilation or tachycardia. As a result, stroke volume is reduced, and fewer red blood cells are available to transport needed oxygen.

High-altitude illness is a collective term for the syndromes that affect unacclimatized individuals shortly after their ascent to high altitude. The term encompasses the primary cerebral syndromes of acute mountain sickness (AMS) and high-altitude cerebral edema as well as the pulmonary syndrome high-altitude pulmonary edema. Both high-altitude cerebral edema and high-altitude pulmonary edema occur much less frequently than AMS, but these two syndromes are potentially fatal. Risk factors for developing high-altitude illness include the rate of ascent, the altitude reached, and the individual's susceptibility (21).

Acute Mountain Sickness

Altitude sickness is a disorder related to **hypoxia** at high altitudes. Predisposing factors include cold temperatures, strenuous exercise, use of cigarettes or alcohol, respiratory infections or a blunted ventilatory response, the water-retaining phase of the menstrual cycle, and a family history of AMS. The mildest form of altitude sickness, AMS arises after rapid ascent (i.e., <24 hours) to altitudes above 8,200 feet (2,500 m). A time lag of 6 to 36 hours occurs between arrival at the altitude and onset of symptoms (17).

SIGNS AND SYMPTOMS. Signs and symptoms are directly proportional to the rapidity of the ascent and both the duration and degree of physical exertion, and they are inversely proportional to acclimatization and physical conditioning. Symptoms usually start 6 to 8 hours after arrival at high altitude. Headache is the cardinal symptom but may not be sufficiently distinctive to differentiate it from other causes of headache. Other symptoms include dizziness, fatigue, nausea, vomiting, suppressed appetite, insomnia, dyspnea, decreased urine output, and tachycardia during physical exertion. Appetite suppression can be severe during the onset of a high-altitude stay, and this suppression can result in an average reduction of energy intake by approximately 40%, with an accompanying loss of body mass. The nonspecific symptoms of AMS can result in diagnostic confusion with those of other disorders, such as exhaustion, dehydration, hypothermia, alcohol hangover, and migraine headache (21).

MANAGEMENT. Acclimatization and physical conditioning can enhance altitude tolerance, reduce the severity of AMS, and decrease the physical performance decrements that occur during the early stages of altitude sickness. In addition, diets that are high in carbohydrates (i.e., >70% of total kilocalories) and low in salt can lessen the impact of AMS. If AMS occurs, treatment involves a reduction in altitude, physical rest, eating frequent small meals, avoiding alcohol, and taking acetaminophen for the headache. Recovery normally is seen within a few days, with no residual effects.

High-Altitude Cerebral Edema

High-altitude cerebral edema, often thought of as the end stage of AMS, rarely occurs below 10,000 feet. It usually happens in people who ascend rapidly to significant altitudes.

SIGNS AND SYMPTOMS. Several days after the onset of mild AMS, increased brain cell volume leads to a severe headache, nausea and vomiting, ataxia, impaired judgment, inability to make decisions, irrational behavior, and in some cases, altered consciousness, which may progress to coma and death caused by brain herniation.

MANAGEMENT. An immediate descent is mandatory. High-flow supplemental oxygen or a portable hyperbaric bag should be used while descending or if descent is delayed.

High-Altitude Pulmonary Edema

For unknown reasons, some individuals experience a severe aspect of AMS at altitudes greater than 9,000 ft. The condition is referred to as high-altitude pulmonary edema. Individuals at greatest risk include those who ascend rapidly, perform strenuous exercise on arrival, are obese, are male, and have a previous history of pulmonary edema (17). High-altitude pulmonary edema may develop during the first exposure but often develops after descent and reascent or occurs during the second night after ascent. The lungs accumulate fluid within the alveolar walls that may progress to pulmonary edema.

SIGNS AND SYMPTOMS. Initial signs and symptoms include **tachypnea** and shortness of **dyspnea** on exertion and reduced exercise tolerance greater than expected for the altitude (21). A dry cough with substernal chest pains becomes productive, with blood-stained sputum, later in the illness. During rest, headache, decreased concentration, fatigue, tachycardia, and abnormal breath sounds (i.e., **rales**) in the middle right lobe also may be present. Later, **cyanosis**, extreme weakness, mild fever (rarely exceeding 38.3°C [101°F]), productive cough with bloody, frothy sputum, irrational behavior, and coma may occur.

MANAGEMENT. A rapid return to a lower altitude is imperative. The individual should be given oxygen as soon as possible. Exertion should be kept to a minimum. If oxygen is unavailable and descent impossible, treatment in a portable hyperbaric chamber may be lifesaving, although the recumbent position that is necessary for operation of the chamber may not be tolerated by the individual. The condition resolves rapidly.

Preventing Altitude Illness

Acclimatization is the single most important factor in preventing the onset of altitude sickness. In general, the length of the acclimatization period depends on the altitude. Individuals who are native to areas of high altitude have a larger chest capacity, more alveoli, more capillaries that transport blood to tissues, and a higher red blood cell level. As a result, these individuals have an advantage in endurance activities at higher altitudes. Training for aerobic activities (i.e., events lasting longer than 3 or 4 minutes) at altitudes above 6,800 feet (2,000 m) requires acclimatization for 10 to 20 days for maximal performance. Highly anaerobic activities at intermediate altitudes do not require arrival in advance of the event (17). The benefits of acclimatization probably are lost within 2 to 3 weeks after returning to sea level.

Air Pollution and Exercise

Chemicals that make up air pollution typically are classified as either primary pollutants (i.e., those emitted directly into the environment) or secondary pollutants (i.e., those that develop from the interactions of the primary pollutants). Most primary pollutants essentially come from the combustion of petroleum-based fuels, including carbon monoxide, sulfur oxides, nitrogen oxides, hydrocarbons, and particulates. Secondary pollutants include ozone, peroxyacetyl nitrate, sulfuric acid, aldehydes, and sulfates. Smog usually contains both primary and secondary pollutants. Certain individuals are more susceptible to the adverse effects of air pollution. Even what would be subthreshold concentrations of air pollutants for healthy adults can compromise respiratory and cardiovascular function in children and elderly people. Others who are more affected by air pollution include individuals with respiratory disorders (e.g., asthma or chronic obstructive pulmonary disease) and heart disease.

Carbon Monoxide

The most frequent air pollutant is carbon monoxide. It is a colorless, odorless gas that reduces the ability of hemoglobin to transport oxygen and restricts the release of oxygen at the cellular level. In an individual who smokes cigarettes, carbon monoxide reduces both aerobic power and the ability to sustain strenuous, submaximal exercise. It not only interferes with maximal performance during exercise but also can impair attentiveness, decision making, and psychomotor, behavioral, or attention-related tasks, and it may result in higher core temperatures during prolonged exercise. The major group at risk from carbon monoxide exposure includes individuals with cardiovascular disorders (e.g., angina pectoris, ischemic cardiovascular disease, and intermittent **claudication**), pulmonary diseases (e.g., chronic bronchitis and emphysema), or anemia.

Sulfur Oxides

Sulfur oxides are produced from burning coal or petroleum products. They include sulfur dioxide, sulfuric acid, and sulfate, with 98% of the sulfur released into the atmosphere being in the form of sulfur dioxide. By itself, sulfur dioxide has little effect on lung function in normal individuals, but it can be a potent bronchoconstrictor in those with asthma. Exposure to just a trace amount of the gas during brief periods of strenuous exercise (i.e., 10 minutes) can produce a marked decrease in airway conductance in people with asthma. Individuals with asthma can prevent problems in breathing by using disodium cromoglycate before exposure or by breathing through the nose.

Nitrogen Oxides

Nitrogen oxide is a combination of nitrogen and oxygen that develops from high-temperature combustion. It is seen in several forms—namely, nitrous oxide, nitric oxide, nitrogen dioxide (NO_2), dinitrogen dioxide, dinitrogen pentoxide, and nitrate ions. Oxide levels in the air are particularly high during peak traffic periods, at airports, and in the smoke associated with cigarette smoking and firefighting. High NO_2 levels (i.e., 200–4,000 ppm) can cause severe pulmonary edema and even death. In lower concentrations (i.e., 2–5 ppm), NO_2 increases airway resistance and reduces pulmonary diffusion capacity. Although normal ambient air concentration generally is less than 1 ppm, the elderly show a reduced tolerance to NO_2, and people with chronic obstructive pulmonary disease or other respiratory diseases show a reduced pulmonary function when exposed for 4 hours to 0.3 ppm of NO_2 (17).

Ozone

Ozone (i.e., triatomic oxygen) is a complex union of oxygen, nitrogen oxides, hydrocarbons, and sunlight and, therefore, designated a photochemical oxidant. Ozone is classified as either ground

TABLE 24.4 Ozone Levels	
LEVEL	**ACTIVITY PRECAUTIONS**
Low	No precautions are necessary.
Moderate	Individuals with respiratory conditions should minimize outdoor exposure and decrease prolonged exercise or work.
High	Individuals with respiratory conditions should stay indoors. Individual without respiratory conditions should minimize outdoor exposure.

level or atmospheric. Atmospheric ozone is produced naturally and protects the earth from the sun's ultraviolet waves. The ozone that interferes with functional capacity is ground level, which stays close to the earth's surface and originates in automobile and factory emissions. Ground-level ozone is an irritant that can exacerbate existing respiratory conditions, such as emphysema and asthma. The effects of ground-level ozone normally are short term, but they can diminish work production and may produce shortness of breath and early fatigue. When maximal exertion is required, ozone may lead to coughing, chest tightness, shortness of breath, pain during deep breaths, nausea, eye irritation, fatigue, and lowered resistance to lung infections.

Ozone levels are indexed as low, moderate, or high (Table 24.4). The ozone index can be found on the weather page of most newspapers or on the web (e.g., www.weather.com). Individuals who reside in regions of high ozone levels may become desensitized to the irritating effects after repeated exposures and, as such, do not develop symptoms or changes in functional abilities.

Primary Particulates

Primary particulates, which include dust, soot, and smoke, can impair pulmonary function when inhaled into the lungs. The fine dust from charcoal and cigarette smoke increases airway resistance and reduces forced expiratory volume. The ability of fine dust to infiltrate the lungs depends on the particle size, amount of air inspired and expired in a single breath (i.e., **tidal volume**), frequency of breathing, and whether the particle was inhaled nasally or orally. During strenuous exercise, the breathing rate significantly increases, and breathing tends to be oral. Therefore, exercise likely increases the impact of these pollutants on breathing effectiveness.

Exercising in Thunderstorms

Another environmental threat is inclement weather conditions, such as rain, lightning, and thunderstorms. Most organized outdoor sport practices and competitions are held between 3:00 PM and 9:00 PM, which are peak periods for the development of thunderstorms and lightning. If the lightning (flash) to thunder (bang) occur within 30 seconds, all outdoor activities should end, and all participants should seek shelter, preferably in a sturdy building.

Lightning Injuries

Lightning poses a triple threat of injury—namely, burns from the high temperature of the lightning strike, injury caused by the elicited mechanical forces activated by the intense levels of electricity (electromechanical forces), and the resulting concussive forces that can propel objects through the air, causing blunt trauma (e.g., fracture and concussion). Lightning injuries usually are the result of five different mechanisms (22):

1. Direct strike

2. Contact injury

3. Side flash (splash)

4. Ground current (step voltage)

5. Blunt trauma

SIGNS AND SYMPTOMS. The most common burn from lightning is a Lichtenberg Figure, which resembles a feathering pattern on the skin. A Lichtenberg Figure is not actually a burn; rather, it is a pattern on the skin from the electron avalanche that strikes the body hit by lightning, causing an inflammatory dermal response (23). The pattern is transient and fades after 24 hours.

Direct strikes are the most deadly, particularly when the person is in contact with metal (e.g., golf club, shoe cleats, belt buckle, bra clips, watch band, or metal bleachers), with the burn normally appearing where the person's body is in contact with that metal object. Additional symptoms are cardiac asystole (cardiac standstill) and respiratory arrest. Fortunately, the heart is likely to restart spontaneously if the victim is not experiencing respiratory arrest. The most critical factor in determining morbidity and mortality associated with a lightning strike is the duration of **apnea** rather than cardiac asystole. It is not uncommon for a person to become unconscious or confused or to develop amnesia following a lightning strike. Other medical conditions that have been reported include blunt trauma, including fractures and internal organ damage; brain lesions because of hypoxia caused by cardiac asystole; ruptured tympanic membranes; ocular problems, including hyphemas as well as fixed and dilated pupils; seizures; subdural and epidural hematomas; anterior compartment syndromes; and transitory lower extremity paralysis (23).

> **EMS** If an individual is not breathing and is in cardiac arrest, the emergency plan, including summoning EMS, should be activated. Rescue breathing and cardiopulmonary resuscitation should be initiated. Unless ruled out, a cervical spine injury should always be suspected, and treatment should proceed accordingly. Any person struck by lightning should be immediately transported to the nearest medical facility.

MANAGEMENT. Lightning strikes claim the lives of approximately 100 people each year (24). If the person is conscious and has normal cardiorespiratory function, a secondary assessment should be conducted to determine if burns, fractures, or other trauma have been sustained.

Lightning Safety Policy

As mentioned, most organized outdoor sport practices and competitions are conducted between the hours of 3:00 PM and 9:00 PM, when risk of thunderstorms is greatest; 70% of all lightning injuries and fatalities occur in the afternoon (25). Thunderstorms can become threatening within 30 minutes of the first sign of thunder. All coaches, athletic trainers, athletic directors, athletic supervisors, managers, and physically active individuals should understand the development of thunderstorms and lightning strikes. Organizations or institutions should develop a policy within guidelines that can be implemented when conditions are favorable for thunderstorm and lightning activity (26). This lightning safety policy can decrease the risk of injury and death as well as protect the organization or institution from litigation if the policy is referred to and heeded.

> See *Lightning Safety Policy for All Outdoor Activities, Including Swimming,* available on the companion website at thePoint.

> *Before the start of the lacrosse game, the athletic trainer should review the school's lightning safety emergency plan, determine who will serve as the designated weather watcher, and meet with the game officials and visiting team's athletic trainer (or coach) to explain the lightning safety plan. The game should be suspended if the "flash-to-bang" is within 30 seconds or if a thunderstorm appears imminent.*

SUMMARY

1. The body generates heat by cutaneous vasoconstriction, increasing the metabolic heat production by shivering or physical activity, and the increase of the hormone thyroxine during gradual, seasonal changes. The body loses heat through respiration, radiation, conduction, convection, and evaporation.

2. During exercise, the body gains heat from external sources (e.g., environmental temperatures) or internal processes (e.g., muscle activity).

3. During rest, approximately two-thirds of the body's normal heat loss results from conduction, convection, and radiation. As air temperature approaches skin temperature and exceeds 30.6°C (87°F), evaporation becomes the primary means of heat dissipation.

4. Sweating places a high demand on the body's fluid reserves and can create a relative state of dehydration. If sweating is excessive and fluids are not continually replaced, plasma volume falls, and core temperature may rise to lethal levels.

5. Acclimatization and proper hydration are among the most critical factors in preventing heat illness. Minerals lost through sweating generally can be replaced through the diet. During prolonged exercise, a small amount of electrolytes added to a rehydration beverage replaces fluids more effectively than drinking plain water.

6. To prevent dehydration, fluids must be ingested and absorbed by the body. Cold liquids, especially water, empty from the stomach and small intestines faster than warm fluids do.

7. Exercise-associated muscle (heat) cramps are caused by excessive loss of water and electrolytes during and after intense exercise in the heat. Treatment involves passive stretching of the involved muscles and ice massage over the affected area. The individual also should drink fluids containing an electrolyte solution to beyond the point of satisfying thirst.

8. Exercise (heat) exhaustion is a functional illness and is not associated with organ damage. Treatment involves moving the individual to a cool place and rapidly cooling the body. The individual also should drink fluids containing an electrolyte solution to beyond the point of satisfying thirst. Intravenous fluids may need to be administered if the dehydrated state is moderate to severe.

9. Exertional heat stroke signifies a significantly elevated core temperature and dehydration. The emergency plan, including summoning EMS, should be activated, because the individual may require airway management, intravenous fluids, and in severe cases, circulatory support. While waiting for EMS to arrive, the individual should be moved to a cool place, and efforts should be made to rapidly cool the body. Immersion in ice water is the most effective method to cool the body; however, to avoid hypothermia, the core temperature should not fall below 38°C (101°F). If conscious, the individual should drink copious amounts of fluid.

10. In the prevention of cold-related injuries, the principle of layering clothing has proven to be effective through providing several thin layers of insulation. In addition, a ski cap, face mask, and neck warmer can protect the face and ears from frostbite.

11. Frostbite occurs when the core temperature remains relatively constant but the shell temperature decreases. Superficial frostbite is treated by moving the individual indoors and rapidly rewarming the involved body part in water heated to between 39 to 42°C (102–108°F) for 30 to 45 minutes. Deep frostbite is best rewarmed under controlled conditions in a hospital. The emergency medical plan should be activated.

12. Hypothermia occurs when both core and shell temperatures decrease, leading to general body cooling. If hypothermia is mild, the individual can be rewarmed; if hypothermia is moderate to severe, on-site rewarming should not be attempted. The emergency plan, including summoning EMS, should be activated.

13. Altitude sickness may involve AMS, high-altitude pulmonary edema, or high-altitude cerebral edema. The latter two conditions can lead quickly to death; therefore, oxygen therapy and immediate descent are mandatory.

14. Carbon monoxide, the most frequent air pollutant, interferes with the ability of hemoglobin to transport oxygen to the cells. Other air pollutants that can affect sport performance include sulfur oxides, nitrogen oxides, ozone, and primary particulates.

15. Lightning poses a double threat of injury—namely, burns from the high temperature of the lightning strike and concussive injuries caused by the elicited electromechanical forces.

16. Most thunderstorms occur between 3:00 PM and 9:00 PM. Schools and sport organizations should have a detailed lightning safety policy to prevent injury or death from storms.

REFERENCES

1. Murray R. Dehydration, hyperthermia, and athletes: science and practice. J Ath Train 1996;31(3):248–252.
2. Moran DS. Potential applications of heat and cold stress indices to sporting event. Sports Med 2001;31(13): 909–917.
3. Binkely HM, Beckett J, Casa DJ, et al. National Athletic Trainers' Association position statement: exertional heat illnesses. J Ath Train 2002;347(3):329–343.
4. Inter-Association Task Force on Exertional Heat Illnesses consensus statement. NATA News 2003;6:24–29.
5. Mellion MB, Shelton GL. Safe exercise in the head and heat injuries. In: Mellion MB, Walsh WM, Madden D, Putukian M, Shelton GL, eds. The Team Physician's Handbook. Philadelphia: Hanley & Belfus, 2002.
6. Casa DJ, Armstrong LE, Hillman SK, et al. National Athletic Trainers' Association position statement: fluid replacement for athletes. J Ath Train 2000;35(2):212–224.
7. Gatorade Sports Science Institute. Dehydration & Heat Injuries: Identification, Treatment, and Prevention. Chicago: Gatorade, 1997.
8. Shi X, Gisolfi CV. Fluid and carbohydrate replacement during intermittent exercise. Sports Med 1998;25(3): 157–172.
9. American College of Sports Medicine. Position stand on exercise and fluid replacement. Med Sci Sports Exerc 1996;28(1):i–vii.
10. Myer F, Bar-Or D, MacDougall D, Heigenhauser G. Drink composition and electrolyte balance of children exercising in the heat. Med Sci Sport Exerc 1995;27(6):882–887.
11. Wexler RK. Evaluation and treatment of heat-related illnesses. Am Fam Physician 2002;65(11):2307–2314.
12. Hadad E, Rav-Acha M, Heled Y, et al. Heat stroke: a review of cooling methods. Sports Med 2004;34(8):501–511.
13. Coris EE, Ramirez AM, Van Durme DJ. Heat illness in athletes: the dangerous combination of heat, humidity and exercise. Sports Med 2004;34(1):9–16.
14. Armstrong LE, Crago LE, Adams AE, et al. Whole-body cooling of hyperthermic runners: comparison of two filed therapies. Am J Emerg Med 1996;14(4):355–358.
15. Sandor RP. Heat illness: on-site diagnosis and cooling. Phys Sportsmed 1997;25(6):35–40.
16. Leshaw SM. Itching in active patients: causes and cures. Phys Sportsmed 1998;26(1):47–53.
17. Montain SJ, Freund BJ. Environmental considerations for exercise. In: Zachazewski JE, Magee DJ, Quillen WS eds. Athletic Injuries and Rehabilitation. Philadelphia: WB Saunders, 1996.
18. Bowman WD. Safe exercise in the cold and cold injuries. In: Mellion MB, Walsh WM, Madden C, Putukian M, Shelton GL, eds. The Team Physician's Handbook. Philadelphia: Hanley & Belfus, 2002.
19. Biem J, Koehncke N, Classen D, Dosman J. Out of the cold: management of hypothermia and frostbite. CMAJ 2003;168(3):305–311.
20. McCullough L, Arora S. Diagnosis and treatment of hypothermia. Am Fam Physician 2004;70(12):2325–2332.
21. Basnyat B, Murdoch DR. High-altitude illness. Lancet 2003;361(9373):1967–1974.
22. Whitcomb D, Martinez JA, Daberkow D. Lightning injuries. South Med J 2002;95(11):1331–1334.
23. Walsh KM, Hanley MJ, Graner SJ, et al. A survey of lightning policy in selected Division I colleges. J Ath Train 1997;32(3):206–210.
24. Cherington M, Yarnell P, Wappes JR. Lightning strikes: how to lower your risk. Phys Sportsmed 1997;25(5): 129–130.
25. Uman MA. All About Lightning. New York: Dover, 1996.
26. Bennett BL. A model lightning safety policy for athletics. J Ath Train 1997;32(3):251–253.

Common Infectious Diseases

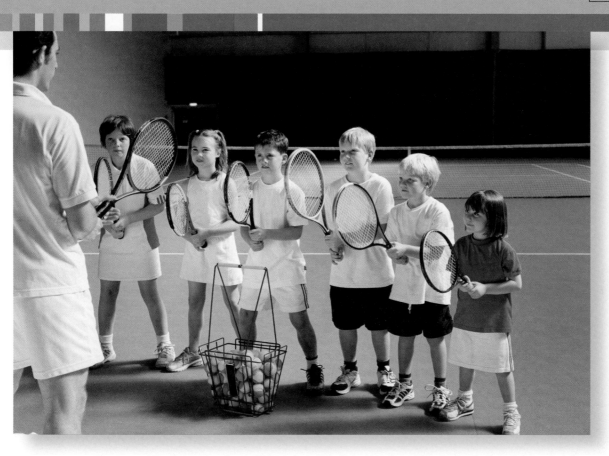

STUDENT OUTCOMES

1. Identify the common childhood diseases that can be prevented through early vaccinations.

2. Describe the characteristic lesions and associated symptoms of specific childhood diseases.

3. Explain the mode of transmission, incubation period, common signs and symptoms, and treatment of infectious mononucleosis.

4. Describe the signs and symptoms of viral meningitis.

5. Differentiate the signs and symptoms of the common sexually transmitted diseases, and describe the treatment for these conditions.

6. Identify the five different classifications of hepatitis, and differentiate the modes of transmission for each.

8. Describe the early signs and symptoms of hepatitis, and explain the progression of severity of symptoms.

9. Identify the common signs and symptoms of acquired immunodeficiency syndrome.

10. Explain the safety precautions that can be taken to minimize the transmission of highly infectious diseases.

ROLE DELINEATION COMPETENCIES

The following Performance Domains and Tasks defined in the National Athletic Trainers' Association Board of Certification *Role Delineation Study*, 5th Edition are addressed in this chapter:

BOC COMPETENCIES

I.   Prevention

   A. Educate the appropriate individual(s) about risks associated with participation and specific activities using effective communication techniques to minimize the risk of injury and illness.
   B. Interpret preparticipation and other relevant screening information in accordance with accepted guidelines to minimize the risk of injury and illness.
   G. Monitor participants and environmental conditions by following accepted guidelines to promote safe participation.

II.   Clinical Evaluation and Diagnosis

   E. Formulate a clinical impression by interpreting the signs, symptoms, and predisposing factors of the injury, illness, or condition to determine the appropriate course of action.
   F. Educate the appropriate individual(s) regarding the assessment by communicating information about the current or potential injury, illness, or health-related condition to encourage compliance with recommended care.
   G. Share assessment findings with other health care professionals using effective means of communication to coordinate appropriate care.

III.   Immediate Care

   A. Employ life-saving techniques through the use of standard emergency procedures in order to reduce morbidity and the incidence of mortality.
   B. Prevent exacerbation of non–life threatening condition(s) through the use of standard procedures in order to reduce morbidity.
   C. Facilitate the timely transfer of care for conditions beyond the scope of practice of the athletic trainer by implementing appropriate referral strategies to stabilize and/or prevent exacerbation of the condition(s).

IV.   Treatment, Rehabilitation, and Reconditioning

   D. Administer treatment for general illness and/or conditions using standard techniques and procedures to facilitate recovery, function, and/or performance.
   E. Reassess the status of injuries, illnesses, and/or conditions using standard techniques and documentation strategies in order to determine appropriate treatment, rehabilitation, and/or reconditioning and to evaluate readiness to return to a desired level of activity.
   F. Educate the appropriate individual(s) in the treatment, rehabilitation, and reconditioning of injuries, illnesses, and/or conditions using applicable methods and materials to facilitate recovery, function, and/or performance.
   G. Provide guidance and/or counseling for the appropriate individual(s) in the treatment, rehabilitation, and reconditioning of injuries, illnesses, and/or conditions through communication to facilitate recovery, function, and/or performance.

Although it is not the intention of this chapter to discuss all infectious diseases to which sport and physical activity participants may be exposed, several common diseases may confront the athletic trainer. For some childhood diseases, vaccines exist that can prevent infection. In older populations, however, individuals may not have received the necessary booster shots to prevent the onset of various illnesses. Chickenpox, mumps, measles (i.e., rubeola), rubella (i.e., German measles), and influenza are among the more commonly transmitted infections.

   Sexually transmitted diseases (STDs) continue to be a major concern for health care providers, particularly clinicians working with teenagers and college students, because many individuals in these populations are sexually active. Chlamydia, candidiasis, and trichomoniasis are common STDs that can affect sport and physical activity performance. If diagnosed and treated early, these conditions tend to be more annoying rather than troublesome. Several serious STDs, however, such as hepatitis and acquired immunodeficiency syndrome (AIDS), deserve special attention.

This chapter addresses the signs and symptoms, identification, and treatment of common childhood diseases, STDs, and other common infectious conditions. Although definitive diagnosis and treatment are completed by a physician, it is critical that the athletic trainer recognize a potential condition and immediately refer the individual to the primary care physician or team physician.

COMMON CHILDHOOD DISEASES

Q *In reviewing the medical history of high school students planning to participate in the upcoming fall sport season, what information would identify an increased risk for contracting influenza?*

Most bacterial and viral infectious diseases of childhood are prevented through a series of early vaccinations given between birth and 18 months of age. A vaccine is a suspension of infectious agents, or some part of them, that are given to establish resistance to an infectious disease. Vaccines are divided into four general classes:

1. Those containing living infectious organisms, which are either disabled or otherwise nonvirulent strains.

2. Those containing infectious agents killed by physical or chemical means.

3. Those containing solutions of toxins from microorganisms that may be used directly but that usually are treated to neutralize their toxic potential.

4. Those containing substances extracted from a portion of an infectious agent. Effective antiviral vaccines often are made by extracting only a small portion of the virus' protein coat.

Whatever its makeup, the vaccine stimulates the body to develop specific defensive mechanisms that result in near-permanent protections from the disease. Booster shots are given on entry into school (age, 4–6 years) and again in adolescence (age, 11–12 and/or 14–16 years). Maintaining immunity against diphtheria and tetanus requires booster vaccinations be given every 10 years. Because of its bloodborne transmission and significance to athletic trainers, however, hepatitis is discussed in more detail later in the chapter.

Bacterial Childhood Diseases

In the United States, infants are immunized against diphtheria, tetanus, and pertussis (DTP) and against *Haemophilus influenzae* type b (Hib). Even so, a few cases of diphtheria and tetanus are reported each year in nonimmunized or partially immunized adults. *Haemophilus influenzae* type b is one of the leading causes of invasive bacterial disease in children younger than 5 years and is the leading cause of meningitis in this age group (1).

Diphtheria

Diphtheria, which is caused by the organism *Corynebacterium diphtheriae,* is an acute, life-threatening, infectious disease that invades the upper respiratory region. The bacterium has an incubation period of 2 to 5 days. As it multiplies along mucous membrane surfaces, the organism irritates the tissue producing a very distinctive, leathery, blue-white pseudomembrane (i.e., false membrane) that is composed of bacteria, necrotized tissue, inflammatory cells, and fibrin. This membrane may grow to the extent that it impairs respiratory function.

SIGNS AND SYMPTOMS. The characteristic symptom is a thick, patchy, gray or blue-white membrane that forms over the mucous membranes of the pharynx, larynx, tonsils, soft palate, and nose (Fig. 25.1). Other symptoms include a mild

 FIGURE 25.1 Diptheria.

fever (100–101°F), sore throat, rasping cough, hoarseness, and enlarged, tender cervical lymph nodes. There may be a strong, foul odor to the breath. If untreated, the pseudomembrane, along with swelling, may occlude the air passages, leading to death by suffocation, or the infection may spread throughout the body, leading to death from its adverse effects on the heart (i.e., myocarditis), nerves (i.e., neuritis), and kidneys. Transmission is by direct contact, droplet spread, and indirect contact with articles soiled by discharges from infected persons.

MANAGEMENT. Immediate referral to a physician is warranted. Treatment involves administration of a diphtheria antitoxin and antibiotics to destroy the organism. The individual must be isolated, and bed rest is required. A soft or liquid diet is recommended.

Tetanus (Lockjaw)

The tetanus bacillus, *Clostridium tetani,* grows in the absence of oxygen in soil, dust, feces, and saliva. Tetanus spores invade the body, usually through a puncture wound or through lacerations, burns, trivial or unnoticed wounds, or injected contaminated street drugs. The spores produce a powerful toxin that attacks the central nervous system, which acts directly on voluntary muscles to produce contraction. The disease may affect anyone at any time, but children are at greater risk because of their tendency to develop skin wounds as a result of play activities.

SIGNS AND SYMPTOMS. The onset of symptoms may be gradual or abrupt. Abdominal rigidity usually is followed by painful muscle contractions, primarily of the masseter and neck muscles, although the trunk muscles also may be involved. Later, in the most common manifestation of tetanus, the jaws become rigidly fixed (i.e., lockjaw). In addition, the voice is altered, and the facial muscles contract, contorting the individual's face into a grimace. Finally, muscles in the back and extremities may become rigid, or the individual may experience extremely severe convulsive spasms of the muscles. The final phase of the disease may be accompanied by tachycardia, profuse sweating, high fever, and intense pain (2).

MANAGEMENT. Because of the serious nature of tetanus, all wounds should be cleansed thoroughly following standard protocol (see Chapter 6). In puncture wounds, bite wounds, and more significant lacerations or burns, a booster shot is recommended as soon as possible (within 72 hours) if the time from the previous booster is greater than 5 years. The toxin is neutralized if the tetanus antitoxin is administered before the toxin becomes attached to nerve tissue. Muscle relaxants also may be prescribed.

Pertussis (Whooping Cough)

Pertussis is caused by the bacillus *Bordetella pertussis* and has an incubation period of 7 to 10 days. It is an extremely contagious respiratory infection that is common in children, yet it remains the most common of all the diseases that can be preventable by routine childhood immunization (3).

SIGNS AND SYMPTOMS. Whooping cough occurs in three stages—namely catarrhal, paroxysmal, and convalescent. The catarrhal state begins with an insidious onset of an irritating cough, particularly at night, which may be accompanied by anorexia, sneezing, listlessness, conjunctivitis, and low-grade fever. The cough becomes progressively more irritating, violent, and eventually, paroxysmal within 1 to 2 weeks. The repeated episodes of violent coughing are interspersed with inhalations that feature a crowing or high-pitched whoop. In older children and adults, the whoop may be absent, but persistent coughing spells are present. These attacks frequently end with the expulsion of clear mucus followed by vomiting caused by choking on mucus. The coughing can be violent enough to cause nosebleed, detached retina, and hernia. During this stage, the child also is highly susceptible to secondary infections, such as otitis media, pneumonia, or encephalopathy. This stage lasts from 3 to 4 weeks. The final stage, the convalescent stage, may last from 1 to 2 months, with even a mild upper respiratory infection triggering symptoms.

MANAGEMENT. Immediate referral to a physician is warranted. Antibiotics are only effective during the early stages (i.e., before the persistent coughing spells); if administration is delayed past this stage, antibiotics have little effect.

Haemophilus Influenzae *Type B*

In children younger than 5 years, Hib is one of the leading causes of invasive bacterial disease and the leading cause of meningitis in this age group. The disease also can cause pneumonia, cellulitis, septic arthritis, otitis, sinusitis, and bronchitis. The bacteria are transmitted through respiratory droplets or other person-to-person contact. Groups at high risk include:

- Those older than 65 years

- Those with chronic disorders of the pulmonary or cardiovascular system, including those with asthma

- Those with chronic metabolic diseases (e.g., diabetes), renal dysfunction, or immunosuppression

- Children and teenagers receiving long-term aspirin therapy (i.e., risk of Reye's syndrome)

Infections have decreased by 95% since introduction of the Hib vaccine in 1988 (1).

■■■■ FIGURE 25.2 *Haemophilus influenzae* **type b.**

SIGNS AND SYMPTOMS. Symptoms usually come on rapidly, and they can include headache, muscle soreness, fatigue, loss of appetite, nasal congestion, sore throat, cough, and chest pains (Fig. 25.2). The virus also can lead to pneumonia and encephalitis, an infection of the meninges of the brain. If the organism leads to meningitis, the symptoms generally include fever, chills, malaise, headache, and vomiting. As the meninges become more irritated, other signs and symptoms occur, such as a stiff neck, exaggerated deep tendon reflexes, and back spasm in which the back arches backward so that the body rests on the head and heels.

MANAGEMENT. When the condition is identified, immediate referral to a physician is warranted. Typically, antibiotics are administered intravenously for at least 2 weeks, followed by oral antibiotics. Prophylactic treatment of close contacts with rifampin also is indicated.

Viral Childhood Diseases

In 1955, Jonas Salk introduced the first killed-virus vaccine for poliomyelitis, one of the most feared diseases of the time because of its potential for permanent crippling, disability, and death. Shortly thereafter, Albert B. Sabin introduced the first live-virus vaccine for polio, and because of its widespread success, this vaccine became the preferred protection against polio. By 1969, vaccines also were available for measles, mumps, and rubella. Vaccines for chickenpox and influenza soon followed. Table 25.1 summarizes the incubation period, signs and symptoms, and duration of the more common viral childhood diseases.

Poliomyelitis (Polio)

Polio is an inflammation of the gray matter of the spinal cord. It often results in spinal and muscle paralysis. The virus is spread by direct contact via fecal–oral and oral–oral routes.

SIGNS AND SYMPTOMS. The site of paralysis depends on the location of nerve cell destruction in the spinal cord or brainstem. Muscle paralysis may involve only one leg, leading to visible muscle wasting (Fig. 25.3). Sensation, however, may be intact, or the individual may have progressive paralysis that affects the vital organs and leads to death. In general, the infection has four possible outcomes (1):

- Asymptomatic illness occurs in 90% of poliovirus infections.

- Minor illness with fever, headache, malaise, sore throat, and vomiting occurs in approximately 5% of the population.

■■■■ FIGURE 25.3 **Polio.**

TABLE 25.1 Common Viral Infections

DISEASE	TRANSMISSION	INCUBATION PERIOD	CLINICAL SYMPTOMS	DURATION
Chickenpox (varicella)	Direct contact with respiratory secretions and fluid from lesions	13–17 days	Fever, headache, profuse rash on trunk and oral mucosa that leads to blisters that turn cloudy and become encrusted with scabs	1–2 weeks
Influenza	Airborne droplets; indirect contact with contaminated objects	1–5 days	Chills, fever, headache, muscle aches and pains, nonproductive cough, sore throat, hoarseness, rhinitis	2–7 days
German measles (rubella)	Nasopharyngeal droplets; direct contact with throat and nasal secretions of infected person	14–23 days	Light rash on face that spreads to trunk and extremities, low-grade fever and enlarged lymph nodes; can cause congenital heart defects in an infant if acquired by the mother during the first trimester of pregnancy	1–5 days
Measles (rubeola)	Airborne droplets; direct contact with nasal and throat secretions of infected person	7–18 days	Fever, photophobia, malaise, rhinitis, Koplik's spots, swollen throat, progressive brownish-pink rash on face and body	4–7 days
Mumps	Airborne droplets; direct contact with saliva of infected person	18 days	Enlarged salivary glands, fever, headache, malaise, and males may have swollen and tender testes	10 days

See *Vaccines and Toxoids Recommended for Adults in the United States*, which identifies the vaccines and booster shots recommended for adults, by age groups, in the United States, at the companion website at thePoint.

- Nonparalytic poliomyelitis with back pain and muscle spasms in addition to symptoms of minor illness occurs in 1 to 2% of the population.

- Paralytic polio with spinal and/or cranial paralysis occurs 3 to 4 days after minor illness has subsided in 0.1 to 2% of infected individuals.

MANAGEMENT. Although the disease has been eradicated in the Western hemisphere by widespread immunization, poliomyelitis remains a potentially serious disease in developing countries. Other than analgesics to relieve pain, no treatment exists for polio.

Chickenpox (Varicella)

Most individuals have chickenpox by age 10. It is a mild, but very contagious, disease in children. In adults, however, the disease can have severe effects. Chickenpox is caused by the human herpes virus 3 (varicella zoster). The incubation period may be 2 to 3 weeks, but it generally runs from 13 to 17 days. The disease is spread by direct contact with respiratory secretions and fluid from lesions of the infected person. It may be communicable from 5 days before to 5 days after the appearance of the first vesicles.

SIGNS AND SYMPTOMS. Chickenpox has a sudden onset of slight fever, mild headache, malaise, and loss of appetite for approximately 24 to 36 hours before the skin rash appears. The rash begins as flat, red spots (macules) that develop on the trunk and scalp and that, in a day or two, develop into raised papules and then clear vesicles containing a clear fluid surrounded by a red base (Fig. 25.4). Within 24 to 48 hours, the blisters turn cloudy and encrusted with a granular scab. They erupt in crops so that all three stages are present at the same time, beginning first on the back and chest and then spreading to the face, neck, and limbs.

MANAGEMENT. Immediate referral to a physician is warranted. Treatment is limited to relief of the symptoms, because no cure exists for chickenpox. Isolation is important during the infectious period,

FIGURE 25.4 **Varicella.**

usually until all the scabs disappear. Bicarbonate of soda baths, calamine lotion, or antihistamine lotions may help to relieve the pruritus. Scratching the lesions should be avoided. In severe cases, an antiviral agent, acyclovir, may be used. Because of its association with an increased incidence of Reye's syndrome, aspirin should not be used to treat fever in cases of chickenpox among children and adolescents.

Mumps

Mumps is most prevalent in the 5- to 9-year-old age group. In contrast to chickenpox, mumps is characterized by swelling of the salivary glands near the neck. The incubation period generally is 18 days, and the disease is communicable from 6 days before symptoms appear to as long as 9 days after symptoms appear. Mumps is spread by airborne droplets and by direct contact with the saliva of an infected person.

SIGNS AND SYMPTOMS. The classic symptoms of mumps are unilateral or bilateral swollen parotid glands (Fig. 25.5). Initially, there may be loss of appetite, headache, discomfort, and mild fever. These signs are followed by earache, salivary gland swelling, and temperature of 38.3 to 40°C (101–104°F) (5). The glands may become so swollen that it hurts to drink sour liquids or chew food. Complications, which tend to occur more frequently in males, may include epididymitis, meningitis, and rarely, a number of other serious illnesses, such as pancreatitis and various central nervous system manifestations.

MANAGEMENT. Immediate referral to a physician is warranted. Because of the viral nature of the disease, antibiotics are ineffective. Analgesics, fluids, and rest are the main forms of treatment.

Measles (Rubeola)

Measles is known to spread rapidly among unimmunized individuals and those who have not received booster shots against the childhood disease. It is spread by airborne droplets, direct contact with the nasal or throat secretions of infected individuals, and articles that have been freshly contaminated. The incubation period generally ranges from 7 to 18 days (usually 14 days to the onset of rash).

SIGNS AND SYMPTOMS. The onset of symptoms usually is gradual. Early symptoms include fever, photophobia, malaise, conjunctivitis, rhinitis, and cough. The disease is characterized by small spots (i.e., Koplik's spots) inside the cheeks that appear 4 to 5 days after the initial symptoms and 1 to 2 days before the onset of rash. Koplik's spots are found on the oral mucosa opposite the molars (Fig. 25.6A). They look like tiny, bluish-gray specks surrounded by a red halo. Throat swelling is present. The temperature may rise to 39.4 to 40.6°C

FIGURE 25.5 **Mumps.**

FIGURE 25.6 Rubeola (measles). A, Koplik's spots. **B,** Rash gives skin a blotchy appearance.

(103–105°F). The rash first appears as irregular, brownish-pink spots around the hairline, ears, and neck. Within 24 to 48 hours, it spreads to the body, arms, and legs, giving the skin a blotchy appearance (Fig. 25.6B). In certain areas, the lesions may be clustered so densely that the skin surface appears generally swollen and red. Within 3 to 5 days, the fever decreases, and the spots flatten, turn a brownish color, and begin to fade. Encephalitis is the most serious complication.

MANAGEMENT. Immediate referral to a physician is warranted. Treatment is symptomatic. Bed rest, usually in a darkened room to alleviate the discomfort of photophobia, is indicated. Fluids and acetaminophen are recommended for fever. Aspirin is not recommended for children because of the chance of developing Reye's syndrome. The individual should be kept isolated until the rash disappears.

Rubella (German Measles)

Normally, rubella is a mild disease in both children and adults, with one attack giving lifelong vaccination, but the disease can be extremely dangerous for an unborn child when a woman is infected during the first trimester of pregnancy. Birth defects may include heart disorders, eye clouding (i.e., cataracts), deafness, and mental retardation. The disease is transmitted by droplets or direct contact with the throat and nasal secretions of infected individuals. The incubation period ranges from 14 to 23 days, and the disease is communicable for approximately 1 week before and at least 4 days after the onset of the rash.

SIGNS AND SYMPTOMS. Rubella is marked by fever, symptoms of a mild upper respiratory tract infection, malaise, headache, swollen lymph nodes, joint pain, and a fine, red rash on the face that spreads to the body (Fig. 25.7). The rash is composed of pale-red, slightly elevated, discrete papules, or the rash may be highly diffuse and bright red. The rash begins on the face, spreads rapidly to other portions of the body, and usually fades so rapidly that the face may clear before the extremities are affected. The symptoms usually last only 2 to 3 days except the joint pain, which may last longer or return.

MANAGEMENT. Referral to a physician is warranted. Treatment is symptomatic. Bed rest is indicated. Topical antipruritic or warm-water baths may be recommended to relieve itching.

FIGURE 25.7 Rubella.

In reviewing the medical history of high school students planning to participate in the upcoming fall sport season, the following conditions would indicate an increased risk for contracting influenza: chronic disorders of the pulmonary or cardiovascular system (e.g., asthma); chronic metabolic diseases (e.g., diabetes), renal dysfunction, or immunosuppression; and long-term aspirin therapy (i.e., risk of Reye's syndrome).

INFECTIOUS MONONUCLEOSIS

What is the inherent danger associated with participation in contact or collision sports for an individual diagnosed with infectious mononucleosis?

The Epstein-Barr virus, which is in the herpes family, causes infectious mononucleosis, an acute viral disease manifested by a general feeling of malaise and fatigue. Commonly called the kissing disease, mononucleosis is transmitted in saliva by the oral–pharyngeal route. It also may be spread by sharing the drinking container of an infected individual. Infectious rates are highest among individuals between 15 and 25 years of age; after age 40, the condition is rare. The incubation period for infectious mononucleosis is 4 to 6 weeks. "Chronic fatigue syndrome" and Epstein-Barr virus have similar signs and symptoms, but the association of the two continues to be debated.

Signs and Symptoms

Initial symptoms include headache, malaise, and fatigue. After 3 to 5 days, fever, swollen lymph glands, and a sore throat develop. Individuals often describe the sore throat as "the worst sore throat I've ever had." In 10 to 15% of patients, jaundice and a rubella-like rash also may be present. Complications may arise if enlarged tonsils or adenoids obstruct the airway or if neurologic or cardiac changes occur.

Management

An individual suspected of having mononucleosis should be immediately referred to a physician.

Anti-inflammatory medication may be used to control headaches, fever, and general muscle aches and pains. Lozenges, saltwater gargles, and viscous lidocaine (Xylocaine) can ease throat pain. The overwhelming majority of individuals recover uneventfully. Corticosteroid therapy (prednisone) is only used for individuals with severe cases or specific indications, such as imminent airway obstruction or severe mono-hepatitis, or in the presence of neurologic, hematologic, or cardiac complications.

Individuals with mononucleosis should not participate in any contact or collision activities during which trauma could rupture the enlarged and vulnerable spleen. In some individuals, an ultrasonograph may be indicated to better assess the size of the spleen. Enlarged spleens have been known to rupture up to 3 weeks after initial symptoms appear. If the spleen is not markedly enlarged or painful, and if liver function is normal, as determined by appropriate laboratory tests, limited physical training may be resumed 3 weeks after onset of the illness, with strenuous exercise and return to contact activities occurring in another 1 to 2 weeks. A flak jacket can be worn to protect the spleen from injury.

The inherent danger associated with participation in contact or collision sports for an individual diagnosed with mononucleosis is the risk of splenic rupture. Enlarged spleens have been known to rupture up to 3 weeks after appearance of the initial symptoms of mononucleosis.

VIRAL MENINGITIS

What practices should be followed to reduce the risk of athletic team members contracting viral meningitis?

Viral infections of the nervous system are rare in athletes. Athletes and physically active individuals are at a greater risk for viral meningitis, however, when poor hygienic measures are used with drink-dispensing machines, water bottles, and water coolers.

Signs and Symptoms

Signs and symptoms of viral meningitis include fever, headache, nausea, vomiting, **myalgia**, neck pain, **nuchal rigidity**, decreased coordination, malaise, photophobia, and altered mental status. Because the meninges are inflamed, stretching them through neck flexion produces pain.

Management

The most important step in treating this condition is immediate referral to a physician for an accurate diagnosis. Drug therapy is used to control symptoms. The condition usually resolves on its own.

The individual should not return to activity until 2 to 3 weeks after symptoms have eased. Activity should be resumed in a gradual progression. If symptoms recur, the virus is still present, and activity should cease until the individual has been reevaluated by a physician.

A *In an effort to reduce the risk of athletic team members contracting viral meningitis, practices should be employed that ensure proper hygienic measures are used with drink dispensing machines, water bottles, and water coolers.*

SEXUALLY TRANSMITTED DISEASES

Q *Why is the diagnosis of STDs more complicated with female patients?*

Infections of the genital tract are called STDs. They affect more than 12 million Americans every year, with transmission being most common in those between 15 and 19 years. Furthermore, more than 80% of college students report being sexually active, and nearly one-fifth of these report at least one past STD episode (6). Chlamydia, the most common bacterial STD in the United States, is the leading STD in college students, with a reported incidence rate of 10 to 20% annually (7). In a recent study of 100 female athletes at Division 1 universities, 11% reported having an STD. Thirty-seven percent of those individuals reported having chlamydia and 18% gonorrhea or genital warts (8). Unlike herpes and the human papillomavirus, chlamydia is highly preventable, because transmission can be interrupted through the use of condoms. In addition, chlamydia is easily treated with antibiotic therapy. In females, chlamydia often is asymptomatic and undiagnosed, leading to potentially dangerous health and fertility problems. Some experts suggest that chlamydia screening should become a routine part of annual gynecologic examinations.

 See *Common Sexually Transmitted Diseases,* found on the companion website at thePoint, for a summary of the modes of transmission, incubation periods, signs and symptoms, and general treatments of the more common STDs.

Gonorrhea, the second most common STD in the United States, is characterized in males by a pungent, thick, milky yellow or greenish discharge and a burning sensation during urination. In women, the condition often is asymptomatic until it progresses to pelvic inflammatory disease. Genital ulcers commonly result from herpes, syphilis, and chancroids (Fig. 25.8). Herpes simplex affects nearly 20% of young adults.

A *In women, many STDs are asymptomatic, and they remain as such until a more serious disease develops. An undiagnosed STD can lead to potentially dangerous health and fertility problems.*

HEPATITIS

Q *What is the mode of transmission for hepatitis B?*

Hepatitis is divided into six types, each of which is caused by a different virus. Table 25.2 compares the five major hepatitis viruses. Hepatitis G virus has been discovered, but little is known about the virus, which is a bloodborne RNA virus. The American Medical Association, American Academy of Family Physicians, and American Academy of Pediatrics advocate that all children should receive a complete series of hepatitis B virus (HBV) vaccinations during the first 18 months of life. Vaccination as a prophylactic measure is required of an employer at no cost to an employee if that employee may

FIGURE 25.8 **Symptoms of sexually transmitted diseases.**

be exposed to bloodborne pathogens. An accelerated, two-dose series for adolescents between 11 and 15 years was approved in 1999, but only when using Recombivax HB (Merck) (9).

All older children and adolescents at high risk for HBV infection, in addition to those listed in Box 25.1, should receive a complete series of the vaccination. Although not specifically mentioned, coaches, referees, officials, recreational sport supervisors, and personal trainers also should be vaccinated, because they often are first on the scene of an acute injury involving hemorrhage.

TABLE 25.2 Major Viruses Known to Cause Hepatitis in Humans					
	HEPATITIS A	**HEPATITIS B**	**HEPATITIS C**	**HEPATITIS D**	**HEPATITIS E**
Transmitted	Fecal–oral; contaminated food and water (epidemics)	Bloodborne; sexual contact; contaminated needles	Bloodborne; sexual contact	Bloodborne	Fecal–oral
Incubation period	15–50 days	45–160 days	15–150 days	30–60 days	20–60 days
Special features	Immunoglobulin prophylaxis is effective	Pre-exposure and postexposure prophylaxis available	Asymptomatic in many; main cause of posttransfusion hepatitis; often becomes chronic	Coinfection with active hepatitis B virus or infection superimposed on chronic hepatitis B	High mortality in pregnant women. Large epidemics caused by contaminated water supplies

Adapted from Bartlett JB. Pocket Book of Infectious Disease Therapy. Baltimore: Williams & Wilkins, 1997; with permission.

Box 25.1 Individuals at Risk for Infection with Hepatitis B Virus and Human Immunodeficiency Virus (HIV)

- All health care workers, including athletic trainers, athletic training students, nurses, and physicians
- Caregivers of the developmentally disabled
- Patients undergoing dialysis
- Injection drug users
- Gay men
- Persons with multiple sex partners
- Inmates in correctional facilities
- Anyone who has resided in Haiti or Central Africa (HIV)
- Household contacts of adoptees who are surface antigen positive

FIGURE 25.9 Jaundice in the eyes.

Hepatitis B, the most common form of viral hepatitis, has an incubation period of 45 to 160 days and is transmitted by blood or blood products (i.e., post-transfusion hepatitis), semen, vaginal secretions, and saliva. Manual, oral, or penile stimulation of the anus is strongly associated with the spread of this virus. It is possible that an individual who is infected with HBV will exhibit no signs or symptoms, and the virus may go undetected. The HBV antigen is still present, however, and can be transmitted unknowingly to others through exposure to blood and other body fluids or through sexual contact. Hepatitis B virus can survive for at least 1 week in dried blood or on contaminated surfaces.

Signs and Symptoms

Hepatitis primarily attacks the liver, severely impairing its function. Early symptoms include mild, flu-like symptoms, such as malaise, fatigue, and loss of appetite. Progressive signs include severe fatigue, anorexia, nausea, vomiting, diarrhea, general muscle and joint pain, high fever, vomiting, severe abdominal pain, and dark urine. The most notable signs include a yellowing of the whites of the eyes and a yellowish or jaundiced skin appearance in light-complexioned individuals (Fig. 25.9). Hepatitis may increase the risk of developing cancer of the liver. In rare cases, hepatitis is fatal.

Management

Immediate referral to a physician is warranted if the individual has been exposed, or is suspected of having been exposed, to the virus. Currently, no specific drug therapy exists that will cure viral hepatitis. Postexposure vaccination also is available when individuals have come into direct contact with the body fluids of an infected person. Bed rest and adequate fluid intake can prevent dehydration, but the disease must run its course.

 Hepatitis B is transmitted by blood or blood products, semen, vaginal secretions, and saliva. Manual, oral, or penile stimulation of the anus is strongly associated with the spread of this virus.

ACQUIRED IMMUNODEFICIENCY SYNDROME

Should an individual who has tested positive for infection with human immunodeficiency virus (HIV) be permitted to participate in an organized sports program?

Acquired immunodeficiency syndrome results from infection with the HIV, which falls within a special category called **retroviruses**. An individual can be HIV-positive and, as such, infectious for years before any signs of AIDS appear. Human immunodeficiency virus attacks and destroys cells in the body's immune system, particularly the lymphocyte known as the helper T cell. In a healthy

Box 25.2   Common Signs and Symptoms Associated with Acquired Immunodeficiency Syndrome

- Persistent fever or night sweats
- Unexplained weight loss and loss of appetite
- Extreme fatigue not explained by physiologic activity or mental depression
- White spots or unusual blemishes in the mouth

- A persistent, dry cough unrelated to smoking
- Persistent, unexplained diarrhea or bloody stools
- Easy bruising or atypical bleeding from any body opening
- Blotches or bumps on or under the skin
- Persistent, severe headaches

individual, these cells stimulate the immune system to fight disease. In an infected individual, a gradual deterioration of the immune system leaves the body vulnerable to a variety of infections and cancers, such as herpes, oral candidiasis, pneumonia, encephalitis, and retinitis.

Currently, HIV has only been found to be transmitted in blood, semen, and vaginal secretions. In sports, the risk of AIDS is rare. In boxing, football, or wrestling, where participants may have a bloody nose or open cuts, close contact with the competitor may pose a health risk. To date, however, no documented case of HIV transmission through participation in sport has been published. Small amounts of bloodstain on a uniform do not require removal of the participant from the game or a uniform change; however, uniforms that become saturated with blood should be changed before returning to participation.

Signs and Symptoms

Signs and symptoms of AIDS vary, depending on the degree to which the immune system is impaired. Common symptoms include those listed in Box 25.2. Some researchers suggest that AIDS is more severe in women, with HIV infection progressing much faster.

Management

Immediate referral to a physician is warranted if the individual has been exposed, or is suspected of having been exposed, to the virus. To date, no effective cure or vaccine exists for AIDS. Various drug therapies have been developed for controlling the symptoms and decreasing the progression of the disease, but the success of drug therapy appears to be related to the stage of the virus and the time at which the drug therapy was initiated. Healthy HIV-positive athletes and those with AIDS may continue physical activity. The Americans with Disabilities Act of 1991 states that individuals infected with HIV cannot be discriminated against and may be excluded from participation only on sound medical grounds. In some cases, fatigue may not allow participation in intensive exercise or competition. The best defenses against the virus remain education about safe-sex practices and use of condoms as well as practicing universal precautions when dealing with blood and blood products (see Field Strategy 6.1).

 The Americans with Disabilities Act of 1991 states that athletes infected with HIV cannot be discriminated against and may be excluded from participation only on sound medical grounds.

SUMMARY

1. Childhood diseases can be prevented by early immunization (between birth and 18 months of age). Booster shots are given on entry into school and at adolescence.

2. Childhood bacterial diseases that can be prevented through vaccinations include diphtheria, tetanus, pertussis (whooping cough), and Hib. Childhood viral diseases that can be prevented

through vaccinations include poliomyelitis (polio), chickenpox (varicella), mumps, measles (rubeola), rubella (German measles), and hepatitis.

3. Adults from 18 to 24 years of age should receive booster shots for measles, mumps, rubella, varicella, and tetanus. Diphtheria and tetanus shots should be repeated every 10 years.

4. Mononucleosis is transmitted in saliva. Infection rates are highest among individuals aged 15 to 25 years. Signs and symptoms include headache, fatigue, loss of appetite, enlarged lymph nodes, swollen glands, and an enlarged spleen.

5. Individuals are at a greater risk of viral meningitis when poor hygienic measures are used around water bottles and watering stations.

6. Chlamydia is the most common bacterial STD in the United States, followed by gonorrhea and genital ulcers from herpes, syphilis, and chancroids. In males, common signs and symptoms of an STD include a mild itching and burning during urination and a discharge from the penis. In females, a vaginal discharge may be present, but many STDs are asymptomatic until the more serious pelvic inflammatory disease occurs.

7. Hepatitis B is the most common form of viral hepatitis, but it can be prevented with proper vaccination. The condition primarily attacks the liver, severely impairing function. Signs and symptoms include severe fatigue, malaise, and loss of appetite progressing to anorexia, nausea, vomiting, high fever, and a jaundiced appearance.

8. AIDS results from infection with HIV, which has been found to be transmitted in blood, semen, and vaginal secretions.

9. Most common viral diseases, including hepatitis and AIDS, can be prevented in the settings of athletics and physical activity by following universal precautions when dealing with blood and blood products.

10. If an individual is suspected of contracting an infectious disease, a physician referral is always recommended so that drug therapy can be prescribed along with other treatment. If the infection can be spread from person to person, individuals who are infected should be isolated from others until the physician determines that cross-infection is no longer possible.

REFERENCES

1. U.S. Department of Health and Human Services. Clinician's Handbook of Preventive Services. Washington, DC: U.S. Government Printing Office, 1994.
2. Tamporo CD, Lewis MA. Diseases of the Human Body. Philadelphia: FA Davis, 2000.
3. Bentsi-Enchill A. The return of the 100-day cough: resurgence of pertussis in the 1990s. Can Med Assoc J 1998; 159(6):695–696.
4. Bartlett JB. Pocket Book of Infectious Disease Therapy. Baltimore: Williams & Wilkins, 1997.
5. Benenson AS, ed. Control of Communicable Diseases Manual. Washington, DC: American Public Health Association, 1995.
6. Zinner SH, McCormack WM. Three decades of research on sexual behavior, and sexually transmitted pathogens in college students. Med Health 1997;80(10):338–340.
7. Sawyer RG, Moss DJ. Sexually transmitted diseases in college men: a preliminary clinical investigation. College Health 1993;42:111–115.
8. Watson A, Martin M, Hunt H. Incidence of sexually transmitted diseases and the need for sexual education for female collegiate athletes. J Ath Train 1998;33(2 Suppl): S–61.
9. Wilson T, Olson-Burgess C. Are you up to date on immunizations? Nurse Pract 2004;29(9):33–43.

Conditions of the Female Athlete, Disabled Athlete, and Senior Athlete

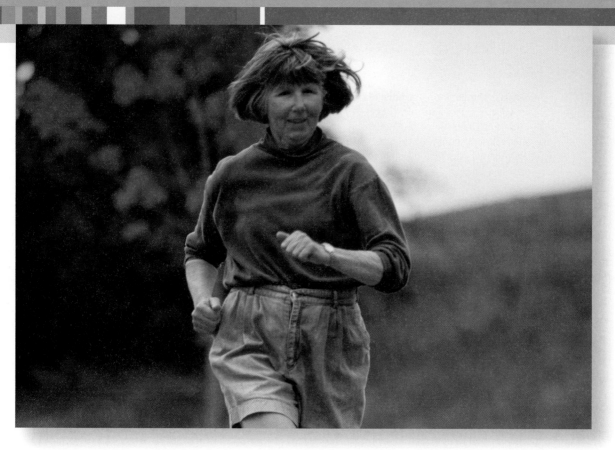

STUDENT OUTCOMES

1. Identify menstrual irregularities, and explain the implications that each irregularity can have on participation in sport and physical activity.

2. Describe the potential effects of oral contraceptives and other commonly used birth control methods on physically active females.

3. Describe the postural and musculoskeletal issues that can affect a pregnant female, including the implications of each condition on participation in sport and physical activity.

4. State the indications and contraindications for participation in sport and physical activity during pregnancy.

5. Identify the categories of eating disorders, and describe the general signs and symptoms of each disorder.

6. Explain the effect of osteoporosis on participation in sport and physical activity.

7. Identify the components of the Female Athlete Triad, and explain the impact of this condition on health and physical activity performance.

8. Describe injuries and medical conditions commonly sustained by wheelchair sport participants.

9. Identify the special considerations associated with physical activity for athletes with amputations, athletes with cerebral palsy, and athletes with visual impairments.

10. Describe the common injuries and medical conditions sustained by senior athletes.

ROLE DELINEATION COMPETENCIES

The following Performance Domains and Tasks defined in the National Athletic Trainers' Association Board of Certification *Role Delineation Study*, 5th Edition are addressed in this chapter:

BOC COMPETENCIES

I.   Prevention

   A. Educate the appropriate individual(s) about risks associated with participation and specific activities using effective communication techniques to minimize the risk of injury and illness.
   B. Interpret preparticipation and other relevant screening information in accordance with accepted guidelines to minimize the risk of injury and illness.
   G. Monitor participants and environmental conditions by following accepted guidelines to promote safe participation.

II.   Clinical Evaluation and Diagnosis

   E. Formulate a clinical impression by interpreting the signs, symptoms, and predisposing factors of the injury, illness, or condition to determine the appropriate course of action.
   F. Educate the appropriate individual(s) regarding the assessment by communicating information about the current or potential injury, illness, or health-related condition to encourage compliance with recommended care.
   G. Share assessment findings with other health care professionals using effective means of communication to coordinate appropriate care.

III.   Immediate Care

   A. Employ life-saving techniques through the use of standard emergency procedures in order to reduce morbidity and the incidence of mortality.
   B. Prevent exacerbation of non–life threatening condition(s) through the use of standard procedures in order to reduce morbidity.
   C. Facilitate the timely transfer of care for conditions beyond the scope of practice of the athletic trainer by implementing appropriate referral strategies to stabilize and/or prevent exacerbation of the condition(s).

IV.   Treatment, Rehabilitation, and Reconditioning

   D. Administer treatment for general illness and/or conditions using standard techniques and procedures to facilitate recovery, function, and/or performance.
   E. Reassess the status of injuries, illnesses, and/or conditions using standard techniques and documentation strategies in order to determine appropriate treatment, rehabilitation, and/or reconditioning and to evaluate readiness to return to a desired level of activity.
   F. Educate the appropriate individual(s) in the treatment, rehabilitation, and reconditioning of injuries, illnesses, and/or conditions using applicable methods and materials to facilitate recovery, function, and/or performance.
   G. Provide guidance and/or counseling for the appropriate individual(s) in the treatment, rehabilitation, and reconditioning of injuries, illnesses, and/or conditions through communication to facilitate recovery, function, and/or performance.

As more children, females, seniors, and people with varying levels of physical ability participate in sport and physical activity, increasing levels of knowledge and clinical skills are required to meet the needs of these participants. This chapter focuses on considerations regarding these special populations. Issues specific to physically active females are discussed, followed by the special concerns of athletes with disabilities. Finally, special considerations for the senior athlete are presented.

SPECIAL CONCERNS OF THE FEMALE ATHLETE

Q *A lean, 16-year-old distance runner reports that she has not had a menstrual period in 3 months and is concerned she may be pregnant. What other menstrual irregularities could account for this absence of menses, and what recommendations should the athletic trainer make to the runner?*

As more and more females of all ages participate in sport and physical activity, an increasing understanding of the unique physical nature of females is required to meet the needs of this population. This section addresses gynecologic irregularities, birth control and physical activity participation, pregnancy and physical activity, eating disorders, osteoporosis, and the Female Athlete Triad.

The Uterine (Menstrual) Cycle

The **uterine**, or **menstrual**, **cycle** is a series of cyclic changes that the inner lining of the uterus (i.e., the endometrium) goes through each month as it responds to varying levels of hormones in the blood. It coincides with the **ovarian cycle**, which is associated with the maturation of an egg. The ovarian cycle is divided into two phases. The **follicular phase** (i.e., days 1–14) is the period of follicle growth; a follicle is a spheroidal cell cluster in the ovary that contains an ovum or egg. **Ovulation**, or release of the egg, occurs midcycle, when the ballooning ovarian wall ruptures and expels the egg. The **luteal phase** (i.e., days 14–28) occurs after ovulation. The ruptured follicle collapses and forms a new endocrine gland, called the corpus luteum, that begins to secrete progesterone and some estrogen. If pregnancy does not occur, the corpus luteum begins to degenerate in approximately 10 days, and its hormonal output ends. In contrast, if the egg is fertilized and pregnancy ensues, the corpus luteum persists until the placenta is ready to take over its hormone-producing responsibility in approximately 3 months. The menstrual cycle follows three distinctive phases, as depicted in Figure 26.1.

1. **Menstrual Phase (Days 1–5):** In this phase, the uterus sheds all but the deepest portion of the endometrium. As the endometrium detaches from the uterine wall, it often is accompanied by bleeding for 3 to 5 days. The tissue and blood pass out through the vagina as the menstrual flow.

2. **Proliferative Phase (Days 6–14):** During this phase, the endometrium rebuilds itself. The basal layer, influenced by rising blood levels of estrogen, generates a new functional layer. As this new layer thickens, the glands of the endometrium enlarge, and its spiral arteries increase in number. As a result, the endometrium once again becomes thick and well vascularized. Also during this phase, estrogen induces synthesis of progesterone receptors in the endometrial cells, readying them for interaction with progesterone. Ovulation occurs in the ovary at the end of this stage.

3. **Secretory Phase (Days 15–28):** In this phase, the endometrium prepares for implantation of an embryo. Rising levels of progesterone act on the estrogen-primed endometrium, causing the spiral arteries to coil more tightly and convert the functional area to a secretory mucosa. The uterine glands enlarge, coil, and begin secreting nutritious glycoproteins into the uterine cavity. These nutrients can sustain an embryo until it becomes implanted into the blood-rich endometrial lining. If fertilization does not occur, the corpus luteum begins to degenerate toward the end of the secretory phase. Progesterone levels fall, depriving the endometrium of hormonal support, and the spiral arteries kink and go into spasm. Without oxygen and nutrients, the endometrial cells begin to die and the functional layer to self-digest, setting the stage for menstruation to begin on day 28.

Non–physically active females experience **menarche** at an average age of 12.8 years, whereas the average age for physically active females ranges from 13.5 to 15.5 years. The normal cycle is 28 days, but the cycle can range from 25 to 35 days. Menarche continues throughout a female's life until menopause, which is the cessation of menstrual function and the subsequent decline in ovarian

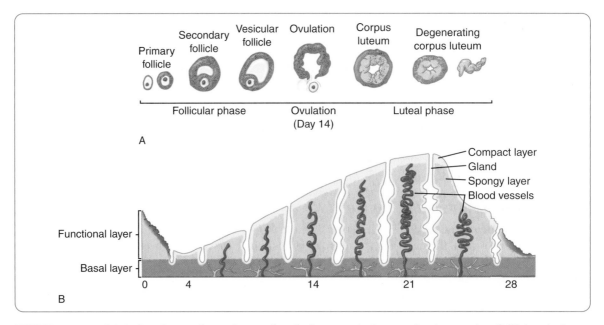

FIGURE 26.1 Ovarian and uterine cycle. A, Structural changes in the ovarian follicles during the 28-day ovarian cycle correlate with changes in the endometrium of the uterus during the uterine cycle. **B,** The uterine cycle has three stages: menstrual, proliferative, and secretory. The first phase (menstrual) is a shedding, and the second phase (proliferative) rebuilds the endometrium. Both of these events occur before ovulation. The final phase (secretory) involves enriching the blood supply and providing nutrients that prepare the endometrium to receive a fertilized egg.

hormone production. Although the average age for menopause is approximately 51 years, a gradual change occurs in reproductive function, called the **climacteric phase,** that ranges from age 46 to 55. During this period, called the **perimenopausal** years, the menstrual cycle may shorten and become irregular in both frequency and bleeding. After 56 years of age, a female is said to be postmenopausal.

Gynecologic Irregularities

Many females at one time or another are affected by gynecologic irregularities. Vaginitis is the most frequent gynecologic diagnosis encountered by physicians who provide primary care to females. Menstrual irregularities may include dysmenorrhea, menstrually induced leg pain, anovulatory oligomenorrhea, luteal phase deficiency, and exercise-associated amenorrhea. Each of these conditions can be identified and managed, but without early detection and proper treatment, some of these irregularities can lead to long-term health problems, including chronic stress fractures, osteoporosis, endometriosis, and infertility.

Vaginitis

Vaginitis, or inflammation of the vagina, occurs when the normal vaginal flora has been altered, either by the introduction of pathogens or by changes in the environment that allow pathogens to proliferate. The condition is difficult to assess, because symptoms may result from fungal, bacterial, or protozoal infections; atrophic vaginitis; cervicitis; genital ulcers; vulvar intraepithelial neoplasia; vestibulitis; and allergic and contact reactions. Infectious causes are predominantly secondary to bacterial vaginosis, vulvovaginal candidiasis, and trichomoniasis. Diagnosis is difficult, because females rarely present with classic symptoms, frequently are asymptomatic, or have more than one cause of their symptoms. Risk factors include douching, use of an intrauterine device, orogenital sex, previous pregnancy, and being from a nonwhite race (1).

SIGNS AND SYMPTOMS. Vaginal discharge, itching, frequent urination, and/or vaginal irritation are common signs and symptoms. Depending on the cause of the inflammation, the vaginal discharge has specific characteristics. **Bacterial vaginosis,** the most common cause of vaginitis, produces a thin, off-white discharge with a "fish" odor that increases in intensity after intercourse. **Candidal vaginitis** produces a thick, white, "cottage cheese" discharge with no odor. Vaginal **pruritus** and **dysuria** also may be present. **Trichomonal vaginitis** presents with a malodorous, yellow-green or discolored discharge as well as with pruritus and vaginal irritation.

MANAGEMENT. Females suspected of having vaginitis should be immediately referred to their primary care physician for early diagnosis. A history and physical examination should include an analysis of the vaginal discharge. In treating bacterial vaginitis, the Centers for Disease Control and Prevention (CDC) recommend the use of metronidazole, 500 mg orally twice a day for 7 days, or clindamycin or metronidazole vaginal cream. If the infection stems from *Candida* sp., a topical antifungal agent or a one-time dose of a 150-mg oral capsule of fluconazole is recommended. Trichomonal vaginitis is a vaginitis for which the sexual partner also needs to be treated. The CDC recommends a 2-g oral dose of metronidazole in a single dose for acute treatment (1).

Menstrual Disorders

Physically active females tend to have a higher degree of menstrual disorders compared with non–physically active females. These disorders include dysmenorrhea, menstrual-induced leg pain, anovulatory oligomenorrhea, luteal phase suppression, and exercise-associated amenorrhea.

DYSMENORRHEA. Menstrual cramps, or **dysmenorrhea**, usually are caused by an overproduction of prostaglandins, a group of chemicals acting as local hormones that are produced in the body and synthesized in all tissues. Uterine prostaglandins cause the muscles of the uterus to contract. Under most conditions, the contractions are minor and go unnoticed. More severe myometrial contractions and the resulting myometrial ischemia, however, lead to the severe abdominal pain associated with dysmenorrhea. This condition is the leading cause of recurrent, short-term school absence in adolescent girls (2).

Pain is localized in the lower abdomen but may radiate into the back, hip, and thighs. The condition usually begins with the onset of menses, continuing through the first days of the menstrual cycle, but tends to decrease in intensity as the individual ages. Other symptoms include bloating, nausea, vomiting, diarrhea, headache, breast tenderness, fatigue, irritability, and nervousness.

Regular exercise and a diet high in fluids and fiber but low in salt can alleviate the bloating and swelling caused by water retention. Nonsteroidal anti-inflammatory drugs (NSAIDS) are the recommended initial therapy for dysmenorrhea (3). These medications have a direct analgesic effect through inhibition of prostaglandin synthesis, which decreases myometrial contractions and the volume of menstrual flow. Ice massage to the low back, application of heat packs, and acupressure also can help to relieve pain. Severe or persistent discomfort may necessitate referral to a physician to rule out pelvic inflammatory disease, benign uterine tumors, obstruction of the cervical opening, and **endometriosis.** Endometriosis is a condition in which endometrial cells from the uterine lining implant themselves in the abdominal and uterine cavities and, occasionally, in the ovarian lining. Hormone therapy is a common method of treatment to decrease pain, discomfort, and other unwanted signs and symptoms associated with dysmenorrhea.

MENSTRUALLY INDUCED LEG PAIN. Some females report leg pain induced by physical activity during the week before their menstrual cycle. This leg pain is associated with females who are ovulating and normally have premenstrual fluid retention. The fluid retention is thought to allow less room for muscle hypertrophy during exercise, resulting in exertional compartment-like symptoms. Females with menstrually induced leg pain can be treated with oral contraceptives that suppress ovulation and decrease fluid retention. Conversely, some females report exertional compartment leg pain after using hormonal therapy as a means of contraception. The progesterone in birth control pills appears to increase the likelihood of fluid retention, resulting in the induced leg pain. Changing the birth control pill to one containing lower progesterone levels often brings relief. Females with menstrually induced exertional compartment-like symptoms should be questioned about their menstrual cycle and use of oral contraceptives.

ANOVULATORY OLIGOMENORRHEA. Anovulation, which is the cessation of ovulation, is associated with chronic, unopposed production of estrogen that leads to continuous endometrial stimulation and lower levels of progesterone. Several different patterns of irregular bleeding range from short (i.e., <21 days) to long (i.e., 35–90 days) cycles with between bleeding (4). The longer pattern is associated with **oligomenorrhea**. Oligomenorrhea refers to infrequent menstrual cycles (i.e., six to nine cycles per year), and it often is associated with a combination of strenuous exercise and significant weight loss. As such, oligomenorrhea and amenorrhea are more prevalent among runners (10–50%) than among the general population (2–5%) (4). During anovulatory oligomenorrhea, bleeding can be very heavy (i.e., menorrhagia), at times leading to iron depletion and anemia, both of which may affect performance in sport and physical activity. Management includes referral to a physician to rule out endometriosis. Monthly progesterone therapy usually is indicated.

LUTEAL PHASE SUPPRESSION. The luteal phase of the ovarian cycle extends from ovulation until the onset of the next menstrual bleeding, normally approximately 12 to 17 days. The hormone progesterone is produced only after ovulation. Luteal phase deficiency is characterized by shortened length of the luteal phase and insufficient production of progesterone. The menstrual cycle usually is normal but occurs more frequently. In runners, more miles per week parallels greater shortening of the luteal phase (1).

EXERCISE-ASSOCIATED AMENORRHEA. The absence of menstruation, or **amenorrhea**, is more prevalent among physically active females, particularly runners, compared with the general population. Amenorrhea is a symptom, not a disease, and it has been linked to prepubertal exercise, premature ovarian failure, central nervous system tumors, infections, hypothalamic–pituitary–ovarian hormonal imbalances, chronic diseases, osteoporosis, and malnutrition. Other related causes include weight loss, low levels of body fat, loss of specific fat stores (particularly femoral adipose tissue stores), excessive exercise, and being a vegetarian. Exercise-associated amenorrhea has been reported in females participating in virtually every sport, and particularly in females who began physical training at a young age. Several risk factors can predispose a female to the condition (Box 26.1).

Primary amenorrhea is the absence of menstruation by age 16 in a girl with secondary sex characteristics. Secondary amenorrhea is the absence of menstruation for three or more consecutive menstrual cycles after menarche. This can result from pregnancy or dysfunction in the ovaries, endometrium, pituitary gland, or hypothalamus.

Box 26.1   Risk Factors for Amenorrhea

- Young age (may have immature hypothalamic–pituitary–ovarian axis)
- Higher activity level (runners, cyclists, swimmers)
- Higher intensity (more strenuous or longer exercise period)
- History of menstrual irregularity
- Prepubertal training
- Delayed menarche
- Low body weight/weight loss or low body fat/fat loss
- Never having given birth
- Never having used oral contraceptive pills (twice as likely to suffer a stress fracture as those who use them)
- Diet lacking in protein and total calories (poor nutrition may be the most important factor to increase the risk of amenorrhea)
- Eating disorders
- Psychological stress (study results are contradictory)
- Genetic/hereditary factors (may play a role in the age of menarche)
- Total number of risk factors (the more risk factors, the more likely the individual will have exercise-related menstrual dysfunction)

Amenorrhea and decreased circulating levels of estrogen are commonly accepted as predisposing females to reduced bone density, leading to an increased risk of osteopenia and stress fractures, particularly in the lumbar vertebrae and lower extremities, as well as increased risk of musculoskeletal injuries. Within the first 3 months of amenorrhea, a female should be fully evaluated to rule out pregnancy, counseled regarding the risks of bone density loss, and encouraged to alter training regimens. Decreasing training, increasing food intake, and administrating hormone therapy have been used to manage amenorrhea.

Research suggests that menses returns in some females with amenorrhea after they gain weight, decrease exercise, or both. This is accomplished by reducing the number of training days, mileage, or intensity. Diet should be evaluated to ensure an adequate caloric intake that matches the high energy output. Hormone therapy, including oral contraceptives and cyclic estrogen/progesterone therapy, does not increase bone mass, but it can prevent further bone loss, vaginal and breast atrophy, and osteopenia. An individual may choose not to take oral contraceptives, however, because of the side effects, which include increased incidence of vaginitis, weight gain, acne, breast tenderness, and mood alterations. Females who remain amenorrheic should be examined annually.

GENERAL MANAGEMENT OF MENSTRUAL DISORDERS. Females experiencing any type of menstrual dysfunction should be referred to a physician, preferably a gynecologist. The referral should include a pelvic examination and, in some cases, blood tests to determine if the menstrual dysfunction is related to exercise or some pathologic condition. In addition, females with oligomenorrhea or amenorrhea should have an annual history and physical examination. Management of menstrual dysfunction often depends on the type of dysfunction. Hormone therapy, including both progesterone and estrogen protocols, often is the treatment of choice, but some side effects may result from the drug therapy. Estrogen therapy would not be indicated for females with hypertension, diabetes mellitus, migraine headaches, fibrocystic breast disease, or gallbladder disease.

Endometriosis

Endometriosis is characterized by the presence of uterine endometrial tissue outside of its normal location. Abnormal locations include the pelvic peritoneum, the ovaries, the rectovaginal septum, and more rarely, the pericardium, pleura, and even the brain. The prevalence of pelvic endometriosis ranges from 6 to 10% in the general female population; in females with pain, infertility, or both, the incidence ranges from 35 to 50% (5).

SIGNS AND SYMPTOMS. When endometrial tissue grows outside of the endometrial cavity, dysmenorrhea, oligomenorrhea, severe pelvic pain, and pain on defecation can occur. Endometriosis may develop asymptomatically, leading to eventual infertility.

MANAGEMENT. Management consists of gynecologic referral for a laparoscopic examination. Treatment focuses on relieving pain, ameliorating infertility, or both. Depending on the level of severity, drug therapy or surgical intervention often is indicated. No contraindications to exercise exist for females who develop endometriosis.

Ovarian Cysts

Benign cysts around the ovary stem from the corpus luteum, a small, yellow structure formed in the ovary at the site of a ruptured ovarian follicle immediately after ovulation. These cysts may occur at any time from puberty to menopause.

SIGNS AND SYMPTOMS. Nonneoplastic cysts usually are small and produce few symptoms. True ovarian neoplasms may be benign, malignant, cystic, or solid. Large cysts may produce pelvic pain, low back pain, and **dyspareunia**. Some cysts are mobile and can twist, resulting in acute spasmodic abdominal pain. Urinary retention also can result if a large, fluid-filled cyst presses on the area near the bladder.

MANAGEMENT. Referral to a physician is necessary for visualization of potential ovarian cysts through laparoscopy or sonography. Treatment varies depending on the type and size of the cyst.

Box 26.2 Symptoms Associated with Premenstrual Syndrome

Physical Symptoms		Psychological Symptoms	
Headache	Changes in appetite	Irritability	Difficulty in concentrating
Bloating	Vasomotor flushing	Depression	Forgetfulness
Breast tenderness	Heart palpitations	Fatigue	
Gastrointestinal upset	Dizziness		

Small cysts may disappear spontaneously by reabsorption or silent rupture; others may require drug-induced ovulation therapy or surgical resection. If concerns exist regarding malignancy, surgery is necessary for proper diagnosis and treatment.

Premenstrual Syndrome

Menstruating females often suffer from **premenstrual syndrome** (PMS), a common cyclic disorder of females across the life span. Symptoms often can become debilitating, interfering with physical training and competition. Fatigue may result in subpar performance and increased rate of injuries. The causes of PMS vary, but fluctuations in hormone levels during the menstrual cycle appear to be the most common cause.

SIGNS AND SYMPTOMS. Headaches, breast tenderness, back pain, bloating, irritability, depression, fatigue, and certain food cravings are all symptoms that may occur during the luteal phase (i.e., days 15–28) of the menstrual cycle. Premenstrual syndrome symptoms frequently are divided into physical and psychological, but a female must consistently exhibit a combination of one psychological change and one physical symptom during the luteal phase to be diagnosed with PMS (6) (Box 26.2).

MANAGEMENT. Regular exercise, particularly aerobic activities, and an overall healthy diet with a reduction in salt intake can help to alleviate some symptoms. Dysmenorrhea and headaches associated with PMS can be treated with NSAIDs. Hormonal therapy may be used, but this should be done on an individual basis. If self-help techniques do not alleviate symptoms, or if symptoms involve moderate to severe psychological problems, referral to a physician is warranted.

Birth Control and Participation in Sport and Physical Activity

Contraceptive choices available to females include steroid contraceptives, intrauterine devices, barrier methods, spermicides, natural family planning, male and female sterilization, and emergency contraceptives. Steroid contraceptives are the most frequently used reversible method in the United State by females under the age of 35 (7). Oral contraceptives prohibit ovulation, reduce dysmenorrhea, and decrease the amount and duration of the menstrual flow.

Certain contraindications to the use of oral contraceptives exist. These contraindications include:

- Hypertension (diastolic pressure > 90 nn Hg)

- Migraine headaches

- Depression

- Hepatitis or impaired liver function

- Oligomenorrhea or amenorrhea

- Abnormal glucose tolerance

- Recent major elective surgery (<4 weeks postoperative)

In addition, some medications, such as antibiotics, analgesics, antihistamines, and drugs used to treat tuberculosis, epilepsy, and depression, can interfere with the effectiveness of oral contraceptives.

The choice of birth control depends on coital frequency, exercise habits, lifestyle, medical history, fertility plans, and potential benefits. Most side effects associated with the amount of estrogen versus progestin and other compounds found in the various oral contraceptives are counteracted by exercise. Regular exercise increases the protective high-density lipoprotein cholesterol, reduced the deleterious low-density lipoprotein cholesterol, lowers the total triglyceride levels, and activates the fibrinolytic system that is responsible for converting fibrin to soluble products. In addition, most physically trained females have lower arterial blood pressure, lower body fat, and higher lean body weight and do not smoke. Each of these factors puts sedentary females at risk for complications. As such, for healthy, active young females, the benefits of oral contraceptives outweigh the risks.

Pregnancy and Sport Participation

The impact of exercise on a pregnant female and her developing fetus is an area of concern, particularly because chemicals and nutrients pass freely in the placental blood flow. Certainly, any factors that compromise the fetal blood supply would be important in counseling a pregnant female regarding exercise during pregnancy. Gains in body weight and fat accumulation are obvious adaptations to pregnancy that can have some effect on weight-bearing exercise. The hormones progesterone and relaxin increase joint laxity, making articulations wider and more mobile during the later stages of pregnancy; as such, ballistic movements must be avoided during daily activities and exercise. Exercise should be an important normal part of pregnancy for the active female and has been shown to have several benefits (Box 26.3).

Postural and Musculoskeletal Issues

Postural adaptations to compensate for the weight of the uterus lead to increased lordosis and upper spine extension. The female's center of gravity shifts upward and forward, often leading to lower back pain. Exercises to strengthen the abdominal and hip extensors (i.e., hamstrings and gluteus maximus) as well as to relax and/or stretch the erector spinae and hip flexors (i.e., iliopsoas, pectineus, and rectus femoris) can relieve some of this pain. Proper lifting techniques to relieve stress on the low back should be incorporated in daily activities. For a previously active, healthy female during an uncomplicated pregnancy, moderate aerobic exercise does not produce circulatory alterations that compromise fetal oxygen supply or lactation. Studies examining fetal development, fetoplacental growth, prematurity, fetal stress/distress, and condition during labor and at birth have found that females who exercise regularly do not experience an increase in abortion, congenital abnormalities, abnormal placentation, premature rupture of the membranes, or preterm labor. Although increases were found in fetal heart rate after exercise, no adverse effects were demonstrated. Exercise and adequate diet also were found to decrease the risk of preeclampsia, a common disorder of pregnancy whereby the normal hemodynamic response to pregnancy is compromised, and to have affect mammary gland development, milk volume, and milk composition (8,9).

Exercise Considerations

Pregnant females should be aware of the potential for fetal hypoglycemia during exercise. Under prolonged exercise, maternal blood sugar may decrease. The pregnant female needs to consume

---

Box 26.3 Benefits of Exercise During Pregnancy

- Maintenance or improvement of maternal fitness
- Control of excess weight gain
- Improved posture and appearance
- Increased energy
- Improved sleep
- Decreased incidence of low back pain
- Improved self-image and self-esteem
- Decreased incidence of varicose veins
- Decreased water retention
- Decreased level of tension
- Possible decrease in complications during labor and shortened labor
- More rapid postpartum recovery

extra calories to meet the demands of both pregnancy and an exercise regime. Furthermore, after the fifth month of pregnancy, maternal hypotension can develop if exercises are performed in a supine position. In this position, the uterus compresses the vena cava, slowing venous return and leading to a decrease in fetal circulation as well as to maternal hypotension. Absolute medical conditions for which exercise is contraindicated (4) include:

- Cardiovascular disease

- Significant anemia

- Premature rupture of membranes

- Persistent second- or third-trimester bleeding

- Preterm labor during the previous or current pregnancy (or both)

- Incompetent cervix or cerclage

- Uncontrolled hypertension, anemia, renal disease, and diabetes mellitus

Exercise programs need to be individualized in consultation with the supervising physician or obstetrician. In January 2002, the American College of Obstetricians and Gynecologists recommended that in the absence of either medical or obstetric complications, pregnant females should complete 30 minutes or more of moderate exercise each day (10). The primary goal with exercise during pregnancy is safety. Females who exercise regularly can participate in several aerobic activities, such as walking, bicycling, aerobic dance, water aerobics, swimming, jogging, cross-country skiing, ice or roller skating, and tennis. Aerobic classes should be modified to decrease the amount of ballistic movements, and exercising in a supine position should be avoided. A 5- to 10-minute warm-up period can be followed by 30 to 60 minutes of exercise at 65 to 85% of maximum heart rate three to five times per week. Elite athletes can exercise for 60 to 90 minutes at 75 to 85% of maximum heart rate four to six times per week (4). The exercise period should be followed by an appropriate cool-down and stretching period.

See *Recommendations for Pregnant Females with Exercise Problems*, available on the companion website at thePoint, for a summary of problems pregnant females can encounter during exercise and suggested recommendations.

Weight training with light weights and higher repetitions can be continued during pregnancy when the goal is strength maintenance rather than gain. Proper lifting and breathing techniques, such as exhaling during exertion, must be practiced consistently. Free-weight exercises that place the joints in a traction position, thereby stressing ligamentous structures, should be avoided.

In running programs, the distance and intensity of workouts should be decreased as the pregnancy progresses. Because many physiologic and morphologic changes of pregnancy persist for 4 to 6 weeks postpartum, exercise routines should be resumed gradually after the sixth-week postpartum medical check-up in consultation with the supervising obstetrician.

Eating Disorders

Clinically, an eating disorder may entail refusal to maintain a healthy body weight (i.e., 85% of expected body weight), dramatic weight loss, fear of gaining weight even when underweight, preoccupation with food, abnormal patterns of food consumption, or recent binge-eating behaviors associated with loss of control and feelings of guilt. Eating disorders are becoming more prevalent in both competitive and recreational sport participants, affecting both females and males. The prevalence of eating disorders at progressively younger ages has become a growing concern. It is estimated that 0.5% of adolescent females in the United States have anorexia nervosa, that 1 to 5% meet the criteria for bulimia nervosa, and that as much as 5 to 10% of all cases of eating disorders occur in males (11). These disorders often are linked to activities that stress leanness (e.g., gymnastics, distance running, swimming, diving, rowing, ballet, cross-country skiing, and wrestling), but no sport is exempt. The incidence of eating disorders is difficult to pinpoint because of the secretive nature of those with the disorders.

Eating disorders are divided into three diagnostic categories—namely, atypical eating disorders, bulimia nervosa, and anorexia nervosa. Anorexia and bulimia account for approximately 66% of all eating disorders. In addition to these three categories, a subclinical eating disorder has recently been termed **disordered eating**, which classifies individuals who demonstrate significant signs and symptoms of eating disorders but do not meet the diagnostic criteria for an eating disorder (12).

Atypical Eating Disorders

Many physically active females and males show signs of disordered eating habits but do not meet the established criteria for bulimia nervosa or anorexia nervosa. For example, the individual's weight may be just above the diagnostic threshold for anorexia nervosa, or a female may continue to have normal menstruation. In addition, an individual may have extreme dietary restraint, pronounced excessive exercising, occasional binge eating, and low to normal body weight. Many of these individuals may have had anorexia nervosa or bulimia nervosa and exhibit certain physical features, as well as psychological and behavioral symptoms, that indicate continued disordered eating characteristics, such as those listed in Box 26.4.

Bulimia Nervosa

Bulimia nervosa is characterized by normal body weight for age and height and having a minimum average of two binge-eating episodes per week for at least 3 months (12). The person with bulimia maintains a cyclical pattern of ingesting large quantities of food, often 1,000 to 10,000 calories, during a few minutes to several hours. Purging may or may not occur; if purging does occur, it is referred to as the "binge–purge cycle." The individual often has significant fluid and electrolyte abnormalities that can result in cardiac arrhythmias, hypotension because of low blood volume, metabolic acidosis caused by laxative-induced diarrhea, and cardiomyopathy. Gastrointestinal complications include esophagitis, possible esophageal perforation, pancreatitis, and constipation secondary to chronic laxative abuse. Rather than amenorrhea, as seen in those with anorexia, irregular menses is common. The three most common physical signs associated with bulimia are:

- Russell's sign, which is a lesion on the dorsum of the hand caused by repetitive trauma to the area during self-induced vomiting. This elongated ulceration, or hyperpigmented callus or scar, is visible on the metacarpophalangeal joint.

Box 26.4   Signs and Symptoms of a Possible Eating Disorder

Physical Features

- Weight that is too low for athletic performance, or extreme fluctuations in weight
- Swollen salivary glands (e.g., puffy cheeks or jaw just in front of the ear)
- Amenorrhea
- Sores or calluses on knuckles or back of hand from inducing vomiting
- Hypoglycemia
- Cardiac arrhythmias or bradycardia
- Gastrointestinal complaints
- Headaches, dizziness, muscle cramps, and weakness resulting from electrolyte disturbances
- Renal dysfunction resulting from electrolyte disturbances
- Tendency toward stress fractures
- Loss or thinning of the hair

Psychological and Behavioral Symptoms

- Excessive dieting and guilt about eating
- Excessive eating without weight gain
- Excessive exercise that is not part of the training program
- Claiming to feel fat when at normal weight despite reassurance from others
- Preoccupation with or hoarding of food
- Avoidance of eating in public or denial of hunger
- Frequent weighing
- Evidence of binge eating or self-induced vomiting
- Use of drugs to attempt to control weight (e.g., abuse of laxatives, diet pills, diuretics, emetics)

■ Hypertrophy of the salivary glands, particularly the parotid glands. The individual often has a chipmunk-like face.

■ Dental erosion caused by acidic gastric secretions that decalcify the teeth during recurrent episodes of vomiting.

Symptoms of depression and anxiety disorders often are prominent, and as with anorexia nervosa, a subgroup of individuals engages in substance misuse, unprotected sexual activity, self-mutilation, and suicide attempts (13,14).

Anorexia Nervosa

Anorexia nervosa is defined as a refusal to maintain body weight over a minimal normal weight for age and height, with body weight being 15% below what is expected (12). The disorder typically is seen in females during adolescence, although it has been known to occur after menopause. These individuals usually are easy to identify because of severe weight loss over a period of time.

Individuals with anorexia have a distorted body image and, even though they are underweight, maintain a great fear of gaining weight. They view themselves as fat and equate body appearance with self-worth. An obsessive–compulsive nature for perfection and achievement leads many individuals to develop into obsessive exercisers. Amenorrhea often occurs before significant weight loss and continues for at least 3 consecutive months. The individual has a desire to control the body and eating and to remain in a prepubertal state, resulting in near-starvation behavior. Many individuals with anorexia complain of being cold even on hot days; others suffer from severe constipation because of poor food intake. Symptoms of depression and anxiety disorders, irritability, mood swings, impaired concentration, loss of sexual appetite, and obsessional features are frequent accompaniments (13).

Because of the deteriorated physical state of the individual, detection of anorexia is easier than detection of bulimia nervosa. Table 26.1 compares bulimia nervosa with anorexia nervosa.

General Treatment of Eating Disorders

Treatment for both bulimia nervosa and anorexia nervosa involves a three-pronged approach that includes referral to a physician, a mental health professional (e.g., psychologist, mental health counselor, or social worker), and a nutritionist. The mental health professional will explore any underlying emotional issues as well as use more immediate behavioral approaches to increase the patient's comfort with eating and maintaining normal body weight. If a personality disorder is present, an extensive rehabilitation program of psychological and pharmacologic intervention is necessary. If recognized early enough, behavioral and psychoeducational intervention with individual counseling

TABLE 26.1 Comparison of Bulimia Nervosa and Anorexia Nervosa		
FACTOR	**BULIMIA NERVOSA**	**ANOREXIA NERVOSA**
Weight	Normal for age and height	15% below expected
Weight loss	Fluctuations are common	Loss is gradual
Age	Females in the teens and twenties; also seen in male wrestlers	Females in the teens and twenties
Body image	Distorted for body shape and weight	Distorted, person feels fat even when emaciated
Eating habits	Recurrent binge eating, followed by fasting	Near-starvation commonly is seen
Purging	May or may not occur; laxatives, diuretics, and self-induced vomiting may be used	Not common
Self-esteem	Low; depression is common; obsessive–compulsive behavior	Low; obsessive–compulsive behavior for perfection
Menses	Irregular menses is common	Amenorrhea is common

can be advantageous. Nutritional supervision and guidance can help the patient to overcome myths about eating and instill factual knowledge while focusing on the direction of proper nutrition. The nutritionist can assist with caloric and nutritional assessment, food diary instruction, nutritional education, and menu planning. Bulimia nervosa and anorexia nervosa may not be curable, but they can be managed with a well-structured, supervised rehabilitation program (14).

Osteoporosis

Osteoporosis is a serious condition of decreased bone mass and strength greater than expected for a person's sex, age, and race. Age-related osteoporosis causes loss in both trabecular and cortical bone, which often leads to fractures. These fractures commonly occur in the vertebral bodies, proximal femur, and distal radius. Cortical bone reaches its peak density at approximately 40 years of age; trabecular bone (e.g., hip, spine, and femur) density peaks in the mid-20s. Subsequently, bone density decreases at a rate of 1% per year. Forty percent of postmenopausal females and 12.5% of men older than 50 years suffer at least one osteoporotic fracture in their lifetime (15). Identifiable risk factors include:

- Low calcium intake

- Sedentary lifestyle

- Tobacco use

- Being underweight

- Amenorrhea related to bone density loss

- Estrogen deficiency

- Decreased bone-mass mineral content, as detected by a bone-mass density test

Estrogen and calcium are needed to develop strong bone. A decrease in the level of estrogen in postmenopausal females places them at greater risk for developing osteoporosis compared with any other population. Primary prevention includes adequate calcium intake (i.e., 1,500 mg/day), maintaining adequate circulating estrogen levels, regular weight-bearing exercise, and avoiding smoking and too much alcohol. Rich sources of calcium include milk, yogurt, cheese, ice cream, spinach, and baked beans. Vitamin D is required to help the body absorb calcium. Although some foods, such as margarine and cereals, contain vitamin D, the major source comes from the action of sunlight on the skin. The National Osteoporosis Society recommends 15 minutes of activity in sunlight each day to provide adequate amounts of vitamin D without exposing the individual to the risk of skin cancer (16).

The important preventative measure is maintaining adequate circulating estrogen. If an individual is amenorrheic, even in the face of proper calcium intake and exercise, then loss of bone density is likely. A sedentary, but normally menstruating, female is likely to have a higher bone density level than an active female with amenorrhea, even though both females are below the optimum of the active female with **eumenorrhea**. Because females can only add to their bone mass between puberty and approximately 40 years of age, periods of amenorrhea may produce long-term harm by introducing osteoporosis prematurely.

Inadequate estrogen levels may be caused by metabolic conditions such as athletic amenorrhea, menopause, or excessive prolactin. Prolactin is a protein that stimulates the secretion of milk, which normally occurs during pregnancy but is an abnormal sign at other times. Other causes of poor estrogen levels may be related to malnutrition, chronic illness, renal insufficiency, connective tissue disorders, abnormal thyroid, connective tissue disorders, or malignancy. Excessive exercise can adversely affect bone remodeling and increase the risk of osteoporosis. Secondary prevention can include estrogen therapy started at menopause or within 5 to 6 years. Weight-bearing exercise and estrogen therapy can prevent bone loss in postmenopausal females.

The Female Athlete Triad

In 1992, the American College of Sports Medicine gathered a panel of experts to discuss a triad of disorders commonly seen in adolescent and young adult female athletes—namely, disordered eating, altered menstrual function, and abnormalities in bone mineralization (17). The Female Athlete Triad—or Female Triad, as it also is called—is particularly common among females participating in sports that require an ideal body weight or optimal level of body fat for achievement (e.g., gymnastics, figure skating, cross-country running, diving, swimming, and ballet).

Each of these three conditions has potentially serious effects on health and sport performance. When seen together, however, they often accelerate each other, producing even more devastating effects on both the quality and the longevity of life. The long-term effects of disordered eating often alter menstrual function, which in turn increases the onset of osteoporosis.

Studies have confirmed that individuals who have experienced stress fractures are more likely to have low bone mass density and dietary calcium intake, menstrual irregularities, and lower use of oral contraceptives (18,19). The results of these studies suggest that amenorrhea is associated with eating disorders, low estrogen levels, and increased risk of lowered bone mass density, which brings the Female Triad full circle. Females who remain amenorrheic continue to lose bone mass; however, once menses resumes, increase in bone mass, particularly in the vertebra, also returns.

A *The distance runner who reported the absence of a menstrual period for 3 months and concern about being pregnant could be experiencing exercise-induced amenorrhea. The individual should be referred to a physician.*

ATHLETES WITH DISABILITIES

Q *As the director of athletic training health care service for the Paralympics being held in Florida during late July, what guidelines should be followed to reduce the incidence of heat-related injury and illness?*

In the United States, between 2 and 3 million people with disabilities participate in recreational and organized sports. Although one might suspect that individuals with disabilities are at a greater risk for physical injury, this is not true. In fact, the percentage of injuries is no higher among sport participants with disabilities. For the most part, the types of injuries sustained by the disabled athlete are similar to those in athletes who are not disabled; the majority involve soft-tissue injuries. This section focus on injuries and medical conditions that are associated with neurologic or neuromuscular involvement pertaining to the disabled sport participant.

Wheelchair Athletes

Individuals with spinal cord injuries, spina bifida, postpolio paralysis, and amputations often are identified as wheelchair athletes. Wheelchair athletes most commonly participate in track, road racing, and basketball, but others may participate in tennis, field events, bowling, archery, slalom skiing, table tennis, swimming, and other sports. Wheelchair designs have changed dramatically over the past two decades. The overall mass of the chair has greatly decreased, and the seat and back rest have been lowered, the wheels cambered, and the size of the push rims modified to suit the needs of individual events.

Injuries to Wheelchair Athletes

Altered patterns of muscle strength and flexibility can change the biomechanical forces that are applied to muscle and joints, making some individuals more susceptible to injury because of repetitive wheelchair propulsion movements. The greatest velocity of ambulation is attained with rapid, rather than long, strokes on the push rims of the chair. The arms operate with a lower mechanical efficiency than the legs, in part because effort is expended in stabilizing the trunk during arm work. Efficiency is particularly poor for individuals with high-level spinal cord injuries. For these reasons, the majority of injuries commonly occur in the upper extremities. The most frequent injuries include:

- Muscular injuries
- Soft-tissue injuries (sprains, strains, tendinitis, or bursitis)
- Blisters and calluses
- Lacerations, abrasions, and cuts (including skin infections)

- Pressure sores
- Arthritis and joint disorders
- Fractures
- Hand weakness or numbness
- Problems with hyperthermia or hypothermia

Constant compression of the heel of the hand on the push rim of a wheelchair also can lead to carpal tunnel syndrome. In addition, constant pressure from sitting can lead to pressure-related sores on the hips and buttocks region. Because of the very nature of their condition, many wheelchair athletes do not have sensation in the lower extremities (i.e., paraplegia). Extreme caution should be directed toward the feet and toes, which can become scraped or dragged on concrete or other hard surfaces during an event, resulting in abrasions or lacerations.

Although some injuries may be related to accidents inherent in the operation of a wheelchair at high speeds, others often are overuse in nature and associated with an increased training load. Gloves should be worn to prevent soft-tissue injuries and pressure-related injuries to the hands. If more padding is needed, layers of athletic tape can be applied to areas of high pressure. To decrease the risk of pressure injuries or irritation occurring in the buttocks and hips area, athletes should shift their weight every 30 minutes. Individuals with open pressure sores should stop physical activity to prevent additional pressure damage. Training progression, along with flexibility and warm-up, are critical to decrease the incidence of musculotendinous injuries; these should be done before and after both training and competition. Some wheelchair athletes suffer from chronic pain in the upper extremities that is related to the nature of their disability; however, this chronic pain should not be mistaken for acute or chronic injury. When treating injuries in this population, cold and heat modalities must be applied with caution, because most of these individuals lack sensation in various extremity areas and cannot feel when a modality is too hot or cold, resulting in the risk of skin irritation or burning.

Environmental Considerations

Wheelchair sport participants are at a greater risk for environment-related conditions, such as heat illness and hypothermia. Spinal cord injuries, especially lesions above the first thoracic vertebra, compromise the parasympathetic nervous system, which affects circulating blood volume and sweat production, and can adversely influence thermoregulation (20). As a result, individuals with quadriplegia do not perspire below the site of the spinal cord lesion and cannot effectively cool the body. Extra precautions must be used when these individuals participate in warm environments. Practice and competitions should be limited when temperatures exceed 85°F and humidity is 70% or greater. The same fluid hydration and rehydration guidelines for athletes without disabilities should be followed (see Chapter 24), but small modifications are needed. For example, rather than ingesting a large amount of a carbohydrate sports drink before exercise, it has been reported that frequent ingestion of smaller amounts of a sports drink is the best strategy for low-lesion paraplegic athletes competing in wheelchair endurance events (21). Although ingesting smaller doses more often during exercise may momentarily disrupt the rhythm and momentum of the individual, it appears that this practice avoids the possibility of an associated decline in plasma glucose concentration during exercise. Water should be sprayed frequently on the skin, and water carriers with bottles should be mounted on wheelchairs so that fluids are readily available. In addition to concerns about dehydration, those with spinal cord injury have decreased sensory distribution and circulatory changes and are at a greater risk for sunburn during sun exposure. Sport participants should wear appropriate sunblock and move to a shaded area before participation, during breaks, and after participation.

In the same manner, wheelchair athletes are at greater risk for cold-induced conditions. Retaining body heat becomes problematic when the temperature drops to approximately 50°F. Wheelchair athletes should wear adequate insulating clothing in the winter, especially on inactive parts (e.g., amputation stumps).

Bladder Dysfunction

Incomplete or lack of proper emptying of the bladder, bladder infections, bladder stones, and bladder obstructions occur in individuals with a neurogenic bladder. Wheelchair sport participants often have to use an indwelling or intermittent catheter to drain the bladder. Catheters increase the risk of bladder and urine infections if not cleaned and used properly. To flush the bladder, individuals must drink 2 liters of water per day. It is imperative that wheelchair sport participants drink plenty of water and properly care for their catheters to decrease the risk of bladder dysfunction. If an individual develops a bladder infection, an antibiotic usually is prescribed. Return to physical activity generally occurs within 8 hours after starting antibiotic treatment. If a fever is present, return to activity should be delayed until at least 24 hours after body temperature returns to normal.

Orthostatic Hypotension

Orthostatic hypotension caused by prolonged sitting or sudden and rapid shifts in body position results from the inability of the sympathetic nervous system to adjust to rapid changes in body position. Individuals with orthostatic hypotension feel light-headed or faint. The individual should be placed in a recumbent position (e.g., tipping the wheelchair backward) and instructed to breathe deeply; this helps to return blood flow to the brain. If a wheelchair sport participant develops a pounding headache, flushed face, and heavy perspiration on the face and neck, the individual may be experiencing **autonomic dysreflexia**, which disturbs the regulation of blood pressure and heart rate.

 Autonomic dysreflexia, a rare but dangerous condition, commonly is triggered by an obstructed bowel or bladder and is a medical emergency. As such, the emergency plan, including summoning emergency medical services, should be activated.

Safety and the Wheelchair Athlete

Because many wheelchair athletes take a variety of drugs for infection, abnormal muscle tone, seizures, and other neurologic conditions, it is important to be alert for drug reactions. It is important to know the medications an individual is taking and to avoid giving any over-the-counter medications before referral to a physician. In addition, several steps can be taken to ensure the safety of a wheelchair sport participant during both practice and competition (Box 26.5). Although many of these steps are dependent on the individual, the athletic trainer must emphasize safety during participation.

Athletes with Amputations

The most common problem for athletes with amputations is irritation at the junction of the amputated limb and prosthetic device. This is more of a problem with limbs of the lower extremity because of weight-bearing forces. The athletic trainer should work closely with the appropriate specialist (e.g., physical therapist or orthopaedist) to resolve any problems quickly. Because of lack of sensation, initial problems may go unnoticed and become infected. Observation of the juncture reveals redness, skin irritation, and occasional swelling. Infections can lead to potentially serious complications, such as osteomyelitis of the underlying bone. A proper fit between the prosthetic and the limb is required to avoid problems. If the fit is too loose, friction occurs; if the fit is too tight, vascular function can be impaired. Treatment of stump irritation involves properly cleansing the area and applying protective padding. If the irritation is severe, the individual may have to limit or even discontinue use of the prosthetic and reduce his or her physical activity.

Box 26.5 Safety Points When Training Wheelchair Athletes

- Use protective devices (e.g., gloves, pressure wraps, cushions).
- Monitor environmental conditions.
- Provide plenty of fluids (e.g., water bottle holders on wheelchairs).
- Provide ample opportunity for emptying catheters.

- Protect against sunburn.
- Protect the feet and toes from abrasions.
- Be alert for drug reactions.

Cerebral Palsy

Cerebral palsy involves uncontrolled muscle spasticity, which can range from mild to severe. Because of the increased load on the musculotendinous units resulting from the constant spasticity and a limited joint range of motion (ROM), muscle strains are a common injury. A flexibility program, including proprioceptive neuromuscular facilitation stretching, and a free-weight, progressive resistance training program should be initiated to decrease the incidence of muscular injuries. The goal of the strength program should be to develop muscle balance between the agonist and antagonist muscles (22). In some cases, athletes with cerebral palsy have elected to undergo Achilles tendon and hamstring surgery to increase ROM and better accommodate any muscle spasticity.

Visual Impairment

Sport participants with visual impairments have a serious problem with unseen barriers. The lack of visual cues, such as visualizing road surface conditions, walls, curbs, and other competitors, often puts the visually impaired individual at a greater risk for lower extremity injuries caused by failure to respond to varying surface conditions. In addition, visually impaired sport participants are speculated to expend more energy and to be likely to fatigue more quickly, increasing the risk of chronic overuse injuries in the lower extremity. It is suggested that a guide be used to provide auditory assistance to the visually impaired participant during training sessions and competition.

A *As the director of athletic training health care service for the Paralympics being held in Florida during late July, the following guidelines should be considered to reduce the incidence of heat-related injury and illness: practices and competitions should be limited when the temperature exceeds 85°F and humidity greater than 70%; athletes should follow the same fluid hydration and rehydration guidelines as athletes without disabilities; water should be sprayed frequently on the skin of wheelchair athletes, and water carriers should be mounted to their wheelchairs; and athletes should be provided with an appropriate sunblock.*

THE SENIOR ATHLETE

Q *A female preparing to compete in badminton during the Senior Olympics reports chronic shoulder pain. What conditions might predispose this individual to a shoulder injury, and what signs and symptoms indicate a subacromial impingement syndrome?*

As the U.S. population continues to age, it is estimated that more than 60% of adults age 65 and older participate in physical activity. Subsequently, this age group has an increasing need for strength, conditioning, and care of athletic-related injuries. The aging process plays a major role in skeletal and neuromuscular function. As mentioned, bone mass decreases with aging, although physical activity can delay this process. Aging decreases the density of collagen, which lowers tissue elasticity; however, physical activity stimulates collagen production, which in turn helps to maintain elasticity. Aging also causes deterioration of type I and type II muscle fibers, but activity maintains these fibers for longer periods of time. Activity also stimulates and maintains chondrocyte activity, which helps to maintain the status of menisci and cartilage tissue.

As individuals age, muscles tend to become shortened and weak, which can lead to muscle imbalance. This often is caused by chronic injury, postural adaptations to gravity, neuromuscular and neurologic dysfunction, and overall body fatigue. The very nature of the aging process increases the risk of injury for the senior sport participant (Box 26.6). In fact, most injuries in this population are a direct response to the effects of aging on the musculoskeletal system. The key to treating an older active individual, as with any active individual, is to enable the person to continue participating as pain-free as possible. This section focuses on special musculoskeletal considerations for this population. The reader should refer to the relevant condition chapters for more information on specific injuries and conditions.

Upper Extremity and Spinal Considerations

Adhesive capsulitis, subacromial bursitis, and subacromial impingement syndrome are common injuries in older athletes. These conditions are seen frequently in individuals with kyphosis, which

Box 26.6 Common Injuries in the Senior Athlete

- Adhesive capsulitis
- Subacromial bursitis
- Subacromial impingement syndrome
- Strains of the hamstrings, quadriceps, and triceps surae
- Trochanteric bursitis

- Degenerative meniscal tears
- Achilles tendon rupture
- Posttraumatic ankle instability
- Plantar fasciitis

often leads to structural alterations, biomechanical changes, and muscle imbalances in the shoulder region. Each condition may cause referred pain to the lateral arm.

Adhesive capsulitis occurs when the glenohumeral capsular lining tightens or develops adhesions. The condition is more common in females than in males and is found with progressive rotator cuff lesions. Signs include acute, intense pain with passive and active movement in the terminal ROMs. Limitations in ROM are most noticeable during glenohumeral flexion, abduction, and external rotation. Night pain often is a complaint. The first steps in managing the condition are to identify the capsular pattern of restricted movement, then to apply thermotherapy (e.g., ultrasound), NSAID therapy, and mobilization techniques that focus on the terminal ranges. A full rehabilitation program should be developed to complement the thermotherapy. If the person ignores the restricted ROM and continues activity, additional damage to surrounding soft tissue will result.

Subacromial bursitis often is associated with subacromial impingement syndrome. Predisposing factors include a calcific rotator cuff tendon and poor biomechanical alignment and function of the glenohumeral joint. Pain is reported as being intense, constant, acute, or dull and to increase with terminal glenohumeral flexion and abduction. During the acute phase, subacromial bursitis should be treated with cryotherapy, NSAIDs, and application of a sling along with controlled ROM exercises. During the chronic phase, thermotherapy may be used in combination with appropriate rehabilitation exercises. In some cases, an injection of corticosteroids may be administered by a physician to complement traditional therapeutic techniques.

A kyphotic spinal alignment, muscle imbalances of the shoulder, and past tears or chronic tendinitis of the rotator cuff are predisposing factors for subacromial impingement syndrome. Pain is isolated in the anterolateral shoulder, with referred pain to the lateral arm extending distally to the elbow. The onset of pain usually is gradual and increases with glenohumeral abduction, flexion, and external rotation. Management involves rest, NSAIDs, and avoiding aggravating activities. Ultrasound and friction massage frequently are used with rehabilitative exercises. Corticosteroid injections sometimes are indicated. If the impingement is associated with degenerative lesions, healing is extremely slow and, in some cases, does not occur because of poor blood flow and continued stress on the shoulder.

Lumbar disk herniations are more common during middle age but may occur in senior sport participants. Lumbar disk disease is more common in seniors. Because of aging, the disks become avascular and lose water content. Degeneration of the viscoelastic and structural properties predisposes many individuals to degenerative disk disease.

Lower Extremity Considerations

Poor flexibility and aging changes in soft tissue put the senior sport participant at increased risk for strains of the hamstrings and quadriceps muscle groups. These injuries most often are associated with "power" sports, such as running, sprinting, field events, soccer, and basketball. Acute strains occur more frequently than chronic strains. Signs, symptoms, and management are the same as those for strains occurring in younger populations, but because of the aging process, the injury may take longer to heal.

Weak hip abductors and lack of flexibility in the iliotibial band also increase the risk of trochanteric bursitis in this age group. Hallmark signs include an insidious onset of pain at the lateral hip extending to the lateral thigh and pain when rolling over on the affected hip. Pain increases with resisted hip abduction, jumping, running up inclines, and climbing stairs. Management includes application of cryotherapy, use of NSAIDs, and limitation of aggravating activities. A biomechanical analysis should be conducted to determine if aspects of the individual's gait increase stress on the iliotibial band and greater trochanter. Non–weight bearing activities (e.g., swimming) may need to be substituted during the healing phase of injury. A physician referral is warranted if the condition does not improve with therapy and rest.

Degenerative meniscal tears of the knee (i.e., wearing away of meniscal cartilage), which result from a constant grinding motion between the tibia and femur, do not resemble injuries seen in the knees of younger athletes. Degenerative meniscal tears normally occur in individuals who participate in sports that require large weight-bearing forces (e.g., running, jumping, or twisting). Pain usually is at the medial joint line. A history of "catching" or inability to extend the knee is reported, and there may be joint instability because of the lack of a full meniscal cartilage. Acute management includes cryotherapy and partial weight bearing with crutches. Referral to a physician is warranted if the individual appears to have instability or limited motion.

Partial tears of the gastrocnemius–soleus complex (i.e., triceps surae) are the second most common muscle strain in experienced senior athletes (23). The tear normally occurs in the muscle belly, often with a popping or snapping sound. The individual feels immediate, intense pain, and a palpable defect in the muscle often can be found. The individual is not able to push off with the involved foot. Management includes ice, rest, and limited weight bearing with crutches. Following the acute phase, ultrasound is suggested, with rehabilitation exercises and gradual return to activity.

Rupture of the Achilles tendon occurs during push-off while the knee is extended, as in jumping (e.g., volleyball or basketball) or sprinting (e.g., tennis or soccer). As with the triceps surae strain, the individual feels a popping or snapping sensation and is unable to bear weight while standing on the toes of the affected leg. An observable and palpable defect is present, and the Thompson test is positive (see Chapter 18). Application of ice, a posterior splint, crutches, and referral to a physician are necessary.

Repeated sprains to the collateral ligaments of the ankle in combination with osteoarthritis may predispose the senior sport participant to posttraumatic ankle instability. Limited dorsiflexion is associated with osteophyte development on the anterior portion of the talus. Instability usually is in an anterior direction and is evaluated with a positive anterior drawer test (see Chapter 18). Treatment primarily focuses on rehabilitation of the supportive musculature. If treatment is unsuccessful in providing enough stability, reconstructive surgery is indicated.

Plantar fasciitis occurs in all ages but is more common among older individuals because of a tight heel cord and calcaneal spurs. Pain often is greatest during the morning, decreases during the day, and then increases at the end of the day or during weight-bearing activities. Pain generally is localized on the plantar surface of the calcaneus. Palpation reveals a tight plantar fascia with or without defects. Acute management includes cryotherapy, NSAIDs, and a heel lift to reduce tension on the Achilles tendon. Stretching exercises of the heel cord, plantar fascia, and hamstrings are suggested. If the individual has excessive foot pronation, an orthosis may be required.

The senior athlete with shoulder pain is predisposed to subacromial impingement syndrome if any of the following conditions are present: kyphotic spinal alignment, muscle imbalance of the shoulder complex, or history of chronic rotator cuff tendinitis. Additional signs and symptoms indicating the syndrome include gradual onset of pain in the anterolateral shoulder region that increases with glenohumeral abduction, flexion, and external rotation.

SUMMARY

1. Menstrual dysfunctions include dysmenorrhea, menstrually induced leg pain, anovulatory oligomenorrhea, luteal phase deficiency, and exercise-associated amenorrhea.

2. Endometriosis involves tissue growth outside of the endometrial cavity, which can lead to dysmenorrhea, oligomenorrhea, severe pelvic pain, and pain on defecation. In extreme situations, endometriosis can lead to infertility.

3. Premenstrual syndrome is associated with the luteal phase (i.e., days 15–28) of the menstrual cycle. Signs and symptoms of PMS include headaches, breast tenderness, back pain, bloating, irritability, depression, fatigue, and certain food cravings.

4. Exercise programs for the pregnant female must be individualized in consultation with the supervising physician. A 5- to 10-minute warm-up period and 30 to 60 minutes at 65 to 85% of maximum heart rate three to five times per week is recommended for a recreational athlete or regular fitness exercises. Each exercise period should be followed by a cool-down and stretching period.

5. Eating disorders manifest as a refusal to maintain a healthy body weight (i.e., 85% of expected body weight), dramatic weight loss, fear of gaining weight even when underweight, preoccupation with food, abnormal food-consumption patterns, or recent binge-eating behaviors associated with loss of control and feelings of guilt. Treatment involves a three-pronged approach that includes referral to a physician, a mental health professional, and a nutritionist.

6. Osteoporosis results from a decrease in bone mass and strength, which predisposes the individual to fractures. Primary prevention includes adequate calcium intake, circulating estrogen levels, and weight-bearing exercise. The most important of these is adequate levels of circulating estrogen.

7. The combination of disordered eating habits, amenorrhea, and osteoporosis commonly is referred as the Female Triad. When seen together, they often accelerate each other, producing even more devastating effects on the quality and longevity of life.

8. Disabled sport participants are no more prone to athletic injuries than nondisabled sport participants. The most common injuries seen in wheelchair sport participants are strains and sprains; bursitis of the upper extremity; soft-tissue injuries, such as blisters, abrasions, lacerations, and cuts; carpal tunnel syndrome; and pressure-related injuries of the hands, hips, and buttocks. In addition, wheelchair sport participants are at a higher risk of sunburn, dehydration, hyperthermia and hypothermia, bladder dysfunction, and hypotension.

9. Common injuries in the senior sport participant include adhesive capsulitis, bursitis, muscle strains, plantar fasciitis, degenerative conditions, and decreases in flexibility, strength, and balance.

REFERENCES

1. Lipsky MS. Vaginitis: case reports and brief review. AIDS Patient Care and STDs 2002;16(8):367–373.
2. French L. Dysmenorrhea. Am Fam Physician 2005;71(2):285–291.
3. Proctor M, Farguhar C. Dysmenorrhea. Br Med J: Clin Evid 2002;(7):1639-1653.
4. Joy EA, Macintyre JG. Women in sports. In: Mellion MB, Walsh WM, Madden C, Putukian M, Shelton GL, eds. The Team Physician's Handbook. Philadelphia: Hanley & Belfus, 2002.
5. Giudice LC, Kao LE. Endometriosis. Lancet 2004; 364(9447):1789–1799.
6. Dickerson LM, Mazyck PJ, Hunter JG. Premenstrual syndrome. Am Fam Physician 2003;67(8):1743–1752.
7. Naz RK. Contraceptive vaccines. Drugs 2005;665(5):593–603.
8. Yeo S, Davidge ST. Possible beneficial effect of exercise, by reducing oxidative stress, on the incidence of preeclampsia. J Womens Health Gend Based Med 2001;10(10):983–989.
9. Carey GB, Quinn TJ. Exercise and lactation: are they compatible? Can J Appl Physiol 2001;26(1):55–74.
10. American College of Obstetricians and Gynecologists Committee Obstetric Practice. ACOG Committee Opinion, No 267, January 2002: exercise during pregnancy and the postpartum period. Obstet Gynecol 2002;99(1):171–173.
11. American Academy of Pediatrics. Identifying and treating eating disorders. Policy Statement: Committee on Adolescence. Pediatrics 2003;111(1):204–211.
12. American Psychiatric Association. Diagnostic and Statistical Manual of Mental Disorders, 4th Ed. Washington, DC: American Psychiatric Association, 2000.
13. Fairburn CG, Harrison PJ. Eating disorders. Lancet 2003;361(9355):407–416.
14. Kaplan Seidenfeld ME, Sosin E, Rickert VI. Nutrition and eating disorders in adolescents. Mt Sinai J Med 2004; 71(3):155–161.
15. Campion JM, Maricic MJ. Osteoporosis in men. Am Fam Physician 2003; 67(7):1521–1526.
16. Silverwood B. Building healthy bones. Paediatr Nurs 2003; 15(5):27–30.
17. Otis CL, Drinkwater B, Johnson M, et al. American College of Sports Medicine position stand: the female athlete triad. Med Sci Sports Exerc 1997;29(5):i–ix.
18. Kadel NJ, Teitz CC, Kronmal RA. Stress fractures in ballet dancers. Am J Sports Med 1992;20(3):445–449.
19. Licata AA. Stress fractures in young athletic women: case reports of unsuspected cortisol-induced osteoporosis. Med Sci Sports Exerc 1992;24(8):955–957.
20. Kahanov L, Roberts J, Mazza J. Heat illness: wheelchair athletes with spinal-cord injury. Ath Ther Today 2004; 9(2):26–27.
21. Spendiff O, Campbell IG. Influence of timing of glucose drink ingestion on selected responses of wheelchair athletes. Adapt Phys Act Quart 2004;21(1):50–62.
22. Morton JF, Brownlee M, McFadyen AK. The effects of progressive resistance training for children with cerebral palsy. Clin Rehab 2005;19(3):283–289.
23. Scott WA, Couzens GC. Treating injuries in active seniors. Phys Sport Med 1996;24(5):63–68.

Pharmacology

STUDENT OUTCOMES

1. Define the term pharmacokinetics.

2. List the five major principles associated with pharmacokinetics.

3. Describe the two common routes of drug administration—namely, enteral and parenteral.

4. Explain the factors that affect a drug's absorption rate in crossing cell membranes.

5. Explain the distribution, metabolization, and excretion of drugs from the body.

6. Describe the factors that influence the therapeutic effects produced by a drug.

7. Explain the importance of potentially dangerous drug interactions.

8. State the adverse side effects of common therapeutic medications.

9. Describe the process of naming drugs.

10. List the general guidelines for documentation and storage of therapeutic medications.

11. Describe the use of the *Physician's Desk Reference* and other references to access information regarding common therapeutic medications.

12. Identify the common therapeutic medications used to treat soft-tissue injuries.

13. Describe the uses and adverse effects of common performance-enhancing substances.

14. Describe the methods of drug testing.

ROLE DELINEATION COMPETENCIES

The following Performance Domains and Tasks defined in the National Athletic Trainers' Association Board of Certification *Role Delineation Study*, 5th Edition are addressed in this chapter:

BOC COMPETENCIES

I. Prevention

A. Educate the appropriate individual(s) about risks associated with participation and specific activities using effective communication techniques to minimize the risk of injury and illness.

B. Interpret preparticipation and other relevant screening information in accordance with accepted guidelines to minimize the risk of injury and illness.

G. Monitor participants and environmental conditions by following accepted guidelines to promote safe participation.

II. Clinical Evaluation and Diagnosis

E. Formulate a clinical impression by interpreting the signs, symptoms, and predisposing factors of the injury, illness, or condition to determine the appropriate course of action.

F. Educate the appropriate individual(s) regarding the assessment by communicating information about the current or potential injury, illness, or health-related condition to encourage compliance with recommended care.

G. Share assessment findings with other health care professionals using effective means of communication to coordinate appropriate care.

III. Immediate Care

A. Employ life-saving techniques through the use of standard emergency procedures in order to reduce morbidity and the incidence of mortality.

B. Prevent exacerbation of non–life threatening condition(s) through the use of standard procedures in order to reduce morbidity.

C. Facilitate the timely transfer of care for conditions beyond the scope of practice of the athletic trainer by implementing appropriate referral strategies to stabilize and/or prevent exacerbation of the condition(s).

IV. Treatment, Rehabilitation, and Reconditioning

D. Administer treatment for general illness and/or conditions using standard techniques and procedures to facilitate recovery, function, and/or performance.

E. Reassess the status of injuries, illnesses, and/or conditions using standard techniques and documentation strategies in order to determine appropriate treatment, rehabilitation, and/or reconditioning and to evaluate readiness to return to a desired level of activity.

F. Educate the appropriate individual(s) in the treatment, rehabilitation, and reconditioning of injuries, illnesses, and/or conditions using applicable methods and materials to facilitate recovery, function, and/or performance.

G. Provide guidance and/or counseling for the appropriate individual(s) in the treatment, rehabilitation, and reconditioning of injuries, illnesses, and/or conditions through communication to facilitate recovery, function, and/or performance.

VI. Professional Responsibility

A. Demonstrate appropriate professional conduct by complying with applicable standards and maintaining continuing competence to provide quality athletic training services.

B. Adhere to statutory and regulatory provisions and other legal responsibilities relating to the practice of athletic training by maintaining an understanding of these provisions and responsibilities in order to contribute to the safety and welfare of the public.

In a national study of 13,914 student-athletes by the National Collegiate Athletic Association (NCAA), the majority of respondents reported the regular use of alcohol (80.5%), followed by marijuana (28.4%), smokeless tobacco (22.5%), psychedelics (5.6%), ephedrine (3.5%), amphetamines (3.1%), cocaine (1.5%), and anabolic steroids (1.1%) (1). It was discouraging to note that 38% of anabolic steroid users reported obtaining them from a physician other than the institution's team physician (1). The results of this survey and other data sources demonstrate the importance of the athletic trainer understanding both performance-enhancing substances and the therapeutic medications used in the treatment of injuries, including their effects, indications, and contraindications.

This chapter examines the process of a drug's journey through the body. It begins with a discussion of pharmacokinetics and is followed by information regarding factors that contribute to the therapeutic effect of a drug, drug interactions, drug reactions, guidelines for use of therapeutic medications, and common medications used in the management of sports injuries. With the exception of nonsteroidal anti-inflammatory drugs (NSAIDs), only over-the-counter (OTC) therapeutic medications are presented. Finally, information is presented concerning performance-enhancing substances (i.e., ergogenic aids) and drug testing.

PHARMACOKINETICS

Q ▶ *Why might an individual be given an enteric-coated medication?*

A **drug** is a chemical agent that affects living processes. The effects can be beneficial or harmful. A drug is effective only when it reaches a particular site and interacts at the cellular level. This interaction may result in the reduction or enhancement of chemical processes in the body. This interaction can help to restore an impaired body function or prevent a disease process from occurring. The effects can be local, systemic, or both. Some medications result in only a local effect, as occurs when ulcer drugs block the production of stomach acid. Other medications, such as oral decongestants, produce both positive and negative effects throughout the body (i.e., systemically), even though the desired effect is to open the nasal passages. Undesirable or negative effects are characterized as side effects of the medication.

Pharmacokinetics is the study of the movement of a drug through the body to produce the desired effects. Movement of the drug through the body involves five steps (Fig. 27.1):

1. Administration
2. Absorption
3. Distribution
4. Metabolism
5. Excretion

Each step can affect the concentration of a drug when it reaches the desired target. The amount of a drug's concentration when it reaches the target site within a certain time frame is referred to as the **bioavailability** of a drug. The bioavailability of a drug is influenced by two of the pharmacokinetic processes—namely, the route of drug administration and absorption. When the drug reaches the target site, the drug–receptor interaction either facilitates or inhibits a sequence of biological

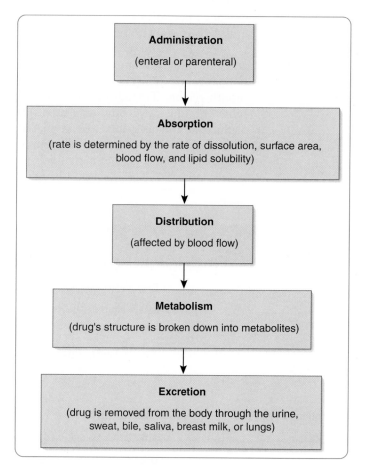

■■■■ **FIGURE 27.1 Pharmacokinetics.** Movement of the drug through the body involves five steps—namely, administration, absorption, distribution, metabolism, and excretion.

changes that ultimately alters the function of the cell, tissue, or organ. Drugs that facilitate or produce a change are called **agonists**; drugs that inhibit or block effects are **antagonists**.

Drug Administration

The means by which a drug is administered often determines its **absorption rate**. The absorption rate is the amount of time that it takes to move into the tissues to produce a therapeutic effect. Two general routes of drug administration exist—namely, enteral and parenteral. Each route is further divided into subroutes.

Enteral Route

Enteral routes (i.e., oral, sublingual, or rectal) use the gastrointestinal (GI) tract for entry into the body. These are the most commonly used routes for drug administration. Medications that use enteral routes are combined with substances called **vehicles** that facilitate entry into the body. These vehicles include tablets, capsules, liquids, powders, suppositories, enteric-coated preparations, and sustained-release preparations.

Enteric-coated preparations are drugs that are covered by acid-resistant materials (e.g., fatty acids, waxes, and shellac) that protect the drug from the acid and pepsin in the stomach. The drug passes through the stomach and is dissolved in the intestine, preventing stomach and duodenal irritation. An enteric-coated medication, such as Ecotrin aspirin, may be used if an individual has GI sensitivity to aspirin. Other enteric medications also are available.

Sustained-released preparations are capsules or tablets filled with tiny spheres that contain the drug. These spheres are coated and designed to dissolve at variable rates. Sustained-released preparations can reduce the number of daily doses and provide a relatively steady drug level for an extended period of time (i.e., usually 8–24 hours). Short-acting medications, such as antihistamines and decongestants, are offered as sustained-released preparations.

Oral medications are absorbed within the stomach, small intestine, or large intestine and can enter the bloodstream within 30 minutes after ingestion. Drugs placed under the tongue (i.e., sublingual route) are quickly absorbed through the oral mucosa into the venous system that drains the mouth region. This allows the medication to avoid initial metabolism in the liver. Nitroglycerin tablets are the most commonly used sublingual medication. This route also is used when drugs, such as those in smokeless tobacco, are placed in the **buccal** region of the mouth (i.e., the space between the lip and gum). Suppositories and enemas are examples of drugs that enter the body through the rectal route; this route is used in individuals who have trouble holding down foods or liquids and in unconscious patients. Table 27.1 lists advantages and disadvantages of enteral routes for drug administration.

TABLE 27.1 Enteral Routes of Drug Administration

ROUTE OF ADMINISTRATION	ADVANTAGES	DISADVANTAGES
Oral	Easy and convenient to administer	Rates of absorption vary
	Relatively inexpensive	Difficult to control concentrations
	Usually safe	Must undergo initial liver metabolism (first-pass effect)
	Avoids sudden increases in plasma levels	Requires patient compliance
		May cause local stomach and duodenal irritation
Sublingual	Rapid onset	Must be absorbed by oral mucosa
Rectal	Alternative to oral medications	Can be poorly and incompletely absorbed
	Used for unconscious patients or in those who have trouble holding down foods or liquids	May cause rectal irritation

Parenteral Route

Parenteral routes do not use the GI tract as entry to the body but, rather, use other methods, both invasive and noninvasive. Invasive avenues include intravenous, intra-arterial, intramuscular, and subcutaneous injections, whereas noninvasive methods include inhalation, topical, and transdermal application.

Intravenous and intra-arterial injections put the drug directly into the bloodstream, where it is instantaneously absorbed. Drugs used for anesthesia before surgery and fluids given through an intravenous drip are examples of these routes. Pain medications often are injected intramuscularly, whereas local anesthetics and insulin are injected subcutaneously. Drugs that are given through intramuscular or subcutaneous means are absorbed at variable rates (i.e., rapid and slow) through capillary walls.

Inhaled drugs are rapidly absorbed through the lungs or sinus passages and should not irritate the nasal cavity, bronchial tubes, or lungs. Bronchial inhalers for exercise-induced bronchial spasms are an example of an inhaled drug.

Antibiotic, antifungal, and anesthetic ointments are applied topically. They penetrate the superficial layers of the skin and underlying tissue, but they do not provide deep skin penetration. Unlike inhaled and topical drugs, drugs administered with a transdermal patch provide a more controlled, slow release of medication into the body. Similar to topical medications, transdermal drugs must be capable of penetrating the skin. Examples include nicotine patches, medicated patches for motion sickness, and drugs used in iontophoresis. Table 27.2 lists advantages and disadvantages of parenteral routes of drug administration.

Drug Absorption

Drug absorption is the movement of a drug from its site of administration into the blood. The rate of absorption determines the onset of the effect of the drug (i.e., the amount of absorption determines

TABLE 27.2 Parenteral Routes of Drug Administration		
ROUTE OF ADMINISTRATION	**ADVANTAGES**	**DISADVANTAGES**
Intravenous/intra-arterial	Instantaneous/complete absorption Rapid onset (10-15 seconds) Controlled dosage Allows administration of large volumes of fluid	Irreversible once in body Can overload the body with fluids Relatively expensive
Intramuscular/subcutaneous	Complete absorption Controlled dosage	Inconvenient Can produce local soreness
Inhalation	Quick absorption Rapid onset (58 seconds)	Patient compliance Can produce tissue irritation
Topical	Local effects Noninvasive Easy to administer Relatively safe	Only effective in treating outer layers of skin Can produce skin irritation
Transdermal	Local effects Noninvasive Easy to administer Relatively safe	Must be capable of passing through dermal layers of skin Can produce skin irritation

the intensity of the effects). Several factors affect the absorption rate of drugs, including the rate of dissolution, surface area, blood flow, and lipid solubility.

Factors Affecting Drug Absorption

The dissolution rate of a drug refers to the length of time that it takes for a drug to dissolve. The more rapidly a drug dissolves, the faster the onset of effects. As such, a liquid medication typically has a more rapid onset of effects compared with an enteric-coated preparation that dissolves more slowly.

The surface area in which a tablet or capsule dissolves also plays a major role in its absorption rate—that is, the larger the surface area, the faster the absorption rate. For example, most oral medications are absorbed in the small intestine, which has a larger surface area than the stomach. Drugs that are inhaled are absorbed into the lungs, which also have a large surface area.

The blood flow in an area also influences the absorption rate. A drug is absorbed more rapidly when administered in areas of high blood flow. As such, drugs administered intravenously are absorbed more quickly than drugs administered orally.

A drug must pass through various cell membranes to reach the blood. Membranes that surround cells are called cytoplasmic membranes and are composed primarily of a double layer of phospholipids, or simple fats. The **blood-brain barrier** also is composed of highly phospholipid materials. Drugs that are lipid soluble have the ability to cross cell membranes readily and enter the blood quickly; therefore, they are absorbed more quickly than other drugs. When it enters the blood, a drug is carried throughout the body to the target sites. This concept of **lipid solubility** explains the difference between water- and fat-soluble vitamin absorption. Fat-soluble vitamins are absorbed better than water-soluble vitamins and can accumulate in the body as a result of their increased ability to cross cell membranes.

Crossing Cell Membranes

For a drug to reach the target site, it must cross the cell membrane using one of three methods. First, a drug can cross via channels and pores; however, drugs are small enough in chemical structure for entry into the membrane by this method. Second, a drug may cross cell membranes via a transport system that uses natural body chemicals as carriers to move the drugs from one side of the membrane to the other. These body chemicals are extremely selective regarding which drugs they carry; as a result, few drugs cross cell membranes using the transport system. The most common method of crossing cell membranes is through direct penetration. As mentioned, cell membranes are phospholipids. A drug that crosses cell membranes through penetration must be lipid soluble and have the ability to dissolve into the lipid membrane. These drugs move from an area of high lipid concentration to an area of low lipid concentration.

Drug Distribution

Following absorption, a drug is distributed throughout the body and may be influenced by several factors. In the same manner that blood flow affects the rate and amount of drug absorption, it also affects drug distribution. For example, blood flow to the heart, kidneys, liver, and brain is much greater than blood flow to the muscles or skin. Because tissue normally is well perfused, regional blood flow rarely is a limiting factor in drug distribution.

Exiting the Vascular System

Following distribution of a drug to a target site, it must be capable of exiting the vascular system and entering the cell membrane via a transport system or through lipid solubility. Most drugs leave the blood at the capillary beds, providing little or no resistance to the drug's exit. In the brain, a drug must pass from the blood through the blood-brain barrier. It must be lipid soluble to cross the barrier in significant quantities; however, some drugs do not exit the blood. A drug that binds to proteins, particularly albumin, cannot leave the blood, because the albumin molecule is too large. Therefore, the drug never gets distributed to target sites and remains in the blood. Only free-floating (unbound) drug molecules can exit the blood to produce a therapeutic effect.

Receptorless Drugs

For most drugs to exert a therapeutic effect, absorption and distribution must occur at a **receptor,** or target site. A receptor is a functional macromolecule in a cell to which a drug binds to produce its effects; however, some drugs do not need to attach to a receptor to produce a therapeutic effect. These drugs produce their effects by acting through physical or chemical interactions. An example of a receptorless drug is an antacid, which decreases gastric acidity by direct chemical reaction with stomach acids. Antiseptics also are receptorless, because their effects are produced by direct physical and chemical reactions with the skin.

Drug Metabolism

Drug metabolism, or biotransformation, is the enzymatic alteration of the structure of a drug, whereby the original drug is broken down into **metabolites.** Most drug metabolism takes place in the liver via hepatic enzymes. This is called the **first-pass effect.** Metabolism in the liver can increase or decrease the therapeutic action as well as the toxicity of a drug. Many drugs are given by nonoral routes to avoid the first-pass effect, avoiding the loss of effectiveness once it has been metabolized. Not all drugs are metabolized, however. For example, aminoglycoside antibiotics (e.g., gentamicin) are excreted in the urine almost unchanged. Because the body does not have a mechanism to break down the drug, toxicity can occur with these types of medications. Drugs that are highly lipid soluble often cannot be excreted by the kidneys. During metabolism, however, the liver can convert drugs into less lipid-soluble compounds, which can accelerate renal drug excretion. Drug metabolism also can inactivate a drug.

Many drug metabolites have the same effect as the original medication. As such, medications may be active before metabolization, after metabolization, or both. Some medications are specifically designed to become active after being metabolized; others become inactive and ineffective once metabolized. Drugs that are inactivated by the liver cannot be taken orally.

Metabolism also can be affected by the condition of the liver and other medications. Individuals with hepatic diseases may metabolize drugs slower or faster than a healthy individual does. Alcohol, cigarette smoking, and other medications may affect enzymes that speed or slow metabolism of specific medications.

Drug Excretion

Drug excretion is the process by which a drug is removed from the body through the urine, sweat, bile, saliva, breast milk, or lungs. Most drugs are excreted in the urine by the kidneys. The rate at which a drug is excreted is significantly determined by the quantity and frequency of the drug dosage. As with metabolism, kidney function is very important to the ability of the body to excrete the medication and/or metabolites at the proper rate. Individuals with reduced kidney function are at risk for toxicity from many medications and must either avoid certain medications or use lower dosages. Some medications (i.e., diuretics) may increase excretion, resulting in the need to alter dosage. Box 27.1 provides two examples of the pharmacokinetic process.

 Enteric-coated medications are used to prevent stomach and duodenal irritation. The individual may have GI sensitivity to a certain medication.

FACTORS CONTRIBUTING TO THE THERAPEUTIC EFFECT OF A DRUG

 What factors contribute to the therapeutic effect of a drug during the pharmacokinetic process? Does taking more medication increase its effectiveness?

Subsequent to absorption and distribution in the body, various factors contribute to the therapeutic effects of a drug. These include blood plasma levels, therapeutic range, half-life, dose response, and potency.

Box 27.1 Examples of the Pharmacokinetic Process

Aspirin
- Administered orally.
- Quickly absorbed in stomach and small intestine.
- Once in the blood, 80 to 90% binds to plasma proteins; the remaining 10 to 20% is free floating.
- Free-floating aspirin exits the blood and exerts therapeutic effects.
- Metabolism begins in the blood, where it is converted into salicylic acid, and continues in the liver.
- Excreted via the kidneys.

Acetaminophen (e.g., Tylenol)
- Administered orally.
- Quickly absorbed in the upper gastrointestinal tract.
- Once in the blood, 20 to 50% binds to plasma proteins; the remaining portion is left free floating.
- Free-floating acetaminophen exits the blood and exerts therapeutic effects.
- Metabolized in the liver.
- Excreted via the kidneys.

Blood Plasma Levels

In most cases, a direct correlation exists between the therapeutic and toxic response of a drug and the concentration level of a drug in the blood plasma. As a result, drug dosing objectives (i.e., frequency and quantity of the drug to be taken) often are referred to in terms of achieving specific blood plasma levels. There are two basic drug plasma levels:

1. **Minimum effective concentration (MEC)** refers to the minimum concentration that must be present for the drug to be effective.

2. **Toxic concentrations** reflect drug levels in blood plasma that are too high and, therefore, increase the risk of toxic effects.

Therapeutic Range

The range between the MEC and the toxic concentration is referred to as the **therapeutic range** of a drug. The objective of drug dosing is to maintain plasma levels within the therapeutic range. The wider this range, the safer the drug. For example, because acetaminophen has a toxic concentration range that is 30-fold greater than the MEC, it is considered to be a safe drug. In comparison, lithium has a much narrower toxic concentration range of only threefold greater than the MEC and, therefore, is not considered to be as safe a drug (2).

Medications with a very narrow therapeutic range often require monitoring of blood levels. The asthmatic medication theophylline, for example, is a drug with a narrow therapeutic range. If the dose is too low, the patient runs the risk of an asthma attack; if the dose is too high, the extreme result can be arrhythmias or convulsions. A slight alteration in the dose or a change in absorption, distribution, metabolism, or excretion can easily result in the blood level falling below, or rising above, the therapeutic range of the drug.

Dosing Intervals and Plasma Concentrations

Drug concentrations in the blood rise during metabolism and decline during excretion. Because an adequate response to a drug cannot occur until plasma levels meet the MEC, a latency period occurs between the time of drug administration and the onset of effects. The extent of this delay is determined by the absorption rate. Because injected drugs are absorbed and enter the blood rapidly, they produce more rapid effects. In contrast, drugs that are taken orally usually require approximately

30 minutes before the onset of effects is noted. Time-release medications are examples of drugs that maintain an average plasma level over a period of time. As a result, the effects of time-release medications do not decline before the next dose. The effects continue throughout the dosing schedule. As long as plasma levels remain above the MEC, the therapeutic response continues. Once plasma levels drop below the MEC, however, the therapeutic response gradually diminishes. As metabolism continues, drug levels decline until excretion eliminates the drug from the body.

Maximal Efficacy

Maximal efficacy is the dose at which a response occurs and continues to increase in magnitude before reaching a plateau, or threshold. Once the response reaches the threshold, the increase in response does not continue, even if more medication is given. Maximal efficacy serves as an index for the maximal response that a drug can produce. This explains why taking more than the recommended dose of a drug does not produce increased effects. In fact, taking more than the recommended dose can lead to toxicity.

Half-Life

The time required for the amount of a drug in the body to reduce by 50% is called the drug's **half-life**. Half-lives can be as short as a few minutes or as long as a week. The longer the half-life of a drug, the slower it leaves the body. For example, acetaminophen has a half-life of 2 hours. Therefore, every 2 hours, 50% of the acetaminophen in the body is excreted. As such, 2 hours after ingesting 200 mg, approximately 100 mg remain, and after another 2 hours, 50 mg remain. If acetaminophen is administered with repeated doses over a period of time, it accumulates in the blood and reaches a threshold. This threshold declines if the dosing is diminished or discontinued. It must be noted that not all drugs have a half-life. For example, alcohol is excreted by the body at a constant rate regardless of the amount present. One aspirin tablet generally is five grains or 325 mg, with a half-life of approximately 3.15 hours. Although the half-life of a drug depends on its volume distribution as well as its clearance, a single aspirin can remain in the body for several hours after ingestion.

See *Half-Life of Aspirin*, available on the companion website at thePoint.

Potency

When comparing two similar drugs, the drug that is more potent requires a lower dosage to produce the same effects. Potency serves as an index for the amount of drug that can be administered to elicit a desired response; it is not synonymous with maximal efficacy. Achieving pain relief with acetaminophen requires a higher dosage than that with morphine, because morphine is much more potent than acetaminophen, requiring less dosage to elicit a given response. The more potent medication, however, is not necessarily the best medication. A variety of factors must be considered, such as side effects, dosing, other available medications, and the patient's specific health factors.

 For a drug to exert a therapeutic effect, it must reach a certain blood plasma level. This level is considered to be the therapeutic range, or the range between minimal effective concentration and toxic concentration. Maximal efficacy is the maximal response of a drug, no matter how much more of the drug is taken. Some drugs are more potent than others. A drug that requires a lower dosage for desired effects is more potent than a similar drug that requires a higher dosage.

DRUG INTERACTIONS

Q *Why is drug interaction a major consideration in the pharmacokinetic process?*

It is not unusual for an individual to use two or more drugs simultaneously, leading to the potential for a **drug interaction**, which refers to the ability of one drug to alter the effects of another drug. Such an interaction may intensify (synergistic action), or reduce (inhibit) the effects of the drug. In some cases, a drug interaction may become life-threatening. Individual response to a drug interaction can be influenced by several factors, many of which alter pharmacokinetic processes (i.e., absorption, distribution, metabolism, and excretion). These factors include:

- Genetics and age
- Current illness or disease
- Quantity of drug ingested
- Duration of the drug therapy
- Time interval between taking two or more drugs
- Which drug is taken first

For example, if an individual is taking a muscle relaxant for a low back spasm and drinks alcohol, the depressant effects of both the muscle relaxant and the alcohol intensify, leading to increased drowsiness. In contrast, if two stimulants are combined, such as a nasal decongestant and caffeine, an increased central nervous system (CNS) stimulation effect may result in nervousness, heart palpitations, and even insomnia. Some drugs, such as the H_2-antagonist cimetidine (e.g., Tagamet), which is used to promote stomach ulcer healing by suppressing secretion of gastric acid, can reduce the hepatic (liver) metabolism of many drugs. Taken with NSAIDs, Tagamet may intensify the side effects of the NSAIDs.

Although most medications are not affected by food, drug interactions with food also may occur. Some drugs (e.g., tetracycline antibiotics) should not be taken with milk or milk products, because calcium combines with the medication and inactivates it. Other medications, such as NSAIDs, should be taken with food or plenty of fluids to reduce stomach irritation. Some antifungal medications require food to increase absorption of the medication. As such, it is always important to ask the physician or pharmacist for instructions on taking a medication.

Individuals often find themselves taking more than one drug at a time. Drug interaction refers to the ability of one drug to alter the effects of another drug. The resultant interaction could intensify or reduce the effects of a drug. Drug interactions can alter pharmacokinetic processes (i.e., absorption, distribution, metabolism, and excretion). In some cases, drug interaction may become life-threatening.

ADVERSE DRUG REACTIONS

A college athlete takes a medication prescribed by a physician. The athlete develops hives and problems with his breathing. What condition might the athlete be experiencing, and what is the appropriate management of this condition?

EMS
Severe reactions are life-threatening and are characterized by respiratory depression, rash (e.g., hives or urticaria), allergic reactions (e.g., anaphylaxis), and shock. If a severe reaction occurs, the emergency plan, including summoning emergency medical services, should be activated.

Prescription and OTC medications have the potential to produce adverse reactions. Adverse drug reactions range from mild to severe. Mild reactions are associated with side effects such as drowsiness, nausea, and an upset stomach. These reactions often are temporary and can be tolerated for short periods of time. If the reactions do not dissipate in a few days, a physician should be contacted immediately.

Adverse drug reactions often are immediate and may be local or systemic. Local reactions are isolated to a limited area and often are associated with topical medications. Systemic reactions affect the entire body, such as heart palpitations and acute bronchospasm. Adverse drug reactions that do not occur immediately usually are associated with long-term use of a drug, such as GI irritation from long-term use of some NSAIDs.

Certain drugs, such as tetracycline, sulfa drugs, and even NSAIDs, may make an individual more susceptible to ultraviolet rays from the sun, resulting in a decreased exposure interval needed to develop a sunburn, rash, or allergy to the sun. These reactions can occur with the first dose or up to 1 week after taking the medication. Other drugs may increase an individual's risk of heat illness or dehydration. Diuretics also can lead to dehydration in an exercising individual. Before participation in physical activity, it is important to know if a medication increases the risk of sun sensitivity, heat illness, or other complications. This information is available from a pharmacist.

Unlike prescription medications, most OTC medication labels identify the risk of adverse drug reactions; however, a physician or pharmacist should be consulted before taking two or more drugs simultaneously. Depending on the severity of the adverse reaction, the individual should be taken to the nearest medical facility. Most adverse reactions subside once the medication is discontinued.

A *The athlete is having a severe, adverse reaction to the medication. Management of this condition includes checking and monitoring the vital sign, treating for shock, and activating the emergency plan, including summoning emergency medical services.*

DRUG NAMES

Q *Are there differences in the effectiveness of brand name and generic drugs?*

The U.S. Food and Drug Administration (FDA) is responsible for supervising the manufacturing, labeling, and distribution of chemical substances, including therapeutic medications. Drugs are classified either as prescription or as nonprescription/OTC products. Prescription medications must be prescribed by a licensed practitioner and generally are dispensed by pharmacists. Over-the-counter drugs, which can be purchased directly by the consumer, usually are used to treat minor problems. Unlike prescription medication, containers holding OTC medication provide a variety of critical information (Box 27.2).

Every medication has a chemical, generic, and brand name. The **chemical name** describes the actual scientific compound; because of the complexity of chemical names, they are seldom used. The **generic name** is considered to be a drug's official name and is preferred over brand names for general use. **Trade names**, or **brand names**, are specific names used by the individual manufacturer. They are created by drug companies for ease of use by consumers and physicians, and they generally are shorter than the generic name, are capitalized, or carry the registered trademark symbol ($^{®}$). In addition, generic drugs can appear under more than one trade name. For example, the common OTC medication acetaminophen can be identified with the following names:

Chemical name	4′-hydroxyacetanilide
Generic name	acetaminophen
Trade or brand name	Tylenol; Panadol

Generally, the OTC products are of lower strength than their respective prescription counterparts. Use of doses higher than those indicated on OTC medication labels is not wise unless prescribed by

---

Box 27.2 Information Found on Medication Containers

Prescription Medication Container
- Patient name
- Pharmacy name, address, and telephone number
- Name of medication
- Dose information and directions for use
- Number of refills (if any)
- Warnings for use (if any)
- Date prescription filled
- Practitioner who prescribed the medication
- Additional information depending on individual state laws

Over-the-Counter Medication Container
- Product name
- Manufacturer name and address
- Net contents
- Directions for safe and effective use
- Name of habit-forming drugs
- Cautions and warnings
- Name and quantity of active ingredients

a physician or other licensed practitioner, because this increases the risk of side effects and adverse reactions. In most cases, the prescription generic drug is therapeutically equivalent to, but is less expensive than, the primary brand-name drug.

Drugs differ not by generic or brand names but, rather, by the route of administration and the rate and extent of absorption. Drug names are used for written and verbal communication and for verifying the contents of drug containers.

> **A** *In most cases, a generic drug provides the same therapeutic effects as the brand-name equivalent. The generic form usually is less expensive.*

GUIDELINES FOR THE USE OF THERAPEUTIC MEDICATIONS

> **Q** *A college basketball team is preparing to take a 4-day, out-of-state trip for a tournament. Some of the athletes are taking prescription medications. What instructions should be provided to the athletes traveling with prescription medications?*

State laws vary tremendously regarding who can prescribe, administer, and dispense medications; therefore, legal ramifications also vary. In general, prescription medications can be prescribed only by a licensed practitioner and dispensed only by a registered pharmacist. Depending on state regulations, only authorized persons (e.g., nurses, physician assistants, or physicians) can administer medications. **Administration of medication** is defined as providing one dose of a medication to an individual. **Drug dispensing** is defined as providing more than one individual dose.

Certified athletic trainers cannot administer or dispense prescription medications, nor should they be assigned duties that may put them in a situation to do so. Physicians cannot delegate the duties associated with prescription drug control or dispensing to certified athletic trainers. These duties extend beyond the role delineation and employment requirements of a certified athletic trainer and put the athletic trainer at risk for legal liability (3).

Using Over-the-Counter Medications

Depending on state regulations, athletic trainers may be authorized to administer OTC medications. Before providing someone with an individual dose, however, the athletic trainer should have reason for doing so based on a written protocol developed in concert with the supervising team physician. These drug protocols should be part of the athletic training policy and procedures manual and should be readily available and used as a reference when administering any OTC medication. The drug protocols should include:

- Identification of the medical condition
- Screening questions that should be asked to identify the potential for any adverse effects
- General signs and symptoms of the condition
- Suggested treatment
- Suggested OTC medication
- Banned substance note
- Approval signature/date of the supervising physician

Before administering an OTC medication, it is important to determine if the individual is allergic to any type of medication (e.g., aspirin, sulfa drugs, and penicillin). The response should be noted and documented. When furnishing medication, both written and oral directions for the use of the medication should be provided to the individual. Following administration of medication, the athletic trainer should keep a written record, or "medication log," of the transaction, including the date, name of the individual, sport/activity, name of the medication, manufacturer, dosage, lot number (if available), expiration date of the medication, reason for administering the medication, and signature of the person administering the drug (3). All drug distribution records should be maintained in accordance with appropriate legal guidelines.

See *Example of a Drug Protocol*, available on the companion website at thePoint, for an example of developing a drug protocol for a specific condition.

Box 27.3   Tips for Proper Use of Medications

- Use only as directed.
- Keep medication in the original container; do not alter the label.
- Do not use if the container has been tampered with.
- Do not use the medication if discolored or if the expiration date has passed.
- Measuring spoons or cups should be used when measuring liquid medication.
- Never share your medication with another person.
- When directed, oral medications should be taken with food.
- If a corticosteroid is injected into a joint, do not stress the joint too soon following the injection, because pain will be masked.
- If an overdose occurs, immediately contact the nearest poison control center, and transport the individual to the nearest medical facility.

In addition, the athletic trainer should follow up with the individual to make sure that the medication is working and that the individual is following the appropriate drug dosing regimen. This is especially important when taking antibiotic and antifungal agents. Incomplete therapy can result in developing a resistance to the medication or a recurrence of the infection. Even though an individual may be feeling fine, the infection is not necessarily gone. The entire course of the prescribed treatment must be completed. Box 27.3 lists tips for proper use of medications.

Poison Control Plan

In addition to having drug protocols developed and implemented, it is equally important to have a poison control plan that is readily available at all times. This plan should be part of the athletic training policies and procedures manual. Poison control centers are available in every state and can be contacted through the local health department. Proper procedures and protocols should be discussed for various poison situations. These procedures should be developed in written form, posted in the athletic training facility, and practiced on a regular basis. Box 27.4 lists information that should be provided over the phone to the poison control center if a potential medical poisoning occurs.

Traveling with Medications

It is important to plan ahead when traveling to ensure that an adequate supply of a particular medication is available in case of emergency (Box 27.5). If an individual forgets a medication or if a medication is depleted, it is not easy to obtain a refill. Each state has specific rules and regulations concerning the prescription and refill of medications. Physicians usually cannot prescribe

Box 27.4   Steps for the Management of a Medication Poison Situation

- Call the nearest poison control center.
- Provide the poison control center the following information:
  - Your name and location
  - Name, age, and approximate weight of the person who has taken the medication
  - Name and dosage of the medication
  - Approximate time the medication was taken
  - Any signs and symptoms of the individual, including vital signs
- Proceed with the directions provided by the poison control center.

medications from state to state, nor can pharmacists fill out-of-state prescriptions. If an individual needs prescription medication while traveling, seeking assistance from the host team physician may be warranted. Another solution is to have the individual's personal physician call the host team physician to discuss the situation. In either case, prescription medications should remain in the original containers and be kept either by the individual or by the athletic trainer.

Storing Medications

All prescription and OTC medications should be kept in the original container and stored in a locked cabinet or other secure place. They should be kept away from heat, direct light, dampness, and freezing temperatures. A dry environment with temperatures between 15 to 31.7°C (59–86°F) is suggested (3). All stocked medications should be examined at regular intervals, and expired medications should be discarded. If medications are kept in athletic training, emergency, or travel kits, they should be routinely inspected for medication quality and security. When stocking medications, it is important to avoid overstocking. Overstocking often is determined by the quantity of expired medications in stock and by the quantity of medications in stock relative to the amount actually used during a given period. Overstocking wastes both medication and money.

Physician's Desk Reference

When questions may arise concerning prescription medications, a *Physician's Desk Reference* (PDR), along with other drug reference guides, can be a valuable resource for obtaining drug information. Drug references are typically divided into various sections. A PDR for prescription drugs provides comprehensive information regarding these agents, whereas a PDR for nonprescription drugs contains information on OTC drugs. These references can be quite complicated. They typically include a manufacturers' index; product chemical, generic, and brand names; category index; active ingredient index; product identification guide; and detailed product information. The references also can provide general information, including the generic and brand name of a drug, indications for use, contraindications to use, warnings, dosing protocols, side effects, and other notes, such as identification of banned substances. If a drug is not listed in a PDR, that drug likely has only recently entered the market.

The *Book of Facts and Figures* is continually updated and is the most current source of drug information. This book typically is on file at an area pharmacy and can be referenced by the pharmacists. The Food and Drug Information (www.nal.usda.gov/fnic) is an Internet source for drug information and provides consumer guidelines for drug use. A current list of banned substances can be retrieved from the NCAA (www.ncaa.org) and U.S. Olympic Committee (USOC; www.olympic-usoc.org) websites.

A ▶ *In preparing to take a 4-day, out-of-state trip for a college basketball tournament, the athletes taking prescription medications should be provided with the following instructions: ensure an ample supply of medication for the entire trip, do not place medication in checked luggage, take a copy of your written prescription, keep medications in a safe and secure location, and keep medications in their original containers.*

COMMON MEDICATIONS USED TO TREAT SPORT-RELATED INJURIES

 Following a head-first slide into second base, a softball player sustains an abrasion to the left forearm. What is the treatment for this injury, and what medication should be used as part of the treatment protocol?

A variety of different types of medications are used to treat soft-tissue injuries in sports. The more common medications include **analgesics** and **antipyretics**, NSAIDs, corticosteroids, anesthetics, antiseptics, topical antibiotics, and antifungal agents.

Analgesics and Antipyretics

Two of the more common analgesic–antipyretic medications are acetaminophen (e.g., Tylenol) and aspirin. Acetaminophen inhibits the synthesis of prostaglandins in the CNS but does not inhibit their synthesis in peripheral tissues. As a result, it acts as an analgesic and reduces fever, but it has no anti-inflammatory or antiplatelet (i.e., anticlotting) properties. Because it does not cause GI irritation, acetaminophen often is used as a replacement for aspirin. Overdosage of this medication can lead to liver damage and death.

Aspirin (i.e., acetylsalicylic acid) is a commonly used analgesic, antipyretic, and anti-inflammatory medication. Unfortunately, its use can lead to GI bleeding, nausea, vomiting, and development of gastric ulcers. In high doses, **tinnitus** and dizziness may result. Regardless of the circumstances, most practitioners prefer that no individual under the age of 18 years receive aspirin. If aspirin is used in a child under age 18 during chickenpox or influenza, the risk of **Reye's syndrome** increases. This is a severe disorder characterized by recurrent vomiting that begins a week after onset of the condition, from which the child either recovers rapidly or lapses into a coma, with the possibility of death. Individuals who are intolerant to aspirin, particularly asthmatics, may have an anaphylactic reaction to it. In addition, because aspirin prolongs blood clotting time, it should not be used by individuals who engage in contact sports.

Nonsteroidal Anti-Inflammatory Drugs

Nonsteroidal anti-inflammatory drugs are aspirin-like drugs that suppress inflammation and pain, produce analgesia, and reduce fever. They are among the most commonly used drugs in the treatment of soft-tissue injuries and are distributed as both OTC and prescription medications. Use of OTC NSAIDs can, at times, be high. In a recent study, nearly 75% of high school football players who were surveyed reported using OTC NSAIDs daily without adult supervision (4).

Nonsteroidal anti-inflammatory drugs were developed in an attempt to decrease the GI and hemorrhagic effects produced by aspirin. Most NSAIDs produce the same effects as aspirin but without many of the side effects. Individuals may respond differently to various types of NSAIDs, which differ chemically and pharmacokinetically based on their duration of action, potency level, OTC and prescription status, and dosing regimen.

Therapeutic Effects

Nonsteroidal anti-inflammatory drugs interfere with the biosynthesis of prostaglandins and other related compounds by inhibiting cyclooxygenase (COX), an enzyme responsible for the synthesis of prostaglandins. Prostaglandins are lipid-like compounds produced by almost every living cell, with the exception of red blood cells (RBCs). Under normal conditions, these lipid-like compounds regulate cell function. During inflammation of a soft tissue, increased prostaglandin activity seems to mediate inflammation by increasing blood flow, capillary permeability, and the permeability effects of histamine and bradykinin. Because NSAIDs inhibit prostaglandin activity, they reduce inflammation and pain. The anti-inflammatory effects of NSAIDs result from the inhibition of COX-2. The adverse GI reactions are caused by inhibition of COX-1. More recent NSAIDs (e.g., celecoxib and rofecoxib) appear to inhibit the COX-2 enzyme without inhibiting the COX-1 enzyme. The more traditional NSAIDs (e.g., naproxen and ibuprofen) reduce pain and inflammation by blocking COX-2, but unlike celecoxib and rofecoxib, they also inhibit COX-1. This inhibition of COX-1 can lead to stomach irritation and ulcers (2).

Nonsteroidal anti-inflammatory drugs provide analgesia without sedation or the euphoria that often is associated with narcotic analgesics, such as morphine, meperidine (e.g., Demerol), codeine, oxycodone (e.g., Percodan and Tylox), and propoxyphene (e.g., Darvon and Darvocet). Narcotic analgesics have the potential to produce physical dependence and tolerance; nonnarcotic analgesics, such as NSAIDs, do not normally produce dependence.

Nonsteroidal anti-inflammatory drugs may reduce fever without reducing normal body temperature. The hypothalamus has a set point that determines body temperature; if this set point is elevated by fever-promoting substances (e.g., endogenous pyrogens), fever develops. Nonsteroidal anti-inflammatory drugs inhibit prostaglandins and, as a result, lower the set point of the hypothalamus and reduce fever. In addition, NSAIDs have some antiplatelet (i.e., anticlotting) properties. In contrast to the strong antiplatelet properties of aspirin, however, the effects of NSAIDs are much lower in intensity. They are considered to be safe when used to treat acute soft-tissue injuries.

Adverse Effects

Side effects of NSAIDs can include GI irritation, renal impairment, hypersensitivity reactions (e.g., asthma, urticaria, and rhinitis), and toxicity. Other side effects can be seen in Box 27.6. Nonsteroidal anti-inflammatory drugs should be taken with food, milk, or a glass of water to decrease the risk of GI irritation. Alcohol should never be taken with NSAIDs, because it increases the risk of GI irritation and development of gastric ulcers. In the elderly, NSAIDs should be used cautiously, because the risk of serious ulcer disease in adults older than 65 years is increased with higher doses of NSAIDs.

The risk of renal impairment is relatively low with most NSAIDs. Signs of renal impairment include reduced urine output and rapid increase in serum creatinine and blood urea nitrogen. Signs and symptoms of a hypersensitive reaction or toxicity include dyspnea, rapid and irregular heartbeat, hematuria, upper abdominal tenderness, and jaundice. If any of these signs and symptoms develop, immediate medical attention is required.

Use and Availability

Nonsteroidal anti-inflammatory drugs are used to treat mild to moderate pain associated with joints, muscles, and headaches. In addition, they often are used to treat inflammation associated with rheumatoid arthritis, tendinitis, and bursitis conditions. They are not, however, effective for the relief of severe pain.

Nonsteroidal anti-inflammatory drugs are available in both OTC and prescription strengths and are routinely taken orally. Prescription strength NSAIDs can only be prescribed by a licensed

---

Box 27.6 General Adverse Reactions to Nonsteroidal Anti-Inflammatory Drugs

- **Gastrointestinal:** nausea, vomiting, diarrhea, constipation, epigastric pain, indigestion, intestinal ulceration, jaundice, bloating, and dry mouth
- **Central nervous system:** dizziness, anxiety, light-headedness, vertigo, headache, drowsiness, insomnia, depression, and psychic disturbances
- **Cardiovascular:** congestive heart failure, decreased or increased blood pressure, and cardiac arrhythmias
- **Renal:** hematuria, cystitis, elevated blood urea nitrogen, polyuria, dysuria, oliguria, and acute renal failure in those with impaired renal function
- **The senses:** visual disturbances, blurred or diminished vision, diplopia, swollen or irritated eyes, photophobia, reversible loss of color vision, tinnitus, taste change, and rhinitis
- **Skin:** rash, erythema, irritation, skin eruptions, exfoliative dermatitis, Stevens-Johnson syndrome, ecchymosis, and purpura
- **Metabolic/endocrinologic:** decreased appetite, weight increase or decrease, hyperglycemia, hypoglycemia, flushing, sweating, menstrual disorders, and vaginal bleeding
- **Other:** thirst, fever, chills, and vaginitis

Adapted from Roach S. Pharmacology for Health Professionals. Philadelphia. Lippincott Williams & Wilkins, 2005; with permission.

practitioner. These NSAIDs are prescribed on a case-by-case basis and should not be shared among individuals with similar soft-tissue injuries or conditions. Sharing medication is not recommended, because individuals respond differently to the same medication. Nonprescription NSAIDs include ibuprofen (e.g., Advil, Motrin, and Nuprin), ketoprofen (e.g., Orudis KT and Actron), and naproxen sodium (e.g., Aleve).

Pain relief usually is noted within 30 minutes after ingestion and lasts for several hours, depending on the dosage and duration of the particular NSAID. Both OTC and prescription products should be used only for short-term (i.e., 10 days maximum) treatment of inflammation and pain associated with soft-tissue injuries. When used as an antipyretic, NSAIDs should only be used for 3 days (2). If pain, inflammation, or fever does not subside or increases within these time periods, consult a physician immediately.

As with most medications, and as mentioned previously, NSAIDs should not be used in combination with alcohol. A physician or pharmacist should be consulted before combining NSAIDs with other medications.

> See *Common Nonsteroidal Anti-inflammatory Medications,* available on the companion website at thePoint, for a listing of the common NSAIDs used in treating soft-tissue injuries among sport participants.

Corticosteroids

Corticosteroids are steroid hormones that are produced naturally within the adrenal cortex but that also can be produced synthetically. They are powerful drugs that affect nearly the entire body.

Therapeutic Effects

Corticosteroids are lipid soluble and block the body's natural response to inflammation by inhibiting the synthesis of chemical mediators (e.g., prostaglandins, leukotrienes, and histamine). As a result, swelling, warmth, redness, and pain associated with inflammation are decreased. The manner in which corticosteroids suppress inflammation, however, is much broader in scope than the manner in which NSAIDs do so. Corticosteroids inhibit prostaglandin synthesis, as do NSAIDs, but corticosteroids also act in several other ways to decrease inflammation.

Adverse Effects

Side effects of corticosteroids, which often resemble those of the condition for which they are prescribed to treat, include itching, burning, dry skin, and fluid retention. Side effects that are rare include an increase or decrease in appetite, dizziness, restlessness, facial or body hair growth, GI irritation, menstrual irregularities, and optic pain. Most of these side effects disappear soon after the medication is discontinued. Because oral NSAIDs and corticosteroids have similar effects on the GI tract, concurrent use severely increases the risk of GI irritation and ulceration. In addition, chronic use of corticosteroids can suppress the body's immune system, making the user more susceptible to infection.

Availability and Use

Corticosteroids are indicated for skin disorders, nasal inflammation, rheumatic disorders (e.g., bursitis, arthritis, and tendinitis), and skin infections. They are administered through oral and nasal inhalation, intra-articular injection, subcutaneous injection, intravenous injection, topically, and orally.

Corticosteroids should not be used by individuals who are infected with human immunodeficiency virus (HIV) or have acquired immunodeficiency syndrome, heart disease, hypertension, diabetes, gastritis, peptic ulcers, lupus, or other infections (e.g., bronchitis or flu). By reducing inflammation and pain, corticosteroids also may delay exercise-induced pain, placing an individual at increased risk for further injury. Corticosteroids are not banned by the NCAA, but the USOC bans all types, with the exception of most topical (e.g., ear, eye, and skin) agents. The USOC allows inhaled, local, or intra-articular injections if written permission is provided (5).

> See *Common Corticosteroids,* available on the companion website at thePoint, for a list of the common corticosteroids administered through oral and nasal inhalation or injections.

Local Anesthetics

Anesthetics, frequently called "pain killers," inhibit the activity of sensory nerve receptors in the skin. Under normal conditions, the skin does not respond well to aspirin or other oral analgesics.

When irritated, the same sensory nerve endings in the skin can lead to **pruritus** from a weak stimulation or to skin pain from a strong stimulation. The skin responds more readily to topical medications. Local anesthetics are categorized by route of administration and may be injectable, topical, or sprayed. Injectable anesthetics are prescription medications that can only be administered by a licensed professional (i.e., physician, physician assistant, nurse practitioner, or nurse).

Injectable Anesthetics

In the treatment of sports-related injuries, injectable anesthetics most commonly are used for **infiltrative anesthesia**, a process that produces numbness by interfering with nerve function in a localized, subcutaneous, soft-tissue area. Infiltrative anesthesia commonly is used for the treatment of soft-tissue injuries, such as hip pointers and turf toe. In addition, they are used as an anesthetic before minor surgical procedures, such as suturing or aspiration of bursal or joint fluid. They are classified by the duration of action—namely, short-, intermediate-, and long-term action. Side effects are minimal when used as directed. Large quantities of the drugs must be absorbed to produce any associated side effects, such as tremors, drowsiness, hypotension, or hypersensitivity and anaphylactic reactions.

Topical Anesthetics

Topical anesthetics are OTC and prescription medications that are applied to the skin. Topical anesthetics or analgesics often are used to relieve pain associated with musculoskeletal injury (e.g., strains, sprains, tendinitis, and bursitis). When used for these purposes, topical medications are called **counterirritants**. These medications stimulate nerve endings in the skin that respond to pain and to warm and cold sensations, which in theory distracts the user from the original pain or itching. Essentially, these products irritate the skin to relieve pain and itching. Counterirritants come in various forms, including lotions, rubs, liniments, and creams. Popular examples include Ben-Gay, Mineral Ice, Flex-All 454, Menthol, Absorbine Jr, wintergreen oil, and Icy Hot. The U.S. FDA suggests that these drugs are safe when applied three to four times per day, but they are not suggested for long-term use. If pain persists after 7 days, a physician should be consulted immediately.

In addition to the counterirritant properties, topical anesthetics can further be classified according to whether they reduce itching, pain, or both. Most topical anesthetics are easily identified in their brand names by the suffix "-caine" (e.g., Americaine, Lanacane, Xylocaine, and Solarcaine).

Spray Anesthetics

In addition to creams, lotions, and liniments, a few spray anesthetics are on the market (e.g., Aerofreeze, ethyl chloride, and fluoromethane). These products temporarily freeze the skin in an effort to decrease pain; however, the duration of action is quite limited and only lasts for approximately 1 minute. These products are not recommended for use, because the freezing action can damage the skin and delay healing.

Adverse Effects

Topical anesthetics are relatively safe when used as directed. Common side effects are limited to skin irritation (e.g., rashes or hives). These normally disappear once use of the product is stopped. Systemic absorption can occur if large amounts of these products are used over a large surface area or if used on deep wounds. Systemic absorption is toxic and may produce convulsions and paralysis of the CNS.

Individuals who are allergic to aspirin should not use methyl salicylate products, because the body may absorb the salicylate, the major ingredient in aspirin. In addition, products that produce warm sensations should never be used in combination with a heating pad or occlusive dressing. This may increase systemic absorption and result in skin and muscle necrosis. These products should never be used before exercise in hot, humid conditions or immediately following exercise. Application is appropriate after the body cools down. The NCAA and USOC permit the use of topical anesthetics; the NCAA also permits intra-articular injections of local anesthesia when medically justified (3).

Muscle Relaxants

Unlike local anesthetics that inhibit sensory nerve receptors in the skin and subcutaneous tissue, muscle relaxants actually block afferent messages that travel from the muscles to the brain. Skeletal muscle relaxants are classified as either central or direct acting. Central agents exert their effects within the spinal cord, whereas direct-acting muscle relaxants affect the skeletal muscle cell. Both types are available by prescription only. Muscle relaxants prescribed for muscle spasms associated with musculoskeletal injury are central acting. They decrease local pain, spasm, and tenderness and, in doing so, allow increased range of motion. Examples of common muscle relaxants are chlorzoxazone (e.g., Parafon Forte and Paraflex), cyclobenzaprine (e.g., Flexeril), diazepam (e.g., Valium), methocarbamol (e.g., Robaxin), and orphenadrine (e.g., Norflex). These drugs often are used in combination with rest and physical therapy (e.g., thermotherapy, cryotherapy, and electrotherapy) to relieve pain from acute muscle spasms associated with musculoskeletal conditions. Because central-acting muscle relaxants produce their effects by acting on the CNS, they often produce a general depression of CNS functions. As a result, common side effects include dizziness, drowsiness, and sedation. Muscle relaxants are not banned by either the NCAA or the USOC; however, they may be prohibited by international federations of certain sports.

> See *Common Muscle Relaxant Medications,* found on the companion website at thePoint, for a list of the common muscle relaxants and their possible side effects.

Topical Antibiotics

Antibiotics are substances that kill disease-producing bacteria and are used to prevent and treat infections. Two basic types of bacteria cause most skin infections, namely *Streptococcus* and *Staphylococcus.* Because it is difficult to predict which type of bacteria may be producing a skin infection, most topical antibiotics contain several active ingredients that treat both organisms. Topical antibiotics are used on small open wounds, such as abrasions, and can be purchased as creams, ointments, or powders. Bacitracin, Neosporin, Neomycin, and Polysporin are examples of OTC topical antibiotics. These products are not designed to be used on deep wounds, because internal absorption of some of these antibiotics can be toxic. Topical antibiotics should be used in small amounts, generally three times daily, and for not more than 1 week (2). Topical antibiotics are not banned by the NCAA or USOC.

> See *Common Topical Antibiotics,* found on the companion website at thePoint, for a list of the common topical antibiotics and their possible side effects.

Antiseptics and Disinfectants

The terms antiseptic and disinfectant sometimes are used interchangeably, but they are not the same. **Antiseptics** are applied to living tissue to stop growth of microorganisms or destroy bacteria on contact and prevent infection. They are most appropriate in the cleansing and treatment of large, open skin wounds and come in sprays, powders, and swab-on liquids. Isopropyl alcohol, Betadine, and tincture of iodine are common OTC antiseptics. Antiseptics are for external use only and are not banned by the NCAA or USOC.

Disinfectants are chemical agents applied to nonliving objects. They most commonly are used to disinfect surgical instruments and cleanse medical equipment and facilities. Common disinfectants used in athletic training are alcohol products, Versa-Quat, and Iso-quin. The companion website on thePoint provides information about disinfecting techniques used in the athletic training room to prevent the spread of infectious diseases related to bloodborne pathogens.

Antifungal Agents

Tolnaftate (e.g., Tinactin), miconazole nitrate (e.g., Micatin), and clotrimazole (e.g., Lotrimin and Mycelex) are agents that treat infections caused by fungal cells. In humans, fungal cells are either molds or yeasts. Tinea pedis, tinea cruris, and tinea corporis are caused by fungal molds, whereas candidiasis and moniliasis are caused by fungal yeasts. Products used to treat fungal molds usually are applied twice daily, with symptoms disappearing within a few days of initial treatment. Following disappearance of symptoms, the molds often can still be found within skin cracks and nail beds. For this reason, physicians suggest regular, continued application of antifungal agents as

See *Common Antifungal Agents*, found on the companion website at thePoint, for a list of these agents and their possible side effects.

part of a preventive protocol. Before applying antifungal agents, the infected area should be cleansed thoroughly with mild soap and water. If the infection does not clear within 1 week (e.g., tinea cruris) or 1 month (e.g., tinea pedis and corporis), another antifungal agent should be used or a physician should be consulted.

Historically, drugs used to treat vaginal yeast infections were by prescription only, but a variety of antiyeast agents can now be purchased over the counter. Examples include clotrimazole (e.g., Gyne-Lotrimin, Mycelex-7, and Mycelex-G), miconazole nitrate (e.g., Monistat), and tioconazole (e.g., Vagistat-1). Approximately 25% of females of childbearing age will develop a yeast infection. Predisposing factors include pregnancy, obesity, diabetes, debilitation, and the use of certain drugs (e.g., oral contraceptives and systemic antibiotics). Depending on the product, it should be used once daily for 1 to 14 days. If a course of treatment does not resolve the problem, the possibility exits that some other microorganism is present, and a physician should be consulted immediately.

Antifungal agents are relatively safe when used as directed. Some can be toxic if they are absorbed systemically and, as such, should be for external use only. Side effects usually resemble a worsening of the condition being treated, including increased redness, irritation, and itching. These products are not banned by the NCAA or USOC.

A *Treatment for the softball player who sustained an abrasion to the left forearm should include initiating proper first-aid care for an open wound using universal precautions, cleaning the abrasion with an antiseptic (e.g., Betadine), and applying a topical antibiotic, (e.g., Bacitracin, Neosporin, or Neomycin).*

PERFORMANCE-ENHANCING SUBSTANCES (ERGOGENIC AIDS)

Q *Ephedrine is found in many OTC sinus and cold medications. What adverse affects are associated with the use of ephedrine?*

Ergogenic aids are substances taken in nonpharmacologic doses specifically to enhance energy production, energy use, or recovery to provide a competitive edge. A substance is considered to be performance enhancing if it benefits sport participation by increasing strength, power, speed, or endurance or by altering body weight or composition. Even substances that change behavior, arousal level, and/or perception of pain should be considered as performance enhancing (6). Some substances are legal and may be a part of one's normal diet (e.g., caffeine, alcohol, and tobacco). Taken in excess, however, even these substances can produce adverse effects in a healthy individual.

Caffeine

Coffee, tea, chocolate, and coca drinks are common beverages and foods found in the American diet. Each contains caffeine—the most widely abused drug in the world. Caffeine is a low-level CNS stimulant that increases alertness and feelings of well-being. It is used as a stimulant in fatigue states (e.g., Vivarin and NoDoz), in combination with analgesic compounds (e.g., Excedrin and Anacin), and in diet pills. Caffeine also is found in many new products, including energy drinks, sport gels, and alcoholic beverages.

Caffeine is rapidly absorbed, with peak levels being achieved in 30 to 60 minutes and a half-life of 3.5 hours (7). Caffeine stimulates the secretion of adrenaline (epinephrine) and, except in the renal afferent artery, causes vasoconstriction. This response could produce a number of secondary metabolic changes that could promote an ergogenic action, such as enhancing the contractility of skeletal and cardiac muscle and assisting in fat metabolism (8). Therefore, caffeine is considered to be an ergogenic aid for prolonged endurance exercise activities in doses of approximately 3 to 6 mg/kg body mass (9). Ergogenic dose effects are found at approximately half the banned dose level, which equals three cups of coffee or six to eight caffeinated soft drinks (10). Many individuals take caffeine in pill form.

When used in large doses (15–30 mg/kg), caffeine overdose may lead to agitation, delirium, seizures, dyspnea, cardiac arrhythmia, myoclonus, nausea, vomiting, hyperglycemia, and hypokalemia. With lower doses of caffeine, such as those via coffee consumption, adverse reactions may include tachycardia, palpitations, insomnia, restlessness, nervousness, tremor, headache, abdominal pain, nausea, vomiting, diarrhea, and diuresis (11). Caffeine is considered by the NCAA and International Olympic Committee (IOC) to be a "restricted or controlled drug" when urine levels exceed 15 and 12 µg/ml, respectively (9). Similar to most stimulants, caffeine does produce tolerance and can be addictive, with users experiencing withdrawal symptoms on cessation of use.

Tobacco

Tobacco is a low-level CNS stimulant and is widely used in the United States. Nicotine is the stimulating chemical and addictive substance in the product. Methods of consumption include cigarettes, cigars, and smokeless tobacco (i.e., loose-leaf tobacco [chewing], moist or dry powdered tobacco [snuff or "dipping"], and compressed tobacco ["plug"]). Nicotine is absorbed in the lungs when using cigarettes and cigars and through the oral mucosa when using smokeless tobacco.

Initially, small doses of nicotine stimulate, and then large doses depress, the autonomic ganglia and myoneural junctions. The amount of nicotine in tobacco products varies widely. On average, one cigarette contains 1 mg of nicotine, and a pinch of smokeless tobacco contains 35 mg. Contrary to popular belief, smokeless tobacco is not a safe alternative to cigarette smoking, because the nicotine is more swiftly absorbed into the bloodstream, resulting in a more immediate stimulant effect.

Major League Baseball imposed a ban on the use of smokeless tobacco products in the minor leagues, and the NCAA has an all-sport ban on the use of smokeless tobacco during NCAA practices and games. The use of smokeless tobacco by adults has slowly declined since the late 1990s and rapidly declined in adolescents and teens during this same time period (12). Side effects associated with the use of smokeless tobacco are similar to those of other products that contain nicotine, including feelings of well-being, increased heart rate, increased blood pressure, and addiction (13). The use of smokeless tobacco also can lead to **halitosis**, permanently discolored teeth, oral abrasions, periodontal bone disease, tooth loss, and **leukoplakia**. Leukoplakia is a disease of the mouth characterized by white patches and oral lesions on the cheeks, gums, and/or tongue, which can lead to oral cancer.

Alcohol

Alcohol is the most abused recreational drug in the United States, and it is the number one drug of choice among intercollegiate athletes (3). Alcohol is involved in more than one-third of the deaths attributed to unintentional injury, homicide, and suicide, which together account for 76% of mortality in the 15- to 19-year-old age group. More than half (58%) of 12th-grade students and one fifth (20%) of eight-grade students report having been drunk at least once in their life (14).

When ingested, alcohol is rapidly absorbed, unaltered, into the body. Most absorption takes place in the stomach and small intestine. Absorption rates depend on several factors:

- Type and concentration of the alcohol
- The rate at which the beverage is consumed
- Current stomach contents
- Factors influencing the emptying of the stomach (e.g., levels of carbonated beverages, food, and emotional state)
- Body weight
- Gastric mobility

Unlike other drugs, alcohol is metabolized at a constant rate, typically 1 ounce of alcohol per hour. This equals one 12-ounce beer (excluding lagers and malt liqueurs), 2.5 ounces of wine, or 1 ounce of distilled spirits. The rate of metabolism is related to the actions of liver enzymes, which can vary between individuals. Factors influencing these enzymes include age, menstrual cycle, heredity, race, liver disease, and previous experience with alcohol consumption (15,16).

Alcohol is lipid soluble. As such, it quickly crosses the blood-brain barrier and instantly acts as a CNS depressant. Alcohol is distributed unmodified throughout body fluids, tissues, and organs. The majority of alcohol is metabolized in the liver (90%), with the remainder being excreted through urine, sweat, and one's breath.

Unlike other ergogenic aids, alcohol rarely is used as such. In a 1982 American College of Sports Medicine Position Statement on alcohol use in sports, it was found that:

1. Alcohol in small (i.e., 1.5–2.0 oz) to moderate (i.e., 3–4 oz) amounts has negative effects on psychomotor skills, including reaction times, hand–eye coordination, accuracy, balance, and complex coordination.

2. Alcohol has little or no benefit regarding energy metabolism or oxygen consumption.

3. Alcohol does not improve muscular work capacity and may decrease performance levels as well as impair temperature regulation during prolonged exercise in cold environments.

Therefore, it has been concluded that alcohol lacks ergogenic properties for the majority of sport-related activities. Alcohol may be an ergogenic aid in some aiming sports; however, no conclusive evidence has appeared to support this theory. Alcohol is considered to be an NCAA-banned substance in riflery but not in other NCAA sports.

Marijuana

Marijuana is a naturally occurring cannabinoid that contains the active ingredient δ9-tetrahydro-cannabinol (THC). Although currently an illegal drug, it has been used as an antiemetic agent in conjunction with chemotherapy for patients with cancer and for lowering intraocular pressure in patients with glaucoma. It is used recreationally as a euphoriant.

The active ingredient THC primarily affects the CNS and cardiovascular system. Adverse effects to the CNS include impaired motor coordination, decreased short-term memory, difficulty concentrating, and decline in work performance. Adverse effects to the cardiovascular system include tachycardia and changes in blood pressure (e.g., systolic blood pressure increases in a supine position and decreases in a standing position). The effects depend on the route, dose, setting, and previous experience of the user. Adverse effects on sport and physical activity performance include reduction of maximal exercise performance, with premature achievement of VO_{2max}, and no appreciable effect on tidal volume, arterial blood pressure, or carboxyhemoglobin compared to controls. Marijuana can inhibit sweating, leading to an increase in core body temperature.

Marijuana is not banned by the IOC but is considered a street drug by the NCAA and is prohibited. Because of its high lipid solubility, marijuana can be detected for up to 2 to 4 weeks by drug testing.

Diuretics

Diuretics, commonly known as "water pills," help to rid the body of unneeded water and salt through the urine, allowing the heart to pump blood more freely. In general, diuretics are used to treat high blood pressure, heart failure, kidney and liver problems, and glaucoma. Diuretics are categorized as:

- Carbonic anhydrase inhibitors

- Loop diuretics

- Osmotic diuretics

- Potassium-sparing diuretics

- Thiazides and related diuretics

Carbonic anhydrase inhibitors prevent the action of carbonic anhydrase, an enzyme that produces free hydrogen ions, which are then traded for sodium ions in the kidney tubules. As a result, sodium, potassium, bicarbonate, and water are excreted in the urine. Carbonic anhydrase inhibitors (e.g., acetazolamide and methazolamide) often are used to treat glaucoma, because these agents can decrease the production of aqueous humor in the eye, which in turn decreases intraocular pressure.

Loop diuretics (e.g., furosemide and ethacrynic) are more powerful. These agents are especially useful during emergencies, such as in the treatment of edema associated with chronic heart failure, cirrhosis of the liver, and renal disease.

Osmotic diuretics (e.g., mannitol and urea) are used to promote diuresis in the prevention and treatment of the oliguric phase (i.e., low urine production) of acute renal failure. These agents also are used to reduce cerebral edema as well as intraocular pressure before and after eye surgery.

Potassium-sparing diuretics work in two ways. First, certain medications (e.g., triamterene and amiloride) depress the reabsorption of sodium in the kidney tubules and, in doing so, increase sodium and water excretion. Second, they depress the excretion of potassium, hence the name potassium-sparing. For example, spironolactone, another potassium-sparing diuretic, acts on the hormone aldosterone, which enhances the reabsorption of sodium in the distal tubules of the kidney. When this action is blocked, sodium (but not potassium) and water are excreted. Potassium-sparing diuretics are used in the treatment of chronic heart failure and hypertension.

Thiazides and related diuretics inhibit the reabsorption of sodium and chloride, leading to moderate increases in the excretion of sodium, chloride, and water. They often are used in long-term treatment of hypertension, edema caused by chronic heart failure, hepatic cirrhosis, corticosteroid and estrogen therapy, and renal dysfunction.

Use of diuretics should be closely monitored by a physician. Abuse of diuretics can impair thermoregulation; exacerbate exercise-related dehydration; decrease stroke volume; increase arrhythmia; cause a reflex increase in total peripheral resistance, which may decrease muscle blood flow; and contribute to electrolyte depletion (17). In addition, adverse reactions may involve fever, rash, photosensitivity, blurred vision, nausea, vomiting, headaches, vertigo, and diarrhea (2).

Anabolic-Androgenic Steroids

Anabolic-androgenic steroids include more than 30 natural and synthetically made derivatives of testosterone. They most commonly are used to stimulate growth and accelerate weight gain. When naturally secreted from the pituitary gland (men, 4–10 mg/day; women, 1 mg/day) testosterone produces secondary sex characteristics. Tetrahydrogestinone (THG) has received considerable media attention as a performance-enhancing substance. Although difficult to detect, there have been various reports of its use by high-profile athletes in several sports, including track and field, football, tennis, and baseball. After developing a way to detect THG in the urine following the 2004 Olympics, both the U.S. FDA, Major League Baseball, and the World Anti-Doping Agency have banned this substance (18).

Physiologically, anabolic steroids promote rapid synthesis of protein in the body by binding to androgen receptors at the cellular level, stimulating the production of ribonucleic acid, which in turn increases the synthesis of protein. In healthy individuals who do not exercise, steroids increase appetite and feelings of well-being but have no effect on muscle size or strength. Among individuals who are involved in high-intensity training, anabolic steroids can increase body weight, lean body mass, and muscle size as well as strength (19); however, anabolic steroids provide little benefit in terms of aerobic capacity. Other adverse effects include bouts of uncontrolled anger and explosive behavior, increased appetite and sexual desires, and a lowered tolerance to pain (20,21). Short- and long-term physical effects, such as those listed in Box 27.7, are dependent on the type of steroid

---

Box 27.7   Physical Effects of Anabolic Steroid Use

Short Term	Long Term
Acne	Cardiovascular disease
Gynecomastia	Liver disease
Male pattern baldness	Testicular atrophy
Enhanced facial and body hair growth	Impotence/sterility
Menstrual irregularities	Decrease in sperm
Decreased breast development in women	Enlargement of clitoris
Deepening of the voice	Uterine atrophy
Increased risk of muscles strains/ruptures	Early closure of physis in children (shorter adult height)

used, the frequency of use, and the age of initiation (22). Some of these effects are irreversible even after discontinuation of steroid use.

Anabolic steroids most commonly are used in 6- to 12-week cycles with pyramid or stacking techniques (22). The term stacking denotes the simultaneous use of two or more types of anabolic steroids, which could include both oral and intramuscular injections, and the pattern of increasing a dose through a cycle is referred to as pyramiding. An individual using the pyramid technique begins with a lower daily dose, then moves to a higher dose in the middle of a cycle, and then ends with a lower dose at the end of a cycle. Pyramiding may lead to doses 10- to 40-fold greater than those used for medical indications. A common belief is that pyramiding and stacking maximize steroid receptor binding and minimizes toxic side effects. These benefits have not been substantiated scientifically, but this has not appreciably influenced dosing patterns.

Human Growth Hormone

Human growth hormone (hGH) is a popular antiaging drug and commonly is used to enhance muscular strength and growth as well as for its musculoskeletal healing properties. Human growth hormone is used in growth hormone–deficient children (to stimulate skeletal and soft-tissue growth), growth hormone–deficient adults, the elderly, children with chronic renal failure, and children with large cutaneous burns (to accelerate wound healing). It also is used to increase lean body mass and decrease fat in patients postoperatively and is approved for treatment of wasting syndrome secondary to HIV infection (7).

In its natural form, hGH is secreted from the anterior pituitary gland and mediates a plethora of metabolic and growth processes, with effects on the majority of body tissues. The hormone increases protein synthesis by enhancing uptake and transport of amino acids. Synthetic or recombinant hGH is administered intramuscularly or subcutaneously, with a typical dose being 0.30 mg/kg per week (23).

The most common side effect of hGH is **acromegaly,** a condition described as gigantism and characterized by costal and mandibular growth; vertebral, phalangeal, and frontal bone overgrowth; widening of joint spaces; accelerated osteoarthritis; and soft-tissue swelling. As little as a twofold increase in recommended dosage may result in acromegaly, which leaves a narrow therapeutic window. The risk of acromegaly is significant for individuals consuming up to 20 mg/day. Other side effects include hypertension, hyperglycemia, glycosuria, diabetes, arthritis, menstrual irregularities, vision loss, sleep apnea, ventricular hypertrophy, myopathies, and characteristic coarsening of bones in the face, hands, and feet (7,18).

In the athletic environment, hGH often is used in combination with various testosterone derivatives and is extremely difficult to detect in routine urine drug tests. Therefore, it is becoming increasingly popular among athletes. Efforts are being made, however, to develop a noninvasive technique to detect the use of hGH.

Amphetamines

Amphetamines are powerful CNS stimulants that are banned by the NCAA and IOC. They are used for therapeutic purposes to treat a variety of conditions, such as refractory obesity, narcolepsy, attention deficit disorder, and severe depression. Sport participants may use amphetamines to mask fatigue and pain and to improve certain mental tasks (24,25).

Classified as sympathomimetics, amphetamines influence involuntary actions of the CNS (i.e., heart rate and blood pressure). Most users take amphetamines orally, but injectable and inhaled forms (e.g., cocaine and crack) also are available. Serious side effects include a lowered threshold for arrhythmias and provocation of angina, which may lead to sudden cardiac death, stroke, tremors, insomnia, psychosis, psychological addiction, and rhabdomyolysis. Little evidence suggests that many sport participants use amphetamines, but evidence does clearly indicate the use of less potent amphetamine-like products, such as ephedrine. Amphetamines are readily detected by urine tests, because both unchanged amphetamines and metabolites appear in the urine.

Ephedra

Derived from the ancient Chinese herb ephedra, or ma huang, the ephedrine alkaloids (e.g., pseudoephedrine, norephedrine, methylephedrine, methylpseudoephedrine, and norpseudoephedrine) can have powerful effects on the body. Ephedra is a CNS stimulant that increases serum levels of norepinephrine and can, directly or indirectly, increase blood pressure, heart rate, cardiac output, and peripheral vascular resistance (18). Traditionally used as a bronchodilator and nasal decongestant, ephedra is found in many OTC sinus and cold medications. It is used therapeutically to treat chronic postural hypotension, enuresis, and narcolepsy. Ephedra is a common ingredient in weight loss and energy-boosting products, and it is available OTC in 25-mg tablets.

Side effects of ephedra can be life-threatening, because it increases heat production and body temperature and, as such, increases the risk of heat illness, especially in warm environments. Mild adverse effects include heart palpitations and irregular heart beats, dizziness, headache, insomnia, nervousness, and skin flushing or tingling. Moderate to severe adverse reactions include tachycardia, life-threatening arrhythmias, hypertension, stroke, seizures, and death (26). Recently, ephedra has been shown to be ergogenic for anaerobic exercise, especially when taken with caffeine; however, the potential for toxicity is high (27). It is important to note that synthetic ephedrine derivatives are used to produce the street drugs ecstasy and methamphetamine, which are used as stimulants. Ephedra is banned by the IOC, NCAA, and National Football League.

Blood Doping and Erythropoietin

The primary purpose of blood doping and use of erythropoietin is to stimulate the production of RBCs so that more oxygen is available for use during long-distance aerobic activities (e.g., cycling) to enhance oxygen-carrying capacity and skeletal muscle performance. Before the increased popularity of erythropoietin, two techniques were used to produce the desired effects of blood doping:

1. Homologous transfusions use blood from another person or donor and transfuse it into the identified individual. Two major concerns with this procedure are the compatibility of the transfusion between the donor and recipient and the risk of contracting HIV and hepatitis.

2. Autologous transfusions remove blood from the individual, freeze the blood, and reinfuse the blood several weeks later, after the recipient's body has had ample time to make new RBCs. Following the transfusion, the recipient has an increased concentration of RBCs.

Transfusions can improve performance during endurance exercises by increasing hemoglobin concentration, which leads to increased maximal oxygen consumption and total exercise time as well as improved tolerance in some extreme environmental conditions (7). The IOC bans blood doping, but enforcement is limited by the lack of effective techniques for detection.

Intravenous use of recombinant human erythropoietin stimulates RBC production within days, and effects can be seen for as long as 3 to 4 weeks. Erythropoietin is used therapeutically in several conditions, including anemia secondary to end-stage renal disease; anemias secondary to prematurity, multiple myeloma, and cancer; and acquired immunodeficiency syndrome treated with zidovudine. Its use also increases the yield of autologous blood donors both safely and effectively over a 21-day period and can reduce the need for transfusions in patients undergoing hip replacement. Miscalculations in dosing and dehydration may result in a hematocrit level as high as 80% and can cause severe hyperviscosity leading to encephalopathy, stroke, seizures, and tissue hypoxia (18). Rapid clotting also may lead to pulmonary embolism, myocardial infarction, and peripheral clot formation (i.e., vascular thrombosis). In addition, intravenous use increases other inherent risks (e.g., infection with hepatitis, infection with HIV, and endocarditis).

The prevalence of erythropoietin use is unknown. Various media reports concerning its use among athletes have appeared, but no scientific reports indicate its prevalence. According to the position statement of the American College of Sports Medicine on "Use of Blood Doping as an Ergogenic Aid," any blood-doping procedure used to enhance athletic performance is unethical, unfair, and exposes the individual to serious health risks (28). Darbepoetin, a related substance, causes similar effects and was detected during the 2002 Winter Olympics in cross-country skiers, who subsequently were disqualified. Because recombinant human erythropoietin and darbepoetin can now be detected, newer strategies to evade detection and boost performance are likely to be used in the near future.

Creatine

Creatine is a nonessential dietary element found in protein-rich sources, such as meat and fish. It is the most widely used and marketed nonsteroidal, nonstimulant ergogenic aid in young athletes, and it has been reported to be used in 41% of 219 Division I intercollegiate athletes (29). It is synthesized primarily in the liver and is stored predominantly in skeletal muscle. Hydrolysis of muscle phosphocreatine results in rapid production of adenosine triphosphate (ATP), which is needed for muscle contraction. As muscle stores of phosphocreatine become depleted, performance decreases. Oral creatine supplementation can increase muscle phosphocreatine stores by 6 to 8% and, in doing so, causes faster regeneration of ATP. This can result in shorter recovery periods and increased energy for repeated bouts of exercise. Increased muscle creatine also buffers the lactic acid produced during exercise, delaying muscle fatigue and soreness (10). In anaerobic exercise, creatine depletion is a limiting factor (30).

The total daily requirement of creatine is 2 g/day, approximately half of which comes from in vivo production and the other half from dietary sources (30). Supplemental dosing varies. One method involves ingesting loading doses of 20 g daily, divided in four doses, for 5 to 10 days, followed by a maintenance dose of 5 g/day. Another method eliminates the loading phase and involves ingesting 3 g/day. Lower doses take longer to reach the desired intramuscular creatine levels (29).

Creatine purports to be a safe ergogenic aid in adults. The adverse effects are few and dose dependent, including weight gain and GI distress (e.g., nausea, bloating, cramping, and diarrhea). Although increased muscle cramping originally was thought to be a side effect of creatine use, recent studies with college football players showed that creatine supplementation did not appear to increase the incidence or injury or cramping and, when combined with resistance and anaerobic training, may positively affect cell hydration status and enhance performance variables further than the augmentation that is seen with training alone (31,32). No other serious long-term, detrimental effects in the absence of other nutritional supplements have been consistently documented (33). Several areas of concern, however, include the potential for renal damage in those with preexisting renal dysfunction, rhabdomyolysis, cardiovascular impact if the creatine is taken up by the myocardium, increased risk of heat illness because of potential dehydration, and increased risk of exertional compartment syndrome as a result of fluid retention that may accompany loading doses of the substance (34). In the most recent position statement on creatine use, the American College of Sports Medicine discouraged creatine use in people less than 18 years of age because of unknown potential adverse health effects (34).

A *Even though ephedrine is found in many OTC sinus and cold medications, adverse effects are associated with its use. The mild adverse effects of ephedrine include heart palpitations and irregular heart beats, dizziness, headache, insomnia, nervousness, and skin flushing or tingling. Moderate to severe adverse reactions to ephedrine include tachycardia, life-threatening arrhythmias, hypertension, stroke, seizures, and death. Combining caffeine with ephedra greatly increases the severity of side effects.*

DRUG TESTING

In 1965, Beckett developed the first chromatographic drug testing procedures for the Tour of Britain cycling competition. Three years later, the IOC drug testing program was implemented during the 1968 Summer Olympic Games. Following the lead of the IOC, the NCAA began drug testing at championship events in 1986. The intent of drug testing programs is threefold:

1. Drug testing discovers those individuals who may be experiencing problems.

2. Testing is performed to screen participants for evidence of drug use/abuse.

3. Drug testing protects individuals from injury or from causing injury to others.

Various drug testing methods (e.g., urine tests, blood tests, human hair tests, and radioimmunoassay) are available. Urine testing is the method of choice. It is noninvasive, and large volumes of urine can be collected easily. Analysis for the presence of drugs and their metabolites is usually seen in high concentrations in the urine. Two disadvantages of urine testing are the ease of tampering with the sample and the potentially humiliating experience for the individual.

Current drug testing uses gas chromatography/mass spectrometry (GC/MS). Factors influencing test accuracy include individual urine output/volume, urine pH, dosage, timing and formulation of used substances, occasional or chronic substance use, substances taken simultaneously, variability of testing equipment, individual metabolism, recent trauma, and shock. Although GC/MS may approach 100% accuracy, individuals have attempted to avoid detection using several methods:.

- **Masking agents.** Diuretics often are used to counteract steroid-induced fluid retention and reduce the concentration of banned substances (35).

- **Determination of drug half-life.** If drug testing is announced, individuals can determine the length of time during which a specific drug can be detected in the urine.

- **Substitution of urine.** Several methods can be used to substitute "clean" urine (e.g., self-catheterization and innovative "delivery systems"). In efforts to eliminate this problem, collection is conducted under constant supervision and close observation.

The NCAA does not require drug testing programs at its institutional membership schools. Many colleges and universities along with professional sport teams, however, have implemented drug testing programs. In addition, the NCAA does perform drug testing at NCAA championships events and randomly selected regional events. The NCAA also visits all NCAA Division I schools twice per year to randomly drug test selected football and track-and-field athletes. Athletic trainers working with athletes should be familiar with the NCAA, USOC, and IOC banned substance lists. It must be noted that many OTC products and nutritional supplements may have substances that are banned by the NCAA and/or USOC; athletes should always make sure the ingredients in these products are not banned before using them. Information concerning the NCAA drug testing program and the banned substance lists is available on the NCAA website (www.ncaa.org) and the USOC website (www.usoc.org).

> See *Drug Clearance Times*, found on the companion website at thePoint, for specific drugs and their approximate elimination time.

SUMMARY

1. Medications have chemical, generic, and brand names.

2. Pharmacokinetics is the process that explains a drug's entry into the body as well as its absorption, distribution, metabolization, and excretion.

3. The pharmacokinetic process determines the means by which a drug reaches a target site to either facilitate or inhibit an action.

4. The half-life of a drug, lipid solubility, therapeutic range, dosage, potency, and maximal efficacy all play a role in determining the drug's action and effect.

5. Common medications for the treatment of soft-tissue injuries include analgesics and antipyretics, NSAIDs, corticosteroids, muscle relaxants, topical antibiotics, antiseptics, and antifungal agents. Each of these drugs comes in both prescription and OTC forms.

6. Athletic trainers are not allowed to prescribe or dispense prescription medication.

7. Depending on state regulations, athletic trainers may be authorized by the team physician to administer a one-dose pack of an OTC medication when approved protocols warrant their use.

8. When providing OTC medications, a record log should be kept that indicates the individual's name, date, medication administered, reasons for administering the medication, and signature of the athletic trainer administering the medication.

9. Over-the-counter medications should be stored as directed on packaging labels and placed in a secure, locked cabinet.

10. Prescription medications should be kept in a secured and locked location under the direct supervision of a licensed physician or pharmacist.

11. Therapeutic medications, if not used as directed, can cause adverse reactions and, in some cases, toxicity and death.

12. Ergogenic aids are substances or devices that enhance energy production, energy use, or recovery to provide a competitive edge.

13. Current drug testing uses gas chromatography/mass spectrometry.

REFERENCES

1. Green GA, Uryasz FD, Petr TA, Bray CD. NCAA study of substance use and abuse habits of college student-athletes. Clin J Sports Med 2001;11(1):51–56.

2. Roach S. Pharmacology for Health Professionals. Philadelphia: Lippincott Williams & Wilkins, 2005.

3. Klossner D, ed. Dispensing prescription medication. In: 2005–2006 NCAA Sports Medicine Handbook. Overland Park, KS: National Collegiate Athletic Association, 2005.

4. Warner DC, Schnepf G, Barrett MS, et al. Prevalence, attitudes, and behaviors related to the use of nonsteroidal anti-inflammatory drugs (NSAIDs) in student athletes. J Adolesc Health 2002;30(3):150–153.

5. U.S. Olympic Committee. Drug Education Handbook. Colorado Springs, CO: U.S. Olympic Committee, 1996.

6. American Academic of Pediatrics. Policy statement: use of performance-enhancing substances. Pediatrics 2005;115(4):1103–1106.

7. Green GA, Puffer JC. Drugs and doping in athletes In: Mellion MB, Walsh WM, Madden C, Putukian M, Shelton GL, eds. The Team Physician's Handbook. Philadelphia: Hanley & Belfus, 2002.

8. Graham TE. Caffeine and exercise: metabolism, endurance, and performance. Sports Med 2001;31(1):785–807.

9. Bahrke MS, Yesalis CE. Performance Enhancing Substances in Sport and Exercise. Champaign, IL: Human Kinetics, 2002.

10. Ahrendt DM. Ergogenic aids: counseling the athlete. Am Fam Physician 2001;63(5):36–40.

11. Higdon JV, Frei B. Coffee and health: a review of recent human research. Crit Rev Food Sci Nutr 2006;46(2):101–123.

12. Nelson DE, Mowery P, Tomar S, et al. Trends in smokeless tobacco use among adults and adolescents in the United States. Am J Public Health 2006;96(5):897–905.

13. Cassisi NJ. Smokeless tobacco: is it worth the risk? NCAA Sports Science Education Newsletter 2000;Spring.

14. Johnson LD, O'Malley PM, Bachman JG, Schulenberg JE. Monitoring the Future National Survey Results on Adolescent Drug Use: Overview of Key Findings, 2003. Bethesda, MD: National Institute on Drug Abuse; 2004.

15. Chen YC, Lu EB, Peng GS, et al. Alcohol metabolism and cardiovascular response in an alcohol patient homozygous for the ALDH2*2 variant gene allele. Alcoholism. Clin Exp Res 1999;23(12):1853–1860.

16. Diamond I, Jay CA. Alcoholism and alcohol abuse. In: Goldman L, Bennett JC, eds. Cecil Textbook of Medicine. Philadelphia: WB Saunders, 2000.

17. Anish EJ. The senior athlete. In: Mellion MB, Walsh WM, Madden C, Putukian M, Shelton GL, eds. The Team Physician's Handbook. Philadelphia: Hanley & Belfus, 2002.

18. Dhar R, Stout W, Link MS, et al. Cardiovascular toxicities of performance-enhancing substances in sports. Mayo Clin Proc 2005;80(10):1307–1315.

19. Hartgens F, Kuipers H. Effects of androgenic-anabolic steroids in athletes. Sports Med 2004;34(8):513–554.

20. Pope HG, Kouri EM, Hudson JI. Effects of supraphysiologic doses of testosterone on mood and aggression in normal men. Arch Gen Psychiatry 2000;57(2):133–140.

21. Thiblin I, Petersson A. Pharmacoepidemiology of anabolic androgenic steroids: a review. Fundam Clin Pharmacol 2005;19(1):27–44.

22. Llewellyn W. Anabolics 2000. Aurora, CO: Williams Llewellyn, 2000.

23. Windisch PA, Papatheofanis FJ, Matuszewski KA. Recombinant human growth hormone for AIDS-associated wasting. Ann Pharmacother 1998;32(4):437–445.

24. Dekhuijzen PH, Machiels HA, Heunks LM, et al. Athletes and doping: effects of drugs on the respiratory system. Thorax 1999;54(11):1041–1046.

25. Mattay VS, Callicott JH. Effects of dextroamphetamine on cognitive performance and cortical activation. Neuroimage 2000;12(3):268–275.

26. Munson BL. About ephedrine use. Nursing 2003;33(4):81.

27. Jacobs I, Pasternak H, Dell DG. Effect of ephedrine, caffeine, and their combination on muscular endurance. Med Sci Sports Exerc 2003;35(6):987–994.

28. American College of Sports Medicine. Position stand on the use of blood doping as an ergogenic aid. Med Sci Sports Exerc 1996;28(6):i–viii.

29. Metzl JD, Small E, Levine SR, Gershel JC. Creatine use among young athletes. Pediatrics 2001;108(2):421–424.

30. Trojian T, Pengel B, Anderson JM. Sports supplements. In: Mellion MB, Walsh WM, Madden C, Putukian M, Shelton GL, eds. The Team Physician's Handbook. Philadelphia: Hanley & Belfus, 2002.

31. Greenwood M, Kreider RB, Melton C, et al. Creatine supplementation during college football training does not increase the incidence of cramping or injury. Mol Cell Biochem 2003;244(1–2):83–88.

32. Bemben MG, Bemben DA, Loftiss DD, Knehans AW. Creatine supplementation during resistance training in college football athletes. Med Sci Sports Exerc 2001;33(10):1667–1673.

33. Mayhew D, Mayhew JL, Ware JS. Effects of long-term creatine supplementation on liver and kidney functions in American college football players. Int J Sport Nutr Exerc Metab 2002;12(4):454–460.

34. Tjerung RL, Clarkson P, Eichner ER, et al. The physiological and health effects of oral creatine supplementation. Med Sci Sports Exerc 2000;32(3):706–717.

35. Ventura R, Segura J. Detection of diuretic agents in doping control. J Chromatogr B Biomed Appl 1996;687(1):127–144.

Dermatology

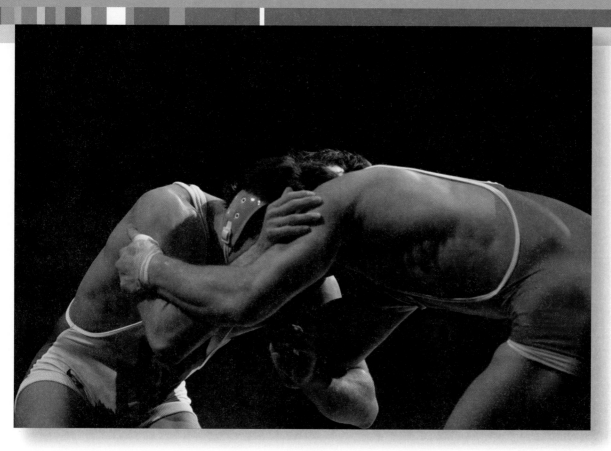

STUDENT OUTCOMES

1. Describe the common skin lesions.

2. List the signs and symptoms of an abscess, acne, onychia, paronychia, folliculitis, furuncles, carbuncles, cellulitis, and impetigo contagiosa.

3. List the signs and symptoms of tinea unguium, tinea pedis, tinea cruris, tinea corporis, tinea capitis, tinea versicolor, and candidiasis.

4. List the signs and symptoms of herpes gladiatorum, herpes zoster, verrucae, and molluscum contagiosum.

5. Describe the general management of bacterial, fungal, and viral skin infections.

6. Describe the common skin irritations caused by mechanical reactions, such as intertrigo, athlete's nodules, acne mechanica, and striae distensae, and explain the management of each condition.

7. List the signs and symptoms of sunburn, pernio, miliaria, eczema, psoriasis, and hyperhidrosis, and explain the management of each condition.

8. List the signs and symptoms of bites or stings from a mosquito, bee, wasp, ant, spider, flea, tick, and lice.

9. Explain the management of an insect bite or sting.

10. Differentiate between allergic contact dermatitis and irritant contact dermatitis, and explain the management of both conditions.

11. Describe the three types of urticaria, and explain the management of each.

ROLE DELINEATION COMPETENCIES

The following Performance Domains and Tasks defined in the National Athletic Trainers' Association Board of Certification *Role Delineation Study*, 5th Edition, are addressed in this chapter:

BOC COMPETENCIES

I.   Prevention

    A. Educate the appropriate individual(s) about risks associated with participation and specific activities using effective communication techniques to minimize the risk of injury and illness.

    B. Interpret preparticipation and other relevant screening information in accordance with accepted guidelines to minimize the risk of injury and illness.

    G. Monitor participants and environmental conditions by following accepted guidelines to promote safe participation.

II.   Clinical Evaluation and Diagnosis

    E. Formulate a clinical impression by interpreting the signs, symptoms, and predisposing factors of the injury, illness, or condition to determine the appropriate course of action.

    F. Educate the appropriate individual(s) regarding the assessment by communicating information about the current or potential injury, illness, or health-related condition to encourage compliance with recommended care.

    G. Share assessment findings with other health care professionals using effective means of communication to coordinate appropriate care.

III.   Immediate Care

    A. Employ life-saving techniques through the use of standard emergency procedures in order to reduce morbidity and the incidence of mortality.

    B. Prevent exacerbation of non–life threatening condition(s) through the use of standard procedures in order to reduce morbidity.

    C. Facilitate the timely transfer of care for conditions beyond the scope of practice of the athletic trainer by implementing appropriate referral strategies to stabilize and/or prevent exacerbation of the condition(s).

IV.   Treatment, Rehabilitation, and Reconditioning

    D. Administer treatment for general illness and/or conditions using standard techniques and procedures to facilitate recovery, function, and/or performance.

    E. Reassess the status of injuries, illnesses, and/or conditions using standard techniques and documentation strategies in order to determine appropriate treatment, rehabilitation, and/or reconditioning and to evaluate readiness to return to a desired level of activity.

    F. Educate the appropriate individual(s) in the treatment, rehabilitation, and reconditioning of injuries, illnesses, and/or conditions using applicable methods and materials to facilitate recovery, function, and/or performance.

    G. Provide guidance and/or counseling for the appropriate individual(s) in the treatment, rehabilitation, and reconditioning of injuries, illnesses, and/or conditions through communication to facilitate recovery, function, and/or performance.

Dermatology is the study of the skin. Any individual can occasionally contract skin conditions, but several are more commonly seen in the physically active population. Skin infections may be caused by bacteria, fungi, or viruses. Related inflammatory skin conditions may result from mechanical, environmental, allergic, or chemical skin reactions. Early identification of the ensuing lesions and specific treatment minimizes the healing time and prevents both the spread and the recurrence of the condition.

This chapter first provides an overview of the various types of skin lesions and then discusses the more common skin infections and conditions that are seen in the physically active population. When appropriate, individual management plans are provided. Many of these conditions can be seen in the color plates included with this chapter. It is important to note that many systemic diseases are manifested in skin lesions or rashes. Therefore, it is critical for the athletic trainer to identify potentially serious lesions and refer the individual immediately to a physician, particularly if any uncertainty exists regarding the nature of the skin lesion.

TYPES OF SKIN LESIONS

Q *A soccer player has a transient, elevated lesion caused by local edema. What type of skin lesion is suggested, and what are the potential causes of this type of lesion?*

The skin is the largest organ of the body. It serves four major functions:

1. The skin protects the body from bacteria, fungi, various viruses, and other germs in the outside environment.

2. The skin helps to regulate body temperature.

3. The skin prevents the loss of fluids and nutrients through the cutaneous surface.

4. The skin aids in the transmission of information from the outside environment to the brain.

The outer layer of skin, called the **epidermis**, contains the germinal layer, in which the production of new skin cells occurs and **sebum** is produced. The underlying **dermis** contains the sweat glands, hair follicles, sebaceous glands, blood vessels, and a complex array of nerve endings (see Fig. 6.6). The deepest layer, called the subcutaneous tissue, is composed primarily of fat (for insulation and energy storage).

The skin can be damaged by direct trauma, allergic reactions, chemical irritants, heat, cold, bacteria, fungi, and viruses. Whenever the skin is damaged, a lesion appears. These lesions are identified by their size and by their depth (Table 28.1).

A *The soccer player has a transient, elevated lesion caused by local edema. This indicates a possible wheal. The wheal could be a common allergic reaction to an insect bite, sunlight, or pressure.*

SKIN INFECTIONS

Q *A wrestler received treatment for an open sore on the right thigh. Three days later, observation reveals a honey-colored crust with surrounding erythema. Impetigo is suspected. What signs and symptoms would confirm this suspicion?*

Skin infections may stem from bacteria, fungi, or viruses. Bacterial or fungal infections can cause pustules on or within the skin or its associated structures, such as the sweat glands and the hair follicles. Although most infections tend to be painful, superficial irritations also can be extremely itchy. The three main bacteria are staphylococci, streptococci, and bacilli. Staphylococci commonly appear in clumps on the skin, in upper respiratory tract infections, and in lesions which contain pus. Streptococci are associated with serious systemic diseases, such as scarlet fever. Many bacilli are not pathologic, but some can lead to major systemic diseases, such as tetanus. Fungi, such as yeast and molds, often attack the skin, hair, and nails. Fungi fall into three basic categories: dermatophytes, candidiasis (moniliasis), and tinea versicolor. Viruses invade the living cells and may multiply until they kill the cell, burst out to reinfect other cells, or lie dormant within the cell without ever causing an infection.

Skin infections can preclude an individual from participating in physical activity. Participation should not be permitted if open wounds or infectious skin conditions cannot be adequately protected, thus preventing exposure to others. The National Collegiate Athletic Association (NCAA) has identified several skin infections that would lead to medical disqualification from practice or competition. These include bacterial infections (i.e., impetigo, erysipelas, carbuncles, staphylococcal disease, folliculitis, and hidradenitis suppurative), viral skin infections (i.e., herpes simples, herpes

TABLE 28.1 Basic Types of Skin Lesions

PRIMARY LESIONS (MAY ARISE FROM PREVIOUSLY NORMAL SKIN)

Circumscribed, flat, nonpalpable changes in skin color	Palpable, elevated, solid masses	Circumscribed, superficial elevations of the skin formed by free fluid in a cavity within the skin layers

Macule—Small, flat spot up to 1 cm (freckle, mole, rubella)

Patch—Flat spot; 1.0 cm or larger

Papule—Solid, elevated lesion less than 10 mm (wart, psoriasis)

Plaque—Elevated superficial lesion 1.0 cm or larger, often formed by coalescence of papules

Nodule—Marble-like lesion; larger than 0.05 cm; often deeper and firmer than a papule (lipoma, cysts, tumors)

Wheal—Transient, irregular superficial area of localized skin edema (mosquito bite, hive, sunlight, or pressure)

Vesicle—Up to 1.0 cm; filled with serous fluid (contact dermatitis, herpes simplex, herpes zoster)

Bulla—1.0 cm or larger; filled with serous fluid (second-degree burn)

Pustule—Elevated lesion containing pus (acne, furuncle [boil], carbuncle)

SECOND LESIONS (RESULT FROM CHANGES IN PRIMARY LESIONS)

Erosion—Loss of the superficial epidermis; surface is moist but does not bleed (moist area after the rupture of a vesicle, as in chickenpox)

Ulcer—Deeper loss of epidermis and dermis; may bleed and scar (stasis ulcer of venous insufficiency, syphilitic chancre)

Fissure—A linear crack in the skin (athlete's foot)

Crust—Dried residue of serum, pus, or blood (impetigo, scab)

Scales—A think flake of exfoliated epidermis (dandruff, psoriasis, tinea versicolor)

zoster [chickenpox], and molluscum contagiosum), fungal skin infections (i.e., tinea corporis), and parasitic skin infections (i.e., pediculosis and scabies) (1).

Bacterial Skin Conditions

Bacterial lesions typically are caused by a staphylococcal or streptococcal infection. Hot tubs or whirlpools that are not adequately chlorinated may harbor *Pseudomonas* sp.; most infections are self-limiting and need no treatment other than regulating pool chlorination. The more common bacterial infections in the physically active population are abscesses, acne vulgaris, onychia and paronychia, folliculitis, furuncles (boils) and carbuncles, hidradenitis suppurative, erysipelas, cellulitis, and impetigo contagiosa.

Abscess

An **abscess** is a circumscribed collection of pus appearing in an acute or chronic, localized infection. The abscess may be a cavity formed by liquefaction necrosis within solid tissue, and it may affect any tissue of the body, such as bone, tooth root, appendix, brain, gums, lungs, abdominal wall, gastrointestinal tract, ears, tonsils, sinuses, breasts, kidneys, and prostate gland.

SIGNS AND SYMPTOMS. An abscess usually is associated with tissue destruction, so the lesion appears as an encapsulated pocket of pus (Fig. 28.1). Pain, redness, swelling, and a fever typically are present.

MANAGEMENT. Applying ice packs or taking a hot bath may relieve the pain. Drinking plenty of clear fluids and bed rest may be helpful. If an abscess is associated with a fever, the individual should be seen immediately by a physician. Some abscesses may need to be treated surgically, but most only require antibiotics.

Acne

Nearly all adolescents experience acne at one time or another, but a few develop a more serious case. Although the etiology is unknown, acne is believed to be caused by excessive sebum production secondary to a hormonal imbalance, abnormal follicular keratinization that results in follicular blockage, proliferation of *Propionibacterium acnes*, and inflammation. At 8 or 9 years of age, the adrenal glands begin to produce increasing amounts of an androgen that causes the sebaceous glands to enlarge and produce more sebum. Sebum secretion peaks during adolescence and declines after the teenage years. Two types of lesions occur in acne: noninflammatory lesions, such as open or closed comedones, and inflammatory (popular, nodular, or cystic) lesions (2).

SIGNS AND SYMPTOMS. The obstructed follicle may become apparent as a blackhead (i.e., open follicle) or whitehead (i.e., closed follicle). The blackhead is not dirt, so scrubbing or washing will not remove it. Whiteheads represent follicles that have become dilated with cellular debris but possess only a microscopic opening to the skin surface. When the oil and other material in the whitehead break through the pore wall and cause irritation under the skin, a pimple results. Pimples can be erythematous papules, pustules, or nodules, and they commonly are seen on the face, neck, and back. Papules and pustules are small (diameter, <5 mm), whereas nodules are larger. The superficial pustules eventually dry, whereas the deeper nodules may become chronic and form disfiguring scars.

MANAGEMENT. No cure exists for acne, but the condition can be controlled with medication. Management usually is symptomatic, with routine cleansing of the inflamed area

FIGURE 28.1 Abscess. This walled-off lesion began as folliculitis that became a furuncle and then an abscess. Note the older scar from previous furuncles and cystic acne lesions.

once or twice a day using a mild soap. To prevent drying and redness, the skin should be allowed to dry for 20 to 30 minutes before applying any medication. Medications are divided into topical and systemic preparations. Topical therapies include benzoyl peroxide, antibiotics, retinoids, and salicylic acid. Common systemic preparations include oral antibiotics and hormonal therapy. The type of medication used is based on the type and number of lesions that are present, the severity of the disease, the extent of the acne, the patient's past experiences with medications, and the physician's personal preference. Most acne treatment is a long-term process, with 6 to 8 weeks needed before any therapeutic benefit is seen. Serious cases may necessitate referral to a dermatologist for treatment.

During the treatment phase, it is important not to pinch, pop, or pick at the acne, because this may cause the pimples to become larger, lengthen the time of appearance, or form a scar. Protective equipment (e.g., helmet or chin strap) and tight clothing may put added pressure on the skin, making acne worse. Cosmetics and moisturizers that contain oils also can aggravate the condition. Young women may notice premenstrual flare-ups. These often are caused by androgenic effects of progesterone, which is dominant during the second half of the menstrual cycle.

Onychia and Paronychia

Onychia is inflammation of the matrix of the nail plate, whereas **paronychia** involves only the lateral border or nail fold (Fig. 28.2). The conditions may develop from staphylococcal, streptococcal, or fungal organisms; with fungal organisms, the infection is called onychomycosis. The conditions also may occur secondary to diabetes, vaginal candidal infection, or occasionally, from endocrine problems, such as hypoparathyroidism, hypothyroidism, and adrenocortical deficiency (3).

SIGNS AND SYMPTOMS. If onychia is present, the nail fold becomes red, swollen, and painful and can produce purulent drainage. Paronychia often follows a hangnail and is seen in individuals whose hands frequently are immersed in water or mud (e.g., football linemen, chefs, and nurses). Occasionally, the feet may be affected if they are immersed frequently. Inflammation and swelling is centralized on the lateral border of the nail plate or nail fold. Small amounts of pus may be extruded from the nail fold, particularly with secondary infection.

MANAGEMENT. Warm-water soaks with a germicide may reduce the inflammation. The individual should keep the hands dry and avoid wearing rubber gloves or dressings that encourage seating. Cotton-lined gloves may be worn for short periods of time. In more severe cases, a physician may recommend systemic antibiotics (e.g., itraconazole, fluconazole, or terbinafine) and drainage of localized pus. Systemic medications may involve 6 weeks to several months of treatment (3). The area should be protected with a dry, sterile dressing. If left unchecked, onychia may lead to yellowing, **onycholysis,** and accumulation of subungual debris under the nail. This condition requires immediate physician referral for possible removal of the nail.

▰▰▰▰ FIGURE 28.2 **Nail conditions. A,** Onycholysis is a painless separation of the distal nail plate from the nail bed. **B,** Paronychia is an inflammation of the proximal and lateral nail folds and may be acute or chronic.

FIGURE 28.3 Folliculitis. A, Folliculitis commonly is called an "ingrown" hair, whereby the hair grows inward and curls up to form an infected nodule. **B,** Pustular rashes can occur where occlusive bathing suits are worn. **C,** Hot tub folliculitis can result from high water temperatures in the presence of staphylococcus.

Folliculitis

Folliculitis is an infection of the upper portion of the hair follicle and surrounding areas caused by staphylococci. Commonly referred to as an "ingrown" hair, the hair grows inward and curls up to form an infected nodule (Fig. 28.3). It tends to occur in areas with short, coarse hair (e.g., facial hair, nape of the neck, chest, back, buttocks, thighs, or skin under protective padding) and can develop from friction with pads or during shaving. Pustular rashes on the trunk have been reported where occlusive bathing suits are worn. Chemical irritants, inadequate chlorination, and superhydration of the skin caused by high water temperatures (i.e., hot tubs) also are causative factors (4).

SIGNS AND SYMPTOMS. The inflammation begins with a pustule forming at the mouth of the hair follicle; a crust forms and, eventually, sloughs off, along with the hair. This relatively painless pustule heals without scarring. If associated with staphylococci, swelling and erythema with or without a pustule may be present on the skin surface. These lesions are painful and may scar. "Hot tub" folliculitis, caused by *Pseudomonas aeruginosa*, may present with multiple pustular lesions on the trunk and extremities within 6 hours to 2 days after exposure (5). Mild fever and malaise also may occur.

MANAGEMENT. Treatment involves eliminating the friction-causing agent and applying mupirocin ointment. In more widespread infection, antistaphylococcal antibiotics (e.g., dicloxacillin and cephalexin) are required three times a day for 10 to 14 days. If the face is involved, shaving should be avoided for several days. For "hot tub" folliculitis, treatment is supportive, with antipruritics administered orally or topically, because the infection is self-limited over a period of 7 to 14 days (5). Acetic acid (5%) compresses applied for 20 minutes twice daily also can be used for symptomatic relief. If systemic manifestations are present (e.g., fever, chills, and lymphadenopathy), a course of oral ciprofloxacin therapy may be warranted (6). Prevention should focus on cleaning the whirlpool or hot tub and maintaining adequate chlorination and control of the pH level in the water.

Furuncles and Carbuncles

Furuncles (boils) and carbuncles are complications of folliculitis that result from friction or repeated blunt trauma. The infection progresses deeper and extends out from the follicle, and the lesions usually contain pus. Common sites include the buttocks, belt line, anterior thigh, back of the neck, face, and axilla.

SIGNS AND SYMPTOMS. Commonly called an abscess or boil, a furuncle is a large, well-defined, deep erythematous nodule that progresses into a pustule of walled-off, purulent material, turning hard and tender when staphylococci invade the subcutaneous tissue (Fig. 28.4).

FIGURE 28.4 Furuncle. This patient has a painful, "pointing" furuncular nodule on the thigh.

FIGURE 28.5 Hidradenitis suppurative. This chronic inflammatory, pus-producing disorder affects the follicles and apocrine sweat glands.

The furuncle develops into a fluctuant mass and, eventually, opens to the skin surface, allowing the purulent contents to drain, either spontaneously or following incision of the furuncle. A carbuncle is several furuncles that have merged.

MANAGEMENT. Treatment requires immediate referral to a physician for incision, drainage, and in severe cases, hospitalization. Warm compresses produce a point on the abscess to allow easier drainage and help reduce symptoms. During treatment, it is best to keep the individual isolated from others while the boil is draining. Antibiotics, although often prescribed, are not required (5). Picking, squeezing, or cutting a boil is not recommended. Physical activity is contraindicated until the infection no longer exists, because trauma can lead to cellulitis or thrombophlebitis.

Hidradenitis Suppurativa

Hidradenitis suppurativa is a potentially serious, chronic inflammatory, **suppurative** disorder affecting the follicles and apocrine sweat glands (Fig. 28.5). The condition is not present before puberty, because the sweat glands are not active. At any later age, however, it can appear. *Staphylococcus aureus* usually is involved in the condition, but in chronic cases, the *Proteus* sp. may be involved. Seen more commonly in women than in men, it develops primarily in the sweat glands located in the armpits, groin, around the breasts, and in the anal region. The condition also is seen at a higher rate in extremely overweight individuals and cigarette smokers (7).

SIGNS AND SYMPTOMS. Stage 1 hidradenitis suppurativa presents with solitary or multiple isolated, firm, red nodules without scarring or sinus tract. In stage 2, pustules and abscesses may discharge pus spontaneously and heal slowly, resulting in scar tissue. Stage 3 is characterized by extensive, multiregion involvement, with multiple interconnected sinus tracts and scarring. The appearance of nodules recurs periodically throughout the year. Heat, perspiration, and being overweight can aggravate the condition.

Pain is a common symptom in chronic conditions. Over time, extensive scarring can lead to restrictive, tight skin and vaginal, urethral, and anal strictures. If the sweat glands in the armpits or groin are involved, this can limit motion of the arms or legs. Secondary bacterial infection with staphylococci, streptococci, pseudomonas, and *Escherichia* sp. is common and produces a foul-smelling odor (7). Infection and inflammation can spread beyond the sweat glands into the deep layers of the skin and muscle tissue, leading to cellulitis. Individuals with hidradenitis suppurativa often feel socially isolated, suffering severe psychological impact because of this physically painful and disabling disease.

MANAGEMENT. Hidradenitis suppurativa is difficult to treat. Early intervention is preferred to prevent scarring, which ultimately will require surgical intervention. For mild to moderate cases, daily use of moist heat with antibacterial soaps or Burow's soaks are used along with topical medication, such as with benzoyl peroxide and a topical retinoid (7). In chronic cases, oral antibiotics are prescribed. In severe cases, surgical removal of scarred skin and underlying diseased tissues may be the only alternative.

Cellulitis

Cellulitis is a painful infection of the deep dermis caused by ?-hemolytic streptococci or *Staphylococcus aureus*.

SIGNS AND SYMPTOMS. The lesion appears as an ill-defined area of tender erythema on the trunk or extremities, usually around a break in the skin, such as surgical wounds, trauma, tinea infections, or ulcerations (Fig. 28.6). Intense pain may be present, as may malaise, fever, and **lymphangitis**. Sport participation is contraindicated, because trauma to the site can cause **bacteremia**. Periorbital cellulitis is of particular concern in children because of the potential meningeal seeding by *Haemophilus influenzae* following bacteremia. The prevalence of *H. influenzae* bacteremia in children, however, has decreased since the introduction of the *H. influenzae* type b vaccine in 1985.

MANAGEMENT. Mild cases of cellulitis are managed with oral antibiotics (e.g., penicillin and amoxicillin), warm tap-water compresses for 15 minutes three times a day, and bed rest with the involved area elevated to reduce edema, pain, and fever. Most cases of superficial cellulitis improve within 1 day; more substantial cases may take 5 to 10 days for recovery (8,9). Antibiotics should be taken for at least 3 days after the resolution of acute inflammation (4). In severe cases, immediate referral to a physician for hospitalization and intravenous antibiotics may be necessary.

FIGURE 28.6 Cellulitis. This painful infection of the deep dermis and subcutaneous tissue usually occurs around a break in the skin.

Erysipelas

Erysipelas is an acute, superficial, bacterial infection of the dermis and hypodermis that characteristically extends into the cutaneous lymphatics. It is considered to be a specific clinical type of cellulitis caused more frequently by streptococcal bacteria (9). The leg is the clinical site most frequently encountered; other common sites are the face, arm, and upper thigh.

Bacterial inoculation into an area of skin trauma is the initial event in developing erysipelas. A common portal of entry is athlete's foot. Other portals include superficial wounds, stasis ulcerations, inflammatory dermatoses, dermatophyte infections, insect bites, and surgical incisions. Other predisposing factors include diabetes, alcohol abuse, infection with the human immunodeficiency virus (HIV), nephrotic syndrome, other immunocompromising conditions, and vagrant lifestyle.

Cases of erysipelas have been reported in all age groups, but it appears that infants, young children, and elderly patients are the most commonly affected groups. The peak incidence has been reported to occur between 60 and 80 years of age, especially in patients who are considered to be high risk and immunocompromised or in those with lymphatic drainage problems (e.g., after mastectomy, pelvic surgery, and bypass grafting) (9).

SIGNS AND SYMPTOMS. Erysipelas is characterized by sudden onset. Individuals often cannot recall an inciting event but may have a history of recent trauma or pharyngitis. Prodromal symptoms, such as malaise, chills, and high fever, often begin before onset of the skin lesions and usually are present within 48 hours of cutaneous involvement. Initially, a small erythematous patch progresses to a fiery-red, indurated, tense, and shiny plaque. Pruritus, burning, and tenderness are typical complaints. A well-demarcated plaque may extend by 2 to 10 cm each day. The infection rapidly invades and spreads through the lymphatic vessels, producing overlying skin "streaking" and regional lymph node swelling and tenderness. Systemic symptoms may include drowsiness or disorientation, tachypnea, tachycardia, hypotension, and oliguria.

MANAGEMENT. As with cellulitis, elevation and rest of the affected limb are recommended to reduce local swelling, inflammation, and pain. Saline wet dressings should be applied to ulcerated and necrotic lesions and changed every 2 to 12 hours, depending on the severity of the infection. Antibacterial medication (e.g., penicillin and erythromycin), administered either orally or intravenously, should produce rapid improvement. Within 24 to 72 hours, fever and pain should decrease as well as skin signs (i.e., borders decrease in size and thickness) (9). When the individual is mobile, it is advisable to wear an elastic stocking for as long as 1 month in previously healthy patients and for the long term in patients with preexisting lower extremity cellulitis. Hospitalization for close monitoring and intravenous antibiotics is recommended in severe cases and in infants, elderly patients, and patients who are immunocompromised.

FIGURE 28.7 Impetigo. This highly contagious skin condition often is seen in wrestlers, swimmers, and gymnasts.

Individuals with recurrent erysipelas should be educated regarding local antisepsis and general wound care. Predisposing lower extremity skin lesions (e.g., tinea pedis or stasis ulcers) should be treated aggressively. Long-term prophylactic antibiotic therapy generally is accepted, but no true guidelines are available.

Impetigo Contagiosa

Impetigo is a highly contagious, bacterial inflammation of the skin most often seen in those who participate in wrestling, football, rugby, swimming, and gymnastics (Fig. 28.7). Caused by *Staphylococcus aureus* either alone or in combination with β-hemolytic streptococci (GABHS), the condition can be transmitted by direct contact or through sharing unclean towels, clothing, and equipment or after a minor skin injury, such as an insect bite, abrasion, or dermatitis (10).

SIGNS AND SYMPTOMS. Impetigo has two different presentations—namely, bullous and nonbullous (5). The bullous type, which is linked to *S. aureus*, begins as multiple, fluid-filled vesicles that either combine or individually enlarge and form blister-like lesions that eventually collapse centrally. The center has the characteristic honey-crusted lesion that when removed, reveals reddened plaques draining serous fluid. Nonbullous impetigo, which is caused by GABHS, begins as small vesicles or pustules with erythematous bases and honey-colored crusts, which also drain fluid. The lesions may itch or burn, but generally are painless. Eventually, the crust disappears, leaving a red mark that heals without scarring. Common sites are the face, buttocks, extremities, or perineum.

Ecthyma, a more serious form of impetigo, occurs when the infection penetrates deep into the skin's second layer (i.e., the dermis). Signs and symptoms include painful, fluid- or pus-filled sores that turn into deep ulcers, usually on the legs and feet. A hard, thick, gray-yellow crust covers the sores. Lymph glands may be swollen in the affected area. Scars may remain after the ulcers heal. Several conditions can be complicated by impetigo, including:

- Abrasions
- Atopic dermatitis:
  - Individuals with a history of asthma, hay fever, or eczema
  - Frequent crusts on the face, popliteal region, or antecubital fossae
  - Contact dermatitis (especially from shoe materials and rubberized pads)
  - Irritant dermatitis (hands chapped from frequent immersion in or handling of irritating substances)

MANAGEMENT. Localized impetigo can be treated with topical mupirocin ointment applied to the skin three times a day for 10 days (10). Gentle cleansing with soap and water helps to remove the crusts and allow full penetration of the topical antibiotic. Treatment for diffuse or multiple areas of impetigo consists of systemic antibiotics rather than topical therapy. It should be emphasized that the entire course of antibiotics be taken—even if the lesions seem to have resolved. With prompt treatment, impetigo usually clears within 7 to 10 days after the initiation of antibiotics (4). Individuals with impetigo should not participate in physical activity until the crusts have dried to a thick, coagulated crust. The NCAA wrestling guidelines require any patient who has impetigo to take oral antibiotics for at least 72 hours and be free from any new skin lesions for 48 hours before being cleared to participate (1).

General Management of Bacterial Infections

Most infectious bacterial skin conditions (e.g., folliculitis, acne, cellulitis, furuncles, and carbuncles) should be cleansed with soap, water, and **astringents** and are treated initially with over-the-counter

FIELD STRATEGY 28.1

Management of Bacterial Skin Conditions

Noninfectious Bacterial Skin Conditions

- Wash the region 4 to 5 times daily and after physical exertion.
- Rinse all soap residues from the region, and completely dry the area by patting gently.
- When dry, apply over-the-counter topical antibacterial agents two to three times daily.
- If the condition is more severe, refer to a physician. Incision, drainage, or débridement may be necessary. Systemic antibiotics may be prescribed for 7 to 10 days.

Suspected Impetigo

- Isolate the infected individual from other players, as well as from athletic clothing and towels, to prevent the spread of the disease.
- Localized impetigo can be treated with mupirocin ointment applied to the skin three times a day.
- With diffuse or multiple areas of impetigo, refer to a physician. Systemic antibiotics may be indicated for 5 to 7 days.
- Gentle cleansing with soap and water helps to remove the crusts.

Participation Guidelines

- Satellite lesions, cellulitis, purulent conjunctivitis, large or multiple honey-crusted lesions, and weeping lesions warrants withholding the athlete from competition.
- With impetigo, no participation until the crusts have dried to a thick, coagulated crust.
- Individuals with cellulitis, furuncles, or carbuncles should not participate in sports because of possible systemic complications, such as bacteremia and progressive soft-tissue infections.

(OTC) topical antibacterial agents that are applied several times per day. A physician referral may be necessary for incision, drainage, and in some instances, débridement. If the condition is more severe, systemic antibiotics may need to be prescribed.

Individuals should be withheld from physical activity and competition if satellite lesions, cellulitis, purulent conjunctivitis, weeping lesions, or large or multiple, honey-crusted lesions are present. Individuals who have cellulitis, furuncles, or carbuncles are not significantly contagious to others but should not participate in sports, because continued trauma to the involved areas can lead to systemic complications, such as bacteremia and progressive soft-tissue infections. Field Strategy 28.1 summarizes the general treatment of bacterial infections.

Fungal Skin Conditions

Fungal skin infections are quite common among physically active individuals. Fungus grows and thrives in dark, warm, moist environments, such as the areas between the toes or between the skin of the groin and scrotum. During activity, perspiration often accumulates in these areas. Augmented with the wearing of constrictive clothing, such as an athletic supporter, tight shorts, or spandex, the perspiration often enhances and encourages fungal growth. In addition, tight garments often cause chafing and irritation.

Fungal infections are identified by small patches of erythema, scaling, and severe itching. Dermatophytes, also known as ringworm (tinea) fungi, and yeasts cause most fungal infections, including tinea unguium (nails), tinea pedis (feet), tinea cruris (groin), tinea corporis (body), tinea capitis (scalp), candidiasis, and tinea versicolor (Fig. 28.8). All but tinea versicolor are contagious and spread from person to person by sharing towels or socks and by walking with no shoes in the locker rooms and shower stalls. Fungal infections can be prevented by taking several precautionary measures (Box 28.1).

FIGURE 28.8 Fungal infections. A, Tinea cruris. **B,** Tinea corporis.

Tinea Unguium

Tinea unguium (nail), or onychomycosis, as it is more properly known, is a fungal infection of the nail beds and nails. It is common among physically active individuals, particularly those who swim in pools, use communal showers, or have chronic tinea pedis and wear occlusive footwear (11). The fungus invades the hyponychium at the most distal attachment of the nail plate or a lateral nail fold. It migrates to the undersurface of the nail plate, leading to a nail bed infection that causes discoloration of the nail plate. The most common form, distal subungual onychomycosis usually is associated with athlete's foot (tinea pedis).

The fingernails are more commonly affected by the fungus *Candida albicans,* which leads to *Candida* onychomycosis. Although the fungus can cause primary nail infection in people with chronic mucocutaneous candidiasis or other immunologic disorders, it usually occurs as a secondary infection in otherwise healthy nails.

SIGNS AND SYMPTOMS. Infections usually start distally, with yellow streaks in the nail plate that gradually extend to include the entire nail. The nails become thickened, with a marked subungual hyperkeratosis that can be painful and can separate the nail plate from the bed. Over time, the nail plate becomes brittle and crumbles. Clinically, *Candida* onychomycosis may be similar in appearance to distal subungual onychomycosis, except that the entire thickness of the nail plate is affected and appears yellow, green, or opaque. The individual usually will complain of pain with activity and have some aesthetic concerns (11).

MANAGEMENT. Treatment varies depending on the type of infection, severity of the nail changes, and personal preference of the supervising physician and patient. For a single-nail-plate infection, a new

Box 28.1   Prevention of Fungal Infections

- Shower after every practice and competition.
- After each shower, thoroughly dry the feet, groin, and areas between the toes as well as under the arms and breasts.
- Apply absorbent antifungal powder to the shoes, socks, feet, between the toes, under the arms and breast, and in the groin area.
- Change socks and underwear daily; allow wet shoes to dry thoroughly before wearing them.
- Wear street shoes that allow some ventilation to the feet.
- Clean and disinfect the floors in the shower room, dressing room, and athletic training room daily.
- Never go barefoot in a shower or locker room.

topical nail lacquer is indicated but requires daily topical application for 6 to 12 months. The nail is cleaned weekly with alcohol, and then, periodically, any unattached infected nail is removed. Potential side effects are localized erythema and mild application-site reactions (11).

Distal subungual onychomycosis may be treated with topical creams only during its early, mild stage. The affected portion of the nail is trimmed away as much as possible, and then a topical antifungal agent is applied several times daily. Newer treatments include itraconazole (200 mg daily for 3–4 months), terbinafine (250 mg daily for 2–4 months), and fluconazole (150 mg once weekly for 10–18 months). Potential side effects of the medications may include liver toxicity and gastrointestinal disturbances (11).

Candida onychomycosis responds well to oral ketoconazole, although it has a greater potential for toxicity. If topical or systemic drug therapy does not resolve the condition, surgical nail avulsion is performed.

Tinea Pedis

Tinea pedis (i.e., athlete's foot) is the most frequent fungal infection in the physically active population. It can spread in the locker room during casual handling of contaminated socks, or it can be picked up by another player on the floor or shower stall. Infection is based on individual susceptibility, however, and may not affect certain people. Although 1 to 3% of the population are carriers of tinea pedis, prepubertal children rarely are affected.

SIGNS AND SYMPTOMS. Tinea pedis is divided into three types. The most common type is found in the intertriginous web spaces as a scaly, peeling eruption with or without erythema, maceration, or fissuring. When the toe webs are **macerated** and infected, *Candida* yeast usually is present in addition to the original dermatophyte. It is common for the eruptions to extend to the plantar or dorsal surface of the toe. The second type includes an eruption of vesicles and bullae on the midfoot. Dry, vesicular lesions may exude a yellowish serum. Scratching the area leads to scaling, peeling, and cracking fissures in the skin, particularly if the condition extends between the toes, and can spread the problem to other parts of the body. The third type produces a hyperkeratotic scale with minimal erythema on the plantar surface. All three types are recognized by extreme **pruritus**, redness, and scaling on the sole of the feet and between the toes.

Tinea Cruris

Tinea cruris (i.e., jock itch) involves the genitalia but often originates in the feet; therefore, the feet should always be examined when this condition is present (12). Although typically seen in obese adult men and male athletes, women are reporting an increase in the incidence of the condition because of the increased use of panty hose, spandex, and other tight, restricting clothing. It rarely is seen in children. *Trichophyton rubrum* is the most common source of tinea cruris.

SIGNS AND SYMPTOMS. Perspiration can accumulate between the genitals and skin of the thigh. The crural or perineal folds between the scrotum and inner thighs usually are the first areas to exhibit small patches of erythema and scaling. Other signs and symptoms include diffuse, thick, dark lesions; weeping vesicles or pustules on the margins of inflammation; and severe itching. The infection can spread to the thighs, perineal area, buttocks, and abdomen. When scrotal redness or scaling occurs, it typically is the result either of an allergic reaction to skin medications used before seeing a physician or of chronic skin inflammation caused by scratching or long-term irritation. It is important to note that an individual with tinea cruris can infect bedding, towels, and clothing; these should be changed daily and thoroughly washed in hot water.

Tinea Corporis

Tinea corporis (i.e., tinea of the body) is caused by dermatophytes, usually of the genus *Trichophyton*. It affects both humans and animals.

SIGNS AND SYMPTOMS. The condition is characterized by one or more circular, pruritic patches that are slightly erythematous, dry, scaly, and usually, hypopigmented (13). The lesions may be slightly elevated at the border, where they are more inflamed and scaly compared with the central part of the lesion.

A well-defined, central ring generally is found on the upper extremities, axillae, and trunk. Certain individuals can carry the spores without the rash; the degree of rash depends on the host's cellular-based immune response, which can vary widely. Tinea corporis is common in prepubertal children, because they often contract the condition from infected pets. Wrestlers are at a high risk for outbreaks because of improper or inadequate cleansing of the mats and uniforms, skin-to-skin contact, occlusive equipment, and macerated skin (14). Among wrestlers, the condition is referred to as tinea gladiatorum.

Tinea Capitis

Tinea capitis, or ringworm of the scalp, is very common in children. Primary sources of the infection are contaminated hair brushes, combs, and animals.

SIGNS AND SYMPTOMS. The condition begins as a small papule on the scalp and then spreads peripherally. The lesions appear as small, gray scales, resulting in scattered bald patches.

Tinea Versicolor

Tinea versicolor, also know as pityriasis versicolor, is one of the most common pigmentary disorders worldwide. It stems from a yeast, known as *Malassezia furfur*, that is a normal part of the skin flora. Excessive heat, humidity, and oily skin promote the growth of this organism in the stratum corneum. It is seen more often on the trunk, primarily the back, and on the upper extremities rather than on the lower extremities. It is commonly seen during adolescence and young adulthood when sebaceous activity is high.

SIGNS AND SYMPTOMS. Referred to as "sun spots," tinea versicolor is best noticed after exposure to the sun. Although the rest of the skin tans, the area with tinea versicolor does not. The individual usually will have many irregularly shaped, slightly scaling macules and patches, generally covering large areas of the body and separated by normal skin. The macules are yellowish-brown, pale yellow, or dark-brown, and occasionally reddish or pinkish, appearing to be either hypopigmented or hyperpigmented (15). In dark-skinned individuals, the infection appears as well-defined, white patches. The area may be asymptomatic or mildly pruritic. Scratching detaches sheets of epidermis, leaving patches of raw base. The patches develop and resolve without treatment. Unlike other fungal infections, it is not contagious.

MANAGEMENT. Treatment involves topical selenium sulfide once daily for 7 days and then on the first and third day of the month for 6 months. It should be left on for 5 to 10 minutes and then washed off (15). Other topical azoles (e.g., clotrimazole, bifonazole, and ketoconazole) for 3 days to 2 weeks also are suitable (11). A daily bifonazole shampoo treatment for 3 weeks is the preferred method for use in children (15). Systemic medication also can be used to treat tinea versicolor. Ketoconazole, itraconazole, and fluconazole are effective. Tinea versicolor often recurs; therefore, periodic treatment is recommended.

Candidiasis

Candidiasis, which is caused by the yeast fungus *Candida albicans*, can produce infections on the skin or mucous membranes or in the vagina. Skin infections tend to be found in skinfolds, such as the axillae, groin, and below the breasts, when friction occurs within a hot, moist, humid environment. The condition is more common in women who wear a swimsuit or a competition uniform for long periods of time.

SIGNS AND SYMPTOMS. The lesion appears as a deep, beefy-red color and is bordered with small, red, satellite pustules. In skinfolds, a white, macerated border may surround the red area. Later, deep and painful fissures may develop where the skin creases. If left untreated, the infection can lead to a life-threatening systemic disease.

MANAGEMENT. The condition can be prevented by showering immediately after exercise, wearing clean briefs made of absorbent fabric, and using absorbent powder in the groin and axillae before workouts. A candidal infection of the mucous membranes of the mouth is called thrush and is treated with oral nystatin. This infection is seen in immunocompromised hosts and in those using inhaled corticosteroids for asthma. The U.S. Food and Drug Administration (FDA) recently approved

FIELD STRATEGY 28.2

Management of Fungal Skin Conditions

- Wash the involved region four to five times daily and after physical exertion.
- Rinse all soap residue from the region, and completely dry the area. With dry tinea infections, apply antifungal powder liberally before an exercise period.
- Apply topical antifungal agents, such as Halotex, Lotrimin, Mycelex, and Tinactin, twice daily for 1 month.
- If the condition does not clear up, see a physician to rule out candidiasis, dermatitis, psoriasis, or other skin disorders.
- In resistant infections, prescribed allylamines, such as terbinafine, butenafine, or naftifine, may be used twice daily for 2 to 4 weeks.
- Follow proper personal hygiene as listed in Box 28.1.

Eraxis (i.e., antifungin) to treat certain infections caused by *Candida* sp. Administered intravenously, Eraxis is intended to be used to treat infections in the esophagus (i.e., candidiasis), bloodstream (i.e., candidemia), and other areas, including abdominal abscesses and inflammation of the lining of the abdominal cavity (16).

General Management of Fungal Skin Infections

Treatment of fungal skin infections involves antifungal medication and changing the warm, moist environment. The two main classes of antifungals are allylamines and azoles. Use of either an allylamine or azole antifungal treatment depends on patient compliance and cost; allylamines are more costly but allow shorter treatment periods. Dry infections of athlete's foot, jock itch, and tinea capitis respond well to OTC topical azoles, such as clotrimazole (e.g., Lotrimin and Mycelex), one of the oldest antifungal treatments. Others include miconazole (e.g., Mictrin and Monistat) or tolnaftate (e.g., Tinactin). These typically are applied twice daily for at least 1 month. Moderate cases are best treated with allylamines, such as terbinafine, butenafine, or naftifine, twice daily for 2 to 4 weeks (11,12). Oral therapy with terbinafine (250 mg once daily for 10 days) or itraconazole (100 mg twice daily for 10 days) has been very successful in treating tinea conditions (11). For individuals who continue the type of activity that can lead to the infection, topical treatment should continue for 2 weeks after signs of the infection are gone. During treatment, the area should be kept clean and dry. Loose, absorbent clothing (e.g., cotton socks and underwear) should be worn, and shower and locker rooms should be kept clean.

Individuals with widespread fungal infections (e.g., tinea corporis or tinea capitis) should be treated with griseofulvin, but this agent is not always effective. Resistant cases may respond better to systemic ketoconazole, fluconazole, and itraconazole; however, long-term use of these drugs, especially ketoconazole, may cause liver toxicity. The general management of fungal skin conditions can be seen in Field Strategy 28.2.

Viral Skin Conditions

Skin lesions caused by viruses, such as herpes simplex, herpes gladiatorum, herpes zoster (i.e., shingles), verrucae (i.e., warts), and molluscum contagiosum, can be difficult to treat, because they often require long-term therapy and activity restrictions. Routine hygienic measures, such as showering immediately after activity and keeping individuals with open lesions on exposed skin from participating in contact sports, may reduce or eliminate transmission of these pathogens.

Herpes Simplex

Herpes simplex virus (HSV) actually encompasses more than 80 different viruses and is extremely contagious. The two most common types are HSV-1 and HSV-2. Herpes simplex virus type 1 (i.e., cold sores) normally infects the area of the lips, nose, and chin, and it orally reoccurs, on average,

FIGURE 28.9 Herpes simplex. Lesions are evident on the vermillion border of the lip and beyond.

one to three times per year (Fig. 28.9). It has been known to be transmitted by direct skin-to-skin contact during participation in sports such as wrestling, in which it is called herpes gladiatorum (17). It also causes approximately one-third of new cases of genital herpes and is transmitted most often through oral sex. Herpes simplex virus type 2 causes two-thirds of all new genital herpes cases and 95% of recurrences of genital herpes, and it is the most sexually transmitted disease in the United States (18). Herpes simplex virus type 1 recurs genitally approximately once every other year, whereas on average, HSV-2 recurs genitally approximately five times per year.

SIGNS AND SYMPTOMS. The incubation period for primary infection (2–8 days) usually begins with a burning and stinging pain, tenderness, or itching at the infected site, followed by clusters of vesicles on an erythematous base. The lesions are capable of latency as they migrate to the dorsal ganglions in the spinal cord. There may be no other symptoms, or there may be fever, localized lymphadenopathy, malaise, **myalgia**, dysuria, pharyngitis, or rarely, keratoconjunctivitis. Preexisting abrasions or other underlying skin conditions will increase the likelihood of transmission.

It is critical to identify the condition at an early stage and immediately refer the individual to a physician for care. During the latent state, the individual has no blisters, sores, or other symptoms. During the shedding stage, the virus begins to multiply in the nerves and can enter into body fluids, such as saliva, semen, or vaginal fluids. No symptoms are present at this stage, but the virus can be easily spread during this time.

A tendency exists to recur regularly—even monthly—at the site of the primary lesion. Several factors can trigger recurrences, particularly of the HSV-1 strain. These include sunlight exposure (especially on the lips), stress, fatigue, food allergies, other infections (e.g., cold or influenza), impaired immune system, hormonal changes caused by a woman's menstrual cycle, or pregnancy.

MANAGEMENT. Herpes lesions will dry up and heal without treatment. The virus, however, cannot be eradicated from the body. Treatment with oral antiviral medications, such as acyclovir (e.g., Zovirax), famciclovir (e.g., Famvir), and valacyclovir (e.g., Valtrex), should begin promptly. Options include acyclovir (i.e., 200 mg five times a day for 10 days, or 400 mg two times daily for 7–10 days), famciclovir (i.e., 250 mg for 7–10 days), or valacyclovir hydrochloride (i.e., 1 g for 7–10 days). Once the vesicles are fully formed and ulcerating, the medication is no longer effective. If ulceration has occurred, topical benzoyl peroxide and gentle use of a hair dryer may dry the crusts more rapidly and minimize secondary bacterial infection. Recurrent episodes can be treated with lower doses for 5 days. Prevention includes avoiding contact with vesicles. Vesicular lesions must be dried scabs before patients return to contact sports. The dried scabs may be covered for additional protection.

Herpes Zoster

Herpes zoster, or shingles, as it is more commonly known, is rare. Local trauma that occurs during contact sports occasionally can precipitate reactivation of the varicella virus, which, after a case of chickenpox, can retreat into the nerve roots, where it lies dormant. Participation should be prohibited, both for pain relief and to lessen transmission to others who have never had chickenpox.

SIGNS AND SYMPTOMS. Herpes zoster is characterized by unilateral, blister-like lesions that erupt along dermatomes, usually T_3 to L_3 in the trunk or, less commonly, in the area of the fifth cranial nerve (19). Migrating along the dermatomes, the condition initially causes pain, burning, tingling, or itching, followed by eruptions of fluid-filled vesicles in strips on one side of the body 1 to 3 days later (Fig. 28.10). Other signs and symptoms include headache, malaise, swollen lymph nodes near the site of the eruption, and a low-grade fever. A few days after the vesicles form, they burst and crust over. Fluids from the lesions contain live viruses, so the patient remains infectious until the lesions crust over. The rash and blisters also can occur around the eye, on the face or scalp, inside the mouth, or down an arm or leg. Although the rash and blisters may resemble chickenpox, shingles typically is limited to a small area on one side of the body.

MANAGEMENT. If the condition is identified early (i.e., within 3 days of developing the rash), shingles can be treated effectively with oral antiviral drugs, such as acyclovir (e.g., Zovirax), valacyclovir (e.g., Valtrex), and famciclovir (e.g., Famvir). Antiviral drugs must be taken early, however, or they are not effective. If the condition is not recognized and treated early, the physician likely will advise the individual to let shingles run its course. Although painful, a case of shingles usually heals entirely within a month with or without treatment. Because infection with HIV can precipitate herpes zoster in a young person, an HIV test is appropriate.

FIGURE 28.10 Herpes zoster. These grouped vesicles of various sizes are on an erythematous base.

Verrucae Virus

More than 60 types of the human papilloma virus can lead to a rapid growth of cells on the outer layer of skin, resulting in a wart, of which verrucae plana (i.e., flat wart) and verrucae plantaris (i.e., plantar wart) are only two of the more common ones. Incubation is several weeks to 5 years after exposure.

SIGNS AND SYMPTOMS. The common wart is prevalent on the hands and appears as a small, round, elevated lesion with a rough, dry surface (Fig. 28.11). They do not retain the normal fingerprint lines on the hands and feet that corns and calluses do (20). Pressure on the wart increases the pain. Because of its location, the common wart often is subjected to secondary bacterial infection. A plantar wart, which grows into the thick stratum corneum of the foot, has tiny, dark red or black dots, representing thrombosed capillaries that have been penetrated by the root of the wart. Verrucae plantaris likely is transmitted from swimming pool decks or shower rooms.

MANAGEMENT. Recurrences are frequent, and no single method of treatment is effective for all lesions. Options include mechanical, chemical, or immunologic methods. Within 6 months, most young people develop an immunologic reaction to the virus, and the wart may disappear with or without treatment. For others, any treatment will be ineffective. During the competitive season, a doughnut pad can be worn to alleviate some of the pressure to the area. After the season, under the direction of a physician or podiatrist, treatment may involve injections of interferon-alfa or bleomycin into the wart to kill the virus, cryosurgery (liquid nitrogen), electrocautery, excision, or laser treatment.

FIGURE 28.11 Verrucae virus. A, Verruca vulgaris produces dry, rough warts on the hands. **B,** Verruca plantaris leads to plantar warts.

FIGURE 28.12 Molluscum contagiosum. This highly contagious pox virus produces characteristic dome-shaped, shiny, waxy papules with a central white core.

Immunologic methods used to induce an immune response to suppress warts include injected agents (e.g., *Candida* or mumps antigen), topical agents (e.g., imiquimod), or oral agents (e.g., 30–40 mg/kg per day of cimetidine) (20).

Molluscum Contagiosum

A pox virus, molluscum contagiosum, is commonly reported by swimmers, wrestlers, gymnasts, and younger children who have immature immune systems. The virus is spread by personal contact and by contaminated swimming pools and gymnastic equipment.

SIGNS AND SYMPTOMS. Lesions, which are multiple, pearly papules 3 to 5 cm in diameter, appear flesh-colored to yellow and have a tiny, round spot on the surface (Fig. 28.12). They commonly are found on the trunk, axilla, face, thighs, and genital areas. The condition is primarily a cosmetic problem; however, blunt trauma can rupture a papule, causing a disabling local inflammatory reaction that can mimic cellulitis. It is moderately contagious and is spread by skin-to-skin contact and autoinoculation. The lesions usually resolves in 6 to 12 months.

MANAGEMENT. Treatment involves immediate referral to a physician who may employ a destructive mechanical modality (e.g., curettage, electrotherapy, or cryotherapy with liquid nitrogen), chemical treatments (e.g., physician applied trichloroacetic acid), or immunologic methods (e.g., topically applied immune enhancer that stimulates cytokine [i.e., 5% imiquimod cream]) (20). Full activity can be resumed 2 to 4 days after resolution of the lesions.

A *The open sore that presented on the right thigh of the wrestler 3 days earlier has a honey-colored crust with surrounding erythema. The signs and symptoms that would indicate impetigo include itching or burning, but the area is not usually painful. The sore ruptures quickly, oozing either fluid or pus that forms a honey-colored crust, and eventually, the crust disappears, leaving a red mark that heals without scarring. Common sites for impetigo are the face, most often around the nose and mouth, body folds, and areas subject to friction and occlusion (e.g., thighs and axillae).*

OTHER SKIN REACTIONS

Q *During a summer field-hockey camp for high school girls, one of the players comes off the field and reports being stung by a bee. This is the first time the individual has ever been stung. What signs and symptoms would suggest an allergic reaction to the venom?*

Unlike skin infections caused by bacteria, fungi, and viruses, other skin problems caused by mechanical, environmental, allergic, or chemical reactions are not infectious and generally are mild in nature. Once identified, they can be treated easily with topical medications.

Chafing of the Skin

Chafing of the skin, or **intertrigo,** is a superficial dermatitis more often caused by the friction of fabric rubbing against moist, warm skin rather than by skin rubbing against skin. The condition may occur between the creases of the neck, in the axillary and buttocks area, or beneath large breasts but is seen primarily in the groin region of individuals with muscular thighs or in obese individuals.

Signs and Symptoms

The condition is characterized by erythema, maceration, burning, and itching (Fig. 28.13). In severe cases, the skin becomes eroded and weeping. The condition can be prevented by wearing loose, soft, cotton underwear to keep the skin dry, clean, and free of friction or by wearing shorts with longer legs made of low-friction fabric.

Management

Treatment involves initial application of a cold compress. The area should be cleansed daily with mild soap and water, followed by application of a soothing ointment. Talcum powders should be avoided, because they can be abrasive and do not effectively absorb moisture.

Athlete's Nodules

Also referred to as surfer's nodules, athlete's nodules are asymptomatic, dermal nodules found at various sites of the body that encounter repeated minor trauma, such as the feet of surfers and runners, knees of canoeists, and knuckles of boxers. Protective pads at the trauma sites can help to decrease pain. Otherwise, high-potency topical or intralesional corticosteroids can be applied. If this does not provide relief, the nodules can be incised.

Acne Mechanica

Characterized by a local exacerbation of acne vulgaris caused by heat, occlusion, pressure, and friction, **acne mechanica** presents with erythematous crops of papules and pustules in areas of mechanical trauma.

Signs and Symptoms

Sometimes referred to as football acne, the acne develops wherever skin is exposed to prolonged causative factors, such as under chin straps, forehead bands, shirt collars, football shoulder pads, backpack straps, automobile seats, bras, wide belts, and orthopaedic casts and braces. Like regular acne, the signs are whiteheads, blackheads, and pimples in the affected area (Fig. 28.14). If left unattended, the acne may develop into a cyst—a thick lump beneath the surface of the skin formed by the buildup of secretions deep within hair follicles.

Management

Treatment and prevention includes thoroughly cleansing the area after activity with a mildly abrasive cleanser and back brush. Application of a topical astringent or 10% benzoyl peroxide agent, topical antibiotic, and in severe cases, a systemic antibiotic may be prescribed. The condition usually improves or resolves after the season. Prevention involves wearing a clean, absorbent t-shirt under the football pads and treating any underlying acne vulgaris. If an exercise leotard is worn during exercise, it should be removed immediately after the workout.

Striae Distensae

Stretch marks, or **striae distensae**, often is seen in individuals who participate in high-intensity weight training. Even though the origin is unclear, it most often is seen after rapid growth of a body part, which is believed to result in fragmented elastic skin fibers.

Signs and Symptoms

The condition is characterized by linear pink or flesh-colored patches most often seen on the chest, shoulders, and upper outer arms (Fig. 28.15).

■■■ **FIGURE 28.13 Intertrigo.** Intertrigo, or chafing of the skin, is a superficial dermatitis more often caused by the friction of fabric rubbing against moist, warm skin rather than by skin rubbing on skin. This condition often is confused with tinea cruris and cutaneous candidiasis.

■■■ **FIGURE 28.14 Acne mechanica.** This young male developed acne-like lesions that appeared under his football chin strap. The bacterial culture was positive for *Staphylococcus aureus*.

FIGURE 28.15 Striae. Striae occurs after rapid growth of a body part, such as during high-intensity weight training or during pregnancy. The initial purplish color will fade over time, but the striae are permanent.

Management

No treatment exists for striae distensae.

Sunburn

Sunburn is an inflammatory response of the skin to excessive exposure to the ultraviolet radiation in the sun's rays. Repeated overexposure can lead to an increased risk of premature aging, cutaneous melanoma, and cancer (21). Sunscreens applied to the skin prior to sun exposure can prevent many of the damaging effects of ultraviolet radiation. The effectiveness of the sunscreen is based on the sun protection factor (SPF). For example, an SPF of 15 indicates that an individual can be exposed to ultraviolet light 15-fold longer than without a sunscreen before the skin will begin to burn. Higher numbers provide better protection: SPF 15 is good, SPF 30 is better, and SPF 50 provides a complete sun block. A minimum SPF of 15 is recommended. Sunscreen should be applied liberally over all exposed areas a few minutes before exposure to the sun and reapplied every 2 hours while exposed, after swimming, and if sweating. Acute sunburn (i.e., actinic dermatitis) can be painful and disfiguring and, depending on the severity, can prevent participation in sport and physical activities. The degree of sunburn depends on the length of exposure to the sun, the sun's relative level of intensity, and personal skin type.

Signs and Symptoms

Sunburns are classified as first, second, or third degree. The full extent of the injury may not be assessed until 24 to 48 hours after exposure. First-degree sunburns have mild erythema throughout the area of exposure and may have associated pain and discomfort (Fig. 28.16). Second-degree burns have vesicles or blisters in addition to the erythema. Peeling of the skin usually begins after 2 to 3 days, and the skin is dry and itchy. Third-degree burns will exhibit skin ulcerations. Systemic symptoms of burns, regardless of their degree, include fever, chills, nausea, and exhaustion. Although sunburns are easily treated, it is best to prevent them from occurring (Box 28.2).

FIGURE 28.16 Sunburn. A, First-degree sunburn. **B,** Second-degree sunburn with substantial blisters.

Box 28.2 Prevention of Sunburn

- Use a sunscreen with an appropriate sun protection factor (SPF) for your skin type (preferably one with an SPF of 15 or higher).
- Apply sunscreen 20 to 30 minutes before exposure to the sun.
- Apply sunscreen evenly over all exposed skin to avoid isolated areas of sunburn.
- Reapply sunscreen every 2 to 4 hours, especially if sweating profusely.
- Select sunscreen that has a high rate of efficacy when subjected to moisture.
- Be careful when applying the sunscreen around the eyes.
- Sunscreen sprays work well for the top of the head; lip protectors also should be used.
- Avoid midday exposure to the sun (10:00 AM to 3:00 PM).
- While in the sun, wear loose, woven, light, cotton clothing.
- Hats with brims are much better than caps or visors.
- Sunburn can occur on cloudy days, so sunscreen should be worn at all times.
- Be aware of the reflective photo-energy potential when around water or snow.
- Several medications (e.g., antibiotics, antiseptics, anesthetics, and certain nonsteroidal anti-inflammatory drugs) increase sensitivity to the sun. Read the instructions for use of any medications before sun exposure. If there are questions, consult a pharmacist or physician.
- Drink plenty of nonalcoholic beverages to prevent dehydration.

Management

If sunburn occurs, apply a cold compress, topical hydrocortisone 1% cream or spray, and aloe vera to decrease pain and discomfort. If systemic aspirin or nonsteroidal anti-inflammatory drugs (NSAIDs) are used, they must be taken immediately after exposure to the sun to be effective. Serious second- and third-degree burns require immediate referral to a physician to ensure proper treatment and prevention of infection. Oral corticosteroids may be prescribed to relieve the pain.

Pernio (Chilblains)

Excessive exposure to cold can lead to **pernio**, in which the tissue does not freeze but, rather, reacts with erythema, itching, and burning. This happens especially on the dorsa of the fingers and toes and on the heels, nose, and ears. More commonly seen in young women, the condition often occurs with the first exposure to lower temperatures in highly humid conditions.

Signs and Symptoms

The affected area appears reddish, and it itches and burns (Fig. 28.17). Lesions may be single or multiple and, in severe cases, may appear blistered or ulcerated.

Management

Treatment involves gradual warming of the body part. Topical steroids help to reduce the inflammation, but the potency must be low enough to prevent further vasoconstriction. Heavy woolen socks may need to be worn at all times, including when indoors and while sleeping.

Miliaria Rubra

Miliaria, or "prickly heat," is caused when active sweat glands become blocked by organic debris, leading to an inflamed and

FIGURE 28.17 Chilblains. Excessive exposure to cold can lead to pernio, in which the tissue does not freeze but, rather, appears reddish, itches, and burns.

pruritic skin eruption. It was discussed in detail in Chapter 24. Treatment involves cooling and drying the skin, controlling the itching, and watching for infection. Individuals should avoid occlusive topical ointments and close-fitting, poorly absorbent fabrics on the skin.

Dry (Xerotic) Skin

Dry skin commonly is seen during the winter months. Individuals who must shower frequently are particularly prone to this condition. Xerotic skin can be caused by a number of factors, but decreased skin lipids appear to be the major cause (Box 28.3). In the winter, dry and cold winds increase evaporation from convection, and low temperatures decrease skin flexibility and, in doing so, exacerbate the condition.

Signs and Symptoms

The skin appears dry, with variable erythema and scaling. Usually appearing first on the shins, it also is common on the forearms and dorsum of the hands. For individuals who exercise outdoors in the winter, the face also can be affected. Localized or generalized pruritus is the most common symptom. When severe, the dry skin loses its suppleness, and cracks, fissures, and erythema appear.

Management

Treatment is focused on preventing excessive water loss and replacing water that has already been lost. Tepid, rather than hot, water should be used for bathing, and time spent in the shower should be limited. Moisturizing soaps should be used; however, xerotic areas should be avoided. If possible, use of soap should be limited to the genitalia, underarms, hands, feet, and face. Bubble baths and brisk scrubbing should be avoided. Emollient lotions containing high concentrations of lipids increase and maintain hydration by occluding the skin surface and help to insulate against the cold. They should be applied frequently and liberally, especially after each hand washing and immediately after bathing to minimize water loss from evaporation. Swimmers should moisturize the whole body after bathing. In severe cases, antipruritics may be used to decrease pruritus and scratching, thus enabling the outer skin layer to heal. α-Hydroxy acids and topical corticosteroids can be used to decrease the inflammation associated with fissures and severely dry skin.

Eczema

Eczema is a generic term for acute or chronic inflammatory conditions of the skin. The condition can have an onset during the first 2 years of life, and a history of asthma or hay fever may be reported (22). Eczema can take a physical as well as an emotional toll.

Signs and Symptoms

The condition is characterized by poorly marginated erythema with scaling and exudate (Fig. 28.18). Persistent itching and burning can lead to evidence of **excoriation**. The condition is aggravated by

---

Box 28.3   Causes of Dry (Xerotic) Skin

- Genetic predisposition to dry skin
- Decreased skin lipids because of:
  - Age
  - Chronic illness
  - Malnutrition
- Use of industrial or domestic cleansers or solvents
- Frequent bathing
- Repetitive trauma from scratching already dry skin
- Environmental factors, such as:
  - Decreased humidity
  - Winter weather (dry, cold winds)
  - Indoor heating and air conditioning
  - Dry environments (airplanes)

an increase in body heat and perspiration, both of which occur during physical activity. Patients may report that the itching and scratching disrupt their sleep.

Management

Treatment involves topical corticosteroids in an emollient cream or ointment base to serve as a substitute for soap, bath oils, and moisturizers. These are active ingredients intended to support the dermal layer and reduce itching. The steroid should be applied to the affected area after bathing. Consistent use of the steroid cream is essential for it be effective. Use of very potent steroids applications should not exceed 3 weeks; use of moderate to mild steroid application should not exceed 3 months at a time without reexamination of the affected region (22). Antihistamines may provide relief from the itching, but during acute flares, systemic corticosteroids most often are used.

Psoriasis

Psoriasis is a chronic, distressing skin disorder that can affect the skin, tendons, ligaments, and joints. It is characterized by a rapid buildup of rough, dry, dead skin cells, forming thick scales. Normally, it takes approximately a month for new skin cells to move from the lowest layer of skin, where they first form, to the outermost layer, where they die and scale off in flakes. In psoriasis, however, the life cycle of skin cells speeds up, resulting in a multitude of dead cells on the outermost layer of skin. The scales tend to flare periodically and may go into remission, but they usually remain active for years.

It is estimated that more than 6.4 million Americans have the condition (23). Prevalence is equal in men and women, but more than twice as many whites as blacks or Asians have the disease. Psoriasis can occur at any age, but the onset usually is gradual, with the diagnosis commonly established between 15 and 35 years of age.

Factors that may trigger psoriasis include a systemic infection (e.g., strep throat), an immune system response to disease, injury to the skin, certain medications (e.g., lithium, β-blockers, antimalarial drugs, NSAIDs, and oral steroid withdrawal), alcohol, and environmental factors, such as overexposure to sun or prolonged contact with chemicals (e.g., disinfectants and paint thinners) (24). The most common form of psoriasis, plaque psoriasis, occurs in more than 80% of affected individuals. Guttate psoriasis occurs in approximately 10% of patients, and erythrodermic and pustular psoriasis each occur in fewer than 3% of patients (23).

Signs and Symptoms

Plaque psoriasis is characterized by sharply demarcated, dry, red patches of skin covered with silvery scales that typically affect the elbows, knees, scalp, and intergluteal cleft (Fig. 28.19). Scales from scalp patches of psoriasis may resemble dandruff. In some cases, there may be pitting, ridging, and discoloration of fingernails and toenails. Guttate psoriasis often arises after streptococcal infection and is characterized by the sudden development of numerous erythematous scaling papules on the trunk and extremities. Erythrodermic psoriasis is characterized by generalized inflamed erythema and widespread scaling that may affect the entire body. Individuals lose many of the protective functions of skin, including its ability to protect against infection, regulate body temperature, and prevent loss of fluids and nutrients through the cutaneous surface (23). Generalized pustular psoriasis is characterized by sterile pustules that may cover large portions of the trunk and

FIGURE 28.18 Eczema. This inflammatory condition of the skin is characterized by poorly marginated erythema with scaling and exudate. In this patient, the vesicles are beginning to dry, and the lesions are becoming scaly.

FIGURE 28.19 Psoriasis. This chronic skin condition is characterized by a rapid buildup of rough, dry, dead skin cells forming thick scales.

extremities. As with erythrodermic psoriasis, individuals with pustular psoriasis lose the skin's protective functions.

Management

Psoriasis is difficult to control because of the wide variation in type, severity, and response to treatment. It is a chronic disease without a cure. Three broad categories of treatment options exist, including topical modalities, phototherapy, and systemic therapy. Topical therapies are effective for mild-to-moderate cases, whereas phototherapy and systemic medications are more appropriate for more severe cases. Topical treatments include topical steroids, tar, anthralin, vitamin D derivatives, retinoids (e.g., tazarotene), immunosuppressants (e.g., tacrolimus and pimecrolimus), and salicylic acid. Newer topical treatments (e.g., Elidel cream and Protopic) have been especially effective in treating children with the disorder (25). Phototherapy with broadband ultraviolet B light, narrowband ultraviolet B light, psoralen with ultraviolet A light, and oral acitretin, methotrexate, and cyclosporin also are highly effective. Exposure to moderate sunlight as well as the topical application of coal tar combined with ultraviolet radiation are effective treatments. Physicians sometimes use phototherapy and oral medications in rotation to minimize side effects of both. In 2003, the U.S. FDA approved the immune-suppressing drug alefacept (e.g., Amevive) for the treatment of psoriasis. The drug appears to work through the lymphocytes to slow the proliferation of skin cells. Alefacept is a treatment option for more severe cases of psoriasis or for those cases that do not respond to other treatments. The drug is given by intravenous infusion, usually once per week for 12 weeks, although a second cycle of treatments may be necessary (23).

Hyperhidrosis

Hyperhidrosis is a condition involving excessive perspiration, particularly on the palms and axillary region. The condition can interfere with sports that require holding various objects (e.g., balls, discus, bars, oars, and sticks) or that require gripping (e.g., tennis and racquetball). The plantar sweat glands often are stimulated when the extremities are used and during times of emotional excitement, which also stimulates the axillary apocrine glands.

A number of factors can affect how much an individual sweats and even how the sweat smells. Some people sweat more than others for no apparent reason; however, other factors can cause intense sweating. These may include heredity, certain foods (i.e., spicy foods, hot beverages, and beverages containing caffeine or alcohol), and certain drugs (i.e., some antipsychotic medications, morphine, excess doses of the thyroid hormone thyroxine, and overdoses of analgesics [e.g., aspirin and acetaminophen]). Women going through menopause may experience hot flashes (i.e., a rise in skin temperature accompanied by sweating and a feeling of intense heat) because of a drop in estrogen levels. Some menopausal women also may be awakened at night by soaking sweats followed by chills.

Signs and Symptoms

Patients describe excessive perspiration triggered by emotion that began in childhood or adolescence. It is most likely to occur on the face, underarms, palms, and soles of the feet. Palmar hyperhidrosis usually is accompanied by plantar hyperhidrosis, which is easier to conceal, but may cause **bromhidrosis**, infection, and skin maceration. Excessive palm perspiration can make it difficult to grasp common objects and, if one avoids handshakes or chooses not to touch other individuals, lead to professional embarrassment.

Management

For some individuals, OTC antiperspirants used on the underarms, hands, and feet may limit the production of perspiration. Antiperspirants block the sweat ducts with aluminum salts, thereby reducing the amount of perspiration that reaches the skin. Deodorants, which can eliminate odor but not perspiration, turn the skin acidic, which makes it less attractive to bacteria. Antiperspirants can cause irritation or even contact dermatitis. For more severe cases, an individual may apply, as prescribed, 20% aluminum chloride hexahydrate with anhydrous ethyl alcohol. The solution must be applied to dry skin, typically before sleep, and washed off 6 to 8 hours later (26). Physically active individuals may wish to wear gloves to help absorb the sweat, or they may choose not to participate in activities that require a prolonged hand grip.

If OTC products are not strong enough, a physician may prescribe antiperspirant. For more severe sweating problems, other recommended treatments may include iontophoresis, botulinum toxin (e.g., Botox) injections to block the nerves that trigger the sweat glands, or surgery to remove troublesome sweat glands.

Bites and Stings

Bites and stings come from a variety of insects, including mosquitoes, flies, spiders, ants, bees, fleas, and ticks. Although many are just annoying pests that can be discouraged with standard insect repellent, their bites and stings can be painful or even life-threatening if the individual develops an allergic reaction to the venom (i.e., anaphylaxis).

Anaphylaxis

Anaphylaxis is an immediate, shock-like, and frequently fatal hypersensitivity reaction that occurs within minutes of administration of an allergen unless appropriate first-aid measures are taken immediately. The condition is characterized by contraction of smooth muscle and dilation of capillaries because of the release of pharmacologically active substances (e.g., histamine, bradykinin, and serotonin).

SIGNS AND SYMPTOMS. Signs and symptoms of anaphylactic shock include respiratory distress, cyanosis, weakness, rapid and weak pulse, low blood pressure, localized urticaria or edema, paresthesia, dilated pupils, choking, wheezing, sudden collapse, involuntary loss of bowel and bladder control, headache, dizziness, seizures, and unconsciousness.

MANAGEMENT. An individual with a history of such reactions may wear a medical identification tag and have a self-administered epinephrine device (EpiPen®). An EpiPen Auto-Injector is an epinephrine-delivery system with a spring-activated needle. It is used to treat severe allergic reactions to insect bites or stings, foods, drugs, and other allergens. It also may be used as treatment for basic life support of individuals suffering from a severe asthma attack.

EpiPen comes in two strengths—namely, EpiPen Jr. for children up to 33 pounds and EpiPen Adult. It is best used when injected directly into the skin, preferably the thigh, but it can be injected through clothing if necessary. Once in the system, epinephrine constricts blood vessels to improve blood circulation and blood pressure and relaxes smooth muscles to improve breathing. Epinephrine also stimulates the heartbeat and reverses swelling and hives. The effects of epinephrine take place within seconds and can last for 10 to 20 minutes. EpiPen should not be stored in extreme heat or direct sunlight, be refrigerated, or be used if the liquid is cloudy or discolored or the expiration date has expired. Field Strategy 28.3 describes the proper use of a self-administered epinephrine device.

FIELD STRATEGY 28.3

Use of an EpiPen Auto-Injector

1. Check the expiration date to make sure the pen is usable.
2. Check the fluid for cloudiness or discoloration (discard if cloudy or discolored).
3. Remove the gray safety cap.
4. Hold the EpiPen firmly with the black tip against the skin of the thigh.
5. Push the pen into the thigh, and apply moderate pressure for 10 seconds to inject the fluid.
6. Discard the used pen using universal precautions.
7. Call emergency medical assistance to provide further care for the injured party.

Mosquitoes, Gnats, and Flies

Mosquitoes, gnats, and a variety of flies feed on human blood and are considered to be biting insects.

SIGNS AND SYMPTOMS. Most bites appear as erythematous, macular or papular, pruritic, painful lesions. The lesion may not be apparent immediately but, rather, may appear as a delayed hypersensitive response to the saliva of the biting organism.

MANAGEMENT. Immediate application of a cold compress can relieve pain, or an OTC topical corticosteroid or systemic antihistamine may be used. Systemic corticosteroids are used in severe cases. Once a lesion has appeared, it should be monitored closely for secondary infection.

Bees, Wasps, and Ants

It is estimated that more than 20% of the U.S. population is allergic to the hymenopteran venom from bees, wasps, and ants, which in turn carries a higher risk of allergic and anaphylactic reactions. Individuals involved in outdoor activities are at special risk for insect stings. Yellow jackets and honeybees, for example, are fond of sweets and can be drawn to rehydration stations stocked with sugar-containing sport drinks. Fire ants, especially in the southern United States, can be found on practice and game fields where individuals may sit on the ground.

SIGNS AND SYMPTOMS. The sting results in a painful wheal or hive caused by the venom. The site rapidly becomes pruritic, and itching can last for several hours. Occasionally, an exaggerated local reaction can occur in which the swelling and itching extend beyond the sting site to the involved extremity and may be associated with dyspnea, tachycardia, hypotension, and anaphylaxis.

MANAGEMENT. This situation may result in a medical emergency. When a sting occurs, the guidelines in Field Strategy 28.4 should be followed.

Spiders

The venom from several spiders also can lead to painful lesions (Fig. 28.20). Black widow spiders are found throughout the United States; however, only the female—a dark-black, globular-shaped spider with the characteristic ventral, reddish marking (typically an "hourglass") on her abdomen—is large enough to bite through human skin. Because the webs typically are built in relatively undisturbed, protected areas, most sport-related bites occur in storage areas for equipment (27). The bite often is felt as a "pinprick" and may be slightly red. Significant symptoms usually start 1 hour after the bite, with the most common symptom being spasmodic muscle pain. The spasms may progress to regional muscle groups of the trunk, with pain and spasm lasting from 12 to 48 hours.

■■■■ FIGURE 28.20 **Spider bites. A,** This spider bite resulted in a large, fluid-filled bullous. **B,** Necrotizing skin damage resulted from a brown recluse spider bite.

FIELD STRATEGY 28.4

Management Algorithm for a Bee Sting

Prevention Note

For sensitive athletes who participate outdoors, suggest that they:

1. Refrain from wearing bright, colorful, or floral clothing.
2. Refrain from using scented soaps, lotions, or aftershaves.

After Sustaining a Bee Sting

1. Immediately refrain from strenuous exercise.
2. Remove the stinger with a fingernail. Do not squeeze it, because this will inject more venom
3. Apply ice to the site.
4. Systemic antihistamines may help with local reactions.
5. Observe closely for signs of anaphylactic shock:

   - Faintness, deteriorating consciousness, or other signs of shock
   - Generalized urticaria or edema
   - Paresthesia
   - Choking or signs of laryngeal edema
   - Pupillary dilation
   - Wheezing, coughing, or difficulty breathing

If Anaphylaxis Occurs

Activate the emergency plan, including summoning emergency medical services

EMS

1. Place the individual supine with the feet elevated.
2. Apply a constricting band a few inches proximal to the sting site that:

   - Occludes superficial venous and lymphatic return.
   - Does not obstruct arterial flow.

3. Continue ice application to further reduce venom absorption.
4. Check for a medical identification tag.
5. If the person has an EpiPen or other allergy kit, inject the epinephrine into the thigh as instructed.
6. If respiratory or cardiac arrest occurs, begin cardiopulmonary resuscitation.

Other reactions may include an increased respiratory rate, tachycardia, hypertension, fever, headache, nausea, vomiting, restlessness, and anxiety.

The brown recluse spider is found predominantly in the southern and midwestern United States. They are not aggressive and tend to avoid humans, but they will bite if threatened or injured (28). Bites from a brown recluse spider cause the most severe form of arthropod-induced tissue necrosis, yet these bites are relatively painless at first and may go undetected. In the ensuing hours, the site becomes pruritic, red, and mildly swollen. Local pain, resulting from vasospasm and ischemia, begins within 2 to 8 hours. After 12 to 18 hours, a small, central vesicle develops, surrounded by an irregular border of erythema, ecchymosis, and edema. If the blister ruptures, the erythema darkens and may spread distally. After 5 to 7 days of progressive aseptic necrosis, the bite area becomes depressed and covered with a black crust that eventually sloughs off, leaving an open ulcer that tends to heal over a period of several weeks. Healing is slow, requiring 2 to 4 months (28).

The bark scorpion, which is native to Arizona and adjacent regions, is a nocturnal spider that tends to hide in dark areas during the day. The small tooth at the base of its stinger distinguishes the bark scorpion from other, less toxic species. Individuals involved with outdoor activities are most at risk. For instance, rock climbers often put their hands into blind spots on overhead ledges. Campers and hikers need to be cautious about turning over stones and logs. They also should inspect footwear before slipping their feet into the shoes, because scorpions may hide in the shoes during the night. Individuals who are stung by a scorpion feel immediate, intense pain that significantly worsens with light pressure over the site. The pain may radiate throughout the extremity. Systemic reactions include restlessness, hypersalivation, dysphagia, visual changes, roving eye movements, respiratory distress (with stridor or wheezing), hypertension, fever, loss of bowel or bladder control, muscle spasms, and paralysis.

MANAGEMENT. The majority of spider bites and stings occurring in healthy young adults can be managed on-site. Management includes cleaning the site with soap and water, application of ice, elevation of the affected limb to approximately heart level, and administration of aspirin or Tylenol as needed for minor discomfort. Application of ice or cold packs to bite sites has been shown to significantly reduce inflammation and slow the evolution of the lesion (28). Prophylactic antibiotics usually are given to prevent secondary infection. Antihistamines are administered mainly to relieve pruritus and swelling. Children who have been stung or any individual who is experiencing severe symptoms, such as respiratory distress, should be transported immediately to the nearest medical facility for evaluation and management.

Fleas and Ticks

Bites from fleas cause only minor discomfort. Most fleas bite in patterns of three and tend to attack the ankle and foot. Scratching the area could complicate the condition by developing a secondary infection. Treatment is limited to applying an antipruritic lotion over the area.

Ticks are parasites that attach their heads onto people or animals and then absorb blood. They are frequent carriers of Rocky Mountain spotted fever and **Lyme disease**. Rocky Mountain spotted fever usually begins 5 to 7 days after inoculation. Common symptoms include generalized malaise, myalgia (especially in the back and legs), fever, frontal headaches, nausea, and vomiting. Other symptoms may include nonproductive cough, sore throat, pleuritic chest pain, and abdominal pain (29). Initially, lesions appear on the palms, soles, wrists, ankles, and forearms and are pink and macular but fade with applied pressure. The rash then extends to the axilla, buttocks, trunk, neck, and face. The lesions may form large areas of ecchymosis and ulceration. Respiratory and circulatory failure, although rare, as well as neurologic compromise may occur (29). Treatment involves the use of antimicrobial agents, such as tetracycline, doxycycline, and chloramphenicol, for a minimum of 7 days.

Deer ticks carry Lyme disease, but the tick needs to stay attached for 24 to 36 hours to transmit the disease-causing bacteria (30). The disease occurs in three stages. Stage 1 occurs 7 to 10 days after a tick bite and is characterized by a bull's-eye rash appearing 3 days to 1 month after infection. It is a round ring with central clearing that may expand to a diameter of up to 50 cm (Fig. 28.21). Common sites are the thigh, groin, trunk, and armpits. Other symptoms may include low-grade fever, fatigue, headache, arthralgia, cough, and regional lymphadenopathy.

Stage 2 occurs a few weeks after the initial infection. Symptoms include multiple secondary cutaneous annular lesions, fever, cough, pharyngitis, adenopathy, and central nervous system symptoms. For dark-complexioned individuals, the rash looks like a bruise. If a rash is present, it is wise to take a picture of it, because some physicians require evidence of the rash before prescribing medication.

Stage 3 symptoms include chronic arthritis, central nervous system impairment, dermatitis, and keratitis (29). Not all rashes occurring at the site of a tick bite are indicators of Lyme disease. An allergic reaction to tick saliva often occurs at the bite site. The resulting rash usually occurs within hours to a few days after the tick bite, usually does not expand, and disappears within a few days.

■■■■ FIGURE 28.21 **Lyme disease.** The characteristic bull's-eye rash appears 3 days to 1 month after infection and presents itself as multiple annular lesions of erythema with central clearing.

MANAGEMENT. The tick should be removed by applying a substance that blocks the tick's access to the air (e.g., petroleum jelly, mineral oil, or fingernail polish). The substance should make the tick withdraw their head. No attempt should be made to pull the tick from the body, because doing so may leave the head embedded under the skin. If signs and symptoms of Rocky Mountain spotted fever or Lyme disease appear, the individual should be referred immediately to a physician for treatment. Routine antibiotic prophylaxis is not indicated; however, if symptoms develop, antibiotic treatment for 14 to 21 days is curative in most cases (29).

Scabies

Scabies is a skin disease caused by a tiny, eight-legged burrowing mite, *Sarcoptes scabiei*, that produces severe, intensely itching lesions in the area of its burrows. The condition can lead to a "miniepidemic" in sports that involve physical contact, such as

FIGURE 28.22 Scabies. Scabies is caused by a burrowing mite, which produces severe, intensely itching lesions in the area of its burrows.

wrestling, rugby, or football. The mite can be spread on towels, uniforms, or equipment. Once on the skin surface, the mite burrows into the epidermis, but symptoms may not arise until 3 to 4 weeks after exposure (11). Because of the contagious nature, physicians often recommend treatment for entire families, sexual partners, athletic teams, groups, or school classes to eradicate the mite.

SIGNS AND SYMPTOMS. Signs and symptoms include intense itching, which often is severe and usually is worse at night. The affected area appears as small, dark burrows and tiny vesicles in a linear distribution between the fingers and in toe web spaces, in axillary skinfolds, around the waist, or on the elbows, wrist, ankles, lateral foot, breasts, buttocks, periumbilical skin, and genitalia (Fig. 28.22). In first-time infections, pruritus may not develop for several weeks, whereas recurring infections may lead to symptoms within 24 hours (14).

MANAGEMENT. Immediate referral to a physician is essential. Treatment involves eliminating the scabies infestation with medications. Topical creams and lotions, such as permethrin (e.g., Acticin) and lindane (e.g., Kwell), can be applied over the body and left on for 8 to 12 hours before being washed off. Lindane is not recommended for infants, small children, women who are pregnant or nursing, or people who have seizures or other neurologic disorders. The locker room and game equipment should be disinfected. Bedding and clothing must be washed daily in hot water. Although these medications kill the mites, the itching may not subside for several weeks. According to the 2005 NCAA guidelines, wrestlers must have a negative scabies test at meet or tournament time to return to play (1).

Lice (Pediculosis)

Pediculus corporis (i.e., body lice), pediculus capitis (i.e., head lice), and pediculus pubis (i.e., genital lice) affect 6 to 12 million people each year and are spread by close physical contact, which makes outbreaks among those who participate in physical activities and sports problematic (11).

SIGNS AND SYMPTOMS. Once infected, it can take up to 10 days for the nit (louse egg) to hatch. Based on the location of the infestation, patients may describe nighttime itching and, through subsequent scratching, pustules and excoriation. Head lice cause itching when they bite the skin of the scalp and neck. Egg sacks, or nits, can adhere firmly to the hair shafts and be seen behind the ears, on the back of the neck, and on the head. Body lice (length, 2–4 mm) are clearly visible, live in the folds of clothing, and tend to bite in areas of close contact with clothing. Pubic lice (e.g., crab lice [length, 1–2 mm]) typically are seen in the genitals, anal region, and lower abdomen but also can be found on the chest or axillary hair (Fig. 28.23).

FIGURE 28.23 Lice. Pubic lice is a small, brown, living crab louse that can be seen here at the base of the pubic hairs (arrow).

MANAGEMENT. Treatment of head and pubic lice involves a 7-day regimen of permethrin lotion (either 1% or 5%), lindane 1% shampoo, petrolatum for eyelashes, and/or shampoo containing pyrethrin and piperonyl butoxide. Nit combs are available to help remove nits from hair, and all clothing, bed linens, and sporting equipment should washed in boiling water and dried in a hot dryer or discarded.

Contact Dermatitis

Contact dermatitis is classified as either allergic or irritant dermatitis (Fig. 28.24). **Allergic contact dermatitis** results when a substance comes in direct contact with the skin leading to a simple inflammatory reaction. In contrast, **irritant contact dermatitis** results when the substance causes direct skin damage, pain, or ulceration. Contact dermatitis affects only the area in direct contact with the causative agent, leading to a sharp line of demarcation between normal skin and affected skin. For example, reacting to a watch band or swimming goggles leads to characteristic patterns of erythema and irritation.

Allergic Contact Dermatitis

Allergic dermatitis accounts for 20 to 30% of all contact dermatitis. Common agents that contribute to the condition include adhesive tape, rubber articles (e.g., straps, pads, swim goggles, swim fins, swim caps, and shoes), tape adherent and remover, soap, detergent, and deodorant. Allergic dermatitis remains localized to the affected area and is identified by dry vesicles that are accompanied by pain, erythema, and pruritic conditions. Heat, whether internal or external (e.g., hot bath), intensifies symptoms and accelerates the skin's reaction.

Irritant Contact Dermatitis

Irritant dermatitis also presents with erythema, pruritus, pain, and swelling. It often occurs secondary to physical and mechanical agents, such as burns from dry ice, abrasions from artificial turf, friction burns caused by poorly fitted equipment, **striae**, or increased sweating between skinfolds (e.g., groin or under breast tissue), as well as during skin loss secondary to an application of a causative agent (e.g., adhesive tape). Diagnosis of either type of contact dermatitis relies on the history and distribution of the rash.

Management of Contact Dermatitis

During acute reactions, a cold compress should be applied to the affected area. Systemic antihistamines are used to reduce itching and inflammation along with topical agents (e.g., corticosteroids)

FIGURE 28.24 Contact dermatitis. A, Allergic contact dermatitis results when a substance comes in direct contact with the skin leading to a simple inflammatory reaction. **B,** Irritant contact dermatitis results when the substance causes direct skin damage, pain, or ulceration, such as with tight shoes or prolonged used of latex gloves.

for acute cases. Topical antihistamines and benzocaine products never should be used for these conditions. In more severe cases with vesiculation and blistering, oral prednisone therapy (1 mg/kg per day for ~7–10 days) may be prescribed (6). The causative agent should be identified and contact with the agent eliminated. Disqualification from activity is dependent on the degree of skin involvement, severity of symptoms, and type of sport (i.e., contact versus noncontact).

Urticaria

Urticaria (i.e., hives) usually is systemic in origin. It is caused by a hypersensitivity to foods or drugs, infection, physical agents (e.g., heat, cold, light, and friction), or psychic stimuli (Fig. 28.25). The condition may present with superficial swellings of the dermis, called **wheals,** or deeper swellings of the dermis, subcutaneous, or submucosal tissues, known as **angioedema.** Wheals are smooth, slightly elevated areas on the body that appear red with a pale center and are accompanied by severe itching. They may mature into pink, superficial plaques that usually resolve within 24 hours without sequela. Angioedema tends to be pale and painful and to last longer than wheals, and it also may affect the mouth and, rarely, the bowel (32). Urticaria commonly is seen in allergies to mechanical or chemical irritants.

FIGURE 28.25 Urticaria. Hives may result from hypersensitivity to foods or drugs, infection, physical agents, or psychic stimuli.

Cholinergic Urticaria

Cholinergic urticaria, also known as generalized heat urticaria, is a common type of urticaria. Lesions occur within 15 minutes of sweat-inducing stimuli, such as physical exertion, a hot bath, fever, alcohol, or sudden emotional stress. Clinical presentation reveals small papules that appear first in the upper thorax and neck, then spread inferiorly to involve the entire body. Systemic symptoms, although rare, include generalized sweating, abdominal cramps, dizziness, wheezing, and bradycardia. The inner aspects of the arms, legs, and lateral flanks are common sites. Currently, no cure is available, but antihistamines, such as hydroxyzine and cyproheptadine, generally are used to relieve symptoms. While individuals are symptomatic, they may wish to avoid physical activity and sports participation.

Exercise-Induced Urticaria

Some medical experts believe that **exercise-induced urticaria** may be a variation of cholinergic urticaria, but the lesions are much larger. Systemic signs are limited to wheezing and hypotension. Unlike cholinergic urticaria, exercise-induced urticaria can be successfully treated with prescribed antihistamines, anticholinergics, or β-agonists. Epinephrine generally is the treatment of choice when systemic signs are present.

Cold Urticaria

Cold urticaria is very common in those who are physically active, is nonallergic, and is characterized by localized or generalized wheals that develop in minutes in response to cold exposure. The condition often becomes apparent when a cold pack is placed on an individual who is hypersensitive to cold. The condition responds well to small doses of oral corticosteroids.

Management of Urticaria

Based on the cause, aggravating factors should be identified and eliminated. Simple cooling lotions, such as menthol in aqueous cream, often are used. Avoid NSAIDs and aspirin in favor of acetaminophen, because analgesics can aggravate the symptoms (31). If necessary, oral antihistamines may reduce the itch, quantity and duration of the wheals.

If the field-hockey player is having an allergic reaction to the venom, she could experience anaphylactic shock. The signs and symptoms of anaphylaxis include respiratory distress, cyanosis, weakness, rapid and weak pulse, low blood pressure, localized urticaria or edema, paresthesia, dilated pupils, choking, wheezing, sudden collapse, involuntary loss of bowel and bladder control, headache, dizziness, seizures, and unconsciousness. This condition is life-threatening and represents a medical emergency.

SUMMARY

1. Whenever skin is damaged, a lesion appears. Skin lesions are identified by their size and depth. Recognizing the type of lesion can help to identify the cause of the skin damage.

2. Skin infections may stem from fungi, bacteria, or viruses.

3. Bacterial lesions typically are caused by a staphylococcal or streptococcal infection. Impetigo is highly contagious and is characterized by small vesicles that form pustules and, eventually, honey-colored, weeping crustaceans. Bacterial skin conditions are treated with OTC antibacterial topical agents.

4. Fungi thrive in dark, warm, moist environments and often attack the fingernails, toenails, foot, groin, body, and scalp. Common signs and symptoms include pruritus, redness, and scaling. Antifungal medication is used to treat the condition.

5. Viral skin conditions can range from the common wart to the highly contagious herpes gladiatorum and molluscum contagiosum, which can infect an entire team. Any lesions on the trunk, axilla, face, and thigh should be referred immediately to a physician.

6. Sunburns are classified as first, second, or third degree. Prevention involves using a sunscreen with an SPF of 15 or higher and avoiding exposure to the sun during the midday.

7. Miliaria, or prickly heat, occurs when active sweat glands become blocked by organic debris. Treatment involves cooling and drying the skin, controlling the itching, and watching for secondary infection.

8. Bites and stings from insects can be painful and itchy. Immediate application of cold can relieve pain, or a topical corticosteroid or systemic antihistamine may be used. In severe cases, systemic corticosteroids are used. The individual should be watched carefully for signs of anaphylactic shock.

9. Allergic contact dermatitis results when a substance comes in direct contact with the skin and causes a simple inflammatory reaction. Irritant contact dermatitis results when the substance causes direct skin damage, pain, or ulceration. Treatment involves removal the substance, application of a cold compress, possible use of topical corticosteroids, and systemic antihistamines to reduce itching and inflammation.

10. Urticaria, or hives, is caused by hypersensitivity to foods or drugs, infection, physical agents, or psychic stimuli. The resulting wheal is accompanied by severe itching and is treated with antihistamines, anticholinergics, or β-agonists.

REFERENCES

1. Klossner D, ed. Skin infections in wrestling. In: 2005–2006 NCAA Sports Medicine Handbook. Overland Park, KS: National Collegiate Athletic Association, 2005.
2. Frith M, Harmon CB. Acne scarring: current treatment options. Dermatol Nurs 2006;18(2):139–142.
3. Watkins J. Independent nurse: clinical—management guide—chronic paronychia. Gen Pract 2006;Feb 17:101.
4. Stulberg DL, Penrod MA, Blatny RA. Common bacterial skin infections. Am Fam Physician 2002;66(1):119–124.
5. Dexter W. Common bacterial dermatoses. Phys Sportsmed 2004;32(6):33–39.
6. Freiman A, Barankin B, Elpern DJ. Sports dermatology. Part 2: swimming and other aquatic sports. Can Med Assoc J 2004;171(11):1339–1340.

7. Trent JT, Kerdel FA. Tumor necrosis factor alpha inhibitors for the treatment of dermatologic diseases. Dermatol Nurs 2005;17(2):97–108.

8. Miller KE. Short-course treatment for uncomplicated cellulitis. Am Fam Physician 2005;71(11):2188–2189.

9. Bonnetblanc JM, Bédane C. Erysipelas: recognition and management. Am J Clin Dermatol 2003;4(3):157–163.

10. Studdiford J, Stonehouse A. Bullous eruption on the posterior thigh. J Fam Pract 2005;54(12):1041–1044.

11. Winokur RC, Dexter WW. Fungal infections and parasitic infestations in sports. Phys Sportsmed 2004;32(10):23–33.

12. Nadalo D, Montoya C. What is the best way to treat tinea cruris? J Fam Pract 2006;55(3):256–258.

13. Tosanger M, Crutchfiled CE III. Tinea corporis. Dermatol Nurs 2004;16(5):453.

14. Adams BB. Dermatologic disorders of the athlete. Sports Med 2002;32(5):309–321.

15. Schwatz TA. Superficial fungal infections. Lancet 2004;364(9440):1173–1182.

16. Another option for fungal infections. FDA Consumer 2006;May–June:7.

17. Landry GL, Chang CJ., Harmon KG, Rubin A. Herpes and tinea in wrestling. Phys Sportsmed 2004;32(1):34–42.

18. U.S. Preventive Services Task Force. Screening for genital herpes: recommendation statement. Am Fam Physician 2005;72(8):1557–1561.

19. Snow M. Shutting down shingles. Nursing 2006;36(4):18–19.

20. Cyr PR, Dexter W. Viral skin infections. Phys Sportsmed 2004;32(7):33–38.

21. Rager EL, Bridgeford EP, Ollila DW. Cutaneous melanoma: update on prevention, screening, diagnosis, and treatment. Am Fam Phys 2005;72(2):269–276.

22. Peter J. Managing mild to moderate eczema. Practice Nurse 2006;31(6):24–28.

23. Lebwohl M. Psoriasis. Lancet 2003;361(9364):1197–2004.

24. Luba KM, Stulberg DL. Chronic plaque psoriasis. Am Fam Physician 2006;73(4):636–644.

25. Petrou I. Managing psoriasis in pediatric cases. Dermatol Times 2006;27(4):38.

26. Eisenach JH, Atkinson JLD, Fealey RD. Hyperhidrosis: evolving therapies for a well-established phenomenon. Mayo Clin Proc 2005;80(5):657–666.

27. Norris RL. Managing arthropod bites and stings. Phys Sportsmed 1998;26(7):47–58.

28. Leach J, Bassichis B, Itani K. Brown recluse spider bites to the head: three cases and a review. Ear Nose Throat J 2004;83(7):465–470.

29. Bratton RL, Corey GR. Tick-borne disease. Am Fam Physician 2005;71(12):2323–2330.

30. Hathaway LR. Lyme disease. Nursing 2005;35(4):44–45.

31. Guldbakke KK, Khachemoune A. Classification and treatment of urticaria: a brief review. Dermatol Nurs 2005;17(5):361–364.

GLOSSARY

A

A-angle The angle between a vertical line dividing the patella in half and a second line drawn from the tibial tubercle to the apex of the inferior pole of the patella. An angle of 35° or greater has been linked to increased patellofemoral pain.

Abscess A circumscribed collection of pus appearing in an acute or chronic, localized infection.

Abscessed tooth A painful infection at the root of a tooth or between the gum and a tooth.

Absorption Occurs when an electrical wave passes through a medium and its kinetic energy is either partially or totally assimilated by the tissue.

Absorption rate How quickly a drug gets into the tissues to produce a therapeutic effect.

Accessory movements Movements within a joint that cannot be performed voluntarily by the individual.

Acclimatization Physiologic adaptations of an individual to a different environment, especially climate or altitude.

Acne mechanica A local exacerbation of acne vulgaris caused by heat, occlusion, pressure, and friction.

Acromegaly A disorder marked by progressive enlargement of peripheral parts of the body, especially the head, face, hands, and feet.

Active inhibition A technique whereby an individual consciously relaxes a muscle before stretching.

Active movement Joint motion performed voluntarily by the individual through muscular contraction.

Acute injury An injury with rapid onset because of a traumatic episode but with short duration.

Adhesions Tissues that bind the healing tissue to adjacent structures, such as other ligaments or bone.

Adhesive capsulitis A condition whereby the glenohumeral capsular lining tightens or develops adhesions; seen more commonly in older individuals.

ADLs Activities of daily living.

Administration of medication Providing one dose of a medication to an individual.

Afferent nerves Nerves carrying sensory input from receptors in the skin, muscles, tendons, and ligaments to the central nervous system.

Affective Pertaining to feelings or a mental state.

Agonist muscles Muscles that perform the desired movement; primary movers.

Albuminuria Protein in the urine.

Allergic contact dermatitis Results when a substance comes in direct contact with the skin and leads to a simple inflammatory reaction.

Alveoli Air sacs at the terminal ends of the bronchial tree where oxygen and carbon dioxide are exchanged between the lungs and surrounding capillaries.

Amenorrhea Absence or abnormal cessation of menstruation.

Amplitude A measure of the force, or intensity, that drives an electrical current; the maximum amplitude is the top or highest point of each phase.

Analgesia A conscious state in which normal pain is not perceived, such as a numbing or sedative effect.

Analgesic An agent that produces analgesia.

Anaphylaxis An immediate, shock-like, frequently fatal, hypersensitivity reaction that occurs within minutes of administration of an allergen unless appropriate first-aid measures are taken immediately.

Anastomosis A network of communicating blood vessels that supply a joint.

Anatomic position Used as a universal reference to determine anatomic direction, it is a position whereby the body is erect, facing forward, with the arms at the side of the body and the palms facing forward.

Anatomical snuffbox Site directly over the scaphoid bone in the wrist; pain here indicates a possible fracture.

Androgen A class of hormones that promote development of male genitals and secondary sex characteristics and that influences sexual motivation.

Anemia Abnormal reduction in red blood cell volume or hemoglobin concentration.

Anesthesia Partial or total loss of sensation.

Anesthetic An agent that produces anesthesia.

Angle of inclination Angle of depression formed by the meeting of a line drawn through the shaft of the femur with a line passing through the long axis of the femoral neck; normally about 125° in the frontal plane.

Angle of torsion In the transverse plane, the relationship between the femoral head and the femoral shaft, which normally is rotated 15°.

Anisocoria A condition in which the two pupils are not of equal size.

Anisotropic Having different strengths in response to loads from different directions.

Annulus fibrosus The ring of fibrocartilage and fibrous tissue forming the circumference of the intervertebral disk.

Anorexia athletica Classification of athletes who demonstrate significant signs and symptoms of eating disorders but who do not meet the American Psychological Association criteria for anorexia or bulimia.

Anorexia nervosa A personality disorder manifested by extreme aversion toward food, resulting in excessive weight loss, amenorrhea, and other physical disorders.

Anovulation Suspension or cessation of ovulation.

Antacid An agent that neutralizes stomach acid.

Antagonist muscles Muscles that oppose or reverse a particular movement.

Antalgic gait A noticeable limp.

Anterograde amnesia Loss of memory of events following a head injury.

Anteversion Forward displacement or the turning forward of a body segment without bending.

Antibiotic A soluble substance derived from a mold or bacterium that inhibits the growth of other microorganisms.

Antihistamine A medication used to counteract the effects of histamine; one that relieves the symptoms of an allergic reaction.

Antipyretic A medication used to relieve or reduce a fever.

Antiseptic A substance that inhibits the growth of infectious agents.

Apnea Temporary cessation of breathing.

Apneustic breathing Characterized by prolonged inspirations unrelieved by attempts to exhale, which indicates trauma to the pons.

Aponeurosis A flat, expanded, tendon-like sheath that attaches a muscle to another structure.

Apophysis An outgrowth or projection on the side of a bone; usually where a tendon attaches.

Apophysitis Inflammation of an apophysis.

Appendicitis Inflammation of the appendix.

Arrhythmia Disturbance in the heart beat rhythm.

Arthralgia Severe joint pain.

Arthrogram Diagnostic tool whereby a radiopaque material is injected into a joint to facilitate obtaining a radiograph.

Arthrokinematics Accessory motion, or an involuntary joint motion, that occurs simultaneously with physiologic motion but that cannot be measured precisely.

Arthroscopy A diagnostic tool whereby the inside of a joint is viewed through a small camera lens (arthroscope) to facilitate surgical repair of the joint and/or joint structures.

Aseptic necrosis The death or decay of tissue because of a poor blood supply in the area.

Asthma A disease of the lungs characterized by constriction of the bronchial muscles, increased bronchial secretions, and mucosal swelling, all leading to airway narrowing and inadequate airflow during respiration.

Astringent An agent that causes contraction of the tissues, arrest of secretion, or control of bleeding.

Ataxia Inability to coordinate the muscles in the execution of voluntary movement.

Ataxic (Biot's) breathing Characterized by unpredictable irregularity, whereby breaths may be shallow or deep and stop for short periods, indicating respiratory depression and brain damage, typically at the medullary level.

Atherosclerosis A condition whereby irregularly distributed lipid deposits are found in the large and medium-sized arteries.

Atrophy A wasting away or deterioration of tissue because of disease, disuse, or malnutrition.

Aura A peculiar sensation that precedes an epileptic attack.

Auricular hematoma Ear injury caused when repeated blunt trauma pulls the cartilage away from the perichondrium; "cauliflower ear."

Auscultation Listening for sounds, often with a stethoscope, to denote the condition of the lungs, heart, pleura, abdomen, and other organs.

Autogenous Originating within the body.

Autoinoculation Spreading of an infection from one body part to another by touching the lesion and then scratching or rubbing somewhere else.

Autonomic dysreflexia A rare but dangerous condition in wheelchair athletes; commonly triggered by an obstructed bowel or bladder, which disturbs the regulation of blood pressure and heart rate.

Axial force Loading directed along the long axis of a body.

Axonotmesis Damage to the axons of a nerve followed by complete degeneration of the peripheral segment, without severance of the supporting structure of the nerve.

B

Bacteremia The presence of viable bacteria in the circulating blood.

Ballistic stretch Increasing flexibility by using repetitive bouncing motions at the end of the available range of motion.

Bankart lesion Avulsion or damage to the anterior lip of the glenoid as the humerus slides forward in an anterior dislocation.

Battery Unpermitted or intentional contact with another individual without his or her consent.

Battle's sign Delayed discoloration behind the ear because of basilar skull fracture.

Bending Loading that produces tension on one side of an object and compression on the other side.

Benign pain Pain characterized as dull, generalized, not lasting long after exertion, and not associated with swelling, localized tenderness, or long-term soreness.

Bennett's fracture Fracture-dislocation to the proximal end of the first metacarpal at the carpal-metacarpal joint.

Bimalleolar fracture Fractures of both the medial and the lateral malleolus.

Bioavailability The amount of the drug's concentration when it reaches the target site within a certain time frame.

Bipartite Having two parts.

Blood-brain barrier The barrier that protects the brain against toxic substances.

Blowout fracture Fracture of the floor of the eye orbit, without fracture to the rim; produced by a blow on the globe, with the force being transmitted via the globe to the orbital floor.

Boutonnière deformity Rupture of the central slip of the extensor tendon at the middle phalanx, resulting in no active extensor mechanism at the proximal interphalangeal joint.

Bowler's thumb Compression of the digital nerve on the medial aspect of the thumb, leading to paresthesia in the thumb.

Boxer's fracture Fracture of the fifth metacarpal, resulting in a flexion deformity because of rotation of the head of the metacarpal over the neck.

Brachial plexus A complex web of spinal nerves (C_5–T_1) that innervate the upper extremity.

Bradykinin Normally present in blood; a potent vasodilator. Increases blood vessel wall permeability, and stimulates nerve endings to cause pain.

Bradypnea Abnormal slowness of respiration.

Break test Used to test resistance, an overload pressure is applied in a stationary or static position.

Bronchitis Inflammation of the mucosal lining of the tracheobronchial tree characterized by bronchial swelling, mucus secretions, and dysfunction of the cilia.

Bronchospasm Contraction of the smooth muscles of the bronchial tubes causing narrowing of the airway.

Buccal Pertaining to, adjacent to, or in the direction of the cheek.

Bucket-handle tear Longitudinal meniscal tear of the central segment that can displace into the joint, leading to locking of the knee.

Bulimia nervosa A personality disorder manifested by episodic bouts of bingeing on large amounts of food followed by purging and feelings of guilt, self-disgust, and depression.

Burner Burning or stinging sensation characteristic of a brachial plexus injury.

Bursa A fibrous sac membrane containing synovial fluid typically found between tendons and bones; acts to decrease friction during motion.

Bursitis Inflammation of bursae.

C

Calcific tendinitis Accumulation of mineral deposits in a tendon.

Call person During an emergency, the person responsible for providing assistance, relaying messages to the sideline, and obtaining additional help if necessary.

Callus Localized thickening of skin epidermis because of physical trauma. Fibrous tissue containing immature bone tissue that forms at fracture sites during repair and regeneration.

Cancellous tissue Bone tissue of relatively low density.

Cardiac asystole Cardiac standstill.

Cardiac tamponade Acute compression of the heart because of effusion of fluid or blood into the pericardium from rupture of the heart or penetrating trauma.

Carpal tunnel syndrome Compression of the median nerve as it passes through the carpal tunnel, leading to pain and tingling in the hand.

Carrying angle The angle between the humerus and ulna when the arm is in anatomical position.

Cathode Negatively charged electrode in a direct current system.

CAT scan Computed axial tomographic scan; a computer-assisted x-ray tomogram that provides detailed images of tissue based on their density.

Cauda equina Lower spinal nerves that course through the lumbar spinal canal; resembles a horse's tail.

Cauliflower ear A hematoma that forms between the perichondrium and cartilage of the auricle (ear) because of repeated blunt trauma.

Causalgia Persistent, severe, burning sensation of the skin, usually following direct or indirect (vascular) partial injury of a sensory nerve and accompanied by cutaneous changes (temperature and sweating).

Cavitation Gas bubble formation because of nonthermal effects of ultrasound.

Celiac plexus Nerve plexus that innervates the abdominal region.

Charge person During an emergency, the most medically trained individual who controls the scene and supervises the care of the athlete until the assessment is complete and the athlete is safely moved.

Chemosensitive Sensitive to chemical stimulation.

Cheyne-Stokes breathing Periods of deep breathing alternating with periods of apnea.

Chondral fracture Fracture involving the articular cartilage at a joint.

Chondromalacia patellae Degenerative condition in the articular cartilage of the patella caused by abnormal compression or shearing forces.

Chronic injury An injury with long onset and long duration.

Chyme A semifluid mass of partly digested food passed from the stomach into the duodenum.

Circumduction Movement of a body part in a circular direction.

Cirrhosis Progressive inflammation of the liver, usually caused by alcoholism.

Claw toes Toe deformity characterized by hyperextension of the metatarsophalangeal joint and hyperflexion of the interphalangeal joints.

Climacteric phase The perimenopausal years, ranging from age 46 to 55, when the menstrual cycle may shorten and become irregular in both frequency and bleeding.

Clonic Movement marked by repetitive muscle contractions and relaxation in rapid succession.

Close-packed position Joint position in which contact between the articulation structures is maximal.

Closed-cell foam Foam material whereby air cannot pass from one cell to another, allowing the material to rebound and return to its original shape quickly but offering less cushioning at low levels of impact.

Coach's finger Fixed-flexion deformity of the finger caused by dislocation at the proximal interphalangeal joint.

Coarctation A constriction, stricture, or stenosis.

Coccygodynia Prolonged or chronic pain in the coccygeal region because of irritation of the coccygeal nerve plexus.

Cognitive The quality of knowing or perceiving.

Cognitive model A model that seeks to explain how an athlete approaches the rehabilitation process and encompasses personal factors, such as performance anxiety, self-esteem/motivation, extroversion/introversion, psychological investment in the sport, coping resources, history of past stressors, and previous intervention strategies.

Cold diuresis Excretion of urine in cold weather because of blood being shunted away from the skin to the core to maintain vascular volume.

Cold urticaria Condition characterized by redness, itching, and large, blister-like wheals on skin that is exposed to cold.

Collateral ligaments Major ligaments that cross the medial and lateral aspects of a hinge joint to provide stability from valgus and varus forces.

Colles' fracture Fracture involving a dorsally angulated and displaced, and a radially angulated and displaced, fracture within 1.5 inches of the wrist.

Commission Committing an act that is not legally your duty to perform.

Comparative negligence The relative degree of negligence on the part of the plaintiff and the defendant, with damages awarded on a basis proportionate to each person's carelessness.

Compartment syndrome A condition in which increased intramuscular pressure brought on by activity impedes blood flow and function of tissues within that compartment.

Compression A pressure or squeezing force directed through a body in such a way as to increase density.

Concentric A shortening of the muscle fibers decreases the angle of the associated joint.

Concussion Violent shaking or jarring action of the brain, resulting in immediate or transient impairment of neurologic function.

Conduction The direct transfer of energy between two objects in physical contact with each other.

Conductors Mediums that facilitate the movement of ions, such as water, blood, and electrolyte solutions (e.g., sweat).

Congenital Existing at birth.

Conjunctivitis Bacterial infection that leads to itching, burning, watering, and inflamed eye; pinkeye.

Constipation Infrequent or incomplete bowel movements.

Contracture Permanent muscular contraction because of tonic spasm, fibrosis, loss of muscular equilibrium, or paralysis.

Contraindication A condition that will be adversely affected if a particular action is taken.

Contralateral Pertaining to the opposite side.

Contranutation Anterior rotation of the ilium on the sacrum, indicating anterior torsion of the joint, or posterior rotation of the sacrum on the ilium on one side; the limb on that side probably is medially rotated.

Contrecoup injuries Injuries away from the actual injury site because of rotational components during acceleration.

Contusion Compression injury involving accumulation of blood and lymph within a muscle; a bruise.

Convection The transfer of energy between two objects via a medium, such as air or water, as it moves across the body, creating temperature variations.

Conversion Involves the changing of another energy form (e.g., sound, electricity, or a chemical agent) into heat.

Coordination The body's ability to execute smooth, fluid, accurate, and controlled movements.

Cortical tissue Compact bone tissue of relatively high density.

Cosine law As the angle deviates from 90°, the energy varies with the cosine of the angle: effective energy = energy × cosine of the angle of incidence.

Counterirritant A substance causing irritation of superficial sensory nerves to reduce pain transmission from another underlying irritation.

Coup injuries Injuries at the site where direct impact occurs.

Coxa valga Alteration of the angle made by the axis of the femoral neck to the axis of the femoral shafts so that the angle exceeds 135°; the femoral neck is in more of a straight-line relationship to the shaft of the femur.

Coxa varum Alteration of the angle made by the axis of the femoral neck to the axis of the femoral shaft so that the angle is less than 135°; the neck becomes more horizontal.

Cramp Painful involuntary muscle contraction either clonic or tonic.

Crepitus Crackling sound or sensation characteristic of a fracture when the bone's ends are moved.

Cruciate ligaments Major ligaments that crisscross the knee in the anteroposterior direction, providing stability in that plane.

Cryokinetics Use of cold treatments before an exercise session.

Cryotherapy Cold application.

Cubital fossa Relating to the anterior elbow.

Cubital recurvatum Extension beyond 0° at the elbow.

Cubital tunnel syndrome Entrapment of the ulnar nerve in the cubital tunnel at the elbow.

Cubital valgus At the elbow, a valgus angle of greater than 20°.

Cubital varus At the elbow, a valgus angle of less than 10°.

Current The actual movement of ions.

Curvatures A bending, as in the spine (kyphosis, scoliosis, or lordosis).

Cyanosis A dark-blue or purple skin color because of deficient oxygen in the blood.

Cyclist's nipples Nipple irritation because of the combined effects of perspiration and wind chill, producing cold, painful nipples.

Cyclist's palsy Seen when a biker leans on the handlebar an extended period of time, resulting in paresthesia in the ulnar nerve distribution.

Cystitis Inflammation of the bladder.

D

Dead arm syndrome Common sensation felt with a recurrent anterior shoulder subluxation and multidirectional instability.

Decerebrate rigidity Extension of all four extremities.

Decompression Surgical release of pressure from fluid or blood accumulation.

Decorticate rigidity Extension of the legs with flexion of the elbows, wrists, and fingers.

de Quervain's tenosynovitis An inflammatory stenosing tenosynovitis of the abductor pollicis longus and extensor pollicis brevis tendons.

Dermatome Region of skin supplied by cutaneous branches of a single spinal nerve.

Dermis Corium of the skin that contains blood and lymphatic vessels, nerves and nerve endings, glands, and except for glabrous skin, hair follicles.

Detached retina A condition in which the neurosensory retina is separated from the retinal epithelium by swelling.

Detraining Loss of the benefits gained in physical training, which can occur after only 1 to 2 weeks of nonactivity, with significant decreases measured in both metabolic and working capacity.

Diabetes mellitus A metabolic disorder characterized by near or absolute lack of the hormone insulin, insulin resistance, or both.

Diabetic ketoacidosis A condition whereby an excess of ketoacids in the blood can lower the blood pH to 7.0; manifested by ketones in the breath, blood, and urine.

Diagnosis The definitive determination of the nature of the injury or illness made by a physician.

Diarrhea Loose or watery stools.

Diastolic pressure Arterial blood pressure reached either during or as a result of diastole; lowest level of any given ventricular cycle.

Diathermy Local elevation of temperature in the tissues produced by therapeutic application of high-frequency electrical current, ultrasound, or microwave radiation.

Diffuse injuries Injury over a large body area, usually because of low velocity–high mass forces.

Diplopia Double vision.

Disinfectant A chemical agent applied to nonliving objects; most commonly used to disinfect surgical instruments and cleanse medical equipment and facilities.

Disposition The immediate and long-term management of an injury or illness.

Diuretic A chemical that promotes the excretion of urine.

Drug A therapeutic agent used in the prevention, diagnosis, cure, treatment, or rehabilitation of a disease, condition, or injury.

Drug dispensing Providing more than one individual dose to a person.

Drug interaction The ability of one drug to alter the effects of another drug; it may either intensify (synergistic action) or reduce (inhibit) the effects of the other drug.

Drug metabolism The enzymatic alteration of a drug's structure whereby the original drug is broken down into metabolites (an altered product of metabolism).

Dural sinuses Formed by tubular separations in the inner and outer layers of the dura mater, these sinuses function as small veins for the brain.

Duty of care The standard of care measured by what is learned, or should have been learned, in the professional preparation of an individual charged with providing health care.

Dysesthesia A disagreeable sensation or a sensation short of anesthesia produced by ordinary stimuli.

Dysmenorrhea Difficult or painful menstruation; menstrual cramps.

Dyspepsia Gastric indigestion.

Dysphagia Difficulty in swallowing.

Dysplasia Abnormal tissue development.

Dyspnea Labored or difficult breathing.

Dysrhythmia Serious irregularity of the heart rate.

Dysuria Pain during urination.

E

Eccentric Movement in which the muscle resists its own lengthening so that the joint angle increases during the contraction.

Ecchymosis Superficial tissue discoloration.

Echocardiogram Ultrasonic record obtained by echocardiography in the investigation of the heart and great vessels.

Ecthyma A more serious form of impetigo, which occurs when the infection penetrates deep into the skin's second layer (dermis).

Ectopic bone Proliferation of bone ossification in an abnormal place.

Edema Swelling from a collection of exuded lymph fluid in interstitial tissues.

Effective radiating area In ultrasound, the portion of the transducer's surface area that actually produces the ultrasound wave.

Efferent nerves Nerves carrying motor impulses from the central nervous system to the muscles.

Effleurage Superficial, longitudinal massage strokes used to relax the patient.

Effusion The escape of fluid from blood vessels into the surrounding tissues or joint cavity.

Elastic limit A material's yield point.

Elasticity The ability of a muscle to return to normal length after either lengthening or shortening has taken place.

Electrocardiogram A graphic record of the heart's action currents obtained with an electrocardiograph.

Electromagnetic radiation Energy emitted by an object.

Electromagnetic spectrum A graphic presentation of electromagnetic radiation based on its wavelength or frequency.

Embolism Obstruction or occlusion of a vessel by bacteria or other foreign body.

Emergency medical services A well-developed process that activates the emergency health care services of the athletic training facility and community to provide immediate health care to an injured individual.

Emesis Vomiting.

Emmetropia 20/20 vision, indicating that the light rays are focused precisely on the retina.

Encephalitis Inflammation of the brain, especially of the cerebral hemisphere, cerebellum, or brainstem, caused by a viral infection.

End feel The sensation felt in the joint as it reaches the end of the available range of motion.

Endometriosis Ectopic occurrence of endometrial tissue, frequently forming cysts containing altered blood.

Enteric coated Drugs covered by acid-resistant materials (e.g., fatty acids, waxes, and shellac) that protect the drug from the acid and pepsin in the stomach.

Epicondylitis Inflammation and microrupturing of the soft tissues on the epicondyles of the distal humerus.

Epidermis The outer epithelial portion of the skin.

Epilepsy Disorder of the brain characterized by recurrent episodes of sudden, excessive discharges of electrical activity in the brain.

Epiphyseal fracture Injury to the growth plate of a long bone in children and adolescents; may lead to arrested bone growth.

Epistaxis Profuse bleeding from the nose; nosebleed.

Erb's point Located 2 to 3 cm above the clavicle at the level of the transverse process of the C_6 vertebra; compression over the site may injure the brachial plexus.

Erythema Inflammatory redness of the skin.

Erythropoietin A hormone produced in the kidneys that stimulates bone marrow to increase production of red blood cells.

Estrogens Hormones that produce female secondary sex characteristics and that affect the menstrual cycle.

Excitability A muscle's ability to respond to a stimulus; irritability.

Excoriation A scratch mark; a linear break in the skin surface, usually covered with blood or serous crusts.

Exculpatory waiver Based on the athlete's assumption of risk, a release that is signed by the athlete, or by the parent of an athlete under the age of 18, that releases the physician from liability of negligence.

Exercise-induced urticaria Hives brought on by exercise; a variation of cholinergic urticaria, but with lesions that are much larger.

Expressed warranty A written guarantee that states the product is safe for consumer use.

Extensibility The ability of a muscle to be stretched or to increase in length.

Extensor mechanism A complex interaction of muscles, ligaments, and tendons that stabilize and provide motion at the patellofemoral joint.

Extrasynovial Structures found outside the synovial cavity and synovial fluid.

Extrinsic Origination outside the part where it is found or on which it acts; denoting, especially, a muscle.

Extruded disk A condition in which the nuclear material bulges into the spinal canal and runs the risk of impinging adjacent nerve roots.

Extruded tooth A tooth driven in an outwardly direction.

Exudate Material composed of fluid, pus, or cells that have escaped from blood vessels into the surrounding tissues following injury or inflammation.

F

Facet joint A joint formed when the superior and inferior articular processes mate with the articular process of adjacent vertebrae.

Failure Loss of continuity; rupture of soft tissue or fracture of bone.

Fasciitis Inflammation of the fascia surrounding portions of a muscle.

Female athlete triad A combination of three disorders commonly seen in adolescent and young adult female athletes: disordered eating, amenorrhea, and osteoporosis.

Fibroblast A cell present in connective tissue and capable of forming collagen fibers.

Fibrositis Inflammation of fibrous tissue.

First-pass effect Drug metabolism that takes place first in the liver via hepatic enzymes.

Fistulas Abnormal passage from a hollow organ to the surface or from one organ to another.

Flatulence Presence of an excessive amount of gas in the stomach and intestines.

Flexibility Total range of motion at a joint; dependent on normal joint mechanics, mobility of soft tissues, and muscle extensibility.

Focal injuries Injury in a small, concentrated area, usually because of high velocity–low mass forces.

Focus The ability to perceive and address various internal (thoughts, emotions, and physical responses) and external (sights and sounds) cues and, when needed, to shift one's attention to other cues in a natural, effortless manner.

Follicular phase Days 1 to 14 of the ovarian cycle, in which the follicle (spheroidal cell cluster in the ovary contain an ovum or egg) grows.

Foot strike hemolysis A condition in which red blood cells are thought to be destroyed by repetitive, hard foot strikes.

Foreseeability of harm A condition whereby danger is or should have been apparent, resulting in an unreasonably unsafe condition.

Fracture A disruption in the continuity of a bone.

Freiberg's disease Avascular necrosis that occurs to the second metatarsal head in some adolescents.

Friction Deepest form of massage, consisting of deep, circular motions performed by the thumb, knuckles, or ends of the fingers at right angles to the involved tissue.

Frontal plane A longitudinal (vertical) line that divides the body or any of it parts into anterior and posterior portions.

G

Gamekeeper's thumb Sprain of the metacarpophalangeal (MP) joint of the thumb when it is in near extension and the thumb is forcefully abducted away from the hand, tearing the ulnar collateral ligament at the MP joint.

Ganglion cyst Benign tumor mass commonly seen on the dorsal aspect of the wrist.

Gangrene Necrosis because of obstruction, loss, or diminution of blood supply; may be localized to a small area or involve an entire extremity or organ.

Gastritis Inflammation, especially mucosal, of the stomach.

Gastrocolic reflex Propulsive reflex in the colon that stimulates defecation.

Gastroenteritis Inflammation of the mucous membrane of the stomach and/or small intestine.

Genu recurvatum A condition of hyperextension of the knee.

Genu valgum A deformity marked by abduction of the leg in relation to the thigh; knock-knee.

Genu varum A deformity marked by adduction of the leg in relation to the thigh; bow-leg.

Gestation Pregnancy.

Gingivitis Inflammation of the gums.

Glenoid labrum Soft-tissue lip around the periphery of the glenoid fossa that widens and deepens the socket to add stability to the joint.

Glucagon A polypeptide hormone secreted by pancreatic alpha cells. It activates hepatic phosphorylase, thereby increasing glycogenolysis; decreases gastric motility and gastric and pancreatic secretions; and increases urinary excretion of nitrogen and potassium.

Goniometer Protractor used to measure joint position and available joint motion (range of motion).

Graves' disease Toxic goiter characterized by diffuse hyperplasia of the thyroid gland; a form of hyperthyroidism.

Gross negligence Committing, or not committing, an act with total disregard for the health and safety of others.

Grottus-Draper law An inverse relationship exists between the amount of penetration and absorption. The more energy absorbed by superficial tissues, the less energy is available to be transmitted to the underlying tissues.

Gynecomastia Excessive development of the male mammary glands.

H

Half-life The period during which an agent decreases to half its original strength. The longer the half-life of an agent, the slower it leaves the body.

Halitosis Bad breath.

Hallux The first toe, or great toe.

Hammer toes A flexion deformity of the distal interphalangeal joint of the toes.

Harmful pain Pain that is sharp, localized to the injury site, experienced during and persisting after exertion, and usually associated with swelling, localized tenderness, and prolonged soreness.

Heat cramps Painful, involuntary muscle spasms caused by excessive water and electrolyte loss.

Heel bruise Contusion to the subcutaneous fat pad located over the inferior aspect of the calcaneus.

Hemarthrosis Collection of blood within a joint or cavity.

Hematemesis Vomiting of blood.

Hematocele A rapid accumulation of blood and fluid in the scrotum around the testicle and cord.

Hematoma A localized mass of blood and lymph confined within a space or tissue.

Hematuria Blood or red blood cells in the urine.

Hemoglobinuria Hemoglobin in the urine; in sufficient quantities, hemoglobin results in the urine being colored from light red-yellow to fairly dark red.

Hemophilia A bleeding disorder characterized by a deficiency of selected proteins in the body's blood-clotting system.

Hemorrhoids Dilations of the venous plexus surrounding the rectal and anal area that can become exposed if they protrude internally or externally.

Hemothorax A condition involving loss of blood into the pleural cavity but outside the lung.

Heparin An anticoagulant that is a component of various tissues and mast cells.

Hepatitis Inflammation of the liver.

Hernia Protrusion of abdominal viscera through a weakened portion of the abdominal wall.

High-density material Materials that absorb more energy from higher impact intensity levels through deformation, thus transferring less stress to a body part.

Hill-Sachs lesion A small defect usually located on the posterior aspect of the articular cartilage of the humeral head and caused by the impact of the humeral head on the glenoid fossa as the humerus dislocates.

Hip pointer Contusions caused by direct compression to an unprotected iliac crest that crushes soft tissue and, sometimes, the bone itself.

Histamine A powerful stimulant of gastric secretion, constrictor of bronchial smooth muscle, and vasodilator (capillaries and arterioles) that causes a fall in blood pressure.

Homeostasis The state of a balanced equilibrium in the body's various tissues and systems.

Hydrocele Swelling in the tunica vaginalis of the testes.

Hyperemia Increased blood flow into a region or body part once treatment has ended.

Hyperesthesia Excessive tactile sensation.

Hyperglycemia Abnormally high levels of glucose in the circulating blood that can lead to diabetic coma.

Hyperhidrosis Excessive or profuse sweating.

Hyperhydrate Overhydration; excess water consumption of the body.

Hypermetropia Farsightedness; occurs when the light rays are focused at a point behind the retina.

Hypermobile patella Movement of the patella equal to three or more quadrants of the patella, indicating laxity of the restraints, which can predispose an athlete to a laterally subluxating or dislocating patella.

Hypermobility Increased motion at a joint; joint laxity.

Hyperplasia An increase in the number of cells in a tissue or organ, excluding tumor formation; overgrowth of the endometrium.

Hyperreflexia A condition in which the reflexes are exaggerated.

Hypertension Sustained elevated blood pressure above the norms of 140 mm Hg systolic or 90 mm Hg diastolic.

Hyperthermia Elevated body temperature.

Hypertrophic cardiomyopathy Excessive hypertrophy of the heart, often of obscure or unknown origin.

Hypertrophy A general increase in the bulk or size of an individual tissue not resulting from tumor formation.

Hyphema Hemorrhage into the anterior chamber of the eye.

Hypoesthesia Decreased tactile sensation.

Hypoglycemia Abnormally low levels of glucose in the circulating blood that can lead to insulin shock.

Hypomobile patella Movement of the patella equal to one quadrant or less.

Hypomobility Decreased motion at a joint.

Hyponatremia Abnormally low concentrations of sodium ions in the circulating blood.

Hypotension Characterized by a fall of 20 mm Hg or more from a person's normal baseline systolic blood pressure.

Hypothalamus A region of the diencephalon forming the floor of the third ventricle of the brain and responsible for thermoregulation and other autonomic nervous mechanisms underlying moods and motivational states.

Hypothenar The fleshy mass of muscle and tissue on the medial side of the palm.

Hypothermia Decreased body temperature.

Hypovolemic shock Shock caused by a reduction in blood volume, as from hemorrhage or dehydration.

Hypoxia Having a reduced concentration of oxygen in air, blood, or tissue, short of anoxia.

I

Idiopathic Of unknown origin or cause.

Impetigo A highly contagious bacterial infection characterized by small vesicles that form pustules and, eventually, honey-colored, weeping crustations.

Impingement syndrome Chronic condition caused by repetitive overhead activity that damages the supraspinatus tendon, glenoid labrum, long head of the biceps brachii, and subacromial bursa.

Implied warranty An unwritten guarantee that the product is reasonably safe when used for its intended purpose.

Indication A condition that could benefit from a specific action.

Infarcts Clumping together of cells that block small blood vessels, leading to vascular occlusion, ischemia, and necrosis in organs.

Infectious mononucleosis An acute illness associated with the Epstein-Barr herpetovirus and characterized by fever, sore throat, enlargement of the lymph nodes and spleen, and leukopenia that changes to lymphocytosis.

Infiltrative anesthesia A process that produces numbness by interfering with nerve function in a localized, subcutaneous, soft-tissue area. Commonly used for the treatment of soft-tissue injuries or as an anesthetic before minor surgical procedures.

Inflammation Pain, swelling, redness, heat, and loss of function that accompany musculoskeletal injuries.

Influenza An acute, infectious respiratory tract condition characterized by malaise, headache, dry cough, and general muscle aches.

Informed consent Consent given by a person of legal age who understands the nature and extent of any treatment and the available alternative treatments before agreeing to receive treatment.

Innominate Without a name; used to describe anatomic structures.

Inspection Refers to factors seen at the actual site of injury, such as redness, bruising, swelling, cuts, or scars.

Instability A joint's inability to function under the stresses encountered during functional activities.

Interpulse interval The period within a discrete pulse when the current is not flowing. The duration of the intrapulse interval cannot exceed the duration of the interpulse interval.

Intersection syndrome A tendinitis or friction tendinitis in the first and second dorsal compartments of the wrist.

Intertrigo Dermatitis occurring between folds of the skin because of sweat retention, moisture, warmth, and concomitant overgrowth of resident microorganisms.

Intracapsular Structures found within the articular capsule; intra-articular.

Intrinsic In anatomy, denoting those muscles of the limbs for which the origin and insertion are both in the same limb.

Intruded tooth A tooth driven deep into the socket in an inward direction.

Inverse square law The intensity of radiant energy striking the tissues (E) is directly proportional to the square of the distance (D) between the source of the energy (E_S) and the tissues ($E = E_S/D^2$).

Ion An atom or group of atoms carrying a charge of electricity by virtue of having gained or lost one or more electrons.

Iontophoresis A technique whereby direct current is used to drive charged molecules from certain medications into damaged tissue.

Ipsilateral Situated on, pertaining to, or affecting the same side (as opposed to *contralateral*).

Irritant contact dermatitis Results when a substance causes direct skin damage, pain, or ulceration.

Ischemia Local anemia because of decreased blood supply.

Ischemic necrosis Death of a tissue because of decreased blood supply.

J

Jaundice A yellowish discoloration of the skin, sclera, and deeper tissues, often resulting from liver damage.

Jersey finger Rupture of the flexor digitorum profundus tendon from the distal phalanx because of rapid extension of the finger while actively flexed.

Jones fracture A transverse stress fracture of the proximal shaft of the fifth metatarsal.

Joule's law The greater the resistance or impedance, the more heat will be developed. Tissues with a high fluid content, such as skeletal muscle and areas surrounding joints, absorb more of the energy and,

therefore, are heated to a greater extent, whereas fat is not heated as much.

K

Kehr's sign Referred pain down the left shoulder; indicative of a ruptured spleen.

Keloids A nodular, firm, movable, often linear mass of hyperplastic scar tissue.

Ketoacidosis A condition caused by excess accumulation of acid or loss of base in the body; characteristic of diabetes mellitus.

Ketonemia A recognizable concentration of ketone bodies in the blood plasma.

Ketonuria Enhanced urinary excretion of ketone bodies.

Kienböck's disease Avascular necrosis of the lunate, often seen in young athletes and thought to be caused by repetitive trauma or an unrecognized lunate fracture.

Kinematic chain A series of interrelated joints that constitute a complex motor unit so that motion at one joint produces motion at the other joints in a predictable manner.

Kinematics The study of the spatial and temporal aspects of movement.

Kinesthesia The sensation of position, movement, tension, and so on of parts of the body as perceived through nerve end organs in the muscles, tendons, and joints.

Kinetics The study of the forces causing and resulting from motion.

Kyphosis Excessive curve in the thoracic region of the spine.

L

Laryngospasm Spasmodic closure of the glottic aperture, leading to shortness of breath, coughing, cyanosis, and even loss of consciousness.

Laxity The amount of "give" within a joint's supportive tissue.

Legg-Calvé-Perthes disease Avascular necrosis of the proximal femoral epiphysis, seen especially in young males ages 3 to 8.

Leukoplakia A disease of the mouth characterized by white patches and oral lesions on the cheeks, gums, and/or tongue that can lead to oral cancer.

Licensure Act that gives permission for an individual to practice a profession by a governmental body.

Lipid solubility Fat soluble; denoting the ability of fat-soluble vitamins to be absorbed better than water-soluble vitamins and to accumulate in the body because of their increased ability to cross cell membranes.

Lisfranc injury Involves disruption of the tarsometatarsal joint, with or without an associated fracture caused by a severe twisting injury. The first metatarsal typically is dislocated from the first cuneiform, whereas the other four metatarsals are displaced laterally, usually in combination with a fracture at the base of the second metatarsal.

Little league elbow Tension stress injury of the medial epicondyle; seen in adolescents.

Little league shoulder Fracture of the proximal humeral growth plate caused by repetitive rotational stresses during the act of pitching; seen in adolescents.

Loose-packed position Resting position where the joint is under the least amount of strain.

Lordosis Excessive convex curve in the lumbar region of the spine.

Low-density material Materials that absorb energy from low impact intensity levels.

Lumbar plexus Interconnected roots of the first four lumbar spinal nerves.

Luteal phase Phase of the ovarian cycle extending from ovulation until onset of the next menstrual bleeding, normally about 12 to 17 days. During this period, both estrogen and progesterone levels are high.

Lyme disease An inflammatory disorder that typically occurs during the summer months and is characterized by a specific lesion and accompanied by fever, malaise, fatigue, headache, and stiff neck.

Lymph nodes Small lymphatic organs that filter lymph; contain macrophages and lymphocytes.

Lymphangitis Inflammation of the lymphatic vessels.

M

Macerated To soften skin with moisture by steeping or soaking.

Macrotrauma When a single force produces an acute injury.

Magnetic resonance imaging A diagnostic technique using magnetism to produce high-quality, cross-sectional images of organs or structures within the body without x-rays or other radiation.

Maisonneuve fracture An external rotation injury of the ankle with an associated fracture of the proximal third of the fibula.

Malaise Lethargic feeling of general discomfort; out-of-sorts feeling.

Malfeasance Committing an act that is not your responsibility to perform.

Mallet finger Rupture of the extensor tendon from the distal phalanx because of forceful flexion of the phalanx.

Mallet toe A toe in neutral position at the metatarsophalangeal and proximal interphalangeal joints but flexed at the distal interphalangeal joint.

Malocclusion Inability to bring the teeth together in a normal bite.

Malpractice Committing a negligent act while providing care.

Marfan's syndrome An inherited connective tissue disorder affecting many organs but commonly resulting in dilation and weakening of the thoracic aorta.

Mast cells Connective tissue cells that carry heparin, which prolongs clotting, and histamine.

Maximal efficacy The drug dose at which a response occurs and continues to increase in magnitude before reaching a plateau, or threshold.

McBurney's point A site one-third of the distance between the anterior superior iliac spines and umbilicus that with deep palpation, produces rebound tenderness indicating appendicitis.

Mechanosensitive Sensitive to mechanical stimulation.

Menarche The onset of menses.

Meninges Three protective membranes that surround the brain and spinal cord.

Meningitis Inflammation of the meninges of the brain and spinal column.

Menisci Fibrocartilaginous disks found within a joint that serve to reduce joint stress.

Menorrhagia Prolonged or profuse menses.

Menstrual phase Phase in the menstrual cycle when the thickened vascular walls of the uterus, the unfertilized ova, and blood from damaged vessels are lost during the menstrual flow.

Metabolites Any altered product of metabolism, especially of catabolism.

Metatarsalgia A condition involving general discomfort around the metatarsals heads.

Microalbuminuria Minute particles of albumin in the urine, signifying the first stage of kidney disease.

Microtrauma Injury to a small number of cells because of accumulative effects of repetitive forces.

Miliaria An eruption of minute vesicles and papules that occurs when active sweat glands become blocked by organic debris; prickly heat.

Minimum effective concentration The minimum concentration of a drug that must be present for that drug to be effective.

Misfeasance While committing an act that is your responsibility to perform, following the wrong procedure or performing the right procedure in an improper manner.

Mitral valve prolapse A condition in which redundant tissue is found on one or both leaflets of the mitral valve. During a ventricular contraction, a portion of the redundant tissue on the mitral valve pushes back beyond the normal limit and, as a result, produces an abnormal sound, followed by a systolic murmur as blood is regurgitated back through the mitral valve into the left atrium; often called a click-murmur syndrome.

Modality A therapeutic agent that promotes optimal healing while reducing pain and disability.

Menorrhagia Abnormal, heavy menstrual bleeding.

Multivalvular disease Acquired valvular heart disease stemming from a defect or insufficiency in more than one heart valve; manifested as either valvular stenosis or regurgitation.

Muscle cramps A painful, involuntary contraction that may be clonic (alternating contraction and relaxation) or tonic (continued contraction over a period of time).

Muscle spasms An involuntary contraction of short duration caused by reflex action biochemically derived or initiated by a mechanical blow to a nerve or muscle.

Myalgia Pain in a muscle.

Myelogram A radiograph of the spinal cord taken after the injection of an opaque substance that shows contrast on the developed photograph.

Myocardial infarction Heart attack.

Myocarditis An inflammatory condition of the muscular walls of the heart that can result from a bacterial or viral infection.

Myopia Nearsightedness.

Myositis Inflammation of connective tissue within a muscle.

Myositis ossificans Accumulation of mineral deposits within muscle tissue.

Myotome A group of muscles primarily innervated by a single nerve root.

N

Near syncope A sense of impending loss of consciousness or weakness.

Necrosis Death of a tissue resulting from deprivation of blood supply.

Negligence Breach of one's duty of care that causes harm to another individual.

Neoplasm Mass of tissue that grows more rapidly than normal and that may be benign or malignant.

Nephropathy Any disease of the kidney.

Neuralgia Pain of a severe throbbing or stabbing character in the course or distribution of a nerve.

Neurapraxia Injury to a nerve that results in temporary neurologic deficits followed by complete recovery of function.

Neuroma A nerve tumor.

Neurotmesis Complete severance of a nerve.

Nightstick fracture Fracture to the ulna because of a direct blow; commonly seen in football players.

Nociceptor A receptor that is sensitive to potentially damaging stimuli that result in pain.

Nonfeasance Failing to perform one's legal duty of care.

Nonunion fracture Failure of normal healing of a fractured bone.

Nuchal rigidity Stiffness in the nape or back of the neck.

Nucleus pulposus The soft fibrocartilage in the central portion of the intervertebral disk.

Nutation The backward rotation of the ilium on the sacrum. When occurring on only one side, the anterior superior iliac spine is higher and the posterior superior iliac spine is lower on that side, resulting in an apparent or functional short leg on the same side.

Nystagmus Abnormal jerking or involuntary eye movement.

O

Observation Visual analysis of overall appearance, symmetry, general motor function, posture, and gait.

Ohm's law Current (I) in a conductor increases as the driving force (V) becomes larger or as resistance (R) is decreased ($I = V/R$).

Oligomenorrhea Infrequent menstrual cycles or menstruation involving scant blood flow.

Omission Failure to perform a legal duty of care.

Onychia Inflammation of the nail matrix.

Open-cell foam Foam with cells that are connected to allow air passage from cell to cell, allowing the foam to deform quickly under stress, which limits its shock-absorbing qualities.

Organomegaly Abnormal enlargement of an organ.

Orthostatic hypotension Low blood pressure caused by a sudden change in body position, such as moving from a lying to a standing position.

Osgood-Schlatter's disease Inflammation or partial avulsion of the tibial apophysis because of traction forces.

Osteitis pubis A stress fracture to the pubic symphysis caused by repeated overload of the adductor muscles or repetitive stress activities.

Osteochondral fracture A fracture involving the articular cartilage and underlying bone.

Osteochondritis dissecans A localized area of avascular necrosis resulting in complete or incomplete separation of joint cartilage and subchondral bone.

Osteochondrosis Any condition characterized by degeneration or aseptic necrosis of the articular cartilage because of limited blood supply.

Osteolysis Softening, absorption, and destruction of bony tissue.

Osteomyelitis Inflammation or infection of the bone and bone marrow.

Osteopenia A condition of reduced bone mineral density that predisposes the individual to fractures.

Osteoporosis A pathologic condition of reduced bone mass and strength.

Otitis externa A bacterial infection involving the lining of the auditory canal; swimmer's ear.

Otitis media A localized infection in the middle ear secondary to upper respiratory infections.

Ovarian cycle Cycle associated with the maturation of an egg.

Overload principle Physiologic improvements occur only when an individual physically demands more of the muscles than is normally required.

Ovulation Release of the egg occurring at midcyle, when the ballooning ovarian wall ruptures and expels the egg.

P

Painful arc Pain located within a limited number of degrees in the range of motion.

Palpitations Perceptible, forcible pulsation of the heart, usually with an increase in frequency or force, with or without irregularity in rhythm.

Papules Small, red, elevated, painful bump on the skin.

Paresis Partial paralysis of a muscle, leading to a weakened contraction.

Paresthesia Abnormal sensations, such as tingling, burning, itching, or prickling.

Paronychia A fungal/bacterial infection in the folds of skin surrounding a fingernail or toenail.

Parrot-beak tear A horizontal meniscal tear, typically in the middle segment of the lateral meniscus.

Passive movement Movement of an injured limb or body part through the range of motion with no assistance from the injured individual.

Patella plica A fold in the synovial lining that may cause medial knee pain without associated trauma.

Patellofemoral joint Gliding joint between the patella and patellar groove of the femur.

Patellofemoral stress syndrome Condition whereby the lateral retinaculum is tight or the vastus medialis oblique is weak, leading to lateral excursion and pressure on the lateral facet of the patella, causing a painful condition.

Pathology The cause of an injury, its development, and the functional changes that result.

Pericardial tamponade Compression of venous return to the heart because of increased volume of fluid in the pericardium; usually results from direct trauma to the chest.

Perilunate dislocation Dorsal dislocation of the lunate relative to the other carpals.

Perimenopausal The period of time between ages 46 to 55 when the menstrual cycle may shorten and become irregular in both frequency and bleeding; precedes menopause.

Periodontitis Inflammation of the deeper gum tissues that normally hold the teeth in place.

Periorbital ecchymosis Swelling and hemorrhage into the surrounding eye lids; black eye.

Periostitis Inflammation of the periosteum (outer membrane covering the bone).

Peristalsis Periodic waves of smooth muscle contraction that propel food through the digestive system.

Peritonitis Irritation of the peritoneum that lines the abdominal cavity.

Pernio Chilblain, a condition in which the tissue does not freeze but, rather, reacts with erythema, itching, and burning.

Pes cavus High arch.

Pes planus Flat feet.

Pétrissage A massage technique that consists of pressing and rolling the muscles under the fingers and hands.

Phagocytosis The process by which white blood cells surround and digest foreign particles, such as bacteria, necrotic tissue, and foreign particles.

Pharmacokinetics The study of how a drug moves through the body to produce the desired effects.

Pharyngitis A viral, bacterial, or fungal infection of the pharynx, leading to a sore throat.

Phlebothrombosis Thrombosis, or clotting, in a vein without overt inflammatory signs and symptoms.

Phonophobia Morbid fear of one's own voice or of any sound.

Phonophoresis The introduction of anti-inflammatory drugs through the skin with the use of ultrasound.

Photophobia Abnormal sensitivity to light.

Plantar fascia A specialized band of fascia that covers the plantar surface of the foot and helps to support the longitudinal arch.

Plyometric training A type of explosive exercise that maximizes the myotactic on-stretch reflex.

Pneumothorax A condition whereby air is trapped in the pleural space, causing a portion of a lung to collapse.

Polydipsia Frequent drinking because of extreme thirst.

Polyphagia Excessive hunger and food consumption; gluttony.

Polyuria Excessive excretion of urine, leading to a huge urinary output of water and electrolytes and, in turn, to decreased blood volume and further dehydration.

Postconcussion syndrome A delayed condition characterized by persistent headaches, blurred vision, irritability, and inability to concentrate.

Premenstrual syndrome A series of physical and psychological symptoms, such as headaches, breast tenderness, back pain, bloating, irritability, depression, fatigue, and certain food cravings, that occurs during the luteal phase (days 15–28) of the menstrual cycle.

Prodromal symptoms An early symptom of a disease.

Progesterone The hormone responsible for thickening the uterine lining in preparation for the fertilized ovum.

Progressive resistance exercise A method to improve strength by increasing resistance using the overload principles as the individual's strength increases.

Prolapsed disk A condition in which the eccentric nucleus produces a definite deformity as it works its way through the fibers of the annulus fibrosus.

Proliferation phase In the menstrual cycle, days 6 to 14, when the endometrium rebuilds itself.

Pronation Inward rotation of the forearm; the palms face posteriorly. At the foot, combined motions of calcaneal eversion, foot abduction, and dorsiflexion.

Pronator syndrome A condition in which the median nerve is entrapped by the pronator teres, leading to pain on activities involving pronation.

Prophylactic To prevent or protect.

Proprioceptive neuromuscular facilitation Exercises that stimulate proprioceptors in muscles, tendons, and joints to improve flexibility and strength.

Prostaglandins Active substances found in many tissues, with effects such as vasodilation, vasoconstriction, and stimulation of intestinal or bronchial smooth muscle.

Proteinuria Abnormal concentrations of protein in the urine.

Pruritus Intense itching.

Pseudo-boutonnière deformity A flexion deformity of the proximal interphalangeal joint, which resembles a boutonnière deformity, but the central slip of the extensor tendon is not involved.

Pulmonary contusion Contusion to the lungs because of compressive force.

Pulmonary embolism A blood clot that travels through the circulatory system to lodge in the lungs.

Pupillary light reflex Rapid constriction of pupils when exposed to intense light.

Purulent Containing, consisting of, or forming pus.

Pyarthrosis Suppurative pus within a joint cavity.

Q

Q-angle The angle between the line of quadriceps force and the patellar tendon.

R

Raccoon eyes Delayed discoloration around the eyes from a fracture of the anterior cranial fossa.

Radial tunnel syndrome A condition caused by direct trauma or entrapment at the elbow as the radial nerve passes anterior to the cubital fossa, pierces the supinator muscle, and runs posterior again into the forearm.

Radiation The transfer of energy in the form of infrared waves (radiant energy) without physical contact.

Rales Abnormal breath sounds.

Rate of dissolution A condition by which the more rapidly a drug dissolves, the faster the onset of its effects will be; for example, drugs that dissolve quickly (liquid medications) have a more rapid onset of effects compared with drugs that dissolve more slowly (enteric-coated preparations).

Raynaud's disease A condition characterized by intermittent bilateral attacks of ischemia of the fingers or toes and marked by severe pallor, numbness, and pain.

Receptor The functional macromolecule, or target site, to which a drug binds to produce its effects.

Reciprocal inhibition A technique using an active contraction of the agonist to cause a reflex relaxation in the antagonist, allowing it to stretch; a phenomenon resulting from reciprocal innervation.

Referred pain A type of visceral pain that travels along the same nerve pathways as somatic pain and that is perceived by the brain as somatic in origin.

Reflection Occurs when an energy wave strikes an object and is bent back away from the material, as in an echo.

Reflex An action involving stimulation of a motor neuron by a sensory neuron in the spinal cord without involvement of the brain.

Reflex sympathetic dystrophy syndrome Complex regional pain syndrome in which pain is associated with findings such as abnormal skin color, temperature changes, abnormal sweating, hypersensitivity in the affected area, abnormal edema, and often significant impairment of motor function.

Refraction The deflection of an energy wave because of a change in the speed of absorption as the wave passes between mediums of different densities.

Registration Used in some states, it requires that individuals who wish to practice a profession within the state must register with a governmental agency.

Regurgitation A backward flow, as of blood through an incompetent heart valve; the return of contents in small amounts from the stomach.

Resilience The ability to bounce or spring back into shape or position after being stretched, bent, or impacted.

Resistors Media that inhibit the movement of ions, such as skin, fat, and lotion.

Resting position A slightly flexed position of a joint that allows maximal volume to accommodate any intra-articular swelling.

Retinopathy A noninflammatory, degenerative disease of the retina.

Retrograde amnesia Forgetting events that occurred before an injury.

Retroversion A turning backward; a decreased angle between the femoral condyles and femoral head, usually <15°.

Retroviruses Any virus of the family Retroviridae known to reverse the usual order of reproduction within the cells they infect.

Reverse piezoelectric effect In ultrasound, the conversion of electrical current into mechanical energy as it passes through a piezoelectric crystal (e.g., quartz, barium titanate, lead zirconate, or titanate) housed in the transducer head.

Reye's syndrome A severe disorder of young children following an acute illness, usually influenza or varicella infection, and characterized by recurrent vomiting beginning within a week after onset of the condition, from which the child either recovers rapidly or lapses into a coma with intracranial hypertension; death may occur because of edema of the brain and resulting cerebral herniation.

Rhabdomyolysis An acute, fulminating, potentially fatal disease of skeletal muscles that entails destruction of skeletal muscles, as evidenced by the release of myoglobin into the blood and urine.

Rhinitis Inflammation of the nasal membranes with excessive mucus production resulting in nasal congestion and postnasal drip.

Rhinorrhea Clear nasal discharge.

Rotator cuff The SITS muscles (supraspinatus, infraspinatus, teres minor, and subscapularis) hold the head of the humerus in the glenoid fossa and produce humeral rotation.

Runner's anemia Exercise-induced hemolytic anemia, which occurs when the red blood cells are destroyed and the hemoglobin is liberated into the medium in which the cells are suspended.

Runner's nipples Nipple irritation resulting from friction as the shirt rubs over the nipples.

S

Sacral plexus Interconnected roots of the L_4–S_4 spinal nerves that innervate the lower extremities.

Saddle joint A biaxial-like condyloid joint with both concave and convex areas but with freer movement; the carpometacarpal joints of the thumbs.

Sagittal plane A longitudinal (vertical) line that divides the body or any of it parts into right and left portions.

Salicylates Any salt of salicylic acid; used in aspirin.

Scapulohumeral rhythm Coordinated rotational movement of the scapula that accompanies abduction and adduction of the humerus.

Scheuermann's disease Osteochondrosis of the spine because of abnormal epiphyseal plate behavior that allows herniation of the disk into the vertebral body, giving a characteristic wedge-shaped appearance.

Sciatica Compression of a spinal nerve because of a herniated disk, annular tear, myogenic or muscle-related disease, spinal stenosis, facet joint arthropathy, or compression from the piriformis muscle.

Scoliosis Lateral rotational spinal curvature.

Scope of care The roles and responsibilities of an individual in a profession; delineates what should be learned in the professional preparation of that individual.

Screwing-home mechanism Rotation of the tibia on the femur at the end of extension to produce a "locking" of the knee in a close-packed position.

Sebum Secretions of the sebaceous glands; oily substance that binds epidermal cells.

Secretory phase Phase in the menstrual cycle, usually days 15 to 28, during which the endometrium prepares for implantation of an embryo.

Seizure Abnormal electrical discharge in the brain.

Seizure disorder Recurrent episodes of sudden, excessive charges of electrical activity in the brain, whether from known or unknown (idiopathic) causes.

Sequestrated disk The nuclear material from an intervertebral disk is separated from the disk itself and potentially migrates.

Serous otitis Fluid buildup behind the eardrum associated with otitis media and upper respiratory infections.

Sever's disease A traction-type injury, or osteochondrosis, of the calcaneal apophysis seen in young adolescents.

Shear force A force directed parallel to a surface.

Shin bruise A contusion to the tibia; sometimes referred to as tibial periostitis.

Shock Collapse of the cardiovascular system when insufficient blood cannot provide circulation for the entire body.

Sickle cell anemia Abnormalities in hemoglobin structure, resulting in a characteristic sickle- or crescent-shaped red blood cell that is fragile and unable to transport oxygen.

Sign An objective, measurable physical finding that you can hear, feel, see, or smell during the assessment.

Sinding-Larsen-Johansson's disease Inflammation or partial avulsion of the apex of the patella because of traction forces.

Sinusitis Inflammation of the paranasal sinuses.

SLAP lesion An injury to the superior labrum that typically begins posteriorly and extends anteriorly, disrupting the attachment of the long head of the biceps tendon to the superior glenoid tubercle.

Smith's fracture Volar displacement of the distal fragment of the radius; sometimes called a reversed Colles fracture.

Snapping hip syndrome A snapping sensation either heard or felt during motion at the hip.

Snowball crepitation Sound similar to that heard when crunching snow into a snowball; indicative of tenosynovitis.

Solar plexus punch A blow to the abdomen with the muscles relaxed, resulting in an immediate inability to catch one's breath.

Somatic pain Pain arising from the skin, ligaments, muscles, bones, and joints.

Spasm Transitory muscle contractions.

Spear tackler's spine A condition caused by a history of using a spear-tackling technique, whereby the athlete uses the top or crown of the helmet as the initial point of contact, placing the cervical spine at risk for serious injury because of excessive axial loading.

Spina bifida occulta A spinal defect characterized by the absence of vertebral arches in which there is no protrusion of the cord or its membrane.

Spinal stenosis A loss of cerebrospinal fluid around the spinal cord because of deformation of the spinal cord or narrowing of the neural canal.

Spondylolisthesis Anterior slippage of a vertebrae resulting from complete bilateral fracture of the pars interarticularis.

Spondylolysis A stress fracture of the pars interarticularis.

Sports medicine The area of health and special services that applies medical and scientific knowledge to prevent, recognize, manage, and rehabilitate injuries related to sport, exercise, or recreational activity.

Sprain Injury to ligamentous tissue.

Sprengel's deformity Congenital elevation of the scapulae; an undescended scapulae.

Stage model Emotional stages that an individual progresses through when confronted with grief, including denial and isolation, anger, bargaining, depression, and acceptance.

Static stretch Slow and deliberate muscle stretching used to increase range of motion.

Standard of care What another minimally competent professional who is educated and practicing in the same profession would have done in the same or similar circumstance to protect an individual from harm.

Static stretch Stretching movement that is slow and deliberate and lasts for at least 15 seconds.

Status epilepticus A condition in which one major attack of epilepsy succeeds another with little or no intermission.

Stenosing Narrowing of an opening or stricture of a canal; stenosis.

Step deformity A change in direction resembling a stairstep in a line, a surface, or the construction of a solid body.

Steroids A large family of chemical substances, including endocrine secretions and hormones.

Sticking point Insufficient strength to move a body segment through a particular angle.

Stitch in the side A sharp pain or spasm in the chest wall, usually on the lower right side, during exertion.

Strain Amount of deformation with respect to the original dimensions of the structure; injury to the musculotendinous unit.

Stress The distribution of force within a body; quantified as force divided by the area over which the force acts.

Stress fracture A fracture resulting from repeated loading with relatively low-magnitude forces.

Striae distensae Bands of thin, wrinkled skin, initially red but becoming purple and white, that commonly occur on the abdomen, buttocks, and thighs during and following pregnancy and that result from atrophy of the dermis and overextension of the skin.

Strict liability Manufacturer's absolute liability for any and all defective or hazardous equipment that unduly threatens an individual's personal safety.

Subconjunctival hemorrhage Minor capillary ruptures in the eye globe.

Subcutaneous emphysema The presence of air or gas in subcutaneous tissue; characterized by a crackling sensation on palpation.

Subungual hematoma Hematoma beneath a fingernail or toenail.

Sudden death A nontraumatic, unexpected death that occurs instantaneously or within a few minutes of an abrupt change in an individual's previous clinical state.

Supination Outward rotation of the forearm, with the palms facing forward. At the foot, combined motions of calcaneal inversion, foot adduction, and plantar flexion.

Supraventricular tachycardia Rapid beating of the heart, proximal to the ventricles, in the atrium or atrioventricular node.

Sustained release A capsule or tablet filled with tiny spheres that contain a drug. The sphere is coated and designed to dissolve at variable rates, ranging from 8 to 24 hours.

Sustentaculum tali The anteromedial surface of the calcaneus that largely supports the talus.

Symptom Subjective information provided by an individual regarding his or her perception of the problem.

Syncope Fainting or lightheadedness.

Syndrome An accumulation of common signs and symptoms characteristic of a particular injury or disease.

Systolic pressure Pressure exerted by blood on the blood vessel walls during ventricular contractions.

T

Tachycardia Rapid beating of the heart; usually applied to rates over 100 beats per minute.

Tachypnea Rapid breathing.

Tackler's exostosis Irritative exostosis on the anterior or lateral humerus.

Tapotement Massage technique that uses sharp, alternating, brisk hand movements, such as hacking, slapping, beating, cupping, and clapping, to increase blood flow and stimulate peripheral nerve endings.

Tendinitis Inflammation of a tendon.

Tendinosis A tendinous condition associated with degeneration rather than with inflammation.

Tenosynovitis Inflammation of a tendon sheath.

Tensile force A pulling or stretching force directed axially through a body or body part.

Tension pneumothorax Condition in which air continuously leaks into the pleural space, causing the mediastinum to displace to the opposite side, compressing the uninjured lung and thoracic aorta.

Testosterone The primary androgen produced by the testes. Testosterone stimulates the growth and maturation of the internal and external genitalia at puberty and is responsible for sexual motivation.

Thenar The fleshy mass of muscle and tissue on the lateral palm; the ball of the thumb.

Therapeutic drugs Prescription or over-the-counter medications used to treat an injury or illness.

Therapeutic range The range between the minimum effective concentration and toxic concentration.

Thermoregulation The process by which the body maintains body temperature; primarily controlled by the hypothalamus.

Thermotherapy Heat application.

Thoracic outlet syndrome Condition whereby nerves and/or vessels become compressed in the root of the neck or axilla, leading to numbness in the arm.

Thrombophlebitis Acute inflammation of a vein.

Tibiofemoral joint Dual condyloid joints between the tibial and femoral condyles that function primarily as a modified hinge joint.

Tidal volume The amount of air inspired and expired in a single breath.

Tinea Ringworm; fungal infection of the hair, skin, or nails characterized by small vesicles, itching, and scaling; types include tinea pedis (athlete's foot), tinea cruris (jock itch), and tinea capitis (ringworm of the scalp).

Tinnitus Ringing or other noises in the ear because of trauma or disease.

Todd's paralysis Paralysis of temporary duration (normally not more than a few days) that occurs in the limb or limbs involved in epilepsy after the seizure.

Tomogram A cross-sectional image of an organ or body part at various depths of field produced by an x-ray technique.

Tonic Steady, rigid muscle contractions with no relaxation.

Torque A rotary force; the product of a force and its moment arm, or moment.

Torsion force Twisting around an object's longitudinal axis in response to an applied torque.

Tort A wrong done to an individual whereby the injured party seeks a remedy for damages suffered.

Torticollis A congenital or acquired spasm of the sternocleidomastoid muscle; "wry neck."

Toxic concentration Concentration of drug levels in the blood plasma that are too high and, therefore, increase the risk of toxic effects.

Toxic synovitis Occurring largely in children, a transient, inflammatory condition characterized by a painful hip joint accompanied by an antalgic gait and limp.

Translation Anterior gliding of the tibial plateau on the femur.

Transverse plane A horizontal line that divides the body into superior and inferior portions.

Traumatic asphyxia A condition involving extravasation of blood into the skin and conjunctivae because of a sudden increase in venous pressure.

Triage Assessing all injured individuals to determine priority of care.

Trigger An event or system in which a relatively small input hastens, worsens, or lengthens the duration of a condition, the magnitude of which is unrelated to the magnitude of the input.

Trigger finger Condition whereby the finger flexors contract but are unable to re-extend because of a nodule within the tendon sheath or the sheath being too constricted to allow free motion.

Tunics Three layers of protected tissues that surround the eye.

U

Unconsciousness Impairment of brain function wherein the individual lacks conscious awareness and is unable to respond to superficial sensory stimuli.

Urethritis Inflammation of the urethra.

Urticaria Hives; an eruption of itching wheals, usually of systemic origin; may result from a state of hypersensitivity to foods or drugs, infection, physical agents, or psychic stimuli.

Uterine cycle The menstrual cycle; a series of cyclic changes that the inner lining of the uterus (endometrium) goes through each month as it responds to varying levels of hormones in the blood.

V

Vaginitis Inflammation of the vagina.

Valgus An opening on the medial side of a joint caused by the distal segment moving laterally.

Valsalva maneuver Holding one's breath against a closed glottis, resulting in sharp increases in blood pressure.

Valvular stenosis A narrowing of the orifice around the cardiac valves.

Varicocele Abnormal dilation of the veins of the spermatic cord, leading to engorgement of blood into the spermatic cord veins when standing.

Varus An opening on the lateral side of a joint caused by the distal segment moving medially.

Vasoconstriction Narrowing of the blood vessels; the opposite of vasodilation.

Vasodilation Enlarging of the blood vessels; the opposite of vasoconstriction.

Vehicles Substances combined with medications that use enteral routes to facilitate entry into the body; may include tablets, capsules, liquids, powders, suppositories, enteric-coated preparations, and sustained-release preparations.

Vertigo A balance disturbance characterized by a whirling sensation of one's self or external objects.

Vibration A massage technique using finite, gentle, and rhythmic movement of the fingers to vibrate the underlying tissues for relaxation or stimulation.

Visceral pain Pain resulting from disease or injury to an organ in the thoracic or abdominal cavity.

Viscoelastic Responding to loading over time with changing rates of deformation.

Volkmann's contracture Ischemic necrosis of the forearm muscles and tissues caused by damage to the blood flow.

Voltage The force that causes ions to move.

W

Watt A unit of electrical power. For an electrical current: watts = voltage × amperage.

Wedge fracture A crushing compression fracture that leaves a vertebra narrowed anteriorly.

Wheal A smooth, slightly elevated area on the body that appears red or white and is accompanied by severe itching; commonly seen in allergies to mechanical or chemical irritants.

Wolff's law A law that states that bone and soft tissue will respond to the physical demands placed on them, causing the formation of collagen to remodel or re-align along the lines of stress, thus promoting healthy joint biomechanics.

Wrist drop Weakness and/or paralysis of the wrist and finger extensors because of radial nerve damage.

Y

Yield point (elastic limit) The maximum load that a material can sustain without permanent deformation.

Z

Zone of primary injury The region of injured tissue before vasodilation.

Zone of secondary injury The region of damaged tissue following vasodilation.

INDEX

Page numbers followed by f denote figures and those followed by t denote tables; page numbers followed by b indicate boxed material and those followed by fs indicate Field Strategies.

A

A-angle, 581, 581f
AAROM. *See* Active assisted range of motion (AAROM)
Abdomen, auscultation of, 385
Abdominal cavity, 353–354
Abdominal pain, nonmusculoskeletal sources of, 380, 381t
Abdominal protection, equipment for, 55, 55f
Abdominal strengthening exercises, 346fs
Abdominal wall, conditions of, 369–372, 371f
  contusions, 370
  hernias, 371–372, 371f
  muscle strains, 370
  skin wounds, 370
  solar plexus contusion, 370–371
Abduction
  hip, 536
  knee, 584
Abduction (valgus stress) test, in injury assessment, knee, 622–623, 622f
Abrasion, corneal, 262
ABS, life expectancy of, 49
Abscess(es), 877, 877f
Absorption
  drug, 849–850
  of electromagnetic energy, 164, 164f
Abuse
  drug, sudden cardiac death due to, 772
  substance, sudden cardiac death due to, 772
Acceleration, in throwing, 401, 401f, 402t
Accessory movements, 103
Acclimatization, in heat tolerance modification, 791, 792b
Acetaminophen
  indications for, 189
  pharmacokinetic process of, 852b
Achilles tendon
  disorders of, 670–671
  rupture of, 671, 671f
    Thompson's test for, 691, 691f
  taping of, 73, 73f
ACL braces, 57–58, 58f
Acne, 877–878
Acne mechanica, 891
Acquired immunodeficiency syndrome (AIDS), 822–823, 823b
Acquired valvular heart disease, sudden cardiac death due to, 719
Acromegaly, 868
Acromioclavicular distraction-compression, 431, 432f
Acromioclavicular joint
  anatomy of, 396, 396f
  instability of, tests for, 429, 431, 432f
  sprains of, 407–409, 410t, 411t
  taping of, 80, 80f
  tests of, 431t
ACSM. *See* American College of Sports Medicine (ACSM)
Active assisted range of motion (AAROM), 210
Active inhibition, 210, 211b
Active movements, in injury assessment
  cervical and thoracic spine, 294–295

elbow, 471–472, 472f
knee, 618–619, 619f
lower leg, ankle, and foot, 688
lumbar spine, 328, 329f, 330f
pelvic, hip, and thigh, 560, 560f
shoulder, 427, 427f, 428f
wrist and hand, 514, 514f
Active range of motion (AROM)
  in injury assessment, 91fs, 101
    emergency, 116
  restoration of, 211
Activities of daily living (ADLs)
  described, 96
  low back injuries in, prevention of, 131b
Activity restriction, in soft-tissue injury care, 203–204, 204fs
Activity-specific functional tests, in injury assessment, 91fs, 111
  elbow, 477, 477b
  knee, 631
  lower leg, ankle, and foot, 692–693
  pelvic, hip, and thigh, 570
  shoulder, 439–440
  spinal
    cervical and thoracic, 301–302
    lumbar, 342
  wrist and hand, 519
Acute compartment syndrome, 542, 661
Acute inflammatory process, 144f
Acute injury, 88, 132
Acute mountain sickness, 804–805
Adam's position, 325
Adduction
  hip, 536
  knee, 584
Adduction (varus stress) test, in injury assessment, knee, 622f, 623
Adductor (groin) strain, 548
Adductor stretch, in pelvic, hip, and thigh injury prevention, 538fs
Adherence confidence, 196
Adhesion(s), 146
Adhesive capsulitis, 842, 842b
ADLs. *See* Activities of daily living (ADLs)
Administration, organization and, domain of, 3, 6
Administration of medication, defined, 856
Adrenocorticosteroid(s), indications for, 189
Adson's test, in shoulder injury assessment, 431t, 437, 438f
Aerobic capacity, 219–220
Affective filters, 158
Afferent (sensory) nerves, 155
Age, in heat tolerance modification, 793–794
Agility, in PPE, 40
Agonist(s), defined, 209, 848
Agonist muscles, 209
AIDS. *See* Acquired immunodeficiency syndrome (AIDS)
Air pollution, exercise and, 806
Alcohol, as performance-enhancing substance, 865–866
Allen test
  in shoulder injury assessment, 431t, 437, 438f
  in wrist and hand injury evaluation, 518
Allergic contact dermatitis, 902, 902f
Allergic rhinitis (hay fever), 750
Alphabet, ankle, 655fs

Alternate arm and leg extension on all fours, 345fs
Alternate arm and leg lift, 345fs
Altitude disorders, 804–806
  acute mountain sickness, 804–805
  high-altitude cerebral edema, 805
  high-altitude pulmonary edema, 805
  prevention of, 805–806
AMA. *See* American Medical Association
Ambulatory assistance, in injury assessment, 122
Amenorrhea, 34, 152, 678
  defined, 830
  exercise-associated, in female athletes, 830–831
  in female athletes, risk factors for, 830–831, 830b
American Academy of Neurology Concussion Grading Scale, 239, 239t
American Academy of Pediatrics Committee on Sports Medicine, guidelines for participation, 41
American College of Obstetrician and Gynecologists, 834
American College of Sports Medicine, 837, 869
American College of Sports Medicine (ACSM)
  in cardiovascular endurance, 220
  risk factors for coronary artery disease of, 720t
  26th Besthesda Conference of, 724–725
American Dental Association, 53
American Hospital Association, athletic trainers recognition by, 4
American Medical Association (AMA), athletic trainers recognition by, 4
American Society for Testing and Materials (ASTM), in protective equipment regulations, 48
Americans with Disabilities Act of 1990, 724
Americans with Disabilities Act of 1991, 823
Amnesia(s)
  anterograde, 241, 723
  retrograde, 241, 723
Amphetamine(s)
  as performance-enhancing substance, 868
  sudden cardiac death due to, 722
Amplitude, of current, 180
Amputation(s), athletes with, 840
Anabolic-androgenic steroids, as performance-enhancing substance, 867–868, 867b
Analgesic(s), for sport-related injuries, 859
Analgesic effect, of cold therapy, 166
Analgesic rebound headache, 732
Anaphylactic shock, 712b
Anaphylaxis, 897, 897f
Anastomosis, defined, 451
Androgen(s), defined, 356
Anemia(s), 704–707, 705b, 707f
  hemolytic, exercise-induced, 706
  iron-deficiency, 706
  predisposing factors for, 705, 705b
  runner's, 706
  sickle cell, 706–707, 707f
  stages of, 705